GENERAL AND ORAL PATHOLOGY
for the Dental Hygienist

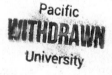

GENERAL AND ORAL PATHOLOGY
for the Dental Hygienist

Leslie DeLong
Lamar Institute of Technology
Beaumont, TX

Nancy W. Burkhart
Baylor College of Dentistry
Texas A&M Health Science Center
Dallas, TX

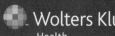 Wolters Kluwer | Lippincott
Health | Williams & Wilkins

Acquisitions Editor: Barret Koger
Managing Editor: Kevin Dietz
Marketing Manager: Nancy Bradshaw
Production Editor: Gina Aiello
Designer: Risa Clow
Compositor: Maryland Composition
Cover photo courtesy of Dr. Valerie Murrah

351 West Camden Street   530 Walnut Street
Baltimore, MD 21201   Philadelphia, PA 19106

Printed in the United States

9 8 7 6 5 4 3 2 1

Library of Congress Cataloging-in-Publication Data

DeLong, Leslie.
  General and oral pathology for the dental hygienist / Leslie DeLong, Nancy Burkhart.
    p. ; cm.
  Includes bibliographical references.
  ISBN-13: 978-0-7817-5546-7
  ISBN-10: 0-7817-5546-8
  1. Mouth--Diseases. 2. Teeth--Diseases. 3. Pathology. 4. Dental hygienists. I. Burkhart, Nancy. II. Title.
  [DNLM: 1. Mouth Diseases. 2. Dental Hygienists. 3. Tooth Diseases.
WU 140 D361g 2008]
  RK307.D43 2008
  617.5'22--dc22
                                                                        2007025134

To purchase additional copies of this book, call our customer service department at (800) 638-3030 or fax orders to (301)
223-2320. International customers should call (301) 223-2300.

Visit Lippincott Williams & Wilkins on the Internet: http://www.lww.com. Lippincott Williams & Wilkins customer service

To my father and mother, Earl and Muriel Yarrington. You always told me I could do anything I put my mind to. I wish you could have seen the completed project. To my husband Richard and my son Brian. You are never-ending sources of strength and encouragement, and I thank you for having patience with me while I worked on this project.

Leslie DeLong

I would like to dedicate my work and efforts in this book to two people.

First to my husband Alan, who displayed true courage during his treatment of oral cancer and his subsequent recovery—you have been admirable. Thank you for the support and encouragement that you have provided me while writing this book. The second dedication is to Mr. Vernon B. Strickland who believed in me and encouraged me throughout my life. Thank you for the many years of being a true role model and mentor to me.

I offer my sincere thanks to Dr. Terry Rees, Dr. John Jacoway, and Dr. Jeff Burkes. My interests in oral disease/pathology would not have occurred if you had not been mentors to me. Thank you for supporting me and above all, teaching me. As an educator, I know that nothing takes the place of experience.

Nancy Burkhart

Preface

General and Oral Pathology for the Dental Hygienist is a comprehensive study of the general concepts of pathophysiology as they relate to systemic and oral conditions. The material in the first part of the book is organized by major determinants of disease and then by a quasi systems approach, whereby different systems are looked at from the viewpoint of a practicing dental hygienist reviewing a medical history. The second part of the book focuses on oral pathology. The different disorders are organized into distinct clinical/radiographic features of oral lesions. Students do not see immunity lesions or genetic lesions, they see red lesions, white lesions, raised lesions, radiolucent lesions, etc. The student needs a recognizable characteristic in order to group diseases/lesions of varying causes into categories that can be easily identified. When students see an ulcer, they can go back into their memories and pull out the things that look like ulcers. White lesions do not look like ulcers, neither do soft tissue enlargements; therefore, they do not need to consider these. They still know what causes the lesions, but they will not have to sift through numerous dissimilar lesions to get to the lesion that is most likely present. It is hoped that this organization strategy will assist the students in their efforts to learn the important and exciting subject of Oral Pathology. This book has been developed with many unique features that will enhance learning and practical application of the material.

FEATURES:

1. Chapter Outline. Each chapter begins with an outline to make locating material within the chapter easier.
2. Learner Objectives and Key Terms. Learner objectives and a listing of key terms are also located at the beginning of each chapter. Learner objectives help students focus on the key elements of the material in the chapter. Key terms are bolded and defined within the text, in addition to being listed in a comprehensive glossary at the end of the book.
3. Disease Lists. The information related to specific oral and systemic diseases/conditions is organized in a similar manner throughout most of the book. The template facilitates the learning process by allowing students to study the material in an organized fashion. The information is organized into the following categories:

- Name. Each disorder may be called by different yet similar names in older texts, by different instructors or clinicians, or in different regions of the country or world. The most common names and some of the less common or outdated names of the disorders are listed, enabling the student to identify them when necessary.
- Etiology. The etiology of each disorder, if known, is identified in this section. In instances where the etiology is unknown, the prevailing theories of the etiology may be stated with information on the current focus of research.
- Method of Transmission. This section contains a concise description of how the disorder is transmitted. If appropriate, this includes the method of transmission of infectious organisms and inheritance patterns or genetic transmission.
- Epidemiology. Basic statistical information, such as incidence and prevalence, and information about the epidemiological aspects of each condition, such as age, sex, ethnicity, and geographical location, are essential for students to know in order to develop an understanding of the disorders and to develop an appropriate differential diagnosis for a patient.
- Pathogenesis. Students need to know the why and the how of the disorders they are learning about in order to understand how the concepts of pathophysiology relate to them. As the students understand more, less memorization will be required. This section focuses on a brief description of how the disease/condition develops. What happens on a cellular, tissue, or organ level? How is the general health of the individual affected?
- Extraoral Characteristics. Dental hygienists treat patients who have the potential to present with a myriad of health problems. In order to properly assess the patient and plan for appropriate dental hygiene care, the modern hygienist must be familiar with signs and symptoms of disease that may present in any area of the body. Clinically observable characteristics associated with the lower and upper body, and the head and neck area, are described in this section.
- Perioral and Intraoral Characteristics. The perioral and oral manifestations of each disorder are compre-

hensively described in this section. In many instances, these manifestations are linked to systemic manifestations. As stated previously, lesions with similar perioral and/or oral characteristics are grouped together in the chapters dealing with oral lesions.

- Distinguishing Characteristics. This section identifies manifestations and sometimes microscopic features that may only be associated with a specific disorder. This information is useful when adding/eliminating conditions from a differential diagnosis.
- Significant Microscopic Features. Many of the conditions include a description of the histological appearance of the affected tissues and/or cells. Often this information is crucial in helping the student understand the pathological basis for the disorder. In addition, it is important for the student to know that the microscopic examination of most lesions is our only means of obtaining a definitive diagnosis.
- Dental Implications. This section focuses on patient management issues that are associated with the specific diseases/conditions. Information related to patient assessment, treatment modifications, potential medical emergencies, homecare recommendations, and other topics enables the student to be conscious of not only the specific disorder, but also the impact that the disorder may have on dental/dental hygiene treatment and on the individual's ability to perform self-care procedures.
- Differential Diagnosis. A differential diagnosis has been developed for many of the disorders. The differential diagnosis includes the names of the disorders that may have similar manifestations and a reference to the chapter that discusses these disorders. At times, a brief explanation of why the condition is listed in the differential diagnosis is included. This is an excellent clinical reference for the student and practicing clinician.
- Treatment and Prognosis. The discussion of each disease/condition concludes with possible treatment methods and the prognosis associated with the disorder. The dental implications of specific therapeutic regimens may also be described in this section.

4. Applications. Applications are specific for each chapter and relate didactic knowledge to clinical practice. The applications may accomplish one or more of the following:
   - Describe how information just learned is encountered in everyday situations.
   - Expand on information for those who might be interested in more detail.
   - Suggest management techniques for patients who present with specific problems.
   - Relate systemic pathology to oral conditions and oral conditions to systemic pathology.
   - Discuss controversial or emerging issues and topics.
   - Suggest methods to educate patients about specific disorders.
5. Critical Thinking Activities. These activities are included in each chapter and encourage the student to reach beyond memorizing the material to consider how the information will impact their practice of dental hygiene.
6. Case Studies. The case studies associated with each chapter were developed to encompass all aspects of dental hygiene care, and require the student to "put it all together."
7. Portfolio Possibilities. More and more dental hygiene programs are requiring their students to produce portfolios showcasing self-evaluation and the achievement of specific program competencies. Therefore, each chapter includes suggestions for student-directed projects that would be useful in showing progress toward meeting competencies associated with patient care, health promotion, and disease prevention or professionalism.
8. Clinical Protocols. References to numbered Clinical Protocols are made throughout the book. Clinical protocols address the management of specific clinical or patient problems. They are excellent practice guidelines and references for the student and/or practicing clinician. The Clinical Protocols are found in the back of the book.

Student Resource Center

The Student Resource Center has review questions with answers and rationales and additional case studies associated with each chapter.

Instructor Resource Center

The Instructor Resource Center has numerous aids for instructors:

- Image bank containing all of the images included in the text.
- Additional case studies that may be used for quizzes, tests, or classroom discussion.
- Classroom discussion points for the Critical Thinking Activities, case studies, and other chapter content.
- Test bank questions that can be used to generate quizzes, tests, and final examinations.

The authors and publisher acknowledge the contributions of the following reviewers for their valuable comments and suggestions.

Sharon Barbieri, MS,
The University of Texas Health Science Center at San
    Antonio
Department of Dental Hygiene
San Antonio, TX

Arthur DiMarco, DMD
Dental Hygiene Department
Eastern Washington University
Spokane, WA

Stephen Holliday, DDS
Allied Health Technologies
Sinclair Community College
Dayton, OH

Nikki Honey, DDS, MS
Dental Hygiene Department
Shoreline Community College
Seattle, WA

Debby Kurtz-Weidinger
Dental Hygiene Dept
Phoenix College
Phoenix, AZ

Brad Neville, DDS
Professor, Division of Oral Pathology
Medical University of South Carolina
Charleston, SC

Virginia Wagner, CDA, RDH, BHS
Dental Health Programs, Tallahassee Community College
Tallahasse, FL

Katherine A. Woods, RDH, MPH
St. Petersburg College
School of Dental Hygiene
Pinellas Park, FL

Acknowledgments

Many individuals were involved in the development of this book. We extend our thanks to all who supported our efforts in completing this project. We would especially like to thank these individuals for their generous contributions.

- The following individuals contributed an enormous amount of time and effort to this project by writing chapters related to their areas of expertise.
  - Dr. Harvey Kessler, Professor of Oral Pathology in the Department of Diagnostic Sciences, Baylor College of Dentistry, Texas A & M Health Science Center, Baylor College of Dentistry, Dallas, Texas
  - Dr. Valerie Murrah, Professor and Chair of Diagnostic Sciences, The University of North Carolina School of Dentistry, Chapel Hill, North Carolina
  - Dr. Jacqueline Plemons, Professor in the Department of Periodontics, Baylor College of Dentistry, Texas A & M Health Science Center, Baylor College of Dentistry, Dallas, Texas
  - Dr. John Wright, Regents Professor and Chair, Diagnostic Sciences Department, Texas A & M Health Science Center, Baylor College of Dentistry, Dallas, Texas
- The following colleagues contributed clinical photographs and radiographs, or wrote clinical protocols related to their area of expertise. We extend our gratitude for their generosity and support.
  - Dr. Celeste Abraham, Professor, Baylor College of Dentistry, Dallas, Texas
  - Dr. Doron Aframian, Professor of Oral Medicine, Hebrew University, Hadassah School of Dental Medicine, Jerusalem, Israel
  - Dr. Ibtisam Al-Hashimi, Professor, Baylor College of Dentistry, Dallas, Texas
  - Dr. Craig Baumgartner, Professor and Chairman, Department of Endodontology, School of Dentistry, Oregon Health and Sciences University, Portland, Oregon
  - Dr. Carolyn Bentley, Former Professor, The University of North Carolina School of Dentistry
  - Dr. Michael Bornstein, Professor, Department of Oral Surgery and Stomatology, University of Bern, Bern, Switzerland
  - Dr. Michael Brennan, Professor and Oral Medicine Residency Director, Director, Sjogren's Syndrome and Salivary Disorders Center, Carolinas Medical Center, Department of Oral Medicine, Charlotte
  - Dr. Jeff Burkes, former Professor, Department of Diagnostic Sciences, The University of North Carolina School of Dentistry, Chapel Hill, North Carolina
  - Dr. William Carpenter, Professor and Chair of the Department of Diagnostic Sciences, University of the Pacific School of Dentistry, San Francisco, California.
  - Dr. Marco Carrozzo, Professor of Oral Medicine School of Dental Sciences, The University of Newcastle upon Tyne.
  - Dr. Yi-Shing Lisa Chenge, Diagnostic Sciences, Baylor College of Dentistry, Dallas
  - Dr. Douglas Damm, Professor, Department of Oral Health Science/Oral Pathology, University of Kentucky School of Dentistry, Lexington, Kentucky
  - Dr. Charles Dunlap, Chair, Department of Oral Pathology, Medicine and Radiology, University of Missouri-Kansas City.
  - Dr. Faiez N. Hattab, Consultant, Family Dental Clinic, Doha, State of Qatar
  - Dr. Wendy Hupp, Assistant Professor of Oral Medicine, Department of Diagnostic Sciences, Prosthodontics, Restorative Dentistry, University of Louisville School of Dentistry, Louisville, Kentucky
  - Dr. Peter Jacobsen, Professor Department of Diagnostic Sciences, University of the Pacific School of Dentistry, San Francisco, California.
  - Dr. John Jacoway, former Professor, Department of Diagnostic Sciences, The University of North Carolina School of Dentistry, Chapel Hill, North Carolina
  - Dr. Michael Kahn, Professor, The Tufts University School of Dental Medicine, Boston, Massachusetts
  - Dr. Michael Krakow, Professor, The University of Medicine & Dentistry of New Jersey, Newark, New Jersey
  - Dr. Robert Langlais, University of Texas Health Science Center at San Antonio

- Dr. Michael Lewis, Professor of Oral Medicine, University of Wales College of Medicine, Heath Park, Cardiff, UK
- Dr. Peter Lockhart, Chair, Department of Oral Medicine, Carolinas Medical Center, Charlotte, North Carolina
- Dr. Denis Lynch, Professor, Associate Dean, Marquette University School of Dentistry, Milwaukee, Wisconsin
- Dr. Shabnum Meer, Professor, Division of Oral Pathology, University of Witwatersrand, Johannesburg, South Africa
- Dr. Lynn Douglas Mouden, Director, Office of Oral Health, Division of Health, Arkansas Department of Health and Human Services
- Dr. Mel Mupparapu, Professor, The University of Medicine & Dentistry of New Jersey, Newark, New Jersey
- Jill Nield-Gehrig, Asheville-Buncombe Technical Community College, Asheville, North Carolina
- Dr. A. Yusuf Oner, Gazi University School of Medicine, Department of Radiology, Ankara, Turkey
- Frieda Pickett, Former Associate Professor, Caruth School of Dental Hygiene, Baylor College of Dentistry, Dallas Texas.
- Dr. Enrique Platin, Professor, The University of North Carolina School of Dentistry, Chapel Hill, North Carolina
- Dr. John Preece, Department of Dental Diagnostic Science, University of Texas Health Science Center at San Antonio
- Dr. Terry Rees, Professor and Director of The Stomatology Clinic, Department of Periodontics, Baylor College of Dentistry, Texas A & M Health Science Center, Baylor College of Dentistry, Dallas, Texas
- Dr. Michael Roberts, University of North Carolina School of Dentistry, Chapel Hill, North Carolina
- Dr. Sumner M. Sapiro, Private Practice and Retired, Tampa, Florida Dr.
- Dr. Kathryn Savitsky, Private Practice, Charlotte, North Carolina
- Dr. James Sciubba, Professor, The John Hopkins School of Medicine, Baltimore, Maryland
- Dr. Maria Siponen, Department of Diagnostics and Oral Medicine, Institute of Dentistry, University of Oulu, Finland
- Dr. Kurt Summersgill, Professor in the Department of Diagnostic Sciences, University of Pittsburgh, Pittsburgh, Pennsylvania
- Dr. John A. Svirsky, Professor, Department of Oral Pathology, Virginia Commonwealth University School of Dentistry, Richmond, Virginia
- Dr. Géza Terézhalmy, Division of Oral Diagnosis/ Oral Medicine, Department of Dental Diagnostic Science, University of Texas Health Science Center at San Antonio
- Dr. Frank Varon, Private Practice, Omaha, Nebraska.
- Dr. Saman Warnakulasuriya, Professor of Oral Medicine, King's College, London
- Dr. David Wray, Professor of Oral Medicine, University of Glasgow, Glasgow, UK
- We would like to thank the following individuals for contributing personal photographs and/or radiographs for use in the text:
  - Chelsea Justice, dental hygiene student at Lamar Institute of Technology
  - Tirza Jo Ochrack-Konradi
  - Jay, Lisa and Jesse Waters
- Ms. Carmen Banks (Dallas, Texas) for her wonderful illustration
- Mr. Dan Bruneau at the United States Department of Veteran's Affairs for his help in obtaining permission to use a number of images critical for the text.
- Special thanks to Ruth Fearing-Tornwall, R.D.H., M.P.H. (Lamar Institute of Technology) and Maria Fiocchi, D.D.S., M.S. (University of Texas Health Science Center at Houston), who always took the time to encourage and motivate us.
- Finally, our sincere thanks to John Goucher, Kevin Dietz, Robyn Alvarez and Marilee LeBon from Lippincott Williams & Wilkins, without whose limitless patience, support, and guidance this book would never have been completed.

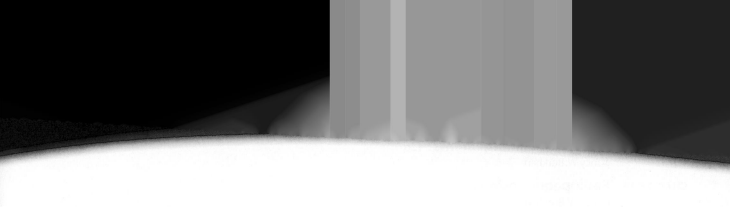

1 General Pathology

Introduction to General and Oral Pathology

Key Terms

- Abrasion
- Amalgam tattoo
- Atypical
- Benign
- Biopsy
- Bulla
- Circumscribed
- Coalesced
- Convergent
- Corrugated
- Crusted
- Definitive diagnosis
- Differential diagnosis
- Divergent
- Endogenous
- Endophytic
- Erosion
- Erythematic
- Exogenous
- Exophytic
- Fissured
- Fluctuant
- Generalized
- Homeostasis
- Indurated
- Lesion
- Localized
- Lymphadenopathy
- Macule
- Malignant
- Melanoma
- Mixed
- Multilocular
- Nodule
- Papillary
- Papule
- Patch
- Pedunculated
- Plaque
- Pseudomembrane
- Purulent exudate
- Pustule
- Radiolucent
- Radiopaque
- Resorption
- Sessile
- Tumor
- Ulcer
- Unilocular
- Vesicle

Learning Objectives

1. Define and use the key terms in this chapter.
2. Discuss the concept of "wellness."
3. Describe the changing roles of the patient and the clinician.
4. State the objectives of the clinical evaluation.
5. Describe the elements of an extraoral and intraoral examination or oral cancer screening.
6. List observations that might suggest that a lesion is benign or malignant.
7. Note the elements of a complete clinical description.
8. List the elements that should be included in a description of radiographic findings.
9. Write a complete clinical description of a sample case study.
10. Describe the steps involved in reaching a differential diagnosis.
11. Describe possible ways of determining a definitive diagnosis.

Chapter Outline

HEALTH AND WELLNESS

Pathology is defined as the study of disease. However, before learning about disease it is necessary to have a clear definition of health. In 1948 the World Health Organization defined health as "a state of complete physical, mental, and social well-being—not merely the absence of disease or infirmity." Almost 50 years later, *Stedman's Concise Medical Dictionary for the Health Professions,* 5th edition, defines health as "A state characterized by anatomical, physiological, and psychological integrity, ability to perform personally valued family, work, and community roles; ability to deal with physical, biological, psychological and social stress; a feeling of well-being; and freedom from the risk of disease and untimely death." The definition and concept of health comprises a wide range of physical, emotional, and spiritual components.

The concept of healthcare has rapidly evolved over the past several decades, and many paradigms or models for healthcare have been examined and modified or eliminated. The role of the healthcare provider has changed from dictator to advisor and facilitator. The role of the patient has also changed. No longer do patients have to be passive participants; they can be dynamic partners in their own healthcare. The internet has added a new dimension to the concept of access to healthcare information, enabling people to become informed consumers of healthcare if they so desire. People everywhere are looking at different methods of achieving "health" as it is defined today. They are seeing that many alternative and complementary forms of medicine have a place in the healthcare system. The concept of "wellness" places a strong focus on the active role of the patient and the importance of the total well-being of the person. The United States government proposed two goals in its report on the state of health in America, *Healthy People 2010.* Those goals are (1) to increase the quality and years of healthy life and (2) to eliminate health disparities among Americans. *Healthy People 2010* reflects the changing attitudes of Americans and encourages establishing a sense of personal responsibility as the key to good health. Students pursuing a career in healthcare study the healthy body in anatomy and physiology and other subjects throughout their formal education. This text draws on this knowledge extensively to provide a study of disease states.

DISEASE

The definition of disease is simpler than that of health. *Stedman's Concise Medical Dictionary for the Health Professions,* 5th edition, defines disease as "An interruption, cessation, or disorder of body functions, systems, or organs," or "A morbid entity characterized usually by at least two of these criteria: recognized etiologic agent(s), identifiable group of signs and symptoms, or consistent anatomical alterations." The discussion of disease does not specifically refer to an infection with a microorganism; it includes any instance in which there is a change or alteration in **homeostasis** or balance within the systems of the body. Knowledge of the processes associated with disease is an essential part of the practice of dental hygiene. As healthcare practitioners, dental hygienists must be aware of the impact that disease has on the functioning of the human body.

For years the dental profession has known that the mouth is not divorced from the rest of the body, rather it is an integral part of it. In the year 2000 the Surgeon General of the United States released "Oral Health in America: A Report of the Surgeon General." This report is the first of its kind, and its intent is to alert Americans to the full meaning of oral health and its importance to general health and well-being (HHS, 2000). Boxes 1.1 and 1.2 summarize the major findings of the report and the major functional and social implications of oral and craniofacial diseases that are identified in the report. What happens in the mouth can and does affect the rest of the body. Research supports the concept that periodontal infections have an impact on heart disease, stroke, diabetes, respiratory disease, and preterm low-birth-weight babies. Many pathologic conditions and diseases have oral manifestations that appear in the early stages of the illness, possibly prior to any other symptoms. Healthcare professionals are entrusted with the difficult task of helping patients remain in an optimal state of health.

The dental hygienist is the prevention specialist of the dental team and, as such, is uniquely qualified to make observations regarding a patient's total health as it relates to oral health and vice versa. The dental hygienist is also in a position to develop strategies directed toward education and the early detection and prevention of disease. Patients schedule preventive appointments two to four times per year; therefore, the dental hygienist is in a key position to recognize abnormalities, sometimes before the patient even knows that they exist, and to call attention to these abnormalities. Following collaboration with the

Box 1.1 MAJOR FINDINGS OF "ORAL HEALTH IN AMERICA: A REPORT OF THE SURGEON GENERAL"

• Oral diseases and disorders in and of themselves affect health and well-being throughout life.
• Safe and effective measures exist to prevent the most common dental diseases—dental caries and periodontal diseases.
• Lifestyle behaviors that affect general health such as tobacco use, excessive alcohol use, and poor dietary choices affect oral and craniofacial health as well.
• There are profound and consequential oral health disparities within the U.S. population.
• More information is needed to improve America's oral health and eliminate health disparities.
• The mouth reflects general health and well-being.
• Oral diseases and conditions are associated with other health problems.
• Scientific research is key to further reduction in the burden of diseases and disorders that affect the face, mouth, and teeth.

From U. S. Department of Health and Human Services. Oral health in America: a report of the Surgeon General. Rockville, MD: U. S. Department of Health and Human Services, National Institute of Dental and Craniofacial Research, National Institutes of Health, 2000.

dentist, the dental hygienist may be the person who assists the patient in obtaining the care that is needed. Although the importance of oral health in the context of total health is known, many patients and most of the public are just beginning to understand the total body "wellness" concept. It will be up to the individual hygienist to decide how big a role to play in the endeavor to spread this information to the general public.

OBJECTIVES OF THE CLINICAL EVALUATION

It is imperative that each patient be thoroughly assessed for any indication of medical and/or oral problems prior to the initiation of any dental or dental hygiene treatment plan. The extraoral and the intraoral examinations compose a large portion of this assessment, and while they are generally referred to as the extraoral and intraoral examinations, together they make up the oral cancer screening examination. Although these examinations can involve the least amount of time compared with a periodontal examination or a dental charting, they are extremely important. Information from these examinations will be essential in determining whether there is any indication of a deviation from normal, not only in the oral cavity but also in the body as a whole. Many of the conditions or characteristics of conditions that are discussed in this text are referred to as **lesions**. A lesion is a wound or a distinct area

Box 1.2 FUNCTIONAL AND SOCIAL IMPLICATIONS OF ORAL AND CRANIOFACIAL DISEASES AS REPORTED IN "ORAL HEALTH IN AMERICA: A REPORT OF THE SURGEON GENERAL"

• Oral health is related to well-being and quality of life as measured along functional, psychosocial, and economic dimensions. Diet, nutrition, sleep, psychological status, social interaction, school, and work are affected by impaired oral and craniofacial health.
• Cultural values influence oral and craniofacial health and well-being and can play an important role in care utilization practices and in perpetuating acceptable oral health and facial norms.
• Oral and craniofacial diseases and their treatment place a burden on society in the form of lost days and years of productive work. Acute dental conditions contribute to a range of problems for employed adults, including restricted activity, bed days, and work loss, and school loss for children. In addition, conditions such as oral and pharyngeal cancers contribute to premature death and can be measured by years of life lost.
• Oral and craniofacial diseases and conditions contribute to compromised ability to bite, chew, and swallow foods; limitations in food selection; and poor nutrition. These conditions include tooth loss, diminished salivary functions, oral–facial pain conditions such as temporo-

mandibular disorders, alterations in taste, and functional limitations of prosthetic replacements.
• Oral–facial pain, as a symptom of untreated dental and oral problems and as a condition in and of itself, is a major source of diminished quality of life. It is associated with sleep deprivation, depression, and multiple adverse psychosocial outcomes.
• Self-reported impacts of oral conditions on social function include limitations in verbal and nonverbal communication, social interaction, and intimacy. Individuals with facial disfigurements due to craniofacial diseases and conditions and their treatments may experience loss of self-image and self-esteem, anxiety, depression, and social stigma; these in turn may limit educational, career, and marital opportunities and affect other social relations.
• Reduced oral-health-related quality of life is associated with poor clinical status and reduced access to care.

Taken from U. S. Department of Health and Human Services. Oral health in America: a report of the Surgeon General. Rockville, MD: U. S. Department of Health and Human Services, National Institute of Dental and Craniofacial Research, National Institutes of Health, 2000.

in which a pathologic change has taken place. Findings can be suggestive of oral or pharyngeal cancer or of many systemic conditions that may manifest in the oral cavity. Presently, most oral cancer lesions are diagnosed during the late stages, making treatment difficult and survival rates low (i.e., a 59% 5-year survival rate (ACS, 2006)). If more of these cancers were found at an earlier stage, the survival chances of patients would increase. The most common locations for oral cancers are on the tongue, lips, and the floor of the mouth. The American Cancer Society estimates that 30,990 individuals in the United States will be diagnosed with oral or oropharyngeal cancer in 2006, and an estimated 7,320 will have died from the disease in 2005 (ACS, 2006).

Positive findings during this examination can prompt the dental team to order additional tests or procedures to determine a diagnosis for the condition. The dental hygiene appointment may have to be postponed to obtain a medical consultation based on findings during this examination (see Box 1.3 for a listing of objectives of the clinical evaluation).

Some positive findings may cause the dental professional to suspect intentional trauma or neglect. Refer to the application at the end of this chapter and to Clinical Protocol 15 for more information on family violence and suggestions for recognizing and managing this situation.

Performing an Extraoral Examination

The extraoral component of the examination should include a general assessment of the patient, an assessment of all visible areas of skin, and an assessment of the head and neck area. This assessment can start as the patient is walking to the dental chair with the dental hygienist observing the gait and posture of the patient, listening to the patient's speech, and watching as he or she sits in the chair to determine whether there are any physical disabilities. While gathering medical and dental history information one must observe all visible areas of the patient's skin. Any abnormalities should be addressed using follow-up questions. The answers to these follow-up questions will determine the next course of action. Patients will respond to most questions that are asked in a professional manner, and most are very willing to discuss their physical status, especially when informed of the necessity for the information.

There is no set sequence for performing a head and neck examination; however, it should be done the same way every time. A systematic procedure for these examinations increases the amount of attention paid to what is being examined, instead of what should be examined next, and possibly wondering if something was omitted. A systematic approach will also make the examinations faster and more reliable. Always look first and then palpate, press the tissue between fingers or against a firm structure such as bone in every area examined, even if there are no visible abnormalities. The head and neck area should be examined for symmetry by observing the patient from all angles including the supraorbital area (Fig. 1.1). The patient's profile should be classified as mesognathic, prognathic, or retrognathic. Observe the skin of the face, look for acne, moles (nevi), lumps or bumps, or roughened areas of skin. The more the hygienist observes over time, the more observant he or she will become. With experience, the hygienist will see things that do not cause alarm as well as noticing the things that do.

The following is a suggested order for performing the extraoral examination:

- Observe the eyes and the pupils. Figure 1.2 depicts an abnormal area at the inner canthus of the eye. This is called a pterygium and may be caused by excessive exposure to sunlight or may be associated with lichen planus (Chapter 14) or other skin disorders. This type

Box 1.3   OBJECTIVES OF THE CLINICAL EVALUATION

1. Oral cancer screening
2. Determine whether the patient is well enough to continue dental treatment
3. Determine the need for medical or other consultations
4. Enable early diagnosis of pathology
5. Determine possible treatment modifications
6. Prepare and record baseline patient assessment information
7. Review and update baseline assessment information
8. Determine whether additional diagnostic procedures are necessary

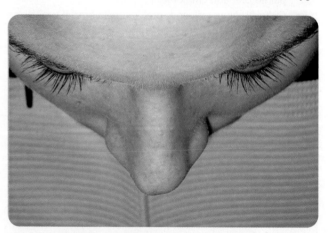

Figure 1.1. Supraorbital. Facial symmetry observed from the supraorbital aspect.

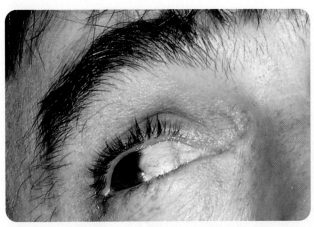

Figure 1.2. Pterygium. A pterygium is an overgrowth of tissue.

of finding should be noted, and the patient should be questioned about it for a possible referral. Hold up the eyelids in older adults so that the entire eyelid can be observed (Fig. 1.3).

- Look at the ears and the skin in back of the ears because patients are not able to see this area themselves, and it can be easily forgotten. Also check the area at the back of the neck, which can be observed while the lymph nodes are being palpated.
- Palpate the occipital, auricular, buccal, submandibular, submental, supraclavicular, and cervical chain, including the deep, superficial, and posterior lymph nodes. Figure 1.4 shows the locations of these lymph nodes. Findings that should be noted are **induration** or hardening, tenderness, mobility or movability, and, if abnormal, whether one or more nodes are involved. Another term that is used to describe enlarged, indurated, and sometimes tender lymph nodes is **lymphadenopathy**. Figure 1.5 shows clinically visible cervical lymphadenopathy.
- While palpating the nodes be aware of the salivary glands in the area and extend the palpations to the parotid and under the mandible for the submandibular.

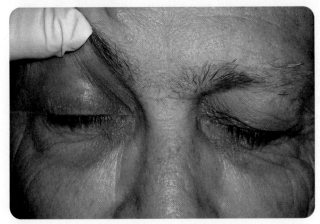

Figure 1.3. Examine the upper eyelid. Stretch the upper eyelid so that you can observe all areas of the lid.

Look for areas of swelling, induration, or tenderness.
- Examine the thyroid gland by pressing one side of the gland against the thyroid cartilage while holding the other side of the gland (Fig. 1.6). Then check to make sure there is symmetrical movement of the thyroid cartilage during swallowing.
- Bilateral palpation of the temporomandibular joints should be done next. The function of the joint is best observed from a supraorbital position while the patient is opening and closing the mouth and moving the jaw from side to side (Fig. 1.7). In addition, examine the patient for any limitations in opening the mouth or for any joint sounds. Ask about joint tenderness or modifications in food choices made to accommodate painful joint function.

Any abnormalities should be accurately and completely recorded in the patient's record. Writing the descriptions of abnormal conditions is presented following the discussion of the intraoral examination.

Performing an Intraoral Examination

The intraoral examination is a continuation of the extraoral examination and may overlap in several areas, especially near the lips and buccal mucosa. As with the extraoral examination, the sequence of the examination is not as important as the routine systematic approach. Repeating the same steps over and over again will increase the accuracy of the examination and decrease the chance that anything will be missed. The oropharynx is a common place to start. The following lists the recommended sequence for performing the intraoral examination:

Make sure the entire area of the oropharynx is observed. There may be only one chance to see the area because some patients have a problem with gagging and after they realize what is being done they may become "difficult," even though they have been informed of the procedures prior to the start of the examination. Figure 1.8 depicts the oropharyngeal area of a patient who has a problem with the retention of food particles within the surface tissues of the tonsils. She complained of a bad mouth odor and stated that occasionally she was able to remove the packed food from these areas with a toothbrush.

Next, visualize and palpate the soft and hard palates and the maxillary tuberosity.

Stretch out the buccal mucosa (Fig. 1.9) and roll the labial mucosa over your fingers and thumbs so that you can visualize the entire surface of each. Palpate all of the soft tissues after they have been observed.

Examine the mandible; stretch the alveolar mucosa at the floor of the mouth to see any areas that may be hiding under the inferior border of the mandible. Palpate the entire mandible from the inferior border to the angle of the mandible.

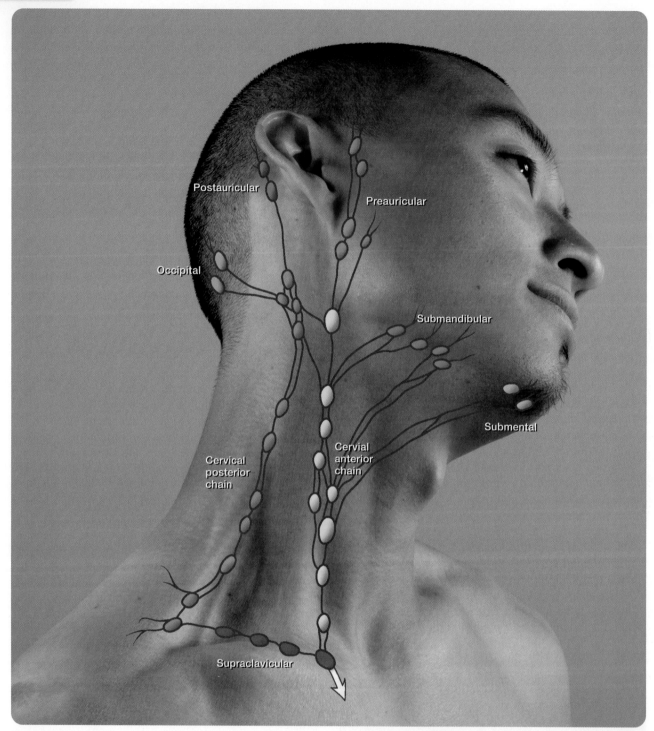

Figure 1.4. Lymph nodes of the head and neck. The location of the lymph nodes that should be palpated during the extraoral examination.

Next examine the floor of the mouth; use bimanual palpation to press the structures against the fingers of your extraoral hand (Fig. 1.10). Look for any areas of color change, tenderness, induration, or masses.

Hold the tongue with a gauze square and gently roll the tongue over on one side to observe the lateral border, then repeat for the other side.(Fig. 1.11). Observe the dorsal and ventral surfaces and then palpate the entire tongue. After removing the gauze, observe the tip of the tongue.

Finally, observe and palpate the attached gingiva on both the maxillary and mandibular arches.

Assess the amount and quality of saliva by observation and by milking the parotid gland. Remember that thick foamy saliva is usually a sign of a very dry mouth.

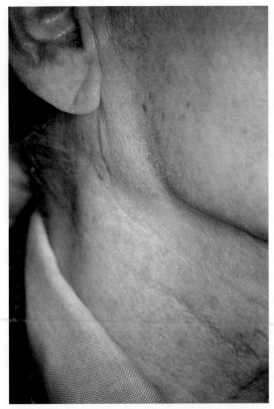

Figure 1.5. Lymphadenopathy. Clinically visible enlarged cervical lymph node. (Courtesy of Dr. Carolyn Bentley.)

Parafunctional habits such as bruxism (grinding) or clenching also need to be assessed and noted in the record if present.

Describing and Recording Clinical Findings

When recording the description of an abnormality there must be enough detail presented to provide another professional the patient may need to see with enough information to decide whether the abnormality is resolving or

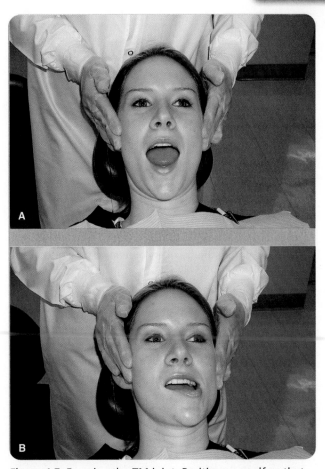

Figure 1.7. Examine the TM joint. Position yourself so that you can observe the mouth opening and closing and moving side to side from the supraorbital aspect while you bimanually palpate the TMJ. **A.** Opening and closing. **B.** Moving from side to side.

becoming worse. Remember that the record is a legal document and should be able to stand up to legal scrutiny if it ever becomes necessary. In many practices intraoral photographs are being used to provide an adjunct to the written description for future comparison, but there must

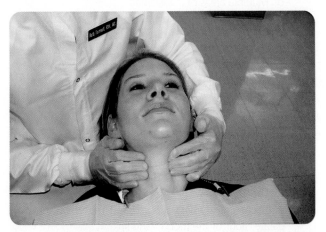

Figure 1.6. Examine the thyroid gland. Gently press the thyroid gland against the thyroid cartilage with the fingers of one hand while you hold the other side of the gland steady against the cartilage.

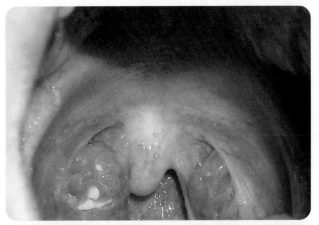

Figure 1.8. Examine the oropharynx. Get a good look at the entire oropharynx as quickly as possible. Notice the yellowish areas of food debris stuck in the craters of the tonsillar tissue.

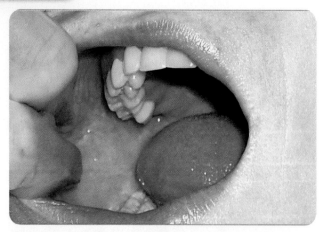

Figure 1.9. Examine the buccal mucosa. Stretch the buccal mucosa away from the maxillary and mandibular arches to examine the entire surface.

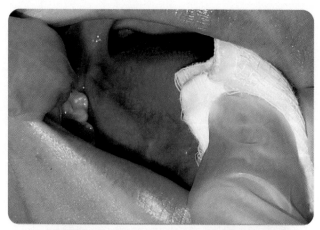

Figure 1.11. Examine the lateral borders of the tongue. Turn the tongue over rather than pulling the tongue out. It is not as uncomfortable and more can be seen than if the tongue is straight.

always be a written description in the patient's record. Certain observations will cause the dental hygienist more concern than others. Some findings will be indicative of very aggressive, **malignant** or cancerous conditions, while others will indicate relatively **benign** or noncancerous and less aggressive conditions. Box 1.4 lists the observations that are more indicative of a benign condition and those that might imply a more serious or malignant condition. The description of unknown lesions or other abnormalities should include the following:

• History—Very often there is no history of an oral condition because the patient is unaware of having it. Sometimes the medical/dental history will provide some clues to the history of the problem through notations about chronic conditions such as diabetes, recent illnesses, and medications. The patient should be asked about pain in the area or feelings of paresthesia (numbness, tingling, or other altered sensations). If there is pain, additional information such as the level of pain, whether it is sharp or dull, whether it is constant or occasional can help begin the process of determining what is happening.

• Location—An accurate description of the location of the lesion must be recorded. Some dental charts will have a diagrammatic representation of the areas in the mouth where a facsimile of the lesion can be drawn. If not, the location of the lesion needs to be described using appropriate terminology. Use terms such as inferior, superior, lateral, medial, anterior, posterior, distal, and mesial to denote location. Always try to pick a fixed point of reference that is close to the lesion to

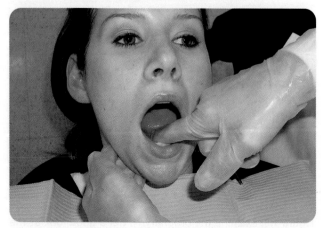

Figure 1.10. Examine the floor of the mouth. Use the fingers of your intraoral hand to press the tissues of the floor of the mouth against the fingers of your extraoral hand.

Box 1.4   **OBSERVATIONS THAT MIGHT INDICATE THE AGGRESSIVENESS OF A PARTICULAR ABNORMALITY**

1. Observations that imply a more benign condition
   a. Nonulcerated lesions
   b. Bilateral involvement
   c. Sharply demarcated borders
   d. Multiple areas of involvement
   e. Elevated, soft and movable lesions
   f. Lesions that have a direct cause and effect relationship
2. Observations that imply a more aggressive, possibly malignant condition
   a. Paresthesia
   b. Single area of involvement
   c. Ill-defined and ragged borders
   d. Flat, indurated, and fixed lesions
   e. Alteration of the periodontal ligament space and/or lamina dura
   f. Mixed red and white lesions and velvety red lesions
   g. Lesions on the lateral borders of the tongue, soft palate, floor of the mouth, and lip
   h. Radiographic evidence of bone expansion or root erosion, displacement, or resorption

APPLICATION

Some may believe that the importance of the clinical evaluation is being overstated or that the authors are overly passionate in their beliefs, but most hygienists will have the opportunity to save someone from disfiguring surgery or to save someone's life by performing a thorough cancer screening examination on each and every patient. Almost every year students or instructors have discovered an extraoral or intraoral suspicious lesion that has turned out to be malignant. For example, a student found a squamous cell carcinoma on her grandmother's arm. In another case, an instructor found a basal cell carcinoma at the corner of a student's eye during a preclinic demonstration of the extraoral examination. Also, a student was doing an extraoral examination on a relative and discovered a thyroid thickening that turned out to be a recurrence of thyroid cancer. The dental hygienist is part of a team of individuals that is working to provide care and education for patients to help them achieve optimal oral and general health. Every person that examines the patient is important because what one misses, the others might not. Two separate studies, done recently, one by Alice Horowitz et al. and one by Jane Forrest et al.

found that dental hygienists did not consistently provide oral cancer screening examinations for their patients even though most of them knew it should be done. Many stated such things as not having enough time or feeling inadequately trained as excuses for not providing this essential service (Horowitz, 2002; Forrest, 2001). In March 2004, Case Western Reserve University's School of Dental Medicine presented the results of a similar survey to the annual research meeting of the American Dental Education Association. The study found that although hygienists placed a high value on oral cancer screening, only 53% actually did the examinations on their patients. It was also reported that the level of knowledge about oral cancer, specifically the causes, appearance, and risk factors, among the dental hygienists surveyed was comparable to that of the general dentists surveyed 1 year earlier in 2003 (Cancer Weekly, May 11, 2004). Almost 84% of patients surveyed by Sandra Johns and reported in the *Journal of Dental Hygiene* in Fall 2001 stated that they had never had an extraoral examination (Johns, 2001). That is why it is important to make sure that the patient knows what is being done for them and why.

start the location description, such as, adjacent to tooth 29 on the buccal mucosa or located in the middle one third of the tongue, or 2 mm left of the midline. Use a probe to measure distances from the point of reference to the lesion and to measure the size of the lesion itself.

- Distribution and definition—Terms that describe distribution include
  - **Localized**, or found in one area only. The term "focal" can also be used (Fig. 1.12).
  - **Generalized**, or located in most of the tissues in one area. The term "diffuse" is also used sometimes (Fig. 1.13).
  - "Single lesion" (Fig. 1.12) or "multiple lesions" (Fig. 1.13) further define the distribution.

- If there are multiple lesions, are they distinct and separate or are they **coalescing** or growing together and becoming one large lesion (Fig. 1.14).
- Margins define the extent of the lesion and are either "well defined" or **circumscribed** (Fig. 1.15) or "ill-defined" and vague. Ill-defined margins are difficult to determine, and the dental hygienist may not be sure where the lesion ends and where normal tissue begins (Fig. 1.16).
  - Well defined margins may be "regular" (Fig. 1.15) or "irregular" (Fig. 1.13) in shape.

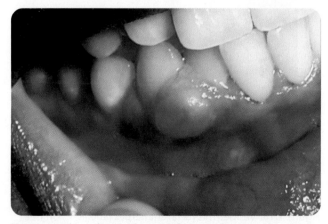

Figure 1.12. Localized. This nodule is confined to the gingival tissues between the canine and the premolar.

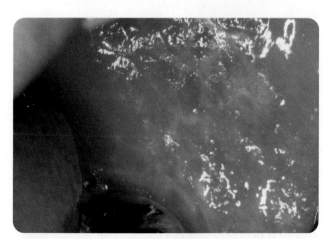

Figure 1.13. Generalized with irregular margins. This white lesion of lichen planus (see Chapter 14) called Wickham's striae covers the entire right and left buccal mucosal surfaces with an irregular lacy pattern.

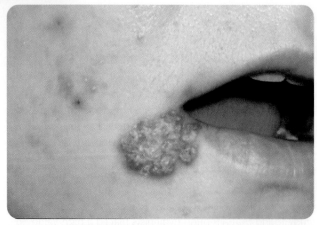

Figure 1.14. Coalescing lesions. This recurrent herpes labialis lesion consists of separate vesicles that have begun to coalesce or grow together.

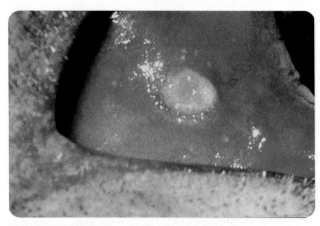

Figure 1.15. Well circumscribed with regular margins. This granular cell tumor is well defined within the tissues. Note the yellow papules called Fordyce's granules (see Chapter 14). (Courtesy of the U. S. Department of Veteran's Affairs.)

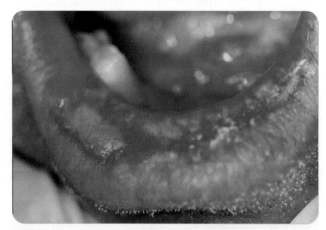

Figure 1.16. Ill-defined margins. Sun exposure has caused actinic keratosis or cheilitis on the lower lip. Some of the central areas are obvious, but it is difficult to determine exactly where the lesion ends, as it extends away from the central area. (Courtesy of the U. S. Department of Veteran's Affairs.)

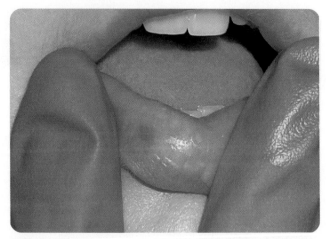

Figure 1.17. Macule. This flat lesion is differentiated from the surrounding tissue by color alone.

- Size and shape—Note the general shape and measure the size of the lesion with a probe. Measure the diameter of round lesions and the width and length of square, rectangular, and oval lesions. When writing the numbers for length and width, the width will come first; for example, a 5 inch by 7 inch frame will be 5 inches wide and 7 inches long. The size of a very large lesion might have to be related to the area that it covers, such as the entire left lateral border of the tongue from the tip to the circumvallate papilla. If the lesion has any height, this must be noted also. Height is listed after the length of the lesion.
  - A flat lesion that is differentiated from the surrounding tissue by color alone is called a **macule** (Fig. 1.17) if it is less than 1 cm in diameter and a **patch** if it is more than 1 cm. A patch may also describe an area that has a different surface texture with or without a color change.
  - An elevated lesion may be a **vesicle** (Fig. 1.18) if it is 1 cm or less and is filled with a clear fluid. If it is larger than 1 cm, it would be called a **bulla**.
  - A **pustule** is a raised lesion that is filled with pus or **purulent exudate**.

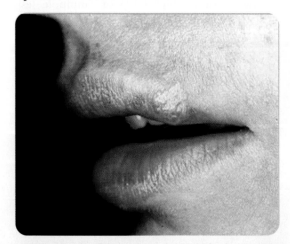

Figure 1.18. Vesicle. This recurrent herpes labialis lesion (see Chapter 11) is in the vesicular stage. The outlines of the smaller vesicles that have coalesced into this larger lesion are still visible.

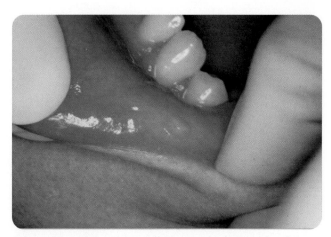

Figure 1.9. Papule. This small fibroma (see Chapter 17) is the appropriate size to be described as a papule.

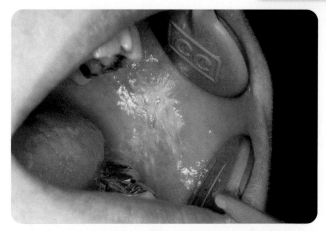

Figure 1.21. Plaque. The slightly raised and flat configuration of this white lichen planus lesion that covers a relatively broad area is indicative of a plaque.

- A raised lesion with no fluid inside is called a **papule** (Fig. 1.19) if it is less than 5 mm in diameter; a slightly larger, less than 2-cm, raised lesion is called a **nodule** (Fig. 1.20), and anything larger than that is called a **tumor**.
- If the area is broad, slightly raised, has a flat top, and looks pasted on, it is called a **plaque** (Fig. 1.21).
- A growth can be attached to the surrounding tissues by a broad or **sessile** base, as illustrated by the fibromas in Figures 1.19 and 1.20, or by a stalk, **pedunculated** (Fig. 1.22).
- Depressed lesions can either be **ulcers** (Fig. 1.23), which extend through the epithelium into the dermis, or **erosions** (Fig. 1.24), which do not extend through the epithelium. Erosions can also be called **abrasions**.
- Two other terms are used to describe the general direction of growth of a lesion. **Exophytic** lesions grow outward from the surface of the tissue like the fibromas in Figures 1.19 and 1.20, and **endophytic** lesions grow into the surrounding tissues and present as palpable masses with or without any noticeable swelling.
- Color—Abnormal areas may be the same color as the surrounding tissues or they could be white, **erythematic** (red), yellow, or pigmented.

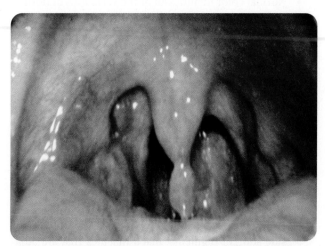

Figure 1.22. Pedunculated. The uvula seen in this picture has a long pedunculated growth extending from its tip. (Courtesy of Jill Nield-Gehrig.)

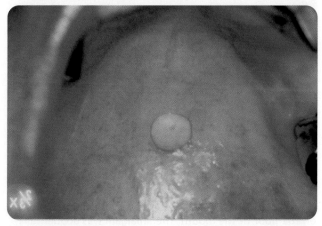

Figure 1.20. Nodule. This larger fibroma on the hard palate is described as a nodule.

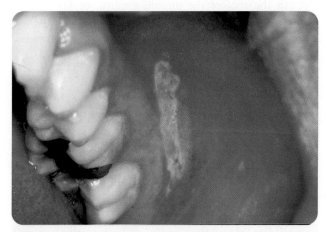

Figure 1.23. Ulcer. This ulcer exhibits the classic features of a central depressed area surrounded by an erythematic ring and covered by a white pseudomembrane. (Courtesy of Dr. Terry Rees.)

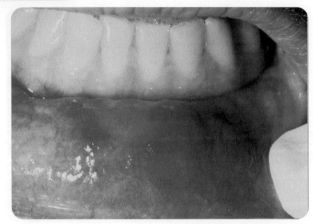

Figure 1.24. Erosion. Just the surface epithelium has been destroyed, leaving a diffuse area of erythema in these erosive lichen planus lesions of the lower lip.

- Normal color includes all of the variations of normal and normal physiologic pigmentations (Fig. 1.25).
- White lesions that cannot be wiped off (Fig. 1.21) usually indicate excess keratin in the tissues, making them more opaque, like a callus on the hand.
- Erythematic areas (Fig. 1.26) usually indicate thinning of the epithelium allowing the more vascular subepithelial or submucosal tissues to be seen, or erythema may indicate an increased blood flow into the area due to an inflammatory reaction (see Chapter 3).
- Yellow can indicate the presence of purulent exudate or adipose tissue (fat) (Fig. 1.27).
- Other pigmentations include brown, black, and blue. These colors can represent either **endogenous** (from within the body) or **exogenous** (from an outside source) pigments. Black macules that are adjacent to teeth with amalgam restorations are very often caused by pigments from the amalgam, accidentally introduced into the soft tissues, leaching into the surrounding tissue, resulting in an **amalgam tattoo** (Fig. 1.28). Smaller black macules in the roof of the mouth, gingiva, or lips can be

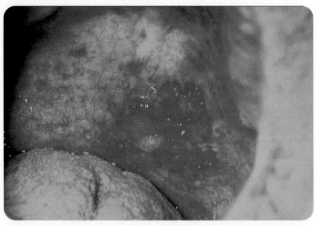

Figure 1.26. Erythema. This red lesion with poorly defined margins was found to be an invasive squamous cell carcinoma. (Courtesy of the U. S. Department of Veteran's Affairs.)

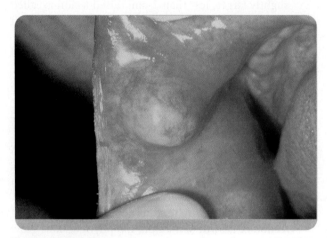

Figure 1.27. Yellow. Adipose tissue often gives a yellow hue to tissues as seen in this lipoma, which is a benign neoplasm of adipose tissue. (Courtesy of the U. S. Department of Veteran's Affairs.)

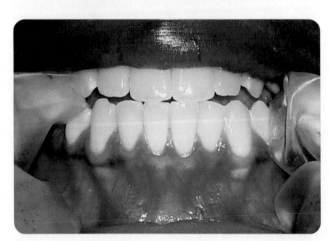

Figure 1.25. Physiologic pigmentation. Normal melanin pigmentation of the gingival tissues.

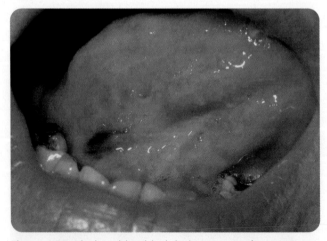

Figure 1.28. Black or blue/black lesion. An amalgam tattoo on the floor of the mouth. The amalgam was accidentally introduced into the soft tissues when an amalgam restoration was being placed. (Courtesy of Dr. Peter Jacobsen.)

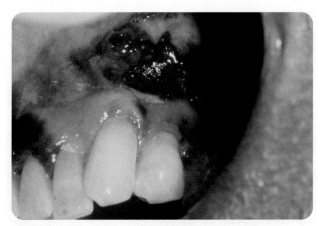

Figure 1.29. Labial varices. This older gentleman has a bluish vascular lesion on the upper lip.

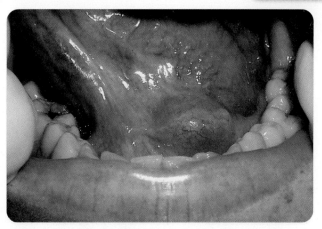

Figure 1.31. Smooth surface texture. This swelling on the floor of the mouth depicts a normal smooth surface texture.

caused by a pencil lead being stabbed into the tissues. This is usually accidental and occurs when children run or play with a pencil in their mouth. The patient may or may not remember the incident. Another cause of a black macule is **melanoma**, a cancer of the pigment-producing cells or melanocytes (see Fig. 15.5A in Chapter 15). Melanoma is very serious and very difficult to treat. Blue lesions are most likely vascular, such as labial varicosities (Fig. 1.29) but they can also be melanomas. Brown lesions usually contain melanin pigments and can be part of normal physiologic pigmentation, an intraoral nevus (Fig. 1.30), or a melanoma. Any black, blue, or brown pigmented lesion is cause for concern, and an explanation for its presence should be determined. The options for follow-up on lesions such as this are discussed in Chapters 5 and 15.

- Consistency—Consistency refers to how something feels when pressed on. Students and clinicians often confuse the terms used for consistency and those used for surface texture. Try to remember that consistency is determined by how the area feels when pressed on, not what it feels like when a fingertip is rubbed across its surface. Most of the case studies in this book provide a description of consistency, since consistency cannot be seen.

- The consistency of soft tissue abnormalities is often soft or normal feeling.
- Indurated soft tissue lesions, such as an inflamed lymph node, feel quite hard.
- **Fluctuant** is used to describe a fluid-filled lesion that moves fluid from one area to another when the lesion is pressed.
- Surface texture—The surface texture of an intraoral lesion is determined by how it feels when the pad of a fingertip is run across it and what it looks like. "Smooth" and "rough" are the main descriptive categories.
  - A smooth surface texture is usually found when there is submucosal swelling and the surface of the lesion is covered by normal mucosal epithelium (Fig. 1.31).
  - Rough surface textures are described by how they feel and how they look. Common terms to describe roughness include
    - **Papillary**, consisting of fingerlike projections (Fig. 1.32)

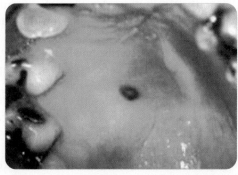

Figure 1.30. Nevus. Blue nevus of the hard palate. (Courtesy of Marquette University School of Dentistry.)

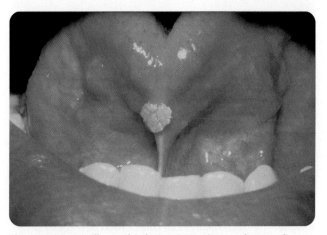

Figure 1.32. Papillary. This lesion is made up of many fingerlike projections as its name papilloma suggests. (Courtesy of the U. S. Department of Veteran's Affairs.)

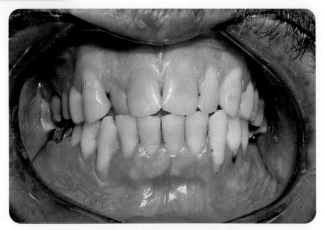

Figure 1.33. Corrugated. The white corrugated lesions extending from the buccal mucosa through the mucobuccal fold up into the attached gingival are characteristic of those caused by spit tobacco use.

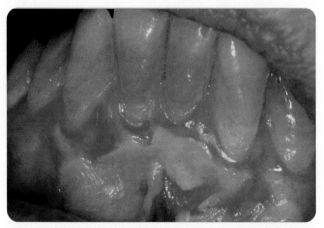

Figure 1.35. Pseudomembrane. The white surface membrane characteristic of pseudomembranous candidiasis leaves a sore erythematic area behind when it is wiped off with gauze.

- **Corrugated**, rippled or washboard-like (Fig. 1.33)
- **Fissured**, consisting of many deep crevices (Fig. 1.34)
- **Crusted** or covered with a scab may also be used to describe perioral lesions (Fig. 1.14). The intraoral counterpart of a crust is a **pseudomembrane** or false membrane that covers the surface of a lesion and can be wiped off (Fig.1.35).

Description of Radiographic Findings

Radiographs are an integral part of most dental examinations. Diagnostic radiographs may be exposed as part of a routine dental examination or they may be exposed to obtain more information about an abnormality that has been discovered through observation or palpation of the intraoral or perioral tissues. Radiographic abnormalities are very often discovered by accident when there are no clinically observable signs or symptoms. A brief description of

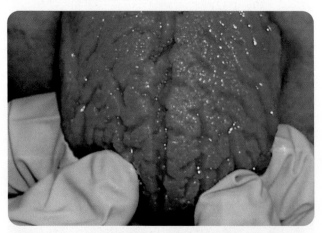

Figure 1.34. Fissured. This is a classic example of a fissured tongue. The deep fissures can collect food debris and provide a perfect environment for the growth of dental biofilm. The fissuring is not usually seen in children and worsens as the individual ages.

radiographic findings should be recorded in the patient's record in case the radiographs become misplaced. The features that should be described include the following:

- History—The patient should asked whether he or she is aware of the area in the radiograph or not. If the patient is aware, ask what he or she was told it was, how long it has been present, and if there are any symptoms associated with it. The most common symptoms associated with bone lesions are pain and paresthesia. Very often there is no history, and the dental team will have to start the process of determining the cause of the lesion.
- Location and size—Determining the location of a radiographic finding is often made difficult by the radiographic technique used for exposing the film. Radiographs that are taken with excessive or inadequate vertical or horizontal angulation will not reflect the true location of the anomaly. Panoramic radiographs may also distort the true position of an anomaly. Care must be taken to use every means to accurately locate the abnormality. In most instances when there is any doubt about the location, multiple radiographs will be taken from different aspects and with different angulations to more accurately place the anomaly. Size can be recorded in millimeters or centimeters and, if large, relative to the structures involved.
- Distribution—Distribution describes the number of anomalies and how they are positioned within the hard tissues.
  - "Single" is used to describe one lesion.
  - More than one lesion is described as "multiple lesions."
    - "Localized" or "focal" describes a clustered group of lesions.
    - "Generalized" or "diffuse" describes multiple findings in a large area of bone.
- Radiographic features—There are terms that are used specifically to describe radiographic findings. These terms include the following:

APPLICATION

Refer to Figure 1.31 for a photo of the soft tissue description developed in this section.

History: The patient was unaware of this lesion until 2 days ago. She reports no history of trauma, and there are no significant findings on the medical or dental histories.

- Location: Floor of the mouth (FOM) 5 mm to the left of the lingual frenum at the level of the sublingual caruncle
- Distribution and definition: Single, localized, and well circumscribed
- Size and shape: Round nodule 18 mm in diameter 10 mm in height, sessile base
- Color: Slightly bluish with an erythematic ring around the base
- Consistency: Soft and fluctuant
- Surface texture: Smooth

Description: Single, well-circumscribed, bluish nodule approximately 18 mm in diameter and 10 mm in height, surrounded by an erythematic ring, soft and fluctuant with a smooth surface and sessile base, located on the FOM, 5 mm to the left of the lingual frenum at the level of the sublingual caruncle. Patient reports that she became aware of the swelling 2 days ago, no report of trauma, no significant findings on the medical or dental histories

---

- Whether a radiographic anomaly is **radiopaque** (whiter than the normal radiographic appearance of the bone), **radiolucent** (darker than the normal radiographic appearance of bone), or **mixed** (consisting of both radiopaque and radiolucent areas) is one of the characteristics that will exclude many conditions from a list of possible diagnoses. A radicular cyst (see Chapter 20) would not be considered as a possible diagnosis if the spherical lesion at the apex of a tooth were radiopaque. Condensing osteitis (see Chapter 19) would be much more likely because its normal presentation is radiopaque (Fig. 1.36), while that of a radicular cyst is radiolucent (Fig. 1.37).

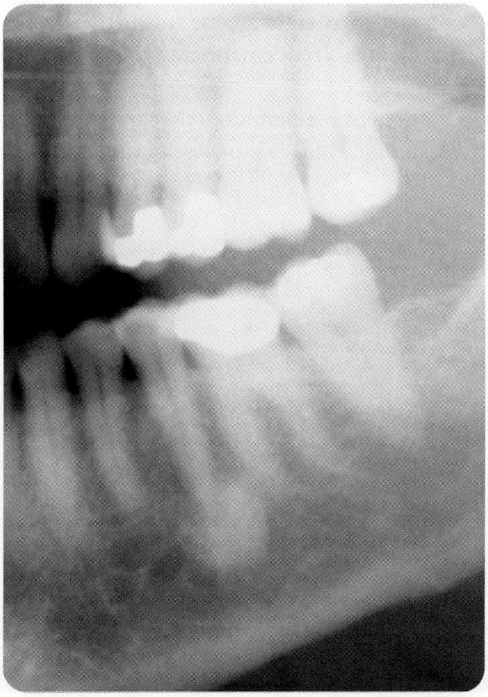

- Many lesions present as a single or **unilocular** radiopaque or radiolucent area, while others look as if there are compartments within the lesion. A radiolucent lesion made up of these compartments is said to be **multilocular**, and they are often described as having a "soap bubble" appearance (Fig. 1.38).

- It is important to determine the clarity of the margins of a radiographic anomaly. Lesions with clearly defined or well-demarcated margins (Fig. 1.39) are much more likely to be benign and less aggressive entities. Indistinct margins should be described as ill-

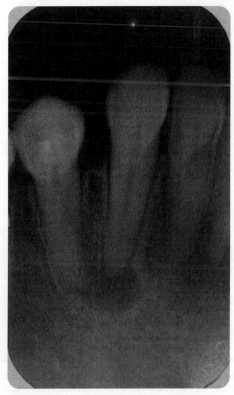

Figure 1.36. Radiopaque. Note the well-defined spherical radiopaque area of condensing osteitis at the apex of the root of the second premolar.

Figure 1.37. Radiolucent. Note the well-defined spherical radiolucent area apical to the canine.

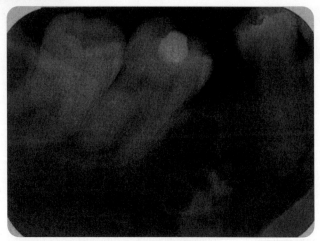

Figure 1.38. Multilocular. The multilocular radiolucent lesion in this radiograph was discovered during a routine radiographic survey. Note also the radiopaque area at the periphery of the lesion.

defined" or "irregular". Ill-defined margins will appear fuzzy or ragged and it is difficult to determine where the abnormal hard tissue ends and the normal tissue begins (Fig.1.40). Ill-defined margins are much more indicative of an aggressive or malignant condition.

• The appearance of the surrounding tissues is also important, and close attention must be paid to this area.

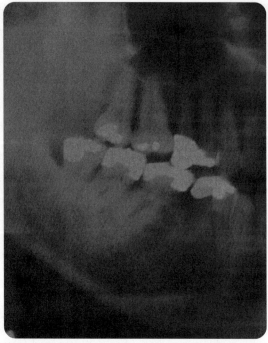

Figure 1.40. Ill-defined margins. Note the radiopaque area surrounding the first and second molars and the slightly opaque areas that seem to be extending toward the anterior region. It is difficult to determine the extent of this osteogenic sarcoma (bone cancer) because of the poorly defined borders. (Courtesy of the U. S. Department of Veteran's Affairs.)

• If the abnormality involves the roots of any teeth, it is important to determine if it is causing **resorption** or destruction of the roots (Fig. 1.41) or causing them to move out of the way through **convergence** (movement toward each other) or **divergence** (movement away from each other) (Fig. 1.42).
• Changes in the periodontal ligament space such as widening (Fig. 1.43) or loss of the space should be noted.

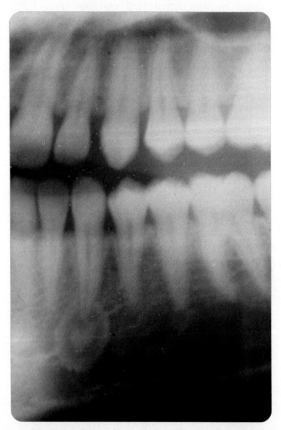

Figure 1.39. Well-defined margins. The cementoblastoma (see Chapter 20) at the apex of the canine is an example of a lesion that has well-defined radiographic margins. (Courtesy of Dr. John Jacoway.)

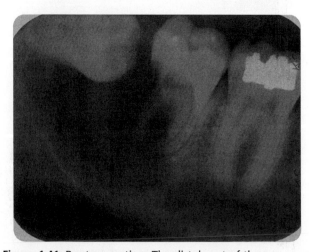

Figure 1.41. Root resorption. The distal root of the mandibular second molar has been severely resorbed by the pathologic lesion surrounding the unerupted third molar.

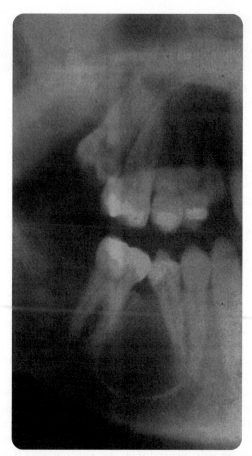

Figure 1.42. Divergence. This odontogenic keratocyst (see Chapter 20) has caused the premolar and molar roots to spread apart. (Courtesy of the U. S. Department of Veteran's Affairs.)

• The lamina dura should be observed to determine whether there have been any changes in its structure or if it is missing altogether.

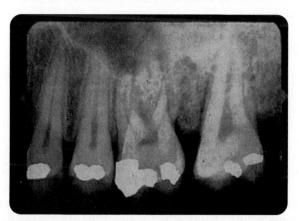

Figure 1.43. Widening of the periodontal ligament space. This radiograph is of a 34-year-old woman who was incorrectly treated for periodontal disease. Note the widened periodontal ligament space around the first molar. There is a separation between the 1st and 2nd molar, and the interproximal alveolar bone has a mottled atypical appearance compared to what would be expected. A biopsy of the area between the two molars found osteogenic carcinoma. (Courtesy of Dr. John W. Preece.)

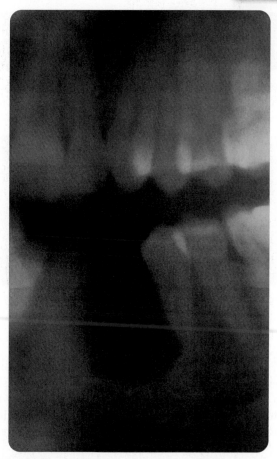

Figure 1.44. Cortical bone destruction. The central giant cell granuloma (see Chapter 18) pictured in this radiograph has eroded through the cortical bone in the edentulous mandibular area. (Courtesy of the U. S. Department of Veteran's Affairs.)

• If the cortical bone can be seen, it should be noted if there have been any changes, specifically if the lesion has been able to erode through the cortical bone (Fig. 1.44) or if there has been expansion of the bone in the surrounding area (Fig. 1.45).

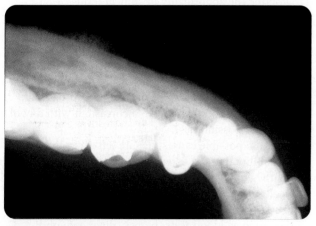

Figure 1.45. Bone expansion. This is an occlusal view of an osteogenic sarcoma (see Chapter 18). Note the sunburst pattern of abnormal bone and expansion that are characteristic of this tumor. (Courtesy of the U. S. Department of Veteran's Affairs.)

APPLICATION

Refer to Figure 1.46 for the panoramic radiograph depicting the radiopaque object that is used as the example for developing the following radiographic description.

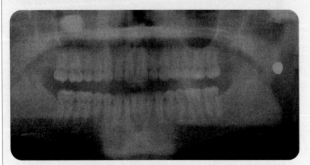

- Location: Left ramus of the mandible just inferior to the condyloid process
- Size: Round, approximately 1 cm in diameter (in the original film)
- Distribution: Single
- Margins: Well defined
- Opacity: Radiopaque

Description: A single, well-defined, 1-cm diameter, round radiopaque object located slightly inferior to the left condyloid process

Figure 1.46. Application. Radiopaque object.

DETERMINING A DIAGNOSIS

Creating a differential diagnosis for a particular lesion can be very interesting and educational. Exploring the outermost boundaries of the scope of dental hygiene practice can provide intellectual stimulation and create career satisfaction.

Differential Diagnosis

A **differential diagnosis** is a listing of the probable causes of a particular disease manifestation or group of manifestations. There is a process involved with creating a differential diagnosis, and it should be followed more or less every time something is seen that cannot be identified. The steps to creating a differential diagnosis are as follows:

1. Describe the abnormality in clinical terms.
2. Determine a list of diseases that present with similar abnormalities.
3. Eliminate some of the possible causes already listed by adding other factors that could be involved with the abnormality (chronic health condition, medications, patient age, and whether the patient has any other manifestations that are inconsistent with any of the listed possibilities).
4. Rank the possible causes that are left according to the probability that the listed cause is what actually causing the condition.
5. Decide what type of additional information might be necessary to eliminate more of the listed possibilities, such as blood tests, biopsy, diagnostic radiographs, cultures of oral microbes, and medical consultations.

It may be decided that treating the lesion as the manifestation of the most likely cause is the best course of

action. For example, if the most likely cause of a lesion is a fungal infection, and it is treated for 10 days with a topical antifungal medication resolving the lesion, it was most likely a fungal infection. A second possibility is that it resolved on its own, and no one will ever be sure of the actual cause. If it did not resolve, more specific diagnostic procedures are appropriate. It is not within the scope of practice of a dental hygienist to order any of these tests or to recommend some therapies, but it is appropriate to be aware of what the options are and thus be able to have some input as a valuable member of the dental team. If a definitive diagnosis is not determined by the additional information obtained, then the list of conditions that remains is the differential diagnosis.

DEFINITIVE DIAGNOSIS

A definitive diagnosis is determined when all of the suspected causes on the list except one have been eliminated. That one cause is the definitive diagnosis. It would be difficult for the dental hygienist to repeat this process every time an abnormal area in or around the oral cavity was discovered. Fortunately, such a lengthy process is not necessary. Many of the most common abnormalities have such distinguishing characteristics that unlikely causes can be eliminated solely through observation of the abnormality. Some of the conditions that are discussed in this book are **atypical**, or variations of normal, and not pathologic. By observing these conditions clinically, the dental hygienist will become very familiar with them and will know immediately if there is something else happening. Conditions such as leukoedema and tori can be clinically diagnosed because they have been seen, and there is no doubt about what they are. Some pathologic conditions such as caries can

APPLICATION

The following is a simple example of how to create a differential diagnosis. The possible causes listed in the differential diagnosis are described in detail in Chapter 12. Refer to this chapter if necessary for a more complete description of why a condition is eliminated from the list of possibilities. Refer to Figure 1.47 for this application.

1. Clinical description and history: Single, well-defined ulcer covered by a white pseudomembrane and surrounded by an erythematic ring; the ulcer is oval, approximately 4 mm × 3 mm, firm and slightly rough to the touch, located on the lower labial mucosa adjacent to tooth 27 at the margin of the labial mucosa and the extraoral lip tissue. The patient is 10 years old and has no significant medical or dental findings other than the report of slight pain in the lip on function.

2. The following are considered as part of the differential diagnosis:
   - Reiter syndrome (Chapter 12)
   - Syphilis (Chapter 12)
   - Erythema multiforme (Chapter 12)
   - Traumatic ulcer (Chapter 12)
   - Recurrent aphthous ulcer (Chapter 12)

3. Rationale for excluding some elements of the differential diagnosis
   - Reiter syndrome usually occurs in males in their 30s and normally manifests with concurrent generalized arthritis. This young man is 10 and reports no significant medical findings such as arthritis. Thus Reiter syndrome can be eliminated as a possibility.
   - Primary syphilis is a sexually transmitted disease that presents with a large ulcer-like chancre at the initial point of contact. This patient is most likely not sexually active at age 10, but the possibility of sexual abuse would have to be ruled out. The clinical appearance of this lesion is much too small to be a chancre, and there would be no pain associated with a chancre, so this can also be eliminated.

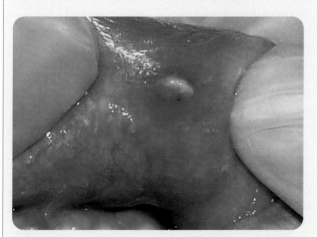

Figure 1.47. Application. Sample differential diagnosis.

- Erythema multiforme is an immune response that presents with skin and mucous membrane lesions. The absence of skin lesions and the fact that this is a solitary lesion probably indicates that this disorder can be eliminated.
- Traumatic ulcers look like this lesion, and they are often found on the lip, tongue, cheeks, and other areas that are subject to frequent trauma. This diagnosis is highly likely.
- Recurrent aphthous ulcers look like this lesion and present on the moveable mucosa; in addition, they can be precipitated by trauma to the tissues. It is not known whether this patient has had this type of ulcer before. Without more information, this diagnosis must also be considered likely.

4. A ranking of the remaining possibilities is difficult in this case because there is an equal probability that it could be either one. In this case, more information is needed. It is necessary to ask a few more questions, such as the following:
   - When did you notice the ulcer?
     Answer: About 2 days ago.
   - Have you ever had ulcers like this on your lip or in your mouth before?
     Answer: I had one on my gums after I hit myself with a toothbrush.
   - Do you remember doing anything to cause the ulcer?
     Answer: Yeah, I bit my lip!

5. These questions have clarified the circumstances that occurred prior to the development of the ulcer. The following must be considered before eliminating either of the possibilities.
   - Only one other ulcer located on the attached gingival surface occurred previous to this ulcer, and that ulcer was also associated with trauma.
   - Recurrent aphthous ulcers do not normally affect the attached gingiva, indicating that the previous ulcer was probably not recurrent aphthous.
   - Causal relationships are important, and in this case the patient has supplied the cause.

6. The only possible way to obtain a definitive diagnosis of this lesion would be to biopsy the lesion, which may not provide anything more than to describe the lesion as containing inflammatory cells, which would be likely in either case. The cause-and-effect relationship between the trauma of biting the lip and the appearance of the ulcer and the fact that there is no previous report of aphthous ulcers supports the diagnosis of a traumatic ulcer. The clinical manifestation of the ulcer would be treated the same way for either diagnosis. The only consideration would be to alert the patient of the possibility that more ulcers occurring in the absence of trauma might indicate recurrent aphthous ulcers.

be diagnosed from their characteristic radiographic appearance. The danger arises when the dental team starts assuming that everything that is seen is a variation of normal. Often there is concern that the patient might be subjected to undue stress about something that is most likely benign. An effort must be made to determine the cause of all suspicious areas that are identified. In many cases this will require a visit to an oral surgeon for a biopsy; or the biopsy, exfoliative cytology, or brush

biopsy may be performed in the general dental office. Some patients may be unduly alarmed by a referral for a biopsy of what turns out to be an amalgam tattoo, but the alternative diagnosis of a melanoma must be considered until ruled out. Many of the conditions throughout this book include a differential diagnosis or listing of other conditions that can cause similar lesions. Attention should be paid to these and they should be incorporated into the student's dental hygiene education.

APPLICATION

FAMILY VIOLENCE: RECOGNITION AND APPROPRIATE INTERVENTION

The epidemic of family violence (the abuse or neglect of children, adults, or the elderly) continues to grow in the United States and elsewhere, with as many as 10 million victims each year in the United States alone. The dental team faces two challenges in dealing with the full spectrum of family violence: (1) the magnitude of the family violence problem and (2) the apparent lack of involvement from dental professionals. The size of the family violence epidemic is constantly growing, but is difficult to measure. Recent statistics have shown that the incidence of child abuse and neglect, the only universally reportable forms of family violence, continues to rise. Typical data show as many as 3 million children each year are reported to child protective service (CPS) agencies in the United States.[1] Moreover, as many as 5000 children are fatalities of abuse and neglect each year.[2]

The incidence of intimate partner violence (IPV) and elderly abuse is even larger, although difficult to quantify. (Note: The term "intimate partner violence" is the current terminology for what was previously known as "domestic violence" or "spousal abuse." Also, some states' statutory language uses "domestic violence" to refer to victims of any age.) Estimates from various sources show that these forms of family violence are as pervasive as child maltreatment. Elderly abuse is at least as common as child abuse, and IPV is more common than child abuse.[3,4] Dr. Donna Shalala, former U.S. secretary of Health and Human Services, has put the magnitude of the IPV epidemic into perspective by stating that it is "as common as birth in the U.S., four million occurrences each year."

Obviously, the size and seriousness of these epidemics are staggering, but dentistry's major involvement has traditionally focused on child abuse and neglect. However, dentistry's commitment to preventing child maltreatment is not commensurate with the epidemic. Although up to 75% of child abuse injuries occur to the head, neck, and face, few dentists apparently ever recognize or report a case of child maltreatment.[5] A protocol for helping professionals identify family violence will most certainly ameliorate this discrepancy as it relates to victims of any age.

IDENTIFICATION

Many of the steps in identifying family violence are applicable to victims of any age. Safety planning must be a consideration for any possible family violence intervention. Safety planning must include protocols to maintain confidentiality for victims, procedures for summoning the police or other emergency aid to the office, and plans for how to protect both victims and office staff from violence. Literature about community resources to help victims should be made available. This information could be discretely placed in the ladies' restroom as opposed to the reception area. A victim may be more comfortable reading or taking this information while she is in the privacy of the ladies' room.

Even though the potential for violence within the dental office is minimal, understand that perpetrators might want to stop interventions on behalf of the victim. Every office should have a "safe room." A safe room must have a sturdy door that can be locked from the inside, have an outside telephone line, and be large enough for the staff and patient to stay until help arrives.

Recognizing family violence can be facilitated by following a simple protocol (Table 1.1). Start by doing a general physical assessment of the patient. While a physical examination is not appropriate in all healthcare settings, the practitioner can always observe the patient for signs that may be consistent with trauma or show obvious delay in seeking treatment.

A patient's behavior may also indicate a history of violence. While everyone's behavior is unique, patients tend to behave differently in the clinical setting than outside this environment. Certain behaviors may lead one to suspect violence. Judge your patients' behavior in light of their maturity and the current setting (see Clinical Protocol 15).

All patients undergo a health history that is updated at each appointment. Especially when dealing with children, it may be useful to get one history from the adult and another, in a separate setting, from the child. Histories about an injury that do not match may indicate violence. Separate dual histories may also be important when dealing with adults or the elderly, since victims will often not answer honestly in the presence of the perpetrator.

continued

Application, cont.

Table 1.1	PHYSICAL AND BEHAVIORAL INDICATORS OF ABUSE AND NEGLECT	
Type of CA/N	**Physical Indicators**	**Behavioral Indicators**
Physical Abuse	*Unexplained Bruises and Welts:* • face, lips, mouth • torso, back, buttocks, thighs • various stages of healing • clustered, regular patterns • reflecting shape of article used to inflict (e.g. buckle) • on several different areas • regular appearance after absence, weekend, vacation *Unexplained Burns:* • cigarette, cigar burns, esp. on soles, palms, back, buttocks • immersion burns (sock or glove-like, circular, on buttocks or genitalia) • patterned: electric burner, iron • rope burns on arms, legs, or torso *Unexplained Fractures:* • skull, nose, facial structures • in various stages of healing • multiple or spiral fractures *Unexplained Laceration or Abrasion:* • to mouth, lips, gingiva, eyes • to external genitalia	• Wary of adult contacts • Apprehensive when others cry • Behavioral extremes: • aggressive • withdrawn • Frightened of parents • Afraid to go home • Reports injury by parents
Physical Neglect	• Constant hunger, poor hygiene, inappropriate dress • Consistent lack of supervision, esp., in dangerous situations or for long periods • Unattended physical problems or medical/dental needs • Abandonment	• Begging, stealing food • Extended stays at school, early arrival, late departure • Constant fatigue, falling asleep in class • Alcohol or drug abuse • Delinquency (e.g. thefts) • Says there is no caretaker
Sexual Abuse	• Difficulty in walking or sitting • Torn, stained, bloody underwear • Pain or itching in genital area • Bruises or bleeding on external genitalia, vaginal, or anal areas • Venereal disease, esp. in pre-teen • Pregnancy	• Unwilling to change for PE • Withdrawal, fantasy or infantile behavior • Bizarre, sophisticated sexual knowledge or behavior • Poor peer relationship • Delinquency; runaways • Reports sexual assault by caretaker

(continued)

Examination of the oral cavity and surrounding structures can identify signs of family violence including injuries to the teeth and supporting structures. Perioral lesions, including lacerations, contusions, pattern injuries or oral lesions of sexually transmitted diseases, may also indicate family violence (Figs. 1.48, 1.49, and 1.50).

In some cases, it may be useful to consult with the patient's physician. Confidential consultation between healthcare pro-

Application, cont.

Table 1.1	PHYSICAL AND BEHAVIORAL INDICATORS OF ABUSE AND NEGLECT, CONT.	
Type of CA/N	**Physical Indicators**	**Behavioral Indicators**
Emotional Maltreatment	• Speech disorders • Lags in physical development • Failure to thrive	• Habit disorders (sucking, biting, rocking, etc.) • Conduct disorders (antisocial, destructive) • Neurotic traits (sleep disorders, inhibited play) • Psychoneurotic behaviors (hysteria, phobia, obsession, compulsion, hypochondria) • Behavior extremes: • Compliant, passive • Aggressive, demanding • Overly adaptive behavior: • Inappropriately adult • Inappropriately infantile • Developmental lags (physical or mental) • Attempted suicide

©Lynn Douglas Mouden, Telephone: (501) 661-2595; e-mail: Lynn.Mouden@arkansas.gov, December 1992.

fessionals is important for a variety of conditions, and family violence suspicions can be strengthened or alleviated by this personal contact.

APPROPRIATE INTERVENTION

When a healthcare provider makes the decision to intervene in suspected family violence situations, one must take action appropriate to the age of the victim, the situation, and the statutory requirements. Healthcare providers in all states are required to report suspected cases of child abuse or neglect, consistent with state law. Carefully document physical and behavioral indicators of abuse or neglect in the patient's chart. Also report, verbatim, statements of history when the histories do not match. It is useful to have a witness in the operatory during the child's examination and history, and that person should cosign the child's chart.

Call the appropriate child protective services agency for your jurisdiction. Reporting agencies are specific to states and counties and may include not only social service agencies but

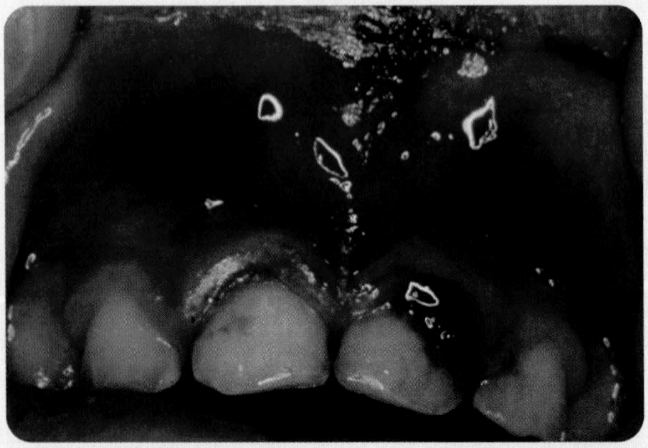

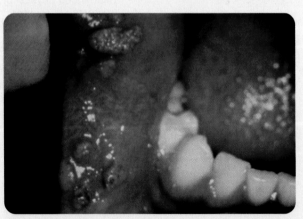

Figure 1.48. Family violence. Multiple oral injuries, including lacerated lip, torn frenum, bruised vestibular tissue, and subluxated central incisor, all caused by an open-handed slap. (Courtesy of Lynn Douglas Mouden.)

Figure 1.49. Family violence. Condyloma acuminatum (venereal warts) contracted during an oral rape. (Courtesy of Lynn Douglas Mouden.)

Application, cont.

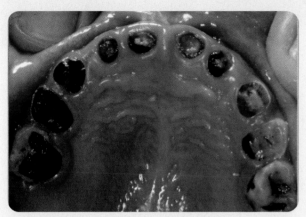

Figure 1.50. Dental neglect. Untreated gross caries with multiple draining abscesses. (Courtesy of Lynn Douglas Mouden.)

also law enforcement agencies. Be sure to know your reporting requirements and keep the reporting number easily available. The person taking information will guide the reporting process and ask for identifying information. That information may include the child's name and address, age, siblings, the nature of the current condition, and other useful information including the name of the suspected perpetrator. While reports can be accepted from anonymous sources, healthcare professionals should identify themselves so that follow-up inquiries are possible when necessary.

When providing assistance for adult or elderly victims, one must also know the statutory requirements specific to the jurisdiction. State laws on reporting adult and elderly victims of family violence vary widely and must be understood before the situation arises. Remember that the patient's health and safety must be your first concern, and inappropriate intervention or reporting when not required may actually place the patient at higher risk.

When dealing with adult victims, healthcare professionals must learn that their role is to serve as facilitators providing information, support, and encouragement. Therefore, providers must learn to communicate respect for all their patients, support their patients' decisions, and be knowledgeable about available community resources. Provide adult victims the opportunity and resources to change their lives. Every healthcare provider must develop attitudes that will allow them to assist all victims of family violence, such as attitudes of urgency, respect, concern, and community.

THE DENTAL PROFESSIONS' RESPONSE TO THE PROBLEM

Several initiatives in recent years have helped healthcare professionals and others deal with family violence. The most no-

table program is the Prevent Abuse and Neglect through Dental Awareness (P.A.N.D.A.) Coalition. P.A.N.D.A., which began with the model program in Missouri, is now in place in 46 U.S. states and 10 international coalitions. Individuals in the remaining U.S. states and many countries are working to form the public/private partnerships that make the P.A.N.D.A. program work. Putting together the resources of healthcare, education, public health, insurers, and social services has been the key to the program's effectiveness. Not only is the dental profession more aware of the problems of family violence in P.A.N.D.A. states, these coalitions have proved their effectiveness. P.A.N.D.A. has shown notable success. Although nationally, the total reports of suspected child abuse and neglect have continued to rise approximately 6% each year, following the first year of P.A.N.D.A.'s educational and awareness campaign in Missouri, the number of reports made by dentists rose by 60%.[6] After 4 years of the P.A.N.D.A. program, the reporting rate by dentists has now risen by 160%.[7] In Illinois, the reporting rate rose an astounding 800% after 5 years of the P.A.N.D.A. program.

Every healthcare professional must not only understand the symptoms of family violence but also be familiar with local resources to help stop the violence. Every professional must take steps to deal with suspected victims: (1) know and understand the applicable state, tribal, or federal laws, (2) learn what is available to help victims in your own community, (3) get involved with P.A.N.D.A. or similar programs, (4) seek out educational opportunities to prepare yourself, and most importantly (5) show concern for every patient's total health and demonstrate your willingness to help. Remember that victims of family violence fall into only two categories, those who survive and those who do not.

References

1. National Center on Child Abuse Prevention Research. Current trends in child abuse reporting and fatalities. National Committee for the Prevention of Child Abuse, Chicago, IL; April 2003:2.
2. U.S. Advisory Board on Child Abuse and Neglect. A nation's shame: fatal child abuse and neglect in the United States. U.S. Department of Health and Human Services, Washington, D.C.; 1995:9.
3. McDowell JD. Domestic violence: recognizing signs of abuse in patients. Dental Teamwork May–June 1994;7(3):23–27.
4. Strauss MA. Wife beating: how common and why. Victimology 1977–78;3–4:443–458.
5. da Fonesca MA; Feigal RJ; ten Besel RW. Dental aspects of 1248 cases of child maltreatment on file at a major county hospital. Pediatr Dent 1992;14(3):152–157.
6. Mouden LD. The role Tennessee's dentists must play in preventing child abuse and neglect. J Tenn Dent Assoc April 1994;74(2):17–21.
7. Mouden LD. Dentistry addressing family violence. Mo Dent J; Nov–Dec 1996;76(6):21–27.

This section was written by Lynn Douglas Mouden, DDS, MPH, FICD, FACD, Director, Office of Oral Health in the Arkansas Department of Health and Human Services and founder of the P.A.N.D.A. program. For more information, you may contact Dr. Mouden at 501-661-2595 or Lynn.Mouden@arkansas.gov.

SUMMARY

- The concept of health comprises a wide range of physical, emotional, and spiritual components.
- Individuals are being encouraged to take charge of their lives and establish a sense of personal responsibility for their own health.
- Patients are expected to take a dynamic role in their health care. Healthcare providers are not only expected to provide treatment but also to facilitate this new active role by helping to direct and educate the patient in ways of attaining total body wellness.
- Oral health is an integral part of total body health, and the dental team is responsible for helping the patient achieve and maintain good oral health.
- The oral cancer screening examination is an important element in determining the oral health of the patient.

- Oral cancers are usually diagnosed in the late stages, and early diagnosis and treatment will decrease the incidence of disfiguring surgery and increase cancer survival rates.
- It is necessary to write an accurate and complete description of abnormal clinical or radiographic findings in the patient's dental record so that the proper follow-up can be accomplished.
- An exciting aspect of oral pathology is first creating a differential diagnosis and then determining a definitive diagnosis based on the elimination of improbable elements of the differential diagnosis.
- A definitive diagnosis should always be obtained for unknown oral or perioral abnormalities.

PORTFOLIO POSSIBILITIES

1. Take photographs of a clinical patient who has a pathologic or interesting atypical condition or copy several pictures of oral lesions from books and write a complete clinical and/or radiographic description of each one. Use your imagination to fill in the elements of consistency and size if necessary. Ask for your instructor's feedback on your project.

2. Write a fact sheet for your patients about why the cancer screening examination (extraoral and intraoral examinations) is done and some examples of what you are looking for.

Critical Thinking Activities

1. You have taken a position as a dental hygienist in an established practice. You are told what you are expected to accomplish during an initial appointment, maintenance appointments, and special appointments for sealants and periodontal debridement. You notice that nothing has been said about a cancer screening examination. You ask if this is an oversight and are told that only the dentist performs the cancer screening examination. What are your initial thoughts about this? Do you think that this is a good protocol for a dental practice? If yes, justify your answer. If no, what

would you do to try to change it? Research your state's dental practice act and report on what the responsibility of the hygienist is in regards to this situation.

2. Refer to Figure 1.31 for this activity. The patient has given you the following additional information: She states that she has experienced frequent dull aching sensations from the area that get sharper just before, during, and for a short time after she eats. Does the additional information bring you any closer to a definitive diagnosis of the lesion? If so, what direction is it leading you in?

Case Study

Refer to Figure 1.51 for this case study. This panoramic radiograph was taken as part of an initial examination of a 25-year-old woman.

1. Write a radiographic description of the anomaly seen in the mandibular right posterior region. (Size is approximately 6 mm diameter.)

2. Based on the radiograph alone, what are some questions that you might want to ask this patient to try to determine a differential diagnosis?

3. How would you clinically evaluate the area?

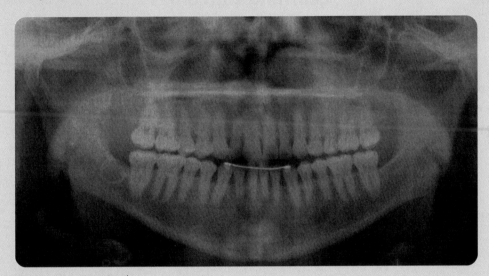

Figure 1-51. Case Study

REFERENCES

Coleman GC, Nelson JF. Principles of oral diagnosis. St. Louis: Mosby-Year Book, 1993:44–159, 267–277.

Dental school survey shows dental hygienist's role in catching cancer. Cancer Weekly May 11, 2004. Available at: http://www.NewsRx.com. Accessed summer 2004.

Forrest JL, Horowitz AM, Shmuely Y. Dental hygienists' knowledge, opinions, and practices related to oral and pharyngeal cancer risk assessment. J Dent Hyg Fall 2001;75(IV):271–281.

Horowitz AM, Siriphant P, Canto MT, Child WL. Maryland dental hygienists' views of oral cancer prevention and early detection. J Dental Hyg Summer 2002;76(III):186–191.

Ibsen OAC. A full investigation: a complete medical, dental, and family history can provide important clues in the oral pathology diagnostic process. Dimensions Dent Hyg May 2004;2(5):36–38.

Ibsen OAC. Putting the pieces together: The diagnostic process used in oral pathology requires a methodical approach. Dimensions Dent Hyg March 2004;2(3):32–34.

Johns SG. The extraoral examination from the perspective of the patient. J Dent Hyg Fall 2001;75 (IV):282–289.

Newland JR, Meiller TF, Wynn RL, Crossley HL. Lexi-Comp's clinical reference library, oral soft tissue diseases: a reference manual for diagnosis and management. Hudson, OH: 2001:4–11.

Regezi JA, Sciubba JJ, Jordan RCK. Oral pathology: clinical pathologic correlations. 4th ed. St. Louis: WB Saunders, 2003.

Risbeck CA. Case study: identifying risk factors for systemic disease. Accessed March 2004;18(3):20–25.

Surveillance, Epidemiology, and End Results (SEER) Program. (www.seer.cancer.gov) SEER* Stat Databases: Incidence—SEER 11 Regs + AK Public-Use, Nov 2003 Sub for Expanded Races (1992–2001) and Incidence—SEER 11 Regs Publuc-Use, Nov 2003 Sub for Hispanics (1992–2001), National Cancer Institute, DCCPS, Surveillance Research Program, Cancer Statistics Branch, released April 2004, based on the November 2003 submission. Available at: http://canques.seer.cancer.gov/cgi-bin/cq_submit?dir=seer2001&db=4&rpt=TAB&sel=1^ . Accessed summer 2004.

Wilkins EM. Clinical practice of the dental hygienist. 9th ed. Baltimore: Lippincott Williams & Wilkins, 2004:174–188.

Langlais RP, Miller CS. Color atlas of common oral diseases. 3rd ed. Baltimore: Lippincott Williams & Wilkins, 2003:2–21.

Ibsen OAC, Phelan JA. Oral pathology for the dental hygienist. 4th ed. St. Louis: WB Saunders, 2004:1–33.

Alonge OK, Narendran S. Opinions about oral cancer prevention and early detection among dentists practicing along the Texas–Mexico border. Oral Dis 2003;9:41–45.

Centers for Disease Control and Prevention. Measuring healthy days. Atlanta, GA: CDC, November 2000:4.

Centers for Disease Control and Prevention. Promoting oral health: interventions for preventing dental caries, oral and pharyngeal cancers, and sports-related craniofacial injuries: a report on recommendations of the Task Force on Community Preventive Services. MMWR 2001:50(no. RR-21):2.

2

Basic Pathology

Key Terms

- Abscess
- Apoptosis
- Atrophy
- Caseous necrosis
- Coagulative necrosis
- Complication
- Dysplasia
- Etiology
- Exacerbate
- Exocrine system
- Free radical
- Goiter
- Hyperplasia
- Hypertrophy
- Hypoxia
- Idiopathic
- Incubation period
- Integumentary system
- Ischemia
- Latent period
- Liquefactive necrosis
- Manifestation
- Metaplasia
- Morbidity
- Mortality
- Necrosis
- Neoplasia
- Pathogenesis
- Pathology
- Prognosis
- Psychogenic
- Relapse
- Resistance
- Resolution
- Risk factor
- Sequela
- Sign
- Stress
- Susceptibility
- Symptom
- Xerostomia

Learning Outcomes

1. Define and use the key terms in this chapter.

2. List the different types of etiologies and give an example of each.

3. Determine whether an etiology is intrinsic or extrinsic.

4. List the major risk factors affecting the resistance of the host and state examples of each.

5. Describe how stress can affect the body.

6. Describe the elements that may be seen in the pathogenesis of a condition.

7. Explain the three major ways that cells react to conditions that are not normal.

8. Determine the type of cellular adaptation that has occurred, given certain characteristic features.

9. Differentiate between cellular adaptation, injury, and death.

10. List the most common mechanisms of cellular injury.

11. Identify instances in which apoptosis would most likely occur.

12. Describe the three different types of necroses.

13. Identify the type of necrosis that causes abscess formation.

Chapter Outline

CONCEPTS OF THE PATHOLOGIC PROCESS

Pathology is the study of disease or, more specifically, the study of abnormal conditions that may result from one or more of the following: disease, traumatic injury, structural or biochemical errors, genetic abnormalities, and so on. To study the disease process, the student must be aware of several factors. These factors include

- The causes or **etiology** of the disease or pathologic entity
- The events or characteristics that make certain individuals more susceptible or resistant to disease
- The manner in which the disease progresses, or **pathogenesis**
- The possible manifestations of disease on a cellular, tissue, and organ basis

This discussion not only involves disease as we know it, but also describes other types of pathology, such as cuts, burns, acne infections, and arthritis.

Etiology

The first element in the development of disease or pathology is the causative factors, or the etiology. There can be a single cause, as in tuberculosis, or a multifactorial etiology, as in hypertension or heart disease. The first step in disease research is directed toward finding the etiology. Prior to knowing what the cause is, only the signs and symptoms of the disease can be treated. For example, as soon as acquired immune deficiency syndrome was recognized, researchers began looking for the cause. Until it was found, physicians could only treat the opportunistic infections or conditions associated with the syndrome. As

---

APPLICATION

Consider, for example, an elderly woman who has enlarged knuckles on some of her fingers and pain when she first uses her hands in the morning. It is obvious that she has some sort of arthritis, but does she have a disease? As another example, a patient complains of a very sore and swollen palate. The patient does not remember doing anything to cause the soreness. The hygienist examines the palate and finds a small torus palatinus. The surface of the torus is abraded, red, and looks like it would be very sore. Does she have a disease?

In the first example, the elderly woman most certainly has a disease. Osteoarthritis is a degenerative disease that could affect the entire skeletal system. The fact that it is affecting only the hands does not make it any less of a disease. There are two conditions in the second example. The torus palatinus is considered a variation of normal with hereditary tendencies; as such, it is not considered a disease or pathology. On the other hand, the traumatic injury to the gingival surface is considered a pathologic lesion, but it would not be considered a disease.

---

soon as the cause was determined to be viral and that virus was identified, finding a "cure" became possible. Current therapies stress slowing down the replication of the virus, specifically inhibiting the ability of the virus to create proteins that are essential for its replication. The cause of most diseases can be classified as either extrinsic (of external origin), intrinsic (of internal origin), or a combination of both. Table 2.1 provides a list of intrinsic and extrinsic causes and examples.

A disease state that is brought on by conscious or subconscious reactions or attitudes is considered to be **psychogenic**. The physical manifestations of psychogenic illnesses are very often real and can prove incapacitating or fatal. No discussion of etiologies would be complete without the inclusion of the **idiopathic** etiology. When disease or pathology is determined to be of idiopathic origin, the causative agent or event has not been discovered. In many instances it is not possible to name one etiologic agent or event as the cause of a particular pathologic process. Often there are several factors working together to produce disease in an individual. When there is more than one causative factor, the condition is said to have a multifactorial etiology. Multifactorial etiologies usually have a combination of extrinsic and intrinsic features. Heredity plays an important part in most of these conditions.

Resistance and Susceptibility

Why does one person develop an illness when others do not, even when they are exposed to the same conditions? The answer to this question lies within the realm of host

Table 2.1	EXTRINSIC AND INTRINSIC CAUSES AND EXAMPLES	

Category	Etiology	Examples
Extrinsic	Pathologic organisms	Bacteria, virus, protozoa, fungus
	Physical agents	Temperature, electricity, radiation
	Chemical agents	Poison, acid, venom, drugs
	Mechanical injury	Gunshot wound, motor vehicle accident
	Nutritional	Deficiency—scurvy, rickets
		Excess—obesity
	Iatrogenic	Infective endocarditis, hospital staphylococcus infection
Intrinsic	Genetic	Sickle cell disease, cystic fibrosis, some types of breast cancer
	Immunologic	Autoimmune—systemic lupus erythematosus
		Hypersensitivity—allergies
		Immunodeficiency—acquired immunodeficiency syndrome
	Degenerative	Osteoporosis, osteoarthritis

resistance and susceptibility. **Resistance** is the natural ability of an organism to remain unaffected by pathogenic or toxic agents. **Susceptibility** is the exact opposite, conditions within or around the organism or host that do not inhibit the action of pathogenic agents. Resistance is affected by many **risk factors** or predisposing conditions. Box 2.1 lists major groups of risk factors.

GENETIC

Genetic influences play an undeniable role in whether or not a person is susceptible to certain conditions and diseases. In fact, it can be safely said that inheritance affects every aspect of our health. Some individuals have a limited genetic lineage, meaning that their ancestors may have the same ethnic or religious background or come from the same geographic area. Often individuals in these groups have a higher risk of developing a disease than someone from another group. Families that do not have a limited genetic lineage may still carry genetic risk factors for certain conditions that will place them at a higher risk of developing conditions than families that do not have the risk factor. Tay-Sachs disease is a fatal genetic disorder that affects individuals of Jewish descent more frequently than any other group. Tay-Sachs disease is characterized by the excess storage of lipids in the cells and tissues of the brain. This process eventually causes destruction of the cells and death of the child, usually within a few years. Sickle cell anemia is found most often in those with an African-American genetic lineage. Sickle cell anemia is the most common fatal genetic disorder among African Americans and is discussed in detail in Chapter 9. Often, inherited traits will decrease the resistance of an individual to certain diseases or conditions. Fair-skinned individuals are at a higher risk of skin cancer than darker-skinned individuals. Higher risks of developing certain conditions such as breast cancer, heart disease, and high blood pressure have also been found in family lineages.

Box 2.1 MAJOR GROUPS OF RISK FACTORS

1. Genetic
2. Immune system dysfunction
3. Compromised first line defenses
4. Age
5. Lifestyle
6. Stress
7. Environment
8. Preexisting conditions

IMMUNE SYSTEM

A deficit in any part of the immune system will cause a decrease in the resistance of the host. Some defects are more serious than others. Loss of the tonsils will cause a defect in the body's ability to fight off infection. However, this is minor in comparison to being born without the ability to manufacture white blood cells that function correctly. The defect in this individual will cause severe **morbidity**, or disease, and most likely an early death from an infectious disease.

FIRST-LINE DEFENSE SYSTEMS

The first-line defense systems include the integumentary system and the exocrine system. The specific actions of this system are discussed in Chapter 3. The **integumen-**

tary system includes the skin, hair, nails, and sweat and sebaceous glands. Damage to the skin can cause severe problems and even death. Burns on over 20% of the total body surface area are considered major burn injuries and result in massive fluid losses, electrolyte imbalances, and a decrease in blood volume, leading to shock and hypotension. In this case, the body is unable to maintain homeostasis because there is no external barrier protection in the area of the burns. The **exocrine system** comprises glands that excrete their products through a duct onto the surface of the skin or other organ. The exocrine system includes sweat glands, sebaceous glands, salivary glands, and glands of the gastrointestinal and respiratory systems. The secretions from some of these glands contain antibodies that help to destroy invading organisms before they are able to cause any damage. The high pH of gastrointestinal secretions destroys many of the contaminants that we ingest. Damage that occurs to any of the major salivary glands can result in **xerostomia** (inadequate salivary flow). As a dental professional, you must be aware of the multiple problems associated with xerostomia to be prepared to assist the patient with adequate measures to minimize discomfort and maintain health. Xerostomia is discussed in detail in Chapter 17.

AGE

The body is less able to adapt to physical, biologic, and mental stresses at the beginning of life and in the later years of life. The infant's ability is impaired because the body's defense systems are not fully developed. The older adult's ability is impaired because of the decline in function of body systems seen with advancing age. The results in both cases are similar; the individual is not able to adapt to stress, resulting in the development of disease or pathology. Biologic and behavioral variations during different phases of life put an individual at risk for developing conditions at specific times during the life cycle. Osteoporosis is found more often in postmenopausal women because of decreased levels of the hormone estrogen (see Chapter 10). Middle ear infections are found more often in small children because of the structure of their ear. Car accidents were the leading cause of death for 15- to 20-year-olds in the year 2000, based on data from the National Center for Health Statistics. This is a higher statistic for this age group than for any other age group. Teenagers accounted for 10% of the U.S. population in 2002 and 14% of motor vehicle deaths (DOT HS 809619, 2002).

LIFESTYLE

Lifestyle choices have a direct effect on resistance to disease. For example, smoking, in addition to the well-known consequences of heart and lung diseases, directly assaults the immune system, decreasing its effectiveness and leaving the smoker at a higher risk for many other types of problems. One such problem is periodontal disease. Dietary choices may increase the risk of cardiovascular disease and cancer. Frequent exposure to ultraviolet light, whether by choice or because of occupation, increases the risk of skin cancer. The abuse of alcohol and/or recreational drugs is a problem that crosses all segments of society in the United States. Risky sexual behaviors can result in contact with the human immunodeficiency virus, syphilis, and/or gonorrhea, among others. Consequences of inappropriate lifestyle choices and behaviors are mirrored in the health of the body and the mind.

STRESS

Stress can be defined as anything, physical or psychologic, that causes the body to initiate the stress response. This is also known as the "fight-or-flight response." Many bodily functions are altered during this response. Box 2.2 lists physiologic changes that occur during the stress response. The stress response is intended to be a short-term action. For example, when individuals are startled, their hearts will beat faster to circulate more blood, they will start breathing faster to increase the amount of oxygen in the body, they become very alert to their surroundings, and so on. When they realize that nothing is wrong, everything starts to go back to normal. This type of stress reaction is beneficial. Stress becomes harmful when the reaction is long term. Chronic stress produces the full range of actions summarized in Box 2.2, but to a lesser degree, over a longer time period. Eventually the body exhausts itself trying to keep up this heightened level of activity, exposing the individual to a higher risk for many

---

Box 2.2 PHYSIOLOGIC RESPONSES TO STRESS

1. Increased blood flow to the heart

2. Increased blood pressure

3. Decreased blood flow to the extremities and to the stomach

4. Airways dilate to increase oxygen supply to blood

5. Increased amount of glucose available for energy

6. Increased mental alertness

7. Decreased unnecessary body functions such as digestion

8. Inhibition of some immune system cell functions

9. Increased fat generation and retention in the cells of the face and trunk

conditions and diseases, such as cardiovascular diseases, musculoskeletal disorders, psychologic disorders, gastrointestinal disorders, and many others.

ENVIRONMENT

The environment can also be a risk factor for developing a disease or condition. For example, someone living in the tropics is at a higher risk of developing a parasitic infection than someone residing in a cold climate. Family members living with a smoker are at higher risk of developing smoking-associated illness than those in a nonsmoking environment (ALA, 2006).

Environmental exposure to toxic substances is a major concern in our world. In the 1960s and 1970s, families living in Love Canal, a neighborhood in Niagara Falls, New York, were exposed to a myriad of toxic substances that were buried under the ground on which their homes and an elementary school were built. During the early and late 1970s, residents reported strange odors and substances that surfaced in their yards and seeped into their basements. The neighborhood had a very high rate of cancer and an alarming number of birth defects. Children that attended the school were always ill. This was the first case concerning hazardous waste disposal and possible health effects that received national attention in the media and at the highest level of government. The residents were relocated, some after years of legal battles. Most of the Love Canal site was eventually decontaminated, and a new community called Black Creek Village now stands on the land, but there is still an area that will not be habitable in any of our lifetimes (Love Canal Collection, 2006).

PREEXISTING CONDITIONS

When an individual is compromised by one disease or condition, there is a much higher risk of developing a second disease or condition. Lesions of psoriasis, if scratched open, can become infected by bacteria. A person with diabetes mellitus is more likely to contract a bacterial infection than a nondiabetic individual. Someone who is debilitated by cancer or cancer treatments is more likely to contract bacterial and viral infections. Someone with emphysema is more likely to develop pneumonia than someone who does not have a chronic lung condition.

MULTIPLE RISK FACTORS

Risk factors may be found alone or in combination with others. As would be expected, the more risk factors involved, the higher the potential for developing a disease or condition. For example, we know that tobacco use increases the risk for oral cancer, but if you add alcohol use, the risk for developing oral cancer increases dramatically. Likewise, an individual with diabetes who also smokes has a very high risk of developing periodontal disease, much higher than those with either risk factor alone.

Pathogenesis

Every disease or abnormality has a specific process of development or pathogenesis. Pathogenesis refers to the sequence of events during which cells or tissues respond to an etiologic agent. One may find individual variations under certain circumstances, but on the whole, the pathogenesis of a particular disease is usually the same from individual to individual. The pathogenesis of a disease may be very specific for that disease or it may be similar to that of other diseases or conditions. For example, the pathogenesis of syphilis is unique to this disease. No other disease mimics the primary, secondary, and tertiary stages of the disease process. Any stage taken alone can be mistaken for another process, but when viewed as a whole, there is no other condition that is similar. Chapter 12 provides more information on syphilis. The pathogenesis of measles (rubeola) and German measles (rubella) (see Chapter 11) are very similar to each other. Both diseases are viral; both are transmitted through respiratory secretions and infect the respiratory epithelium. Both cause coldlike symptoms with the addition of fever and a disseminated red rash. However, rubeola tends to be more serious and can be fatal in the young, elderly, or immunocompromised. Rubella, on the other hand, is less severe but has the distinction of being able to cause devastating birth defects, including spontaneous abortion or miscarriage. Laboratory tests and the clinical appearance of the rashes differentiate between the two; however, they are very similar.

A general understanding of some specific terms is helpful when discussing the pathogenesis of disease.

- The **incubation period** of a disease refers to the time in which the disease is developing but there are no overt signs or symptoms.
- A **sign** is an objective observation usually made by a clinician and sometimes a patient about the clinical manifestations of the disease process. Examples of signs include: fever, rash, low blood pressure, and low red blood cell count.
- A **symptom** is a more subjective report of what a client is feeling such as fatigue, headache, and nausea among others. In conversation, sign and symptom are often used interchangeably; however, an awareness of the difference is important in professional discussions.
- A **manifestation** is an observable or quantifiable characteristic associated with a specific type of pathology. Manifestations include: signs, symptoms, results of laboratory tests, radiographs, and so on.
- A **latent period** is a time during disease development when there are no overt manifestations of the disease, although the disease can be found by using other means such as laboratory tests or radiographs. Herpes simplex (see Chapter 11) is an excellent example of a disease with latent periods. Following the

primary infection, the virus lies dormant in the sensory ganglia of the trigeminal nerve in the head and neck area until an event activates it again. At this point the virus manifests as a vesicular lesion, usually near the lips.

- **Exacerbation** refers to the worsening of a disease condition. For example, eating hot and spicy foods will exacerbate the pain of an oral ulcer.
- **Resolution** occurs when the affected individual or part returns to normal.
- A **sequela** of a disease is a condition or pathology that occurs as a result of that disease. Male sterility is sometimes a sequela of mumps or acute viral sialadenitis (see Chapter 17).
- **Morbidity** refers to the illness or disability associated with a disease. Morbidity is used more often in statistical discussions about the impact of a disease on a population.
- **Mortality** or death can also occur as a consequence of a disease process.
- A **complication** of a disease is an additional disease process or condition occurring at the same time and resulting from the conditions associated with the first disease process. For example, a bacterial sinus infection can be a complication of a cold. The bacterial infection would not have occurred if the cold had not produced the necessary environment of copious secretions and injured mucosal cells.
- A **relapse**, or flare-up of a disease, occurs weeks or months after the pathology was thought to be gone.
- The **prognosis** is an estimate of the most likely outcome of a disease, such as the likelihood that the individual will survive or that the pathology will resolve. The prognosis is based on many factors. For example, the pathogenesis of the disease, the condition of the individual, and the medical therapies that are available will all influence the prognosis.

Disease manifestations usually begin to be apparent as a disease or condition develops.

Disease Manifestations

Disease occurs in many forms, both visible and invisible. Some diseases affect the entire body, and others affect only small areas of the body. No matter what the cause or manifestation of a disease, it all begins on a cellular basis. The extent of a disease is related to how many cells of the body are affected. The seriousness of a disease may be related to exactly which cells are affected. Because every disease is a manifestation of some sort of cellular change, disease should be studied by looking at what occurs on a cellular level. Cells react to conditions that are not normal by adapting to the change (cellular adaptation), becoming injured (reversible injury), or dying (irreversible injury).

CELLULAR ADAPTATION

Changes inside the cell or in the area surrounding the cell can occur as a result of normal or pathologic processes. Normal changes can have as much of an effect on the individual cell as pathologic changes. For example, all of the changes associated with pregnancy and the inevitable changes associated with aging are normal changes. Another example of a normal process is the manner in which the body adapts to life at high altitudes. Less oxygen is available to the body at high altitudes, causing the body to compensate by producing more red blood cells to carry more oxygen to the tissues (secondary polycythemia, or erythrocytosis; see Chapter 9). Since this process takes time, travelers to areas of higher altitude experience shortness of breath much more quickly than normal for several days. Erythrocytosis can also be a manifestation of a pathologic condition such as chronic obstructive lung disease (see Chapter 10). In this case the oxygen deprivation is due to a decrease in the transfer of oxygen within the lungs caused by damaged tissues. Pathologic changes are associated with infection, immune system dysfunction, traumatic injury, and many other factors. The adaptive process will continue until the stimulus for the change is removed and the environment returns to normal. If this does not happen, the cell may reach a point at which it can no longer adapt to the continued change, and internal damage will begin to occur. In many cases even this damage is reversible if normal conditions are reestablished. If the damage continues, cell death or irreversible injury will occur. Adaptive cellular changes include atrophy, hypertrophy, hyperplasia, metaplasia, dysplasia, and the intracellular retention of substances that are injurious to the cell (Fig. 2.1). Neoplasia is a continuum of the process of dysplasia, but since neoplastic growth is not considered an adaptive change, it is only mentioned here and is discussed in depth in Chapter 5.

Atrophy. Atrophy is a decrease in the size and function of a cell, tissue, or organ, caused by one or more of the following conditions: reduced functional demand, hormonal stimulation, nutrient supply (including oxygen), and/or the normal process of aging. Reduced functional demand on a cell, tissue, or organ will cause it to decrease in size. For example, when a cast is removed from a broken arm or leg, there is an obvious difference in size between the previously broken limb and the limb that was not broken. This occurs simply because the limb was not allowed to function for a length of time. The same condition occurs with paralyzed body parts, because there is no longer any neural stimulation of the affected area. Musculoskeletal disorders such as carpal tunnel syndrome cause atrophy of the affected areas (Fig. 2.2). Atrophy also occurs in response to a reduction in hormonal stimulation. After menopause the ovaries atrophy because they no longer receive hormonal stimulation from the pituitary gland. Reduced nutrient supply may also cause atrophy. Muscle

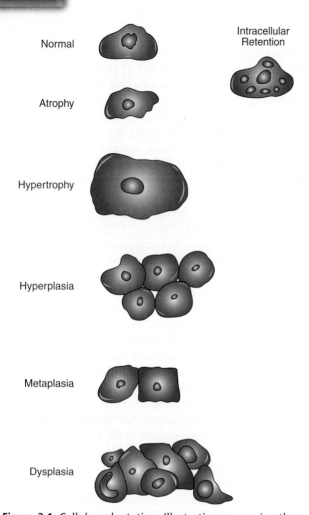

Normal

Atrophy

Hypertrophy

Hyperplasia

Metaplasia

Dysplasia

Intracellular
Retention

Figure 2.1. Cellular adaptation. Illustration comparing the different ways a cell can adapt to changes in its environment. **A.** Normal cell, **B.** Atrophy, **C.** Hypertrophy, **D.** Hyperplasia, **E.** Metaplasia, **F.** Dysplasia, **G.** Intracellular retention of substances.

and organ atrophy is associated with anorexia nervosa and with many cancers. In anorexia nervosa, the cells are not receiving nutrients because they are not getting them from the individual; in cancer, the individual's nutrients are being devoured by the out-of-control demands of the cancerous growth. Atrophy caused by a reduction of nutrients may occur in areas where there is chronic cellular injury, such as areas that are involved with a persistent bacterial infection. A decreased supply of oxygen to the cell, or is-chemia, will cause cell atrophy. This type of atrophy is usually seen around areas where there has been vascular damage, such as the damage done during a myocardial infarction or heart attack (see Chapter 8). Cellular atrophy occurs in the normal process of aging. The best examples of this are seen in the aging heart muscle and brain.

Hypertrophy. **Hypertrophy** is the enlargement of individual cells leading to an increase in the size of the tissue or organ and is commonly caused by increased functional demand or hormonal stimulation. The increase in size may also result in an increase in the functional capacity of the tissue or organ. Hypertrophy caused by an increase in the functional demand placed on the cells is best exemplified by the increase in muscle mass due to weight lifting or exercise. Muscle cells do not replicate, therefore, the increased demand of strenuous exercise will stimulate hypertrophy. Hypertension (see Chapter 8) causes an increased demand on the heart muscle, which in turn causes individual cells to become hypertrophic (Fig. 2.3). The end result in this case is hypertrophy of the left ventricle, which is being overworked to pump blood through

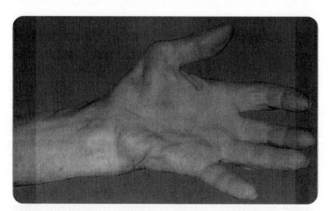

Figure 2.2. Atrophy. Atrophy of the thenar muscles at the base of the thumb due to chronic compression of the median nerve (carpal tunnel syndrome). (From Moore KL, Dalley AF. Clinical oriented anatomy. 4th ed. Baltimore: Lippincott Williams & Wilkins 1999.)

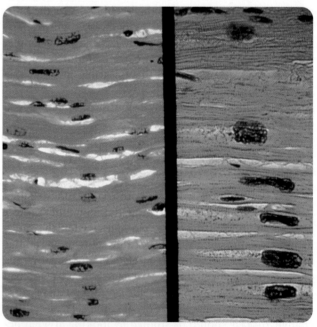

Figure 2.3. Hypertrophy. Myocardial hypertrophy. Compared with a normal myocardium *(left),* the hypertrophic myocardium *(right)* shows thicker fibers and enlarged, hyperchromatic, rectangular nuclei. (From Rubin E, Farber JL. Pathology, 3rd ed. Philadelphia: Lippincott Williams & Wilkins, 1999.)

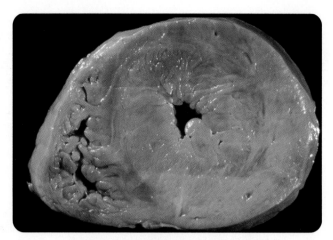

Figure 2.4. Ventricular hypertrophy. Cross-section of the heart of a patient with long-standing hypertension shows pronounced, left ventricular hypertrophy. (From Rubin E, Farber JL. Pathology, 3rd ed. Philadelphia: Lippincott Williams & Wilkins, 1999.)

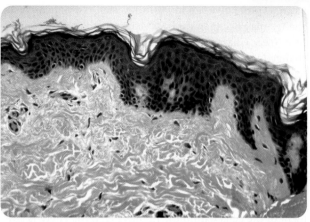

Figure 2.6. Hyperplasia. Normal epidermal tissue is seen on the left, hyperplastic tissue is seen on the right. (From Rubin E, Farber JL. Pathology, 3rd ed. Philadelphia: Lippincott Williams & Wilkins, 1999.)

peripheral arteries that have lost their elasticity (Fig. 2.4). Hypertrophy caused by excessive hormonal stimulation occurs in the thyroid gland when there is an inadequate dietary intake of iodine. The pituitary gland reacts to the low level of circulating thyroid hormones by sending out more TSH, or thyroid-stimulating hormone, to the thyroid gland. This overstimulation will induce the cells of the gland to enlarge to produce more thyroxine, creating a **goiter** (Fig. 2.5).

Hyperplasia. **Hyperplasia** is an increase in the number of cells in a tissue or organ, which results in enlargement of that part. Hyperplasia may be the result of excessive hormone stimulation, chronic cell injury, or extensive cell death. Hormonal stimulation of the uterine lining during pregnancy causes hyperplasia of these cells. The creation of more red blood cells in those living at high altitudes or secondary polycythemia is an example of hyperplasia and

is caused by the increased secretion of the hormone erythropoietin by the kidneys. This hormone is released in response to a decreased level of oxygen in the blood. Constant irritation of epithelial cells in the skin causes a callous or epithelial hyperplasia at the point of friction. Figure 2.6 shows an area of hyperplasia within the epidermis that could have occurred in response to chronic irritation. Liver cells will become hyperplastic to replace cells that are lost because part of the liver is removed. Hyperplasia often occurs in conjunction with hypertrophy in tissues that are able to replicate. For instance, in the goiter example, hypertrophy and hyperplasia usually occur concurrently because the glandular tissue is able to replicate (see Fig. 2.5). Cardiac muscle, on the other hand, will only hypertrophy, because it is not able to replicate.

Metaplasia. **Metaplasia** is the conversion of one differentiated cell type to another. One of the most common examples of this process occurs in smokers. The bronchial epithelium undergoes a metaplastic change from normal cells that have cilia and produce mucus to squamous epithelium that functions as a protective barrier only (Fig. 2.7). This might appear to be in the best interest of the host; however, the metaplastic change compromises the

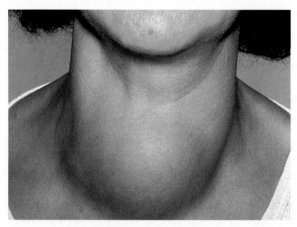

Figure 2.5. Hypertrophy and hyperplasia. Diffuse enlargement of the thyroid gland or goiter usually results from a combination of hypertrophy and hyperplasia. (From Weber J, Kelley J. Health assessment in nursing, 2nd ed. Philadelphia: Lippincott Williams & Wilkins, 2003.)

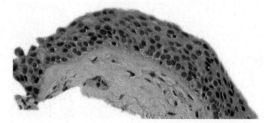

Figure 2.7. Metaplasia. Squamous metaplasia shows squamous epithelial cells lining a portion of bronchial mucosa instead of the normal ciliated cells and mucous secreting goblet cells. (From Cagle PT. Color atlas and text of pulmonary pathology. Philadelphia: Lippincott Williams & Wilkins, 2005.)

natural protective ability of the lungs. A metaplastic change may occur in cases of gastroesophageal reflux disease (see Chapter 10). The esophageal epithelium is changed to a type of gastric mucosa that has more protective ability than the normal lining epithelium. If the cause of the metaplasia is removed, the cells will eventually revert to the normal type. This is an adaptive process; however, dysplastic and even neoplastic changes have been observed in areas of metaplastic change.

Dysplasia. **Dysplasia** refers to the creation of abnormal cells from normal cells. The abnormalities include changes in the size and shape of the cell along with nuclear changes within the cell and the irregular arrangement of the cells within the tissue (Fig. 2.8). There is controversy surrounding dysplasia. Some say that it is an adaptive process; others believe it is not an adaptive process but rather a neoplastic process. Most consider dysplasia to be a premalignant condition and often malignant lesions will have areas of dysplasia surrounding them. Dysplasia is classified as mild, moderate, or severe. Severe dysplasia is so like cancer that in many cases it is assumed to be and treated as such. If the cells are truly dysplastic and the stimulus that caused the dysplasia is removed, the cells will revert to their normal state. If the stimulus is removed and the cells continue to reproduce uncontrollably, then a true neoplastic process is taking place.

Neoplasia. **Neoplasia** is defined as a new growth of cells. Neoplastic growth is not an adaptive change but rather a pathologic growth of cells. Neoplastic cell growth is not regulated by the elements that normally control the growth of cells; thus cell growth continues unchecked. Neoplastic growth is covered in depth in Chapter 5.

Intracellular Retention of Substances. In some cases cells may retain or store certain substances that are either

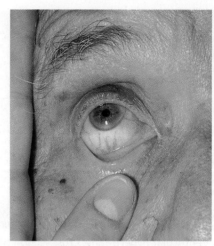

Figure 2.9. Intracellular retention of bilirubin. A yellow sclera and the yellow cast of the skin indicate jaundice. (From Bickley LS, Szilagyi P. Bates' guide to physical examination and history taking, 8th ed. Philadelphia: Lippincott Williams & Wilkins, 2003.)

normally present in smaller quantities or are pathologic. This is also an adaptive process, and if the reason for the storage of these substances is removed, then the cell will return to normal. Hepatitis A infection will cause skin and mucous membranes to turn yellow or become jaundiced. This is due to an excess amount of bilirubin in the affected epithelial cells (Fig. 2.9) . The bilirubin is being stored in the cells because the liver is not functioning correctly because of the hepatitis A infection. When the liver recovers and begins to work correctly, the color dissipates. Many genetic diseases cause errors in the creation or metabolism of important cellular substances. Often these abnormal substances cannot be used by the cells or removed from them, and their accumulation becomes toxic to the cell. The substances accumulate in cells until the cell is no longer able to adapt to the accumulations, at which point the cell dies. Tay-Sachs disease is an uncommon genetic disease that results from the accumulation of an abnormal glycoprotein in the cells of the brain and nervous system (Fig. 2.10). The glycoprotein is toxic to the cells and causes their death. Children with Tay-Sachs disease normally survive little more than 1 year.

REVERSIBLE CELLULAR INJURY

Reversible cellular injury occurs if there is persistent or chronic damage or if the cell is no longer able to adapt to changes in the ways discussed above. This section provides a brief introduction to the mechanisms by which reversible cellular damage occurs, to promote awareness of the current concepts in treatment for various pathologic conditions. Reversible cellular injury most commonly results from free radical injury, hypoxic injury, and/or impairment of calcium balance within the cell.

Free Radical Injury. A **free radical** is a highly reactive class of chemical that is generated by the cell during most

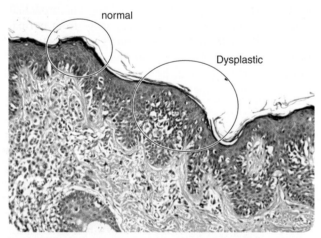

Figure 2.8. Dysplasia. *Left,* An area containing the typical melanin-producing cells of a nevus or mole. *Right,* Proliferation of dysplastic melanin-producing cells of differing size and shape that appear in a disordered arrangement. (From Rubin E, Farber JL. Pathology, 3rd ed. Philadelphia: Lippincott Williams & Wilkins, 1999.)

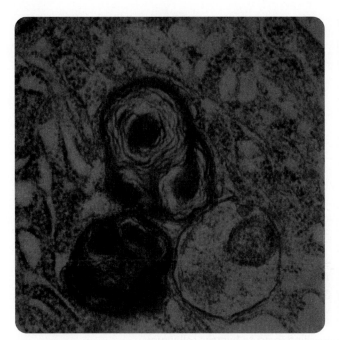

Figure 2.10. Abnormal retention of substances within the cell. Tay-Sachs disease. The cytoplasm of the nerve cell contains lysosomes filled with whorled membranes. (From Rubin E, Farber JL. Pathology, 3rd ed. Philadelphia: Lippincott Williams & Wilkins, 1999.)

APPLICATION

Free radical injury has been associated with many chronic diseases including atherosclerosis, cancer, Parkinson's disease, and Alzheimer's disease. It is also thought that aging may be an accumulation of cellular injuries caused in part by free radicals. The production of free radicals by the cell during metabolism has been compared to the production of ashes when a fire burns; both are the leftovers of oxidation. Our bodies can defend themselves against this injury most of the time by using antioxidants, which are produced by the cells. However, as we age, the abilities of this defense system diminish, manifesting more chronic diseases with aging. Consider the following question being researched today: If oxidation damages our bodies and antioxidants help to protect us from this damage, if we introduce more antioxidants into the equation (through dietary supplementation, for example), will it help to stop or reverse the process? One method of increasing the amount of available antioxidants in the body is to increase the dietary intake of foods high in antioxidants. The most common antioxidants are vitamin C, vitamin E, and β-carotene. Some trace elements have also been recommended including selenium, copper, zinc, and manganese. To date, research has not been favorable for curing the degenerative neurologic diseases such as Alzheimer's or Parkinson's disease. The risk of some cancers, such as colon cancer, may be reduced when more fresh fruits and vegetables are introduced into the diet. However, researchers are not positive that it is the antioxidant properties of these foods that are beneficial. Also, increasing antioxidant ingestion may decrease the formation of atherosclerotic plaques that lead to heart attacks and strokes. The American Heart Association has recommended establishing a balanced diet with an emphasis on antioxidant-rich fruits, vegetables, and whole grains to influence the risk of disease in the general population (AHA, 2006). Many believe that the key to preventing the effects of aging is associated with antioxidants. This raises the question: will antioxidant therapy be the key to the fountain of youth?

of its normal metabolic processes. Oxygen is the most frequent source of free radicals because it has two unpaired outer electrons and is used in almost all of the cell's activities. Normally the cell has built-in defenses against free radical injury; however, when the cell is under stress for any reason, these defenses can become impaired. Impaired defenses against free radical injury allow single-strand breaks in DNA to occur. The phospholipids in the cell membrane and organelle membranes can be destroyed, compromising the integrity of these structures, which impairs the normal function and replicative capabilities of the cell. In addition, cell membrane disruption will upset the balance of calcium within the cell, which causes even more problems.

Hypoxic Cell Injury. In **hypoxic** cell injury, a lack of oxygen to the cells inhibits or stops the production of energy within the cell. Without energy the cell is not able to survive. One of the first manifestations of oxygen deprivation, or ischemia, is an increase in the amount of water in the cell. This occurs because the cell depends on an energy source to actively maintain the sodium/potassium balance within it. If that mechanism is not working because there is no source of energy, then sodium and water will flow unchecked into the cell causing swelling (Fig. 2.11). The imbalance of minerals and water within the cell also allows intercellular substances, usually enzymes, to leak into the surrounding tissues and be picked up by the circulatory system. These substances are markers for cell injury and can be detected in laboratory tests that target their presence. This is an important factor in diagnosing

many conditions that are characterized by cell injury and death. For example, the presence of certain cardiac enzymes in the blood can diagnose a myocardial infarction or heart attack because those enzymes would not be present unless cardiac cells had been destroyed. If hypoxia is severe enough or lasts for a long time, cell death can result. Oxygen deprivation can be partial or total. Partial deprivation occurs in anemia (see Chapter 9) or obstructive lung diseases such as emphysema or chronic obstructive bronchitis (see Chapter 10). Total deprivation occurs when, for example, a blood vessel is completely obstructed during a stroke or a myocardial infarction (see Chapter 8). The type of cell determines how long the cell can go without any oxygen. Cells that are well differentiated, such as brain and heart cells, can withstand only

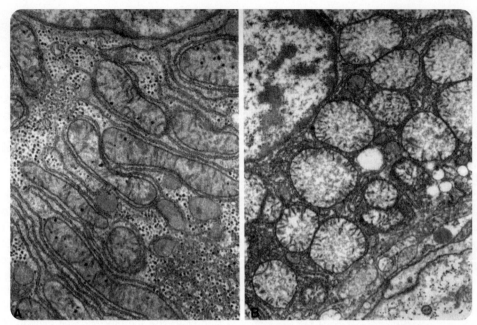

Figure 2.11. Hypoxic cell injury. Mitochondrial swelling in acute hypoxic cell injury. **A.** Normal mitochondria are elongated and display a dense mitochondrial matrix. **B.** Mitochondria from a hypoxic cell are swollen and round and exhibit a decreased matrix density. (From Rubin E, Farber JL. Pathology, 3rd ed. Philadelphia: Lippincott Williams & Wilkins, 1999.)

minutes of complete oxygen deprivation without irreversible damage, while skin cells may survive for hours without oxygen. The ability of the cell to produce energy anaerobically or without oxygen is also important. Skeletal muscle cells can work longer under hypoxic conditions because they can produce energy without using oxygen for short periods of time. If the oxygen supply is reestablished soon enough, cellular damage may be reversible.

Imbalance of Intracellular Calcium. When the system that maintains the sodium and potassium levels in the cells fails, the system that maintains the calcium and magnesium levels will also fail. Normal cells have less calcium inside them than is found in the extracellular environment. When the mechanism that maintains this balance fails, there is an influx of calcium into the cell. Increased levels of calcium activate enzymes that can damage the cell and compromise the cell membrane, eventually causing lysis or death of the cell.

IRREVERSIBLE CELL INJURY

Two basic classifications of cell death include apoptosis and necrosis. **Apoptosis** is cellular self-destruction. It is common knowledge that many tissues of the body are constantly producing new cells; imagine if there was no way to get rid of the old cells. The result would be very large bodies. The average adult produces about 10 billion new cells every day and destroys about the same number. In the process of apoptosis, the cell nucleus

disintegrates and the cell falls apart (Fig. 2.12). The remnants of the cell are digested by phagocytic cells and removed via the lymphatic system. Aging white blood cells are removed from the body through the process of apoptosis. If they were not removed, for instance, a pathologic accumulation of white blood cells, or leukemia, would occur. Epithelial cells that form the lining of the intestines undergo the process of apoptosis. Also, in fetal development the formation of separate digits from webbed fingers is a result of apoptosis. Apoptosis is usually a normal process; however, it can also be triggered by stimuli such as viral infections or mutagenic agents.

Necrosis is another type of cell death. If the cell is unable to adapt to its environment by nonlethal means

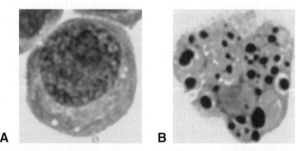

Figure 2.12. Apoptosis. A viable leukemic cell **(A)** contrasts with an apoptotic cell **(B)** in which the nucleus has undergone disintegration. (From Rubin E, Farber JL. Pathology, 3rd ed. Philadelphia: Lippincott Williams & Wilkins, 1999.)

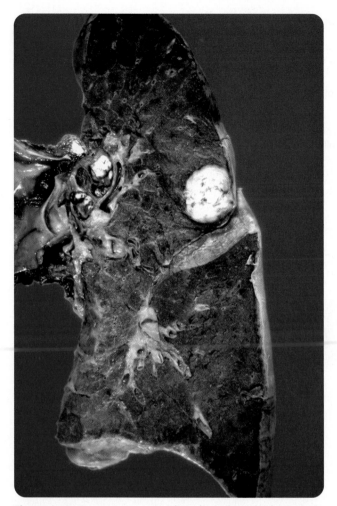

Figure 2.13. Caseous necrosis. The white cheesy substance is the caseous necrosis seen in tuberculosis. (From Rubin E, Farber JL. Pathology, 3rd ed. Philadelphia: Lippincott Williams & Wilkins, 1999.)

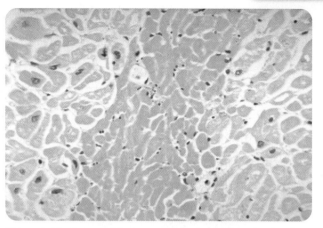

Figure 2.14. Coagulative necrosis. A photomicrograph of the heart in a patient with an acute myocardial infarction. *Center,* The deeply colored necrotic cells have lost their nuclei. The necrotic focus is surrounded by paler-staining, viable cardiac cells. (From Rubin E, Farber JL. Pathology, 3rd ed. Philadelphia: Lippincott Williams & Wilkins, 1999.)

surrounding healthy tissue. The body is unable to remove the debris as fast as it is being produced, resulting in an **abscess**, which is an accumulation of dead cells, dead bacteria, and dead and dying white blood cells. Figure 2.15 shows an abscess in the submental area that was caused by a dental or periapical abscess.

The process of cell injury and death does not occur without a response from the body of the host. Figure 2.16 provides a summary of the process of cellular injury. These responses include the inflammatory response, the immune response, and the process of healing and repair. These topics are discussed in depth in the following chapters.

such as hypertrophy or if the changes are too deleterious to the cell over the long term, the cell will undergo necrosis. Caseous necrosis, coagulative necrosis, and liquefactive necrosis are among several types of necroses. **Caseous necrosis** is specific to the lesions found in the lungs of individuals with tuberculosis. The lesions are called tubercles (Fig. 2.13), and as the cells inside the tubercle become necrotic, they form a thick cheesy, or caseous, material. **Coagulative necrosis** occurs primarily when there has been cell hypoxia or ischemia, as in a myocardial infarction. When the cells die they become firm and opaque. Figure 2.14 depicts the darker streak of necrotic cardiac cells that contain no nuclei and are characteristic of coagulative necrosis. **Liquefactive necrosis** occurs when the body is dealing with a bacterial infection, especially by staphylococci and streptococci. White blood cells that rush to the area are armed with potent enzymes that destroy not only the bacterial invaders but also the cells of the host. This action takes place in an area that is walled off from the

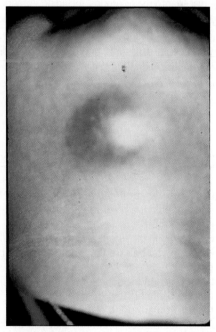

Figure 2.15. Liquefactive necrosis. The periapical abscess is an example of liquefactive necrosis. (Courtesy of Dr. John Jacoway.)

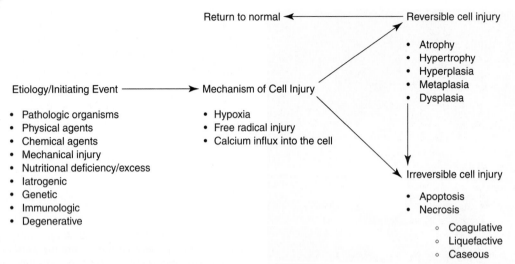

Figure 2.16. Summary of the process of cellular injury.

SUMMARY

- The first element in the study of disease is the etiology. There are intrinsic and extrinsic causes. Pathogenic organisms, physical agents, chemical agents, mechanical injury, and nutritional factors are extrinsic causes. Genetic, immunologic, and degenerative diseases are intrinsic causes.
- Whether or not an individual actually acquires a disease or condition depends on many variables or risk factors that determine resistance and susceptibility. The risk factors can be placed into major groups, including immune system dysfunction, compromised first-line defenses, age, inheritance, risky lifestyle behaviors and choices, undue stress, environmental exposures, and preexisting conditions.
- When an individual does acquire a disease or condition, the sequence of events in the development of the disease is called the pathogenesis.

- All disease manifestations are first evident on a cellular level. The clinical manifestations of the disease or condition will depend on which cells and how many cells are affected.
- The cells can adapt, undergo reversible injury, or die. The cells adapt through atrophy, hypertrophy, hyperplasia, metaplasia, and dysplasia and by retaining certain intracellular substances.
- If reversible injury is not stopped, the cell will die. The normal process of cell death is called apoptosis. Pathologic cell death is necrosis.
- There are several types of necrosis; liquefactive necrosis may lead to the formation of an abscess. Other forms occur in response to ischemia and specific diseases.

Critical Thinking Activities

1. A. If we knew that our integumentary system was totally intact, would we need to wear gloves while performing procedures?
   B. How can you be sure that your skin is totally intact?
   C. How can you be sure that your gloves are totally intact?
   D. What precautions do you take to try to make sure that no contamination reaches your hands even though you are using gloves?
2. A. Construct a list of conditions that you think might be associated in some way with the age of an individual.
   B. Explain why you have included each condition on the list and share your list with your classmates.

   C. Can you think of any reason such a list might be useful in your practice of dental hygiene?
3. A. Consider the lifestyle choices you have made. Categorize them by whether you think they are healthy, unhealthy, or neutral. Think of how you might eliminate or modify some of the unhealthy choices, then think of ways that you can maintain the healthy choices.
   B. Do you think that encouraging patients to examine their lifestyle choices is part of your "job description"? Why or Why not?

Case Study

The patient is a 40-year-old male who has been a patient in your office for several years. You have never seen him for any procedures because he has always come for evening appointments. He has an appointment for dental hygiene care. You review his medical history, take vital signs, and update his personal information. There are no significant findings. Findings from your extraoral examination are normal. As you perform your intraoral examination you see the condition pictured in Figure 2.17. You question the patient about the appearance of his tongue.

1. What type of questions would you like to ask this patient?

2. How would you describe the lateral surface of the tongue?

3. What do you think has caused the condition?

4. What could be done to help resolve the condition and prevent it from recurring?

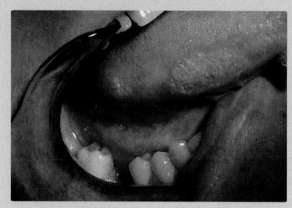

Figure 2.17. Case Study

5. What type of cellular adaptation has most likely occurred within the tissues of the tongue?

REFERENCES

Anderson DM, Keith J, Novak PD, Elliot MA. Mosby's medical, nursing & allied health dictionary. 6th ed. Philadelphia: Mosby, 2002.

Cotran RS, Kumar V, Collins T. Robbins: pathologic basis of disease. 6th ed. Philadelphia: WB Saunders, 1999:1–49.

Stedman's concise medical dictionary for the health professions. 5th ed. Baltimore: Williams & Wilkins, 2005.

Fatality facts: teenagers 2002. Insurance Institute for Highway Safety/Highway Loss Data Institute. Available at *http://www.iihs.org/safety_facts/fatality_facts/teens.htm*. Accessed summer 2004.

Fontera WR, Hughes VA, Krivickas LS, et al. Strength training in older women: early and late changes in whole muscle and single cells. Muscle Nerve 2003;28(5):601–608.

Helwig B. Antioxidants and Exercise. Available at http://www.exrx.net/ Nutrition/Antioxidants/Antioxidants.html. Accessed summer 2004.

Huether SE, McCance KL. Understanding pathophysiology. 3rd ed. St. Louis: Mosby, 2004: 65–104.

Join the Smokefree Air 2010 Challenge. American Lung Association. Available at http://lungaction.org/campaign/smokefree2010. Accessed spring 2006.

Love Canal Collection. University Archives, University Libraries, State University of New York at Buffalo. Available at http://ublib.buffalo.edu/libraries/projects/lovecanal/. Accessed spring 2006.

National Center for Statistics & Analysis of the National Highway Traffic Safety Administration. Traffic safety facts 2002: young drivers. DOT HS 809619.

Porth CM. Essentials of pathophysiology: concepts of altered health states. Philadelphia: Lippincott Williams & Wilkins, 2004:24–35.

Price SA, Wilson LM. Pathophysiology: clinical concepts of disease processes. 6th ed. St. Louis: Mosby, 2003:33–43.

Regezi JA, Sciubba JJ, Jordan RCK. Oral pathology: Clinical pathologic correlations. 4th ed. St. Louis: WB Saunders, 2003:159.

Rubin E, Gorstein F, Rubin R, et al. Rubin's pathology: clinicopathologic foundations of medicine. 4th ed. Baltimore: Lippincott Williams & Wilkins, 2005:4–39.

Stress at work. DHHS (NIOSH) Publication no. 99–101. National Institute for Occupational Safety and Health. Available at: http://www.cdc.gov/niosh. Accessed summer 2004.

Tribble DL. Antioxidant consumption and risk of coronary heart disease: emphasis on vitamin C, vitamin E, and β-carotene: a statement for healthcare professionals from the American Heart Association. Circulation 1999;99:591–595.

Key Terms

- Abscess
- Acute inflammation
- Adhesion
- Agranulocytes
- Alternative pathway
- Alveolar osteitis
- Angiogenesis
- Bacteremia
- Basophils
- Bradykinin
- Cardinal signs of inflammation
- Cascade
- Cellulitis
- Chemical mediator
- Chemokine
- Chemotaxis
- Cicatrix
- Classic pathway
- Clotting system
- Complement system
- Cytokines
- Edema
- Emigration
- Endothelium
- Eosinophils
- Epithelization
- Exudate
- Fibroblasts

- Fibrous repair
- Fistula
- Giant cell
- Granulation tissue
- Granulocyte
- Granuloma
- Granulomatous inflammation
- Histamine
- Hyperemia
- Immunoglobulins
- Interleukin-1 (IL-1)
- Keloid
- Kinin system
- Leukocyte
- Leukocytosis
- Leukotrienes
- Lipopolysaccharides (LPS)
- Lymphadenopathy
- Lymphocytes
- Lysosome
- Lysosomal enzymes
- Macrophage
- Margination
- Mast cell
- Membrane attack complex
- Microcirculation
- Monocyte
- Motile phagocytes

- Opsonins
- Opsonization
- Pavementing
- Permeable
- Phagocytes
- Phagocytosis
- Phagosome
- Plasma cells
- Plasma fluid
- Platelet-activating factor
- Polymorphonuclear neutrophils
- Prostaglandin
- Pyogenic
- Pyrexia
- Pyrogen
- Regeneration
- Repair
- Resolution
- Septicemia
- Serotonin
- Serous exudate
- Transmigration
- Tumor necrosis factor
- Vascular stasis
- Vasoconstriction
- Vasodilation

Learning Outcomes

1. Define the terms used to describe the inflammatory process.

2. Describe the normal sequence of events in the acute inflammatory process.

3. Describe the function of each type of cell that takes part in the acute inflammatory process.

4. Identify and describe the functions of the major chemical mediators involved in the inflammatory process.

5. Identify the two major forms of exudate.

6. List the positive aspects of edema.

7. Identify the expected outcomes of acute inflammation.

8. Describe the chronic inflammatory process.

9. Identify and describe the functions of the cells that take part in chronic inflammation.

10. List the systemic manifestations of inflammation.

11. Define and differentiate between the processes of regeneration and repair.

12. List the sequence of events in the repair process.

13. Identify the major chemical mediators involved in the repair process.

14. Describe healing by primary and secondary intention.

15. List factors that can affect wound healing.

16. List specific ways that tissue can be damaged during the chronic inflammatory process.

17. Identify the complications of wound healing.

18. Describe the clinical characteristics of alveolar osteitis.

19. Describe possible ways to prevent and treat alveolar osteitis.

Chapter Outline

ACUTE INFLAMMATORY PROCESS

Any time that the body is injured by exogenous or endogenous elements, the body must respond. The inflammatory process is the body's mechanism for dealing with the injuries caused by these elements. Most of the time the inflammatory process is considered beneficial to the body, but occasionally, the inflammatory process is the ultimate cause of severe damage to the body and must be held under control. Many of the immune system diseases (discussed in Chapter 4) are the result of an excessive or unnecessary inflammatory process. There are two broad categories of inflammatory processes, acute and chronic. **Acute inflammation** is most often limited in area and duration and is characterized by the **Cardinal signs of inflammation** (Table 3.1). Occasionally, acute inflammation can be very extensive and involve multiple body organs or systems. Chronic inflammation is one of the possible results of acute inflammation and is characterized by a long duration or a history of repeated insults or injuries. Other outcomes are abscess formation, **resolution** of inflammation (reversal of the inflammatory process with return to normal), and healing or **repair** of the area. Although the repair process is discussed at the end of this chapter, repair begins at almost the same time the inflammatory process is activated. That is, they occur simultaneously.

Phases of the Acute Inflammatory Process

There are three phases of the acute inflammatory process. The first phase, or initiation, is activated when the injury occurs. It comprises changes to the structure of the small blood vessels (**microcirculation**) in the area of the injury, leading to loss of fluid from the blood and the movement of white blood cells from the blood vessels to the injured area. The second phase (amplification) involves the action of chemical substances that direct more and different types of white blood cells into the injured area. These act to increase the response and quickly neutralize whatever caused the injury and to clean up the debris resulting from the injury. The third phase (termination) requires that other chemical substances stop or inhibit the inflammatory

Table 3.1   CARDINAL SIGNS OF INFLAMMATION

Cardinal Sign (Latin Term)	Causative Agent in Inflammatory Process
Redness (rubor)	Hyperemia
Heat (calor)	Hyperemia
Swelling (tumor)	Edema
Pain (dolor)	Edema and chemical mediators
Loss of function (functio laesa)	Edema

process; if the inflammatory process continues unhindered, it will produce even more damage then the initial injury.

Understanding the inflammatory process requires an understanding of the events that occur within the tissues on a microscopic level and the stimuli that cause these events. Table 3.2 provides a list of the main events occurring in this process, and Figure 3.1 illustrates the events at the microscopic level. The following is an example of the acute inflammatory process as discussed in Table 3.2.

Imagine that you are working in your yard, cleaning up the debris from a hard winter. It is so wonderfully warm that you have taken your shoes off and are barefoot. Before too long you step on a rusty nail. Your first reac-

tions are to yell with pain and pull the nail out. The following is a description of how your body reacts on a microscopic level.

INITIATION PHASE

The very first reaction during initiation is an immediate constriction of the microcirculation comprising the arterioles, capillaries, and venules known as **vasoconstriction** (event 1). The constriction is very brief, lasting several minutes or less, but it serves the purpose of controlling bleeding, especially in small injuries. When tissue cells are damaged, as the cells of the foot in this situation, they re-

Table 3.2   SUMMARY OF THE ACUTE INFLAMMATORY PROCESS

Event	Stimuli	Description
1. Vasoconstriction	Injured nervous tissue	Brief hemorrhage control
2. Vasodilation	Histamine PAF Bradykinin Prostaglandins (late)	Increases diameter of vessels Hyperemia (increased blood in the area)
3. Increased vascular permeability	Histamine Serotonin PAF Bradykinin Prostaglandins (late) Leukotrienes (late)	Causes gaps in vessel wall between endothelial cells Begins process of exudate formation and vascular stasis
4. Vascular stasis a. Margination	Increased vascular permeability Increased blood viscosity	Increases blood viscosity Leukocytes move to the endothelial walls and begin the process of rolling
b. Adhesion	Tumor necrosis factor Interleukin-1	Leukocytes stick to the vessel walls
c. Transmigration	Complement	Leukocytes squeeze through gaps in endothelial cells
5. Chemotaxis	Leukotrienes Chemokines Complement	Drives PMNs and other leukocytes to the affected area
6. Opsonization	Immunoglobulins Complement	Prepares resistant pathogens for phagocytosis
7. Phagocytosis	Platelet-activating factor	Enables ingestion and digestion of foreign material or cellular debris
8. Termination of process		Removes debris through lymphatic system

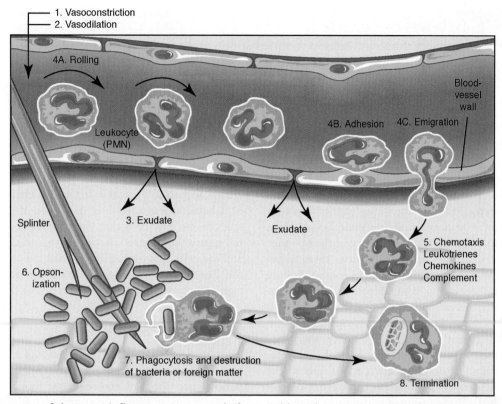

Figure 3.1. Summary of the acute inflammatory process (refer to Table 3.2). **1. Event 1, Vasoconstriction.** Following the injury, there is a brief vasoconstriction that may help to control bleeding. **2. Event 2, Vasodilation.** Chemical mediators released by the injured cells cause dilation of the blood vessels immediately after the vasoconstriction. **3. Event 3, Increased vascular permeability.** Increased vascular permeability allows plasma fluid (exudate) to leave the vessels and the blood flow to slow, causing vascular stasis. **4. Vascular Stasis. Event 4A, Margination.** Leukocytes (PMNs) move to the vessel walls and begin the process of rolling. **Event 4B, Adhesion/Pavementing.** Leukocytes (PMNs) stick to the vessel walls. **Event 4C. Emigration.** Leukocytes (PMNs) squeeze through the gaps in the endothelial cells. **5. Event 5, Chemotaxis.** Chemical mediators released by the injured cells and bacteria drive leukocytes (PMNs) toward the area of injury. **6. Event 6, Opsonization.** Opsonins prepare resistant microbes and/or other matter for phagocytosis, if necessary. **7. Event 7, Phagocytosis.** Microbes or other matter are phagocytized and digested by the leukocytes (PMNs). **8. Event 8, Termination.** Leukocytes remove digested matter through the lymph system.

lease substances that start the inflammatory process. These substances are called **chemical mediators.** The first action of these chemical mediators is to cause the blood vessels in the area to undergo **vasodilation** (event 2), or increase in diameter, so that more blood (**hyperemia**) and nutrients can be brought into the area. Some of the chemical mediators cause the blood vessels to become more **permeable** (event 3). When this occurs the chemical mediators affect the cells of the blood vessel walls, causing them to separate slightly, forming microscopic gaps between the cells. This allows **plasma fluid** and white blood cells in the vessels to travel out of the vessels and into the area where the injury occurred. The plasma fluid and white blood cells are necessary to clear the area of dead or injured cells and any foreign material that entered with the nail.

At this point you notice that your foot is becoming red, warm to touch, and swollen around the injury. The increased blood flow from the dilation of the blood vessels causes the redness and heat; and the plasma fluid flowing out of the now more permeable vessels causes the

swelling. Heat, redness, and swelling are all components of the cardinal signs of inflammation. The fluid that came from the blood vessels into the injured tissue is called **exudate.** There are several types of exudate; in this case, **serous exudate** is present. Table 3.3 gives a description of the different types of exudates. The exudate contains more chemical mediators that enhance the inflammatory process. It also contains nutrients for the white blood cells that are being called to the area by these chemical mediators. Exudates dilute toxic substances and contain enzymes that can neutralize these toxic substances. A large amount of exudate in the tissues is known as **edema.**

When the amount of plasma fluid in the blood decreases as a result of the formation of exudate, the blood becomes thicker or more viscous. This results in **vascular stasis** (event 4) or slowing of the blood through the vessels in the affected area. Vascular stasis allows more nutrients to be removed from the blood and brought into the tissues, but it also allows the blood to become stagnant and slows the removal of waste products. Vascular stasis allows the next step in the inflammatory process to begin.

Table 3.3	TYPES OF EXUDATE	
Type of Exudate	**Description**	**Example**
Serous	Thin and clear Few cells	Blisters from a second-degree sunburn
Purulent or suppurative (commonly called "pus")	Somewhat thick and white or yellowish Many polymorphonuclear neutrophils	Pustules of acne Periodontal abscess

Slower blood flow causes the red blood cells to move toward the center of the blood vessel while white blood cells, or **leukocytes**, move to the lining of the vessels or the **endothelium**. The move toward the endothelial cells is called **margination** (event 4A). As they move they bounce against the endothelial surface, which causes them to begin to rotate. This motion is referred to as rolling. Rolling exposes the surface of the white blood cell to the endothelium, which activates the white blood cell so that it can stick to the endothelium in a process called **adhesion** or **pavementing** (event 4B) (Fig. 3.2). When the white blood cells are firmly attached to the endothelial cells, they squeeze through the gaps between the cells in the vessel wall created when the vessel became more permeable. This process is called **transmigration** or **emigration** (event 4C) (Fig. 3.3). After the leukocytes leave the blood vessels they migrate to the injured area by following a chemical path in a process known as **chemotaxis** (event 5). Chemotaxis is a result of the action of chemical mediators released by cells that were damaged during the initial injury that "drive" the leukocytes to the injured area and the cells that originally released the chemical mediator. The leukocytes are ready to destroy and remove foreign substances and dead or injured host cells.

AMPLIFICATION PHASE

The amplification phase begins as the first leukocytes gather in the area of the injury. Referring back to the scenario, when the nail entered your foot it brought microorganisms and bits of dirt and rust with it. All of this foreign matter needs to be removed from the tissues.

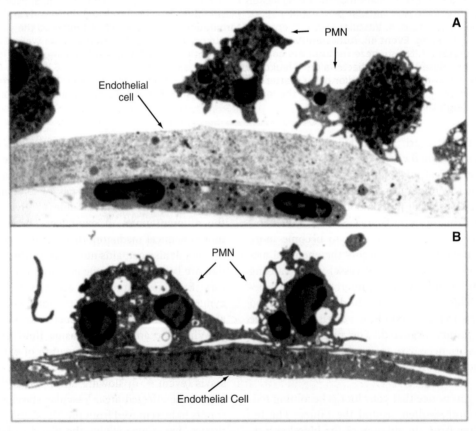

Figure 3.2. Adhesion. A. The surface of a PMN is exposed to chemical mediators on and near the surface of the endothelial cells as it rolls along the endothelial surface. **B.** The chemical mediators enable firm adhesion of the PMN to the endothelial cell surface.

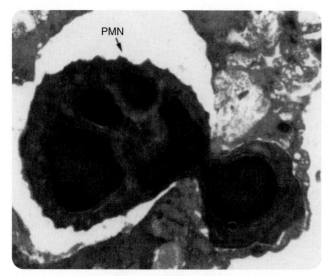

Figure 3.3. Leukocyte emigration/transmigration. The PMN is exiting through the gap in the endothelial cells.

Many pathogenic organisms have created defense mechanisms that make them difficult for the leukocytes to destroy and remove from the area. Opsonization (event 6) enables the leukocytes to destroy and remove these resistant organisms. During **opsonization**, the resistant organisms are prepared for destruction by chemical substances called **opsonins** that are found in the exudate that has collected within the injured area. An example of one type of opsonin are **immunoglobulins**, which are natural antibodies produced by the immune system. If opsonization is necessary, the organisms will be coated with opsonins to prepare them for removal by the leukocytes. Foreign matter is eliminated by leukocytes when they ingest and digest it during a process called **phagocytosis** (event 7) (Fig. 3.4). If the extent of the injury is great and there is much debris that can not be phagocytized by the leukocytes, the inflammatory process will be amplified by more chemical mediators and different types of leukocytes will be called into action from the surrounding tissue and blood vessels.

TERMINATION PHASE

During the termination phase, the foreign material and cellular debris that resulted from the injury and the action of the inflammatory process will be removed from the body through the lymphatic system (event 8). Other chemical mediators will inhibit or stop any further action by the inflammatory process, and the area will complete the healing or repair process. If the inflammatory process is not halted for some reason, the process will become long term and result in more damage to the tissue instead of healing.

The "nail-in-foot" scenario describes how the inflammatory process is carried out by both cellular and chemical components. These components are described below in more detail to examine how they are interrelated.

CELLULAR COMPONENTS OF THE INFLAMMATORY PROCESS

The main cellular components of the inflammatory reaction are white blood cells or leukocytes, which are illustrated in Figure 3.5. Each type of leukocyte plays a vital role in accomplishing the actual work that is done during the inflammatory process. Leukocytes are divided into two major classes, **granulocytes**, which include polymorphonuclear neutrophils, eosinophils, and basophils; and **agranulocytes**, which include lymphocytes and monocytes. Lymphocytes or lymphoid cells play a specific role in the immune system and are discussed in Chapter 4. Mast cells also play a role during the inflammatory process. The **mast cell** is not a leukocyte but does exhibit some of the same properties as the basophil. The mast cell is very important to the immune system (see Chapter 4), and because the immune system plays an important role in the inflammatory process, the mast cell is included in this list.

Granulocytes

The **polymorphonuclear neutrophil** (PMN) is the most active granulocyte in the inflammatory process. The PMN follows an elaborate plan to eliminate or neutralize the initial cause of the inflammatory process, whether it is foreign material, microbes, or injured host cells that no longer function correctly. PMNs are **motile phagocytes** that can move independently within the tissues and carry out the process of phagocytosis of whatever material they are sent to eliminate. The PMNs are attracted to an area by chemotactic factors and are active in fighting bacterial and fungal infections. It is important to remember that they are the first cells to arrive in an area of acute inflammation.

Basophils and **eosinophils** play a role in inflammation related to allergic reactions. In addition, eosinophils are also active in fighting off parasitic infections especially of the helminthic (tapeworm) type.

Agranulocytes

While granulocytes are active during the initial stages of inflammation, the agranulocytes are more active during the later stages of the acute inflammatory process. The agranulocytes are longer-lived (i.e., several months as opposed to 6 to 9 hours) and much slower to respond to the direction of chemical mediators. There are two types of agranulocyte, monocytes (macrophages) and lymphocytes.

Monocytes circulate within the bloodstream until they enter a specific tissue and become "fixed." This monocyte differentiates into a **macrophage** that is specific for that particular tissue. There are many different types of macrophages, for example, a monocyte that becomes fixed in the liver is called a Kupffer cell. A monocyte that becomes fixed in connective tissue becomes a histiocyte, or tissue macrophage. Histiocytes are very important not

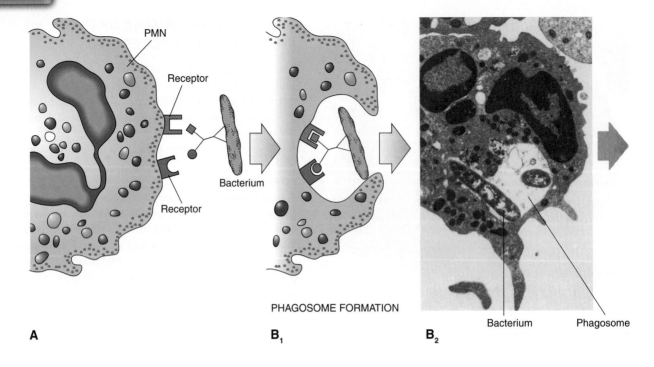

PHAGOSOME FORMATION

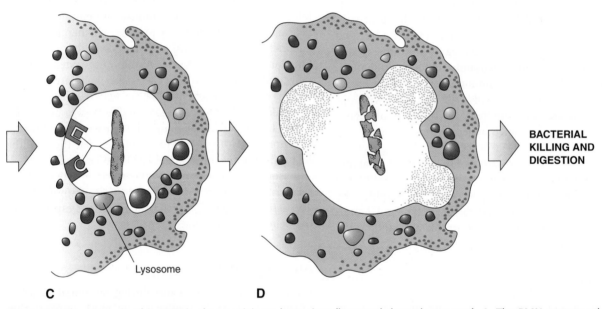

BACTERIAL
KILLING AND
DIGESTION

Figure 3.4. Phagocytosis. This PMN is phagocytizing a bacterium (long rod-shaped structure). **A.** The PMN captures the bacterium. Receptors on the surface of the PMN are attracted to substances (opsonins) on the surface of the bacterium. **B1.** The PMN forms a phagosome around the bacterium. **B2.** Micrograph of an actual phagosome containing a long rod-shaped bacterium. **C.** Lysosomes fuse with the surface of the phagosome and release lysosomal enzymes into the phagosome. **D.** The bacterium is destroyed and digested by the PMN. (From Rubin E, Farber JL. Pathology. 4th ed. Philadelphia: Lippincott Williams & Wilkins, 2005.)

only for the inflammatory process but for the immune system as a whole. Macrophages are one type of cell that can introduce foreign substances to the immune system and thus provides a cellular link between the inflammatory process and immunity (see Chapter 4). Box 3.1 lists the functions of macrophages.

If the material that needs to be removed is too large for a single macrophage or the microbe is highly resistant to phagocytosis, several will join together to form a **giant cell** (Fig. 3.6) . Giant cells can digest larger matter or destroy resistant microbes, such as the fungus *Candida,* because together they produce a more highly toxic enzyme than a

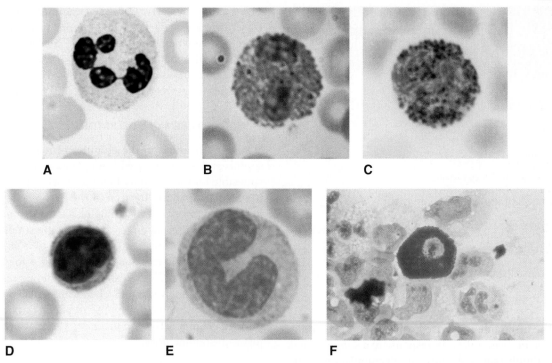

Figure 3.5. Cells that take part in the inflammatory process. **A.** Polymorphonuclear neutrophil. **B.** Eosinophil. **C.** Basophil. **D.** Lymphocyte. **E.** Monocyte. **F.** Mast cell. (From Rubin E, Farber JL. Pathology. 4th ed. Philadelphia: Lippincott Williams & Wilkins, 2005.)

single macrophage can. A giant cell that forms in response to foreign material is called a foreign body giant cell. Langhans giant cells are formed in response to a tuberculosis infection and Aschoff cells are formed during rheumatic fever.

Lymphocytes are leukocytes found in the lymph system. Lymphocytes play a central role in the function of the immune system and are discussed in detail in Chapter 4.

Mast Cells

The mast cell is not a leukocyte. It is created in the bone marrow and then travels through the circulatory system to a tissue site where it matures. The mast cell stays in connective tissue close to vessels of the circulatory system and epithelial tissues of the integumentary system including the respiratory and gastrointestinal tracts. Both the mast cell and the basophil have granules in their cytoplasm that contain **histamine**, an important chemical me-

Box 3.1 FUNCTIONS OF MACROPHAGES

1. Removal of dead and dying cells

2. Removal of damaged tissues

3. Removal of inhaled particles

4. Removal of foreign bodies

5. Primary defense against some microorganisms; for example, *Mycobacterium tuberculosis*

6. Processing of antigens for presentation to T cells (see Chapter 4)

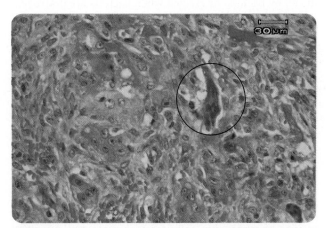

Figure 3.6. Giant cell. Note the large multinucleated giant cell in the center of the photo. (Courtesy Yi-Shing Lisa Cheng.

Box 3.2 STIMULI THAT CAUSE BASOPHILS AND MAST CELLS TO DEGRANULATE

1. Mechanical trauma
2. Heat
3. Ultraviolet radiation
4. Bacterial and fungal toxins
5. Elements of the complement system
6. Enzymes released by injured cells
7. Substances released from PMNs
8. Specific allergens

diator. The histamine is released when the cell's granules break open, or degranulate, in response to a stimulus. Box 3.2 lists stimuli that will cause the degranulation or release of histamine from basophils and mast cells.

CHEMICAL MEDIATORS

Chemical mediators are molecular substances that direct the actions of the cells that take part in the inflammatory and other processes. Chemical mediators recruit cells into an area of injury and determine what specific action is required of them, where the action will take place, and how long the action will be maintained. Chemical mediators can be either exogenous (produced outside of the body) or endogenous (made within the body).

Exogenous Chemical Mediators

Exogenous chemical mediators include the toxins produced by bacteria or created when bacteria are destroyed. For example, **lipopolysaccharide (LPS)** is a component of all gram-negative bacterial cell walls. When gram-negative bacteria are destroyed, they release LPS. LPS is an important chemical mediator that is associated with the chronic inflammation seen in periodontal disease. Chemical irritants, such as the substance that is released into tissues when a mosquito bites or the oil from a poison ivy plant are also considered exogenous chemical mediators.

Endogenous Chemical Mediators

Endogenous chemical mediators are produced by the body. These chemicals can be produced by a complex sequence of events that activates a physiologically inactive form of a substance or precursor that is circulating in the blood plasma or they can be produced by specific cells.

These cells may carry preformed chemicals in intracellular storage areas, such as the granules in mast cells, and secrete them when stimulated or the cells may synthesize the chemicals when told to do so by other chemical mediators. Endogenous mediators can be divided into three categories: preformed, synthesized, and plasma derived.

PREFORMED CHEMICAL MEDIATORS

Histamine is found in the granules of mast cells and basophils and is also released from platelets. Histamine is responsible for the dilation of blood vessels and the increase in vascular permeability seen in the first phases of the inflammatory process. Histamine also causes smooth muscle contraction in the lungs and gastrointestinal tract and stimulates nasal mucus production, all of which are important in allergic reactions. See Chapter 4 for a detailed discussion of the role of histamine in allergic reactions.

Serotonin is a preformed chemical mediator that is released from platelets in response to platelet-activating factor (see below). Serotonin increases vascular permeability just as histamine does.

SYNTHESIZED CHEMICAL MEDIATORS

Platelet-activating factor (PAF) is derived from the cell membranes of neutrophils, eosinophils, basophils, mast cells, monocytes, platelets, and endothelial cells. PAF causes the aggregation (sticking together) of platelets and the release of serotonin from the platelets. PAF is a potent chemical and can increase vasodilation and vascular permeability 100 to 10,000 times more than histamine can. PAF also interacts with phagocytes such as neutrophils and monocytes/macrophages to increase their phagocytic action.

Prostaglandins are synthesized by all types of leukocytes in response to a stimulus. The prostaglandins cause vasodilation, increased vascular permeability, and increased feelings of pain. They also cause bronchoconstriction and smooth muscle contraction and play a part in elevating body temperature. The prostaglandins are responsible for the sustained effects of vasodilation and vascular permeability seen in the later stages of inflammation. In addition, prostaglandins are associated with the tissue destruction seen in periodontal disease.

The **leukotrienes** are synthesized by all types of leukocytes and mast cells. Leukotrienes increase vascular permeability and act as chemotactic agents to bring inflammatory cells into an area. Along with the prostaglandins, leukotrienes are responsible for the sustained effects of vasodilation and vascular permeability seen in the later stages of inflammation.

Cytokines are produced by macrophages and some types of lymphocytes. Examples of cytokines that are active in the inflammatory process are chemokines, tumor necrosis factor, and interleukin-1. The **chemokines** are very strong chemotactic agents for the cells involved in the inflammatory process. **Tumor necrosis factor (TNF)** and **interleukin-1 (IL-1)** have numerous effects during all stages of the inflammatory process. They produce fever, increase the need for sleep, and decrease the appetite. TNF and IL-1 also increase leukocyte adherence, prostaglandin synthesis, and fibroblast production. These substances are also involved with the tissue destruction that occurs in periodontal disease.

PLASMA-DERIVED CHEMICAL MEDIATORS

Three major plasma protein systems are involved in the mediation of the inflammatory process. These systems include the complement system, the clotting system, and the kinin system. These systems consist of a series of inactive enzymes. Once the first enzyme in a series is activated, it initiates the next in a series of reactions in which the product of the last reaction is the initiator of the next reaction. This type of process is called a **cascade.**

The Complement System. Activation of the complement system is important in both the inflammatory process and in immunity. The **complement system** comprises a complex series of reactions between plasma proteins. The end product of this cascade is a substance called the **membrane attack complex (MAC)** that actually punches a hole in the cell membrane of microbes that are targeted for destruction by the immune system. Other substances that are produced in the cascade influence events in the inflammatory process, including vascular effects, leukocyte activation, adhesion and chemotaxis, and the enhancement of microbial phagocytosis. Products of the complement system cause mast cells to release their histamine. The vascular effects of histamine are described above in this chapter. Other products cause leukocytes to become more active and increase adherence to endothelial cells. The substances that enhance the action of leukocytes are also very strong chemotactic agents that stimulate leukocytes to travel to the area that has been injured or compromised. Still another product of the complement cascade is a type of opsonin that can attach to the cell wall of microbes, making them easier for the leukocytes to phagocytize (opsonization).

The complement cascade can be triggered by two different pathways, the classic and the alternative pathway. The **classic pathway** is triggered, or started, by antibodies that are created specifically for the agent causing the inflammatory process. This pathway requires the production of a specific antibody for the offending agent and can take time. The **alternative pathway** can be triggered by bacterial lipopolysaccharides or aggregates (clumps) of preformed immunoglobulins that are already circulating through the body. The alternative pathway is of much greater importance in an immediate inflammatory process because no time is needed to produce a specific antibody.

The Clotting System. The **clotting system** cascade is activated when a plasma protein called the Hageman factor comes in contact with cellular debris from an en-

dothelial or vessel injury. Although best known for its blood clotting effects, which will be involved in the repair process, the clotting system is involved in activation of both the kinin system and the complement system. Thus the clotting system is an important factor in the inflammatory process.

The Kinin System. Activation of the **kinin system** cascade results in the formation of the chemical mediator **bradykinin.** Bradykinin is capable of causing vasodilation, increased vascular permeability, and pain. The kinin system is activated by the same substance that activates the clotting system.

Now that more details have been provided regarding the elements of the acute inflammatory process, refer back to the "nail-in-foot" scenario and replace some of the broader terms such as "chemical mediators" with the names of the specific chemical mediator involved in the action. The same can be done with the broader term "leukocytes." Again, Table 3.2 can be used to complete this exercise. In addition to a localized reaction, you may see systemic manifestations of inflammation in some cases.

SYSTEMIC MANIFESTATIONS OF INFLAMMATION

The systemic manifestations of inflammation function to help control the injury and encourage the removal of the offending agents and debris associated with the inflammatory process. Systemic manifestations also help to start the repair process. Systemic involvement does not occur every time the inflammatory process is initiated; it depends on the extent of the process and how long it has been present, among other factors.

One of the hallmarks of systemic involvement is fever, or **pyrexia.** Chemical agents that cause pyrexia are called **pyrogens.** Common pyrogens are the cytokines that are produced by leukocytes during the inflammatory process and some of the substances released by bacteria. The pyrogens stimulate the production of prostaglandins, which activate the thermoregulatory center in the hypothalamus, thereby causing an elevation in temperature. An elevated temperature can be important because many pathogens have a very narrow temperature range within which they operate, and even a slight rise in temperature may help to destroy them. Pyrexia can also be caused by noninfectious agents. For example, pyrexia can be caused by an excess of thyroid hormones, severe dehydration, and cancer.

Leukocytosis, an increase in the number of white cells in the blood, is another systemic effect of inflammation. Normal white blood cell counts range from 4,000 to 10,000 per mm^3; however, during leukocytosis, white blood cell counts run up to 100,000 per mm^3. Neutrophils or PMNs will be increased in bacterial infections, in inflammatory disorders, and in response to certain drugs. Lymphocytes are the primary responders in viral infections, and monocytes predominate in chronic infections.

The lymphatic system is very important in draining the edema fluid or exudate and clearing the cellular debris and foreign matter from the affected area. **Lymphadenopathy**, enlargement of the lymph nodes, is another common systemic manifestation of the inflammatory process. The lymph nodes become enlarged, firm, and tender. Lymphadenopathy can present as a localized or generalized involvement. In a localized involvement, one or more of the nodes in the area of the infection or inflammation will become swollen and tender, such as when a streptococcal infection in the throat causes the cervical lymph nodes to become involved. In generalized involvement, nodes all over the body become swollen and tender; for example, the persistent generalized lymphadenopathy (PGL) seen in HIV infection (see Chapter 22). The lymphatic system is responsible for removing all of the waste products from the inflamed area before the area can heal. If this cannot be accomplished, or if for some other reason the inflammatory process cannot be halted, the reaction will continue into a chronic phase.

CHRONIC INFLAMMATION

Chronic inflammation is one of the possible results of acute inflammation, and it is often difficult to determine where the acute inflammatory process ends and the chronic inflammatory process begins. Acute inflammation should resolve in about 2 weeks. Anything that lasts longer than 2 weeks is most likely chronic. The purpose of chronic inflammation is to contain or remove a foreign substance or pathologic agent that the acute inflammatory process failed to remove from the tissue. However, chronic inflammation can occur without a preceding acute stage, as may occur in some of the autoimmune diseases discussed in Chapter 4. Chronic periodontitis may also occur without a preceding acute inflammatory process. Chronic inflammation is characterized by a large number of mononuclear cells in the tissue, tissue destruction, and ongoing unsuccessful attempts by the tissue to heal.

The major cells seen in chronic inflammation are macrophages, lymphocytes, and less frequently, plasma cells. Macrophages are driven to the inflamed area by chemotactic agents released by the neutrophils that are already working in the area and by chemical mediators released by some lymphocytes. Once there, macrophages secrete chemokines that recruit additional monocytes from the blood vessels to the injured site, where they differentiate into macrophages. Other chemical mediators released by the macrophages stimulate lymphocytes or enhance their actions. Macrophages have the major role in chronic inflammation. Macrophages are so powerful that they often cause significant amounts of tissue destruction while they are doing their job. Tissue destruction is one of the characteristic features of chronic inflammation.

Lymphocytes are present in all cases of chronic inflammation because almost all of the agents that can cause chronic inflammation are also recognized by the immune system as something it should react against. Lymphocytes initiate the immune process that occurs in conjunction with chronic inflammation. **Plasma cells** are also involved in the immune system response and may be seen in areas of chronic inflammation. Plasma cells are a form of lymphocyte that produce antibodies. Chapter 4 discusses how the immune system functions in conjunction with the inflammatory process. It is important to note that chemical mediators released by lymphocytes can stimulate or enhance the action of macrophages. The simultaneous stimulation of both macrophages and lymphocytes by each other enables the persistence of chronic inflammation.

The tissue destruction seen in chronic inflammation is caused by chemicals released from the cells that are attempting to eliminate the offending agent or substance from the area. Many of these chemical substances are found within the **lysosomes** of these cells. Lysosomes are organelles that contain strong digestive enzymes, called **lysosomal enzymes**, which are associated with the digestion or elimination of phagocytized foreign matter. When a phagocytic cell traps a foreign substance, it creates an intracellular space or vacuole called a **phagosome** to hold it in (Fig. 3.4). Chemicals that are released when the phagosome is being created drive the cell's lysosomes to the surface of the phagosome. The lysosomes fuse with the phagosome and release all of their lysosomal enzymes into it, enabling the digestion of the foreign matter. Problems occur when lysosomal enzymes find their way out of the cells and into the tissues. The enzymes may leak from the cell as it is digesting a foreign substance or all of the intracellular substances may be released when the cell dies. The lysosomal enzymes can destroy normal cells in the area. They can also destroy collagen fibers and activate osteoclasts. The osteoclasts will cause bone destruction. The destruction that occurs during chronic adult periodontitis is a good example of this process. While these destructive processes are occurring, the tissue is trying to heal itself.

Chronic inflammation has been described as "frustrated healing" by many, because everything that is needed for repair, such as **fibroblasts** (immature connective tissue cell that can differentiate into cells that produce collagen and other tissues) and small blood vessels, is present in the affected tissues. Chronic inflammation will only resolve when all of the agents that caused it are eliminated. Box 3.3 presents a list of factors that can contribute to the development and maintenance of chronic inflammation.

Granulomatous Inflammation

Granulomatous inflammation is a subset of chronic inflammation and is characterized by the formation of

FACTORS CONTRIBUTING TO THE DEVELOPMENT AND MAINTENANCE OF CHRONIC INFLAMMATION

1. Infectious agents in the area of inflammation
2. Remains of partially digested organisms in the tissues
3. Foreign material in the inflamed tissues
4. Substances produced by the body as part of an abnormal process, which remain in the tissues (e.g., the urate crystals in gout)
5. Incomplete drainage of an abscess
6. Presence of dead or necrotic tissues in the inflamed area
7. Insufficient stability or too much motion of the injured part
8. Physical or mechanical irritation of the injured part

granulomas. The **granuloma** comprises large macrophages called giant cells and other chronic inflammatory cells surrounding some type of foreign matter. The purpose of the granuloma is to form a wall around the foreign substance and prevent its spread (Fig. 3.7). A periapical granuloma will form at the apex of a nonvital tooth in response to the substances produced by necrotic dental pulp tissue (see Chapter 21). Another example is the granuloma produced in the lung in response to *Mycobacterium tuberculosis*. Granulomas can heal only after all the stimuli that initiated the inflammatory process are eliminated. For example, the periapical granuloma will heal after endodontic therapy removes the necrotic dental pulp.

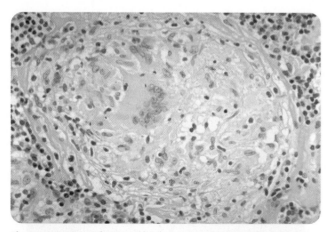

Figure 3.7. Granuloma. A higher-power photomicrograph of a single granuloma in a lymph node depicts a multinucleated giant cell amid numerous pale epithelioid cells. A thin rim of fibrous tissue separates the granuloma from the lymphoid cells of the node. (From Rubin E, Farber JL. Pathology. 3rd ed. Philadelphia: Lippincott Williams & Wilkins, 1999.)

OUTCOMES OF ACUTE INFLAMMATION

Chronic inflammation is only one of the possible outcomes of the acute inflammatory process; others include abscess formation, resolution of the inflammatory process, and healing by either regeneration or repair (Fig. 3.8).

Abscess Formation

Abscess formation occurs when **pyogenic**, or pus-producing, organisms such as staphylococci or streptococci are introduced into the tissues. Pyogenic organisms produce chemical mediators that send out a message for every leukocyte, specifically the PMNs, in the area to come to the site of the injury to consume the organisms. A problem occurs when the pyogenic organisms are resistant to phagocytosis. In this case, the neutrophils die trying to eliminate the organisms, and tissues in the area are destroyed because the neutrophils release lysosomal enzymes when they die. All of the resulting debris accumulates in the tissues as purulent exudate or pus, forming the abscess. The abscess can cause significant damage if not treated. A **fistula** can form through soft or hard tissues. Fistulas occur when enzymes that are released by macrophages literally bore a hole through the tissues along the path of least resistance, ultimately allowing the purulent exudate to exit one area and flow into another or find a path to an outer surface. An example of this is a parulis, which is created when an abscessed tooth forms a fistula tract to the surface of the oral mucosa (Fig. 3.9).

Another sequela involves the spread of the bacteria into the surrounding tissues producing **cellulitis** (Fig. 3.10), an inflammation of the connective tissue. In some cases the bacteria enter the blood and produce **bacteremia**, or bacteria in the blood. This can lead to **septicemia**, or blood poisoning, and several other conditions. An abscess needs to be treated quickly before any of these conditions can occur.

Resolution of the Inflammatory Process

In many cases the inflammatory process is not triggered by a traumatic injury or microbial assault. In these cases, because there was no traumatic tissue damage, resolution can take place. When the stimulus that initiated the process, such as pollen in hay fever, is neutralized, the inflammation resolves, and the tissues return to normal. In the case of tissue damage, healing can only be completed when all of the stimuli that initiated the inflammatory process are neutralized or removed.

Regeneration

The most desired outcome of the inflammatory process is **regeneration**. This is the body's attempt to restore itself to

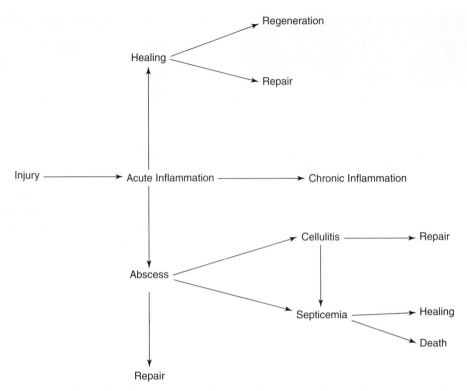

Figure 3.8. Outcomes of the acute inflammatory process. This flowchart shows the possible outcomes of acute inflammation.

its original state. Regeneration occurs when the stimulus that caused the inflammation is completely removed, the vascular system returns to normal, the injured tissue is replaced with the same type of tissues and cells that were damaged, and the area regains full function. Regeneration depends on the type of cell that was damaged and the extent of the injury. The epithelial cells that line the oral cavity will regenerate because they are already constantly replicating themselves to keep the mucosal barrier intact.

Liver cells will regenerate. In transplantations, the liver of the donor will completely regenerate, and the part of the liver that is transplanted into the recipient will regenerate to a more normal size. Brain cells, however, are permanent or nondividing cells; therefore, injured brain cells will not replicate. Some of the lost function may be regained by forming alternative pathways through uninjured brain cells, but the cells that were lost will not regenerate. No matter what type of tissue is involved, if the injured area is large enough, regeneration will not be an option.

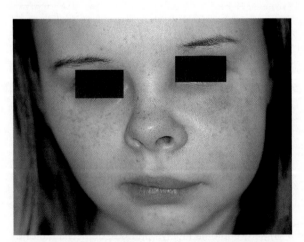

Figure 3.9. Abscess. A parulis that forms as a result of a periapical abscess is an example of an outcome of acute inflammation. (From Fleisher GR, Ludwig S, Baskin MN. Atlas of pediatric emergency medicine. Philadelphia: Lippincott Williams & Wilkins, 2004.)

Figure 3.10. Cellulitis. This child had a painful swollen cheek and infraorbital cellulitis caused by an abscessed tooth. (Courtesy of Dr. Debra Weiner; From Fleisher GR, Ludwig S, Baskin MN. Atlas of pediatric emergency medicine. Philadelphia: Lippincott Williams & Wilkins, 2004.)

Fibrous Repair

If regeneration is not possible then **fibrous repair** will be the final outcome. Fibrous repair results in the creation of a **cicatrix** (scar) that may recreate normal or near-normal tissue formation or architecture but not normal function. Chronic inflammation inevitably resolves with scar formation. This outcome is related to the extended healing time and to the amount of tissue damage usually associated with chronic inflammation. Repair is one of the primary functions of the immune system. The process of repair, like the inflammatory process, requires many chemical mediators that control the timing of the wound healing. Some of these chemical mediators include cytokines and epithelium-, fibroblast-, and platelet derived growth factors.

Remember that the process of repair begins as soon as the inflammatory process is initiated. Almost immediately following an injury, a blood clot forms and fills the wound. The clot provides an area where leukocytes can clean the wound of foreign matter and dead or injured tissue cells. As this is occurring, fibroblasts and vascular endothelial cells begin to appear within the clot. The endothelial cells begin to form new blood vessels in a process called **angiogenesis**, and the fibroblasts start to form collagen fibers. The very fragile vascular tissue that is starting to form is called **granulation tissue** (Fig. 3.11). Granulation tissue forms the framework upon and within which fibrous repair takes place. If the wound appears on a surface of the body, such as the skin or buccal mucosa, epithelialization will most likely occur in conjunction with the formation of granulation tissue. During **epithelialization**, epithelial cells from the lower layer of the epithelium at the edges of the wound start to slide down and across the wound surface beneath the scab. These cells eventually meet and unite, forming a basement membrane and normal stratified squamous epithelium. Eventually the vascular granulation tissue becomes less vascular as

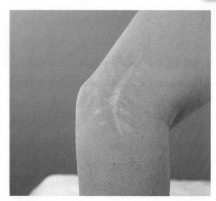

Figure 3.12. Fibrous repair. This scar is an example of fibrous repair. (From Weber J, Kelley J. Health assessment in nursing, 2nd ed. Philadelphia: Lippincott Williams & Wilkins, 2003.)

the fibroblasts create more collagen fibers. In the end, most of the blood vessels in the tissue are resorbed because they are no longer needed to bring nutrients into the area. Fibroblasts disappear, and what is left is a very dense collagenous tissue, or scar, containing very few blood vessels (Fig. 3.12). It is important to note that whenever a scar forms the function of that area of tissue is lost. Loss of function may not be crucial in a small skin wound, but many problems are associated with even small injuries to nervous tissue. Another problem regarding scar formation occurs because the injured tissue will only regain about 70 to 80% of its full strength; in large injuries this could be very significant.

TYPES OF FIBROUS REPAIR

Healing can involve both repair and regeneration, depending on the specific types of tissue and cells that are involved. In the skin and mucous membranes, the epidermal tissues and the blood vessels in the area will regenerate. The dermis or deeper connective tissues will undergo fibrous repair. Healing by primary intention and secondary intention are the main methods whereby surface wounds undergo healing.

Healing by Primary Intention. This type of repair occurs when the margins of the injury are clean and brought together by sutures, bandages, or pressure. The migrating epithelial cells have little distance to travel, and healing may occur with very little or no visible scarring (Fig. 3.13).

Healing by Secondary Intention. Healing by secondary intention occurs when the loss of tissue is significant enough that the edges of the wound cannot be brought together. The process of repair must begin at the base of the injury and proceed from the bottom to the top. Healing by secondary intention will result in scar formation (Fig. 3.14).

FACTORS THAT AFFECT WOUND HEALING

The type, size, and location of the wound will affect how it heals. A sharp, clean wound will heal faster than tissue

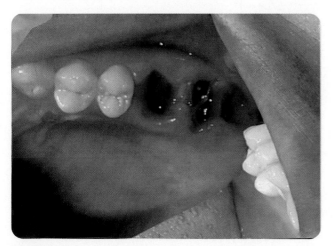

Figure 3.11. Granulation tissue. Granulation tissue is the framework upon which the healing tissue repairs itself. The bottom of this extraction site is filled with granulation tissue.

APPLICATION

The following two scenarios illustrate the difference between healing that occurs in a tissue in which cells replicate and that which occurs in a tissue in which cells do not replicate.

Scenario I: Latoya is a first-year dental hygiene student using an anterior sickle scaler on a "real" patient for the first time. Other than the fact that she is very nervous, she is desperately trying to remember everything that she should do to remove the slightly subgingival calculus from the distal of tooth 25. Latoya gets the side of the tip one third inserted under the calculus and opens the face of the blade to what she thinks is the correct working angulation. What she doesn't know is that she has mistakenly opened the face of the blade too far, and the opposite cutting edge is impinging on the interdental papilla. Latoya activates a working stroke and to her disbelief, does not remove any of the calculus. Even more disconcerting is the fact that when she activated her working stroke, she removed a small portion of the interdental papilla. Although this is traumatic to almost every student the first time it happens, the effect on the patient is very minor. The oral epithelial tissues are made of rapidly dividing epithelial cells, and the area of injury is

very small; therefore, the tissue is more or less regenerated and heals back to its normal size and function. Latoya is relieved to see that the tissue has returned to normal the next time the patient comes in.

Scenario II: Shawn, a friend of Julian, another dental hygiene student, has gone to a piercing parlor to have his tongue pierced. The next day Julian gets a phone call from a very upset Shawn, who is unhappy because the feeling in his tongue does not seem to be returning. Julian suggests that it might just be due to the swelling from the inflammatory process that was triggered by the injury and that Shawn should give it time to heal. Several days later Shawn is still experiencing a loss of sensation in his tongue and some loss of function. After consulting with his dentist, it is determined that a portion of the lingual nerve was most likely damaged during the tongue piercing. The dentist's recommendation is to wait and see if, after time, some of the sensation and function will return, but there is nothing more that can be done. The injury in this case was small, and the lingual nerve was not totally severed. However, nerve tissue is permanent or nondividing and the scar tissue that was produced cannot perform the function of the original tissue.

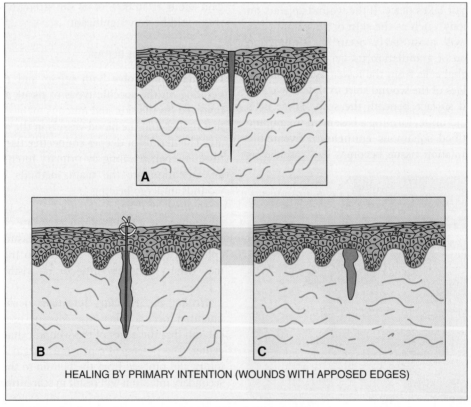

HEALING BY PRIMARY INTENTION (WOUNDS WITH APPOSED EDGES)

Figure 3.13. Healing by primary intention. **A.** There is little loss of tissue in the wound pictured here. In addition, the edges are clean and held closely together by sutures. **B.** This type of damage requires only minimal cell proliferation and the creation of new blood vessels (angiogenesis) to heal. **C.** The outcome of healing by primary intention is a small scar. (From Rubin E, Farber JL. Pathology. 3rd ed. Philadelphia: Lippincott Williams & Wilkins, 1999.)

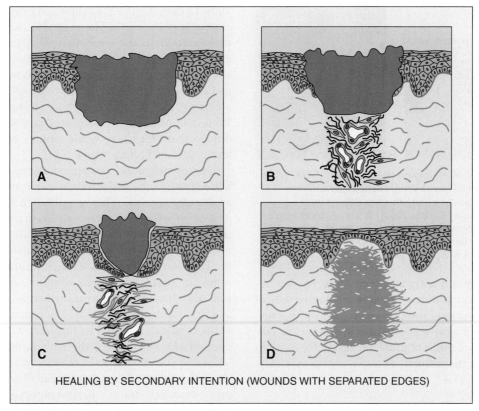

HEALING BY SECONDARY INTENTION (WOUNDS WITH SEPARATED EDGES)

Figure 3.14. Healing by secondary intention. **A.** There is substantial loss of tissue in the wound pictured here; the edges are far apart and cannot be drawn together. A blood clot has filled the wound. **B.** Granulation tissue forms within the wound and is the framework upon which the repair process will take place. Endothelial cells migrate into the area and form new vessels (angiogenesis). **C.** Epithelial cells continue to migrate down into and across the wound until they meet, forming the new basement membrane. Fibroblasts create collagen fibers that are deposited within the granulation tissue. **D.** Granulation tissue is eventually resorbed and replaced by the fibrous tissue that forms a large scar that is often functionally and esthetically unsatisfactory. (From Rubin E, Farber JL. Pathology. 3rd ed. Philadelphia: Lippincott Williams & Wilkins, 1999.)

that is torn apart. A large wound will heal more slowly than a small wound. A wound that involves tissues around a joint will heal more slowly than one located in a nonmoving area. Likewise, a wound in an area that has constant irritation from clothing will heal more slowly than one that is not irritated by clothing.

Wounds in highly vascular tissue will heal faster than those in nonvascular tissues. For example, a wound in the oral cavity will heal faster than one located on the dermal surface, primarily because of the increased vascular supply. This is because vascular tissue is better able to supply the necessary elements for healing than less vascular tissue.

Several other local factors play a part in slowing wound healing. Infection will impair the healing process, as will the presence of a foreign object such as a splinter or shard of glass. Impaired circulation in the area of the wound will delay or prevent healing. This is especially important in older adults and in persons with chronic cardiopulmonary diseases. If an excessive amount of granulation tissue forms in the wound, healing will be delayed because the process of epithelialization will be stopped until the excess tissue is removed.

Systemic factors, such as those occurring in diabetes, can interfere with wound healing. Smokers also have an impaired capacity for wound healing. Many types of nutritional deficiencies, such as starvation, protein malnutrition, and vitamin and mineral deficiencies (especially vitamin C), will delay healing. Healing will be impaired in individuals who have genetic syndromes (see Chapter 6) such as Marfan and Ehlers-Danlos syndromes, which include connective tissue disorders. The systemic effects of certain medications will also impair the healing process. The most important of these are medications that interfere with the inflammatory process or with the immune system, such as corticosteroid, nonsteroidal antiinflammatory, and other immunosuppressive drugs.

COMPLICATIONS OF WOUND HEALING

The most common complications of healing are inadequate scar formation, excessive scar formation, and excessive contracture of the scar tissue. Inadequate scar formation usually occurs as the result of the production of an inadequate amount of granulation tissue. The most serious result of this is the bursting of a wound after surgery; if a wound bursts after abdominal surgery there is a 30% chance of mortality (Rubin, 2005). Excessive scar formation results in a hypertrophic scar, or **keloid** (Fig. 3.15).

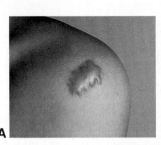
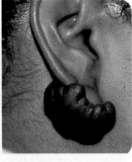

Figure 3.15. Keloid. **A.** Keloid on the shoulder. (From Willis MC. Medical terminology: a programmed learning approach to the language of health care. Baltimore: Lippincott Williams & Wilkins, 2002.) **B.** This is an example of excessive scar formation after having the ear pierced. (From Rubin E, Farber JL. Pathology. 3rd ed. Philadelphia: Lippincott Williams & Wilkins, 1999.)

These are usually unsightly and tend to recur after removal. The last complication is excessive contracture of the edges of the wound causing extensive deformity especially if the area is near a joint where limitations in mobility can cause a significant problem. Severe burns often result in wounds that exhibit excessive contracture (Fig. 3.16).

Tooth Extraction: Bone and Soft Tissue Repair

The repair of an extraction site involves most of the same processes discussed above, with slight variation. The acute inflammatory process is triggered by the injury, and PMNs rush into the area. A blood clot fills the extraction site. As stated above, the inflammatory process and the process of repair are occurring at the same time. As the acute inflammatory process continues, the epithelial cells at the edges of the wound begin the process of epithelialization and completely cover the extraction site in about

10 to 12 days. Figure 3.17 shows an extraction site that is almost fully healed. In the meantime, under the surface, osteoblasts from the bone marrow migrate into the clot and begin to produce new bone. The entire area of the extraction undergoes remodeling. The alveolar process is resorbed because it is no longer needed to maintain a tooth and is replaced with spongy bone. The bone is completely filled in by about 12 weeks postextraction. The same conditions that affect soft tissue wound healing, as stated above, will affect bone repair.

One of the more common problems associated with bone repair in the oral cavity is a dry socket also known as **alveolar osteitis**. This complication is specific to the healing of extraction sites and occurs most often with third molar extractions. Alveolar osteitis occurs when the initial blood clot within the socket is disrupted or lost and the bone surface becomes exposed to the intraoral environment, increasing the risk of infection and causing severe pain. In addition, the exposed bone becomes necrotic and may produce a foul odor. The patient becomes aware of the condition within 2 to 4 days after the extraction. In cases of alveolar osteitis, the necrotic bone must be resorbed by the body, and granulation tissue must form along the walls of the socket instead of within a clot. This process is much slower, often taking several weeks longer, than normal. The risk factors associated with alveolar osteitis include excessive trauma to the bone during extraction, tobacco use, and noncompliance with postoperative instructions (Larsen, 1992). Most cases of alveolar osteitis can be prevented by limiting the amount of trauma during the extraction and by the patient complying with postoperative instructions that focus on maintaining the integrity of the blood clot. For example, the patient should avoid the following:

- Producing a vacuum in the mouth by drinking through a straw or by smoking for at least 24 hours, because this can dislodge the fragile new clot
- Tobacco use, because this will impair circulation in the area

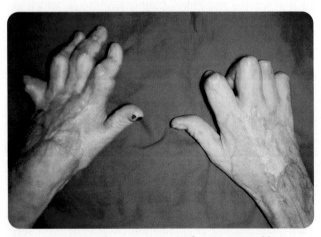

Figure 3.16. Wound contracture. Deformity caused by excessive contracture of scar tissues after severe thermal burns on the hands. (From Strickland JW, Graham TJ. Master techniques in orthopaedic surgery: the hand, 2nd ed. Philadelphia: Lippincott Williams & Wilkins, 2005.)

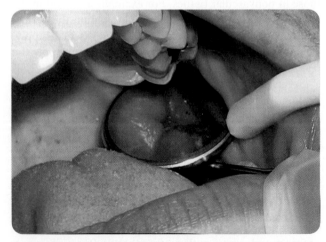

Figure 3.17. Extraction site. Third molar extraction site is almost totally healed after 5 weeks.

- Vigorous rinsing for at least 24 hours, because this can also dislodge the clot
- Eating or drinking hot liquids, which might melt the clot

Alveolar osteitis is treated by gently packing strips of a special type of gauze into the socket. The gauze is treated with an antiseptic to reduce the risk of infection and a medication that can soothe the exposed nerves, such as clove oil. In addition, the physical presence of the gauze reduces the chance that food will become lodged in the area. The patient returns every day or two to replace the packing and to check on the healing process until completed.

Conditions and diseases that manifest as inflammatory processes are caused by hundreds of different stimuli, both endogenous and exogenous. Almost every disorder that can be imagined has inflammatory components within its clinical manifestations. The most common diseases and conditions and those that are important in the practice of dental hygiene are discussed in later chapters, where they are addressed within the context of sharing similar clinical manifestations.

SUMMARY

- The acute inflammatory process is carried out by the body using both cellular and chemical mechanisms.
- There are three phases in the acute inflammatory process, initiation, amplification, and termination.
- Initiation involves changes in the microcirculation in which chemical mediators instruct the blood vessels to briefly constrict, then dilate and become more permeable. The vascular changes enable PMNs to emigrate through the endothelial walls into the connective tissue, where they follow the direction of more chemical mediators to the areas where they are needed. In addition, exudate is allowed to flow from the blood vessels into the surrounding area, creating edema.
- Amplification involves gathering all of the necessary cells into the area to phagocytize all of the microorganisms, foreign matter, or other debris that needs to be removed before healing can take place.
- Termination requires shutting down the inflammatory process through the action of other chemical mediators so that healing can be completed.
- The complement, kinin, and clotting systems are all involved in mediating the inflammatory process.
- During the process of acute inflammation, systemic manifestations such as pyrexia, leukocytosis, and lymphadenopathy may occur.
- Chronic inflammation may result from unresolved acute inflammation or it may occur without this stimulus.
- The chronic inflammatory process is controlled by different cells and chemical mediators that attempt to neutralize whatever stimulus is causing the reaction. Continuation of chronic inflammation leads to significant tissue destruction and delayed or abnormal healing.
- Other outcomes of the inflammatory process include abscesses, fistula formation, and cellulitis.
- Chronic inflammation always stimulates an immune system response.
- Tissue regeneration or repair begins at almost the same time as the inflammatory process and continues in conjunction with it.
- Regeneration occurs when the tissue is repaired with the same type of tissue that was lost and the area regains full function. Anything less then this is considered repair.
- Repair of surface wounds occurs by either primary or secondary intention and involves the production of granulation tissue within the wound. Lost tissue is replaced by newly formed connective tissue, and the blood supply is reestablished through the process of angiogenesis.
- Epithelialization replaces the skin covering the wound. The end product is fibrous repair or scar formation.
- Many factors can affect how a wound heals, including the type, size, and location of the wound; the type of tissue involved; and the health status of the individual.
- Keloids, excessive wound contracture, and wound rupture are complications of the repair process.
- Healing of extraction sites involves bone repair and remodeling in addition to soft tissue healing.
- Alveolar osteitis, a common complication following extraction of third molars, can be prevented by reducing the amount of trauma during the surgery, avoiding tobacco use, and following postoperative instruction.

Critical Thinking Activities

1. What would be the positive and negative aspects of having no inflammatory process?

2. What do you think would happen if the inflammatory process were to run out of control? How would you attempt to control it?

Case Study

Your patient presents complaining of soreness around the distal of #17. She has not been able to eat on the left side for 2 days and has been taking aspirin for the pain but has had no relief. When you perform your intraoral examination you see the condition depicted in Figure 3.18.

1. How would you describe your clinical findings?

2. Which cardinal signs of inflammation are present and what has caused them?

3. Which of the cardinal signs of inflammation would be mediated by histamine?

4. What could have caused the inflammation?

5. What can be done to alleviate the condition?

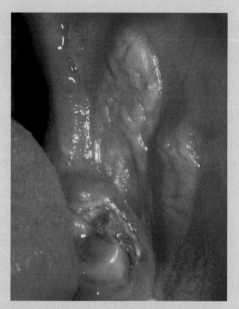

Figure 3.18. Case Study. Pericoronitis with chemical burn. (Courtesy of Dr. John Jacoway.)

REFERENCES

Anderson DM, Keith J, Novak PD, Elliot MA. Mosby's medical, nursing & allied health dictionary. 6th ed. Philadelphia: Mosby, 2002.

Barrett RJ. Chemokines. Blood 1997;90:909–928.

Cotran RS, Kumar V, Collins T. Robbins: pathologic basis of disease, 6th ed. Philadelphia: WB Saunders 1999:50–112.

Dirckx JH, ed. Stedman's concise medical dictionary for the health professions. 3rd ed. Baltimore: Williams & Wilkins, 1997.

Goljan EF. Pathology: Saunders text and review series. Philadelphia: WB Saunders, 1998:38–54.

Huether SE, McCance KL. Understanding pathophysiology. 3rd ed. St. Louis: Mosby, 2004:153–180.

Ibsen OAC, Phelan JA. Oral pathology for the dental hygienist. 4th ed. St. Louis: WB Saunders, 2004:36–85.

Kirshenbaum A. (NIH/NIAD) *AGILFILLAN@niaid.nih.gov*, personal email message March 11, 2004.

Larsen PE. Alveolar osteitis after surgical removal of impacted mandibu-lar third molars. Identification of the patient at risk. Oral Surg Oral Med Oral Pathol 1992;73(4):393–397.

Porth CM. Essentials of pathophysiology: concepts of altered health states, Philadelphia: Lippincott Williams & Wilkins, 2004:150–167.

Price SA, Wilson LM. Pathophysiology: Clinical concepts of disease processes, 6th ed. St. Louis: Mosby, 2003:44–63.

Regezi JA, Sciubba JJ, Jordan RCK. Oral pathology: clinical pathologic correlations. 4th ed. St. Louis: WB Saunders, 2003.

Rubin E, Gorstein F, Rubin R, et al. Rubin's pathology: clinicopathologic foundations of medicine. 4th ed. Baltimore: Lippincott Williams & Wilkins, 2005:41–116.

Stvrtinova V, Jakubovsky J, Hulin I. Inflammation and fever. Available at: *http://www.sovba.sk/logos/books/scientific/Inffever.html*, accessed February 2004.

Ten Cate R. Oral histology: development, structure, and function, 5th ed. St. Louis: Mosby, 1998:421.

Trowbridge HO, Emling RC. Inflammation: a review of the process. 5th ed. Chicago: Quintessence; 1997.

4 The Immune System and Immunity

Key Terms

- Active immunity
- Anaphylactic reaction
- Antibody
- Antigen
- Antigen binding fragment
- Antigen-presenting cell (APC)
- Atopic reaction
- Autoimmune disease
- Cell-mediated reaction
- Contact dermatitis
- Cytokines
- Cytotoxic reaction
- Graft-versus-host reaction
- Haptens
- Immune complex-mediated reaction
- Immunoglobulin (Ig)
- Maculopapular
- Major histocompatibility complex (MHC)
- Memory cell
- Natural killer cell
- Nonspecific immunity
- Opportunistic infection
- Passive immunity
- Plasma cell
- Primary immune response
- Primary immunodeficiency
- Secondary immune response
- Secondary immunodeficiency
- Self-tolerance
- Specific immunity
- Target cells
- T cytotoxic cell
- T helper cell
- Waldeyer's ring

Learning Outcomes

1. Define and use the key terms that describe the immune system.
2. List examples of antigens.
3. Describe the nonspecific immune system.
4. Describe the location and elements of Waldeyer's ring.
5. Describe the immune system cells and their functions.
6. List the names and functions of the major cytokines involved in the immune response.
7. State the ultimate goal of the immune response.
8. Describe and differentiate between humoral and cell-mediated immunity.
9. Discuss how the immune system recognizes, reacts to, and remembers antigenic agents.
10. Describe the characteristics of the five major antibody groups.
11. List the four ways of achieving specific immunity.
12. Discuss and give examples of the four types of hypersensitivity reactions.
13. Identify methods to avoid latex hypersensitivity reactions.
14. Describe the concept of self-tolerance as it relates to autoimmune diseases.
15. Differentiate between primary and acquired immune deficiency diseases.
16. Describe the impact of immune deficiency on an individual and the role that opportunistic infections play in the process.

Chapter Outline

IMMUNITY

The body has many defenses against invaders or substances that can cause disease or injury. The inflammatory process, discussed in Chapter 3, is one of these defense mechanisms. Inflammation is an immediate response that occurs when foreign or injurious agents are allowed into the cells or tissues of the body. Cells and chemical products produced during the inflammatory process are essential in activating another of the body's defenses, the immune system. The goal of the immune system is to prevent foreign substances from entering the body and to establish immunity or resistance to disease-producing agents, such as bacteria and viruses, through the immune response.

Immune System Triggers or Antigens

The agent that triggers the immune response is called an **antigen**. Antigens can be chemicals (natural or synthetic), food proteins, the products of microbes (lipopolysaccharides), the microbes themselves, abnormal human tissue cells, donor tissue cells, or the person's own normal tissue cells. Antigens are usually large-molecular-weight substances, such as proteins and polysaccharides. Smaller-molecular-weight substances, such as some metals, the oils from the poison ivy leaf, and some medications such as penicillin are called **haptens**, and can only exhibit antigenic properties when combined with a larger human protein from the skin, blood, or other tissue. The larger-molecular-weight substances, such as lipopolysaccharides, can trigger the immune response without such help.

The immune system cells need to be able to distinguish self from nonself. The body accomplishes this by "coding" each cell surface with molecules that are the equivalent of an identification tag. These molecular identification tags are called **major histocompatibility complexes (MHC)** and are found on almost every cell that has a nucleus. MHCs may also be called human leukocyte antigens (HLAs). The MHCs play an important role in activating the immune response. Any time there is a change in the MHC of a particular cell, caused by injury, viral infection, or other stimulus, the MHC will become antigenic, and the cell will no longer be recognized by the immune system as self. This change initiates the immune response, which results in destruction of the cell. MHCs play a vital role in organ and tissue transplantation. It is important to match the MHC molecules of organ and tissue transplant recipients and their donors as closely as possible to minimize the potential for rejection of the transplant.

Nonspecific Immunity

Nonspecific immunity (sometimes called innate immunity) comprises defense mechanisms that are nonspecific, meaning they require no previous exposure to the offending agent to accomplish their objective of neutralizing that agent. Examples of nonspecific immunity include the following:

- Physical barriers
  - Integumentary system, skin, and mucous membranes
  - Waldeyer's ring
  - Nasal hairs, sneezing
  - Respiratory tract cilia, coughing
- Chemical barriers
  - pH of the skin
  - Mucous secretions
  - Gastric acids
  - Tears, sweat, and saliva
- Nonspecific phagocytes
  - Monocytes, macrophages, and neutrophils
- Indigenous microbes that compete with pathogens
- The inflammatory response
- The clotting system
- The complement and kinin systems

The inflammatory process, kinin, clotting, and complement systems and the action of some of the phagocytic cells are integral parts of nonspecific immunity. In addition, the chemical mediators involved in these processes or secreted by the phagocytic cells are essential in activating or enhancing the immune process that results in resistance to specific antigens or specific immunity.

Specific Immunity

Another form of immunity that helps maintain the body in a healthy state is **specific immunity** (sometimes called acquired immunity). Specific immunity acts against previously encountered agents with antibodies and activated lymphocytes that are specific for that agent. This is called the immune response, and it is carried out by the immune system. The immune system works in conjunction with the inflammatory and the healing and repair processes of the body to maintain the health of the individual.

ORGANS ASSOCIATED WITH THE IMMUNE SYSTEM

The principal organs of the immune system are the bone marrow, thymus, spleen, lymphatic vessels and nodes, and mucosa-associated lymphoid tissues. The bone marrow produces all of the cells of the immune system from precursor stem cells. The thymus gland educates some of these cells, called T cells, to make them **self-tolerant** (having the ability to recognize the host's own cells as self). The spleen has two functions. It serves as a filter to remove old and damaged red blood cells from the general circulation, and as part of the immune system; it will mount an immune response against any foreign substance presented to it via the same circulating blood. The lymphatic system can initiate an immune response, process some of the immune system cells, called B cells, and remove foreign substances from the host through a system of vessels and nodes placed throughout the body. There are also numerous strategically placed mucosa-associated lymph tissues that are important in maintaining the immune status of the individual by detecting and removing injurious substances before they compromise this defensive barrier. Most of these are located in the gastrointestinal, respiratory, and genitourinary tracts. The most notable in the oral-pharyngeal area is **Waldeyer's ring**, which comprises the adenoid or pharyngeal tonsil and the lingual and palatine tonsils (Fig. 4.1).

CELLULAR AND CHEMICAL COMPONENTS OF THE IMMUNE SYSTEM

The immune system consists of chemical molecules and immune cells that inhabit lymphatic tissue and circulate in body fluids. The cells of the immune system include macrophages and lymphocytes. Chapter 3 describes macrophages as they relate to the inflammatory process. This chapter illustrates the role of macrophages in the immune system response, showing how they are an integral part of both processes. The lymphocytes are white blood cells that are found in lymphoid tissues. Lymphocytes are divided into two categories, B lymphocytes and T lymphocytes. The B lymphocytes are most active in humoral immunity, while the T lymphocytes are most active in cell-mediated immunity, although they are also necessary

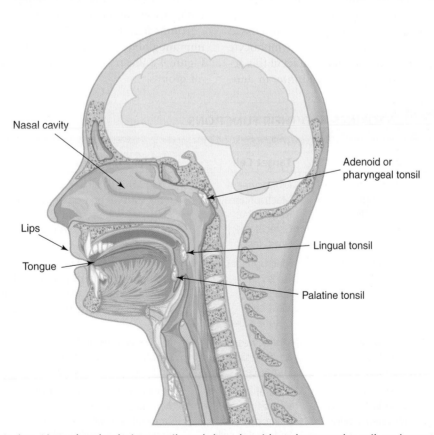

Figure 4.1. Waldeyer's ring. Lingual and palatine tonsils and the adenoid or pharyngeal tonsil are important elements of nonspecific immunity that encounter foreign substances as they enter the body through the oral cavity.

for the optimal functioning of humoral immunity. Lymphocytes are discussed below in this chapter.

A complex system of chemical molecules or **cytokines** produced by the immune cells modulates or regulates how the system responds to a stimulus. Cytokines have various functions, such as carrying messages to and from cells, enhancing cell growth, stimulating chemotaxis, and activating immune cells. Table 4.1 lists specific cytokines, their source, target cells, and actions.

THE IMMUNE RESPONSE

The goal of the immune response is to remove or neutralize antigenic substances. To accomplish this goal, the system must recognize the "invader," react to the invader, and remember the invader. There are two interactive components of this systemic immune response, the humoral response and the cell-mediated or cellular response.

Humoral Immunity

Humoral immunity is provided by the B lymphocytes or B cells. These cells develop in the bone marrow and then mature in lymphoid tissue throughout the body. The maturation process ensures that the surface of each B cell contains an **antibody**, which is a molecule that will react against one or more specific types of antigen. The **antigen-binding fragment** (Fab) is the part of the antibody that combines with or binds to an antigen (Fig. 4.2). The B cell becomes activated when its antigen-binding fragment comes in contact with an antigen that it can bind to. Another type of lymphocyte, the **T helper cell** (discussed in the next section) must also bind to the B lymphocyte before it can become activated. The end product of this activation is the transformation of the B cell into an anti-

body-secreting lymphocyte known as a **plasma cell.** Both B and T cells must function together before a plasma cell can be created and antibodies produced. Plasma cells live for only a few days. The process of B cell activation also stimulates the plasma cells to divide and become more numerous, which increases the amount of antibody produced. In turn, the bone marrow is stimulated to produce more B cells that can become plasma cells upon activation. It takes about 2 to 3 weeks to build up enough circulating antibody to inactivate most antigens after this initial exposure. This process is called the **primary immune response.** The slow production of antibody at the initial exposure results in the host usually showing some overt signs and/or symptoms of the specific pathology or disease associated with that antigen. Another type of B lymphocyte, known as a memory B cell, is created as the primary immune response is terminated. The memory B cells carry the description of the antigen so that it will be recognized more quickly and acted against more rapidly the next time the antigen is encountered.

If the host survives the primary encounter with the antigen, a second exposure will activate the memory B cells, which will initiate an immediate, full immune response to the antigen. This is called the **secondary immune response. Memory cells** can live for decades and be ready to mount an immediate antibody assault when triggered by a "remembered" antigen. The various ways in which antibodies attack circulating antigens such as bacteria, viruses, and toxic substances are listed in Box 4.1.

Antibodies. There are 5 major groups of antibodies or **immunoglobulins (Ig)** produced by the B lymphocytes. Figure 4.3 illustrates the molecular structure of these major groups.

Table 4.1 CYTOKINES AND THEIR FUNCTIONS

Cytokine	Source	Target Cell	Biologic Activities
Interleukin 1 (IL-1)	Lymphocytes Antigen-presenting cells (APCs)	Monocytes Macrophages Neutrophils Osteoclasts Fibroblasts	Chemotactic factor for monocytes and neutrophils Induces fever and other systemic manifestations Increases bone resorption Induces fibroblast proliferation
Interleukins (IL) 2–8	Activated T cells Mast cells	Macrophages T cells B cells Mast cells Natural killer cells	Chemotactic factor for macrophages and neutrophils Promotes growth of B and T cells Growth factor for mast cells and natural killer cells Enhances activation of cytotoxic T cells
Tumor necrosis factor	Macrophages Activated T cells	Monocytes Neutrophils Tumor cells	Mimics actions of IL-1 Cytotoxic to select tumor cells Activates phagocytic cells
Interferon	Leukocytes Fibroblasts Activated T cells	Natural killer cells Viruses Macrophages Endothelial cells	Induces natural killer activity Activates macrophages Antiviral activities Activates endothelial cells

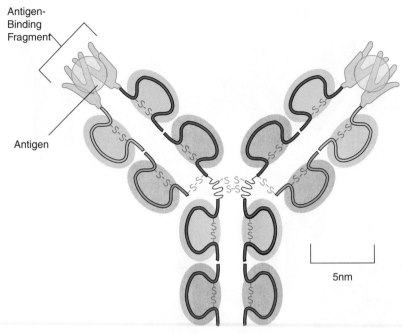

Figure 4.2. Antigen-binding fragment (Fab). The antigen-binding fragment is the area on the immunoglobulin that binds with an antigen.

1. IgG (4 types): IgG (gamma globulin) is a circulating antibody and is directed against common infectious agents such as viruses, bacteria, and toxins. IgG binds to the antigen and then binds to a surface receptor on a phagocytic cell allowing for phagocytosis of the antigen–antibody complex. IgG also activates the classic pathway of the complement system and is active in the secondary immune response. IgG is the only immunoglobulin that crosses the placental barrier and protects the developing child and newborn until his or her own immune system matures. IgG makes up 80% of the circulating antibodies in the adult body.

2. IgM: This antibody is found on the surface of B cells and is the largest of the immunoglobulins. It may have up to 10 antigen-binding fragments available for use. This is the first antibody that is produced in response to an antigen. Its main purpose is to cause clumping,

or agglutination, of antigen proteins during the primary immune response. IgM is more efficient in activating the classic pathway of the complement system than any of the other immunoglobulins.

3. IgA (2 types): IgA is found in secretions such as saliva, tears, and the mucus of the respiratory, gastrointestinal, and genitourinary tracts. IgA is secreted by plasma cells located in the epithelium of the associated tissues. These secretions form part of the primary defense mechanism of the body by preventing the attachment of the pathogens to epithelial cells. IgA can activate the alternative pathway of the complement system. In addition, IgA is found in breast milk and can help protect the newborn infant.

4. IgE: IgE is secreted by plasma cells in the skin and mucous membranes. IgE triggers the release of histamine from mast cells and basophils and is important in the inflammatory response. It is also the antibody that is responsible for the symptoms of immediate hypersensitivity (anaphylactic) allergic reactions. IgE helps to protect the body from some parasitic infections, such as intestinal worms. An antigenic substance on the surface of the worms stimulates the release of histamine from mast cells in the intestinal mucosa. Histamine increases the permeability of the intestinal lining causing a large amount of water to flow into the intestine causing diarrhea, which is meant to result in expulsion of the worms.

5. IgD: IgD is found on B lymphocyte cell surfaces and is usually associated with IgM. It appears to have some regulatory effect on the functioning of the B cell.

The humoral response uses antibodies to accomplish its goals; however, antibodies cannot interact with host

Box 4.1 ANTIBODY ACTIONS AGAINST ANTIGENS

1. Neutralize bacterial toxins
2. Bind with viruses to prevent entrance into cells
3. Cause the agglutination or clumping of antigens to facilitate phagocytosis
4. Bind to the surfaces of the antigen to aid in phagocytosis (opsonization)
5. Bind with an antigen to activate the complement system

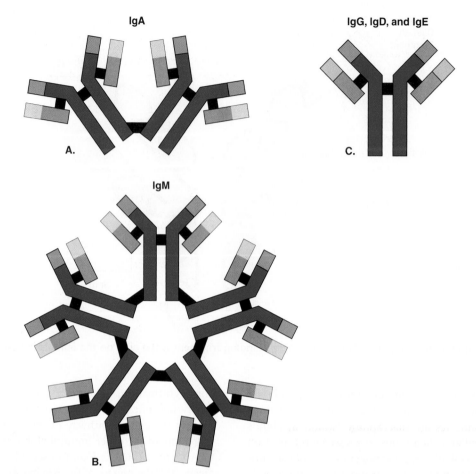

Figure 4.3. Molecular structure of immunoglobulins. The five major groups of immunoglobulin are represented by three different molecular structures. **A.** The molecular structure of IgA. **B.** The molecular structure of IgM. **C.** IgG, IgD, and IgE share the same type of structure.

cells that have become infected with a virus or have become abnormal in any other way. This function is carried out by the other, equally important, component of the immune response, that is, the cellular or cell-mediated response.

Cell-Mediated Immunity

Cell-mediated immunity is specific for host cells (**target cells**) that have become infected with viruses or have mutated and are possible sources of harm for the individual. The end result of the cellular immune response is the destruction of the target cell. Cells involved in this response are always lymphocytes and include the following: T lymphocytes, natural killer cells, and macrophages.

T Lymphocytes. T lymphocytes develop in the bone marrow from the same precursor or stem cells from which B lymphocytes develop. However, instead of maturing in lymphoid tissue, T lymphocytes mature (become self-tolerant) and differentiate (become antigen specific) in the thymus and are stored in lymphatic tissue throughout the body. T cells must be activated to function. Activation usually occurs when an **antigen-presenting cell** (APC) phagocytizes or otherwise binds to an antigen and brings it to the T cell. The most common antigen-presenting cells

are macrophages, monocytes, and B cells. After the APC presents its antigen to the T cell, the T cell is activated against that antigen. Cytokines called interleukins assist in the activation of the T cells. The activation stimulates the T cell to divide and produce several types of T lymphocyte that are specific for the activating antigen. Some T cells can live for long periods of time and maintain their antigenic specificity, becoming T memory cells. The T cell functions are determined by protein molecules carried on their surfaces, which are called clusters of differentiation (CD). There are other types of cluster designations but the following are the most significant:

1. $CD4^+$ or T helper cell: These cells regulate the action of all the other cells of the immune system. They increase or enable the functioning of B lymphocytes, macrophages, natural killer cells, and other T cells by the release of cytokines (see Table 4.1). Humans normally have twice as many $CD4^+$ cells circulating in the blood as $CD8^+$ cells.

2. $CD8^+$ or **T cytotoxic cell:** These cells are able to kill cells that have been recognized as being antigenic, such as cells infected with viruses, cancer cells, and sometimes normal cells that the body has confused as

nonself. The cytotoxic cell must be activated by a T helper cell or macrophage before it can bind to and destroy the antigen. The cytotoxic cells are active in tissue and organ rejection.

Natural Killer Cells. **Natural killer (NK) cells** are similar to the cytotoxic T lymphocytes. The difference is that they do not need to be sensitized to an antigen before reacting with that antigen. In other words, they have the ability to recognize foreign substances without any input from other cells or chemical mediators. These cells recognize virus-infected cells and other abnormal cells and destroy them. NK cells can respond immediately to the presence of one of these cells and thus play a very important role in the immune system. Often NK cell functions are impaired in immune deficiency disorders such as acquired immune deficiency syndrome (AIDS). There is evidence that natural killer and cytotoxic T cells play a part in detecting and eliminating cancer cells before they can multiply. Currently, much more research is being conducted in this area.

Macrophages. As stated in Chapter 3, macrophages provide a crucial cellular link between the inflammatory process and the immune system response. Macrophages are monocytes that have left the circulating blood to enter connective or other tissues where they develop into macrophages. Histiocytes are macrophages found in connective tissue, Kupffer cells are macrophages found in the liver, and Langerhans cells are macrophages found in the epidermis. These are all large, mononuclear, phagocytic cells that are considered part of cell-mediated immunity. They do not have to be sensitized by an antigen to recognize it and destroy it. Like PMNs, macrophages have receptors on their surfaces that recognize opsonized matter. Unlike PMNs, macrophages can be activated to become even more destructive by chemical mediators released by CD4$^+$ T cells, for example, gamma interferon. Activated macrophages are able to secrete many more chemical mediators and have enhanced capabilities related to chemotaxis, phagocytosis, and antigen presentation. In addition, activated macrophages exhibit increased metabolism, size, and ability to adhere to, and spread on, surfaces. When this high level of destruction is no longer necessary, other chemical mediators are released that deactivate the macrophages. After the macrophage destroys the antigen it will present specific proteins from it to a T lymphocyte, thereby activating the lymphocyte and starting the immune response. Macrophages can survive for years, and because they retain no memory of an antigen after it has been destroyed, they must be reactivated when they encounter the same antigen again. The nonspecific nature of the macrophage assists in helping the immune system respond immediately to injurious agents. The cell-mediated immune response results in destruction of the target cells and/or activation of the humoral immune response. Figure 4.4 illustrates the interrelationship between humoral and cell-mediated immunity and the importance of macrophages to both.

TYPES OF SPECIFIC IMMUNITY

The integrated efforts of the two components of the immune system enable the body to mount an immediate response to an antigen the next time it is encountered so that the host is able to avoid any pathology that the antigen would have caused. There are two forms of specific immunity, active and passive.

Active Immunity
Active immunity occurs when antibodies are produced by the body in response to an antigen. This can happen naturally, by an individual having an infectious disease, such as varicella-zoster (chicken pox), or it can occur through artificial means by vaccination. Vaccines are produced with either killed or attenuated (weakened) bacteria or virus or chemically altered toxins. Active immunity produces long-term immunity because the memory cells that are produced in response to the antigen will reproduce for the life of the host. Booster shots are often given just to make sure that the memory stays strong and to strengthen the antibody response. Types of vaccinations include polio, tetanus, hepatitis A and B, measles, mumps, rubella, and so on.

Passive Immunity
Passive immunity occurs when the host does not form his or her own antibodies but is given antibodies derived from another source, either human or animal. This type of immunity is short-lived because there is no memory produced in the individual's own immune system. There are no B cells activated by antigens to produce plasma or memory cells; in other words, the individual is still subject to infection. Passive immunity occurs naturally prior to birth when maternal antibodies are transferred across the placenta to the infant. It also occurs when an individual is given an injection of specific antibodies from a second source, very often a horse. The immunoglobulin used most often for this purpose is gamma globulin (IgG). For example, gamma globulin is given to unvaccinated dental healthcare workers who have a needlestick injury or percutaneous (through unbroken skin) exposure to the hepatitis B virus, as a form of postexposure prophylaxis to try to boost the immune response against any viral particles that may have entered the body.

IMMUNOPATHOLOGY

The previous scenarios depict how the immune system is supposed to function. Many times the immune system does not function the way it should. The problems resulting from dysfunction of the immune system can be grouped into three major categories: hypersensitivity reactions, autoimmune diseases, and immune deficiency diseases.

Hypersensitivity Reactions

Hypersensitivity reactions set the immune system against the host and in many cases become destructive to the in-

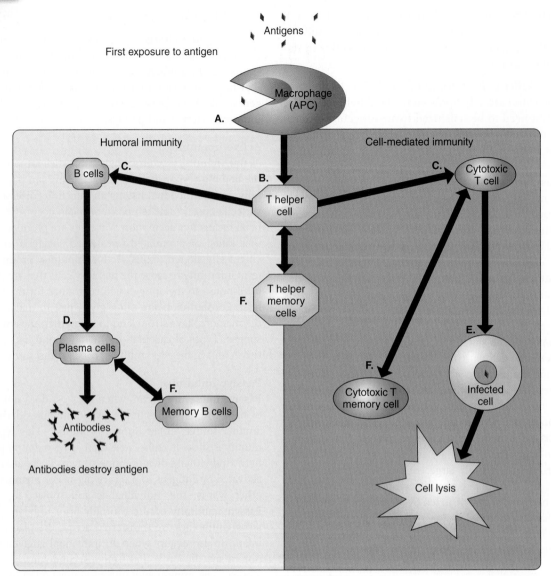

Figure 4.4. Humoral and cell-mediated immune responses and how they relate to each other. **A.** Initial exposure. The antigen is phagocytized by an antigen-presenting cell, in this case, a macrophage. **B.** Antigen presentation. The macrophage or other APC presents the antigen to a T helper cell. **C.** T helper cell activates other lymphocytes. The T helper cell activates B cells and cytotoxic T cells. **D.** Plasma cell formation. Activated B cells produce plasma cells that begin to produce antibodies against the antigen. **E.** Cytotoxic T cell activation. Activated cytotoxic T cells attack cells that are infected with the antigen, causing cell lysis. **F.** Immunity-established. T helper cells create T helper memory cells, plasma cells produce memory B cells, and cytotoxic T cells produce cytotoxic T memory cells. A second encounter with the antigen (not pictured) stimulates the T helper memory cells to activate cytotoxic T memory cells that will cause infected cells to lyse and B memory cells that will begin to produce antibodies specific for the antigen.

dividual. One way to think of these reactions is to imagine the food preferences of a diverse group of individuals. Suppose one person does not like peanut butter and another does not like artichokes. Both avoid contact with the offending food items as much as possible. This is a conscious decision that the individuals made, and if they did eat the items, nothing would result but a bad taste in their mouths. The cells of the body cannot make these types of conscious decisions. Their decisions are preprogrammed by either environmental or genetic factors. Hypersensitivity reactions occur when the body's cells come into

contact with something that they dislike. In many cases the offending agent or antigen is not harmful to the general population. The antigen may even be part of the individual's normal cellular makeup.

There are four types of hypersensitivity reactions that may occur in response to an antigen. The first three types are immediate responses and are mediated or controlled by antibodies; the last type is a delayed reaction and is mediated or controlled by a cellular response. Remember that most of these reactions are self-limiting. When the agent that causes them is gone, the reaction will stop.

APPLICATION

Scenario 1: Mary is 5 years old and goes to day care at a neighbor's house with six other children. She has never been vaccinated for any childhood illnesses. Mary's friend Heather becomes sick with the measles. Mary has come in contact with the rubeola virus. How does the immune system respond?

1. Recognition
   a. B cell surface antibodies come in contact with the virus and bind to it.
   b. The B cell acts as an antigen-presenting cell and binds with a T cell.
   c. The B cell and the T cell are now activated against the rubeola virus.
2. Reaction
   a. The activated B cell produces both plasma cells that secrete antibody specific for rubeola and memory cells that will carry the image of the antigen for future encounters.
   b. The activated T cell produces CD4$^+$ helper cells and CD8$^+$ cytotoxic cells. Using cytokines, the helper cells will enhance the functioning of the B cells and call the macrophages and natural killer cells into action. The cytotoxic cells will begin to destroy any of Mary's cells that have become infected by the virus. The reaction time is slow during this initial encounter with the virus, and 10 to 12 days after Mary came in contact with the virus she begins to show symptoms of fever, upper respiratory congestion, cough, and general malaise. Mary breaks out in a generalized **maculopapular** (erythematic, raised) rash about 2 days after the other symptoms appear. These symptoms are the result of a systemic inflammatory response that has been initiated as a result of both the immune response and activation of the complement system. Four to 7 days later, the symptoms begin to dissipate, and Mary feels much better. Her immune system will remember this encounter.
3. Remember
   a. Mary's immune system has produced both B memory cells and T memory cells that will react faster and to a much higher degree the next time they encounter the rubeola virus. During subsequent exposures, the secondary immune response will stop the virus before it can produce any manifestations of the disease.

Scenario 2: Once again, Mary is 5 years old and goes to day care at a neighbor's house with six other children. However, this time she has been vaccinated for all appropriate childhood illnesses. Mary's friend Heather becomes sick with the measles. Mary has come in contact with the rubeola virus. How does the immune system respond in this situation?

1. Recognition
   a. Mary received her vaccination for measles when she was supposed to.
   b. The vaccination stimulated Mary's immune system to produce B and T cells, including memory cells, which were activated against the rubeola virus.
   c. B and T memory cells come in contact with the rubeola virus at this time, and they know exactly what to do.
2. Reaction
   a. The activated B memory cells initiate the production of enormous amounts of both plasma cells that secrete antibody specific for rubeola and memory cells that will carry the image of the antigen for future encounters.
   b. The activated T memory cells produce CD4$^+$ helper cells and CD8$^+$ cytotoxic cells. Using cytokines, the helper cells will enhance the functioning of the B cells and call the macrophages and natural killer cells into action. The cytotoxic cells will begin to destroy cells that have become infected by the virus, if any. Mary never shows any signs that she has come into contact with this disease. Even though this is the first time she has encountered the viable virus, her immune system was ready for it and treated it as a second encounter. Her vaccine-primed immune system has done its job.
3. Remember
   a. Mary's immune system still has the memory cells, now primed and ready for a third encounter.

TYPE I (ANAPHYLACTIC OR ATOPIC REACTIONS)

Type I hypersensitivity reactions occur immediately (within minutes) after exposure to a previously encountered antigen such as penicillin, cat hair, or pollen. These antigens are usually not harmful to the general population, only to specific individuals. This reaction has two major forms: systemic or **anaphylactic reactions** and **atopic reactions** that include skin reactions, asthma, and upper respiratory manifestations. The systemic form causes the most dramatic reactions. These include reactions to bee stings, peanuts, and latex, which are life altering for those affected by them. Individuals who are allergic to these substances must be on constant alert so that they do not come into contact with them.

In the systemic form, plasma cells produce IgE in response to a particular antigen. IgE attaches to the surface of mast cells throughout the body. When the mast cells encounter the specific antigen again, they release granules that contain histamine, which results in dilation and in-

Box 4.2 — SEQUENCE OF EVENTS IN A SYSTEMIC TYPE I ANAPHYLACTIC HYPERSENSITIVITY REACTION

1. Contact with allergen
2. Release of histamine from sensitized mast cells
3. Blood vessels dilate and exudate forms
4. Blood pressure falls
5. Venous return to the heart decreases
6. Cardiac output decreases
7. Circulation decreases
8. Circulatory system collapse

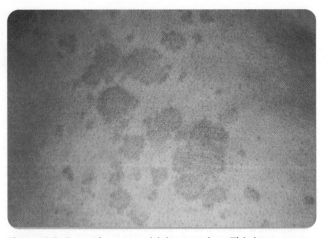

Figure 4.5. Type I hypersensitivity reaction. This is an example of urticaria or hives seen with a type I hypersensitivity reaction. (From Goodheart HP. Goodheart's photoguide of common skin disorders. 2nd ed. Philadelphia: Lippincott Williams & Wilkins, 2003.)

creased permeability of the blood vessels. As a result, blood pressure falls, and the entire circulatory system may shut down. Breathing is also impaired because histamine causes constriction of the smooth muscles in the bronchioles and tissue edema. This is a life-threatening emergency and must be recognized and treated quickly or the individual may die. Many individuals with known allergies wear medical identification tags to alert medical personnel about their allergy should they ever become unable to do so and need medical care. This is especially important if an individual is allergic to drugs or materials such as latex that would be used in a medical emergency.

The most effective treatment for an anaphylactic reaction is injected epinephrine. Epinephrine causes constriction of the dilated blood vessels, which increases blood pressure and causes relaxation of the smooth muscles in the lungs, opening the airways. Individuals who may have severe anaphylactic reactions have access to this medication in the form of an Epi-pen. The Epi-pen carries a single dose of epinephrine that is easily injected by even young children. Other drugs that are used include oral antihistamines and corticosteroids. Box 4.2 describes the sequence of events that may occur in a type I anaphylactic hypersensitivity reaction.

The atopic form of type I reaction is exemplified by hay fever and mold and animal allergies. The symptoms associated with atopic type I reactions depend upon where the antigen comes into contact with the body. If the antigen comes in contact with the skin, hives or urticaria will manifest (Fig. 4.5). Hay fever (sneezing, sinus edema, and watery eyes) will become evident if contact is made in the upper respiratory system. Asthma may be the result if contact is made in the lungs, and diarrhea and vomiting may result if contact is made in the gastrointestinal tract. The localized reactions are usually treated with drugs that control or inhibit the release of histamine (antihistamines) or act on other elements of the immune response, such as the release of leukotrienes or cytokines.

TYPE II (CYTOTOXIC REACTIONS)

Cytotoxic reactions occur when an antibody, usually IgG or IgM, combines with an antigen that is bound to the surface of cells of a specific type. This action can produce several results:

1. It can cause direct lysis or destruction of the affected cells.
2. It can prepare the affected cells for phagocytosis by immune system cells.
3. It can cause the affected cells to malfunction in some way.

The classic example of direct lysis is a transfusion reaction that occurs when an individual is given an incompatible blood type. Another example of this type of reaction occurs in erythroblastosis fetalis. In this disorder the mother is Rh⁻ and the fetus is Rh⁺. Erythroblastosis fetalis occurs during a second pregnancy with an Rh⁺ fetus, since it takes an initial sensitizing exposure or first pregnancy with an Rh⁺ fetus to enable the hypersensitivity reaction. Maternal antibodies against the positive factor cross the placental barrier and destroy the red blood cells of the fetus, necessitating an immediate blood transfusion when the infant is born. This can be avoided if the at-risk mother is identified before the birth of the first child and is given injections of gamma globulin containing Rh antibody. The Rh antibody will prevent the sensitization of the mother and thus prevent problems with a future pregnancy.

Hyperthyroidism, as seen in Graves' disease (see Chapter 7) is an example of a cytotoxic reaction in which the cells remain viable but malfunction and cause excess production of the thyroid hormones. Other forms of cytotoxic reactions occur when something happens that changes the major histocompatibility complexes attached to some of the body's cells. The result is that the immune system thinks that the affected cells are foreign and at-

tacks them. This can also happen in the reverse. A problem in the immune system may cause it to get confused and attack cells that have had no alterations of their MHCs. The event that alters the cells or the immune system is very often unknown or it may be related to a drug or environmental agent. If the problem is related to a drug or known environmental agent, removal of the offending agent should stop the hypersensitivity reaction and the resulting tissue damage. If the cause is unknown, the problem is considered an autoimmune dysfunction. Autoimmunity is discussed below in this chapter. Examples of autoimmune disorders that are considered to be type II hypersensitivity reactions are pemphigus vulgaris (see Chapter 11), cicatricial pemphigoid (see Chapter 11), and acute rheumatic fever (see Chapter 8).

TYPE III (IMMUNE COMPLEX-MEDIATED REACTIONS)

In **immune complex-mediated reactions** IgM, IgA, or IgG form antigen–antibody complexes with circulating antigens. The antigens can be exogenous, such as bacteria, viruses, drugs, or chemicals, or they can be endogenous, created by the body as part of an immune dysfunction. The damage to tissues is done when these antigen–antibody complexes are deposited in a particular part of the body and cause the initiation of the inflammatory response. Chemotactic agents that are released in the inflammatory response cause PMNs to travel to the site or sites and release their destructive enzymes. These enzymes cause either local or systemic tissue destruction. Autoimmune examples of this type of reaction include: systemic lupus erythematosus (see Chapter 12), rheumatoid arthritis (see Chapter 10), and forms of glomerulonephritis (kidney disease).

TYPE IV (CELL-MEDIATED OR DELAYED HYPERSENSITIVITY REACTIONS)

Cell-mediated reactions do not require the action of antibodies; instead they involve specific T cells that have been sensitized to a particular antigen. Type IV reactions are usually delayed and can take 24 to 72 hours or more for the full response to be observed. **Contact dermatitis** is an example of one of the most common forms of type IV hypersensitivity (Fig. 4.6). Haptens, which are very small antigenic molecules, combine with skin proteins and result in a hypersensitivity reaction that will not stop until the antigen is eliminated or the skin is destroyed. Oil from poison ivy and sumac leaves and certain chemicals in rubber are examples of haptens. The type IV hypersensitivity reaction is the result of T lymphocytes reacting with an antigen. The reaction either causes death of the involved cells or initiation of an inflammatory response. The most typical presentation involves the development of an erythematic vesicular rash that is extremely pruritic or itchy. The rash will continue to develop as all areas touched by

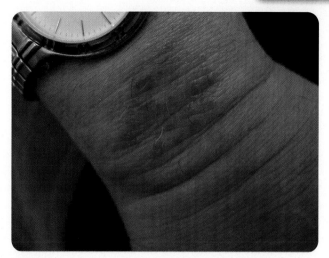

Figure 4.6. Allergic contact dermatitis. This patient was hypersensitive to nickel and formed a pruritic rash under a watch that contained nickel. (Stedman's concise medical dictionary for the health professions. 5th ed. Baltimore: Lippincott Williams & Wilkins, 2005.)

the allergen are involved. Resolution can take several days or several weeks, depending on the antigen and the duration of the exposure. Prior exposure to the antigen is necessary as a sensitizing event, and the reaction is confined to the area that was contacted. The same type of reaction occurs in the mouth. It is called allergic stomatitis and has a variety of possible presentations including diffuse erythema, ulcers, and vesicles. Contact stomatitis is discussed further in Chapter 12. Examples of substances that can cause a contact allergic reaction are poison ivy, metals, cosmetics, and various chemicals, including those used in toothpaste and mouth rinse. Topical corticosteroids and antiitch creams can help alleviate the symptoms associated with cutaneous rashes. Occasionally systemic corticosteroids are used to treat severe reactions. Tissue and organ graft rejection as seen in **graft-versus-host or host-versus-graft reaction** is also a type IV hypersensitivity reaction. This reaction results from an immune response to major histocompatibility complexes that are present on the surface of cells in the donor or recipient tissue. No matter how closely the MHCs are matched, they will not be identical, except in identical twins, and patients must take immunosuppressant drugs for the rest of their lives to control this reaction. Current research supports evidence that Sjögren syndrome is a type IV hypersensitivity reaction that results in salivary and other exocrine gland damage caused directly by T and B lymphocytes (see Chapter 17).

Name: Latex hypersensitivity

Etiology: Contact with natural rubber latex (NRL) proteins causes latex hypersensitivity.

Method of transmission: Latex hypersensitivity is more common among individuals who have allergies to other substances. There is also an increased risk of developing a latex hypersensitivity with continued exposure to the protein.

Epidemiology: Latex hypersensitivity is estimated to occur in 1–5% of the general population. Data suggest that up to 17% of healthcare workers are latex sensitive (Behrman, March 2005). Other populations that are at higher risk for developing latex hypersensitivity include patients with spina bifida, urogenital abnormalities, and those who have had multiple surgeries. Individuals who are allergic to certain foods may also be allergic to latex because the molecular structure of the foods that they are allergic to are very similar to the latex proteins. Box 4.3 lists foods that appear to have molecular structures similar to that of latex. There is equal distribution of this type of hypersensitivity among males and females.

Pathogenesis: Contact with the NRL proteins can occur through the skin or mucous membranes or the proteins can be inhaled or injected. Exposure to the NRL proteins triggers an immediate type I anaphylactic reaction. When mast cells that have been previously sensitized by IgE produced in response to an initial exposure to NRL come into contact with NRL proteins a second time, they release granules that contain histamine. Histamine causes the myriad of symptoms associated with the anaphylactic reaction.

Extraoral characteristics: Symptoms generally appear within minutes of the exposure and include a generalized burning feeling in the skin or mucous membranes, pruritic rash or urticaria, runny nose, watery eyes, and sneezing. Symptoms seen in the most severely hypersensitive individuals may continue to worsen, causing asthma-like breathing difficulties, gastrointestinal cramping and diarrhea, hypotension, and eventual cardiovascular collapse and death.

Perioral and intraoral characteristics: Mucous membranes can become swollen, and the patient may experience burning sensations and/or pruritus. Laryngeal spasms can make speaking and swallowing difficult.

Box 4.3   **FOOD ALLERGIES ASSOCIATED WITH AN INCREASED RISK OF LATEX HYPERSENSITIVITY**

- Banana
- Kiwi
- Avocado
- Chestnuts
- Potatoes

Box 4.4   **DENTAL OFFICE ITEMS/EQUIPMENT THAT MAY CONTAIN LATEX**

- Blood pressure cuffs
- Stethoscopes
- Examination gloves
- Syringes
- Face masks
- Oxygen/nitrous oxide delivery systems
- Handpiece and air/water syringe hoses
- Suction hoses
- Irrigation tubing
- Rubber dams
- Bite blocks
- Prophy cups
- Prophy angles
- Orthodontic elastics
- Protective eyewear
- Interdental stimulators

Distinguishing characteristics: The abrupt immediate manifestation of the symptoms associated with anaphylaxis are somewhat distinguishing.

Significant microscopic features: Not applicable

Dental implications: Latex hypersensitivity has numerous dental implications for not only the patient but also the dental healthcare worker. Many items in the dental office may contain latex and could be the source of an exposure for a hypersensitive person. Box 4.4 lists some common items found in a dental office that may contain latex. Examination gloves worn during dental treatment can be a source of exposure for both the patient and the dental healthcare worker. In fact, continued daily exposure to latex examination gloves increases the risk that an individual will become sensitive to the NRL protein. In addition, powdered latex gloves can contaminate the air with powder that contains molecules of NRL proteins. This powder can come to rest on any surface and be picked up by the skin when someone touches the surface, and it can be inhaled into the lungs. Glove manufacturers have developed low-protein latex gloves that may help to prevent sensitization to the NRL protein but will not eliminate or even minimize a hypersensitivity reaction. Many dental offices have established a latex-free glove policy and have attempted to replace patient care items that contain latex with latex-free items. Box 4.5 lists recommendations for treating the latex-sensitive patient in the dental environment. Even if all precautions are taken, a latex sensitive individual could possibly have a significant latex exposure during dental care. It is essential that the dental professional investigate any possibility of a latex allergy indicated by the patient's health history.

Box 4.5
RECOMMENDATIONS FOR TREATING LATEX-SENSITIVE PATIENTS IN THE DENTAL OFFICE

- Schedule patient for the first appointment of the day
- Have no latex products in the treatment room
- Make sure that instruments have not been handled with latex gloves
- Watch for powder from latex gloves on clothes and equipment
- Have a supply of latex-free supplies stored in a sealed container
- Have the medications and equipment necessary to treat a latex hypersensitivity reaction

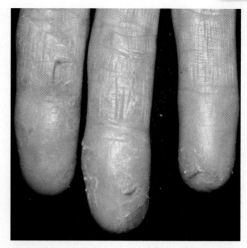

Figure 4.7. Allergic contact dermatitis. ACD associated with chemicals used in manufacturing latex gloves. (From Goodheart HP. Goodheart's photoguide of common skin disorders. 2nd ed. Philadelphia: Lippincott Williams & Wilkins, 2003.)

Differential diagnosis: A type I hypersensitivity reaction can be caused by almost any substance that comes in contact with a susceptible individual. Other conditions that might have similar symptoms include:

1. Asthma (see Chapter 10). The sudden abrupt onset and breathing difficulties experienced during an asthma attack are similar to those seen in anaphylaxis.
2. Acute adrenal insufficiency (see Chapter 7). Symptoms of vomiting, abdominal pain, hypotension, and cardiovascular collapse are similar to those seen in anaphylaxis. This condition can quickly lead to coma and death. Respiratory distress is not a significant feature of this condition, neither is urticaria or runny nose and watering eyes.
3. Hypoglycemia (see Chapter 7). Hypoglycemia or insulin reaction could mimic some of the symptoms of an anaphylactic reaction, specifically, confusion and unconsciousness.

Treatment and prognosis: Prevention is the best policy in cases of latex hypersensitivity, and the best way to prevent the reactions is to avoid all contact with latex. Treatment depends on the severity of the symptoms and usually consists of an injection of epinephrine followed by oral antihistamines. However, care must be taken because occasionally the patient will have a biphasic reaction. A biphasic reaction occurs several hours after the initial hypersensitivity reaction and must be treated with additional injections of epinephrine. This patient should be released into the care of emergency medical services (EMS). Most patients will recover from anaphylactic reactions with no ill effects; however, if treatment is not rendered immediately, these reactions can be fatal.

Allergic Contact Dermatitis (ACD)
ACD is more common than type I latex hypersensitivity. ACD is caused by contact with the residue of chemicals used in manufacturing latex gloves. This is a type IV hy-

persensitivity reaction and is thought to affect about 5 to 20% of dental healthcare workers (DePaola, 2004). This delayed reaction occurs 24–48 hours after exposure of a sensitized individual to these substances. Macrophages (APC) in the epidermis known as Langerhans cells ingest the chemical molecules and present them to the T lymphocytes. The T lymphocytes activate more macrophages and cytotoxic T cells that start destroying cells that have had contact with the allergen. The clinical manifestations of this are erythema and the appearance of a pruritic, vesicular rash. The skin becomes dry and cracked with repeated exposure (Fig. 4.7). ACD can be prevented by avoiding the use of latex gloves and by avoiding contact with other latex containing items. Dental patients who indicate that they have a latex allergy may have this type of reaction instead of the type I hypersensitivity reaction. Questions about the clinical signs and symptoms associated with their allergy should be all that is required to determine the type of reaction they have. If there is any doubt, the patient should be referred to a physician for definitive diagnosis.

Irritant Contact Dermatitis (ICD)
ICD is not a hypersensitivity reaction. ICD is a skin inflammation caused by exposure to caustic chemicals or mechanical irritation of the skin (Fig. 4.8). Many chemicals found in a dental office should only be used when hands are protected by gloves, for example, surface disinfectants such as glutaraldehyde and bleach. Mechanical irritation can be caused by gloves rubbing against the skin or by the powder that is in some of the gloves to make them easier to put on. The symptoms of ICD are similar to those of ACD except for vesicle formation, making it difficult to differentiate between the two. Changing from latex to latex-free gloves may help to determine what type of dermatitis is present.

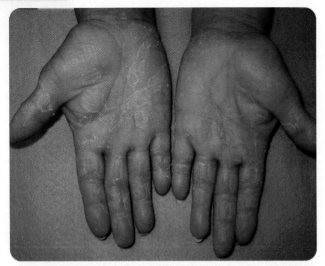

Figure 4.8. Irritant contact dermatitis. This is an example of ICD in a healthcare worker who did not use appropriate protection while using chemical disinfectants. (From Stedman's concise medical dictionary for the health professions. 5th ed. Baltimore: Lippincott Williams & Wilkins, 2005.)

Autoimmune Diseases

As discussed above, the immune system usually functions under the premise of self-tolerance. When the immune system loses the ability to distinguish self from nonself or there is an alteration of the host's cells that changes their makeup, (such as a change in an MHC), the immune system will attack the cells of the host just as if they were foreign matter, and an **autoimmune disease** becomes manifest. The tissue damage that is done in these diseases is the direct result of the actions of the host's own immune and inflammatory responses. The damage may be throughout the body, as in systemic lupus erythematosus (see Chapter 12), or it may occur in a single organ, as in hyperthyroidism (see Chapter 7). Autoimmune diseases are usually chronic conditions that manifest with many exacerbations and remissions often over many years. Most autoimmune diseases present or manifest as type II, III, or IV hypersensitivity reactions. Many of the autoimmune disorders have a genetic predisposition for their occurrence. Table 4.2 lists common autoimmune disorders and the chapters in which they are discussed, based on the clinical appearance of their characteristic oral lesions. The dental hygienist may be the first healthcare professional to observe signs of some of the autoimmune diseases such as pemphigus vulgaris, cicatricial pemphigoid, and oral lichen planus, all of which may present with oral lesions prior to any cutaneous lesions (Fig. 4.9).

Immune Deficiency Diseases

Hypersensitivity reactions and autoimmune disorders are examples of conditions that have their basis in an immune system that is overstepping its boundaries. Immune deficiency disorders occur when the immune system or part of it fails to function. Immunodeficiency diseases fall into two basic categories, primary (congenital) and secondary (acquired).

PRIMARY IMMUNODEFICIENCY DISEASE

Primary immunodeficiency diseases are always caused by a genetic or congenital abnormality. "Congenital" is de-

Table 4.2	CHAPTER LOCATIONS FOR IMMUNE SYSTEM DISORDERS WITH ORAL MANIFESTATIONS	
Immune System Disorder	**Clinical Appearance of the Characteristic Oral Lesions**	**Chapter Location**
Cicatricial pemphigoid	Vesicles	Chapter 11, "Lesions That Look like Vesicles"
Pemphigus vulgaris	Vesicles	Chapter 11, "Lesions That Look like Vesicles"
Bullous pemphigoid	Bulla	Chapter 11, "Lesions That Look like Vesicles"
Aphthous ulcers	Mucosal ulcers	Chapter 12, "Ulcer and Ulcer-like Lesions"
Systemic lupus erythematosus and discoid lupus erythematosus	Mucosal ulcers	Chapter 12, "Ulcer and Ulcer-like Lesions"
Behçet syndrome	Mucosal ulcers	Chapter 12, "Ulcer and Ulcer-like Lesions"
Reiter syndrome	Mucosal ulcers	Chapter 12, "Ulcer and Ulcer-like Lesions"
Erythema multiforme	Mucosal ulcers	Chapter 12, "Ulcer and Ulcer-like Lesions"
Lichen planus	White lesions	Chapter 14, "White Lesions"
Sjögren syndrome	Enlarged salivary glands	Chapter 17, "Soft Tissue Enlargements"
Salivary lymphoepithelial lesion	Enlarged salivary glands	Chapter 17, "Soft Tissue Enlargements"
HIV infection and AIDS	Various	Chapter 22, "HIV and AIDS"

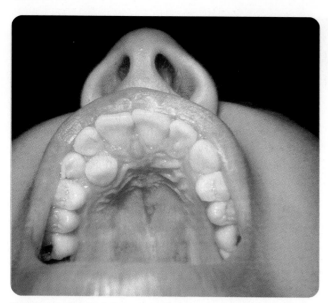

Figure 4.9. Systemic lupus erythematosus. The dental professional may be the first to observe the manifestations of some autoimmune disorders because they may present in the oral cavity prior to any cutaneous manifestations. Ulceration is present on the hard palate in this individual with systemic lupus erythematosus. (From Goodheart HP. Goodheart's photoguide of common skin disorders. 2nd ed. Philadelphia: Lippincott Williams & Wilkins, 2003.)

fined as existing at the time of birth. Congenital abnormalities are not necessarily caused by an inherited trait but may result from a spontaneous genetic mutation or a random developmental defect. The abnormality results in defective functioning of at least one part of the individual's immune system or inflammatory process. The problem may be that the T cells do not function correctly or perhaps the complement system is dysfunctional because a specific protein is not created correctly. In either case, the result is an impaired ability of the host to fight off infection and maintain the health status of the body. There are numerous examples of primary deficiencies; this chapter examines Bruton's disease because it is one of the most common deficiency diseases and DiGeorge syndrome because of the possible perioral abnormalities that may result from this deficiency.

In Bruton's disease, the individual's B cells do not mature correctly and do not produce functioning antibodies. Recurrent bacterial and, to a lesser extent, some viral infections begin to cause problems at about 6 months of age, which corresponds to the time when maternal antibodies are depleted. The child's T cells function normally so that antigens such as most viruses and fungal infections that are normally destroyed through T cell function are still destroyed. Bruton's disease is treated with injections of immunoglobulins, and most of its victims survive into adulthood.

DiGeorge syndrome is a genetic disorder that can be inherited or can result from a spontaneous genetic mutation that occurs in the developing fetus. The problems associated with DiGeorge syndrome are caused by failure of the third and fourth pharyngeal pouches to develop. The thymus, parathyroid glands, and some of the thyroid gland are partially or totally missing, and the face, ears, and mouth may be formed incorrectly. The individual may also be mentally challenged. This disorder affects the T cells and B cells. The T cell level is diminished or altogether absent, making the individual more susceptible to viral and fungal infections. B cell activity, including the production of antibodies, is also diminished because B cells must be activated with the help of CD4$^+$ T helper cells. It is important for the dental hygienist to remember in all instances of immune deficiency, that normal standard precautions for preventing the transmission of disease may not be effective and that any contact with a pathogenic organism may cause a fatal infection.

SECONDARY IMMUNODEFICIENCY DISEASE

Acquired or **secondary immunodeficiency** diseases develop after birth and are not related to genetics. Any of the following conditions can be associated with an acquired immune deficiency: renal disease, cancer, malnutrition, diabetes, immunosuppressive drugs (corticosteroids) or treatments (radiation), advanced age, tuberculosis, HIV infection, and more. One of the most common causes of immune suppression is the use of corticosteroid drug therapy to control the myriad of inflammatory diseases that are found today. Corticosteroids depress the inflammatory response, thereby reducing the damage and symptoms associated with diseases such as rheumatoid arthritis and systemic lupus erythematosus.

Immune deficiency conditions allow **opportunistic infections** to overwhelm the host. Opportunistic infections are caused by organisms that usually pose no threat to the individual with a normal immune system. For example, individuals undergoing chemotherapy for cancer are at a high risk for overgrowth of oral *Candida albicans* (fungus) because their immune systems are not able to control this normally innocuous microorganism that lives with us in a commensal (causing neither harm nor benefit) relationship. The compromised individual is also at risk of having infections such as periodontal disease become more aggressive and severe than they would be in an individual with a normal immune system. The most prominent immune deficiency disease at this time is acquired immune deficiency syndrome, or AIDS. Because of the number of oral and perioral manifestations of AIDS and the fact that most of these are abnormal presentations of diseases discussed in later chapters, AIDS and HIV infection are presented in detail in Chapter 22.

SUMMARY

- Nonspecific immunity provides generic defenses to protect the body, including the first-line defense systems of the body such as the inflammatory response and the integumentary system.
- Specific immunity is designed to provide protection from specific threats to our health. The organs associated with specific immunity include the bone marrow, thymus, and spleen, and lymph nodes, vessels, and tissues scattered throughout the body.
- The immune response is directed against foreign substances or antigens that can be microbes, chemicals, donated organs or tissues, and sometimes the individual's own tissue cells.
- Lymphocytes and macrophages are the main cellular components of the immune system. The lymphocytes are further defined as B or T lymphocytes. B lymphocytes are active in humoral immunity, and T lymphocytes are more active in cell-mediated immunity.
- Cell-mediated immunity is specific for cells that have been infected or that the immune system sees as harmful. Cells active in cell-mediated immunity are the T lymphocytes, natural killer cells, and the macrophages.
- Macrophages or another APC phagocytize an antigen, process it, and present it to a CD4$^+$ T helper cell. With the aid of such cytokines as the interleukins, the T helper cell becomes activated against the antigen that was presented to it. The activated T cell can now enhance the actions of other immune cells against the antigen. It can activate B cells to produce plasma cells and CD8$^+$ cytotoxic T cells to actively search out and destroy the antigen.
- Humoral immunity involves the production of antigen-specific antibodies by B lymphocytes. The B lymphocyte encounters an antigen that can bind to its Fab. A cooperating CD4$^+$ T helper cell also binds with the B cell, and using cytokines in the form of interleukins, activates the B cell for the specific antigen that is bound to it. The end result is the creation of a plasma cell that produces antibody specific for that antigen. The plasma cell divides rapidly and produces more antigen-specific plasma cells that produce more and more antibodies. At the conclusion of this primary immune response, some B cells become memory cells so that the antigen can be remembered and reacted to more quickly during a secondary immune response the next time the body recognizes it.
- Active immunity is produced when the individual makes his or her own antibodies in response to an antigen. Active natural immunity occurs when an individual is exposed to the actual infection; artificial immunity occurs when an individual is vaccinated with a live or attenuated antigen.
- Passive immunity occurs naturally as antibodies are transferred across the placenta and through breast milk to the infant and artificially when a patient receives an injection of IgG after an exposure to hepatitis B virus.
- Hypersensitivity reactions are an abnormal immune response to an antigen that in most individuals is not harmful to the body. There are four types of hypersensitivity reaction: type I anaphylactic or atopic; type II cytotoxic, type III immune complex-mediated, and type IV delayed hypersensitivity reactions.
- Autoimmune diseases result when immune or self-tolerance fails. The immune system can cause direct lysis of the involved cells, initiate an inflammatory response to destroy the cells, or alter the functioning of the cells.
- Most autoimmune diseases are chronic and progressive and have remissions and exacerbations of the signs and symptoms many times over a period of years.
- Immunodeficiency diseases are either primary or acquired. Primary immunodeficiencies are present at birth but may not be caused by inherited traits. These disorders can affect the entire immune system or one or more parts of it.
- Acquired immunodeficiencies occur later in life and can be associated with chronic illness, malnutrition, diabetes, immunosuppressant drug therapy, and other systemic problems.

PORTFOLIO POSSIBILITIES

1. Choose a dental disease associated with the immune system and research the topic on the web. Write a patient fact sheet on the disease that describes the disease in lay terms and presents possible oral manifestations of the disease. Discuss what patients might do to alleviate the oral signs of the disease and what products are available to assist them.
2. Choose a disease associated with the immune system. Using current research, write a chairside reference sheet for your own use that includes a description of typical oral and perioral lesions, systemic manifestations, and health history clues that would alert you to the possibility of this condition. Discuss the implications of the disease for the dental professional, including any treatment modifications or consultations that might be necessary. Make a list of drugs available to treat the disease and their possible side effects, including dental side effects.

Critical Thinking Activities

1. Why do some individuals come into contact with a disease and remain disease free, while others have the same contact with the disease and become ill with it?

2. Explain this statement. "People don't die from immunodeficiency diseases; they always die from some other condition."

Case Study

Mehrnaz, a 19-year-old female, presents to your office for her 6-month "check-up." You review her medical history and discover no significant findings. Mehrnaz's dental history includes the loss of tooth #10 about 1 year ago during a gymnastic accident on the uneven bars. The lateral was replaced temporarily by a removable acrylic partial denture or "flipper" (Fig. 4.10). An extraoral examination yields no significant findings. You observe the condition depicted

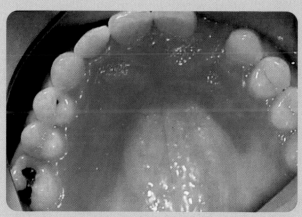

Figure 4.11. Case study. Erythema of the hard palate and gingiva.

in Figure 4.11 when you perform your intraoral examination.

1. How would you describe Mehrnaz's hard palate and lingual attached gingiva?
2. What could you ask Mehrnaz about this area?
3. What do you think is causing the condition?
4. If this is a hypersensitivity reaction, which type of reaction would it be?

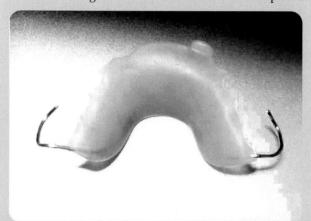

Figure 4.10. Case study. "Flipper" replacing tooth 10.

REFERENCES

Anderson DM, Keith J, Novak PD, Elliot MA. Mosby's medical, nursing & allied health dictionary. 6th ed. Philadelphia: Mosby, 2002.

Avery JK. Essentials of oral histology and embryology: a clinical approach. St. Louis: Mosby-Year Book, 1992:192.

Behrman AJ, Howarth M. Latex allergy. Last update March 2005. e medicine: Instant access to the minds of medicine. Available at: http://www.emedicine.com/emerg/topic814.htm. Accessed summer 2006.

Cotran RS, Kumar V, Collins T. Robbins: Pathologic basis of disease. 6th ed. Philadelphia: WB Saunders, 1999:188–259.

DePaola LG. Latex hypersensitivity and related issues in the dental office. Infect Control Forum 2004;2(3):1–6.

Stedman's concise medical dictionary for the health professions. 5th ed. Baltimore: Lippincott Williams & Wilkins, 2005.

Huether SE, McCance KL. Understanding pathophysiology. 3rd ed. St. Louis: Mosby, 2004:127–152, 181–220.

Joachim G, Acorn S. Life with a rare chronic disease: the scleroderma experience. J Adv Nurs 2003;42(6):598–606.

McKenna S, Mondal D. Immunity. Available at *http://www.liunet.edu/cwis/bklyn/acadres/facdev/FacultyProjects/WebClass/micro-web/html-files/ChapterH-1.htm*. Accessed Spring 2003.

Porth CM. Essentials of pathophysiology: concepts of altered health states. Philadelphia: Lippincott Williams & Wilkins, 2004:134–149, 168–190, 824–825.

Price SA, Wilson LM. Pathophysiology: clinical concepts of disease processes. 6th ed. St. Louis: Mosby, 2003:64–83, 129–189.

Purves WK, Sadava D, Orians GH, Heller HC. Life: The science of biology. 6th ed. Gordonsville, VA: WH Freeman; 2001:354–377.

Regezi JA, Sciubba JJ, Jordan RCK. Oral pathology: clinical pathologic correlations. 4th ed. St. Louis: WB Saunders, 2003:97–100.

Rubin E, Gorstein F, Rubin R, et al. Rubin's pathology: clinicopathologic foundations of medicine. 4th ed. Baltimore: Lippincott Williams & Wilkins, 2005:119–163.

Schindler LW. Understanding the immune system. National Institutes of Health Publication no. 93-529: Revised January 1993.

Trowbridge HO, Emling RC. Inflammation: a review of the process. 5th ed. Chicago: Quintessence; 1997.

Neoplasia

Key Terms

- Acromegaly
- Alopecia
- Anaplasia
- Anemia
- Anorexia
- Benign
- Benign nevus
- Bone marrow suppression
- Cancer grading
- Carcinogenic agent
- Carcinogenesis
- Carcinoma
- Carcinoma in situ
- Caretaker (mutator) gene
- Chemocaries
- Chemotherapy
- Chronic myelogenous leukemia
- Colonoscopy
- Colostomy
- Deoxyribonucleic acid (DNA)
- Differentiation
- Dysphagia
- Embolus (emboli)

- Encapsulated
- Epidermis
- Excisional biopsy
- Fine-needle aspiration
- Giantism
- Hepatocellular carcinoma
- Hormone/antihormone therapy
- Hyperadrenalism
- Hypercoagulation
- Hyperthyroidism
- Hypochromatic nuclei
- Immunotherapy
- Incisional biopsy
- Ionizing radiation
- Keratinocytes
- Labile cell
- Leukopenia
- Malignant
- Mammography
- Metastasis/metastatic/metastasize
- Mitotic figures
- Mucositis
- Needle biopsy

- Neoplastic growth/neoplasm/neoplasia
- Oncogene
- Paraneoplastic syndromes
- Peritoneal cavity
- Permanent cell
- Peutz-Jeghers syndrome
- Philadelphia chromosome
- Pleomorphism
- Pleural cavity
- Polyps
- Primary tumor
- Protooncogene
- Radiation caries
- Radiosensitive
- Sarcoma
- Seeding
- Stable (quiescent) cell
- Thrombocytopenia
- Thrombus (thrombi)
- Translocation
- Tumor markers
- Tumor staging
- Tumor suppressor gene

Objectives

1. Define and use the key terms discussed in this chapter.

2. Describe the difference between labile, stable, and permanent tissues.

3. Describe the basic principles of genetic control over cell growth.

4. Discuss how unregulated growth of cells resulting from genetic changes may occur.

5. Compare and contrast the characteristics of malignant and benign tumors.

6. Discuss genetic changes that have the potential to initiate neoplastic growth.

7. Discuss the five general etiologic factors involved in carcinogenesis.

8. Describe the local growth of malignant neoplasms.

9. Describe three mechanisms of metastasis.

10. List possible symptoms of neoplasia and the methods used to diagnose neoplastic growth.

11. Describe cancer grading and tumor staging and state the importance of each in determining treatment and prognosis.

12. Describe the systemic effects of malignancy.

13. List the different types of cancer therapies available and describe how they work.

14. Describe the potential systemic and oral side effects of cancer therapy.

15. List measures an individual can take to lower the risk of developing cancer.

16. Describe the characteristics of the three most common skin cancers.

17. List screening methods for breast, prostate, and colorectal cancers.

18. Describe the symptoms of lung cancer.

19. Describe the typical appearance of metastatic cancer found in the oral cavity.

20. List the cancers that are most likely to metastasize to the oral cavity.

Chapter Outline

Normal Cell Growth
    Growth Categories
    Growth Regulators
Neoplastic Growth
    Benign Neoplasms
    Malignant Neoplasms
        Carcinogenesis
        Local Growth and Distant Metastasis

Diagnosis
Tumor Grading and Staging
Systemic Effects of Malignancy
Cancer Therapies
    Side Effects of Cancer Therapy
Prevention
Common Cancers
        Basal cell carcinoma (BCC)
        Squamous cell carcinoma (SCC)
        Melanoma
        Breast cancer
        Prostate cancer
        Lung cancer
        Colorectal cancer
        Oral metastatic cancer

NORMAL CELL GROWTH

The cell is the basic unit of life. Cells make up tissues that form organs, which combine to form systems, and finally develop into a living organism. The growth of the organism is evidenced by the multiplication and growth of individual cells within the organism. While all the cells within the body have the genetic ability to reproduce, they are not all allowed to do so. In fact, each type of cell within the body has a specific growth potential that is reached when the cell becomes mature. It will be helpful to review this information before discussing what happens when the mechanisms that regulate cellular growth go awry.

Growth Categories

The tissues of the body can be categorized into three major groups: labile, stable, and permanent, depending on the growth potential of their component cells. **Labile** cells are found in tissues that are constantly undergoing controlled, rapid reproduction to replace cells lost through normal wear and minor injury. The skin, mucous membranes, blood cell-forming tissues, and lymphoid tissues are examples of tissues comprised of labile cells. In the skin and mucous membranes, the epithelial cells rapidly reproduce to replace cells that are lost continuously throughout the day. The life expectancy of a normal red blood cell is approximately 120 days, after which it undergoes apoptosis, is removed from the body, and is replaced by another mature red blood cell that was formed in the bone marrow.

Stable or **quiescent** cells are found in tissues that do not usually undergo reproduction but can be triggered to do so under the right circumstances, such as those that occur in an injury. In this case the cells are stimulated by growth factors manufactured by the injured cells and other cells that surround the injured cells. The liver, kidneys, pancreas, smooth muscles, and vascular endothelium are comprised of stable cells. Liver cells do not usually replicate, but if traumatic damage does occur, the cells are triggered to start reproducing. For example, when an individual receives a liver transplant, he or she receives only a portion of the donor's liver.

Not only does that portion grow to a normal size within the recipient, but also the remainder of the donor's liver regenerates to its normal size.

Permanent cells have reached their final differentiated form and are not capable of reproduction. These cells do not regenerate after injury. The tissues of the heart, skeletal muscle, and nervous system are examples of tissues made up of permanent cells. When the heart undergoes a traumatic event such as a heart attack or myocardial infarction (MI), the cells cannot reproduce to repair the injury. Scar tissue is formed, and the remaining heart muscle must take over the functioning of the damaged area, resulting in increased demand on the remaining tissue. In addition, depending on the extent of the injury, the individual would be at a higher risk for another MI or problems such as congestive heart failure. Currently, researchers are investigating the potential for using stem cells to repair some of these permanent tissues as well as other purposes.

Growth Regulators

The growth potential of labile, stable, and permanent cells is genetically controlled. Genes are the single units of inheritance that make up the chromosome. Genes are comprised of molecules of **deoxyribonucleic acid (DNA)**, a double-stranded molecule made up of up to one million nucleotides. Specific genes called **protooncogenes** act to regulate the growth of the cells in which they are contained. Each cell is also endowed with **tumor suppressor genes** that produce substances that inhibit uncontrolled growth of the individual cells. Additionally, there are genes known as **caretaker or mutator genes** that monitor the structural components of the DNA strand within each cell. If these genes sense that something is not correct in the DNA sequence, they will attempt to repair it. If the error cannot be repaired, the caretaker genes mark the cell for destruction by apoptosis. If something interferes with these genetic controls, then neoplastic or new cellular growth can occur.

NEOPLASTIC GROWTH

Neoplastic or unregulated growth occurs when a genetic change or mutation interferes with the regulation of normal cell growth. Neoplastic growth is not considered hyperplasia because unlike hyperplasia, a permanent change in the regulation of cellular division, growth, or differentiation has occurred on the genetic level. Hyperplasia is a cellular adaptation seen in response to a stressful stimulus; when the stimulus is removed, the process stops and may resolve. Neoplasia occurs in response to a stimulus also but does not stop when the stimulus is removed. In fact, in most cases the stimulus is unknown and may have been encountered many years prior to the growth of the neoplasm. Neoplasms express a wide range of characteristics that can be divided into two basic groups, benign and malignant. Table 5.1 provides a summary of the characteristics of benign and malignant neoplasms.

APPLICATION

There are two types of stem cells, embryonic stem cells that are obtained from the blastocyst (3- to 5-day-old embryo) and adult stem cells or somatic stem cells that are found in the bone marrow and possibly in muscle, brain, and other tissues as well. Embryonic stem cells can differentiate into any of the specialized cells in the body. These cells can be grown in the laboratory and remain undifferentiated for what is thought to be an indefinite amount of time. This enables the production of large amounts of stem cells that can be used for research purposes.

Adult stem cells are thought to be much more directed in their development. In other words, there is a limit as to what type of cell the adult stem cell can differentiate into. For example, a stem cell found in the bone marrow may only be able to differentiate into a blood-forming cell and not a nerve cell. However, recent animal studies have suggested that these adult stem cells may be more flexible than is now thought. If so, this would increase the potential use of these cells. Adult stem cells are much harder to find within the tissues and do not reproduce as rapidly as the embryonic stem cells.

There are numerous potential uses for stem cells. Stem cells could be used to test the effectiveness of drugs or to determine whether drugs could harm specific types of cells. They could be used to develop drugs that target cells of a specific type. Stem cells could be used to generate tissues that could replace or repair damaged or destroyed tissues, such as skin that was destroyed by burns or nerve tissues destroyed by a spinal cord injury. Stem cells could be stimulated to differentiate into cells that secrete essential substances and could be the answer to finding cures for disorders such as Parkinson's disease and diabetes. Research on stem cells could help determine what happens to make a normal cell become malignant or why some birth defects occur. One of the more important questions being looked at now relates to discovering what signals prompt the stem cells to reproduce and then to differentiate. In addition, researchers must discover what causes the stem cell to differentiate into a skin cell as opposed to a nerve cell or liver cell.

Stem cells have been used successfully to treat leukemia for many years (Chapter 9, "Blood Disorders"). Current research is focused on expanding the role that stem cells play in the medical treatment of human disorders (Stem Cell Information, 2006).

APPLICATION

Intraoral examples of the difference between hyperplasia and neoplasia can be seen in the following two cases. Case 1 involves leukoplakia associated with smokeless or spit tobacco and case 2 involves verrucous carcinoma, which is also associated with spit tobacco.

Both cases start as the individual begins to use the product. The mucosal site in which the tobacco is kept begins to undergo a change. The chemicals in the tobacco are toxic, and the body initiates a line of defense against them in the form of cellular adaptation. Eventually, after months or years, depending on the individual, the mucosal tissues in the area where the tobacco is kept start to show a clinical difference from the areas that are not in direct contact with the tobacco. The tissue becomes whiter (hence the name leukoplakia), more leathery, and eventually so thick that the tissue starts to become fissured (Fig. 5.1). Leukoplakia is a clinical description for a white lesion that has not yet been definitively diagnosed by biopsy. In this case, the lesion of leukoplakia is the clinical manifestation of mucosal hyperplasia. As the epithelial cell layer becomes thicker, the tissue becomes less transparent and more opaque or white. At this point the two cases follow different paths.

In the first case, the hygienist discusses the area and the cause with the patient. The patient is shown the area and is asked if he wants to quit tobacco use. The patient decides that cessation is the right thing to do at this time, and with the help of the dental team and support from family and friends, he is successful. The area of leukoplakia is kept under observation at each preventive maintenance appointment for the next 2 years. Slowly the hyperplastic area resolves, and after 2 years, the tissues are no different from the tissues that did not have direct contact with the tobacco. As in a true case of hyperplasia, once the stimulus was removed, the growth stopped and actually resolved over time.

In the second case, the hygienist follows the same protocol, but the patient does not want to stop use of the tobacco. The oral tissues in the area where the tobacco is kept become more and more hyperplastic. Often the hyperplastic change is accompanied by differing degrees of dysplasia. After years of constant tobacco use, the chemicals interfere with one or more genetic controls within the epithelial cells, and a neoplastic change occurs. After several more years, the hygienist notices a distinct change in the appearance of the lesion. It starts to become exophytic and verrucous, or wartlike (Fig. 5.2). The patient is shown the area and asked again if he would like to quit tobacco use. This time he agrees and after months of hard work is successful in his attempt to quit. The dental team monitors the intraoral area for the next several months but does not notice any resolution; to the contrary, the lesion appears to be enlarging and becoming more exophytic. The patient is sent for a biopsy of the area, which returns with a definitive diagnosis of verrucous carcinoma. As expected, removal of the stimulus only stopped the hyperplastic lesion, not the neoplastic lesion. Verrucous carcinoma will be covered in detail in Chapter 16: "Raised Lesions with a Rough or Papillary Surface Texture."

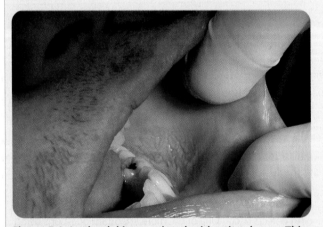

Figure 5.1. Leukoplakia associated with spit tobacco. This picture shows the characteristic white color and fissuring consistent with lesions of this type.

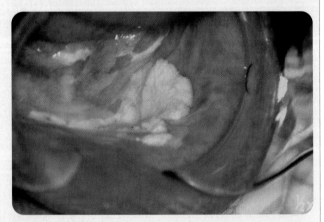

Figure 5.2. Verrucous carcinoma. Verrucous carcinoma associated with long-term spit tobacco use. Note the exophytic, thick, leathery growth and fissuring. (Courtesy of Dr. John Jacoway.)

Benign Neoplasms

Benign neoplasms do not spread into adjacent tissues or metastasize to distant sites. These neoplasms normally, but not always, grow slowly by expansion and put pressure on surrounding structures and tissues. They are usually **encapsulated** (encased in a fibrous capsule) and move freely within the surrounding tissues. The surface of these lesions, if visible, may appear stretched, but it is usually normal in color. Benign neoplasms do not have

Table 5.1 — COMPARISON OF THE CHARACTERISTICS OF BENIGN AND MALIGNANT NEOPLASMS

Characteristic	Benign	Malignant
Cell characteristics	Well-differentiated, resemble normal cells of the tissue of origin	Range of well to undifferentiated with little or no resemblance to the tissue of origin
Tumor growth	Localized expansion, usually encapsulated or otherwise separated from the surrounding tissues	Infiltrates the surrounding tissues, becomes fixed to them and not easily separated
Growth rate	Slow growth, mitotic figures are rare	Varies, the more undifferentiated the cells are the faster the rate of growth, mitotic figures are common
Metastasis	None	Metastasizes through the blood and lymph to distant sites
Damage to adjacent tissues	Not likely unless the tumor interferes with the blood supply to the tissues	Usually causes extensive tissue destruction as it commandeers nutrients from the local blood supply
Systemic effects	Related to the location of the tumor and its interference with vital functions	Weight loss, anemia, fatigue, and more
Mortality	Related to the location of the tumor and its interference with vital functions	Certain death unless the tumor can be controlled

Porth CM, Essentials of pathophysiology: concepts of altered health states. Baltimore: Lippincott Williams & Wilkins: 2004:,68; Table 5-2.

an effect on the host unless they impinge on a nerve or vital organ or become very large, at which time, pain, paralysis, loss of function, or even death may result. For example, a benign brain tumor can prove just as fatal as a malignant tumor, because it displaces and damages vital brain tissues. Often, benign tumors of endocrine glands can cause the gland to hyperfunction and prove damaging to the host. Examples of this are **giantism** and **acromegaly** caused by prepubertal and postpubertal hyperfunction of the pituitary gland, respectively. These endocrine disorders are discussed in Chapter 7, "Endocrine Disorders." A histological study of a benign tumor will usually show well-**differentiated** cells that are the same as, or closely resemble, the cells of origin (Fig. 5.3). Benign neoplastic cells maintain the genetic capability to remain differentiated but have somehow lost the genetic capability to stop unnecessary cellular replication. Terms that denote benign neoplasms usually contain the name of the tissue of origin and end in "-oma." Table 5.2 lists the nomenclature of benign and malignant tumors. Pictures of the following benign growths, fibroma (Fig. 1.20), papilloma (Fig. 1.32), and lipoma (Fig. 1.27), can be seen in Chapter 1, "Introduction to General and Oral Pathology."

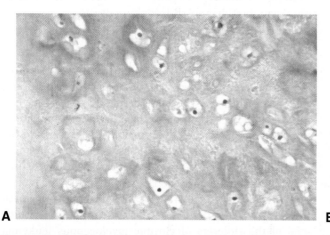
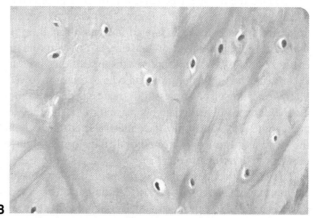

Figure 5.3. Histologic comparison of normal cartilage and a benign chondroma. A benign chondroma **(A)** closely resembles normal cartilage **(B)**. (From Rubin E, Farber JL. Pathology, 3rd ed. Philadelphia: Lippincott Williams & Wilkins, 1999.)

Table 5.2   NOMENCLATURE FOR BENIGN AND MALIGNANT NEOPLASMS

Tissue of Origin	Benign Neoplasm	Malignant Neoplasm
Epithelial		
Epidermis	Squamous papilloma	Squamous cell carcinoma
Glandular	Adenoma	Adenocarcinoma
Melanocytes	Nevus	Melanoma
Nervous		
Nerve sheath	Neurofibroma	Neurofibrosarcoma
Nerve cell	Neuroma	Neuroblastoma
Glial cells	None	Glioblastoma
Blood		
Red blood cells		Erythroleukemia
White blood cells		Leukemia
Connective		
Bone	Osteoma	Osteosarcoma
Cartilage	Chondroma	Chondrosarcoma
Adipose	Lipoma	Liposarcoma
Fibrous	Fibroma	Fibrosarcoma
Blood vessels	Hemangioma	Hemangiosarcoma
Lymph vessels	Lymphangioma	Lymphangiosarcoma
Muscle		
Smooth	Leiomyoma	Leiomyosarcoma
Striated	Rhabdomyoma	Rhabdomyosarcoma

Malignant Neoplasms

Malignant neoplasms or cancers differ from benign neoplasms in many ways. However, the defining characteristics of malignant tumors are their ability to invade local tissues and to **metastasize** to distant sites. Malignant neoplasms usually grow more rapidly, and when they invade the surrounding tissue, it is difficult to determine where the tumor begins and the normal tissue ends. Clinically, the tumor may appear fixed to underlying tissues when palpated, because the tumor has extended into these tissues and has not just pushed them aside. Histologically, the cancer cells may be fairly well differentiated; however, they are often seen as mildly to severely undifferentiated and may bear little resemblance to the tissue of origin. Cancer is asymptomatic in its early stages. When symptoms do appear, they are varied and depend on the location and type of tumor involved. Many cancers can be successfully treated if detected in a timely manner. All malignant neoplasms are fatal if they remain undetected until they have metastasized throughout the body and cannot be treated or if they are allowed to progress with no treatment.

There are two general types of malignant neoplasm, **carcinoma** and **sarcoma**. In cancer nomenclature, carcinoma is applied to cancers arising from epithelial cells, for example, squamous cell carcinoma and basal cell carcinoma. Likewise, sarcoma denotes a growth arising from connective tissues and sarcoma would be added to the name of the specific tissue of origin, for example, os-teosarcoma or osteogenic sarcoma and fibrosarcoma. Cancer nomenclature is not consistent, and there are exceptions to the rules. For example, melanoma is a malignant growth of melanocytes, and a lymphoma is a malignant growth of lymph cells, and neither is benign as their names would appear to signify. The name "leukemia" would imply a white blood cell deficiency, while in fact leukemia is a malignant growth of white blood cells; there is no benign growth of white blood cells. Other cancers are named for the person who first diagnosed them, for example, Thomas Hodgkin (1798-1866), an English physician, first diagnosed Hodgkin's disease.

CARCINOGENESIS

Carcinogenesis is the development or process of cancer growth. Protooncogenes, tumor-suppressor genes, and caretaker or mutator genes are needed to control the cellular growth cycle. If protooncogenes undergo mutation, they become **oncogenes** that encourage or accelerate the growth of a particular cell. The most common protooncogene mutations involve the alteration of just one or two nucleotide base pairs in the DNA strand. Another type of mutation involves the **translocation** of genetic material from one chromosome to a different chromosome. Some 95% of the sufferers of **chronic myelogenous leukemia** (Chapter 9, "Blood Diseases") carry the **Philadelphia chromosome.** This chromosome is the result of the incorrect fusion of parts of two different chromosomes. The fusion separates two genes so that part of each gene is located in the wrong place. The result of this oncogenic mutation is the production of an abnormal protein that actually promotes the overproduction of the white blood cell precursors or myeloid cells seen in this disease. Tumor suppressor genes inhibit the growth of cells and can actually stop the growth of cells that are damaged in some way. When tumor suppressor genes are inactivated by genetic mutation, cell division and growth can proceed unregulated. Caretaker or mutator genes form a line of defense against genetic mutations. They are contained in the genetic material of every cell, where they watch over the integrity of the DNA and regulate the repair or destruction of the involved cells. If these genetic functions are lost, the cells with errors in their DNA will be allowed to replicate. If the errors involve a neoplastic change, neoplastic growth (whether benign or malignant) will be allowed to occur. Genetic mutations are involved in the initiation of neoplastic growth. However, it is just as important to know what can cause the mutations. These causes include:

1. Inherited traits or influences
2. Chemical exposures
3. Environmental insults
4. Viruses
5. Immune system defects

Inherited traits or influences can cause any of the following:
- Benign tumors
- Benign tumors that may become malignant
- Malignant tumors
- Syndromes that carry a high risk of malignant tumors

Mutations in tumor suppressor genes are most often related to inherited forms of cancer. About 50 types of cancer have a genetic predisposition. Breast cancer, for example, is more likely to occur in women who have a history of breast cancer in their families. Individuals who have inherited Gardner syndrome have a higher than normal risk of developing colorectal cancers. Gardner syndrome is discussed in Chapter 19, "Radiopaque Lesions." Children who have inherited the dominant retinoblastoma gene have a 95% chance of developing at least one of these eye tumors.

Chemical agents can cause genetic mutations. In many cases, exposure to the chemical agent is consistent over a long period of time. Smoking exposes the individual to many chemicals that have been proved to cause cancer. Lung and laryngeal cancers are directly related to smoking, while esophageal, pancreas, and bladder cancers have been associated with tobacco use. Many of our food products contain added nitrates as a preservative. There is concern that these nitrates may be converted into nitrosamines in our digestive tracts. Nitrosamines have been implicated in cancer development because they are known to produce cancer in rodents. Many other chemicals have been shown to cause cancers in humans and animals. Box 5.1 provides a list of some of the more common chemical **carcinogenic** (cancer causing) agents.

Box 5.1 — CHEMICALS ASSOCIATED WITH A HIGH RISK OF CANCER

- Alcohol
- Vinyl chloride
- Diethylstilbestrol
- Benzene
- Arsenic
- Formaldehyde
- Nickel compounds

Environmental agents have also been linked to cancer in humans. Many skin cancers are caused by exposure to ultraviolet light from the sun. Ultraviolet radiation causes a specific type of DNA damage that no other carcinogenic agent has been shown to cause. The damage done by ultraviolet radiation is cumulative, and damage done during the early years of life may result in cancer later in life. Asbestos, used for many construction needs from roofing and flooring to insulation, is another example of an environmental agent that causes cancer. Asbestos is associated with mesothelioma, or cancer of the **pleural** (lung) and **peritoneal** (abdominal) cavities. While mesothelioma is rare in the general population, workers who were exposed to large amounts of asbestos over many years have a 3% or more chance of developing this cancer.

Viruses that have the ability to cause cancer are called "oncogenic viruses." Human papilloma virus (HPV), Epstein-Barr virus (EBV), and hepatitis B and C viruses (HBV, HCV) have all been recognized as oncogenic viruses. Viruses enter the host cells and use the cell's replication mechanisms to reproduce viral particles. To accomplish this, the virus integrates some of its DNA into the host cell's DNA. This altered DNA becomes oncogenic, or cancer causing. Certain strains of HPV have been shown to cause cervical and anogenital squamous cell carcinoma. EBV has been associated with several types of cancer including: Burkitt's lymphoma, nasopharyngeal cancer, B-cell lymphoma in immunosuppressed individuals, and Hodgkin's disease. HCV and HBV have both been implicated in hepatocellular carcinoma (liver cancer) when the individual is a chronic carrier of either disease.

Immune system defects may also be associated with a higher risk of cancer. Studies are under way to determine if parts of our immune system can protect us from malignant neoplastic growths. Many of the studies are focusing on the ability of T cells, natural killer cells, and macrophages to destroy tumor cells. An immune defect that affects any of these cells may increase the individual's risk for cancer. Most of the evidence that points toward a possible immune system role in cancer prevention has been associated with the fact that immunocompromised individuals are more likely to develop malignancies than their healthy counterparts. For example, Kaposi's sarcoma and lymphoma are commonly seen in patients with AIDS.

LOCAL GROWTH AND DISTANT METASTASIS

Malignant tumors do not magically appear. They start out with a single cell that has undergone a change. This starts a sequence of changes that very often begins with dyspla-

sia and ends with an invasive neoplasm that eventually metastasizes to distant sites (Fig. 5.4). In the case of epithelial cancer or carcinoma, the dysplastic cells are separated from the surrounding tissues by the basement membrane (Fig. 5.5). While carcinoma is in this early stage, it is called **carcinoma in situ** and can be readily treated and cured. If left untreated, the tumor cells will penetrate the basement membrane using one or more of the mechanisms discussed below and extend into the surrounding

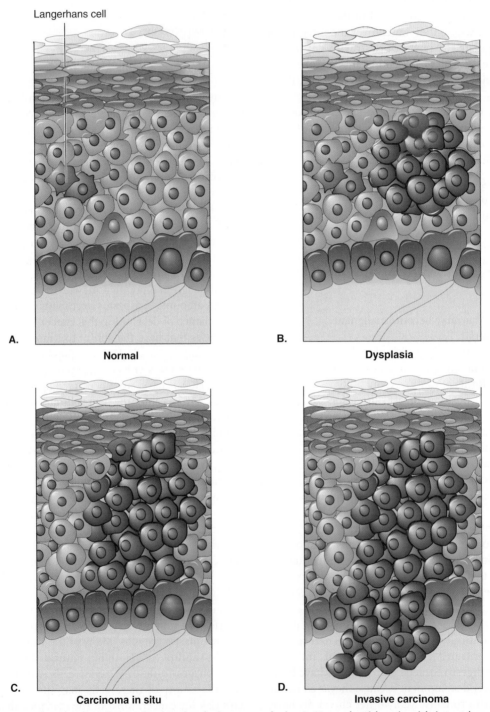

Langerhans cell

A. **Normal**

B. **Dysplasia**

C. **Carcinoma in situ**

D. **Invasive carcinoma**

Figure 5.4. Progressive changes from adaptive dysplasia to neoplasia. A. Normal epidermis with intact basement membrane. B. Epidermis showing dysplastic changes. C. Severe dysplasia or carcinoma in situ. Note that the basement membrane is still intact. D. Invasive neoplasia. The basement membrane has been breached.

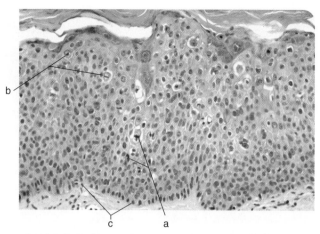

Figure 5.5. Squamous cell carcinoma in situ. The entire epidermis is replaced by atypical keratinocytes. Multinucleation of the keratinocytes *(a)* and numerous mitotic figures *(b)* are apparent, but the basement membrane *(c)* is intact. (From Rubin E, Farber JL. Pathology, 3rd ed. Philadelphia: Lippincott Williams & Wilkins, 1999.)

tissues (Fig. 5.6). Other types of cells, such as connective tissue or nervous tissue cells do not have a defined in situ stage because they do not have a basement membrane. Once any tumor cell has extended into the local tissues, there is an increased risk of lymph node involvement and metastasis to distant sites.

Malignant tumors are able to spread into the surrounding tissues by use of several mechanisms. As the tumors grow, they can exert mechanical pressure on normal cells in the area, disrupt their nutrient supply, and weaken or destroy them, enabling the cancer cells to push into the surrounding tissues. The cancer cells are also able to produce substances that allow them to destroy collagen and in turn weaken the extracellular substances that hold normal tissue cells together, thereby allowing the spread of the cancer cells. Cancer cells do not adhere to each other as tightly as normal cells; therefore they can break off

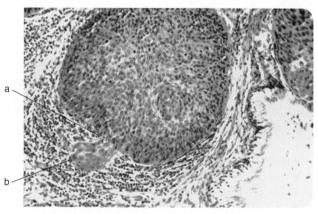

Figure 5.6. Microinvasive squamous cell carcinoma. Cancer cells have used mechanisms to destroy normal cells to breach the basement membrane of this gland *(a)* and spread into the adjacent tissues *(b)*. (From Rubin E, Farber JL. Pathology, 3rd ed. Philadelphia: Lippincott Williams & Wilkins, 1999.)

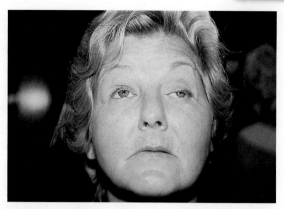

Figure 5.7. Metastatic breast cancer. Breast cancer has metastasized to the area superior to the left orbit, causing ptosis or sinking of the eye. (From Tasman W, Jaeger E. The Wills Eye Hospital atlas of clinical ophthalmology, 2nd ed. Baltimore: Lippincott Williams & Wilkins, 2001.)

from the primary tumor and actually move into the surrounding tissues.

Several events must occur before tumor cells can establish a secondary tumor or metastatic site (Fig. 5.7). The tumor cells must penetrate the basement membrane if there is one, and they must move through the cells of the surrounding tissues until they enter either a lymph or blood vessel. If the tumor cells enter a lymph vessel, they will travel to the regional lymph nodes and may establish a secondary tumor within the node or nodes. Eventually cancer cells will find their way into the circulating blood by way of the venous drainage of the lymphatics. When metastasis occurs through the blood vessels, it is more complicated because the tumor cells must move within the blood vessel until they are able to attach to the vascular endothelium. Next, the cancer cells must exit through the endothelium and begin to multiply in the new site. Body cavities may also provide an avenue for tumor metastasis. When tumors arise in the abdominal organs or the lungs, the cancer cells may break off from the primary tumor and travel through the spaces to grow in adjacent organs. The process of tumor spread through the body's cavities is called **seeding** (Fig. 5.8). The most common method of tumor spread is through the lymphatic system.

Diagnosis

The presence of a neoplasm may be suspected for many reasons. The individual may have symptoms related to the anatomic area in which a tumor is growing. **Dysphagia**, or difficulty swallowing, would occur with an esophageal tumor. Loss of memory might occur with a brain tumor. Other symptoms may relate to the tissue that is affected. A thyroid tumor might cause symptoms of **hyperthyroidism**, excessive production of thyroid hormone, while an adrenal tumor causes symptoms associated with **hyperadrenalism**, excessive production of cortisol (both are discussed in Chapter 7, "Endocrine Disorders"). Small tu-

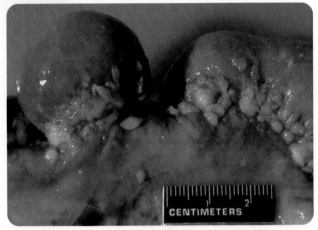

Figure 5.8. Seeding. Metastatic spread of ovarian cancer throughout the peritoneal cavity by means of seeding. Note the multiple small nodules of cancer studding this section of mesentery and small bowel. (From Rubin E, Farber JL. Pathology, 3rd ed. Philadelphia: Lippincott Williams & Wilkins, 1999.)

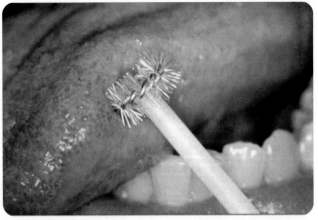

Figure 5.9. Brush biopsy. This is an example of using the brush biopsy technique to obtain cells from a lesion on the lateral border of the tongue. (Photo provided by CDx Laboratories, Inc., Suffern, NY.)

mors may remain undetected until they metastasize and the secondary tumors produce symptoms. Many cancers metastasize to bone tissue; therefore, bone pain may be the initial symptom of a primary tumor unrelated to bone.

Tumors may be discovered through a screening process. Common cancer screening methods include

• Colonoscopy
• Skin examination
• Mammography
• Prostate examination
• Blood tests
• Oral cancer screening

Blood tests are done to detect the presence of **tumor markers.** Tumor markers are chemicals produced by specific types of cancer cells. For example, prostate cancer cells produce prostate-specific antigen (PSA). If an elevated level of this marker is found in the blood, additional testing should be done to determine if a prostate tumor exists. Lung and breast cancers may produce carcinoembryonic antigen (CEA); an elevated level of this substance would require further testing to rule out the presence of cancer in these areas. Some suspicious areas in the oral cavity may be screened using a technique called "brush biopsy," which uses a stiff circular brush to scrape cells from small oral lesions of unknown etiology (Fig. 5.9). The brush is placed firmly on the surface of the lesion and rotated on the lesion until pinpoint bleeding is observed. The bleeding ensures that the brush has reached the deepest layers of the epidermis. The cells are placed and fixed on a glass slide and sent to the company for computer analysis. The software program that is used is said to be able to identify as few as one or two abnormal cells from the sample. If the brush biopsy result is positive, a scalpel biopsy should be done (Gurenlian, 2003).

Another type of oral cancer screening aid has recently become available. ViziLite Plus is a system that was devel-

oped to identify and mark oral lesions. This system is used as an adjunct to conventional visual examinations. Refer to Protocol 12 for a description of these screening methods. Promising new methods of screening are being developed; one method uses saliva to detect oral cancer. The most common sites for oral cancer to develop are listed in Box 5.2. All of these sites are visible to the dental hygienist, and unidentified lesions should be evaluated in office or referred for evaluation by another medical or dental professional. In addition, all patients (especially those patients who are at high risk for developing oral cancer) should be shown how to examine their own mouths for signs of abnormal soft tissues. Clinical Protocol 11 suggests guidelines for training the patient to do this examination. In all cases, regardless of the symptoms or level of tumor markers, the final determination of a benign or malignant tumor must be made at the microscopic level.

There are several methods of obtaining tissue cells for microscopic examination. If the neoplasm is discovered in an early stage and is small enough, an **excisional biopsy** is performed. An excisional biopsy removes the entire neoplasm and a wide margin of normal-appearing tissue sur-

---

Box 5.2   MOST COMMON SITES FOR ORAL CANCER DEVELOPMENT

• Lip* (lower more than upper)
• Tongue (posterior lateral border more often)
• Floor of the mouth
• Buccal mucosa
• Gingiva
• Soft palate

*The lip is the most common site for cancer development in the perioral area; however, the tongue is the most common intraoral site.

rounding the tumor. The entire specimen is sent for microscopic examination, at which time the type of growth will be determined. If it is determined to be malignant, the margins of normal-appearing tissues will be thoroughly examined for any evidence of malignant cells. Whether the surgical margins are or are not found to be clear of cancer cells will affect the course of treatment and the prognosis of the disease. If the tumor is too large to remove without more complicated surgical methods, an **incisional biopsy**, which involves the removal of a small piece of the tumor with some normal-appearing cells, may be done. Other methods of obtaining cells for testing include the **needle biopsy**, in which a core of tissue is removed through a large-bore needle or **fine-needle aspiration**, which involves removal of tumor fluid through a small-diameter needle. Both of these methods are used effectively to diagnose a malignancy, with some limitations. These methods require an adequate and representative sample of the suspect cells. Results that are positive for cancer are usually reliable; however, negative results may have to be followed up with a more invasive procedure to definitively rule out a malignancy.

Benign and malignant neoplasms are definitively diagnosed by microscopic evaluation of their cellular makeup. The cells of benign neoplasms are usually well differentiated and closely resemble the cells of origin. Benign tumors will not exhibit extension into, or fixation to, the surrounding tissues and, by definition, none will have metastasized to distant sites.

The cells of malignant neoplasms manifest a wide range of levels of differentiation from relatively well differentiated to severely undifferentiated, or **anaplastic**. The more anaplastic the cells, the more aggressive the tumor is likely to be. **Pleomorphism** (a change in the size and shape of the cells and their nuclei) and **hyperchromatic nuclei** (darkly stained nuclei) are examples of the types of anaplastic changes seen in malignant cells (Fig. 5.10). In addition, malignant neoplasms will exhibit numerous **mitotic figures**, which signify cellular division and the characteristic rapid growth of these neoplasms (Fig. 5.11). Malignant tumors will extend into the surrounding tissues, and it may be difficult to find any type of boundary between tumor and normal cells. Finally, evidence of tumor cells in the regional lymph nodes or of distant metastasis clearly indicates that the tumor is malignant.

Tumor Grading and Staging

To determine the probable clinical course or outcome of a malignancy and to help choose appropriate therapy, physicians use a **cancer grading** and staging system. Cancer cells are graded according to their level of differentiation and the number of mitotic figures in a given tissue sample. The cells are ranked from grade I to grade IV, with each level representing a greater lack of differentiation, or anaplasia, and increasing numbers of mitotic fig-

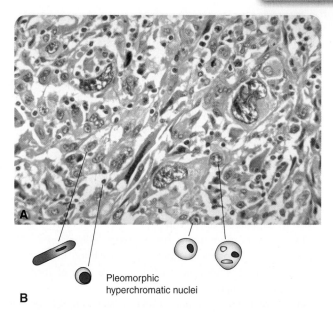

Pleomorphic
hyperchromatic nuclei

Figure 5.10. Anaplastic changes. A. Actual histology slide showing pleomorphic cells with large and hyperchromatic nuclei. (From Rubin E, Farber JL. Pathology, 3rd ed. Philadelphia: Lippincott Williams & Wilkins, 1999.) **B.** Illustration depicting pleomorphism and large hyperchromatic nuclei.

ures. It is presumed that the higher the cancer grade, the more aggressive the tumor will be, but this is not always the case.

Tumor staging is used to determine the extent of the disease. Several cancer staging systems are in use at this time, including the TNM system (T, size of the primary tumor; N, lymph node involvement; M, metastasis) developed by the International Union Against Cancer and the American Joint Committee on Cancer. The TNM system has a specific set of criteria for each organ or cancer site in

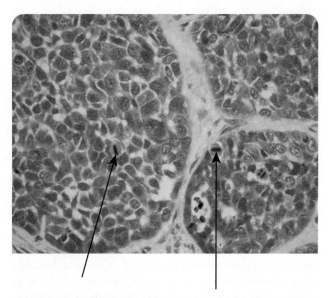

Figure 5.11. Mitotic figures. Numerous mitotic figures signify rapid growth in this squamous cell carcinoma. (Courtesy of Yi-Shing Lisa Cheng.)

Box 5.3   TNM SYSTEM OF CANCER STAGING

Lip and oral cavity (nonepithelial tumors such as those of lymphoid tissue, soft tissue, bone, and cartilage are not included)

Primary tumor (T)

Tis   Carcinoma in situ

T1   Tumor 2 cm or less in greatest dimension

T2   Tumor more than 2 cm but not more than 4 cm in greatest dimension

T3   Tumor more than 4 cm in greatest dimension

T4a   (lip) Tumor invades through cortical bone, inferior alveolar nerve, floor of mouth, or skin of face (i.e., chin or nose)

T4a   (oral cavity) Tumor invades adjacent structures (e.g., through cortical bone, into deep muscles of the tongue, maxillary sinus, skin of face)

T4b   Tumor invades masticator space, pterygoid plates, or skull base and/or encases internal carotid artery

Regional lymph nodes

N0   No regional lymph node metastasis

N1   Metastasis in single lymph node, same side, 3 cm or less in greatest dimension

N2a   Metastasis in single lymph node, same side, more than 3 cm but not more than 6 cm in greatest dimension

N2b   Metastasis in multiple lymph nodes, same side, none more than 6 cm in greatest dimension

N2c   Metastasis in multiple lymph nodes, bilateral or contralateral, none more than 6 cm in greatest dimension

N3   Metastasis in a lymph node more than 6 cm in greatest dimension

Distant metastasis

M0   No distant metastasis

M1   Distant metastasis

Used with permission of the American Joint Committee on Cancer (AJCC), Chicago, Illinois. The original source for this material is the AJCC Cancer Staging Manual, 6th ed. New York: Springer-Verlag, 2002. www.springeronline.com.

creases numerically, the prognosis becomes worse, treatment becomes more difficult, and the treatment options become less numerous (AJCC, 2006). Surgery may no longer be an option if the cancer has invaded vital structures of the head and neck area, and if metastasis has occurred, chemotherapy may be the only option to prolong survival and maintain a good quality of life for as long as possible.

Systemic Effects of Malignancy

Systemic effects of malignancy that are not directly related to tumor invasion or metastasis are collectively called **paraneoplastic syndromes**. These syndromes are not common; however, when they are present they can complicate care for the patient and can have an overwhelming effect on the patient's psychologic outlook and quality of life. One or more of the following elements can occur by itself or in conjunction with any of the other elements. Fever of unknown origin, caused by the release of pyrogens by the tumor cells and interleukins by inflammatory cells in the area, often occurs, especially with osteogenic sarcoma and Hodgkin's disease. Extreme weight loss and **anorexia** are very common to all cancer patients. The reason for this weight loss is not clearly understood but may be associated with an increased metabolic rate that occurs with malignancies. Endocrine imbalances are common and can be caused by hypersecretion of tumors of the endocrine glands or overstimulation of the endocrine glands by tumor byproducts. **Anemia** is another common problem associated with malignancies. Anemia can be caused by chronic bleeding, malnutrition, anticancer therapies, and malignancies of the blood-forming tissues. **Leukopenia**, or a low white blood cell count, can be caused by anticancer therapies and malignancies of the blood-forming tissues. **Thrombocytopenia**, or a low platelet level, can cause severe bleeding with little or no provocation, and to the contrary, **hypercoagulation** problems may cause blood clots or **thrombi** to form that can obstruct vital vessels or produce **emboli** that may obstruct vessels in distant areas. Neurologic problems can result in varying degrees of motor and sensory dysfunction and may cause orthostatic hypotension or syncope. Generalized fatigue is very common in cancer patients, especially while they are undergoing treatment.

the body. Refer to Box 5.3 for the coding information necessary to determine the TNM for epithelial cancers of the lip and oral cavity. The information from the TNM is grouped together and used to determine a cancer/tumor stage. Table 5.3 provides an example of how TNM information is grouped into stages. Stage 0 includes all findings of carcinoma in situ. Treatment for this stage of cancer is rather conservative, depending of the grade of the cancer, and may involve surgical removal including a wide margin of normal tissue along with the tumor. As the stage in-

Cancer Therapies

The major cancer therapies are surgery, radiation, and chemotherapy. The choice of an appropriate therapy or combination of therapies is based on the characteristics of the neoplasm, such as the type (carcinoma or sarcoma), stage, and location; on the characteristics of the patient, such as age, sex, health status; and on the patient's preferences. Determining treatment options for neoplasms in the head and neck area can prove very challenging be-

Table 5.3   USING THE TNM SYSTEM TO DETERMINE STAGE GROUPINGS

Stage Grouping	Primary Tumor	Regional Lymph Nodes	Distant Metastasis
Stage 0	Tis	N0	M0
Stage I	T1	N0	M0
Stage II	T2	N0	M0
Stage III	T3	N0	M0
	T1-3	N1	M0
Stage IVA	T4a	N0	M0
	T4a	N1	M0
	T1-3	N2	M0
	T4a	N2	M0
Stage IVB	Any T	N3	M0
	T4b	Any N	M0
Stage IVC	Any T	Any N	M1

Used with permission of the American Joint Committee on Cancer (AJCC), Chicago, Illinois. The original source for this material is AJCC Cancer Staging Manual, 6th ed. New York: Springer-Verlag, 2002. www.springeronline.com.

cause of the number of vital structures involved, the importance of maintaining adequate function, and sparing tissues to provide adequate opportunities for some degree of aesthetic reconstruction if necessary and possible. Surgery is the initial therapy for many cancers.

If the neoplasm is discovered in an early stage and is small enough, an excisional biopsy might be performed. If it is determined to be malignant, the margins of normal-appearing tissues will be thoroughly examined for any evidence of malignant cells. If none are found, there may not be any further therapy indicated or radiation or chemotherapy might be used to try to ensure complete elimination of any remaining malignant cells. Surgical procedures for larger neoplasms, especially in the head and neck area, can be very complicated and are often combined with other therapies to help ensure that the malignant cells are eliminated if possible.

Radiation therapy is often combined with surgical procedures in the treatment of malignant neoplasms. Radiation therapy is used to destroy cancer cells and to attempt to avoid damage to surrounding normal structures. Ionizing radiation damages the DNA in malignant and normal cells. Rapidly dividing cells, such as cancer cells, are especially **radiosensitive**, or able to be injured or destroyed by radiation. A problem occurs with radiation because other types of rapidly dividing normal cells exist in the body, and if the radiation comes in contact with these normal cells, they will also be affected. Epithelial and mucosal cells are the most likely type of cells to be harmed by ionizing radiation, resulting in many side effects, some irreversible.

Chemotherapy is used to destroy cancer cells in several ways. Some treatments interfere with the production of essential cellular components, and others disrupt DNA in both resting and dividing cells. Most often a combination of chemotherapeutic drugs is used to increase the potential for destroying all of the cancer cells. Like radiation therapy, most chemotherapy drugs target rapidly dividing cells. Chemotherapy drugs are very toxic and will affect both normal and malignant cells. The associated side effects of chemotherapy are often unpredictable and can be very intense. While most of the side effects of chemotherapy are reversible, irreversible damage is possible.

Two other forms of therapy, hormone and immunotherapy, are now being used. **Hormone and antihormone therapy** is being used for tumors that require hormones for growth or for those that will not grow in the presence of specific hormones. For example, some breast cancers depend on estrogen for growth; thus, giving an estrogen-blocking drug can impair growth of the tumor. To the contrary, prostate cancer cells will not grow well in the presence of estrogen and estrogen therapy is often used to stop the growth of these tumors. Much research is being done in a new area of treatment called **immunotherapy**, which takes advantage of the body's own immune system to destroy cancer cells. Tumor-specific vaccines are being developed that will initiate a T cell immune response against the tumor. Research is also using antibodies to target certain proteins found on specific cancer cells. Once the antibodies attach to these proteins, the cell is marked for destruction by the immune system. Targeting only the cancer cells with the specific protein spares normal cells that do not exhibit this protein. Most of the substances being developed for this type of treatment are being tested in combination with standard chemotherapeutic agents to maximize their effects.

Research is being done on the effectiveness of other types of therapy on some forms of cancer. The most promising of these include antiangiogenesis therapy, photodynamic therapy, and hyperthermia (ACS, 2005). Antiangiogenesis therapy prevents or inhibits the growth of blood vessels that supply a tumor with nutrients. Photodynamic therapy uses a light source to activate a chemical substance that was introduced into the cancer cells. The light causes the chemical to react with the oxygen within the cancer cell to create a substance that destroys the cell. Hyperthermia uses directed heat to destroy cancer cells or to make them more vulnerable to chemotherapy or radiation therapy.

Many forms of complementary and alternative therapies can be found that have helped many patients manage their disease on a physical as well as psychologic and spiritual level. Complementary therapies focus on pain relief and managing the side effects of therapy, including the psychologic aspects. Alternative therapies are unproved treatments that are sometimes offered as cures. Some alternative therapies may help patients deal with their disease, but only in combination with accepted treatment methods. Box 5.4 provides examples of some of the more common complementary and alternative therapies that are available.

SIDE EFFECTS OF CANCER THERAPY

Each cancer therapy has many potential side effects. Whether or not an individual experiences specific side effects depends on the extent of the therapy and the individual's response to the therapy. Surgical side effects include complete or partial loss of function, form, or aesthetics, depending on the extent and area of surgical intervention.

Box 5.4 COMPLEMENTARY AND ALTERNATIVE THERAPIES

Complementary Therapies

- Acupuncture
- Meditation
- Massage therapy
- Prayer/spirituality
- Yoga
- Reflexology
- Aroma therapy
- Music therapy

Alternative Therapies

- Herbal medicines
- Homeopathy
- Diet and nutritional changes
- Hypnosis
- Tobacco use cessation

Radiation side effects are related to the area that is irradiated and the amount of radiation received. Because radiation affects rapidly dividing cells, the mucosal cells of the gastrointestinal tract are at high risk. One of the most common mucosal side effects is **mucositis**, which manifests as painful ulcerations. Mucositis can occur anywhere mucosal tissues are found (Fig. 5.12). Mucositis of the esophagus, stomach, and intestines can cause bleeding and possible perforation of the lining of these structures. Infections are more likely in areas affected by mucositis because the mucosal barrier is compromised and normal intestinal flora can invade the tissues.

When mucositis occurs in the mouth, it is very painful and will cause the patient to avoid eating. The oral ulcers can become infected with oral bacteria. Several options are available to help patients who are suffering from oral mucositis to eat, because an adequate diet is essential for positive therapeutic outcomes. Refer to Clinical Protocol 13 for treatment options for mucositis. Radiation permanently destroys both the acinar and mucus-producing cells of the salivary glands that are in the field of radiation. The acinar cells are the first to be destroyed, resulting in the production of very thick, viscous saliva that does not have all of the properties it needs to properly protect the oral structures. Continued radiation will also destroy the mucus-producing cells. Both of these together or alone will result in xerostomia. Xerostomia will result in varying degrees of oral discomfort, taste perversions, an increased risk of caries, and difficulty eating, speaking, and wearing prosthetic appliances. Caries associated with xerostomia caused by radiation are called **radiation caries**. Radiation caries first occur around the cervical one third of the teeth and result from an accumulation of acidogenic bacteria, a decrease in the amount of IgA in the saliva, and an impaired natural cleansing mechanism within the oral cavity (Fig. 5.13). The destruction of the salivary glands in radiation therapy is permanent, and patients must continue to deal with the complications of xerostomia for the rest of their lives. Oral complications due to radiation therapy

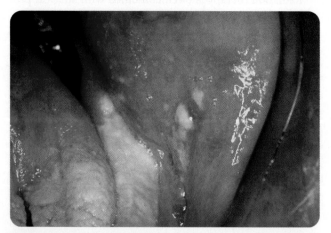

Figure 5.12. Mucositis. Painful oral ulcerations associated with radiation therapy. (Courtesy of Dr. Mike Brennan.)

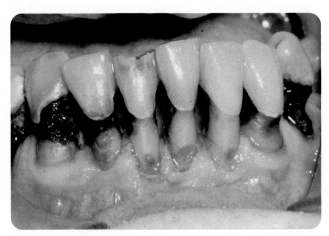

Figure 5.13. Radiation caries. Caries caused by acidogenic bacteria and xerostomia induced by radiation therapy. (Courtesy of Dr. Carolyn Bentley.)

can be controlled and the natural dentition can be maintained if the patient is compliant with a rigorous regimen of fluoride, meticulous homecare, and frequent professional care. Refer to Clinical Protocol 4 for suggestions to help patients with radiation-induced xerostomia.

Radiation therapy that includes the blood-forming bone marrow will cause **bone marrow suppression**, which results in a decrease in white blood cells, red blood cells, and platelets. A decrease in white blood cells increases the patient's risk of acquiring any type of infection. A low red blood cell count results in anemia and fatigue, shortness of breath, and increased demands on the heart and lungs. Drugs are available that will help to increase the number of white blood cells and red blood cells that are produced to help lower the risk of infection and decrease fatigue. A decrease in platelets leaves the patient at risk for uncontrolled bleeding. All patients undergoing radiation therapy have their blood tested routinely for early detection of these deficiencies.

Side effects associated with chemotherapy include most of the same side effects associated with radiation except that they occur in the whole body and not just in the area of the radiation beam. Bone marrow suppression is a side effect of almost all chemotherapeutic agents. The potential for severe depletion of all the different blood cells is high. Therefore, patients are monitored very closely with frequent blood tests and for any symptoms associated with deficiencies. Oral and gastrointestinal mucositis occurs with many chemotherapeutic agents. Nausea and vomiting are almost always expected, and several drugs are available to help counteract this side effect. Severe xerostomia is often a complaint and will cause the same problems as xerostomia associated with radiation therapy; however, unlike the xerostomia caused by radiation, chemotherapy-induced xerostomia will resolve after completion of the therapy. Caries associated with chemotherapy are called **chemocaries**, and the same preventive measures used for radiation caries can be used to control chemocaries. Most chemotherapy patients will undergo

APPLICATION

Aside from providing each patient with a thorough examination to detect possible oral cancers, the dental professional plays an important role in caring for patients who are facing cancer treatment or are undergoing cancer therapy. The extent of this role will be determined in part on the location of the cancer and the type of therapy involved. All cancer patients should have a dental evaluation prior to radiation to the head and neck area and prior to any type of chemotherapy. It is extremely important with any cancer therapy to maintain a healthy oral environment. Healthy oral tissues will decrease the potential for extreme oral side effects and infections resulting from normal oral bacteria. The dental hygienist's main role will be in educating the patient about what to expect and how to deal with some of the oral side effects. In addition, the hygienist may be called upon to help construct custom fluoride trays for the patient. These fluoride trays should be used during chemotherapy and during and after radiation therapy that places the salivary glands in the target area.

temporary **alopecia**, or hair loss, starting within the first 2 to 3 weeks of treatment.

Prevention

Cancer does not have one cause, nor is the risk of getting cancer the same for every individual. Many of the risk factors for cancer are genetic, and many are determined by sex, age, and ethnicity. No one can change these factors. However, some of the risk factors for cancer are modifiable, and each person has the power to decrease or eliminate his or her cancer risk due to these factors. Cancer prevention is not a new concept. For example, tobacco use cessation is the most effective way for individuals to eliminate or decrease their risk of developing many cancers. Refer to Box 5.5 for examples of behaviors that can be modified and may decrease an individual's risk of developing cancer.

COMMON CANCERS

This chapter concludes with a brief description of the most common cancers reported by the American Cancer Society. They include skin (squamous cell and basal cell), melanoma, lung, breast, prostate, and colorectal cancers. Metastatic cancer found in the oral cavity is also discussed. It is hoped that this information will increase the awareness of the dental hygienist about diseases not seen specifically in the oral cavity and that it will aid in patient management. All other oral cancers are discussed in the chapters pertaining to the specific clinical characteristics of the oral lesions. Table 5.4 lists the major forms of oral cancer, the appearance of their characteristic oral lesion, and the chapter in which they are discussed.

- Stop the use of tobacco products
- Proper nutrition
  - Eat a variety of fruits and vegetables every day
  - Reduce the amount of refined grains and sugars consumed
  - Reduce the amount of high-fat red meat consumed
- Maintain a healthy weight throughout life
  - Stay physically active
- Limit alcohol consumption
- Limit sun exposure and use sunscreen or other forms of protection

There are three major forms of skin cancer: basal cell carcinoma, squamous cell carcinoma, and malignant melanoma. Each of these can be visible during the intra- and extraoral examination performed by the dental hygienist. Premalignant sun damage, as well as other visible skin abnormalities, should be brought to the attention of the patient. Any suspicious lesions should be referred for definitive diagnosis by a physician. Clinical Protocol 10 contains suggestions for advising patients about protecting the skin from ultraviolet radiation.

Name: Basal cell carcinoma (BCC)

Etiology: Risk factors associated with BCC include exposure to ultraviolet light, genetic factors, and arsenic ingestion.

Method of Transmission: Not applicable

Epidemiology: BCCs are not reportable for cancer statistics; however, the American Cancer Society estimates that over 1 million cases of BCC and squamous cell carcinoma of the skin will occur in 2005 (ACS, 2005). BCC is the most common skin cancer and accounts for about 75 to 80% of these cases. BCC occurs more frequently in those between 55 and 75 years of age and occurs two times more often in men than in women (ACS, 2005).

Pathogenesis: Basal cell carcinoma starts in the cells of the basal (deep) layer of the epidermis in sun exposed areas. BCC will occur in any area in persons afflicted with nevoid basal cell carcinoma syndrome (Chapter 20, "Radiolucent Lesions") and xeroderma pigmentosum. Xeroderma pigmentosum is an inherited disease in which the person lacks a specific enzyme necessary to repair sun-damaged DNA (Huether, 2004). BCC enlarges slowly, invades the surrounding tissues, and is locally destructive. This type of cancer has a less than 1% metastatic potential (Singh, 2000). There has been at least one published report of a metastatic tumor in recent years (Berlin, 2002).

Extraoral Characteristics: Early BCC presents as a papular growth with a sessile base. As the tumor becomes more nodular in size, features specific to BCC begin to appear. The central area of the nodule becomes depressed, ulcerated, and may become crusted. The borders of the lesion are raised and exhibit a pearly appearance, with a network of small capillaries visible on the surface. The lesions are painless and may have been present for varying lengths of time, depending on the size of the lesion. These tumors are locally destructive and can cause deformities if not treated early (Fig. 5.14).

Perioral and Intraoral Characteristics: BCC rarely appears intraorally. It may appear on the lips or vermilion border where it will have the same characteristic features noted above (Fig. 5.15).

Distinguishing Characteristics: The appearance of this tumor is its most distinguishing feature, the raised

Table 5.4   CHAPTER LOCATIONS FOR THE MAJOR TYPES OF ORAL CANCERS

Type of Cancer	Characteristic Lesion	Chapter
Squamous cell carcinoma	Ulcers and a variety of other presentations	Chapter 12, "Ulcer and Ulcerlike Lesions"
Verrucous carcinoma	Raised, rough	Chapter 16, "Raised Lesions with a Rough or Papillary Surface"
Melanoma	Pigmented	Chapter 15, "Pigmented Lesions"
Mucoepidermoid carcinoma	Soft tissue mass	Chapter 17, "Soft Tissue Enlargements"
Lymphoma	Soft tissue mass and a variety of other presentations	Chapter 9, "Blood Disorders"
Ameloblastoma	Bone enlargement	Chapter 18, "Hard Tissue Enlargements"
Kaposi's sarcoma	Red/purple, raised/flat	Chapter 22, "HIV and AIDS"

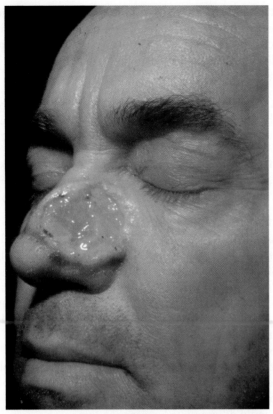

Figure 5.14. Basal cell carcinoma. A neglected basal cell carcinoma of the skin overlying the nose has ulcerated and invaded the deeper tissues. (From Rubin E, Farber JL. Pathology, 3rd ed. Philadelphia: Lippincott Williams & Wilkins, 1999.)

pearly borders with a visible capillary network surrounding a central depressed, crusted area.

Significant Microscopic Features: Not applicable

Dental Implications: When a lesion with the characteristic features of BCC is observed, the patient should be referred to an appropriate physician for evaluation.

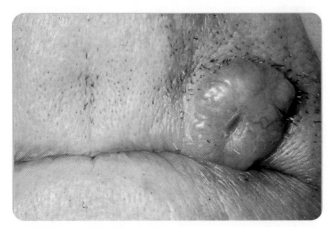

Figure 5.15. Basal cell carcinoma. This tumor on the vermilion border exhibits typical rolled pearly borders with visible capillaries and central ulceration. (From Rubin E, Farber JL. Pathology, 4th ed. Philadelphia: Lippincott Williams & Wilkins, 2005.)

Differential Diagnosis: The following are considerations:

- Actinic keratosis, Chapter 14. This lesion is also caused by sun damage. However, it presents as a plaque or patch of rough scaly skin that appears in a range of colors from yellow to brown or red. Lesions of actinic keratosis do not have rolled pearly borders with visible capillary networks. Advanced actinic keratosis may have a depressed central region, but would still not have the characteristic borders of BCC.
- Keratoacanthoma, Chapter 16. Keratoacanthoma occurs on the sun-exposed skin. It begins as a small red papule that enlarges rapidly over 3 to 6 weeks into a 2- to 3-cm nodule. The rapid development of this lesion along with differences in its appearance differentiates it from BCC.
- Seborrheic keratosis, Chapter 23. Seborrheic keratosis presents in older patients and appears clinically as a scaly brown-to-black plaque with well-defined margins. The lesion looks pasted on and usually has a greasy-feeling crust that can be rubbed off. Seborrheic keratosis does not present with rolled pearly margins that have a visible capillary network like BCC, and BCC does not present with a greasy feeling crust.
- Squamous cell carcinoma. Squamous cell carcinoma of the skin usually occurs on sun-damaged areas. Its early presentation may mimic that of BCC, but it will become ulcerated and scab over as it enlarges. Biopsy is the only way to definitively differentiate between the two.

Treatment and Prognosis: Treatment options for BCC include. surgical excision, laser surgery, cryosurgery (freezing with liquid nitrogen), electrodesiccation (burning), and radiation therapy. Radiation therapy can be used successfully for large tumors, those that involve areas that are difficult to access, or those that present other surgical problems such as tumors on the eyelids. The earlier these cancers are identified, the less invasive the procedures will have to be. The 5-year survival rate for localized BCC is over 99%. If the tumor metastasizes, the 5-year survival rate drops to a dismal 10% (Singh, 2005). Because patients who have had one skin cancer are at a higher risk for another for the rest of their lives, they should be monitored for new lesions on an annual basis.

Name: Squamous cell carcinoma (SCC)

Etiology: Risk factors for squamous cell carcinoma include ultraviolet light, arsenic ingestion, radiation therapy, areas that were previously burned, genetics, and skin diseases or injuries that cause scarring.

Method of Transmission: Not applicable

Epidemiology: SCCs are not reportable for cancer statistics; however the American Cancer Society estimates that over one million cases of SCC and BCC of the skin will occur in 2005. SCC accounts for about 16% of these cases (ACS, 2005). SCC is found most often in fair-skinned older individuals with a history of sun damage to their skin. People living in the sun belt of the United States have a higher risk than those living in areas where the sun's rays are not so intense.

Pathogenesis:
SCC begins in the **keratinocytes** of the outer epidermis. SCC is usually found in areas of sun-damaged skin, and it has an affinity for occurring in lesions of actinic keratosis and in scar tissue caused by burns and some skin diseases, such as discoid lupus erythematosus (Chapter 12, "Ulcer and Ulcerlike Lesions"). Mutations in tumor suppressor gene function are seen in over 90% of SCCs (Regezi, 2003). SCC, like BCC, has a defined in situ stage that may last for many years, increasing the opportunity for early diagnosis. Untreated SCC metastasizes in about 2% of cases, which makes this a more aggressive malignancy than BCC.

Extraoral Characteristics:
SCC often develops in a preexisting actinic keratosis. Early SCC most commonly presents as a painless, nonhealing, rough, erythematic, scaly papule that may cause pruritus or itching. As the lesion enlarges, it becomes indurated because of increased endophytic and exophytic growth. Eventually the surface becomes ulcerated, crusted, and bleeds easily. The surrounding tissues are usually erythematic and inflamed (Fig. 5.16). SCC may not present with these common features. It may look like many nonpathogenic entities or may actually develop within an area affected by another type of lesion. Any area that does not respond to appropriate treatment or does not heal or resolve within a specified time should be biopsied. SCC is as locally destructive as BCC, but because it metastasizes more readily, it is a more dangerous tumor.

Perioral and Intraoral Characteristics:
Perioral lesions of the lip and surrounding area appear the same as described above (Fig. 5.17). Intraoral SCCs are common and are discussed in detail in Chapter 12, "Ulcer and Ulcerlike Lesions."

Distinguishing Characteristics:
Because there is such a range of possible presentations of SCC, any non-healing lesion should be biopsied and identified.

Dental Implications:
Lesions that present as painless, nonhealing ulcers should be suspected as being SCC and should be biopsied.

Differential Diagnosis:
- Actinic keratosis, Chapter 14. Since SCC often develops in a preexisting lesion of actinic keratosis, these lesions should be evaluated by a physician or dermatologist.
- Psoriasis and eczema, Chapter 23. SCC that develops in a person with psoriasis or eczema has often been mistaken for the lesions of these skin diseases. Any lesions from these skin disorders that do not respond to appropriate treatment should be biopsied.
- Basal cell carcinoma. SCC, in its early stages, often looks like BCC, but as SCC grows, the lack of rolled pearly borders with the visible capillary network should differentiate between the two.

Treatment and Prognosis:
Treatment options for SCC include surgical excision, laser surgery, cryosurgery (freezing with liquid nitrogen), electrodesiccation (burning), and radiation therapy. The earlier these cancers are identified, the less invasive the procedures need to be. Radiation therapy can be used successfully for small tumors. It can also delay the growth of large tumors or those that involve areas on which surgery is difficult to perform. Chemotherapy can be used to treat SCC that has metasta-

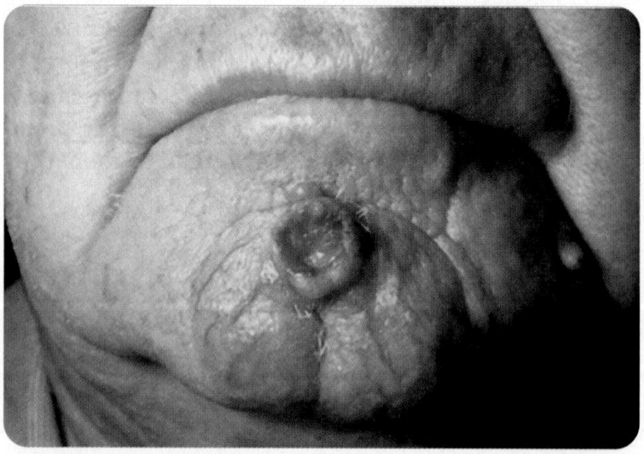

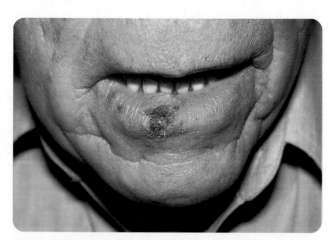

Figure 5.16. Squamous cell carcinoma. Note the exophytic growth and ulceration that this squamous cell carcinoma exhibits. (From Weber J, Kelley J. Health assessment in nursing. 2nd ed. Philadelphia: Lippincott Williams & Wilkins, 2003.)

Figure 5.17. Squamous cell carcinoma. Squamous cell carcinoma presenting as a nodular ulceration of the lip. (From Goodheart HP. Goodheart's photoguide of common skin disorders. 2nd ed. Philadelphia: Lippincott Williams & Wilkins, 2003.)

sized. The 5-year survival rate for localized SCC is over 95%. If the tumor metastasizes, the 5-year survival rate drops to 25% (Singh, 2000). Because patients who have had one skin cancer are at a higher risk for another for the rest of their lives, they should be monitored for new lesions on an annual basis.

Name: Melanoma

Etiology: Refer to Box 5.6 for a summary of the risk factors associated with melanoma.

Method of Transmission: Not applicable

Epidemiology: Only 4% of all skin cancers are melanomas; however, melanoma causes most deaths due to skin cancer. The American Cancer Society estimates that 59,580 new cases of melanoma will be diagnosed in the Unites States in 2005 (ACS, 2005). Most of these will be in 40-to-70-year-olds, but the number of cases in those 20-to-40 years old is increasing. The rate of melanoma development is 10 times higher in Caucasians than in African Americans. Melanoma is most often found on the sun-exposed areas of Caucasians and on non-sun-exposed areas such as the palms and soles of the feet in African Americans (ACS, 2005).

Pathogenesis: Melanoma develops within the melanocytes located deep in the basal layer of the **epidermis** (Fig 5.18) or in a preexisting **benign nevus**, which occurs in approximately 30% of cases. Rarely, melanoma will develop intraorally. Normal melanocytic activity is an innate defense mechanism against ultraviolet radiation damage to nuclear material (DNA) in the skin cells. When

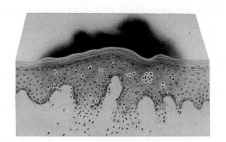

A

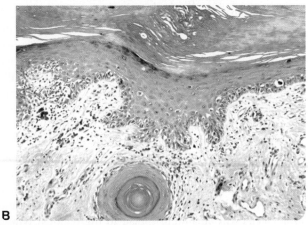

B

Figure 5.18. Melanoma. A. Melanoma develops from melanocytes found in the basal layer of the epidermis. (Provided by Anatomical Chart Co.). **B.** Malignant melanoma. Atypical melanocytes are present along the dermal-epidermal junction, with focal upward growth. (From Rubin E, Farber JL. Pathology, 3rd ed. Philadelphia: Lippincott Williams & Wilkins, 1999.)

Box 5.6 RISK FACTORS ASSOCIATED WITH MELANOMA

Factor	Details
Personal history	A history of dysplastic nevi and/or having a large number of nevi put an individual at a higher risk for melanoma. Individuals who have compromised immune systems and those taking medications that decrease the immune response are also at increased risk
Familial history of melanoma	Even though there is not a strong hereditary association, 10% of cases exhibit defects in two genes, CDKN2A and CDK4, which puts individuals with a family history of melanoma at a higher risk
Ultraviolet radiation	Individuals who work in the sun and/or live in areas that have intense sunlight and those that use tanning beds are at a higher risk for melanoma
Individual characteristics	Fair skin, light hair, blue eyes, and freckles increase an individual's risk up to 2 to 3 times
Previous sunburns	Risk of melanoma increases as the number of severe blistering sunburns that have occurred increases; especially problematic are sunburns that occur at a young age

changes that are associated with known or unknown risk factors occur within the genetic material of the melanocytes, unsuppressed growth of abnormal melanocytes may take place. The growth is initially confined to the epidermis by the basement membrane but will breach the basement membrane eventually. How soon this process will occur depends on the type of melanoma that is developing. There are three major types of melanoma: superficial spreading, nodular, and lentigo maligna. Superficial spreading and lentigo maligna melanomas have two phases of development, radial and vertical. During the radial phase, the tumor spreads out in all directions but remains within the confines of the basement membrane or in situ. Superficial spreading and lentigo melanoma may remain in this phase for years. Eventually a change in the growth potential of some cells will occur, and the major growth pattern will become vertical instead of horizontal. Nodular melanoma has no identifiable radial growth phase. Vertical growth is seen in the initial presentation and throughout the development of the lesion. Nodular melanoma thus has a worse prognosis then either superficial spreading or lentigo maligna melanoma. Vertical growth will breach the basement membrane, and tumor cells will be able to spread to the regional lymph nodes via the lymphatic system. Distant metastases may occur through either the lymphatic or circulatory systems and may present in any area of the body (Fig. 5.19).

Extraoral Characteristics: Melanomas may present with a wide range of clinical characteristics, and many mimic the characteristics of benign pigmented lesions such as the nevus. In its radial phase, the superficial spreading melanoma presents as a variably colored nevus with a slightly raised irregular border. When it enters the vertical phase, growth will occur both through the base-

ment membrane and into the dermis and superior to the basement membrane so that the lesion looks raised. The lesion will start to exhibit a nodular appearance and form raised, variably colored, dome-shaped areas within the original lesion (Fig. 5.20). The lentigo maligna melanoma develops within a preexisting lentigo maligna. Lentigo maligna, sometimes called Hutchinson's melanotic freckle, is a precancerous melanocytic macule that forms on sun-exposed skin and grows slowly over 20 or more years to a large size, often more than 5 cm. The associated melanoma presents as a large, flat, multicolored macule (Fig. 5.21). Although the lentigo maligna melanoma tends to stay in the radial growth phase for many years, it will usually enter the vertical growth phase at some point and exhibit the same dome-shaped nodular formations as in superficial spreading melanoma. The lesions of nodular melanoma exhibit no radial growth phase, and the main focus of growth occurs in the dermis, not the epidermis. Nodular melanoma will form firm dome-shaped lesions that are shiny and blue-black (Fig. 5.22).

Perioral and Intraoral Characteristics: Perioral melanomas will exhibit the same characteristics as those described above. Intraoral lesions are described in Chapter 15, "Pigmented Lesions."

Distinguishing Characteristics: The American Cancer Society has developed an ABCD rule to aid professionals and the general public in identifying suspicious le-

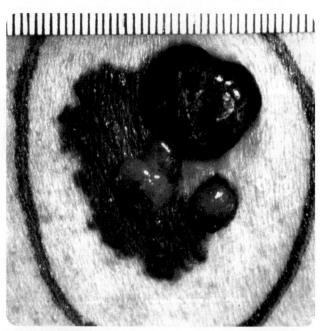

Figure 5.20. Melanoma. Clinically, the radial growth phase in malignant melanoma of the superficial spreading type is represented by the relatively flat, dark, brown-black portion of the tumor. There are three areas in this lesion that are characteristic of the vertical growth phase. All are nodular in configuration; two have a pink coloration, and the largest is rich, ebony black. (From Rubin E, Farber JL. Pathology, 3rd ed. Philadelphia: Lippincott Williams & Wilkins, 1999.)

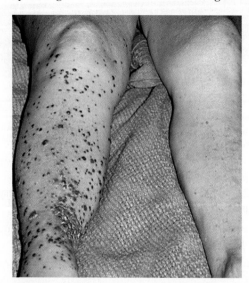

Figure 5.19. Metastatic malignant melanoma. Note the multiple metastatic nodules on this patient's leg. (From Goodheart HP. Goodheart's photoguide of common skin disorders. 2nd ed. Philadelphia: Lippincott Williams & Wilkins, 2003.)

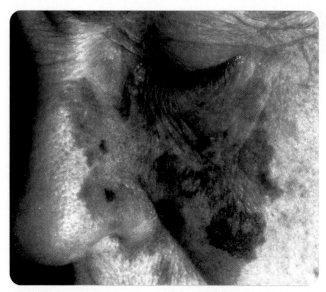

Figure 5.21. Lentigo maligna melanoma. The radial growth phase of lentigo maligna melanoma is shown in this picture. (From Rubin E, Farber JL. Pathology, 3rd ed. Philadelphia: Lippincott Williams & Wilkins, 1999.)

sions (ACS, 2005). See Box 5.7 for an explanation of this rule. If any of the characteristics of a suspicious lesion are similar to those described by the ABCD rule, the lesion should be evaluated by a physician. Patients should also be made aware of the characteristics to observe to monitor their own nevi.

Significant Microscopic Features: Not applicable

Dental Implications: The clinician should observe all visible pigmented areas for the ABCD rule and refer any suspicious areas for evaluation.

Differential Diagnosis: There are many different presentations of melanoma including nonpigmented and red melanomas. Any pigmented lesion that is not identifiable should be biopsied.

- Benign nevus, Chapter 23. Melanoma can mimic a benign nevus. However, a benign nevus will rarely grow

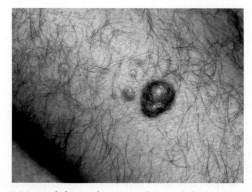

Figure 5.22. Nodular melanoma. This nodule is surrounded with satellite lesions representing local metastasis. (From Goodheart HP. Goodheart's photoguide of common skin disorders. 2nd ed. Philadelphia: Lippincott Williams & Wilkins, 2003.)

after it has reached its mature size, and the borders and colors of the nevus will stay uniform.

- Kaposi's sarcoma, Chapter 22. Kaposi's sarcoma has a more purplish color because of its vascular origin, and there is probably a history of HIV infection or another condition that causes long-term immunosuppression.
- Solar lentigo (liver spot), Chapter 23. The solar lentigo is a hyperpigmented macule that develops on sun-exposed skin. They are usually larger than ephelides, or freckles, but unlike freckles do not fade when not exposed to the sun. Solar lentigines that develop darker pigmentation, thickening, or an irregular border should be evaluated for malignancy.
- Tattoo (pigment introduced into the skin accidentally or by design for body decoration), Chapter 15. The cause for any pigmented area should be determined. Intraoral pigmented lesions may be related to the accidental traumatic introduction of amalgam into the oral mucosa known as an amalgam tattoo.

Treatment and Prognosis: Although melanoma accounts for only 4% of skin cancers, it is responsible for 79% of deaths associated with skin cancer (Melanoma-ASCO, 2005). The prognosis associated with a particular melanoma depends on the thickness of the original, or primary, lesion and whether there has been metastasis to regional lymph nodes or distant metastasis. The thinner and more localized the tumor, the higher the chances of a complete cure. This is why it is so important to identify any suspicious lesion as early as possible. The 5-year survival rate for all melanomas combined is 90%. If the lesion is discovered in the early in situ stage, the 5-year survival rate is 97% (ACS, 2005). Surgery is the treatment of choice for all but the largest or most disseminated cases of melanoma. The smaller tumors are completely excised with a large margin of normal appearing tissue. If the melanoma has spread to even one regional lymph node, all of the nodes in the region must be removed. Radiation therapy is used to increase the quality of life and prolong the life of patients who have advanced metastatic disease. Chemotherapy is used to prolong life and as an adjunct to surgery for tumors that have spread to lymph nodes. Neither radiation nor chemotherapy is used as the primary treatment for melanoma. Other promising treatments being researched at this time include immunotherapy and vaccines that help the immune system identify melanoma cells and destroy them.

Name: Breast cancer

Etiology: Refer to Box 5.8 for a list of risk factors associated with breast cancer development.

Method of Transmission: Not applicable

Epidemiology: The American Cancer Society estimates that approximately 21,240 women in the United States will be diagnosed with invasive breast cancer, and about 40,410 will die from the disease in 2005. An addi-

Box 5.7   ABCD RULE FOR MALIGNANT MELANOMA

Picture	Rule
	Asymmetry One half of the mole does not match the other half.
	Border irregularity The edges of the mole are irregular, ragged, blurred, or notched.
	Color The color over the mole is not the same. There may be differing shades of tan, brown, or black and sometimes patches of red, blue, or white.
	Diameter The mole is larger than 6 mm (about ¼ inch or about the size of a pencil eraser), although in recent years, doctors are finding more melanomas between 3 and 6 mm.

tional 58,490 women will be diagnosed with in situ breast cancer. Most of these women will be over the age of 50. A small number of men are also diagnosed with breast cancer every year. The American Cancer Society estimates that 1,690 men will be diagnosed with breast cancer in 2005 (ACS, 2005).

Pathogenesis: Some 90% of breast cancers begin in the lobules that contain milk glands (lobular carcinoma) or in the ducts that carry the milk to the nipple (ductal carcinoma). Approximately 10% are less common variants of carcinoma, including inflammatory breast cancer and Paget disease of the nipple. Breast cancer probably results from two or three different events occurring throughout the life of the individual. The initial event may involve a change in the DNA structure of the breast cells and may occur very early in the life of the individual, even before the breast develops at puberty or prior to full breast maturity at the end of a successful pregnancy. The second and third events involve chromosomal changes such as

Box 5.8 RISK FACTORS ASSOCIATED WITH BREAST CANCER

Factor	Details
Age	The risk of breast cancer increases with age
Race	More Caucasians are affected than African Americans, but more African Americans die from the disease
Previous history of breast cancer	There is a 3 to 4 times greater risk of breast cancer in the opposite breast after having cancer diagnosed in one breast
Previous history of other hormone-associated cancers	Ovarian and endometrial cancer are examples of other hormone-associated cancers that increase the risk of having breast cancer
Family history of breast cancer	Breast cancer in one primary relative (mother, sister) increases risk; two or more relatives with breast cancer increases that risk even more
Genetic predisposition	Some 2–3% of breast cancers are known to be associated with the BRCA 1 and 2 genes
Estrogen exposure	Early menstruation, late menopause, and the use of hormone replacement therapy increase a woman's overall exposure to estrogen
Lifestyle factors	Obesity, lack of physical activity, and excessive alcohol consumption have all been associated with an increased risk of breast cancer
Radiation	Radiation therapy for other cancers that place the breast in the radiation beam increase the risk for breast cancer in that breast

defective functioning or loss of suppressor genes and/or the creation of oncogenes from protooncogenes. In addition, in approximately 70 to 80% of breast cancers, estrogen exposure is associated with the growth of the tumor. Most tumors occur in the upper outer quadrant of the breast and around the nipple. Local lymph node involvement usually begins with the axial nodes and may extend to the nodes located around the clavicle and the sternum. Common distant metastatic sites include the lungs, kidneys, liver, adrenal glands, ovaries, bones of the spine, ribs, pelvis, and skull, including the maxilla and the mandible.

Extraoral Characteristics: None, unless the clavicular lymph nodes are involved.

Perioral and Intraoral Characteristics: Metastatic breast cancer may present as radiolucent areas in the maxilla or mandible, which may or may not be associated with the roots of a tooth.

Distinguishing Characteristics: Not applicable

Significant Microscopic Features: Not applicable

Dental Implications. These patients should be followed closely to determine the origins of any suspicious intraoral radiographic areas.

Differential Diagnosis: Not applicable

Treatment and Prognosis: Treatment depends on multiple factors including the stage of the disease, familial history, patient preferences, and type of cancer. Most in situ breast cancers are surgically removed during either a lumpectomy or simple mastectomy, removal of just the breast tissue and skin. Invasive or infiltrating cancers are treated with surgery and either chemotherapy, radiation therapy, or both. Often large tumors are treated with chemotherapy to shrink the tumor prior to surgery. Patients who have estrogen-receptive tumors are usually placed on medication that inhibits the production of estrogen by any part of the body for about 5 years following completion of their therapy. The 5-year survival rate for cancer limited to the breast is 97%, 79% if it has spread to the regional lymph nodes, and 23% if it has spread to distant sites (Breast Cancer-ASCO, 2005). It is estimated that 40,410 women and 460 men in the United States will die from breast cancer in 2005 (ACS, 2005).

Name: Prostate cancer

Etiology: The only recognized risk factors at this time are being over 65 years of age, having a family history of prostate cancer, and being of African-American descent.

Method of Transmission: Not applicable

Epidemiology: The American Cancer Society estimates that 232,090 new cases of prostate cancer will occur in 2005. African-American men have a significantly higher incidence than Caucasian men. This is the second leading cause of cancer death in men, with an estimated 30,350 deaths expected in 2005 (ACS, 2005).

Pathogenesis: Most prostate tumors are adenocarcinomas or glandular tumors. Androgens such as testosterone are thought to play a significant role in the development of this cancer. There are no symptoms associated with prostate cancer in the early stages of the disease. More advanced cancers will obstruct the flow of urine from the bladder and cause difficulty in starting or stopping urine flow and in urinary frequency, especially at night. Early detection is the most important factor relative to survival with prostate cancer. It is recommended that men have annual blood tests to detect the prostate-specific antigen (PSA) and an annual digital rectal examination starting at age 50. Examinations should begin even earlier for men at higher risk because of history or ethnicity. An increased level of circulating PSA is associated with progressive disease and also with a recurrence of a treated tumor.

Extraoral Characteristics: None

Perioral and Intraoral Characteristics: None

Distinguishing Characteristics: Not applicable

Significant Microscopic Features: Not applicable

Dental Implications: These patients should be followed closely to determine the origins of any suspicious intraoral radiographic areas.

Differential Diagnosis: Not applicable

Treatment and Prognosis: Treatments include surgery, radiation, chemotherapy, and hormonal therapy. Treatment can lead to temporary or permanent incontinence and varying degrees of sexual dysfunction. The prognosis for prostate cancer found in the early stages is 100% for 5-year survival, 79% for 10-year survival, and 57% for 15-year survival (Prostate Cancer-ASCO, 2005).

Name: Lung cancer

Etiology: Tobacco smoking is the most common cause of lung cancer. Exposure to other occupational or environmental agents can contribute to lung cancer development. Some of these agents include arsenic, radon, asbestos, air pollution, and environmental tobacco smoke.

Method of Transmission: Not applicable

Epidemiology: The American Cancer Society estimates that 172,570 new cases of lung cancer will occur in 2005. Lung cancer is the leading cause of cancer death in both men and women, with 163,510 deaths expected in 2005 (ACS, 2005).

Pathogenesis: Smoking and the associated carcinogens that are contained in the smoke are associated with 80 to 90% of lung cancers. The carcinogens can cause mutations in chromosomes, creation of oncogenes, and defects in tumor suppressor genes. A genetic predisposition is also a factor in the development of lung cancer. Loss of a specific tumor suppressor gene has been determined in 90% of small cell carcinomas (Huether, 2004). Most lung cancers manifest with clinical symptoms such as cough, sputum production, and difficult or painful breathing. These symptoms are associated with most common pulmonary conditions, and most individuals (especially smokers) tend to ignore them until they disrupt their everyday lives. Lung cancer begins in the tissues of the bronchial mucosa and as it grows it will breach the basement membrane and then spread into the local tissues. Eventually, metastasis to the brain, bone marrow, and liver is most likely.

Extraoral Characteristics: Not applicable

Perioral and Intraoral Characteristics: Not applicable

Distinguishing Characteristics: Not applicable

Significant Microscopic Features: Some 95% of primary lung or bronchiogenic cancers comprise four specific histologic types: squamous cell carcinoma, large cell carcinoma, adenocarcinoma, and small cell carcinoma.

Dental Implications: Small cell carcinoma may present with symptoms that are similar to those of Cushing syndrome, in which there is excess production of hormones, specifically cortisol, by the adrenal glands. In lung cancer, these symptoms represent a paraneoplastic syndrome caused by the hypersecretion of adrenal hormones by the tumor cells, not the adrenal glands. This might be important in analyzing health history information and in possible explanations for intraoral and extraoral findings. Specifically, Cushing syndrome presents with muscle weakness, facial edema, hypertension, and increased pigmentation, often around the oral and perioral area. This information added to a history of smoking, chronic cough, and other symptoms might lead to a referral and early diagnosis. Cushing syndrome is discussed in Chapter 7. In addition, dental professionals have the opportunity to help decrease the incidence of lung cancer by providing tobacco cessation information and help during dental appointments. Studies have shown that even brief interventions consisting of the 5 As are effective in helping the individual decide to attempt to quit smoking. The "5 As" of tobacco intervention are listed in Box 5.9.

Differential Diagnosis: Not applicable

Treatment and Prognosis: Treatment options depend on the type of cancer and the stage at which it is diagnosed. Surgery, chemotherapy, and radiation therapy are all possible with combinations of two or more treatments often necessary. Like oral cancer, lung cancer has few if any early symptoms, and by the time symptoms are

Box 5.9   THE "5 As" OF TOBACCO INTERVENTION

The "5 As"	Action
Ask	Ask patients if they use or have used tobacco. Include tobacco use status as a vital sign.
Advise	Advise each tobacco user of the need to stop now, make the message personal and strong. Congratulate nonusers and former users on their tobacco-free status.
Assess	Ask patients if they are willing to quit now or within the next 30 days
Assist	Establish a quit date Provide counseling or arrange for counseling Discuss pharmacotherapeutic options Provide supplementary information and/or materials to help with the quit attempt
Arrange	Follow-up with personal contact by phone or other means to show your interest and concern on the quit date and at weekly or monthly intervals as necessary Provide additional information and referrals Praise patients who are able to stay tobacco-free

From Fiore MC, Bailey WC, Cohen SJ, et al. Treating tobacco use and dependence. Quick reference guide for clinicians. Rockville, MD: U.S. Department of Health and Human Services. Public Health Service. October 2000.

acknowledged, the disease has progressed to more advanced stages. The 1-year survival rate for lung cancer is about 42%; the 5-year survival rate is 15% (Lung Cancer-ASCO, 2005).

Name: Colorectal cancer

Etiology: Risk factors include a history of ovarian, uterine, or breast cancer and a family history of colorectal cancer. Inflammatory bowel disease, smoking, physical inactivity, and obesity may all increase the risk of this cancer.

Method of Transmission: Not applicable

Epidemiology: The American Cancer Society estimates that approximately 145,290 new cases of colorectal cancer will be diagnosed in 2005, and approximately 56,290 people will die of this disease. The highest rate is found in African-Americans, then Caucasians, Asians, American Indians, Alaska natives, and finally Hispanics. The numbers of men and women diagnosed with colorectal cancer are approximately the same. About 90% of colorectal cancers occur in people over the age of 50 (ACS, 2005).

Pathogenesis: Adenomatous **polyps** of the colon and rectum usually precede the development of colorectal cancers. Anything that is associated with the growth of these polyps will be associated with the development of colorectal cancers. Nonsteroidal antiinflammatories,

adequate exercise, and a diet rich in fruits and vegetables and low in red meats may decrease the risk of colorectal cancers.

Extraoral Characteristics: Not applicable

Perioral and Intraoral Characteristics: Peutz-Jeghers syndrome (Chapter 10) is an inherited condition associated with an increased risk of intestinal cancer. Occasionally, these cancers can be found in the colon or rectum (Rubin, 2005). One of the other presenting features of this syndrome is mucosal and perioral brown-pigmented macules, or ephelides. The hands and feet may also be affected by the macular pigmentations.

Distinguishing Characteristics: Not applicable

Significant Microscopic Features: Not applicable

Dental Implications: Oral and perioral melanotic macules in the presence of other historical information such as gastrointestinal problems might lead the clinician to suggest a referral for a definitive diagnosis and appropriate screening examinations.

Differential Diagnosis: Not applicable

Treatment and Prognosis: Surgery is the most common treatment for colorectal cancer. The extent of surgery depends on the extent of the cancer. In situ cancer that is confined to a polyp can be treated by simple removal of the polyp. Cancer that has progressed might necessitate the removal of a portion of the colon or rectum and might require the removal of any involved lymph nodes. As a last resort in extensive disease the surgeon might have to perform a **colostomy** so that wastes can be passed through an opening in the abdomen into a bag. Chemotherapy and radiation therapy can be used in addition to surgical procedures. The 5-year survival rate for cancer that is confined to the bowel wall is 90%, if it has spread to the lymph nodes it is 66%, and if it has metastasized to distant sites it is 9% (Colorectal Cancer-ASCO, 2005).

Name: Oral metastatic cancer

Etiology: Metastatic cancer of any type from any primary tumor. Breast cancer, lung cancer, prostate cancer, and colorectal cancers are the most likely to metastasize to the jaws (Regezi, 2003).

Method of Transmission: Not applicable

Epidemiology: No data available

Pathogenesis: Metastasis to the oral cavity is rare and usually occurs 2 to 3 years after the diagnosis of a primary tumor and completion of appropriate treatment. Metastasis to the mandible is more common than to the maxilla and metastasis to either or both jaw bones is more common than to the oral soft tissues.

Extraoral Characteristics: Not applicable

Perioral and Intraoral Characteristics: Lesions of the jaw bones can present as ill-defined radiolucent or, rarely, radiopaque defects that may or may not be associated with tooth roots Figure 5.23. The patient may experience pain, loosening of the teeth, bone expansion, or growth of a soft tissue tumor. Paresthesia or numbness of the lip or other soft tissue is common, along with an increased risk for pathologic fractures of the jaw.

Distinguishing Characteristics: The ill-defined borders of the lesions is the most significant observation.

Significant Microscopic Features: Not applicable

Dental Implications: Patients who present with a history of cancer should always be examined for any sus-

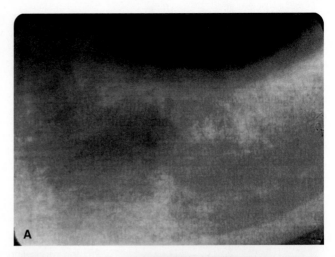
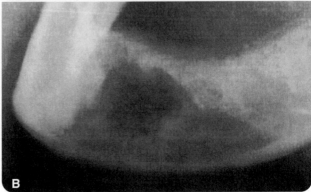

Figure 5.23. Metastatic cancer. Radiograph showing radiolucent lesion with poorly defined margins representing a metastatic breast cancer. (Courtesy of Dr. Robert P. Langlais.)

picious areas in the oral cavity or on any periodic radiographic surveys.

Differential Diagnosis: The differential diagnosis of any of these findings would include primary oral cancer and any similar-appearing bone or oral lesions. Biopsy is necessary for a definitive diagnosis.

Treatment and Prognosis: Treatment for metastatic cancer in the oral cavity is determined by the type of primary tumor and the extent of metastasis. The prognosis for patients with this type of metastasis is very poor, with about 10% reaching 5 years.

SUMMARY

- The three main categories of cells based on their ability to reproduce are labile, stable, and permanent cells. Each cell has a specific growth potential that is genetically determined.
- Some of the genes that control growth include protooncogenes, tumor suppressor genes, and caretaker genes. If a change or mutation occurs in any of these genetic control mechanisms, unregulated growth may occur.
- Genetic mutations initiate the neoplastic process and can cause defective functioning of the tumor suppressor genes and the caretaker genes, resulting in neoplastic growth.
- Protooncogenes can mutate and become oncogenes that also support uncontrolled growth of the affected cells.
- Genetic mutations can be inherited; they can be caused by chemical, environmental, or viral agents; or they can be associated with an immune system defect. There are two types of neoplasia, benign and malignant.
- Benign neoplasms grow locally and are usually encapsulated. They do not metastasize but can still cause death or disability, depending on the location of the tumor.
- Malignant tumors grow by extension into the surrounding tissues. They disrupt the nutrient supply to normal cells and destroy extracellular substances so that tissues in the area are weakened, and the tumor cells can penetrate more easily.
- An epithelial tumor that has not breached the basement membrane is called carcinoma in situ and is highly treatable.
- Cancer cells break off from the primary tumor and move deeper into the tissues, where they spread the disease through the lymphatic and blood vessels to distant sites, in a process called metastasis.
- Cancer can also spread to adjacent organs by movement of the cancer cells through the pleural and abdominal cavities in a process called seeding.
- Neoplasms may be suspected because of symptoms that a patient reports or signs that a healthcare professional observes. Neoplasms may also be detected by one of the many screening methods in use at this time.
- Definitive diagnosis is only made by microscopic examination of tumor cells obtained by excisional, incisional, or other forms of biopsy.
- Benign cells are well differentiated and do not exhibit the structural changes that are seen in malignant cells. Malignant cells exhibit varying degrees of anaplasia, pleomorphism, hyperchromatic nuclei, and other features.
- Pathology reports also define the number of mitotic figures seen in the sample, indicating rapid growth. Other factors are determined during or after surgery or other tests. These factors include whether regional or distant lymph nodes are involved and whether there has been metastasis to a distant site.
- The cancer grading system classifies cells in grades I through IV according to their microscopic features. The higher the cancer grade, the more aggressive a tumor is supposed to be.
- Tumor staging appears to be more reliable in determining probable disease outcomes. Tumor staging systems, such as the TNM system, consider the size of the tumor and whether it has involved the regional lymph nodes and/or has metastasized to a distant site.
- Paraneoplastic syndromes are not common but when present can include some or all of the following: fever of unknown origin, weight loss, anorexia, endocrine imbalances, anemia, leukopenia, thrombocytopenia, blood clots, neurologic problems, fatigue, and pain.
- Surgery is a major form of cancer therapy and is often the initial therapy chosen unless the tumor is too large or is located in an inaccessible area.
- Radiation therapy may be used in conjunction with surgery and/or chemotherapy to help ensure that all cancer cells are eliminated if possible. Radiation affects rapidly dividing cells, which are especially radiosensitive, and either destroys them or destroys their ability to replicate.
- Chemotherapy works in a similar way but may not necessarily target just rapidly dividing cells.
- Hormone therapy can be useful when a tumor depends on a particular hormone for growth or when a tumor will not grow in the presence of a specific hormone.
- Immunotherapy is a relatively new area of treatment that is supposed to enlist our own immune system to destroy the cancer cells and thus spare the body's normal cells.
- Cancer therapies have many associated side effects. Most of the side effects are temporary, but many can be permanent. Surgery can result in loss of function and form. Radiation therapy can cause irreversible damage to salivary glands, reproductive organs, and

(continued)

SUMMARY *(continued)*

other structures. Radiation and chemotherapy cause temporary side effects that increase an individual's risk of getting an infection and can cause oral and gastrointestinal mucositis, caries, nausea, vomiting, and alopecia, among others.

- While many of the risk factors associated with cancer such as age, sex, and ethnicity are unchangeable, many others can be modified, and individuals have the power to decrease their risk of cancer associated with these factors.
- Basal cell carcinoma, squamous cell carcinoma, and melanoma are the three major forms of skin cancer. All forms of skin cancer are associated with UV light damage to the skin.
- Basal cell carcinoma is a slow-growing, locally invasive cancer that appears as a nodular growth with a depressed, ulcerated, or crusted central region surrounded by raised pearly borders that have visible capillaries on their surface.
- Squamous cell carcinoma presents as a painless, nonhealing lesion that may appear as an ulcer, leukoplakia, or erythroplakia, among others. Squamous cell carcinoma is locally destructive and has a high potential for metastasis.
- Melanoma, a less common form of skin cancer, is responsible for the highest number of deaths associated

with any form of skin cancer. Melanomas may be brown, black, red, or unpigmented and may form in a preexisting nevus. The ABCD rule for identifying suspicious pigmented lesions should be used when performing the intra- and extraoral examinations.

- Dental professionals commonly encounter patients who have a history of breast or prostate cancer. It is important to thoroughly examine these patients for any sign of an oral metastatic lesion.
- Lung cancer is the leading cause of cancer death in men and women. Tobacco smoking is the most common cause of lung cancer. Even brief tobacco cessation interventions done in the dental environment may help patients to decide to quit.
- Colon cancer is associated with polyps that form in the colon and rectum. Oral and perioral melanotic macules may indicate Peutz-Jeghers syndrome, which is associated with this type of polyp. Any patient who exhibits this type of oral and/or perioral pigmentation should be referred for medical evaluation.
- Metastatic cancers of any type may manifest in the oral or perioral areas. Any patient with a history of cancer should be thoroughly examined, with any nonhealing or suspicious lesions being referred quickly for evaluation.

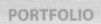

PORTFOLIO ACTIVITIES

1. Make arrangements to visit a support group for cancer patients and/or survivors. Bring information about oral care during and after treatment and be prepared to answer any questions that the participants might have. Talk to the individuals and ask about their dental needs and possible oral side effects of treatment that they are dealing with. Conduct evidence-based research to try to help with

their problems and revisit with them and discuss what you have discovered. Write a short description for your portfolio of your experience, what you think you have learned from the experience, and the individuals with whom you have interacted. How will this experience prepare you for the practice of dental hygiene?

Critical Thinking Activities

1. You have completed an intra- and extraoral examination on an elderly patient and have discovered the lesion depicted in Figure 5.24. Create responses to the following situations:
A. Mr. Nantz is a new patient, and you do not know him at all. Write a dialogue that will not only help you to get to know Mr. Nantz, but will also educate him about suspicious skin lesions and the importance of complying with a referral to a physician.

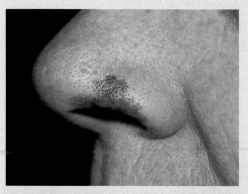

Figure 5.24. Case Study. Lentigo maligna melanoma. Biopsy of this lesion demonstrated invasion into the dermis. (From Goodheart HP. Goodheart's photoguide of common skin disorders. 2nd ed. Philadelphia: Lippincott Williams & Wilkins, 2003.)

B. Mr. Yarrington has been seen in your office every 3 to 4 months for the last 10 years. He is partially deaf, has poor eyesight, and is confined to a wheelchair. He prides himself on his ability to take public transportation to his medical/dental appointments and thus not be as much of a burden on his daughter, who works. This is the first time you have seen Mr. Yarrington in several years. You have looked in his dental record and have found no mention of this obvious lesion. (1) What would be the best way to inform Mr. Yarrington about this suspicious lesion? (2) What can you do to make sure lesions like this are noted in the dental record and that appropriate follow-up procedures are used in the future?

2. This chapter has introduced many cancers that are not included in any area that a dental hygienist might examine. How far do you think a dental professional can go with this knowledge? Can it be used to suggest that patients of a certain age group be screened for prostate cancer, for example? Would you feel comfortable discussing risk factors for breast cancer with your female patients? Write down what you think you could incorporate into your practice of dental hygiene and how you would incorporate it. Share this with the rest of the class and enjoy a good exchange of opinion and ideas.

Case Study

Study Figures 5.25 and 5.26
1. Write a clinical description of the lesions seen in these figures. The consistency for Figure 5.25 is fluctuant, and that of Figure 5.26 is indurated.
2. One of these is a common skin cancer. Pick the one that you think is the cancer and decide which type

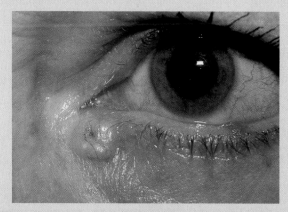

Figure 5.26. Case study. (From Tasman W, Jaeger E. The Wills Eye Hospital atlas of clinical ophthalmology. 2nd ed. Baltimore: Lippincott Williams & Wilkins, 2001.)

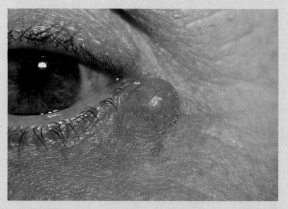

Figure 5.25. Case Study. (From Tasman W, Jaeger E. The Wills Eye Hospital atlas of clinical ophthalmology. 2nd ed. Baltimore: Lippincott Williams & Wilkins, 2001.)

of skin cancer you think it is. What elements of the clinical description were the major factors in your decision?
3. Which of these would you want to refer for a biopsy?

INTERNET RESOURCES

People Living with Cancer
American Society of Clinical Oncology
www.plwc.org/portal/site/PLWC

American Cancer Society
www.cancer.org

Washington Musculoskeletal Tumor Center
www.sarcoma.org

American Joint Committee on Cancer
www.cancerstaging.org

The University of Texas MD Anderson Cancer Center
www.mdanderson.org

Centers for Disease Control and Prevention
www.cdc.gov

Sarcoma Alliance
www.sarcomaalliance.com

Johns Hopkins Medicine
www.hopkinshospital.org/health_info/Cancer/

REFERENCES

American Cancer Society. Cancer Facts and Figures 2005. Atlanta: American Cancer Society; 2005.

American Cancer Society. Cancer Prevention & Early Detection Facts and Figures 2005. Atlanta. American Cancer Society; 2005.

American Cancer Society. American Cancer Society history. Available at *http://www.cancer.org/docroot/AA/content/AA_1_4_ACS_History.asp? sitearea=AA&vie*. Accessed December 13, 2004.

Ames BN, Wakimoto P. Are vitamin and mineral deficiencies a major cancer risk? Nature Rev 2002;2:694–703. Available at *www.nature.com/reviews/cancer*. Accessed June 23, 2004.

Berlin JM, Warner MR, Bailin PL. Metastatic basal cell carcinoma presenting as unilateral axillary lymphadenopathy.   Report of a case and review of the literature. Dermatol Surg 2002;28:1082–1084.

Blackburn GI, Copeland T, Khaodhiar L, Buckley RB. Diet and breast cancer. J Womens Health 2003;12(2):183–192.

Breast cancer. People living with cancer, American Society of Clinical Oncology. Available at. http://www.plwc.org/plwc/cancer_type/cancer_type_print_all_articles/1,2122,1,00.html . Accessed June 13, 2005.

Brody JG, Rudel RA. Environmental pollutants and breast cancer. Environ Health Perspect 2003;111(8):1007–1019.

CancerWise. How to do a skin self-exam. The University of Texas MD Anderson Cancer Center. Available at. http://www.cancerwise.org/May_2002/display.cfm?id=7A03902D-BA4B-43AF-895176704B413D6C&method=displayFull&color=green . Accessed June 5, 2005.

Coleman EA, Hutchins L, Goodwin J. An overview of cancer in the older adult. Medsurg Nurs 2004;13(2):75–109.

Colorectal cancer. People living with cancer. American Society of Clinical Oncology. Available at http://www.plwc.org/plwc/cancer_type/cancer_type_print_all_articles/1,2122,3,00.html. Accessed June 30, 2005.

Cotran RS, Kumar V, Collins T. Robbins pathologic basis of disease. 6th ed. Philadelphia. WB Saunders, 1999:260–327, 741–750, 833–835, 1104–1117, 1027–1033, 1177–1179, 1184–1187.

Ferenczy A, Coutlée F, Franco E, Hankins C. Human papillomavirus and HIV coinfection and the risk of neoplasia of the lower genital tract: a review of recent developments. Can Med Assoc J 2003;169(5):431–434.

Finley RS. Overview of targeted therapies for cancer. Am J Health-Syst Pharm 2003;60(Suppl 9):s4–s10.

Fiore MC, Bailey WC, Cohen SJ, et al. Treating tobacco use and dependence. quick reference guide for clinicians. Rockville, MD: U.S. Department of Health and Human Services. Public Health Service. October 2000.

Goldie MP. Oral cancer. Accessed April 2002, 32–38.

Greene FL, Page DL, Fleming ID, et al. AJCC cancer staging manual. 6th ed. New York: Springer-Verlag, 2002:24–25.

Gurenlian JR. The brush biopsy: a chairside technique for early detection of oral cancer. Access September/October 2003;32–36.

Houghton AN, Guevara-Patino JA. Immune recognition of self in immunity against cancer. J Clin Invest 2004;114(4):468-471.

Huether SE, McCance KL. Understanding pathophysiology. 3rd ed. St. Louis: Mosby, 2004:237–286, 779–782, 919–925, 927–941, 1154–1157.

Key TJ, Allen NE, Spencer EA, Travis RC. The effect of diet on risk of cancer. Lancet 2002;360:861–868.

Lamanna LM. College student's knowledge and attitudes about cancer and perceived risks of developing skin cancer. Dermatol Nurs 2004;16(2):161–176.

Luba MC, Bangs SA, Mohler AM, Stulberg DI. Common benign skin tumors. Am Fam Physician 2003;67(4):729–737.

Lung cancer. People living with cancer, American Society of Clinical Oncology. Available at. http://www.plwc.org/plwc/cancer_type/cancer_type_print_all_articles/1,2122,4,00.html . Accessed June 5, 2005.

Mahon SM. Patient education regarding cancer screening guidelines. Clin J Oncol Nurs 2003;7(5):581–584.

Melanoma. People living with cancer, American Society of Clinical Oncology. Available at. http://www.plwc.org/plwc/cancer_type/cancer_type_print_all_articles/1,2122,46,00.html. Accessed June 5, 2005.

Melanoma skin cancer, American Cancer Society. Available at: http://www.cancer.org/docroot/CRI/content/CRI_2_4_7x_CRC_Melanoma_Skin_Cancer_PDF.asp . Accessed June 5, 2005.

Nonmelanoma skin cancer, American Cancer Society. Available at. http://www.cancer.org/docroot/CRI/content/CRI_2_4_7x_CRC_Non melanoma_PDF.asp . Accessed June 13, 2005.

PLWC feature: understanding targeted treatments. People living with cancer, American Society of Clinical Oncology. Available at. http://www.plwc.org/plwc/Shared/plwc_ArticleViewPrint/1,1890,36762,00.html . Accessed June 13, 2005.

Porth CM. Essentials of pathophysiology. concepts of altered health states. Philadelphia: Lippincott Williams & Wilkins, 2004: 64–83, 367–369, 489–491, 594–597, 623–625, 853–856.

Powe BD, Finnie R. Knowledge of oral cancer risk factors among African Americans. Do nurses have a role? Oncol Nurs Forum 2004;31(4):785–791.

Price SA, Wilson LM. Pathophysiology: clinical concepts of disease processes. 6th ed. St. Louis: Mosby, 2003:109–125, 363–364, 623–628, 975–980, 992–993, 1097–1105.

Prostate cancer. People living with cancer, American Society of Clinical Oncology. Available at. http://www.plwc.org/plwc/cancer_type/cancer_type_print_all_articles/1,2122,5,00.html . Accessed June 12, 2005.

Rankin KV, Jones DL, Redding, SW, eds. Oral health in cancer therapy. 2nd ed. Texas Cancer Council, 2004:43–52.

Regezi JA, Sciubba JJ, Jordan RCK. Oral pathology. Clinical pathologic correlations. 4th ed. St. Louis: WB Saunders, 2003:392–393, 397–399, 409–427.

Rubin E, Gorstein F, Rubin R, et al. Rubin's pathology. Clinicopathologic foundations of medicine. 4th ed. Baltimore: Lippincott Williams & Wilkins, 2005:165–213, 646–654, 727–731, 918–925, 1006–1015, 1247–1255, 1259–1261.

Saliva: A test for oral cancer. J Dent Hyg Spring 2003;77(II):79.

Scarpa R. Advanced practice nursing in head and neck cancer. Implementation of five roles. Oncol Nurs Forum 2004;31(3): 579–583.

Schmitt CA. Senescence, apoptosis and therapy: cutting the lifelines of cancer. Nature Rev 2003;3:286-294. Available at *www.nature.com/ reviews/cancer* . Accessed October 15, 2004.

Sekido Y, Fong KM, Minna JD. Molecular genetics of lung cancer. Annu Rev Med 2003;54:73–87. Available at *http://med.annualreviews.org* . Accessed July 24, 2004.

Sharpless NE, DePinho RA. Telomeres, stem cells, senescence, and cancer. J Clin Invest January 2004;113(2):160–167.

Singh N, Lim RB, Sawyer MA. The cell cycle. Hawaii Med J 2000;59(7):300–306.

Skin cancer (nonmelanoma). People living with cancer, American Society of Clinical Oncology. Available at. http://www.plwc.org/plwc/ MainConstructor/1,1744,_04-0017-00_12-001042-00_21-008,00.asp . Accessed June 3, 2005.

Stedman's medical dictionary for the health professions and nursing. Illustrated 5th ed. Baltimore: Lippincott Williams & Wilkins, 2005.

Stem cell information. The Official National Institutes of Health Resource for stem cell research. Available at. http://www.stemcells. nih.gov/. Accessed May 27, 2006.

TNM Cancer Staging. International Union Against Cancer. Available at. *http://www.uicc.org/index* . Accessed May 28, 2006.

6

Developmental, Hereditary, and Congenital Disorders

Key Terms

- Allele
- Aneuploid
- Anodontia
- Autosomal
- Barr body
- Bossing
- Carrier
- Centromere
- Chromatin
- Chromatid
- Chromosome
- Codominance
- Congenital
- Deletion
- Developmental disorder
- Diploid
- Dominant
- Echocardiogram
- Epicanthal fold
- Euploid
- Expressivity
- Fetus
- Gamete
- Gene
- Genome
- Genotype
- Gorlin's sign
- Haploid
- Hereditary/inherited
- Heterozygous
- Homologous
- Homozygous
- Hyperhidrosis
- Hypertelorism
- Hypodontia
- Hypotelorism
- Intermediate expression
- Inversion
- Karyotype
- Locus
- Macroglossia
- Monosomy
- Morphogenesis
- Mosaicism
- Multifactorial inheritance
- Nondisjunction
- Penetrance
  Complete
  Incomplete
- Periosteum
- Phenotype
- Photophobia
- Polymorphism
- Prognathism
- Pseudoanodontia
- Recessive
- Simian crease
- Somatic
- Telomere
- Teratogen
- Teratology
- Trait
- Translocation
- Trisomy
- Xerophthalmia
- Zygote

Chapter Objectives

1. Define and use the key terms in this chapter.

2. Compare and contrast developmental, hereditary, and congenital disorders.

3. Provide examples of teratogenic agents and describe how a teratogenic agent may affect morphogenesis.

4. Describe the inheritance pattern of autosomal dominant disorders and of autosomal recessive disorders.

5. Describe the inheritance pattern of X-linked disorders.

6. Discuss the concept of multifactorial inheritance.

7. State the etiology, method of transmission, and pathogenesis of the disorders discussed in this chapter.

8. Describe the characteristics of developmental, hereditary, and congenital disorders.

9. Describe the dental implications and appropriate dental care modifications associated with the disorders discussed.

Chapter Outline

The terms "developmental," "hereditary," and "congenital" are often used incorrectly. **Developmental disorders** occur when there is a disturbance in the development of the body that results in an abnormality. The developmental abnormality can be very severe and cause spontaneous abortion or miscarriage or it can be very minor and cause few, if any, problems. **Hereditary** conditions are caused by a genetic abnormality that can be passed from generation to generation. Many hereditary conditions are not compatible with life and result in a spontaneous abortion or early infant death; others can be very mild and not even noticed. **Congenital** abnormalities, sometimes called birth defects, are present at or around the time of birth and can be caused by a variety of factors, as listed in Box 6.1. A congenital abnormality could be hereditary or developmental, as long as it is present at or around the time of birth. Hereditary and developmental conditions not obvious at birth can become manifest later in life. This chapter focuses on an overview of developmental and genetic concepts and a description of the more common developmental and hereditary disorders. Specific dental disorders are discussed in those chapters that are associated with the clinical appearance of the conditions. Table 6.1 lists the most common developmental and hereditary dental disorders and the chapters in which they are found.

Box 6.1 ETIOLOGIES OF CONGENITAL ABNORMALITIES

The etiology of most congenital abnormalities is unknown, with hereditary conditions accounting for the largest number of known causes.

Causes of congenital abnormalities

Unknown	70%
Hereditary	20%
Chromosomal abnormalities	4%
Drugs, chemicals, radiation	2%
Maternal infection	2%
Maternal metabolic factors	1%
Birth trauma and uterine factors	1%

From Rubin E, Gorstein F, Rubin R, et al. Rubin's pathology: clinico-pathologic foundations of medicine. 4th ed. Baltimore: Lippincott Williams & Wilkins, 2005. Figure 6-2, p. 217.

CONCEPTS OF DEVELOPMENTAL ABNORMALITIES

Teratology is the study of developmental anomalies that take place during fetal development (Rubin et al., 2005). The agents that cause developmental anomalies are called **teratogens**. Teratogens can be chemical, biologic, or physical in nature. Table 6.2 lists some of the known teratogenic agents and examples of disturbances they may cause. Many of these abnormalities are due to errors in **morphogenesis**, the differentiation of embryonic cells that determines form and function of organs and parts of the body. The human body is especially vulnerable to teratogenic agents during morphogenesis. Figure 6.1 indicates critical stages in the development of specific organs and systems. Development of the **fetus** technically starts at the end of the 8th week of gestation; prior to that the fetus is called an **embryo**. Errors in morphogenesis occur in-utero and can take many forms such as

- Agenesis: The complete or partial absence of an organ or part of the body
- Dysraphic abnormality: Anomaly caused by the failure of opposing structures to fuse
- Involution failure: The existence of embryologic structures that should have been destroyed by the body at a certain stage of development
- Division failure: The failure of certain structures to divide or cleave during fetal development
- Atresia: Failure of a lumen to form, causing a structure that should be hollow to be constricted or solid
- Ectopia: The development of structures away from the normal site

Table 6.1   DEVELOPMENTAL AND HEREDITARY ORAL DISORDERS

Disorder	Type of Disorder	Chapter
Cherubism	Hereditary	Chapter 10
Epidermolysis bullosa	Hereditary	Chapter 11
Congenital hemangioma	Developmental	Chapter 13
Vascular malformations	Developmental	Chapter 13
Hereditary hemorrhagic telangiectasia	Hereditary	Chapter 13
White sponge nevus	Hereditary	Chapter 14
Neurofibromatosis	Hereditary	Chapter 17
Multiple endocrine neoplasia syndrome	Hereditary	Chapter 17
Lymphangioma	Developmental	Chapter 17
Cervical lymphoepithelial cyst	Developmental	Chapter 17
Thyroglossal tract cyst	Developmental	Chapter 17
Dermoid cyst	Developmental	Chapter 17
Osteopetrosis	Hereditary	Chapter 18
Gardner syndrome	Hereditary	Chapter 19
Hypophosphatasia	Hereditary	Chapter 21
Osteogenesis imperfecta	Hereditary	Chapter 21
Dentinogenesis imperfecta	Hereditary	Chapter 21
Amelogenesis imperfecta	Hereditary	Chapter 21

- Dystopia: The failure of an embryologic structure to move into its final adult position during development

Teratogens can cause multiple abnormalities in multiple organs or systems, depending on whether exposure to them occurs when more than one developmental process is going on. Defects in multiple systems and/or organs can also occur when a single change takes place that affects other developmental processes farther along in time.

Agenesis of the thyroid gland not only affects *embryogenesis*, development of the embryo, and fetal development but causes *congenital hypothyroidism*, a developmental defect that severely stunts growth and causes mental retardation in the child (Chapter 7). The effect of teratogenic agents is greatly reduced after the 12th week of gestation, when most of the crucial morphogenesis is completed.

Chapter 21

Table 6.2   TERATOGENIC AGENTS

Listed are examples of teratogenic agents and some of the congenital abnormalities that they are associated with.

Teratogen	Example
Alcohol	Fetal alcohol spectrum defects
Tobacco	Low birth weight, preterm birth, spontaneous abortion, sudden infant death syndrome
Cocaine	Preterm birth, growth retardation, central nervous system infarctions, seizures, genitourinary and gastrointestinal tract abnormalities
Heroin	Low birth weight, addiction at birth, learning disabilities, personality dysfunctions
Warfarin	Congenital central nervous system defects and nasal hypoplasia
Thalidomide	Absent or flipperlike arms and legs
Accutane (isotretinoin)	Craniofacial abnormalities, cleft lip and/or palate, micrognathia, cardiac and central nervous system abnormalities
Anticancer drugs	Multiple congenital abnormalities, spontaneous abortion
Tetracycline	Inhibits bone growth, intrinsic dental staining
Paramyxovirus (mumps)	Orchitis, oophoritis, male and female sterility
Maternal diabetes	High birth weight, neural tube defects, cleft lip and/or palate, respiratory distress syndrome, congenital heart defects
Maternal folic acid deficiency	Neural tube defects, anemia, cleft lip and/or palate
Systemic lupus erythematosus	Congenital heart block, stillbirth

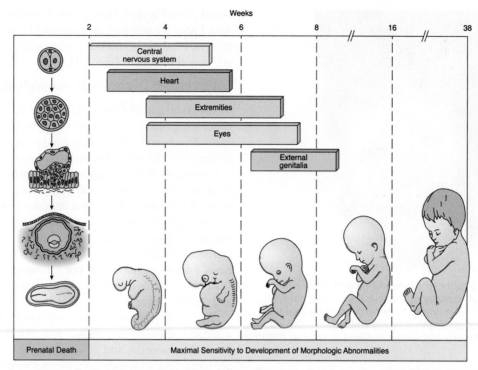

Figure 6.1. Sensitivity of specific organs to teratogenic agents at critical stages of human development. Exposure to teratogenic agents in the preimplantation and early postimplantation stages of development *(far left)* leads to prenatal death. Periods of maximal sensitivity to teratogens *(horizontal bars)* vary for different organ systems but overall are limited to the first 8 weeks of pregnancy. (From Rubin E, Farber JL. Pathology. 3rd ed. Philadelphia: Lippincott Williams & Wilkins, 1999.)

Developmental Disorders

The following are two examples of developmental disorders that may be encountered during dental hygiene practice. Remember that these are not representative of most errors in morphogenesis which can be as harmless as a folded ear or as severe as anencephaly, in which the brain does not develop.

Name: Fetal alcohol spectrum defects (FASD)

Etiology: FASD is an umbrella term describing the range of effects that can occur in a person who was exposed to alcohol, a teratogenic agent, during pregnancy (NOFAS, 2006). This is not a diagnostic term; it encompasses the following diagnoses:
- Fetal alcohol syndrome (FAS)
- Alcohol-related neurodevelopmental disorder (ARND)
- Partial fetal alcohol syndrome (PFAS)
- Alcohol-related birth defects (ARBD)
- Fetal alcohol effects (FAE)

There is no specific amount of alcohol that is known to produce FASD nor is there a safe time to indulge in alcohol ingestion during pregnancy. Each individual is affected by alcohol differently; FASD may affect the child of a mother who only drank three beers a day on the weekends, while another child born to a woman who drank two beers a day throughout her pregnancy is not affected at all.

Method of Transmission: FASD cannot be transmitted from person to person.

Epidemiology: Not all of the diagnoses under FASD have statistical data available. FAS is estimated to occur in 1 to 2 infants in 1000 live births. If this number included the number of children without the syndrome but with fetal alcohol effects (FAE), a milder expression of FAS with fewer abnormalities, the rate would rise to about 1 in 300 births (Dittmer et al., 2004; Lewanda, 2003). The incidence increases in children born to mothers who drink heavily during pregnancy. FAS affects all races but has a significantly higher incidence among Native Americans (Lewanda, 2003).

Pathogenesis: Alcohol crosses the placenta and is maintained at the maternal concentration level for extended lengths of time. The alcohol is also stored in the amniotic fluid, increasing the exposure of the fetus to the alcohol. The exact mechanism responsible for all of the abnormalities that are associated with this syndrome and affect almost every organ and system in the body is not known (Dittmer et al., 2004; Lewanda, 2003).

Extraoral Characteristics: Three general groups of abnormalities must be present for a child to be diagnosed with FAS. The child must have growth problems, characteristic facial features, and neurodevelopmental problems. The list of potential abnormalities is extensive; only the most common and characteristic defects are discussed in

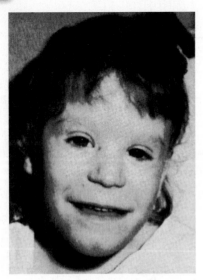

Figure 6.2. Fetal alcohol syndrome. Child with fetal alcohol syndrome illustrating many of the characteristic facial features. These children may also have cardiovascular and limb defects. (Sadler T. Langman's medical embryology, 9th ed. Image Bank. Baltimore: Lippincott Williams & Wilkins, 2003.)

this text. Children with FAS have microcephaly (a small head), are short in length, are underweight at birth, and continue to be significantly shorter in stature than their peers throughout life. The characteristic facial features include narrow eyes with epicanthal folds, short nose with a turned-up end, and thin upper lip with an indistinct flat philtrum area (Fig. 6.2). Neurodevelopmental problems include the following: mild-to-moderate mental retardation (lower IQ), attention deficit and hyperactivity disorders, learning disabilities, language impairment, poor coordination, poor judgment, behavior problems, and poor social skills. Other common problems include seizure disorders, eye disorders, hearing loss, congenital heart defects, and an increased risk for certain cancers (Dittmer et al., 2004).

Perioral and Intraoral Characteristics:
In addition to the characteristic facial features discussed above, cleft lip and/or palate may be present.

Distinguishing Characteristics:
The facial features at birth are distinctive for this syndrome. As the child ages and progresses into adulthood these features become less obvious.

Significant Microscopic Features:
Not applicable

Dental Implications:
Knowledge of the facial features characteristic of FASD is very important. A dental professional may be able to connect the features with observable behavior and facilitate the diagnosis of a previously undiagnosed case. It is crucial to identify these individuals as early as possible to initiate intervention therapies to help them reach their highest potential. In addition, the dental hygienist might be able to counsel pregnant patients about the effects of alcohol on the unborn child. The dental profes-

sional should review the medical/dental history of a patient with FASD for any sign of congenital heart defects and determine what medications are being taken prior to initiating any dental treatment (Box 6.2).

Differential Diagnosis:
Not applicable

Treatment and Prognosis:
The damage done by alcohol exposure is permanent. Congenital defects such as heart defects and oral clefting can be corrected surgically. Behavior modification therapies and a structured learning environment that is sensitive to the needs of these children are crucial. Children are often treated with medications (Ritalin and others) that are used to alleviate behavioral symptoms that are similar to those seen in attention deficit disorder. Working with children who have FASD can be very difficult, but also very rewarding. The prognosis for these children is not measured in terms of life span but in terms of quality of life. Between the ages of 21 and 51, 95% have mental health problems, 55% are incarcerated or institutionalized for substance abuse or mental disorders, 60% are in conflict with the law, 82% cannot live independently, and 50% of men and 70% of women are struggling with their own alcohol or drug abuse problems (Dittmer et al., 2004).

Box 6.2   HEART DEFECTS AND DENTAL CARE

Certain heart defects that change the character of the flow of blood through the heart place the individual who has the defect at a higher risk of developing an infection of the valves and tissues within the heart (endocarditis). The source of this infection is usually bacteria that have found their way into the bloodstream, causing a bacteremia (bacteria in the blood). The oral cavity is a major source of bacteria. The oral environment is normally separated from the blood by the mucous membranes lining the entire oral cavity. When these membranes become compromised or injured because of infection or trauma, bacteria are allowed to pass into the blood. When the dental hygienist performs scaling procedures, the membranes can be compromised. The chance of creating a bacteremia increases when there is periodontal or gingival infection present. For example, it is very easy to create a bacteremia during normal brushing and flossing when infection is present. The American Heart Association has recommended a prophylactic antibiotic regimen to try to prevent the development of endocarditis in susceptible individuals such as those with heart defects. This regimen should be followed prior to providing dental care for patients who are at risk for developing this infection. More on this topic can be found in Chapter 8.

Name: TORCH syndrome

TORCH is an acronym that refers to a number of pathogenic agents that cause similar developmental abnormalities in the embryo or fetus if the mother is infected with the specific organisms during pregnancy.

Etiology: The organisms that cause the following infections are the etiologic agents for the disorders in this syndrome:

T—Toxoplasmosis
O—Other infections such as syphilis, tuberculosis, and Epstein-Barr and varicella-zoster viruses
R—Rubella
C—Cytomegalovirus
H—Herpesvirus

Method of Transmission: These infectious agents are transmitted to the fetus or neonate across the placenta or during passage through the birth canal in all cases except for herpesvirus, which is almost always acquired during birth.

Epidemiology: TORCH organism infections occur in about 1 to 5% of live births and are a major cause of abnormalities and death in neonates (Rubin et al., 2005).

Pathogenesis: Rubella, cytomegalovirus, herpesvirus, Epstein-Barr, and varicella-zoster are all viral infections. Syphilis and tuberculosis are bacterial infections, and toxoplasmosis is caused by a protozoan. The mechanisms responsible for producing the pathology associated with the TORCH syndrome are specific for each of the different organisms and not crucial to understand this syndrome.

Extraoral Characteristics: General characteristics associated with defects caused by most of the TORCH agents include the following: premature birth, encephalitis, microcephaly, hydrocephaly, mental deficiency, hearing loss, visual impairment, enlarged liver, anemia, thrombocytopenia (bleeding disorder), rash, petechiae and bruising, congenital heart diseases, and pulmonary problems (Rubin et al., 2005). There are additional abnormalities associated with each specific organism; however, only those that occur in the oral cavity are mentioned here.

Perioral and Intraoral Characteristics: Congenital syphilis will cause the permanent incisors to have a notched incisal edge, called *Hutchinson incisors*, and the first permanent molars to have an abnormal occlusal surface that looks like a cluster of berries, thus the name *mulberry molars* Figure 6.3. Perinatal herpes infections can present with vesicular lesions on the oral and perioral mucosa.

Distinguishing Characteristics: Not applicable

Significant Microscopic Features: Not applicable

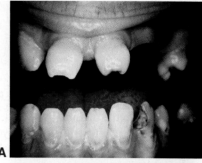
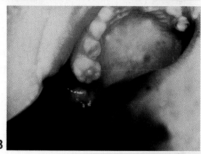

Figure 6.3. Oral manifestations of congenital syphilis, one of the TORCH syndrome disorders. **A.** Hutchinson incisors. **B.** Mulberry molars. (From Sweet RL, Gibbs RS. Atlas of infectious diseases of the female genital tract. Philadelphia: Lippincott Williams & Wilkins, 2005.)

Dental Implications: Dental considerations should focus on prophylactic antibiotic medication for cardiac abnormalities and any other treatment modifications that may be necessary because of elements of the syndrome. Pregnant patients could be counseled about the need for appropriate vaccinations and the need to be cautious around substances that could contain or harbor these organisms, such as cat litter, or sex partners with recurrent herpes infections.

Treatment and Prognosis: The best treatment for this syndrome is prevention. Dental care depends on the specific abnormality involved. Hutchinson incisors can be crowned or otherwise esthetically restored to make them look normal; mulberry molars do not normally require any treatment. Prognosis also depends on the specific abnormality involved, such as mental deficiencies, sensory losses, and heart defects.

OVERVIEW OF GENETIC CONCEPTS

The science and technology of genetics are progressing at a phenomenal pace. More and more information about genes and the human **genome**, the genetic composition of a haploid set of human chromosomes, is being discovered. In 1990 Congress gave 3 billion dollars to the National Institutes of Health (NIH) and the U. S. Department of Energy (DOE) to map the genes in the human body. The Human Genome Project (HGP) was completed in April 2003. The HGP resulted in finding and mapping approximately 20,000 to 25,000 genes to their locations on spe-

Box 6.3 — THE MINIMUM STANDARD FOR GENETICS EDUCATION

The National Coalition for Health Professional Education in Genetics has proposed a minimum standard for current genetics education. The American Dental Hygienists' Association is listed as a Member Organization of this coalition.

Each health-care professional should at a minimum be able to

- Appreciate limitations of his or her genetics expertise
- Understand the social and psychological implications of genetic services
- Know how to make a referral to a genetics professional

Taken from Core competencies in genetics essential for all health-care professions, National Coalition for Health Professional Education in Genetics. Available at: http://www.nchpeg.org/eduresources/core/Corecomps2005.pdf.

cific chromosomes (HGP, 2005). Healthcare professionals are responsible for integrating this information into their specific professions. In 2005 a group called the National Coalition for Health Professional Education in Genetics released a revised set of Core Competencies in Genetics (NCHPEG, 2005). The competencies encompass not only knowledge, but skills and attitudes related to genetics. The curriculum in dental hygiene programs does not allow complete coverage of this topic at this time; however, the Coalition suggests a minimum standard of knowledge as stated in Box 6.3. The information and activities in this text are focused toward helping students to meet this standard.

Chromosomes

People inherit their characteristics from their ancestors through the genetic material contained within the sperm and egg cells contributed by each of their parents. The genetic material is called **chromatin** and is comprised mainly of deoxyribonucleic acid (DNA). This genetic material is found in the nuclei of most human cells. All human cells, other than the sperm and egg cells, divide by mitosis, which results in identical copies of the original cell. Sperm and egg cells divide by meiosis, which results in genetically different cells containing only one half of the genetic material needed for life; the other one half being supplied by the other parent at fertilization. The phases of mitosis and meiosis are depicted in Figure 6.4. Chromatin is replicated during interphase. Prior to cellular division the chromatin forms a tightly coiled structure called a **chromosome**. Each chromosome has a constricted area, called a **centromere**, which is constant for that chromosome. The centromere

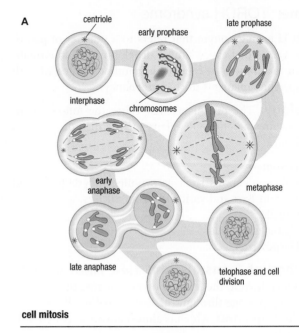

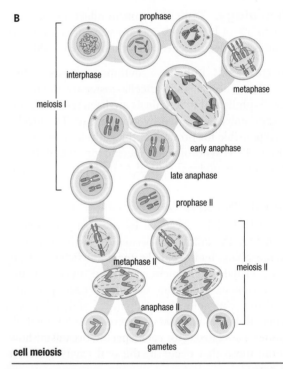

Figure 6.4. Stages of mitosis and meiosis. **A.** Mitosis results in the creation of an identical sister cell. (With permission, from Cohen BJ, Wood DL. Memmler's the human body in health and disease. 9th ed. Philadelphia: Lippincott Williams & Wilkins, 2000.) **B.** Meiosis results in four haploid cells. In the female there is one egg and three polar bodies and in the male there are four sperm cells created.

separates the chromosome into a short arm, or *p-arm*, and a long arm, or *q-arm*. During metaphase, the centromeres of two sister (one original and one replicated) chromosomes will join and attach the chromosomes to the spindle fibers. When joined together, each pair of sister chromo-

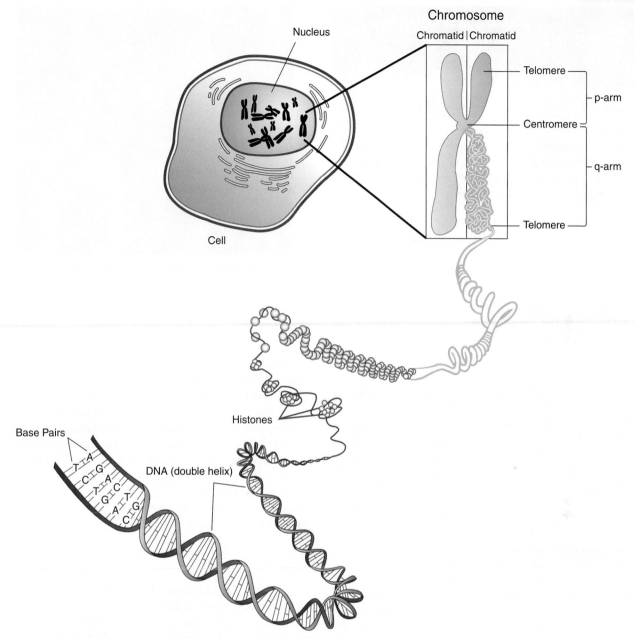

Figure 6.5. The chromosome during mitosis. Chromatin material coils into familiar chromosome structure prior to mitosis. The chromosome is composed of two identical chromatids joined at their constricted areas, or centromeres. The short arm created by the centromeres is the p-arm; the long arm is called the q-arm. The ends of each chromatid are called telomeres. (Courtesy of the National Human Genome Research Institute.)

somes is called a single chromosome and each vertical half of that chromosome is called a **chromatid** (Fig. 6.5). The end of each arm of the chromosome is called a **telomere**, end cap. The telomere appears to have a very important role in the reproductive capacity of most cells. Every time a cell undergoes mitosis, the telomeres get smaller; when they are almost gone, the chromosome's DNA becomes unstable, and the cell ceases to function. Scientists are researching this concept, since it appears that cancer cells have the capacity to repair the telomeres, thereby preventing cell death and enabling uncontrolled reproduction (Huether and McCance, 2004).

Based on the number of chromosomes, human cells can be classified into two main types: **somatic** cells and **gametes.** The human body is comprised of somatic cells from the top of the head to the tip of the toes. Each somatic cell has 46 chromosomes or 23 pairs of chromosomes, one paternal and one maternal set. The 46 pairs of chromosomes make these **diploid** cells. Gametes are the reproductive or sex cells, ovum and sperm. Each gamete has 23 single chromosomes, or half the genetic complement of a somatic cell. The single set of 23 chromosomes makes the gametes **haploid** cells. To further define chromosomal makeup, each somatic cell contains 22 pairs of

Box 6.4	COMPARISON OF GAMETE AND SOMATIC CELLS	

Gamete	Somatic cells
22 autosomal chromosomes	22 pairs of autosomal chromosomes
1 sex chromosome	1 pair of sex chromosomes
Found only as ova or sperm	All cells except ova and sperm

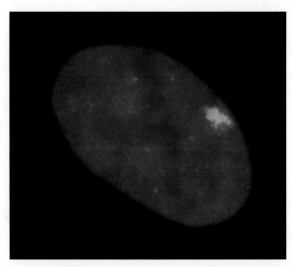

Figure 6.6. Barr body. Every normal female somatic cell contains one Barr body within the nucleus. This is a micrograph of a fibroblast nucleus. The dense spot at the nuclear periphery is the Barr body. The Barr body stains more intensely because the DNA of the inactive X is more compact. (Courtesy of Gayle Pageau.)

autosomal chromosomes that regulate almost everything that the body is and does and one pair of sex chromosomes that not only determine sex but also have a few other important functions. Each gamete has 22 single autosomal chromosomes and a single sex chromosome. Box 6.4 illustrates the chromosomal difference between gametes and somatic cells.

SEX CHROMOSOMES

The sex chromosomes make up one pair of the 23 pairs of chromosomes. Males have one each of the X and Y (XY) chromosomes, while females have two X chromosomes (XX). The female carries two of each gene on the X chromosome. The male, however, carries only one X chromosome and thus has only one copy of the genes on that chromosome. Any **trait** (characteristic or attribute) controlled by a gene that is found on a man's X chromosome will be expressed.

X CHROMOSOME INACTIVATION

As noted above, females normally receive two X chromosomes, and males receive one. It could be presumed that women would therefore have a double dose of functioning genes on those chromosomes. However, this is not the case for most of the genes on the X chromosome. Following research on this topic, in 1961 Mary Lyon proposed that approximately 7 to 14 days after fertilization one of the X chromosomes in each cell becomes inactivated, or turned off, and forms what is called a **Barr body.** This proposal is known as the *Lyon hypothesis* and has been proved correct. The Barr body (Fig. 6.6) is tightly compressed genetic material from the second X chromosome that is found close to the inner wall of the nuclear membrane and can be seen in cytology smears under a microscope but cannot be seen by the naked eye. Normal females have one Barr body per cell, normal males have none. There is no pattern as to which chromosome is inactivated in the cells of the embryo; one cell may inactivate the X chromosome contributed by the mother, while another will inactivate the X chromosome contributed by the father. The inactivation is permanent, and all of the cells that develop from that embryologic cell will have the same inactive X chromosome. That means that an adult woman will have somatic cells that contain either an active X chromosome from her mother or one from her father but not both. To make matters even more interesting, not all of the genes on the inactive chromosome are inactive. There are about 18 genes that are the same on both the X and Y chromosomes. These 18 or so genes remain active in the Barr body and thus allow women to have the same total active gene count as men (Huether and McCance, 2004; Rubin et al., 2005).

Genes

The genetic material in the chromosomes is arranged into areas that function as a unit to create a specific protein or enzyme. This functional unit is called a **gene.** The location of the gene on the chromosome is called the **locus.** Thus the maternal genes for eye color and the paternal genes for eye color would be located at the same locus on opposing chromatids of a chromosome. The gene involved with a specific single gene disorder would be found at the same locus of opposing chromatids as well (Fig. 6.7). Each opposing gene is called an **allele** of the other; together they are called alleles. A **karyotype** is a picture of a collection of the 46 chromosomes from one of an individual's cells. One of the purposes of a karyotype is to show whether an individual has too many or too few chromosomes (Fig. 6.8).

Elements of Genetics

The genetic makeup of an individual consisting of the genes on all 46 chromosomes is called the **genotype** of the indi-

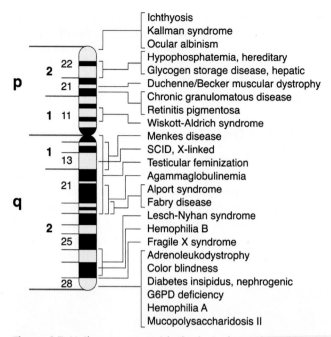

Figure 6.7. X Chromosome with the loci of specific genes identified. The location of representative inherited disorders on the X chromosome. Genes that are located at the same locus on homologous chromatids are called alleles. (From Rubin E, Farber JL. Pathology. 3rd ed. Philadelphia: Lippincott Williams & Wilkins, 1999.)

vidual. How the specific individual's body functions and what the person looks like physically is called the **phenotype**. When the alleles at a specific locus are identical, the individual is said to be **homozygous** for that genetic trait, when they are different, the individual is **heterozygous** for the trait. Some genes are **dominant**, that is they will express the trait whether the individual is homozygous or heterozygous for that trait. To the contrary, identical **recessive** genes must be present in both alleles for a recessive trait to be expressed. An individual who is heterozygous for a particular genetic trait may be a **carrier** of a recessive trait, disorder, or disease. Carriers do not usually exhibit characteristics of the gene in their phenotype, but they are able to transmit the gene to the next generation. If the partner of the carrier is also a carrier, then it is possible to have a child who will exhibit the full phenotypic expression of the recessive trait. Occasionally carriers will benefit from being heterozygous or having one recessive gene and one dominant gene, as is the case with sickle cell trait (Chapter 9).

Intermediate expression occurs when an individual who is heterozygous for a particular trait exhibits neither of the homozygous phenotypes but exhibits a trait somewhere between the two. For example, male voice pitch is controlled by a specific gene; when the alleles are homozygous, the voice is either a high or low pitch, when the alleles are

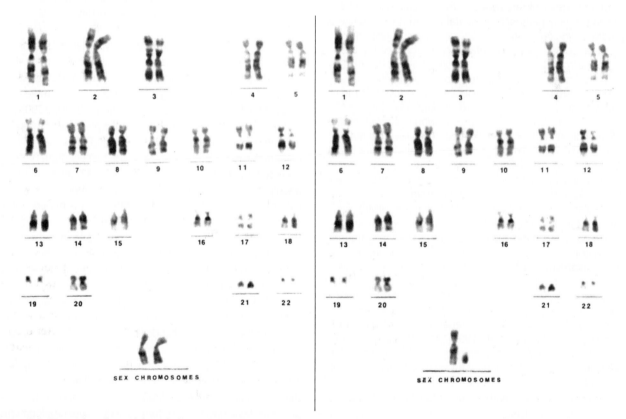

Figure 6.8. Normal male and female karyotypes. Photomicrographs of human chromosomes arranged in a standard classification. If a blood sample is taken from a child or adult and the white blood cells are examined at the mitotic division phase of reproduction, transferred to slides, and photographed under high-power magnification, the individual chromosomes can be cut from the photograph and arranged according to size and shape. **A.** Normal female karyotype. **B.** Normal male karyotype. (From Pillitteri A. Maternal and child nursing. 4th ed. Philadelphia: Lippincott Williams & Wilkins, 2003.)

heterozygous the voice is a baritone or middle range. Both alleles of the same gene can be equally expressed through **codominance.** An example of codominance can be seen in the inheritance of blood type. An individual who has the allele for type A and the allele for type B blood will exhibit type AB blood. Two other concepts that are quite important in understanding how an individual exhibits genetically controlled traits are penetrance and expressivity. **Penetrance** refers to the number of people that have the genotype for a specific trait and who exhibit the expected characteristics or phenotype. *Complete penetrance* describes a genotype that is always portrayed in the phenotype. *Incomplete penetrance* refers to the number of individuals who have the same genotype as above but who do not exhibit the characteristics or the phenotype expected of those who have this genotype. They may transmit the genetic trait to the next generation, who also may or may not exhibit the expected phenotype. **Expressivity** refers to variations with which individuals even within the same family may exhibit the phenotype of an identical genetic trait. Refer to Table 6.3 for an example of how these traits are expressed in the phenotype of individuals.

Hereditary Disorders

There are two potential sources of hereditary disorders, the chromosome and the genes contained within it. Chromosomal abnormalities can involve either the *number* of chromosomes or the *structure* of the chromosome. Disorders caused by gene abnormalities can be inherited from one or both parents, or they can be the result of a spontaneous mutation in a gamete or an early fetal cell.

APPLICATION

Information from the Human Genome Project has an impact on the practice of dentistry. The most obvious use for this information is in research to find ways to eliminate craniofacial, oral, and dental disorders and diseases that are genetic. However, this is not the only use for this information. Dental professionals are aware of the intricate balance between bacterial pathogens in dental biofilm, the presence of predisposing/contributing factors, and the host response in the development of periodontal disease. Some of the predisposing/contributing factors include: smoking, diabetes, nutrition, immune system dysfunction, and genetic predisposition. Some researchers are looking at a cluster of three genes located on the long arm of chromosome 2 in region 13, which they hope will help predict who will develop periodontal disease. The cluster of three genes controls the amount of interleukin-1 (IL-1) that is produced by the body in response to a bacterial challenge. IL-1 is a cytokine that can not only take part in an inflammatory response but can also increase the action of two other enzymes, prostaglandin E_2 (PGE$_2$) and metalloproteinase (MMP). All three of these substances have been associated with the bone and collagen destruction observed in severe periodontal disease. Individuals who do not have a variation, or **polymorphism,** in the IL-1 cluster (IL-1 genotype negative) do not produce an excessive amount of the three enzymes. People who are positive for a variation in the IL-1 cluster (IL-1 genotype positive) will overproduce all of these substances whenever they respond to a bacterial challenge for the rest of their lives (Kornman et al., 1997). As with any new information, more research on using genetic polymorphism as a predictor of periodontal disease needs to be done. Some of the findings of studies done thus far include:

- This gene variation tends to run in families (Kornman and di Giovine, 1998).
- IL-1 genotype positive is a strong predictor of severe periodontal disease in nonsmokers between the ages of 40 and 60 years (Kornman et al.,1997).

- Sixty-seven percent of those that had severe periodontal disease in one study were IL-1 genotype positive (Kornman and di Giovine, 1998).
- Individuals who are IL-1 genotype positive had a higher percentage of virulent periodontal pathogens than those who were IL-1 genotype negative (Socransky et al., 2000).
- Within a population of individuals who had had guided tissue regeneration 4 years previously, 73% of those IL-1 genotype negative had stable postoperative results, while only 21% of those IL-1 genotype positive had stable postoperative results (De Sanctis and Zucchelli, 2000).

Currently there is a genetic test for the presence of this gene called the periodontal susceptibility test (PST). It is used to help determine if individuals are at higher risk for periodontal disease because they are IL-1 genotype positive. DNA testing is done on a sample of buccal cells obtained by rubbing the cheek with a cotton swab. After the sample is obtained, it is mailed to the company and in about 2 days a detailed report is mailed out (Hein, 2005). This information can be used to identify an increased risk for disease, enabling hygienists and other dental professionals to develop individualized education and treatment plans for their patients to help prevent disease. Another area of research focuses on the genetic makeup of the bacteria involved in dental diseases. In fact, an *effector* or mutated strain of *Streptococcus mutans* that does not produce the enamel-dissolving acid that the original strain does has already been developed. The idea is to replace the original strain with the new effector strain that does not produce acid, thereby decreasing the potential for caries (Hein, 2005). It is the responsibility of the dental professional to keep informed about these developments and to bring them into their practices after their validity and usefulness have been determined.

Table 6.3   COMPARISON OF GENOTYPE WITH PHENOTYPIC EXPRESSION

B, Blue hair (dominant) y, yellow hair (recessive)	Genotype	Phenotype
Homozygous dominant	BB	Blue hair
Heterozygous dominant	By	Blue hair
Homozygous recessive	yy	Yellow hair
Intermediate expression (blending)	By	Green hair
Codominance (both B and y are expressed)	By	Blue and yellow hair
Incomplete penetrance	By	Yellow hair
Variable expressivity	BB or By	Navy blue hair Periwinkle hair Sky blue hair

Every time a cell divides there is a potential for something to go wrong. As discussed above, a small number of human cells undergo genetic changes regularly. These cells are usually destroyed by the body or not allowed to replicate; thus there is little chance of catastrophic consequences. However, if that genetic change or mutation occurs in a gamete or in one of the very early cells in the **zygote** or **embryo**, the results can be disastrous, since all of the cells that are generated by the mutated cell will have the same mutation.

ABNORMAL NUMBER OF CHROMOSOMES

A **euploid** cell has the correct number of chromosomes. As mentioned above, autosomal cells have 46 chromosomes (1 pair each of 23 chromosomes) and are called diploid cells. Gametes have 23 single chromosomes and are called haploid cells. Both gametes and autosomal cells with the correct number of chromosomes are considered euploid cells. An autosomal cell with an entire extra set of chromosomes or 69 instead of 46 is a triploid cell; one with four sets or 92 is a tetraploid cell. Most pregnancies affected by either of these abnormalities will result in spontaneous abortion or stillbirth.

In some cases, cells may not have an entire extra set of chromosomes but may have one or more extra individual chromosomes, or they may be missing one or more individual chromosomes. This condition is called aneuploidy, and the abnormal cells are called **aneuploid** cells. **Trisomy** results when there are three of any chromosome (Fig. 6.9),and **monosomy** results when there is only one chromosome instead of two. Monosomy of any of the somatic cells will not support life. Likewise a zygote or cell resulting from conception that contains no X chromosomes will not survive. Generally, missing chromosomal material is much more serious than extra chromosomal material. Abnormalities in the number of chromosomes are usually caused by **nondisjunction**, or failure of paired chromosomes to separate and migrate to opposite poles during anaphase. This process creates monosomy in the cell without the chromosome and trisomy in the cell with too many chromosomes.

ABNORMALITIES IN CHROMOSOME STRUCTURE

Not only can an abnormal number of chromosomes cause disorders, but also the structure of a chromosome can be altered in a way that will cause disease or disorders. Structural abnormalities are caused by chromosome breakage, followed by a rearrangement or loss of the parts that broke off. The cause of these structural abnormalities is mostly unknown, but exposure to radiation, viruses, and other environmental agents is being studied. Several of the more common structural changes that can take place are listed below.

- Deletion—When a portion of a chromosome is lost, it is called **deletion**. Deletion can occur any time there is a break in a chromosome (Fig. 6.10A).

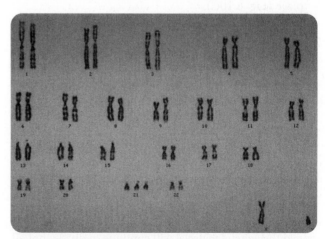

Figure 6.9. Karyotype of Trisomy 21. Trisomy 21 in the karyotype of a child with Down syndrome. All other chromosomes are normal. (From Rubin E, Farber JL. Pathology. 3rd ed. Philadelphia: Lippincott Williams & Wilkins, 1999.)

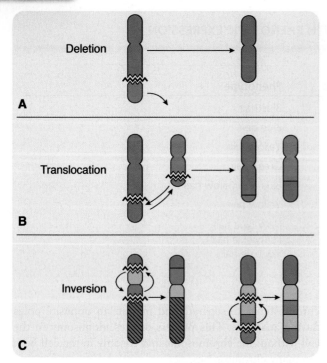

Figure 6.10. Abnormal chromosome structures. **A.** Deletion of genetic material results in a shorter chromosome with missing genetic material. **B.** Translocation occurs when there is a break in two chromosomes and the genetic material is switched between them. **C.** Inversions occur when there are two breaks in the same chromosome and the resulting piece of genetic material is turned upside down and reinserted. (From Rubin E, Farber JL. Pathology. 3rd ed. Philadelphia: Lippincott Williams & Wilkins, 1999.)

- Translocation—**Translocation** occurs when parts of two chromosomes are exchanged (Fig. 6.10B). For example, the short arm of chromosome 4 is exchanged with the long arm of chromosome 5.
- Inversion—An **inversion** occurs when there are two breaks in a chromosome and the resulting piece is inverted or turned around and reinserted in the same place (Fig. 6.10C).

In translocation and inversion there is no loss of genetic material, and the individual will function normally; however, when egg or sperm cells are produced, abnormal cells containing either too little genetic material or too much genetic material will result.

MOSAICISM

When an egg is fertilized, the resulting diploid cell divides into two cells and then again into four cells and so on. Genetic **mosaicism** is created when a cell in the very early development of the embryo loses or gains genetic material. The amount of loss or gain can vary from an entire chromosome to a single gene. The cell that has lost or gained the genetic material will continue to divide, but all of the future cells will have the identical genetic material. Thus an individual born with genetic mosaicism will have a variable percentage of abnormal cells mixed in with nor-

mal cells, depending on when the actual loss or gain of genetic material occurred in the development of the embryo (Fig. 6.11). Mosaicism is a key concept because it accounts for some of the variations that are seen in most genetic disorders. For example, classic trisomy 21, or Down syndrome, occurs when an individual is created from a fertilized egg that has an extra copy of chromosome 21. This individual will express the classic clinical signs of Down syndrome. If, however, the fertilized egg did not contain any extra genetic material but an error occurred in one cell after several divisions, then the individual who

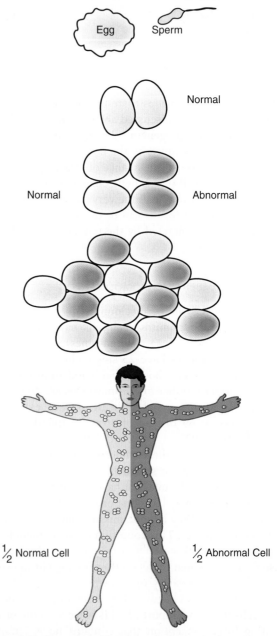

Figure 6.11. Mosacism. Mosaicism is created when an error in early embryologic cell division causes the development of two different genotypes within the same individual. The earlier the error occurs, the higher the number or percentage of abnormal cells.

develops will have a mixture of normal and abnormal cells. This person would likely exhibit milder signs of Down syndrome than one who has all abnormal cells.

Name: Trisomy 21 (Down syndrome, Down's syndrome)

Etiology: Chromosome disorder in which there is either one complete or one partial extra copy of chromosome 21.

Method of Transmission: Nondisjunction during the development of the egg accounts for about 95% of cases of trisomy 21. Translocation of the long arm of chromosome 21 to another chromosome accounts for 3–5%, and mosaicism accounts for 2% or less (Huether and McCance, 2004).

Epidemiology: There were approximately 350,000 individuals with trisomy 21 living in the United States in 2002. Trisomy 21 will occur in one of every 800 to 1000 live births. The incidence of trisomy 21 increases with the age of the mother; at 25 there is a 1:1300 chance of trisomy 21, 1:400 at 35, 1:110 at 40, and 1:35 at 45 (NDSS, 2005). Trisomy 21 does not occur more frequently in males or females and race and social or economic status of the parents do not appear to be factors in the occurrence of this disorder. Once a child with trisomy 21 has been born, there is a 1:100 chance that a future pregnancy will result in another child with the syndrome.

Pathogenesis: The extra genetic material from the third chromosome may cause overproduction of important proteins associated with those genes. Chromosome 21 contains from 200 to 250 genes, and there are more than 9 genes on this chromosome that if overexpressed could lead to the development of the characteristic features seen in trisomy 21 (OMIM #190685 Down Syndrome, 2005).

Extraoral Characteristics: Individuals with trisomy 21 are affected with varying degrees of mild-to-severe mental impairment, which unfortunately progresses as the individual ages. In addition, virtually all individuals will exhibit brain abnormalities consistent with those of Alzheimer disease and over half will manifest clinical signs of dementia as they grow into their 40s and 50s.

Congenital heart defects are seen in at least 33 to 50% of cases. Most of these involve defects between the chambers of the heart and mitral valve prolapse. There appears to be an increased susceptibility to infections, most likely caused by a problem with immune function. Respiratory infections are unusually common and severe in this group; the most common are upper respiratory infections, ear infections, bronchitis, and pneumonia (March of Dimes, Down syndrome, 2005). Some 50 to 90% of affected individuals have varying degrees of hearing and vision problems (March of Dimes, Down syndrome, 2005).

Leukemia is seen 10 to 20 times more often in the trisomy 21 population than in the general population (OMIM Down Syndrome #190685, 2005).

Physically, individuals are shorter than normal, with poor muscle tone and lax joints. Their hands are stubby, with a shorter than normal little finger and a single transverse crease across the palm called a **simian crease**. The face appears flat with a prominent forehead. The eyes are set close together (**hypotelorism**) and slant upward. There is a fold of skin beginning at the root of the nose and extending to the beginning of the eyebrow called an **epicanthal fold** (Fig. 6.12).

Perioral and Intraoral Characteristics: Hypoplasia, or underdevelopment of the midface, is characteristic of trisomy 21. The bridge of the nose is flattened. The frontal and maxillary sinuses may be smaller than normal or entirely absent. Intraorally, the palate is high, narrow, and shortened from anterior to posterior, contributing to the appearance of mandibular **prognathism**, or protrusion, because the mandible has developed normally. Individuals often have posterior crossbites and severe crowding of the anterior teeth. Patients with trisomy 21 have a characteristic open mouth posture that was once thought to be the result of **macroglossia**, enlarged tongue, but is now considered to be the result of a small nasopharynx and enlarged tonsils and adenoids that compromise the upper air passages. While there is no true macroglossia, the tongue does protrude because the mouth is so small. The tongue is usually fissured but has no definable central fissure.

Anterior open bites are very common in this population and are thought to be caused by the lack of lip muscle tone and the pressure of the protruding tongue. Constant mouth breathing and the protruding tongue cause xerostomia and cracking and drying of the lips. Cleft lip and palate have a higher than average incidence in this population.

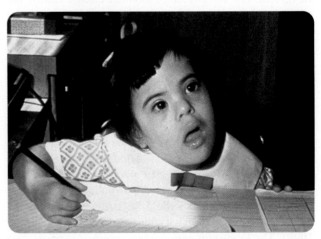

Figure 6.12. Trisomy 21. A young girl exhibits the typical facial features of this syndrome. (From Rubin E, Farber JL. Pathology. 3rd ed. Philadelphia: Lippincott Williams & Wilkins, 1999.)

Abnormalities of the dentition are common and varied. Eruption of the primary and permanent dentition is delayed, and the eruption sequence may be abnormal (Regezi et al., 2003; Pilcher, 1998). Hypodontia, missing one or more teeth, in both primary and permanent dentitions is very common (Pilcher, 1998). Abnormal tooth and root development and enamel hypocalcification is also common. The caries rate in trisomy 21 is approximately the same or slightly lower than that in the general population (Pilcher, 1998).

The incidence of periodontal disease has been reported to range from 60 to 100% in individuals under the age of 30 affected by trisomy 21 (Yoshihara et al., 2005). Decreased immune system function coupled with the presence of important periodontal pathogens is thought to be the underlying cause of the disease in this population.

Distinguishing Characteristics: The appearance of the face is the most distinguishing clinical feature of this syndrome.

Significant Microscopic Features: Not applicable.

Dental Implications: Dental professionals need to be very careful in their initial assessment of the medical history of individuals affected by trisomy 21. Cardiac defects, especially mitral valve prolapse, can develop as the individual ages, so that even if one did not have a defect as a child, it could be present as a adult. The AHA standard antibiotic prophylactic regimen should be followed to prevent infective endocarditis in susceptible individuals (Chapter 8).

Preventive oral hygiene care and frequent preventive care or maintenance appointments should be stressed to minimize the potential for a self-induced bacteremia. Care should also be used in preventing inhalation of oral pathogens to reduce the possibility of acquiring a respiratory infection. Dental care should be regular, and preventive home care methods should be taught to the patient and caregivers. The severity of periodontal disease can be decreased and the process slowed with proper home care and regular periodontal debridement (Yoshihara et al., 2005).

Differential Diagnosis: Not applicable

Treatment and Prognosis: Medical or surgical treatment for conditions such as heart defects is completed as soon as is practical. Cleft lip and palate are treated the same as for any child born with the condition. The child with trisomy 21 needs to be followed closely by a team of healthcare providers including, but not limited to, those in the medical, dental, vision, hearing, and speech fields. Extensive cosmetic, orthodontic, and/or reconstructive treatments should be made available to the person according to what they can manage (Pilcher, 1998). The long-term periodontal prognosis is poor.

Life expectancy of a child born with this syndrome depends on the presence and severity of heart defects. Some 25% of those with significant heart defects die before the age of 10, while only 5% without the defects die before age 10. After this age, the life expectancy is about 20 years less than that in the general population, with only about 10% surviving into their 70s (Rubin et al., 2005).

Name: Klinefelter syndrome (testicular dysgenesis)

Etiology: Classic Klinefelter syndrome is caused by an extra X chromosome in the male genotype (XXY). Variations of this grouping are possible and may include up to four extra X chromosomes.

Method of Transmission: The extra chromosomes seen in Klinefelter syndrome are due to nondisjunction in the egg cell in 50 to 60% of cases. The chances of this occurring increase as the age of the mother increases.

Epidemiology: Klinefelter syndrome occurs in about 1 of every 500 to 1000 live births. It occurs equally across all races. However, by definition, it occurs only in males (Chen, December 2004).

Pathogenesis: The abnormalities seen in Klinefelter syndrome are a result of altered male and female hormone levels. There is a deficit of testosterone, which results in underdevelopment or absence of secondary sexual characteristics at puberty. Because there is no production of testosterone, the levels of luteinizing and follicle-stimulating hormones are elevated. These hormones stay elevated because the negative feedback system keeps telling the hypothalamus that there is no testosterone, and the hypothalamus keeps sending the signal to produce it. The severity of the deficits seen in this syndrome increase with the addition of each extra X chromosome, so that an individual with a XXY genotype will have less severe manifestations than an individual with a XXXXY genotype.

Extraoral Characteristics: Individuals with Klinefelter syndrome are taller than usual, with long arms and legs (Fig. 6.13). Their intelligence is usually normal, but mental retardation has been noted in individuals with more than one extra X chromosome. About half of affected individuals have mitral valve prolapse. The lack of proper sexual development in these individuals is the most obvious characteristic. No matter how many extra Xs are in the genotype, the phenotype will always be that of a male. However, the lack of testosterone results in little or no development of secondary sexual characteristics. Sparse facial and body hair, female pubic hair distribution, high-pitched voice, female fat distribution, small hard testes, and infertility are all characteristic of Klinefelter syndrome. Fifty percent or more have gynecomastia, enlarged breasts, and a 20 times higher chance of developing male breast cancer than normal. Autoimmune disorders such as rheumatoid arthritis, lupus erythematosus, and Sjögren syndrome may be more prevalent because of higher levels of estrogen (Chen, December 2004).

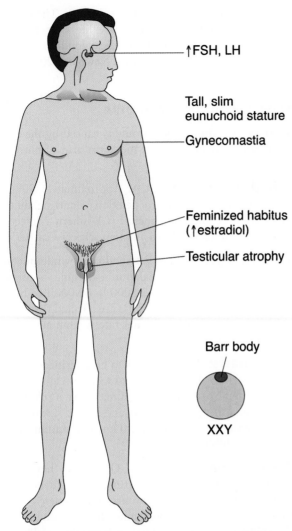

↑FSH, LH

Tall, slim
eunuchoid stature

Gynecomastia

Feminized habitus
(↑estradiol)

Testicular atrophy

Barr body

XXY

Figure 6.13. Klinefelter syndrome. Illustration of patient with Klinefelter syndrome, exhibiting long arms and legs, enlarged breasts, and a feminine body build. (From Rubin E, Farber JL. Pathology. 3rd ed. Philadelphia: Lippincott Williams & Wilkins, 1999.)

Perioral and Intraoral Characteristics: Aside from possible feminization of the facial features, the maxilla may be hypoplastic, and the molars may exhibit taurodontism, enlargement of the pulp chamber, and relative shortening of the root (Chapter 21).

Distinguishing Characteristics: The lack of sexual development is the most obvious feature of this syndrome.

Significant Microscopic Features: Male cells do not normally contain any Barr bodies. Individuals with this syndrome will express one Barr body for each extra X chromosome that is contained in their cells.

Dental Implications: The medical history must be closely examined because of the high probability of mitral valve prolapse. If present, appropriate antibiotic prophylactic medication may be considered. Taurodontism is of no clinical significance and requires no treatment.

Differential Diagnosis: Not applicable

Treatment and Prognosis: This disorder is usually not identified until the lack of sexual development causes concern. Treatment should begin in puberty and focuses on hormone replacement therapy. Testosterone injections promote the development of more masculine features and help to prevent osteoporosis. Mastectomy may be necessary to treat significant gynecomastia. There should be no modifications in dental care unless the patient needs prophylactic antibiotic coverage for mitral valve prolapse. The life span of these individuals is the same as that of the general population.

Name: Turner syndrome (monosomy X)

Etiology: Turner syndrome is caused by monosomy of the X chromosome, resulting in 22 pairs of autosomal chromosomes and one single X chromosome in a female genotype. This is the only monosomy that is compatible with life.

Method of Transmission: Turner syndrome is usually associated with an error in the paternal genetic contribution. About 50% are true monosomies caused by nondisjunction, while the rest are mosaics (XO,XX) or are missing portions of the second X chromosome. Individuals with mosaicism will not exhibit the entire range of abnormalities associated with Turner syndrome.

Epidemiology: Turner syndrome occurs in about 1 of every 2500 live births. All of those affected are women, and all ethnic groups are equally affected.

Pathogenesis: Almost all of the abnormalities seen in Turner syndrome are attributable to the absence of estrogen. Like Klinefelter syndrome, diagnosis of Turner syndrome often does not occur until a girl fails to begin puberty at the normal age.

Extraoral Characteristics: Turner syndrome produces short women (5 feet and under) who have webbing of the neck (Fig. 6.14), a low posterior hairline, and a wide chest with widely spaced nipples. They usually have no ovaries but do have a uterus. Without adequate hormonal replacement therapy they will develop no secondary sexual characteristics. Fifty percent or more will have osteoporosis, even with hormone replacement therapy. Coarctation of the aorta (Chapter 8), aortic valve defects, and hypertension are common. Endocrine disorders (Chapter 7), specifically type II diabetes (30–40%) and hypothyroidism (35%) occur more often in this population than in the general public. Epicanthal folds and other ocular abnormalities as well as vision and hearing defects are common. Most individuals who have Turner syndrome have average or above average intelligence, but many have learning disabilities and a characteristic impairment of spatial and mathematic reasoning skills.

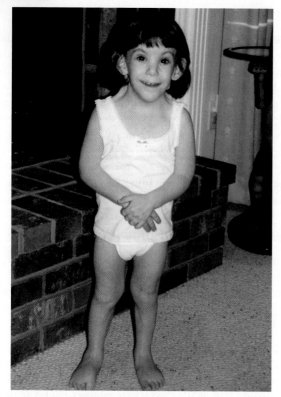

Figure 6.14. Turner syndrome. A 3-year-old with Turner syndrome. Note the webbed neck. (From Nettina SM. The Lippincott manual of nursing practice. 7th ed. Lippincott Williams & Wilkins, 2001.)

Perioral and Intraoral Characteristics: These individuals may have an unusually high number of melanotic macules on their skin in any area. The only noted intraoral finding is the potential for a very high narrow palate.

Distinguishing Characteristics: The short stature, webbed neck, and low hairline are clinically distinguishing characteristics.

Significant Microscopic Features: Not applicable.

Dental Implications: The medical history should be thoroughly reviewed to rule out the presence of heart defects and thus the need for prophylactic antibiotic medication. Undiagnosed girls with the characteristic features of this syndrome should be referred to a physician for evaluation. Girls who do not receive hormone replacement therapy will have the potential for social, psychologic, and medical problems throughout life.

Differential Diagnosis: Not applicable

Treatment and Prognosis: Treatment for Turner syndrome focuses on the clinical features. Growth hormone and androgens given at the appropriate times can increase the height of these girls. Estrogens will cause the development of secondary sexual characteristics. Medications can control hypertension, diabetes, and hypothyroidism. Surgery can correct cardiovascular problems when necessary. Adequate calcium, exercise, and es-

trogen therapy can help prevent osteoporosis. The woman with Turner syndrome has the same life expectancy as anyone else with her particular medical conditions, if any exist (Turner Syndrome, High-Risk Newborn, 2006).

Name: Cri du chat syndrome

Etiology: Cri du chat syndrome is caused by the deletion of genetic material from the short arm of chromosome 5.

Method of Transmission: Approximately 90% of cases result from a de novo deletion occurring during meiosis in the creation of gametes; 10% inherit a defective number 5 chromosome from a parent who is a carrier.

Epidemiology: Cri du chat syndrome, while uncommon, is the most common deletion syndrome, occurring at a rate of about 1 of every 20,000 to 50,000 live births (Campbell et. al, 2005). More girls are affected than boys, but there is no evidence of higher rates within any ethnic groups (Chen, September 2005).

Pathogenesis: There appears to be a "critical region" on chromosome 5 that is associated with the catlike cry of cri du chat syndrome. This region may have a role in the proper development of the larynx and central nervous system, and when it is not present, the manifestations of cri du chat are exhibited.

Extraoral Characteristics: The infant born with this syndrome usually has a distinctive cry that sounds like the mewing of a cat. The cry is considered to be pathognomonic for this syndrome. In addition, infants may exhibit the following: low birth weight, cardiac defects, thymic dysplasia (abnormal thymus gland development), gastrointestinal abnormalities, hypotonia (muscle weakness), and microcephaly. As the infant ages there is growth retardation, severe mental retardation, and chronic medical problems.

Perioral and Intraoral Characteristics: Newborns have round faces with full cheeks, **hypertelorism** (eyes set far apart), epicanthal folds, and downslanting eyes. They also may have a flat nasal bridge and low-set ears (Fig. 6.15).The mandible is micrognathic (small), and the mouth seems to turn down at the commissures. The palate is high vaulted, and cleft lip and/or palate has been associated with the syndrome. The primary teeth are small, and delayed eruption is common. Malocclusion is common in older children.

Distinguishing Characteristics: The catlike cry that this syndrome is named for is its most distinguishing feature.

Significant Microscopic Features: Not applicable

Dental Implications: Medical histories should be reviewed closely to rule out the need for prophylactic an-

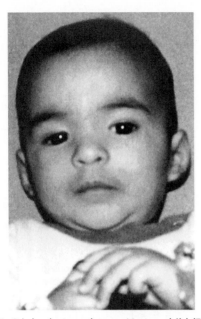

Figure 6.15. Cri du chat syndrome. Young child (5 months) with cri-du-chat syndrome exhibits the characteristic facial features of the syndrome. (From McClatchey KD. Clinical laboratory medicine. 2nd ed. Philadelphia: Lippincott Williams & Wilkins, 2002.)

tibiotic medication. Regular preventive dental care should be performed to decrease the chance of systemic infections and, if at risk, endocarditis.

Differential Diagnosis: Not applicable

Treatment and Prognosis: Treatment for this disorder focuses on managing physical abnormalities. Surgery should be performed to correct cardiac, gastrointestinal, and oral defects, if necessary. Recurring infections are common and should be treated promptly. Early educational and social intervention has shown that these children have a higher capacity for learning than was once thought (Campbell et al., 2005). Six to 8% of the population does not survive childhood, usually because of infections and complications from the heart defects (Chen, September 2005).

SINGLE-GENE OR MENDELIAN DISORDERS

Single-gene abnormalities occur on the molecular level and are not microscopically detectable. The abnormalities usually involve a change in the nitrogen bases of the DNA. This may be a substitution of one base pair for another, or one or more base pairs might be added to the DNA. The exact mechanism is beyond the scope of this text; however, elements that can increase the chance that a mutation will occur are discussed in Chapters 2 and 6.

There is also a small chance that a spontaneous genetic mutation will occur. Single-gene disorders usually affect the structure or presence of a particular protein or enzyme component of the body. These disorders can be divided into four groups:

- Autosomal dominant—Autosomal dominant disorders refer to single-gene abnormalities that are expressed clinically whether the individual is heterozygous or homozygous for the trait (Fig. 6.16A).
- Autosomal recessive—Autosomal recessive disorders are associated with clinical symptoms only when both alleles at a given locus on **homologous**, or like, chromosomes are defective (homozygous). Both parents are usually heterozygous for the trait and appear clinically normal. Rare autosomal recessive disorders are often a product of consanguinity or inbreeding (Fig. 6.16B).
- Sex-linked dominant—A dominant sex-linked disorder will always be expressed whether the individual is heterozygous for the disorder or homozygous. In males, any gene found on the X or Y chromosome, aside from the 18 or so that are duplicated on both genes, will be expressed in the phenotype because there is only one copy.
- X-linked recessive—A recessive X-linked disorder will be expressed in the female only if she is homozygous for the trait, while the male will always express an X-linked recessive trait because he carries only one copy of the X chromosome (Fig. 6.16 C).

Box 6.5 lists examples of common autosomal dominant, autosomal recessive, and major X-linked recessive disorders.

Any trait linked to the Y chromosome and sex-linked dominant traits are very rare and discussion of these is beyond the scope of this text. This discussion focuses on X-linked recessive disorders that are much more common and germane to dental practices.

Refer to Box 6.6 for a listing of the characteristics of inheritance patterns of autosomal dominant, autosomal recessive, and X-linked disorders.

Most of the traits that are observed in an individual's phenotype are not governed by one gene and therefore do not follow the four types of inheritance patterns just discussed. Two other types of inheritance, oligogenic and multifactorial, are also involved the expression of an individual's inherited traits or phenotype. **Oligogenic inheritance** is the result of the interaction of more than one gene found at different loci. The result of the interaction of multiple genes causes the phenotypic expression of a trait or modifies its expression by making it more or less severe. For example, many of the physical characteristics of humans such as eye color, hair color, tooth form, and skin color are the result of oligogenic inheritance (Beales et al., 2003). Autism is one condition that may be oligogenic. Multifactorial inheritance involves the interaction between genetic and environmental factors and is discussed below in this chapter.

Most of the following are common genetic disorders. Remember that individuals with these disorders may or may not express the full range of possible abnormalities.

Name: Marfan syndrome

Etiology: Marfan syndrome is a connective tissue disorder caused by an abnormal gene (FNB1) on chromo-

A Autosomal Dominant

D = Disorder
d = No disorder

1. Heterozygous, displays the disorder

(left axis: Homozygous, does not display disorder)

	D	d
d	DD	dd
d	Dd	dd

50% will display the disorder

2. Heterozygous, displays the disorder

(left axis: Heterozygous, displays the disorder)

	D	d
D	DD	Dd
d	Dd	dd

25% homozygous for the disorder

50% heterozygous for the disorder

25% homozygous for no disorder

B Autosomal Recessive

R = No disorder
r = Disorder

1. Homozygous for the disorder, exhibits the disorder

(left axis: Homozygous, for no disorder, does not exhibit the disorder)

	r	r
R	Rr	Rr
R	Rr	Rr

All offspring are heterozygous for the disorder, not displayed

2. Heterozygous for the disorder does not display the disorder

(left axis: Heterozygous for the disorder does not display the disorder)

	R	r
R	RR	Rr
R	Rr	rr

25% homozygous for nodisorder

50% heterozygous for the disorder, not displayed

25% homozygous for the disorder and display it

3. Heterozygous for the disorder does not display the disorder

(left axis: Homozygous for the disorder, displays the disease)

	R	r
r	Rr	rr
r	Rr	rr

50% heterozygous for the disorder, not displayed

50% homozygous for the disorder and display it

Figure 6.16. Inheritance patterns. **A.** Autosomal dominant inheritance. If an individual who is heterozygous for an autosomal dominant disorder mates with an individual who is homozygous for not having the disorder, you would expect 50% of their offspring to be heterozygous for the disorder and to exhibit it in their phenotype. If both partners are heterozygous for the disorder, then 75% of their offspring would exhibit the phenotype, with 50% having a heterozygous genotype and 50% having a homozygous genotype (25% for the disorder and 25% for not having the disorder). **B.** Autosomal recessive inheritance. If an individual who is homozygous for not having autosomal recessive disorder mates with an individual who is homozygous for the disorder, all of their offspring will have a heterozygous genotype and will have a normal phenotype. If the individuals are both heterozygous for the disorder then 75% of the offspring will not exhibit the phenotype, and 25% will exhibit the disorder. In the case of a homozygous and a heterozygous parent, 50% of the children would express the phenotype, and 50% would not. The heterozygous offspring are carriers of the recessive disorder. *(continued)*

some 15. This gene enables the production of a protein called fibrillin that is essential in providing strength and elasticity to certain connective tissues, especially those of the heart, blood vessels, eyes, and **periosteum** (connective tissue covering bones).

Method of Transmission: Marfan syndrome is transmitted in an autosomal dominant inheritance pattern in about 75% of cases. Spontaneous genetic mutations not associated with hereditary traits account for the other 25% (NMF, 2005).

C X-Linked Recessive

x = carries the disorder

X = does not carry the disorder

Y = does not carry the disorder

1.

Heterozygous female not displaying the disorder

Male with normal X	X	x
X	XX	Xx
Y	XY	xY

25% normal females

25% carrier females

25% normal males

25% males with the disorder

2.

Heterozygous female not displaying the disorder

Male with the disorder	X	x
x	Xx	xx
Y	XY	xY

25% carrier females

25% females with the disorder

25% normal males

25% males with the disorder

Figure 6.16. (continued) Inheritance patterns. **C.** X-Linked recessive inheritance. A heterozygous female and a male whose X chromosome does not carry the disorder will produce male offspring who have a 50% chance of receiving the affected chromosome from their mother and exhibiting the disorder in their phenotype. The daughters have a 50% chance of becoming carriers of the disorder. An affected male and a heterozygous female would produce males who had a 50% chance of exhibiting the disorder just as above. However, now any female offspring have a 50% chance of being homozygous for the disorder and thus exhibiting the disorder.

Epidemiology: Marfan syndrome is one of the more common hereditary connective tissue disorders. Marfan syndrome affects about 1 in every 10,000 Americans (Rubin et al., 2005). Marfan syndrome presents with high, variable expressivity, even within families in which one person might be severely affected and another only slightly. The disorder affects males and females equally and, depending on the severity of the involvement, is di-agnosed at birth up to around puberty. It may be found even later for those with minor expression of the disorder.

Pathogenesis: The genetic mutation causes decreased production of fibrillin, which is a glycoprotein that helps form the extracellular matrices of the connective tissues mentioned above. Without the proper amount of fibrillin, the connective tissues that form are more flex-

---

Box 6.5 COMMON EXAMPLES OF AUTOSOMAL DOMINANT DISORDERS, AUTOSOMAL RECESSIVE DISORDERS, AND X-LINKED RECESSIVE DISORDERS

COMMON EXAMPLES OF AUTOSOMAL DOMINANT DISORDERS

Marfan syndrome

Ehlers-Danlos syndrome

Epidermolysis bullosa

Achondroplastic dwarfism

Hereditary hemorrhagic telangiectasia

Familial hypercholesterolemia

Von Willebrand's disease

Retinoblastoma

Neurofibromatosis

Gardner syndrome

Multiple endocrine neoplasia syndromes I, II

Peutz-Jeghers syndrome

Familial dysplastic nevus syndrome

Huntington's disease

Treacher Collins syndrome

Osteogenesis imperfecta (some types)

COMMON EXAMPLES OF AUTOSOMAL RECESSIVE DISORDERS

Cystic fibrosis

Tay-Sachs disease

Phenylketonuria

Albinism

Severe form of von Willebrand's disease

Severe form of epidermolysis bullosa

Sickle cell anemia

A-thalassemia major

COMMON X-LINKED RECESSIVE DISORDERS

Hemophilia A and B

Duchenne's muscular dystrophy

Red–green color blindness

Fragile X syndrome

Box 6.6   CHARACTERISTICS OF SPECIFIC INHERITANCE PATTERNS

The major inheritance patterns associated with autosomal dominant, autosomal recessive, and X-linked recessive disorders are listed below.

Autosomal dominant
- Males and females are equally affected.
- The trait is expressed in the parents' phenotype whether they are homozygous or heterozygous.
- There is a 50% chance that the offspring will be affected.

Autosomal recessive
- Males and females are equally affected.
- Parents are usually heterozygous and phenotypically normal.
- There is a 25% chance of the offspring exhibiting the trait, and a 50% chance that they will be heterozygous for the trait, or carriers.

X-Linked Recessive
- Males with these disorders cannot transmit them to their sons.
- Women who are carriers (Xx) have a 50% chance of transmitting the trait to their sons, who will be symptomatic. There is also a 50% chance of transmission to their daughters, who will be asymptomatic.
- All daughters of affected men are asymptomatic carriers, but the sons will be free of the abnormality and cannot transmit the disease to their children.
- Symptomatic homozygous females result only from the rare mating of an affected male and an asymptomatic heterozygous or symptomatic homozygous female.

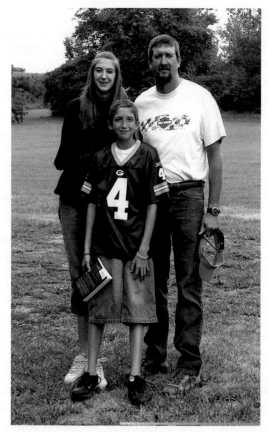

Figure 6.17. Marfan syndrome. Father, son, and daughter with Marfan syndrome. Father is 38 years old and has had his mitral valve replaced. Daughter is 16 and has had surgery to correct a depressed sternum. Son is 10 and has had surgery to remove an extra toe and is restricted in his activities due to joint laxness and a symptomatic mitral valve prolapse. (Courtesy of the Waters' Family.)

ible than they should be. The increased flexibility causes abnormal stretching of the various connective tissues and results in all of the major manifestations of this syndrome.

Extraoral Characteristics: It is thought that Abraham Lincoln might have had Marfan syndrome because he exhibited all of the associated skeletal characteristics. There are three major categories of manifestations: skeletal, ocular, and cardiovascular. Approximately 88% of individuals affected by Marfan syndrome are very tall and slim and have long arms and legs in relation to their torsos (Fig. 6.17). In addition, they usually have very long fingers and toes. They may also have scoliosis or curvature of the spine and either a depressed or protuberant breast bone or sternum. Their bones, especially rib bones, may be deformed, and there is a generalized joint laxness that results in hyperextensibility and potential injury. The unusual length of the bones is due to an overly flexible periosteum that does not restrict the amount of growth. The defective periosteum is also associated with any of the bony malformations or defects that are manifested with the condition. The joint laxity is due to the increased flexibility of the ligaments.

The most common (79%) ocular defect seen in Marfan syndrome is off-center lenses caused by the increased flexibility of the ligaments that should be holding them in place. Myopia and cataracts are also common problems.

The most serious manifestations of Marfan syndrome are found in the cardiovascular system and include weakness of the aorta and heart valve defects, especially of the mitral valve. Some 80% of adults with Marfan syndrome exhibit an enlarged aorta, because of its structural weakness. This can lead to aneurysms or thinning and bulging of the vessel wall and eventually ruptures or dissections as discussed in Chapter 8. Some 80% of children with Marfan syndrome are diagnosed with mitral valve prolapse by the age of 10. Increased elasticity of the muscles that control the function of the heart valves cause the valve defects, which can lead to cardiac hypertrophy, dysrhythmia, tachycardia, shortness of breath, and heart failure (NMF, 2005). These are also discussed in Chapter 8.

Perioral and Intraoral Characteristics: The dental problems most commonly observed in Marfan syndrome are related to the development of the bones of the face. The individual may have a high narrow palate, posterior crossbite, and a class II malocclusion. Patients may also have significant crowding of the teeth due to these abnormalities. The TM joint may be affected by either bone deformity or laxity of the ligaments that control the joint during function. Either of these can cause the individual with Marfan syndrome to be more susceptible to TMJ dysfunction.

Distinguishing Characteristics: The most obvious characteristics are those related to the skeletal system: height, length of arms and legs, etc.

Significant Microscopic Features: Not applicable

Dental Implications: Preventive care should be stressed to limit the potential for creating a bacteremia. Dental treatment modifications should include prophylactic antibiotic coverage per American Heart Association recommendations for those with indications of mitral valve prolapse with regurgitation. In addition, if the patient has had heart valve replacements, blood tests should be done to determine their coagulation status. Regular dental care should be a high priority, and these patients have no more contraindications for dental care than normal patients with the same type of cardiac or skeletal problems. Patients who are aware of their disorder will most likely know whether cardiac defects exist or not. It is the patient who has not been diagnosed that is the problem. The National Marfan Foundation believes that dental professionals should use their knowledge of the physical manifestations of Marfan syndrome to refer suspected patients for further medical evaluation (NMF, 2005).

Differential Diagnosis: Not applicable

Treatment and Prognosis: Medical treatment for those with Marfan syndrome centers on anticipating problems, early intervention, and dedicated follow-up. Many skeletal abnormalities including scoliosis can be corrected with physical therapy and braces. If necessary, surgery can correct skeletal problems that cannot be prevented or that need more aggressive treatment. Ocular defects can usually be treated with glasses and sometimes laser surgery.

Ninety percent of deaths associated with Marfan syndrome are due to cardiovascular events. The individual's cardiovascular status should be monitored closely. Many of these patients are on medication such as beta-blockers, to reduce the strength and number of cardiac contractions and to lower blood pressure, thus putting less strain on the aorta. Since heart valve involvement is common, many affected individuals have had valve replacements. These individuals will be taking anticoagulants for the rest of their lives and must be followed appropriately.

In 1970 the life expectancy of an individual with Marfan syndrome was approximately 30 to 40 years. This increased in 1995 to about the same as a normal individual, or 72 years. The increase is thought to be due to better medical, surgical, and pharmacologic management and early diagnosis of cardiac problems.

Name: Cleidocranial dysplasia (CCD)

Etiology: CCD has been determined to be caused by a deletion of genetic material on the short arm of chromosome 6 in region 21 (6p21). The *CBFA1* gene is a core binding factor that plays a role in osteoblast formation and the differentiation of other cells necessary for normal bone development (Mundlos, 1999).

Method of Transmission: CCD has an autosomal dominant inheritance pattern. About one third of all cases are caused by a spontaneous mutation not related to inheritance.

Epidemiology: CCD occurs equally in males and females and within all racial and ethnic groups.

Pathogenesis: It appears that the *CBFA1* gene actually controls the differentiation of precursor cells into osteoblasts. Without osteoblasts there is no bone matrix and therefore no bone. All of the characteristics of this disorder are associated with this defect.

Extraoral Characteristics: Individuals with CCD are of moderately short stature and are at risk for skeletal problems such as scoliosis. They have underdeveloped, hypoplastic, or missing clavicles which allows them to almost bring their shoulders together in front of them. Characteristic facial features include enlarged rounding, or **bossing**, of the frontal and parietal bones, caused by delayed closure of the sutures and fontanels. The paranasal sinuses may be missing or hypoplastic, and the nose has a wide nasal root and depressed bridge. Other facial bones are hypoplastic, giving the face a small short look. There may also be a wider distance between the eyes, or hypertelorism.

Perioral and Intraoral Characteristics: The most striking intraoral manifestation of this disorder is multiple supernumerary teeth thought to be due to the delayed resorption of the dental lamina, which appears to reactivate when the crowns of the permanent teeth are completely formed (Regezi et al., 2003). While the primary dentition usually develops normally, there is a marked delay in exfoliation and an extreme delay in eruption of the permanent dentition. One cause of this is thought to be a lack of cellular cementum on the roots of the teeth, which is characteristic of CCD. The presence of many supernumerary teeth also interferes with the eruption of the permanent dentition (Fig. 6.18). Often patients will have an extended period of time during which they have few if any erupted teeth or **pseudoanodontia**. The maxilla is hypoplastic and is associated with a high narrow palate. All of these dental anomalies result in severe malocclusion.

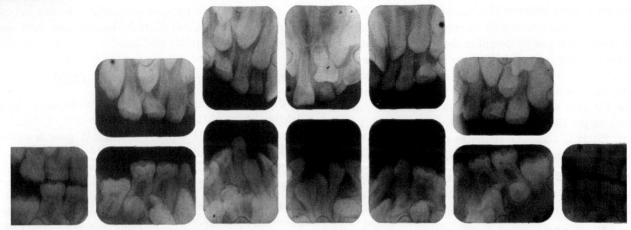

Figure 6.18. Cleidocranial dysplasia. This full-mouth survey shows multiple supernumerary teeth and unerupted teeth in an individual with CCD. (Courtesy Dr. John Jacoway.)

Distinguishing Characteristics: The characteristic appearance of individuals with CCD and the presence of multiple supernumerary teeth are distinguishing features of this disorder.

Significant Microscopic Features: Not applicable

Dental Implications: Delayed exfoliation of the primary dentition, delayed eruption of the permanent dentition, and multiple supernumerary teeth result in many dental abnormalities. Dental treatment should start early, and regular dental care should be a lifelong goal. Orthodontic treatment is usually necessary to establish a stable dentition. Temporary full or partial dentures may need to be constructed over unerupted teeth to enable proper function until the teeth erupt. It may be necessary to extract primary teeth and surgically expose unerupted permanent teeth to assist in the eruption process. If clefting is present, corrective surgery is indicated.

Differential Diagnosis: Other disorders that present with delayed exfoliation of primary teeth, delayed eruption of permanent teeth, and multiple supernumerary teeth that might be considered in a differential diagnosis include

1. Hypothyroidism (Chapter 7). These individuals exhibit delayed eruption of the permanent teeth but do not exhibit the characteristic skeletal features of CCD, and they usually do not present with supernumerary teeth.

2. Cherubism (Chapter 10). Individuals affected by cherubism exhibit delayed eruption of the permanent dentition, but they also present with early exfoliation of the primary dentition which is not consistent with CCD. They also lack the characteristic skeletal deformities.

3. Gardner's syndrome (Chapter 19). Gardner's syndrome presents with multiple supernumerary teeth and multiple osteomas. The osteomas are not consistent with a diagnosis of CCD, and these patients do not have the bone abnormalities associated with CCD.

Treatment and Prognosis: The skeletal defects do not usually interfere with the health of the patient and therefore do not need treatment. An exception to this is if the individual develops scoliosis. It may be suggested that protective head gear be worn, especially by children, to prevent damage if the fontanels are open. Individuals with CCD have every expectation for a normal life span.

Name: Treacher Collins syndrome (TCS) (mandibulofacial dysostosis, Treacher Collins-Franceschetti syndrome)

Etiology: A mutation of the *TCOF1* gene on the long arm of chromosome 5, region 32–33 is believed to be the cause of this syndrome.

Method of Transmission: TCS has an autosomal dominant inheritance pattern with high penetrance and variable expressivity. The disorder becomes more severe as it is passed from generation to generation. About 60% of affected individuals are believed to have had a spontaneous mutation that was not inherited from either parent (Lewanda, 2001).

Epidemiology: This disorder occurs from 1 in 10,000 to 1 in 50,000 live births, occurs equally in males and females, and affects all ethnic groups (Lewanda, 2001).

Pathogenesis: The pathogenesis of this syndrome is unknown.

Extraoral Characteristics: The facial features related to TCS are quite striking and have been called birdlike (Fig. 6.19).The eyes slant downward, and the lower lid is notched and missing most or all of the eyelashes. The zygomatic processes, mandible, and maxilla are hypoplastic. The ears are usually low set and malformed, but may be totally missing, and there is always some hearing loss. Residual ear tags can be located anywhere along the line from the commissures to the angle of the mandible. Sideburns may extend onto the cheek in an oblique direc-

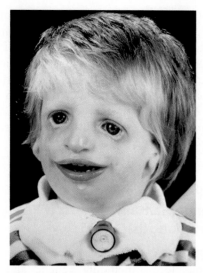

Figure 6.19. Treacher Collins syndrome or mandibulofacial dysostosis. The face is small, but head size is normal. The eyes slant down, and there are underdeveloped or absent malar bones. The zygomatic arch is evident. Lower eyelids show symmetrical defects in the outer one-third and sparse lashes. Ear deformities and conduction deafness are also normally present. The lower jaw is small and angled downward, giving an open bite malocclusion. This child required tracheostomy to manage severe airway problems caused by micrognathia and incorrect development of the tongue. (From Gold DH, Weingeist TA. Color atlas of the eye in systemic disease. Baltimore: Lippincott Williams & Wilkins, 2001.)

tion. There are no mental deficits associated with Treacher Collins syndrome.

Perioral and Intraoral Characteristics: A high vault is normally present, and approximately 30% may have cleft lip and/or palate. All will have mandibular hypoplasia. Severe malocclusion, comprised of an open bite, wide interproximal separations, and displaced teeth, is common in patients who have TCS.

Distinguishing Characteristics: The facial features associated with this disorder distinguish it from other disorders.

Significant Microscopic Findings: Not applicable

Dental Implications: The intraoral and perioral features of this syndrome are significant in that collaboration with several specialists is needed to treat these patients. Regular dental care including adequate home care instruction is crucial because of the extensive treatment and length of time required to complete the treatment.

Differential Diagnosis: Not applicable

Treatment and Prognosis: Treatment focuses on correcting the facial defects by surgical means and the oral defects by surgery and orthodontics. Hearing aids can assist those with partial hearing loss, and those with total hearing loss may be helped with cochlear implants. Individuals with Treacher Collins syndrome have every expectation for a normal life.

Name: Ehlers-Danlos syndrome (EDS)

Etiology: Genetic defects on chromosomes 1, 2, 6, 9, and 17 have been associated with the different types of Ehlers-Danlos syndrome.

Method of Transmission: Most forms of EDS follow an autosomal dominant inheritance pattern; fewer show a recessive pattern, and rarely an X-linked pattern is involved.

Epidemiology: The frequency of Ehlers-Danlos syndrome has been estimated at 1 in every 5,000 to 10,000 live births. There is equal distribution of the dominant and recessive types among males and females. The X-linked type is only expressed fully in males.

Pathogenesis: The defects seen in all types of Ehlers-Danlos syndrome are associated with the production of abnormal collagen and its incorporation into the structures of the body. Collagen is the major structural protein in the body, and use of the defective collagen leads to weakness in structures that are composed of it.

Extraoral Characteristics: There are six major types of Ehlers-Danlos syndrome. All of the various types present with varying degrees of excessively loose joints that tend to dislocate easily; hyperelastic, thin, loose skin; and excessively fragile skin, blood vessels, mucous membranes, and other body tissues. Individuals with this condition have abnormal wound healing and may exhibit thin paperlike scarring, especially over bony prominences such as the knees and elbows. There is excessive bruising of the skin because of the fragility of the blood vessels, and often there is excessive bleeding associated with minor injuries. In one type of the disease the vessels appear very close to the skin because of a lack of subcutaneous fat tissue (Fig. 6.20).

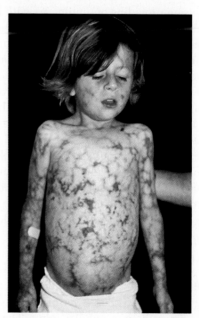

Figure 6.20. Ehlers-Danlos syndrome. Ehlers-Danlos type IV is associated with thin skin and visible veins. (From Gold DH, Weingeist TA. Color atlas of the eye in systemic disease. Baltimore: Lippincott Williams & Wilkins, 2001.)

Blood vessels and hollow organs are at a high risk for rupture, which could cause immediate death. Very often the heart valves become deformed because of the defective collagen, and mitral valve prolapse is very common. Most individuals with Ehlers-Danlos syndrome have chronic joint pain and are at a much higher risk than normal for degenerative bone and joint diseases.

Perioral and Intraoral Characteristics: Individuals with Ehlers-Danlos syndrome may exhibit thin hair, deformed ears, hypertelorism, narrow curved nose, and scarring of the forehead and chin. The TM joint may be prone to dislocation and chronic pain. The tongue is unusually supple and most individuals can touch the tip of their nose with the tip of their tongues (**Gorlin's sign**); only 8–10% of the general population can manage this act (Létourneau et al., 2001). The oral mucosa is fragile and easily torn during eating or dental care. Gingival tissues can be hyperplastic and often bleed easily during home care, even if there is no inflammation. Teeth may be malformed with deep occlusal grooves and higher-than-normal cusps. The roots may be short and/or dilacerated, and the dentin and enamel structure may be abnormal.

Distinguishing Characteristics: Skin hyperelasticity, joint hypermobility, and excessive bruising are all distinguishing characteristics of this disorder.

Significant Microscopic Features: Not applicable

Dental Implications: All dental care should be delayed until the need for prophylactic antibiotic medication is determined. In all types, mucous membrane fragility, poor wound healing, and joint hypermobility could require treatment modifications. Dental treatment should focus on providing optimum care with little to no trauma. Short appointments should be scheduled to avoid damaging the TM joint. The need for surgical procedures should be determined on the basis of anticipated benefits versus the risks of bleeding and inadequate wound healing. Any sutures should be protected by acrylic splints or periodontal dressings to help avoid tearing of the tissues. It is important to identify the rare periodontal form of this disease to start stringent preventive measures. Orthodontic treatment is still possible, but the forces should be adjusted to account for the faster movement of the teeth, and the retention phase would need to be extended to account for the greater potential for relapse because of greater periodontal ligament elasticity.

Differential Diagnosis: Not applicable

Treatment and Prognosis: General treatment for EDS depends on the type and severity of the disorder. Orthopedic braces help to stabilize joints. There is also a special type of finger brace that looks like jewelry but helps to keep the knuckle joints from collapsing as the person is writing or doing other work that requires fine finger motions. Individuals should be cautioned about participating in activities that would put too much stress on the joints. One of the most severe forms of the disorder, the vascular form, has the potential for causing premature death due to organ rupture or large vessel rupture. In fact, about 51% with this type of EDS die before the age of 40. Those with all other types of EDS have relatively normal life expectancies (Létourneau et al., 2001).

Name: Papillon-Lefèvre syndrome (PLS, palmoplantar keratosis (PPK) with periodontitis)

Etiology: PLS is associated with a group of disorders with various forms including genetic and acquired. Papillon-Lefèvre syndrome or PLS has a genetic origin. It can be traced to a gene called Capthasin C on the long arm of chromosome 11q14-21.

Method of Transmission: PLS has an autosomal recessive inheritance pattern.

Epidemiology: PLS is a rare disease, occurring more often in children of consanguineous parents, such as a union between first cousins. PLS occurs in about 1 of 250,000 to 1,000,000 births. The disorder affects all ethnic groups and males and females equally.

Pathogenesis: The pathogenesis of PLS is not well understood, partly because of the infrequency of its occurrence and partly because it is often misdiagnosed. Current research tends to point to defective chemotactic and phagocytic functions in neutrophils and/or a T lymphocyte defect, but the results of these studies are not consistent (Lundgren et al., 2005). In a recent study, the numbers of natural killer cells were found to be consistently and severely depressed in the subjects tested (Lundgren et al., 2005). Whatever the mechanism, the outcome is severe, with aggressive periodontal disease that usually results in loss of both dentitions.

Extraoral Characteristics: The major feature of this disorder is hyperkeratosis comprised of scaly red lesions on the palms of the hands and the soles of the feet (Fig. 6.21). The same lesions can often be found over joints such as the knees and elbows. The individual may exhibit excessive sweating, or **hyperhidrosis**, with associated malodor. Systemically, there may be an increased susceptibility to chronic and recurrent infections such as colds, ear infections, and skin infections.

Perioral and Intraoral Characteristics: Intraoral symptoms do not appear until the first tooth has erupted. Within a short time after eruption signs of gingival inflammation begin to appear, inflammation becomes progressively worse, and attachment loss begins. Loss of alveolar bone and deep pocket formation consistent with severe pe-

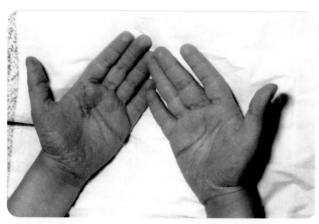

Figure 6.21. Papillon-Lefèvre syndrome. Palms of the hands of the patient in Figure 6.22 showing diffuse erythematous hyperkeratosis, scaling, and fissuring that are characteristic of this disorder. (Courtesy of Faiez N. Hattab.)

riodontal disease are present (Fig. 6.22). Normally the primary teeth are all lost by the age of 5, and the gingiva returns to normal after the loss of the teeth. The permanent teeth erupt at the appropriate time, and the symptoms appear again. Children with PLS usually lose all of their permanent teeth before the age of 15. Some research has identified an increased number of *Actinobacillus actinomycetemcomitans* (AA) and other periodontal pathogens in the subgingival area, which implies a possible immune deficiency.

Distinguishing Characteristics: The anatomic location of the hyperkeratotic lesions and the associated severe periodontal disease are the distinguishing features of this disorder.

Significant Microscopic Features: White blood cell counts, specifically neutrophils and NK cells, may be decreased.

Dental Implications: Severe periodontal disease in a child is almost unheard of, and if a child does present with this disease, PLS should be considered immediately.

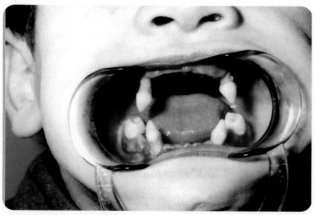

Figure 6.22. Papillon-Lefèvre syndrome. Intraoral view showing generalized severe inflamed and swollen gingiva around the remaining teeth. All primary teeth have been lost prematurely in this 9-year-old girl with Papillon-Lefèvre syndrome. (Courtesy of Faiez N. Hattab.)

Simple observation of the palms of the hands can reveal the other significant feature of this syndrome, hyperkeratosis, which is often misdiagnosed as eczema.

Differential Diagnosis: While there are a group of syndromes that have palmoplantar keratosis as part of their clinical manifestations, PLS is the only one that has severe periodontal disease associated with it. There is one disease, Olmsted syndrome, that is associated with perioral hyperkeratosis, but severe periodontal disease is not part of that syndrome. Other diseases that manifest with severe periodontal infection should be considered, including

1. Hypophosphatasia. Hypophosphatasia is an autosomal recessive disorder that causes a deficiency of alkaline phosphatase, which is essential in the maintenance of bone. This is also one of the few disorders that can cause early exfoliation of the primary dentition. However, the problem is with the structure of the tooth, not with a periodontal infection, and in most cases, only the primary dentition is involved. There is no associated palmoplantar keratosis.
2. Cyclic neutropenia (Chapter 9). Cyclic neutropenia is a blood dyscrasia in which there is a periodic depression of the number of neutrophils in the blood and in the marrow about every 21 days. These individuals are prone to many infections, including periodontal disease. Blood tests aimed at determining the levels of neutrophils present at different times over a period will help to differentiate this disorder from PLS. There is also no associated hyperkeratosis.
3. Ehlers-Danlos syndrome with periodontitis (Chapter 6). EDS with periodontitis can exhibit the same type of severe periodontal disease with complete loss of permanent teeth as PLS, but PLS would not exhibit the skin hyperelasticity seen in EDS. Also, there is no associated fragility of the oral tissues or blood vessels in PLS that is seen in EDS.

Treatment and Prognosis: Treatment for hyperkeratosis consists of oral and possibly topical retinoids, a derivative of vitamin A used to treat severe acne and psoriasis, and sometimes mechanical exfoliation of the scaly lesions (Lee et al., March 2006). Treatment for the periodontal disease focuses on extracting hopeless teeth, with full dentures as the final result. One recent study found that with diligent home care and professional supervision it may be possible to maintain the dentition of those affected by PLS much longer than was ever thought possible (Lundgren and Renvert, 2004). The medical prognosis for these individuals is the same as for the general population.

Name: Gingival fibromatosis

Gingival fibromatosis is included in the clinical manifestations of more than a few syndromes and disorders. It is outside the scope of this text to discuss all of these. Table 6.4 presents an overview of the disorders that are seen in

Table 6.4   DISORDERS ASSOCIATED WITH GINGIVAL FIBROMATOSIS

These are selected examples of a variety of conditions that may present with gingival fibromatosis as one of their elements.

Name	Etiology	Characteristics in Addition to Gingival Fibromatosis
GF[a] with progressive deafness	Unknown	Deafness
GF with hypertrichosis	Autosomal dominant	Excessive hairiness usually on the back and buttocks
Zimmerman-Laband Syndrome	Translocation defect	Structural ear abnormalities, deformed and hypoplastic nails, short fingers, excessive hairiness; hepatosplenomegaly[b]
GF with distinctive facies	Autosomal recessive	Large head, bushy eyebrows, hypertelorism, down-slanting eyes, flat bridge of nose, and high arched palate
Ramon syndrome	Unknown	Cherubism,[c] epilepsy, mental retardation, hypertrichosis, stunted growth, eye abnormalities
GF with hypertrichosis and mental retardation	Unknown	Hirsutism,[d] abnormal appearing ears and nose, epilepsy, possible heart and endocrine defects
Juvenile hyaline fibromatosis	Autosomal recessive	Nodular and papular skin growths on the hands, scalp, and ears and around nose; joint contractures;[e] osteopenia[f]
Congenital generalized fibromatosis	Autosomal recessive	Multiple fibroblastic tumors in skin, muscle, bones and organs; tumors in organs may cause death
Infantile systemic hyalinosis	Autosomal recessive	Joint contractures; red hyperpigmentation over prominent bones; papular and nodular growth on face, scalp, neck and perianal areas; thick skin; osteopenia
Rutherford syndrome	Unknown	Abnormalities of the cornea and delayed tooth eruption

[a]GF, gingival fibromatosis.
[b]Enlarged spleen and liver.
[c]See Chapter 10.
[d]Male-pattern hair growth.
[e]Painful stiffness in a flexed position.
[f]Lower than normal mineral content in the bones but not enough to be considered osteoporotic.

association with gingival fibromatosis. This section specifically discusses hereditary gingival fibromatosis as a separate entity, the clinical aspects of which are consistent with most of these other disorders.

Etiology: Gingival fibromatosis has been associated with genes located on chromosomes 2 and 5 (OMIM #228600 Fibromatosis, juvenile hyaline, 2005).

Method of Transmission: Both autosomal dominant and autosomal recessive inheritance patterns have been observed.

Epidemiology: Unknown

Pathogenesis: Gingival fibromatosis is a slow and progressive collagenous overgrowth of the fibrous connective tissue of the gingiva. It does not normally occur prior to the eruption of teeth.

Extraoral Characteristics: Not applicable

Perioral and Intraoral Characteristics: Gingival fibromatosis can occur in a generalized or localized form. If localized, the maxillary arch is a more common site than the mandible, and the posterior areas are more com-

mon than the anterior areas. Enlargement can begin at any time but normally occurs with the eruption of the deciduous teeth and rarely occurs for the first time after age 20. The tissue can grow over the crowns of the affected teeth and can cause failure or delayed eruption of permanent teeth (Fig. 6.23). The tissue appears normal in color and is firm to the touch. One common presentation involves the posterior palatal area, where gingival overgrowth almost covers the crowns of the teeth and extends toward the midline of the palate, almost touching in some cases. Gingival overgrowth will stop if the patient becomes edentulous.

Distinguishing Characteristics: Hereditary forms of gingival fibromatosis usually present as symmetrical gingival enlargements comprised of normal-appearing tissues. This observation may help to distinguish this from other forms of gingival enlargement, such as the enlargement associated with phenytoin, a medication used to treat seizures, and that associated with biofilm-associated gingivitis.

Significant Microscopic Features: Microscopic examination will show dense collagenous tissue with long thin rete ridges that run deep into the connective tissue.

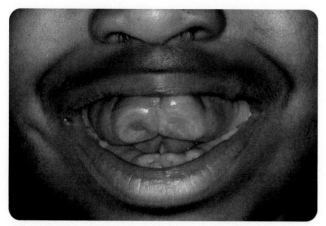

Figure 6.23. Hereditary gingival fibromatosis. Note the thick, normal-colored gingiva enveloping the teeth. The treatment is surgical removal of the excess gingiva, but it always recurs. (Courtesy of Dr. Charles Dunlap.)

Dental Implications: The most important aspect of working with a patient with gingival fibromatosis is to rule out any of the many syndromes that can accompany gingival fibromatosis and to develop treatment and home care plans that can help the individual overcome the difficulties associated with this disorder.

Differential Diagnosis: Gingival hyperplasia due to hormones, medications, and local factors must be considered in a differential diagnosis of gingival enlargement (Chapter 17). The medical history is very important in ruling out medication-induced hyperplasia and hyperplasia due to pregnancy. Even without the medical history information, there are clinically observable differences in these entities. Hyperplasia due to hormonal influences and local factors such as dental biofilm is usually erythematous, is spongy, and bleeds easily. Medication-induced hyperplasia has a very pebbly appearance and is usually firm to the touch.

Treatment and Prognosis: In cases of generalized and in some cases of localized gingival fibromatosis, surgical removal of the excess tissue is often the only way to attempt to control the symptoms. However, the gingiva will continue to grow again, and multiple surgeries will be necessary during the life of the individual. Erupting teeth may need to be "helped" through the thick gingival tissues with surgical crown exposure techniques.

In both localized and generalized forms, it is very important to maintain excellent oral hygiene because any inflammation from infection will only exacerbate the growth of tissue. Dental hygienists have an opportunity to help these patients develop home care regimens that are effective and make compliance as easy as possible. More frequent preventive care appointments are strongly suggested to assist in maintaining healthy tissues.

Name: Ectodermal dysplasia (ED)

There are over 150 different hereditary syndromes associated with ectodermal dysplasia. They follow all inheritance patterns and manifest in a full range of severities. Mutations and deletions associated with ED syndromes have been mapped to the X chromosome and chromosomes 9, 12, 13, and 19. Worldwide, ectodermal dysplasia syndromes occur in about 7 of every 10,000 births. Males and females of all ethnic groups are equally affected by these syndromes, even though several are X-linked. The following discussion focuses on the most common form of ED, X-linked hypohidrotic ectodermal dysplasia (ED1).

Etiology: ED1 is linked to a mutation of the *ED1* gene on the X chromosome.

Method of Transmission: ED1 follows an X-linked recessive inheritance pattern that determines that only the male will exhibit the complete phenotype. There have been reports of an intermediate expression of the disorder in some heterozygous females (Duran-McKinster, 2004; OMIM #305100 Ectodermal Dysplasia, Anhidrotic, 2004). Females only exhibit the full disease if the parents were an affected male and a carrier female.

Epidemiology: The estimated prevalence of ED1 in the United States is 1 in 100,000 births. While all races may be affected, ED syndromes appear to occur more often in Caucasians (Duran-McKinster, 2004).

Pathogenesis: The clinical manifestations of ED1 are the result of abnormal morphogenesis of the tissues that develop from the embryonic ectodermal cells. This includes skin, mucous membranes and associated glands of the oral cavity and upper respiratory system, sweat glands, hair follicles and hair, nails, and teeth.

Extraoral Characteristics: The typical phenotypic expression of this disorder involves sparse or missing hair (entire body), hair and hair follicle defects, absent or few sweat glands, defective mucous glands, and lacrimal gland defects. The skin is thin, smooth, and dry, with a shiny appearance. Characteristic facial features include frontal bossing, midface or maxillary hypoplasia, flattened bridge of the nose or saddle nose, and wrinkled hyperpigmented skin around the eyes. The ears can be large and low set. The nails are normal in ED1. One of the more serious problems associated with ED syndromes is a tendency for high fevers or pyrexia and hyperthermia. These individuals are unable to regulate their body temperature because of the lack of adequate numbers of, or total absence of, sweat glands. Temperature regulation is especially troublesome for infants and children; frequent bouts of hyperthermia can cause seizures, brain damage, and even death. A decreased amount of respiratory secretions and the existence of defective respiratory secretions are believed to impair the host response to respiratory infections, making these individuals susceptible to severe and recurrent respiratory infections. Defective lacrimal glands will cause **xerophthalmia** (dry eyes) and associated **photophobia** (light sensitivity).

Perioral and Intraoral Characteristics: Individuals with ED1 have thick full lips. Their intraoral problems include **anodontia** (missing all teeth) or **hypodontia** (missing some teeth) with hypoplasia and varying degrees of xerostomia. Hypodontia is more common that anodontia. See Chapter 21 for examples of hypodontia associated with ED. There is delayed eruption of teeth that are present, and these teeth are usually small and conical. Xerostomia increases the likelihood for dental biofilm accumulation and increased caries activity. Prosthetic appliances will likewise be more difficult to use and care for. Home care procedures are complicated by the type and number of restorations and prosthetic appliances. Cleft lip and/or palate are not a component of this syndrome but are seen in other ED syndromes.

Distinguishing Characteristics: One of the difficulties associated with ED1 is the relative lack of clinical manifestations in newborns and older infants. ED1 diagnosis is thus often made when the infant is seen to have recurrent problems with pyrexia. In older children and adults, the lack of hair and the dental abnormalities seen with this disorder are distinguishing characteristics.

Significant Microscopic Features: Not applicable

Dental Implications: The dental abnormalities and high probability of severe xerostomia are the most significant factors for dentistry. Missing teeth can be replaced with prosthetic appliances or implants. Hypoplastic teeth can be esthetically restored. Xerostomia can be alleviated with artificial saliva, mechanical stimulation with sugarless gum or candies, and medication, if indicated. Adequate oral hygiene is essential for these patients, and the dental hygienist will be responsible for developing user-friendly home care regimens. Fluoride treatments in the office and at home will be crucial to inhibit caries activity.

Differential Diagnosis: Any of the other ectodermal dysplasia syndromes would need to be ruled out as well as any condition that causes anodontia or hypodontia. Other conditions that might cause anodontia or hypodontia are relatively easy to rule out because of the other elements of the syndrome. However, if a heterozygous female without the classic elements of ED presented with hypodontia of the type seen in this disorder, identification of the problem might be more difficult.

Treatment and Prognosis: Although there is no treatment for this syndrome, the symptoms that it causes can be treated and corrected. No matter how problematic sweating is for most of the human race, it does serve a purpose. Individuals with ED must be advised on how to maintain a proper temperature, including what type of clothing to wear; avoiding activities that would increase the temperature; regulation of home, work, and school environments; and proper hydration. Xerophthalmia and photophobia can be relieved with artificial tears and ointments.

Patients with these syndromes that survive early childhood have a relatively normal life expectancy. Infants and young children have an approximate mortality rate of 30% for all of the ED syndromes, not just ED1. The most frequent causes of death are associated with the sequela of hyperthermia such as seizures and brain damage (Duran-McKinster, 2004; OMIM #305100 Ectodermal Dysplasia, Anhidrotic, 2004).

MULTIFACTORIAL INHERITANCE

Multifactorial inheritance describes a process that reflects the additive effects of a number of genes and environmental factors. Most of our makeup is not determined by the influence of a single gene or even multiple genes, but by the interaction of many genes and the environment. The environment plays a very important role in determining the full expression of our genetic potential. Someone who inherits above-average intelligence but is not exposed to anything but a dark room will not develop to his or her potential. Likewise a boy who grows up with chronic malnutrition will not achieve the 6 foot height he inherited from his grandfather. The mechanisms of inheriting disorders that have been discussed thus far are relatively simple. Most genetic disorders do not follow a simple pattern of inheritance. Many disorders require an environmental trigger or exposure to initiate their expression. Cancer is an example of multifactorial inheritance. As discussed above, a combination of environmental, biologic, and genetic events must occur over time before cancer develops, even though an individual may have a defective tumor suppressor gene or may have developed certain oncogenes. Refer to Box 6.7 for a listing of common disorders that are considered multifactorial. One of the most devastating orofacial disorders that is associated with multifactorial inheritance is cleft lip and/or palate.

Name: Cleft lip and/or palate

Etiology: Cleft lip, cleft palate, and the combination of cleft lip and palate are considered to have a multifactorial cause, including both environmental and genetic elements. Oral clefts have been linked to genes located on more than several chromosomes including 1, 2, 4, 6, and 19, among others (OMIM %119530 Orofacial Cleft 1, 2004). Other genes have been found that are thought to either interfere with the clefting process or enhance it. Clefting has been shown to have a possible association with maternal smoking (especially more than 20/day) and exposure to passive smoke but not with paternal smoking (Shaw et al., 1996). Accutane (the drug used to treat severe cystic acne), anticonvulsants such as phenytoin, warfarin (an anticoagulant), and ethanol (the alcohol in beverages) are known to cause clefting and other craniofacial defects (Czeizel, 2000). Some suggest that a maternal folic acid deficiency might contribute to clefting defects because folic acid has been shown to help prevent neural tube defects such as spina bifida (Czeizel, 2000). In addition, more than 150 different syndromes have cleft lip and/or palate as possible features. Otherwise, the etiology for isolated or nonsyn-

Box 6.7 MULTIFACTORIAL INHERITANCE

Examples of disorders that are commonly considered to be caused by multifactorial inheritance.

ADULTS

Hypertension
Atherosclerosis
Type II diabetes
Psoriasis
Schizophrenia
Ankylosing spondylitis
Gout
Cancer
Obesity
Osteoporosis
Parkinson's disease
Alcoholism

CHILDREN

Pyloric stenosis
Cleft lip and palate
Congenital heart disease
Congenital hip dislocation

dromic cases of clefting that account for about 70% of clefts is unknown at this time (NIDCR, 2006).

Method of Transmission: The method of transmission depends on the specific cause of the clefting. Multifactorial clefts can exhibit evidence of autosomal dominant, autosomal recessive, and sex-linked inheritance patterns or they may be the result of a spontaneous mutation or mutations in one or more genes. While genetic factors appear to predispose an individual for clefting, environmental factors act as a trigger to cause development of the cleft.

Epidemiology: Orofacial clefting of some type occurs in approximately 1 of every 500 to 550 live births in the United States. The frequency and cause of oral clefting is highly related to the sex of the individual and the type of cleft involved. Females who have a bilateral cleft have the greatest number of genetic influences and the lowest number of environmental factors, and males with a unilateral cleft have the lowest number of genetic influences and the highest number of environmental factors (Tolarova, July 2005).

Pathogenesis: Cleft lip/palate occurs when there is incomplete or no fusion of the palate, premaxilla, and related soft tissues during the 6th to 8th week of embryologic development. Multifactorial inheritance implies that changing something in the environment will either interfere with the development of a cleft or enhance the

probability that a genetic predisposition will actually result in clefting.

Extraoral Characteristics: Not applicable

Perioral and Intraoral Characteristics: Refer to Figure 6.24 for examples of cleft lip, cleft palate, and cleft

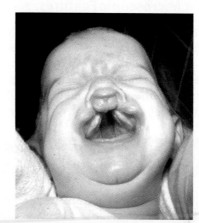
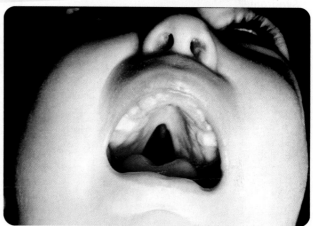
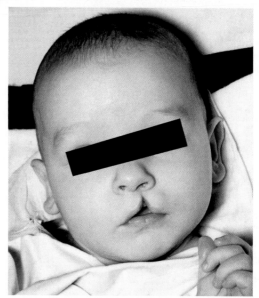

Figure 6.24. Oral clefting. **A.** Bilateral cleft of the lip and palate. (From Rubin E, Farber JL. Pathology. 3rd ed. Philadelphia: Lippincott Williams & Wilkins, 1999.) **B.** Cleft of the hard and soft palates. (Courtesy of R Chase.) **C.** Unilateral cleft of the upper lip. (Courtesy of R Chase.)

lip and palate. Clefting can interfere with proper development of the teeth and alveolar ridges, causing hypodontia, malformed teeth, bony defects of the maxillary alveolar process, and malocclusion.

Distinguishing Characteristics: Not applicable

Significant Microscopic Features: Not applicable

Dental Implications: The dental implications of cleft lip and/or palate depend on the number of dental abnormalities present and the stage of treatment. The dental hygienist can play an important role in managing the care of the individual with a cleft lip and/or palate through education and preventive dental hygiene therapy.

Differential Diagnosis: A cleft lip or palate is either present or not present. However, since 10 to 20% of clefts are part of a syndrome, it is important to rule out the presence of these syndromes. Refer to Table 6.5.

Treatment and Prognosis: Treatment for cleft palate focuses on prevention first. Folic acid has been shown to reduce the occurrence of nonsyndromic cleft lip and/or palate along with neural tube defects such as spina bifida. Because many women are not aware that they are pregnant until after the fetus has passed the 12th week of development, all women of childbearing age who are not actively preventing pregnancy should eat a diet rich in all nutrients, especially folic acid, and take a multivitamin

Table 6.5	HEREDITARY SYNDROMES ASSOCIATED WITH POSSIBLE CLEFT LIP AND/OR PALATE

These syndromes are not discussed in the text, but are associated with cleft lip and/or palate.

Syndrome	Characteristics in addition to cleft lip and/or palate
Pierre-Robin sequence	Micrognathia Posterior soft palate cleft is more likely than any other type Tongue tends to fall back in the throat Feeding and respiratory problems
Craniofacial dysostosis (Crouzon syndrome)	Abnormal head shape Hypoplastic midface Hearing and vision deficits Severe maxillary hypoplasia and malocclusion
Deletion 22q11 syndrome	Congenital heart defects Unique hypoplastic facial features Microcephaly Learning disabilities Thymic hypoplasia
Miller syndrome	Hypoplastic cheeks Micrognathia Small, cup-shaped ears Drooping lower eyelids
Opitz syndrome	Facial abnormalities Hypertelorism Intellectual defects
Stickler syndrome	Cataracts Midface hypoplasia Hearing loss Hypermobile joints
Saethre-Chotzen syndrome	Early fusion of the skull bones Facial abnormalities Short, webbed fingers and toes Small ears with hearing loss Bone abnormalities
Van der Woude syndrome	Lower congenital lip pits
Nager syndrome	Midface hypoplasia Down-slanting eyes with no lower lashes External ear absent or hypoplastic Hypoplastic or absent thumb Short forearm with limited range of motion in the elbows

supplement that contains an appropriate amount of folic acid (Czeizel, 2000). Up to 70% of neural tube defects (March of Dimes, 2005) and a "significant reduction" in cleft lip and/or palate (Czeizel, 2000) could be prevented by folic acid. The dental hygienist can affect many families by educating patients about this simple preventive action.

Numerous surgical and other medical and dental treatments are necessary to correct cleft lip/palate. The surgeries are scheduled starting at about 3 months of age and ending at about 1 year to correct simple clefts. Orthodontic treatment starts as early as age 1 and will continue until all teeth are erupted and into the teen years. Other procedures might include an alveolar bone graft and procedures to correct any nasal deformities (Tolarova, 2005). The prognosis for individuals with a repaired cleft is excellent. Clefts that are not repaired can cause eating, speech, and respiratory difficulties along with severe psychologic and social problems.

SUMMARY

- The etiology of most congenital abnormalities is unknown.
- Teratogens can cause errors in morphogenesis when an embryo or fetus is exposed to them at a crucial time in organ development. Exposure of the embryo or fetus to teratogenic agents after the 12th week of gestation is much less likely to result in the development of abnormalities.
- Fetal alcohol spectrum defects are a group of defects that are associated with the ingestion of alcohol during pregnancy. The amount of alcohol ingested that will result in any of these disorders is unknown and is different for each woman. A diagnosis of fetal alcohol syndrome requires that three criteria be met: growth problems, neurodevelopmental problems, and characteristic facial features. Prophylactic antibiotics might be necessary prior to dental care, because these patients have an increased risk of heart defects.
- The TORCH syndrome is caused by a variety of organisms that are able to affect the developing embryo/fetus in the womb. The general characteristics include heart defects, mental deficiencies, hearing and vision defects, and premature birth. Oral defects associated with TORCH are related to the specific cause and can include oral clefts and abnormally shaped teeth. Prophylactic antibiotics might be necessary prior to dental care because these patients have an increased risk of heart defects.
- Healthcare professionals are responsible for integrating genetic information into their practices.
- Genetic material or chromatin is found in the nucleus of cells and is passed from parents to offspring in the form of chromosomes.
- The structure of each chromosome is unique to that specific chromosome, but each chromosome is made up of a p-arm and a q-arm, a centromere, and two telomeres.
- There are 22 pairs of autosomal chromosomes and 1 pair of sex chromosomes in a diploid cell; haploid cells contain only one of each chromosome.
- The Lyon hypothesis states that the genetic material on the second X chromosome in females is largely inactivated to equalize the genetic activity potential between males that have only one X chromosome and females. The inactive X chromosome material can be seen as the Barr body, lying adjacent to the inner surface of the nuclear membrane.
- The functional unit of genetics is the gene.
- An individual's genotype is not necessarily expressed in their phenotype because of the characteristics of inheritance; for example, dominance, codominance, mosaicism, and variable expressivity.
- Chromosomal abnormalities involve either the number of chromosomes or their structure.
- Trisomy 21 is usually caused by the nondisjunction of chromosome 21 during meiosis. Trisomy 21 causes mental impairment, congenital heart defects, compromised immune system, hearing and vision defects, and other organ/system defects. Flat facial features and epicanthal folds are characteristic of this disorder. There is a myriad of oral problems associated with trisomy 21, including midface hypoplasia, clefts, malocclusion, and a very high risk of periodontal disease. Prophylactic antibiotics might be necessary prior to dental care because these patients have an increased risk of heart defects.
- Klinefelter syndrome is caused by one or more extra X chromosomes in a male genotype. The individual is male but lacks development of secondary sexual characteristics. Mental deficiencies and learning disabilities are seen more often in those who have more than one extra X chromosome. Congenital heart defects such as mitral valve prolapse are common, indicating the possible need for antibiotic prophylaxis.

(continued)

SUMMARY *(continued)*

- Turner syndrome is the only monosomy that is compatible with life. Individuals with Turner syndrome are very short, have a webbed neck, and do not develop secondary sex characteristics. They usually are of average intelligence but may have learning disabilities. Osteoporosis and endocrine disorders as well as a slightly higher risk of heart and vascular defects are characteristic of Turner syndrome. Prophylactic antibiotics might be necessary prior to dental care because these patients have an increased risk of heart defects.

- Cri du chat syndrome is caused by the deletion of genes from chromosome 5. The syndrome is named for the characteristic catlike cry that newborns make. Severe growth retardation, heart defects, mental deficiencies, and chronic medical problems are characteristic of this syndrome. Oral problems include hypodontia, delayed eruption, clefting, and malocclusion. Prophylactic antibiotics might be necessary prior to dental care because these patients have an increased risk of heart defects.

- Single-gene disorders usually result in the creation of abnormal proteins or the absence of an important protein.

- Single-gene disorders follow dominant, recessive, or sex-linked inheritance patterns.

- Most traits that are observed in a phenotype are not linked to one gene but are influenced by several genes working together or oligogenic inheritance.

- Marfan syndrome is an autosomal dominant disorder that causes the production of a defective protein that is essential in making certain connective tissues such as the periosteum and heart and vascular tissues. These patients are very tall and have long arms and legs. Mitral valve prolapse is very common, and many have to have the valve replaced. Dental implications include prophylactic antibiotics if needed, care of the temporomandibular joint, and malocclusion caused by a high arched palate.

- Cleidocranial dysplasia is an autosomal dominant disorder causing bone malformation and agenesis. Multiple supernumerary teeth and delayed eruption as well as pseudoanodontia are common.

- Treacher Collins syndrome is an autosomal dominant disorder that affects the development of the craniofacial structures, causing gross deformities. There are no other organs or tissues involved, and intelligence is normal. There is always some hearing loss.

- Ehlers-Danlos syndrome is usually caused by autosomal dominant inheritance. Ehlers-Danlos syndrome causes the production of an abnormal collagen leading to weakness in the structures that are composed of it. Hyperelastic, thin, loose skin is the characteristic feature of this disorder. Blood vessels, skin, and mucous membranes are very fragile and can be the cause of excessive bleeding after minor trauma. Prophylactic antibiotics might be necessary prior to dental care because these patients have an increased risk of heart defects.

- Papillon-Lefèvre syndrome follows an autosomal recessive inheritance pattern and is associated with severe periodontal disease resulting in the loss of both the primary and permanent teeth several years after they erupt.

- Hereditary forms of gingival fibromatosis are associated with a variety of disorders.

- Forms of ectodermal dysplasia are associated with all types of inheritance patterns. ED1 follows an X-linked recessive pattern and is the most common form. The disorder causes the development of defective tissues that are derived from the embryonic ectodermal cells. This includes skin, sweat glands, salivary glands, hair, nails, and teeth. Temperature regulation, increased incidence of respiratory infections, and photophobia are all characteristic of the disorder. Dental implications include hypodontia or anodontia, and xerostomia.

- Multifactorial inheritance involves the additive effects of a number of genes and environmental factors.

- Cleft lip and/or palate is considered to follow a multifactorial inheritance pattern. They have been associated with numerous genetic syndromes and follow any of the inheritance patterns. Most cases are of unknown origin; however, maternal smoking, alcohol, and certain drugs have been associated with cleft development. In addition, folic acid deficiency may be associated with clefts, indicating the possible need for folic acid supplements prior to and during pregnancy.

PORTFOLIO POSSIBILITIES

1. Get involved with Special Olympics, offer to present an educational session on basic oral hygiene care or help to perform the dental examinations that they offer for the participants. Make sure to get pictures of your adventure and write a summary of your experiences reflecting on what you have learned and how dental hygienists could make a difference in this population.
2. Visit the web page of an organization offering support for a disorder that interests you. Contact them and offer to answer questions on basic oral hygiene care to visitors to the site. You can also offer to research more complex questions or find an appropriate referral for them. Another option would be to ask them what their dental experiences have been, do they have a problem with access to care, have the problems associated with their disorder been adequately addressed, do they have specific needs that have not been addressed? Include copies of your correspondence with these individuals (identifying information blocked out) in your portfolio, with a reflection of your thoughts on what transpired and what the dental hygiene profession might do to improve services to them.

Critical Thinking Activities

1. Extra X chromosomes are found in Klinefelter syndrome, Turner syndrome is caused by the loss of an X chromosome. Why is there no mention of a syndrome that is characterized by a missing Y chromosome?
2. Why must all carriers of recessive traits be heterozygous for those traits?
3. Describe the mechanisms that can modify the phenotypic expression of an individual with a particular genotype. Why doesn't everyone with a particular genotype exhibit the exact same characteristics?
4. When you look at all of the genetic disorders discussed what do you feel are the most important dental/medical concerns that you will be faced with when determining dental hygiene care for these individuals? Why?

Case Study

A 3-year-old child is brought to the dental office for his first dental visit. The medical history is unremarkable, with no systemic problems noted except that the child has had to be brought to the hospital several times for very high temperatures. The extraoral examination notes pale thin skin with sparse, fine, blond hair. Intraorally, the hygienist notes delayed eruption or missing maxillary and mandibular incisors and mandibular molars. The teeth that are present are small and appear to be shaped abnormally.

a. What additional diagnostic information would you like to have and what would it tell you?
b. What additional information would you like to know from the parent?
c. What disorders cause delayed eruption and/or hypoplastic teeth?
d. What disorder do you think this child has?
e. Describe the dental problems that are related to this genetic disorder.

INTERNET RESOURCES

Center for Craniofacial Development and Disorders
www.hopkinsmedicine.org/craniofacial/Home/Index.cfm

FACES: The National Craniofacial Association
www.faces-cranio.org/

Gene Gateway: Exploring Genes and Genetic Disorders
www.ornl.gov/sci/techresources/Human_Genome/
posters/chromosome/index.shtml

National Organization on Fetal Alcohol Syndrome
www.nofas.org/default.aspx

Genes at Work: The Center for Human and Molecular
Genetics
www.umdnj.edu/genesatwork/index.htm

National Human Genome Research Institute
www.genome.gov/10001191

NCBI: Online Mendelian Inheritance in Man (OMIM)
www.ncbi.nlm.nih.gov/entrez/query.fcgi?db5OMIM

March of Dimes
www.marchofdimes.com

The National Marfan Association
www.marfan.org

NCHPEG (National Coalition for Health Professional
Education in Genetics)
http://www.nchpeg.org

Support for People with Oral and Head and Neck
Cancer
www.spohnc.org

REFERENCES

Beales PL, Badano JL, Ross AJ, et al. Genetic interaction of *BBS1* mutations with alleles of other *BBS* loci can result in non-mendelian Bardet-Biedl syndrome. Am J Hum Genet 2003;72:1187–1199.

Brent RL. Environmental causes of human congenital malformations: the pediatrician's role in dealing with these complex clinical problems caused by a multiplicity of environmental and genetic factors. Pediatrics 2004;113:957–968.

Campbell DJ, Carlin ME, Justen JE, Baird SM. Cri-du-chat syndrome: a topical overview. 5p Minus Society. Available at: http://www.fivep-minus.org/online.htm . Accessed January 4, 2006.

Chen H. Cri-du-chat syndrome. Last updated September 30, 2005. e medicine: Instant Access to the Minds of Medicine. Available at: http://www.emedicine.com/ped/topic504.htm. Accessed July 12, 2005.

Chen H. Klinefelter syndrome. Last updated December 17, 2004. e medicine: Instant Access to the Minds of Medicine. Available at: http://www.emedicine.com/ped/topic1252.htm. Accessed June 14, 2006.

Core curriculum for cleft palate and other craniofacial anomalies: a guide for educators. American Cleft Palate-Craniofacial Association 2004. Available at: http://www.acpa-cpf.org/EducMeetings/Core Curriculum2002a.pdf. Accessed July 24, 2005.

Cotran RS, Kumar V, Collins T. Robbins: Pathologic basis of disease. 6th ed. Philadelphia: WB Saunders, 1999:139–187.

Czeizel AE. Primary prevention of neural-tube defects and some other major congenital abnormalities: recommendations for the appropriate use of folic acid during pregnancy. Paediatric Drugs November/December 2000;2(6):437–449.

De Sanctis M, Zucchelli G. Interleukin-1 gene polymorphisms and long-term stability following guided tissue regeneration therapy. J Periodontol 2000;71(4):606–613.

Dittmer CD, Lentz S. Fetal alcohol syndrome. Last updated May 24, 2004. e medicine: Instant Access to the Minds of Medicine. Available at: http://www.emedicine.com/derm/topic767.htm. Accessed June 23, 2006.

Duran-McKinster C. Ectodermal dysplasia syndromes. Last updated January 14, 2004. e medicine: Instant Access to the Minds of Medicine. Available at: http://www.emedicine.com/derm/topic114.htm. Accessed June 23, 2006.

Fetal alcohol information, fetal alcohol syndrome. National Center on Birth Defects and Developmental Disabilities, CDC. Available at: http://www.cdc.gov/ncbddd/fas/default.htm. Accessed January 5, 2006.

Hart TC, Pallos D, Bozzo L, et al. Evidence of genetic heterogeneity for hereditary gingival fibromatosis. J Dent Res October 2000;70(10):1758–1764.

Hein C. The IL-1 polymorphism: the role of genetics in differentiating susceptibility to periodontal disease. Contemp Oral Hyg March 2005;5(3):8–12.

Holzhausen M, Goncalves D, Correa F de O, et al. A case of Zimmerman-Laband syndrome with supernumerary teeth. J Periodontol August 2003;74(8):1225–1230.

Human Genome Program (HGP). How many genes are in the human genome? Human Genome Project information, U. S. Department of Energy Office of Science, Office of Biological and Environmental Research, Human Genome Program. Available at: http://wwwornl/sci/techresources/Human_Genome/faq/genenumber.shtml. Accessed August 15, 2005.

Huether SE, McCance KL. Understanding pathophysiology. 3rd ed. St. Louis: Mosby, 2004:37–63.

Ibsen OAC, Phelan JA. Oral pathology for the dental hygienist. 4th ed. St. Louis: WB Saunders, 2004:216–253.

Kornman KS, Crane A, Wang HY, et al. The interleukin-1 genotype as a severity factor in adult periodontal disease. J Clin Periodontol 1997;24(1):72–77.

Kornman KS, di Giovine FS. Genetic variations in cytokine expression: a risk factor for severity of adult periodontitis. Ann Periodontol 1998;3(1):327–338.

Laufer-Cahana A. Ellis-van Creveld syndrome. Last updated March 8, 2002. e medicine: Instant Access to the Minds of Medicine. Available at: http://www.emedicine.com/ped/topic660.htm. Accessed June 17, 2006.

Lee R, Bowe WP, James WD, et al. Keratosis palmaris et plantaris. Last updated March 23, 2006. e medicine: Instant Access to the Minds of Medicine. Available at: http://www.emedicine.com/derm/topic589.htm. Accessed June 20, 2006..

Leshin L. Trisomy 21: the story of Down syndrome. Down syndrome: health issues. Available at: http://www.ds-health.com/trisomy.htm. Accessed July 23, 2005.

Létourneau Y, Pérusse R, Buithieu H. Oral manifestations of Ehlers-Danlos syndrome. J Can Dent Assoc 2001;67:330–334.

Lewanda AF. Treacher Collins syndrome. January 30, 2001. Center for Craniofacial Development and Disorders, Johns Hopkins University School of Medicine and Johns Hopkins Health System. Available at: http://www.hopkinsmedicine.org/craniofacial/Education/Disorders.cfm?Source=Physician . Accessed June 17, 2006.

Lewanda AF. Crouzon syndrome. June 8, 2000. Center for Craniofacial Development and Disorders, Johns Hopkins University School of Medicine and Johns Hopkins Health System. Available at: http://www.hopkinsmedicine.org/craniofacial/Education/Disorders.cfm?Source=Physician . Accessed June 23, 2006.

Lewanda AF. Fetal alcohol syndrome. Last updated December 16, 2003. Center for Craniofacial Development and Disorders, Johns Hopkins University School of Medicine and Johns Hopkins Health System. Available at: http://www.hopkinsmedicine.org/craniofacial/Education/Disorders.cfm?Source=Physician . Accessed June 2, 2006.

Lundgren T, Parhar RS, Renvert S, Tatakis DN. Impaired cytotoxicity in Papillon-Lefevre syndrome. J D Res May 2005;84(5):414–417.

Lundgren T, Renvert S. Periodontal treatment of patients with Papillon-Lefevre syndrome: a 3-year follow-up. J Clin Periodontol 2004;31:933–938.

Majeski, J. Genetic literacy for dental hygienists. Access January 2004;18(1):18-23.

March of Dimes. Leading categories of birth defects. Available at: http://www.marchofdimes.com/printable articles/680_2164.asp?printable=true. Accessed July 25, 2005.

March of Dimes. Quick reference: Accutane and other retinoids. March of Dimes. Available at: http://www.marchofdimes.com/printable articles/14332_1168.asp. Accessed May 20, 2006.

March of Dimes. Quick reference: chromosome abnormalities. March of Dimes. Available at: http://www.marchofdimes.com/printable articles/14332_1209.asp. Accessed May 20, 2006.

March of Dimes. Quick reference: thalidomide. March of Dimes. Available at: http://www.marchofdimes.com/printable articles/14332_1172.asp. Accessed May 30, 2006.

March of Dimes. Quick reference: Down syndrome. March of Dimes. Available at: http://www.marchofdimes.com/printable articles/14332_1214.asp. Accessed June 5, 2006.

Mayhew SL, Cummings RW, Gonzalez ER. Marfan's syndrome: pathogenesis and management. The U. S. Pharmacist Continuing Education Program February 2003. Available at: http://www.uspharmacist.com/ce/2688/default.htm. Accessed June 23, 2006.

Mone SM, Gillman MW, Miller TL, et al. Effects of environmental exposures on the cardiovascular system: prenatal period through adolescence. Pediatrics 2004;113:1058–1069.

Mundlos S. Cleidocranial dysplasia: clinical and molecular genetics. J Med Genet 1999;36:177–182. Available at: jmg.bmjjournals.com. Accessed June 13, 2006.

Murphy M, Lempert MJ, Epstein LB. Decreased level of T cell receptor expression by Down syndrome (trisomy 21) thymocytes. Am J Med Genet 1990;7:234–237.

National Coalition for Health Professional Education in Genetics (NCHPEG). Core Competencies in Genetics Essential for all Health-care Professions, National Coalition for Health Professional Education in Genetics. Available at: http://www.nchpeg.org/eduresources/core/Corecomps2005.pdf. Accessed July 14, 2005.

National Down Syndrome Society (NDSS). Available at: http://www.ndss.org/content.cfm?fuseaction=InfoRes. Accessed November 23, 2005.

National Institute of Dental and Craniofacial Research (NIDCR). New gene test reported for isolated cleft lip and palate. FACES: The National Craniofacial Association. Available at: http://www.faces-cranio.org/. Accessed June 25, 2006.

National Organization on Fetal Alcohol Syndrome. FAS and FASD clinical indicators. NOFAS. Available at: http://www.nofas.org/healthcare/indicators.aspx. Accessed June 23, 2006.

Noble RL, Warren RP. Altered T-cell subsets and defective T-cell function in young children with Down syndrome (trisomy 21). Immunol Invest August 1987;16(5):371–382.

Online Mendelian Inheritance in Man, OMIM ™, Johns Hopkins University, Baltimore. MIM Number: #123450 Cri-du-chat syndrome: 4/19/2005: Available at: http://www.ncbi.nlm.nhi.gov/entrez/dispomim.cgi?cmd=entry&id=123450. Accessed June 23, 2006.

Online Mendelian Inheritance in Man, OMIM ™, Johns Hopkins University, Baltimore. MIM Number: #154500 Treacher Collins-Franceschetti syndrome TCOF: 5/15/2005: Available at: http://www.ncbi.nlm.nhi.gov/entrez/dispomim.cgi?cmd=entry&id=154500. Accessed June 23, 2006.

Online Mendelian Inheritance in Man, OMIM ™, Johns Hopkins University, Baltimore. MIM Number: #190685 Down Syndrome.: 3/29/2006: Available at: http://www.ncbi.nlm.nih.gov/entrez/dispomim.cgi?id=190685. Accessed June 23, 2006.

Online Mendelian Inheritance in Man, OMIM ™, Johns Hopkins University, Baltimore. MIM Number: #228600 Fibromatosis, juvenile hyaline: 5/3/2005: Available at: http://www.ncbi.nlm.nhi.gov/entrez/dispomim.cgi?cmd=entry&id=228600. Accessed June 23, 2006.

Online Mendelian Inheritance in Man, OMIM ™, Johns Hopkins University, Baltimore. MIM Number: #305100 Ectodermal Dysplasia, Anhidrotic; ED1: 4/22/2004: Available at: http://www.ncbi.nlm.nhi.gov/entrez/dispomim.cgi?cmd=entry&id=305100. Accessed June 23, 2006.

Online Mendelian Inheritance in Man, OMIM ™, Johns Hopkins University, Baltimore. MIM Number: %119530 Orofacial Cleft1: OFC1: 3/15/2004: Available at: http://www.ncbi.nlm.nhi.gov/entrez/dispomim.cgi?cmd=entry&id=119530. Accessed June 23, 2006.

Online Mendelian Inheritance in Man, OMIM ™, Johns Hopkins University, Baltimore. MIM Number: %180900 Rutherford syndrome: 3/17/2004: Available at: http://www.ncbi.nlm.nhi.gov/entrez/dispomim.cgi?cmd=entry&id=180900. Accessed June 23, 2006.

Online Mendelian Inheritance in Man, OMIM ™, Johns Hopkins University, Baltimore. MIM Number: *606847 TCOF-1 Gene: 6/8/2006: Available at: http://www.ncbi.nlm.nhi.gov/entrez/dispomim.cgi?cmd=entry&id=606847. Accessed June 23, 2006.

Patel S, Davidson LE. Papillon-Lefèvre syndrome: a report of two cases. Int J Paediatr Dent 2004;14:288–294.

Pilcher ES. Dental care for the patient with Down syndrome. Down Syndrome Res Pract 1998;5(3):111–116. Available at: http://www.ds-health.com/dental.htm. Accessed June 23, 2006.

Porth CM. Essentials of pathophysiology: concepts of altered health states. Philadelphia: Lippincott Williams & Wilkins, 2004:36–63.

Price SA, Wilson LM. Pathophysiology: clinical concepts of disease processes. 6th ed. St. Louis: Mosby, 2003:8–32.

Questions and answers about . . . Marfan syndrome. NIH Publication no. 02-5000, October 2001.

Regezi JA, Sciubba JJ, Jordan RCK. Oral pathology: clinical pathologic correlations. 4th ed. St. Louis: WB Saunders, 2003.

Rubin E, Gorstein F, Rubin R, et al. Rubin's pathology: Clinicopathologic foundations of medicine, 4th ed. Baltimore: Lippincott Williams & Wilkins, 2005:215–279.

Sakellari D, Arapostathis KN, Konstantinidis A. Periodontal conditions and subgingival microflora in Down syndrome patients: a case-control study. J Clin Periodontol 2005;32:684–690.

Shaw GM, Wasserman CR, Lammer EJ, et al. Orofacial clefts, parental cigarette smoking, and transforming growth factor-alpha gene variants. Am J Hum Genet 1996;58:551–561.

Slavkin HC. The new genetics: genomes, biofilms and their implications for oral health professionals. Dimens Dent Hyg February/March 2003:16–21.

Socransky SS, Haffajee AD, Smith C, et al. Microbiological parameters associated with IL-1 gene polymorphism in periodontitis patients. J Clini Periodontol 2000;27(11):810–818.

Sohrabi F. Ectodermal dysplasia syndromes. February 19, 2004. Center for Craniofacial Development and Disorders, Johns Hopkins University School of Medicine and Johns Hopkins Health System. Available at: http://www.hopkinsmedicine.org/craniofacial/Education/Disorders.cfm?Source=Physician . Accessed June 23, 2006.

Sreedevi H, Munshi AK. Neutrophil chemotaxis in Down syndrome and normal children to *Actinobacillus actinomycetemcomitans*. J Pediatr Dent Winter 1998;22(2):141–146.

Stanier P, Moore GE. Genetics of cleft lip and palate: syndromic genes contribute to the incidence of non-syndromic clefts. Hum Molec Genet 2004;13(Review Issue 1):R73–R81.

Stedman's medical dictionary for the health professions and nursing. 5th ed. Baltimore: Lippincott Williams & Wilkins, 2005.

The Merck Manual, Sec 19, Ch.261, Congenital anomalies. Available at: http://www.merck.com/mrkshared/mmanual/section19/chapter261/2611.jsp. Accessed July 17, 2005.

The National Marfan Foundation (NMF). About Marfan syndrome: what causes the Marfan syndrome? Available at: http://www.marfan.org/nmf/GetContentRequestHandler.do?menu_item_id=2. Accessed Summer 2005.

The National Marfan Foundation (NMF). Marfan syndrome: an overview of related disorders. Available at: http://www.marfan.org/nmf/GetSubContentRequestHandler.do?sub_menu_item_content_id=54&menu_item_id=42. Accessed June 29, 2005.

Tolarova MM. Cleft lip and palate. Last updated July 12, 2005. e medicine: Instant Access to the Minds of Medicine. Available at: http://www.emedicine.com/ped/topic2679.htm. Accessed June 23, 2006.

TORCH Test, Dr. Joseph F. Smith Medical Library. Available at: http://www.chclibrary.org/micromed/00068480.html. Accessed June 3, 2005.

Turbadkar D, Mathur M, Rele M. Seroprevalence of TORCH infection in bad obstetric history. Indian J Med Microbiol. Available at: http://www.ijmm.org/article.asp?issn=0255-0857$_{ear}$=2003;volume=21;issue2$^+$age=108;epage=110;aulast=turbadkar. Accessed July 20, 2005.

Turner syndrome, high-risk newborn. University Health Care, University of Utah Health Sciences Center. Available at: http://uuhsc.utah.edu/healthinfo/pediatric/Hrnewborn/turner.htm. Accessed June 23, 2006.

Wu Q, Niebuhr E, Yang H, Hansen L. Determination of the `critical region' for catlike cry of cri-du chat syndrome and analysis of candidate genes by quantitative PCR. Eur J Hum Genet April 2005;13(4):475–485. Available at: http://www.ncbi.nlm.nih.gov/entrez/query. Accessed June 30, 2005.

Wulfsberg EA. Catch-22. April 9, 2003. Center for Craniofacial Development and Disorders, Johns Hopkins University School of Medicine and Johns Hopkins Health System. Available at: http://www.hopkinsmedicine.org/craniofacial/Education/Disorders.cfm?Source=Physician . Accessed January 7, 2006.

Wulfsberg EA. Cleidocranial dysplasia (cleidocranial dysostosis). April 24, 2003. Center for Craniofacial Development and Disorders, Johns Hopkins University School of Medicine and Johns Hopkins Health System. Available at: http://www.hopkinsmedicine.org/craniofacial/Education/Disorders.cfm?Source=Physician . Accessed June 23, 2006.

Yoshihara T, Morinushi T, Kinjyo S, Yamasaki Y. Effect of periodic preventive care on the progression of periodontal disease in young adults with Down's syndrome. J Clin Periodontol 2005;32:556–560.

Endocrine Disorders

Key Terms

- Acidosis
- Acanthosis nigricans
- Acromegaly
- Adenohypophysis
- Advanced glycation end products
- Autoimmune thyroiditis/ Hashimoto thyroiditis
- Basal metabolic rate
- Dental erosion
- Diabetes mellitus
- Diabetic dermopathy
- Diabetic ketoacidosis
- Exophthalmos
- Fasting plasma glucose test
- Follicles
- Gestational diabetes mellitus
- Gigantism/giantism
- Glycosylation
- Goiter
- Graves' disease
- Hemoglobin A1c (HbA1c)
- Hormone
- Hypercalcemia
- Hyperglycemia
- Hyperglycemic hyperosmolar nonketotic syndrome
- Hyperinsulinism
- Hyperreflexia
- Hypoglycemia
- Hypoglycemic unawareness
- Hypoinsulinism

Objectives

1. Define and use the key terms listed in this chapter.

2. Briefly describe the functioning of the endocrine system.

3. Discuss the function of each organ and name the hormones involved.

4. State the etiology, method of transmission, and pathogenesis of the disorders discussed in this chapter.

5. Describe the extraoral, perioral, and intraoral characteristics of the disorders discussed in this chapter.

6. Note the dental implications and potential dental treatment modifications associated with the disorders discussed in this chapter.

7. Describe the differences between the clinical characteristics of hypothyroidism and hyperthyroidism.

8. Discuss the conditions that can lead to the formation of a goiter.

9. Describe the important epidemiologic factors associated with diabetes mellitus.

10. Describe the hemoglobin A1c test, how it is used, and the significance of the results.

11. Differentiate between hypoglycemia, diabetic ketoacidosis, and hyperglycemic hyperosmolar nonketotic syndrome as they relate to diabetes.

12. Discuss the long-term complications associated with diabetes mellitus.

- Hypophysis
  - Adenohypophysis
  - Neurohypophysis
- Macroglossia
- Macrovascular
- Microangiopathy
- Myxedema
- Negative feedback system
- Nephropathy
- Neurohypophysis

- Neuropathy
  - Autonomic neuropathy
  - Peripheral neuropathy
- Oral glucose tolerance test
- Osteopenia
- Parafollicular cells
- Polydipsia
- Polyphagia

- Polyuria
- Prayer sign
- Prediabetes
- Pseudoanodontia
- Retinopathy
- Striae
- Target cell
- Tetany
- Thyroid storm

13. Describe how the defective host response in diabetes mellitus can lead to periodontal destruction.

14. Identify the two endocrine abnormalities that increase the risk of acquiring an oral fungal infection.

15. Describe the differences and similarities between diabetes insipidus and diabetes mellitus.

16. Describe the proposed relationship between oral infections and premature birth.

Chapter Outline

THE ENDOCRINE SYSTEM

There are two major communications systems within the body, the endocrine system and the nervous system. Both systems are essential to the correct functioning of the body, and each system depends on the other to produce the desired results. The nervous system is responsible for fast processes or immediate actions such as movement, thought, breathing, and heart beat; while the endocrine system is responsible for the slower processes such as growth, metabolism, maintaining electrolyte balance, and the immune response, to name a few. Both systems use chemical messengers to relay information to and from body organs, tissues, and cells.

Organs and Hormones of the Endocrine System

Two types of glands are found in the body, exocrine, and endocrine. Exocrine glands secrete their molecular products onto the surface of skin or mucous membranes by means of a system of ducts. For example, the parotid gland secretes saliva through the parotid duct into the mouth. The endocrine system is comprised of glands that, unlike exocrine glands, secrete their molecular products or chemical messengers directly into the circulatory or lymphatic systems or into local tissues without the use of any ducts. The products that they secrete are called **hormones**. Hormones regulate the functions of the organs and systems in the body. Most hormones affect more than one type of cell or tissue and have different effects on each type of tissue. Some hormones can only function when there are several of them working together to create an effect. Specific hormones will only react with cells that have receptors for that hormone on their cell membranes. Cells that have these receptors are called the **target cells** for that hormone. An entire organ such as the thyroid gland or a specific tissue such as fat tissue will contain cells that all have receptors for one or more specific hormones, thereby creating a target organ or tissue. The hormone stimulates the target cell to do something or to stop doing something, depending on the type of hormone. When that action is complete, hormone release will stop until the body is signaled by another molecular substance, possibly another hormone, which sends the message for that action to occur again. The major endocrine glands and their locations are illustrated in Figure 7.1. To understand the disorders associated with the endocrine system one must understand how the system functions correctly. The following is a brief review of the processes involved in the proper functioning of the endocrine system.

General Function of the Endocrine System

Endocrine functioning begins with the hypothalamus, a gland located superior to the pituitary gland in the area of the midbrain. The hypothalamus serves as the central receiving area for input from the nervous system regarding changes in the environment, such as temperature, or changes in the body, such as pain or feelings of fright or terror. The hypothalamus then relays this information using the hormones listed in Table 7.1 to the next gland in the hierarchy, the pituitary gland or **hypophysis**. The pituitary gland is located directly beneath the hypothalamus in the sella turcica and is connected to the hypothalamus by the pituitary stalk (Fig. 7.2).The pituitary is made up of an anterior portion, or **adenohypophysis**, and a posterior portion, or **neurohypophysis**. The anterior pituitary receives releasing hormones from the hypothalamus by way of the connecting blood flow (Table 7.1). Using thyrotropin-releasing hormone (TRH) as an example, the pituitary gland secretes thyroid-stimulating hormone (TSH), which travels to the thyroid gland, the target organ in this case. The TSH stimulates the cells of the thyroid gland to create thyroid hormones such as thyroxine, which in turn, is secreted by the thyroid gland to travel to all of the cells that have a receptor for thyroxine. Thyroxine stimulates each cell, depending on the type, to start performing or to increase or decrease performance of a specific function. Table 7.2 lists the pituitary hormones,

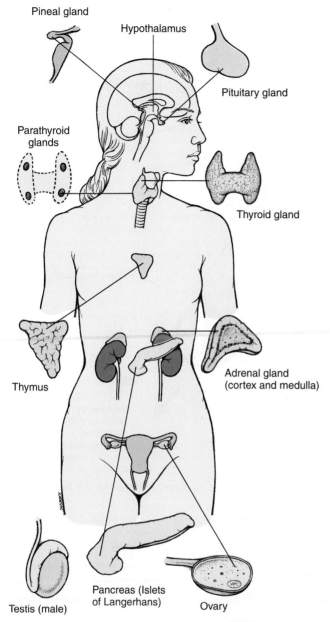

Pineal gland

Hypothalamus

Pituitary gland

Parathyroid glands

Thyroid gland

Thymus

Adrenal gland (cortex and medulla)

Testis (male)

Pancreas (Islets of Langerhans)

Ovary

Figure 7.1. Endocrine glands. Illustration depicting the location of the endocrine glands. (From Stedman's medical dictionary, 27th ed. Baltimore: Lippincott Williams & Wilkins, 2000.)

APPLICATION

Dental professionals must realize that rising levels of a specific type of prostaglandin (Chapter 3) are involved in the determination of when labor should begin. This same type of prostaglandin is created in response to infections, such as gingival and periodontal infections. Thus the proposed relationship between premature birth and periodontal infections is based on excessive production of prostaglandin because of an oral infection that, in turn, causes the level of circulating prostaglandin to rise to a critical point. This stimulates the release of oxytocin from the pituitary, which induces labor, prior to completion of the optimum gestation period.

their target glands or tissues, and their functions. Table 7.3 lists endocrine hormones, their functions, target cells, and the endocrine gland by which they are secreted.

The posterior pituitary receives hormones produced by the neurons of the hypothalamus. These hormones travel along the nerve fibers from the hypothalamus to the posterior pituitary, where they are stored until needed. The hormones secreted by the posterior pituitary are not releasing hormones (see Table 7.1). In other words, they do not stimulate another gland to secrete another hormone; instead, they act directly on the target cells that are designed to provide the desired function. For example, the hypothalamus is signaled by the body that it is time for a pregnant woman's labor to begin. The mechanisms involved in this determination are far outside the scope of this book; however, in response to this stimulus the hypothalamus triggers the posterior pituitary to release oxytocin. The oxytocin is picked up by the circulatory system and is received by receptors on the muscle cells of the uterus, which start to contract and begin labor.

The endocrine system is regulated in most cases by a **negative feedback system**. The negative feedback system works like a thermostat in your home (i.e., when the temperature drops below a set level, the thermostat recognizes it and starts the furnace). When the temperature gets to, or

Table 7.1	HYPOTHALAMIC HORMONES	
Hormone	**Target**	**Action**
Thyrotropin-releasing hormone (TRH)	Anterior pituitary	Stimulates the pituitary to release thyrotropin
Gonadotropin-releasing hormone (GnRH)	Anterior pituitary	Follicle-stimulating, luteinizing
Growth hormone-releasing hormone	Anterior pituitary	Stimulates growth hormone release
Adrenocorticotropin-releasing hormone	Anterior pituitary	Stimulates the release of adrenocorticotropin
Prolactin-releasing hormone	Anterior pituitary	Stimulates the release of prolactin
Oxytocin	Posterior pituitary	Stimulates labor
Antidiuretic hormone (ADH) (vasopressin)	Posterior pituitary	Stimulates the kidney to reabsorb water

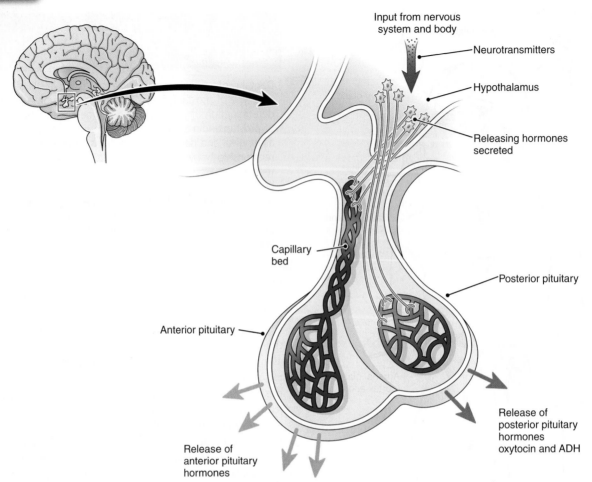

Figure 7.2. Hypothalamus and the pituitary gland. This illustration shows the intimate relationship between the hypothalamus and the pituitary gland.

Table 7.2	PITUITARY HORMONES	
Hormone	**Target Tissue/Cell**	**Function**
Growth hormone (GH)	Bones, muscles, and other tissues	Increases protein synthesis and growth
Adrenocorticotropic hormone (ACTH)	Adrenal cortex	Stimulates the production and release of hormones from the adrenal cortex
Thyroid-stimulating hormone (TSH)	Thyroid gland	Stimulates the production and release of thyroxine
Follicle-stimulating hormone (FSH)	Gonads	Stimulates the growth and maturation of the egg and sperm
Luteinizing hormone (LH)	Gonads	Stimulates the release of sex hormones from the ovaries and testes
Prolactin	Mammary glands	Milk production
Oxytocin	Uterus and breasts	Initiates labor and milk flow
Antidiuretic hormone (ADH)	Kidneys	Increases water retention and raises blood pressure
Endorphins	Neurons in the spinal cord and brain	Decreases pain sensations

Table 7.3 — SELECT ENDOCRINE HORMONES AND THEIR FUNCTIONS

Hormone	Secreting Tissue or Gland	Target Cells or Tissues	Functions
Thyroxine, triiodothyronine	Thyroid	Almost all	Maintains metabolism, is crucial in growth of brain and CNS
Calcitonin	Thyroid	Bones	Stimulates bone formation, regulates the amount of calcium in the blood
Parathormone	Parathyroids	Bones	Resorbs bone, regulates blood calcium levels
Thymosins	Thymus	Immune system cells	Activates T cells in the lymphatic system
Insulin	Pancreas	Muscles, fat, liver, others	Stimulates the uptake and use of glucose, increases the creation of glycogen and fat from glucose
Glucagon	Pancreas	Liver	Increases blood sugar by increasing the metabolism of glycogen
Somatostatin	Pancreas	Digestive system and cells of the pancreas	Inhibits release of insulin and glucagon, decreases all actions of the digestive tract
Epinephrine	Adrenal medulla	Heart, blood vessels	Increases heart rate, increases blood flow to muscles, increases glucose level in the blood, gets person ready for fight or flight response (sympathetic nervous system)
Norepinephrine	Adrenal medulla	Heart, blood vessels	Regulates the normal actions of the heart, blood vessels, etc. (sympathetic nervous system)
Glucocorticoids	Adrenal cortex	Immune system, many others	Antiinflammatory action, affects metabolism of nutrients, maintains blood glucose levels, modifies the effects of stress, involved in growth
Mineralocorticoids (aldosterone)	Adrenal cortex	Kidney	Stimulate excretion of potassium and reabsorption of sodium from the urine
Gastrin	Stomach lining	Stomach	Stimulates release of digestive juices and stomach muscle contractions
Melatonin	Pineal gland	Hypothalamus	Day and night cycles and other biorhythms
Estrogens	Ovaries	Female reproductive organs and other tissues	Female characteristics and sexual behavior
Progesterone	Ovaries	Uterus	Supports pregnancy, maintains female sexual characteristics
Androgens (testosterone)	Testes	Male reproductive organs and other tissues	Male sexual characteristics and behavior, sperm production

slightly above, the set temperature, the thermostat senses this and shuts off the furnace. Thus when the hypothalamus notices a drop in a particular hormone it sends a message to the pituitary gland to secrete the tropic or releasing hormone. The releasing hormone is then received by the target cells in a specific glandular tissue, which stimulates the gland to produce the needed hormone, increasing the level of that hormone. When the level is appropriate, the hypothalamus stops sending out the tropic hormone, and the target cells will not be stimulated to produce the hormone until the level drops again (Fig. 7.3). While the production of most hormones is regulated with a negative feedback system, there are a few examples of positive feedback regulation, occurring mainly in the female reproductive

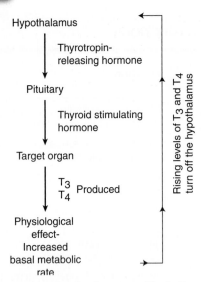

Figure 7.3. Negative feedback system. Illustration of how the negative feedback system functions, using the thyroid gland as an example.

system. In positive feedback regulation, an increasing level of one hormone stimulates the release or increased production of a second hormone. The process is terminated when the original hormone level drops, thereby causing the production of the second hormone to decrease or stop. A properly functioning endocrine system is essential to the well-being of each person. When the system malfunctions, life-threatening disorders occur.

ENDOCRINE SYSTEM DISORDERS

Endocrine disorders can result from numerous abnormalities. The pituitary gland may fail to secrete the appropriate tropic or releasing hormone or it may not receive the appropriate commands from the hypothalamus. The hormone produced could be defective because there is not enough of a crucial ingredient. Likewise, the genetic code for that protein could be defective or the secretory system could be damaged. The blood or lymphatic system may fail to transport the hormone to the target organ or the hormone could be inactivated by a substance or drug in the blood or lymphatic system. There could also be a problem with the receptor cells. The target cells might be blocked from receiving the hormone or the receptor cells could be missing altogether. Growths or tumors can form within the glands and interfere with production or release of the hormones. Tumors can also cause unregulated production and secretion of too much of a hormone. Finally, neoplastic growths can become so anaplastic that even if the tissue of origin is not a glandular tissue, the neoplastic cells can start producing their own hormones. Whatever the cause, the symptoms are usually the result of either too little or too much of a specific hormone, and thus the names of the disorders reflect either hypofunction or hyperfunction of the specific hormone or gland, for example, hyperthyroidism. The following sections discuss information specific to the functioning of each gland and examples of disorders related to them.

Hypothalamus and Pituitary Gland

As previously explained, these two glands work in conjunction to oversee the entire endocrine system. Problems associated with the hypothalamus will manifest as pituitary dysfunction because the role of the hypothalamus is to signal the pituitary to release its hormones. See Tables 7.1 and 7.2 for a listing of the hormones secreted by these glands and their targets and functions. The following conditions are examples of hypothalamic or pituitary disorders.

DIABETES INSIPIDUS

A lower-than-normal level of antidiuretic hormone (ADH), also called vasopressin, causes a disorder known as diabetes insipidus. This is not to be confused with diabetes mellitus, which results from an insulin deficiency or dysfunction. The blood glucose level of an individual with diabetes insipidus should be normal. ADH is synthesized in the hypothalamus gland, stored in the posterior pituitary, and released by the pituitary when signaled to do so by the hypothalamus. ADH controls the reabsorption of water into the body by the kidneys. An inadequate level of ADH causes large amounts of urine to be produced, which quickly leads to dehydration and electrolyte imbalances. Tumors of the hypothalamus or pituitary, head trauma, brain aneurysms, and infections can interfere with the synthesis or transportation of ADH from the hypothalamus or its secretion from the pituitary. Diabetes insipidus can also occur when the target cells in the kidneys do not respond to ADH because of an acquired or genetic kidney disorder. Autoimmune disorders can cause either underproduction of ADH or target tissue response deficiencies. This is a rare disorder that affects males and females equally and can be found in all ages and races.

There are no obvious physical characteristics associated with this disorder. However, affected individuals have intense thirst, or **polydipsia,** and excessive urination, or **polyuria.** In fact, this disorder is called diabetes insipidus because it shares these two universal symptoms with diabetes mellitus. Polydipsia has been generally defined as drinking more than 1 gallon of liquid per day (The Diabetes Insipidus Foundation, 2005). If water intake is inadequate, dehydration will occur rapidly and can be life threatening. The treatment for diabetes insipidus is administration of desmopressin, a synthetic analogue (substance that functions in a similar fashion) of ADH, maintenance of an adequate water intake, and a low sodium diet. In less severe cases, treatment may focus on maintaining an adequate hydration level without the need for supplemental ADH. The prognosis for these individuals is excellent as long as they maintain an adequate water intake.

There has been no evidence of increased dental disease in these patients. However, dehydration is associated with xerostomia, and those who are at risk for xerostomia should have their salivary flow assessed. If insufficient saliva is found, treatment protocols for xerostomia should be followed (Clinical Protocol 4).

HYPOPITUITARISM

Hypopituitarism is a general name given to a deficiency of any of the pituitary hormones. The specific cause of the deficiencies may be related to the hypothalamus or the pituitary gland. By far, the greatest number of these cases are caused by pituitary neoplasms, most often adenomas. Other causes are genetic, infection, radiation therapy to the pituitary or surrounding areas, trauma, and others. Approximately 70 to 90% of the gland must be destroyed for deficiencies to become obvious (Porth, 2004). Hypopituitarism results in the underproduction of a trophic or release-stimulating hormone that in turn will result in a lower level of the target hormone such as growth hormone or thyroid hormone. The characteristics of hypopituitarism are determined by the specific hormones that are affected. For example, if only the thyroid-stimulating hormones are affected, you would expect to see symptoms of hypothyroidism; adrenocorticotropic hormone would cause hypoadrenalism, etc. The age of the individual will also determine the extent and severity of the symptoms. Children need these hormones for their bodies and minds to develop normally; therefore a deficiency in any of these would cause more severe problems in the young than in the adult, who has already matured.

In adults, chronic deficiency of the pituitary hormones will cause a type of premature aging. The skin becomes thin, pale, dry, and winkled and there is little or no sweating. Axial and pubic hair is lost, and the remaining hair becomes soft and fine. Secondary sexual characteristics become less apparent, and sexual libido is lost. Blood pressure and metabolism are low, and the individual tends to be cold intolerant, lethargic, and weak. Life-threatening adrenal crisis can occur if the adrenal glands do not produce enough cortisol (this is discussed below in the chapter). In children, the major presenting symptoms depend on the age and sex of the child. Infants will present with failure to thrive and growth retardation. If the thyroid gland is not functioning, congenital hypothyroidism will cause mental retardation. If the child is older, puberty will not occur. None of the secondary sexual characteristics will develop for either sex. Major hormone deficiencies are usually diagnosed at an early age because of the lack of growth or failure to thrive that is consistent with this type of disorder. Children will tend to have delayed eruption of the primary and permanent teeth, with associated delayed exfoliation of the primary dentition. The abnormal eruption/exfoliation pattern may cause significant malocclusion. The clinician should be prepared to educate the patients and families about this possibility and manage the malocclusion, if any.

Treatment depends on the specific cause and deficiencies that are involved. If the cause is a pituitary tumor, it would be necessary to remove it, if possible. Each deficiency needs to be addressed individually. If there was a deficiency in growth hormone, then a supplement would be prescribed, and so on. If left untreated, there is a high risk of premature death due to adrenal insufficiency. In addition, recent evidence appears to demonstrate an increase in premature adult cardiac deaths in individuals who discontinued the use of supplemental growth hormone after reaching their full linear (height) growth potential at puberty (Hoffman, April 2006).

HYPERSECRETION OF GROWTH HORMONE

Hypersecretion of growth hormone by the anterior pituitary affects patients differently, depending on the individual's age. **Gigantism** is the result of hypersecretion of growth hormone prior to the end of puberty. Gigantism manifests as excessive growth in the skeletal system producing very tall individuals (Fig. 7.4). When hypersecretion of growth hormone occurs after puberty, the disorder is called **acromegaly**. Acromegaly causes enlargement of soft tissues and the bones of the hands, feet, face, and

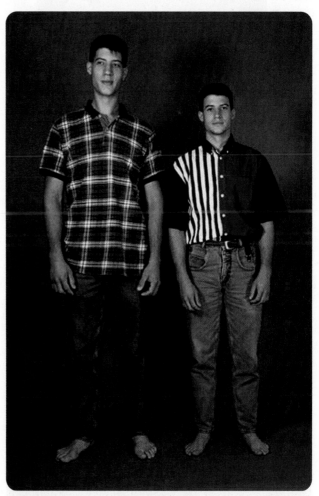

Figure 7.4. Giantism. A 22-year-old man with giantism due to excessive growth hormone is shown to the left of his identical twin. (From Gagel RF, McCutcheon IE. Images in clinical medicine. N Engl J Med 1999;340:524.)

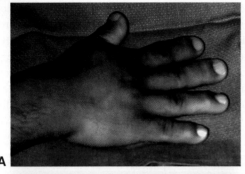

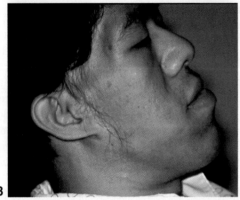

Figure 7.5. Acromegaly. Enlarged hands **(A)** and facial features **(B)** in patient with acromegaly. (Courtesy of Dr. Géza Terézhalmy.)

skull (Fig. 7.5). In addition, internal organs can become enlarged, and nerves can become entrapped and pinched in narrowing foramina.

Respiratory obstructions and sleep apnea, due to excess soft tissue, may interfere with sleep and cause an increased risk for respiratory infections. The facial changes in acromegaly are characteristic for this disease. The face becomes longer with frontal bossing. Enlargement of both maxilla and mandible may result in a class III occlusion and widely separated teeth (Fig. 7.6). The tongue enlarges **(macroglossia)**, and the dorsal surface may become deeply fissured. Dental treatment can be complicated because of the severe malocclusion caused by excessive growth of the jaw bones. Removable prosthetic appliances may be diffi-

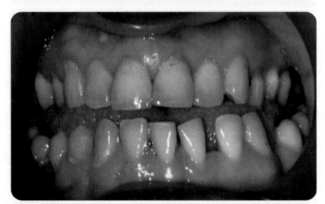

Figure 7.6. Acromegaly. Enlargement of the mandible with interproximal spacing and characteristic class III occlusion. (Courtesy of Dr. Géza Terézhalmy.)

cult for the patient to tolerate because of macroglossia. Medical treatment focuses on removing the cause of the excess growth hormone. In most cases, a pituitary tumor is the cause, and surgical removal is the treatment of choice. Children who are diagnosed with hypersecretion of growth hormone are usually diagnosed quickly because of the very rapid growth that occurs. This rapid diagnosis enables swift medical and surgical treatment, which decreases the chance that they will have any long-term problems associated with giantism or acromegaly.

Thyroid Gland

The thyroid gland develops in the oral cavity at the base of the tongue at the foramen cecum. It migrates into the neck along the thyroglossal duct tract. The thyroid gland is comprised of **follicles**, or microscopic sacs, containing a protein called *colloid*. The cells that make up the walls of these sacs are called follicular cells and produce two types of thyroid hormone, *triiodothyronine* (T_3) and *thyroxine* (T_4). One other type of cell, a **parafollicular** or C cell, populates the thyroid gland. The parafollicular cells produce calcitonin, which inhibits the release of calcium from the bones into the blood and other fluids. The functions of the thyroid hormones are listed in Box 7.1.

Box 7.1   THYROID HORMONE FUNCTIONS

Hormone	Function
Thyroxine and triiodothyronine	• Regulates basal metabolic rate[a] and body temperature • Regulates lipid metabolism • Regulates carbohydrate metabolism • Affects all aspects of linear growth • Crucial in the development of the brain before and after birth • Regulates heart rate, contractibility, and output • Regulates vasodilation • Regulates respiratory rate • Regulates gastrointestinal activity • Affects libido and fertility
Calcitonin	• Decreases blood calcium levels by inhibiting resorption of bone by osteoclasts and reabsorption of calcium and phosphorus in the kidneys

[a]The basal metabolic rate is defined as the amount of oxygen consumed by the body (cells) while at rest (not physically active).

Disorders of the thyroid gland normally manifest symptoms associated with either an excess or deficiency of thyroid hormones. One of the physical manifestations of thyroid disease is called a **goiter**. A goiter is an enlarged thyroid gland caused by hypertrophic or hyperplastic growth. Goiters are not caused by neoplastic growth. If the thyroid gland is not producing enough thyroid hormone or the hormone is defective, the pituitary will continue to release TSH to increase the gland's production of thyroid hormones. The excessive stimulation of the hypofunctioning gland by TSH results in chronic enlargement of the thyroid gland as it attempts to produce enough thyroid hormone to "turn off" the release of TSH by the pituitary. Since the cells that produce the thyroid hormones, T_3 and T_4, are incapable of increased hormone production, they must adapt to the increased demand by becoming hyperplastic or hypertrophic. A goiter can also be observed when there is excessive production of thyroid hormones by the thyroid gland. In this instance, the gland is not "turned off" even though there is an abundance of thyroid hormones circulating through the body. The gland becomes hyperplastic and hypertrophic to enable the uncontrolled production of hormones. Neoplasms of the thyroid gland, benign or malignant, will manifest as an enlarging thyroid gland. However, they are not responding to stimulating hormones from the pituitary gland, and the cells are not hyperplastic or hypertrophic; therefore, these enlargements are not considered goiters. Goiters or other thyroid gland enlargements may be observed by the dental professional during the extraoral examination. The goiter may be large or it may present as a subtle diffuse swelling of the neck just inferior to the thyroid cartilage (Fig. 7.7A and B). The patient should be referred to a physician for evaluation, if the presence of an enlarged thyroid gland is suspected. Thyroid disorders that cause hypofunction or hyperfunction of the gland are common.

Name: Hypothyroidism

Etiology: Internationally, the most common cause of hypothyroidism is an iodine-deficient diet. Without iodine the thyroid hormone that is produced is defective and nonfunctional. In the United States the most common cause of hypothyroidism is **autoimmune thyroiditis**, also known as **Hashimoto thyroiditis**. In this case the body sees the thyroid tissue as an antigen, and a chronic immune reaction occurs that causes progressive destruction of the thyroid tissues, resulting in a gradual decrease in thyroid hormones. Congenital hypothyroidism is seen in infants and can result from a defect in the genes that determine how the gland synthesizes the hormones, resulting in defective hormones or thyroid agenesis.

Method of Transmission:
Genetic transmission of hypothyroidism usually follows an autosomal recessive inheritance pattern. Other forms of hypothyroidism are not transmitted, rather they occur as unrelated events.

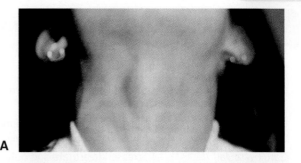
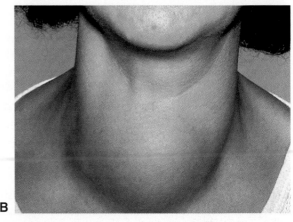

Figure 7.7. Goiter. **A.** Small goiter. (From Moore KL, Dalley AF II. Clinical oriented anatomy. 4th ed. Baltimore, Lippincott Williams & Wilkins 1999.) **B.** Large goiter. (From Weber J, Kelley J. Health assessment in nursing. 2nd ed. Philadelphia: Lippincott Williams & Wilkins, 2003.)

Epidemiology: It is thought that hypothyroidism occurs in approximately 5% of the population. It is most common in Caucasians and least common in African Americans. It is two to eight times more likely that a woman will have hypothyroidism than a man, and the risk of having hypothyroidism increases with age. Hashimoto thyroiditis is the most common cause of this disorder after the age of 6, occurring in 1 of every 5000 children, 3.5 of every 1000 adult women, and 1 of every 1000 adult men (Odeke and Nagelberg, May 2006). Congenital non-iodine-deficient hypothyroidism occurs in about 1 of every 4000 live births (Orlander et al., September 2005). Endemic congenital iodine deficient hypothyroidism occurs in about 5 to 15% of the world's population living in geographic areas that do not have access to natural or supplemental iodine (Postellon, June 2006).

Pathogenesis: Decreased synthesis and release of hormones produced by the thyroid or the production of defective hormones leads to the characteristic clinical manifestations described in the sections below.

Extraoral Characteristics: The general physical characteristics of hypothyroidism are listed in Table 7.4. Individuals with congenital hypothyroidism will exhibit similar symptoms in addition to generalized severe growth retardation, lack of muscle development, and mental retardation. Figure 7.8 shows the typical edema-

Table 7.4   CLINICAL MANIFESTATIONS OF HYPOTHYROIDISM

System	Manifestation
Nervous	Lethargy, memory loss, slowed thinking, depression, hearing loss, night blindness, cold intolerance, and mental agitation
Integumentary	Edema of the face, hands, and feet; skin is dry, rough, pale, and cool to the touch; hypohidrosis; bruises easily and heals slowly; hair is dry and brittle
Cardiovascular	Decreased heart rate and output, edema, atherosclerosis, enlarged heart with dilated chambers
Gastrointestinal	Decreased peristalsis leads to constipation and atrophy of the muscles of the system; anorexia, weight gain
Reproductive	Women: irregular, heavy menstruation, progesterone deficiency and decreased libido Men: decreased libido, erectile dysfunction and low sperm count
Musculoskeletal	Generalized muscle weakness, slowed reflexes, decreased bone formation and resorption and increased bone density, joint pain and stiffness
Pulmonary	Decreased respiratory rate and dyspnea
Blood	Anemia due to inadequate absorption of iron, folate, and/or vitamin B_{12} in the intestinal tract; increased cholesterol levels
Renal	Increased water retention

tous facial features evident in adults with hypothyroidism. This type of edema (**myxedema**) is caused by the accumulation of a substance within the cells of connective tissues all over the body. This substance causes water retention and can interfere with the function of organs such as the heart.

Perioral and Oral Characteristics: In addition to generalized facial edema, there can be puffy lips, enlarged gingival tissues, and macroglossia. Pharyngeal edema may result in a coarse, raspy voice and the individual may experience dysphagia. There will be delayed exfoliation of the primary teeth and delayed eruption of both the primary and the permanent teeth.

Distinguishing Characteristics: Reports of symptoms associated with hypothyroidism coupled with the characteristic goiter or neck swelling and facial edema of this disorder warrants a referral to a physician for a physical evaluation.

Significant Microscopic Features: Not applicable

Dental Implications: The etiology of gingival edema should be investigated. If there is no identifiable cause, the patient should be referred for a medical evaluation, especially if the edema is coupled with other symptoms of this disorder or other disorders. Delayed eruption of the primary and permanent teeth may produce **pseudoanodontia** (the temporary absence of teeth), which may have to be managed with prosthetics, depending on the severity and duration of symptoms.

Differential Diagnosis: Not applicable

Treatment and Prognosis: Treatment focuses on removing the cause of the disorder if possible and then replacing the deficient hormones with oral supplements. Normal function will be achieved shortly after starting the supplemental hormones. Untreated hypothyroidism has a poor prognosis and a high mortality rate (Odeke, Nagelberg, May 2006). If treated, there is every expectation for a normal life. Congenital hypothyroidism results in irreversible damage because thyroid hormones are essential in the proper development of the fetus. If replacement therapy is started at birth the damage can be mini-

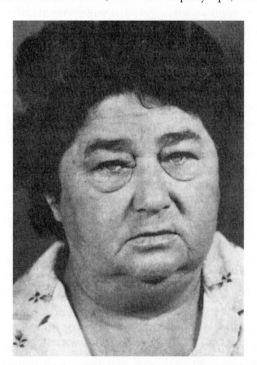

Figure 7.8. Hypothyroidism. Facial features characteristic of hypothyroidism. (From Porth CM. Pathophysiology concepts in altered health states. 6th ed. Philadelphia: Lippincott Williams & Wilkins, 2002.)

mized, but there will still be some lingering evidence of the disorder, at least as far as mental capacity is concerned. Neonatal screening programs in the United States have all but eradicated the effects of this disorder in infants. However, such is not the case in many undeveloped countries or in secluded populations where medical care is inadequate and/or there is an endemic lack of natural or supplemental iodine. In these cases the child is left with profound mental retardation and severe growth retardation resulting in a dwarflike stature.

Name: Hyperthyroidism

Etiology: The most common cause of hyperthyroidism is an autoimmune reaction caused by autoimmune antibodies that bind to TSH hormone receptors and induce the thyroid to create more thyroid hormone. The thyroid enlarges, or becomes hypertrophic, to compensate for this added requirement (Lee, July 2005). This disorder is called **Grave's disease**. Other disorders that can cause hyperthyroidism include inflammation of the thyroid gland or thyroiditis caused by an autoimmune or infectious process, a hyperfunctioning benign glandular tumor or follicular adenoma, and the transformation of a long-standing, nontoxic, multinodular goiter (one that is not secreting too much thyroid hormone) to a toxic, multinodular goiter (one that is hyperactive). Hyperthyroidism, no matter what the cause, presents with similar clinical manifestations. The focus here is on Grave's disease, since it is the most common form of hyperthyroidism.

Method of Transmission: Inheritance appears to have the strongest influence on the development of Grave's disease. It is not known how many genes are involved in the development of Grave's disease, but it is known that it takes more than one and most likely several. Multifactorial inheritance is involved because the rate of hyperthyroidism between identical twins is only about 30 to 50%. The exact environmental causes are unknown, but smoking has been associated with an increased risk of developing this disorder (Rubin et al., 2005).

Epidemiology: In the United States, cases of hyperthyroidism occur in about 1 of every 2000 people. Grave's disease is 5 to 10 times more common in women than in men and usually occurs between the ages of 20 and 40 years. All races are affected, but there is a lower incidence in African Americans than in whites and Asians (Lee, July 2005).

Pathogenesis: All symptoms of hyperthyroidism are caused by the elevated amount of circulating thyroid hormones that reach every cell in the body. This excess triggers an increase in the **basal metabolic rate** (the amount of oxygen consumed while at rest) of each cell, which results in hyperfunction of the cells and excessive body heat production. The results of this increase in metabolic rate are clearly seen in the clinical characteristics of this disorder.

Extraoral Characteristics: The person with long-standing hyperthyroidism typically presents with the general physical characteristics listed in Table 7.5 (Lee, July 2005; Rubin et al., 2005; Porth, 2004; Huther and McCance, 2004). One-third or more of those with Grave's disease will present with some degree of ocular pathology associated with hyperthyroidism. **Exophthalmos**, or protruding eyes, is caused by edema of the muscles and tissues behind the eyeball and is a distinctive feature of this disorder (Fig. 7.9).

Thyroid storm, or crisis, is a life-threatening emergency associated with a hyperactive thyroid. This is a rare

Table 7.5   CLINICAL MANIFESTATIONS OF HYPERTHYROIDISM

System	Manifestation
Nervous	Anxiety, nervousness, tremors of the hand, emotional instability, hyperactivity, insomnia, fatigue, heat intolerance
Integumentary	Warm, smooth, thin skin that may be flushed; hyperhidrosis; may exhibit edema and reddening of the skin of the lower legs; hair is thin, fine, and silky
Cardiovascular	Increased heart rate and output, palpitations, hypertension, atrial dysrhythmia, congestive heart failure, left ventricular hypertrophy
Gastrointestinal	Increased peristalsis and decreased water absorption in the intestines leads to diarrhea; significant weight loss, increased appetite
Reproductive	Women: oligomenorrhea or scanty menstrual flow, amenorrhea Men: impotence, decreased libido
Musculoskeletal	Increased muscle activity, large muscle weakness; increased bone resorption, but decreased bone density is normally only seen in postmenopausal women
Pulmonary	Increased respiratory rate and dyspnea
Blood	Decreased levels of cholesterol

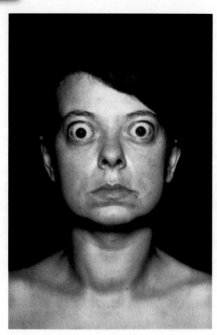

Figure 7.9. Hyperthyroidism (Grave's disease). A young woman with hyperthyroidism with a mass in the neck and exophthalmos. (From Rubin E, Farber JL. Pathology. 3rd ed. Philadelphia: Lippincott Williams & Wilkins, 1999.)

occurrence but may be seen in a patient with undiagnosed disease or in someone who has poorly controlled or inadequately treated disease. It is normally triggered by an infection, such as influenza, or some sort of trauma. It manifests with extreme symptoms of fever, tachycardia (rapid heart beat), angina (heart pain), and central nervous system effects, such as seizures and psychoses (Porth, 2004).

Perioral and Intraoral Characteristics: Intraoral manifestations in children include early exfoliation of the primary dentition and early eruption of the permanent teeth. Adults have an increased risk of **dental erosion**, loss of hard tissue due to acids not associated with bacterial metabolism, and an increased risk for the development or progression of periodontal disease and/or caries. Burning mouth syndrome (Chapter 10) is more common in these individuals as is osteoporosis of the maxilla and mandible (Chapter 10) (Regezi et al., 2003).

Distinguishing Characteristics: The most obvious clinical manifestation of hyperthyroidism is exophthalmos. Note that exophthalmos does not occur in every case and that hyperthyroidism must be confirmed with laboratory tests. In addition, as in hypothyroidism, a goiter may be present.

Significant Microscopic Features: Not applicable

Dental Implications: Oral problems associated with hyperthyroidism should be identified and treated aggressively. Topical fluoride should be used frequently at home to help prevent erosion and caries. Early exfoliation of the primary teeth and early eruption of the permanent teeth should be monitored. Symptoms of burning mouth syn-

drome should always prompt a referral to a physician if the cause can not be identified. Dental treatment modifications include caution using drugs containing epinephrine and atropine, which are contraindicated in poorly controlled hyperthyroidism because of the potential for causing thyroid storm, and using stress reduction protocols during treatment (Regezi et al., 2003).

Differential Diagnosis: Not applicable

Treatment and Prognosis: Treatment for hyperthyroidism is focused on decreasing the amount of thyroid hormone available to the cells. Drugs are available that interfere with the production of these hormones or with the use of them by the cells. The gland or portions of it can be removed surgically or the gland can be destroyed by using radioactive iodine that is injected into the body and is taken up by the thyroid gland. In almost all cases, treatment for hyperthyroidism results in a lifetime need for exogenous thyroid hormone replacement. The prognosis for this disorder is excellent if treated in a timely manner. Untreated hyperthyroidism can result in congestive heart failure, vision loss, musculoskeletal defects, and untimely death.

Parathyroid Gland

The parathyroid glands are found on the posterior surface of the thyroid gland. There are normally four small glands, two on each lobe of the thyroid, one in a superior position, and one in an inferior position, but as many as 12 have been reported (Rubin et al., 2005). The parathyroid glands in conjunction with the parafollicular cells of the thyroid gland regulate the level of calcium in the circulation. While up to 99% of the body's calcium is found in bone and dental tissues, the remaining circulating calcium is essential to the proper functioning of muscles, including the heart, and blood clotting mechanisms. Specialized receptors in the parathyroid gland sense when the amount of calcium in the blood drops below a specific level. When this occurs, the parathyroid gland releases parathyroid hormone (PTH). PTH stimulates release of calcium from bone, increases reabsorption of calcium within the kidney, and stimulates the production of vitamin D within the kidney. Vitamin D facilitates the absorption of calcium through the intestine. Disorders of the parathyroid glands are associated with hypofunction or hyperfunction of the glands.

HYPOPARATHYROIDISM

The most common cause of hypoparathyroidism is removal of the glands during surgical removal of the thyroid gland. Hypoparathyroidism can also be inherited as an element of a multiglandular syndrome or, rarely, by itself. DiGeorge syndrome (Chapter 4) is associated with agenesis of the parathyroid glands. Hypoparathyroidism results in decreased levels of PTHhormone, which leads to hypocalcemia or a low level of calcium in the blood. Hypocalcemia causes hyperexcitable muscle tissues, resulting in muscle spasms (**tetany**), **hyperreflexia** (exaggerated reflexes), convulsions, and respiratory muscle spasms, which could be severe enough to cause asphyxiation and death. Muscle spasms also affect the muscles of the head and neck area (Huether and McCance, 2004). When young children are affected, the developing dentition undergoes hypoplastic changes that can result in pitting of the enamel and abnormal tooth form or number. Treatment is focused on maintaining an adequate blood calcium level with calcium and vitamin D replacements.

HYPERPARATHYROIDISM

There are two main types of hyperparathyroidism, primary and secondary. The cause of most cases of primary hyperparathyroidism is not known. Some have been associated with an autosomal dominant inheritance pattern. Hyperparathyroidism is also seen in multiple endocrine neoplasia syndromes 1 and 2A (discussed in Chapter 17). Parathyroid cancer is rare but does account for some primary cases. The most common cause of primary hyperparathyroidism is adenoma or benign tumor of the parathyroid glands. Secondary hyperparathyroidism is associated with chronic kidney disease.

Excess PTH causes increased resorption of bone, increased reabsorption of calcium from the kidney, and increased production of vitamin D. Findings in the musculoskeletal system include bone pain, bone demineralization, pathologic fractures, and muscle weakness. Kidney stones tend to develop in these individuals because of the high level of calcium in the circulation, or **hypercalcemia** (Rubin et al., 2005). Demineralization in the maxilla and the mandible may present as generalized thinning and loss of trabecular detail as seen radiographically or with a cystic appearance due to replacement of the bone with fibrous tissue. Demineralization associated with this disorder is often observed in panoramic radiographs. Therefore, panoramic radiographs are needed for diagnostic purposes if this condition is suspected. The lamina dura may be partially or totally lost. The teeth may loosen, and in the case of chronic renal disease, the pulp and canals may become completely calcified. Partial or complete absence of the lamina dura noted on radiographs should elicit a referral to a physician for evaluation. The treatment for hyperparathyroidism depends on the cause and severity of the symptoms. Surgery to remove adenomas of the primary disease or hyperplastic glands of secondary disease will resolve the problems associated with hypercalcemia. Medical treatment for those with minor or no symptoms would include monitoring their blood calcium level and level of PTH, limiting intake of calcium, and drastically increasing fluid intake.

Adrenal Gland

The adrenal gland is made up of two very different parts: (1) the *medulla* and (2) the *cortex*. The medulla forms the inner part of the gland and works in conjunction with the sympathetic nervous system. The medulla secretes *epinephrine* (adrenaline) and *norepinephrine*, both of which are also produced within the nervous system. The adrenal cortex forms the outer portion of the gland and is responsible for the production of steroid hormones that are essential for the maintenance of health and life itself. Table 7.6 describes these hormones and their actions. This text concentrates on disorders affecting the adrenal cortex because they are more germane to the clinical practice of dental hygiene. Disorders of the adrenal cortex usually manifest with symptoms associated with either excessive or insufficient levels of the hormones that it secretes.

Name: Adrenocortical insufficiency

Etiology: *Primary adrenal insufficiency,* or *Addison's disease,* is a chronic disorder that occurs when cortical hormones are deficient and adrenocorticotropic hormone levels are elevated because the feedback system is not functioning. This disorder is usually caused by destruction of the adrenal gland. In years past, tuberculosis was the major cause of adrenal destruction in the United States; however, autoimmune destruction appears to be the most common cause at this time (Marzotti and Falorni, 2004). Other causes of adrenal destruction include cancer metastasis, histoplasmosis infection, hemorrhage associated with anticoagulants, opportunistic infections associated with acquired immune deficiency syndrome, and trauma. Rarely, Addison's disease can be associated with an autosomal recessive genetic trait.

Secondary adrenal insufficiency occurs as a result of hypothalamic and/or pituitary disorders or, more commonly, the sudden withdrawal of ingested or injected steroids. Refer to the information on the pituitary gland listed previously for a review of the disorders associated with hypofunction of this gland.

Method of Transmission: In cases other than inherited types, this disorder is not directly transmitted. However, infections that can cause Addison's disease (e.g., tuberculosis, histoplasmosis, and cytomegalovirus) can be transmitted from person to person.

Epidemiology: Primary adrenal insufficiency is a rare disorder with an estimated incidence of 1 per 8000 individuals (Marzotti and Falorni, 2004). It occurs equally among women and men and tends to be diagnosed between the ages of 30 and 50 years. Secondary adrenal insufficiency is much more common and is estimated to affect over 6 million people in the United States (Klauer, April 2005).

Pathogenesis: All of the symptoms of Addison's disease are related to deficiencies in the hormones that the

Table 7.6   HORMONES OF THE ADRENAL CORTEX

Classification	Specific Hormone	Actions
Mineralocorticoids	Aldosterone	• Regulates electrolyte balance by causing kidneys to reabsorb sodium and secrete potassium
Glucocorticoids	Cortisol, cortisone, corticosterone	• Acts as a cardiac stimulant • Induces the release of vasoconstrictive substances • Regulates carbohydrate, lipid, and protein metabolism • Inhibits the effects of insulin • Increases red blood cell and platelet levels • Acts as a strong antiinflammatory agent
Androgens	Dehydroepiandrosterone (DHEA[a]), androstenedione[a]	• Maturation of sex organs • Secondary sex characteristics • Spermatogenesis • Maintenance of various tissues including: nervous, skeletal, muscle, skin, and hair
Estrogen	Estradiol, estrone, estriol	• Maturation of sex organs • Secondary sex characteristics • Maintenance of the menstrual cycle and pregnancy • Maintenance of bone density • Various metabolic effects on numerous systems

[a]Converted to testosterone in peripheral tissues.

adrenal cortex secretes. Secondary adrenal insufficiency is related to pituitary or hypothalamic dysfunction or suppression of the production of glucocorticoids due to therapeutic steroid use. When an individual is taking therapeutic doses of steroid for a medical condition, the adrenal glands stop or slow production of the steroid because the pituitary is no longer sending out adrenocorticotropic hormone. It takes time, sometimes up to 12 months or longer, for the pituitary to recover and release adrenocorticotropic hormone and for the glands to begin production of cortisol and achieve an adequate blood level after withdrawal of the drug (Porth, 2004). Medically supervised withdrawal of these drugs is accomplished with doses decreasing gradually over several days or longer, depending on the length of treatment. If this is not done gradually, hypoadrenalism or adrenal insufficiency will occur.

Extraoral Characteristics: Individuals with Addison's disease present with weakness and fatigue, weight loss, abdominal pain, diarrhea or constipation, and syncope (loss of consciousness and postural tone due to decreased cerebral blood flow). Almost all individuals will exhibit hyperpigmentation of the skin (referred to as "bronzing") in exposed areas and in areas that encounter friction from clothing or function (Fig. 7.10). The color of the hyperpigmented areas gives the individual a tanned look. Hyperpigmentation is caused by elevated levels of adrenocorticotropic hormone (ACTH), which act to stimulate melanocytic production of melanin. Hyperpigmentation does not occur with secondary adrenal insufficiency

because there is no elevation of ACTH in this disorder. **Hypoglycemia,** low blood glucose level, is a common side effect of adrenal insufficiency, and patients must eat regularly scheduled meals to maintain blood glucose levels.

Perioral and Intraoral Characteristics: The most obvious symptom of Addison's disease in this area is hyperpigmentation of the gingival and mucosal tissues and the skin of the face. The color of the gingival/mucosal tissues may range from brown to black or even blue (Fig. 7.11).

Distinguishing Characteristics: Hyperpigmentation of the skin and gingival and mucosal tissues is a dis-

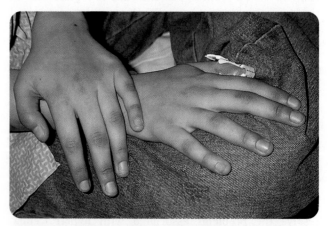

Figure 7.10. Addison's disease. Hyperpigmentation of the skin over the joints of the hands characteristic of Addison's disease. (From Fleisher GR, Ludwig S, Baskin MN. Atlas of pediatric emergency medicine. Philadelphia: Lippincott Williams & Wilkins, 2004.)

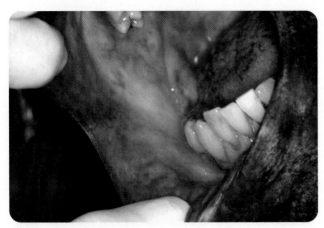

Figure 7.11. Addison's disease. Oral mucosal hyperpigmentation.

tinguishing feature of Addison's disease but not of secondary adrenal insufficiency.

Significant Microscopic Features: Not applicable

Dental Implications: Hyperpigmentation of the oral and perioral tissues should make the dental profession suspect the presence of the primary disorder. In addition, pigmentation of recent origin could be important and might alert the practitioner to the possibility of the disease. Symptoms of weakness, weight loss, and abdominal pain coupled with a history of steroid use would also alert the dental professional to a possible secondary insufficiency. Both instances require a referral to a physician for evaluation.

Differential Diagnosis: Not applicable

Treatment and Prognosis: Treatment for Addison's disease includes replacement of the deficient glucocorticoids with hydrocortisone and maintenance of adequate electrolyte levels in the blood. Secondary adrenal insufficiency also requires hormone replacement therapy until the cause of the problem is corrected, if at all possible. Chronic adrenal insufficiency can be a fatal disease if left untreated; when treated, there is every expectation for a normal life.

ACUTE ADRENAL INSUFFICIENCY OR ADRENAL CRISIS

Acute adrenal insufficiency, or adrenal crisis, is a life threatening condition caused by a sudden physiologically stressful event, such as surgery or trauma, in an individual with chronic adrenal insufficiency or sudden withdrawal of steroid medications after long-term use. Individuals who have used steroids for more than 4 years and those who have deficiencies in sex hormones produced by the adrenal cortex were found to be at the highest risk for an acute episode (Omori et al., 2003). The symptoms are associated with altered electrolyte balances due to mineralocorticoid deficiency and include weakness, vomiting, abdominal pain, confusion, low blood pressure, tachycardia, and

lethargy. Vascular collapse, loss of consciousness, coma, and death will result if this condition is not identified and corrected immediately. Adrenal crisis can be prevented in the dental environment by obtaining a complete medical and dental history as well as a medication history that includes questions regarding steroid use. If a patient has taken or is taking steroids, then questions about length of treatment and dosages are extremely important. Medical consultation should be considered if the patient took doses of more than 20 mg of corticosteroids for longer than 2 weeks within the last 2 years. In cases such as these, supplemental steroids may be needed to create an adequate level of steroid in the blood to avoid an adrenal crisis when dental care, such as extensive surgical procedures, or dental conditions, such as extensive infection, may put undue or unusual stress on the individual.

Name: Hyperadrenalism (Cushing disease or Cushing syndrome)

Etiology: Cushing disease is caused by the hypersecretion of adrenocorticotropic hormone by tumors of the pituitary gland, malignant tumors not of glandular origin (such as small cell carcinoma of the lung), and tumors that secrete corticotropin-releasing hormone that stimulates the production of adrenocorticotropic hormone. Cushing syndrome is most commonly caused by the use of oral or injected steroids for the treatment of medical conditions. Both are characterized by the same symptoms and clinical manifestations.

Method of Transmission: Not applicable

Epidemiology: Cushing disease is a rare disorder affecting about 13 per million individuals in the United States. Most of these cases are due to tumors of the pituitary or adrenal gland. More women than men have these tumors, and they usually occur between the ages of 25 and 40 years. Most nonglandular tumors that produce adrenocorticotropic hormone are related to small cell lung cancers. There is no reliable statistic related to the number of cases of Cushing syndrome caused by the medical use of steroids.

Pathogenesis: The manifestations of Cushing syndrome/disease are caused by the hypersecretion of adrenocorticotropic hormone, which will cause hypersecretion of the adrenal cortex hormones or hypersecretion of the steroid hormones themselves by the adrenal cortex.

Extraoral Characteristics: The classic *cushingoid* features include increased fat in the abdomen, above the clavicles, and in the upper back, which is often referred to as a "buffalo hump." Thinning or atrophy of the skin, rapid weight gain, and collagen deficiencies cause purple **striae**, or stretch marks, to form over the abdomen, upper arms, lower back, buttocks, upper thighs, and breasts (Fig. 7.12).Long-term Cushing syndrome/disease can lead to osteoporosis, diabetes mellitus, and stomach ulcers.

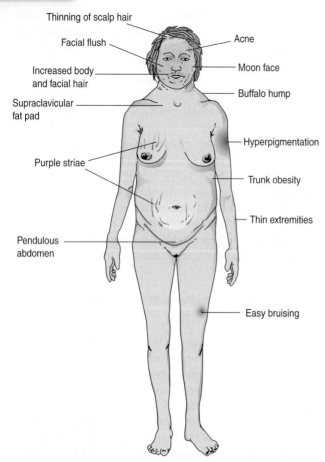

Figure 7.12. Cushing syndrome. The major clinical manifestations of Cushing syndrome. (From Rubin E, Farber JL. Pathology. 3rd ed. Philadelphia: Lippincott Williams & Wilkins, 1999.)

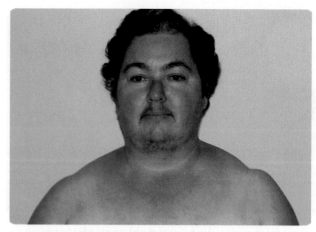

Figure 7.13. Cushing syndrome. Woman with Cushing syndrome associated with long-term use of corticosteroid medications. (From Willis MC. Medical terminology: a programmed learning approach to the language of health care. Baltimore: Lippincott Williams & Wilkins, 2002.)

Distinguishing Characteristics: None of the characteristic manifestations of Cushing syndrome/disease are pathognomonic for this disorder, although obesity and moon face are the most common features. The physical findings can be attributed to many types of disorders. Medical testing is needed to determine the cause of these findings. The most telling finding would be the use of steroids to treat a medical condition.

Significant Microscopic Features: Not applicable

Dental Implications: Any dental care should be prefaced by obtaining a complete medical/dental and drug history. Steroid drug therapy is used in many situations. Common disorders or conditions for which steroid medications are prescribed are listed in Box 7.2. Past and present steroid use should be investigated thoroughly to prevent any problems associated with an inadequate level of

Other problems include an inability to metabolize glucose effectively, leading to **hyperglycemia** (high blood glucose levels), hypertension (Chapter 8), atherosclerosis (Chapter 8), and muscle weakness and wasting. Neurologic findings include depression, emotional instability, and vision abnormalities. Patients may also exhibit steroid acne (on the face, chest, and upper back) caused by an increase in male sex hormones. Women will see an increase and coarsening of facial hair and may see increased hair growth on the neck, chest, and abdomen. Both men and women may experience thinning of scalp hair following male pattern baldness. In addition, Cushing syndrome/disease causes severe growth retardation and lack of sexual development in children.

Perioral and Intraoral Characteristics: Individuals who have Cushing syndrome/disease have a very round full face ("moon face") caused by edema (Fig. 7.13). Individuals suffering from this disorder are at a higher risk of developing oral and oropharyngeal fungal infections than those without the disorder, most likely a result of excessive glucose in the tissues and fluids of the oral environment. *Candida albicans* is the most common cause of this infection (Mann, 2003).

Box 7.2	DISORDERS AND CONDITIONS COMMONLY TREATED WITH CORTICOSTEROID MEDICATIONS

- Arthritis
- Asthma
- Cystic fibrosis
- Eczema
- Hypersensitivity reactions
- Kidney disease
- Leukemia
- Lichen planus
- Organ transplants
- Rheumatoid arthritis
- Sarcoidosis
- Seizures
- Systemic and discoid lupus erythematosus

APPLICATION

No discussion of steroid hormones is complete without mentioning steroid abuse. The specific steroid hormones that are being abused are anabolic–androgenic steroids produced in the adrenal cortex. Medically, these steroids are used to treat hypogonadism in males. Hypogonadism causes a decrease in the amount of testosterone that is produced in the testes. Adequate amounts of testosterone are required for normal growth and development and sexual development and functioning. Anabolic–androgenic steroids are also used to treat some forms of impotence and delayed puberty, to counteract the effects of corticosteroids, to treat anemia that does not respond to normal therapies, and to combat some types of body wasting seen in disorders such as AIDS. Anabolic steroids also cause an increase in skeletal muscle growth and a decrease in body fat.

Steroid abusers desire the latter effects. Weight lifters were the first to start using anabolic steroids to stack the deck in their favor during competitions, but participants in all types of sports are abusing anabolic steroids at this point. Even middle and high school students are abusing these drugs. In a 2004 study entitled "Monitoring the Future," middle and high school students in the United States were surveyed, and an estimated 1.9 to 2.4% of eighth to tenth graders and 3.4% of twelfth graders were found to have taken anabolic steroids at least once. There are no data on anabolic steroid use in adults, but it is suspected that hundreds of thousands of individuals aged 18 and over are abusing. Males are more likely to abuse steroids, but there is a rapidly growing number of females that are currently abusing steroids (NIDA, March 2005).

Anabolic steroids have a number of adverse effects that are seen in both males and females. These effects include heart disease, high blood pressure, stroke, high cholesterol, kidney cancer, liver tumors and cancer, depression, eating disorders, increased risk of blood-borne diseases related to using injectable steroids and a nonsterile technique, and acne. Gender-specific undesirable affects include

Males
- Shrinking of the testicles
- Reduced sperm count
- Infertility
- Male pattern baldness
- Gynecomastia, or breast development
- Increased risk for prostate cancer

Females
- Growth of facial hair
- Loss of scalp hair
- Amenorrhea
- Deepening of the voice
- Enlargement of the clitoris

Teenagers of either sex who take anabolic steroids before they have completed their vertical growth phases risk never attaining their height potential. Some of these effects are reversible, but the longer one abuses steroids, the more likely these will become permanent (NIDA, March 2005).

Aggressive behavior and property crimes (theft and vandalism) appear to be common among steroid abusers. Studies results are ambiguous about whether these behaviors are associated with the steroid itself or with the media attention to this type of behavior as being associated with steroid abuse (NIDA, March 2005). While abusers usually state that they feel good about themselves while on the drugs, depression and violent mood swings commonly occur when the drug is stopped.

Over-the-counter supplements that are touted to promote muscle growth and strength can be found in health food stores and pharmacies across the country. These supplements contain a number of metabolic precursors to testosterone and include: androstenedione, androstenediol, norandrostenedione, norandrostenediol, and dehydroepiandrosterone (DHEA). These compounds are naturally converted into testosterone or similar substances within the body, but there is no evidence that they promote muscle growth, and they may have long-term side effects associated with their use. Extreme care should be taken by individuals using one of these supplements (DEA, March 2004).

Both adults and adolescents who try these drugs may report their use to the dental professional who should be aware of the effects of these drugs and be prepared to discuss their use when indicated. Individuals who report the use of any of the precursor compounds could be attempting to increase their muscle growth and strength and might be open to a discussion about the effects of anabolic steroids on their general health. Above all, the dental professional should be cognizant of the cardiac problems associated with steroid use and be prepared to use treatment modification strategies to prevent emergency situations.

glucocorticosteroids that might occur during stressful dental surgeries and other treatments. Medical consultation might be necessary to ensure the well-being of the patient. Patients presenting with oral fungal infections should be treated aggressively with antifungal agents over the course of 10 to 14 days. Air polishing with a sodium bicarbonate-based polishing agent is contraindicated for patients with Cushing syndrome, because the acid–base

balance may be disrupted when the bicarbonate is introduced into their circulation (Mann, 2003).

Differential Diagnosis: Not applicable

Treatment and Prognosis: Treatment of Cushing disease focuses on the removal of the cause. Surgery to remove pituitary tumors and adrenal tumors is the treatment of choice. As a last resort, complete removal of the adrenal glands could be necessary. Cushing syndrome due to steroid therapy is managed by adjusting dosage amounts, modifying delivery systems to lower systemic exposure, and introducing nonsteroidal drug therapy to limit the use of steroids.

Untreated Cushing syndrome/disease carries a high risk of morbidity from the effects of excess glucocorticoid hormones on the body and a 50% 5-year mortality rate (Adler, 2006).

Pancreas

The pancreas functions as both an exocrine and an endocrine gland. As an exocrine gland, it produces and secretes digestive enzymes via ducts that reduce the acidity of food substances in the duodenum (the first segment of the small intestine), creating an alkaline environment (pH) for proper digestive enzyme function. The endocrine function takes place in the Islets of Langerhans, where hormones that have a regulatory effect on the metabolism of carbohydrates, fat, and protein metabolism are produced and secreted into the bloodstream. The hormones of the pancreas and their actions are listed in Table 7.7.

The most common disorder of the endocrine pancreas is **diabetes mellitus.** Diabetes is made up of a group of metabolic disorders characterized by inappropriate hyperglycemia, which results in chronic microangiopathy (small vessels and capillaries), neuropathic (nerve pathology), and/or macrovascular (large vessel) disease. Hyperglycemia is due to one or both of the following:
- Failure of the β (beta) cells to produce insulin
- Inability of the body to use the insulin produced, due to insulin resistance in muscle, liver, and fat cells

Diabetes mellitus is separated into several etiologic classifications as seen in Table 7.8. The American Diabetes Association estimates that 7% or about 20.8 million people in the United States have diabetes (CDC, 2005). Of these, it is estimated that 30% are not aware that they have the disease. Type 2 diabetes accounts for most of these undiagnosed cases. In addition, it is estimated that 1 in 3 children born in the year 2000 will develop diabetes at some point in their lifetime (Narayan et al., 2003). The incidence of the different types of diabetes is as follows (CDC, 2005):
- Type 1, 5–10%
- Type 2, 90–95%
- All others except gestational diabetes, 1–5%

There are two tests that can be used to diagnosis **prediabetes** (blood glucose level that is higher than normal but not yet high enough to be considered diabetes) or diabetes: (1) the **fasting plasma glucose test** (FPG) or (2) the **oral glucose tolerance test** (OGTT). The results of these tests indicate whether the patient has a normal metabolism, prediabetes, or diabetes. Diabetes is present when the results of these tests indicate hyperglycemia (see Fig. 7.14). There are four primary forms of diabetes that dental professionals will commonly encounter: type 1, type 2, prediabetes, and gestational diabetes (GDM). The characteristics of each are discussed in the following sections.

Name: Diabetes mellitus type 1

Etiology: The *β-cells* in the *Islets of Langerhans* are destroyed by an autoimmune process. There are no known risk factors for type 1 diabetes, and it cannot be prevented.

Method of Transmission: Type 1 immune-mediated diabetes has only slight genetic predisposition, other-

Table 7.7	PANCREATIC HORMONES	
Hormone	**Islets of Langerhans Cells**	**Function**
Insulin	Beta	• Facilitates the entrance of glucose into muscle, fat, and other cells • Stimulates the liver to produce glycogen from glucose • Decreases glucose concentration in the blood • Promotes the synthesis of fatty acids in the liver • Decreases the breakdown of fat in adipose tissues • Increases the uptake of amino acids • Makes many cells more permeable to potassium, magnesium, and phosphate
Amylin	Beta	• Slows nutrient uptake • Suppresses glucagon secretion after eating • Increases feelings of fullness or satiety
Glucagon	Alpha	• Increases blood glucose by stimulating the formation of glucose from glycogen in muscle and fat tissues and in the liver
Somatostatin	Delta	• Regulates α and β cell function in the islets by decreasing the secretion of insulin and glucagon

Table 7.8	ETIOLOGIC CLASSIFICATION OF DIABETES MELLITUS
Type	**Subclassification**
Type 1 β cell destruction, usually leading to absolute insulin deficiency	• Immune mediated • Idiopathic
Type 2 May range from predominantly insulin resistance with relative insulin deficiency to a predominantly secretory defect with insulin resistance	• None

Other types	• Genetic defects of β cell function
	• Genetic defects in insulin action
	• Diseases of the exocrine pancreas
	• Other endocrine diseases
	  o Acromegaly
	  o Cushing syndrome
	  o Hyperthyroidism
	  o Others
	• Drug or chemically induced
	• Infections
	• Uncommon forms of immune-mediated diabetes
	• Other genetic syndromes sometimes associated with diabetes
	  o Down syndrome
	  o Turner syndrome
	  o Others

Gestational diabetes mellitus	

Copyright © 2005. Reprinted with permission from The American Diabetes Association from Diabetes Care 2005;28:S37–S42.

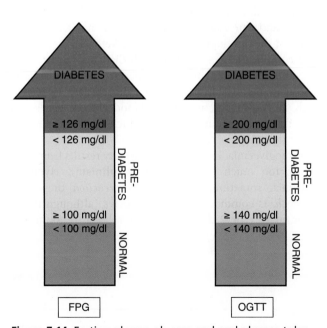

Figure 7.14. Fasting plasma glucose and oral glucose tolerance tests. Glucose levels associated with normal, prediabetic, and diabetic metabolic states. (Copyright © 2006 American Diabetes Association, From http://www.diabetes.org Reprinted with permission from The American Diabetes Association.)

wise it is not transmitted (Porth, 2004; CDC/Diabetes online).

Epidemiology: Type 1 diabetes occurs more frequently in Caucasians and least frequently in African Americans. It can occur at any age, but develops primarily in children, adolescents, and young adults (CDC/Diabetes).

Pathogenesis: Autoimmune destruction of the β cells in the islets of Langerhans causes type 1 immune-mediated diabetes. Approximately 90% of these cells must be destroyed before insulin levels drop enough to cause the blood glucose level to rise (hyperglycemia) and the disease to become clinically apparent. The vast majority of newly diagnosed patients present as a medical emergency (see diabetic ketoacidosis below).

The classic symptoms of diabetes are polydipsia, polyuria, and **polyphagia** (excessive hunger). High blood glucose levels lead to excessive water loss through the urine (polyuria), which leads to dehydration and intense thirst (polydipsia). Insulin is necessary for the metabolism of glucose; therefore, a deficiency of insulin will cause the individual to feel hungry all of the time. Persistent hyperglycemia has different effects on different tissues, but all organ systems are affected. These effects and others lead

Box 7.3   GLYCATED HEMOGLOBIN TEST

Glycosylation is the basis for the glycated hemoglobin test, which measures the amount of glucose that is bound to molecules of hemoglobin A1c. When red blood cells are formed, they do not contain any glucose. As the red blood cells move through the circulatory system, glucose molecules become attached to the hemoglobin contained within them, in the process known as glycosylation. The higher the level of glucose in the blood, the more glucose molecules become attached to the hemoglobin within the red blood cells. Once the glucose is attached to the hemoglobin it stays attached. The amount of glucose that is bound to the hemoglobin reflects the average level of glucose that the cell has been exposed to over time (60 to 80 days), or the glycemic index (Table 7.9). This is a very accurate method of tracking an individuals' control of their glucose levels during the 2 to 3 months prior to the blood test and has been found to be a better predictor of diabetic microvascular complications than the daily blood glucose testing that all patients with diabetes should be performing. Macrovascular complications have been found to be related more to glycemic highs and lows or excursions than to the glycemic index. Researchers are questioning whether or not the glycated hemoglobin test is the best measure of glycemic control (Hirsch and Parkin, 2005), but for now, the HbA1c is the gold standard for assessing glycemic control.

directly to the long-term complications associated with diabetes. For example, in individuals who do not have diabetes, glucose normally binds to proteins, lipids, and nucleic acids in a reversible manner. This process is known as **glycosylation.** In individuals who have diabetes, chronic hyperglycemia leads to permanent binding of glucose to these substances, which causes changes in their normal structure and function. The various substances that undergo this change are collectively called **advanced glycation end products (AGE).** Some of the tissues that are affected by this include components of the lens of the eye and proteins involved in basement membranes, especially in the vascular system. Glucose also binds with the hemoglobin molecules in red blood cells, forming the basis for one of the most accurate tests available to assess an individual's control of their diabetes over a period of time. The **hemoglobin A1c** test measures how much glucose binds to **HbA1c** (a specific type of hemoglobin) during the life of the red blood cell and is currently considered to be the best measure of glycemic control. Box 7.3 describes this test more fully. Table 7.9 lists guidelines for evaluating the results of the HbA1c test using the *HbA1c glycemic index.* HbA1c levels are directly related to the incidence of **microangiopathy** (small blood vessel disorders), but research has not shown a similar relationship to the incidence of **macrovascular** (large blood vessel) disorders (Hirsch, Parkin, 2005).

Extraoral Characteristics: Individuals who have type 1 diabetes are often thin or of normal weight. They usually present with polydipsia, polyuria, and polyphagia. Untreated type 1 diabetics may experience a dramatic weight loss in a relatively short period of time (days or weeks), even if eating more than normal, because they are unable to use glucose or convert it into fat. They may exhibit flulike symptoms: weakness, fatigue, frequent infections, and slow wound healing. The onset of symptoms is abrupt and can quickly lead to death if not treated, because of the development of diabetic ketoacidosis (DKA). The complications associated with diabetes can be separated into acute and chronic manifestations of the disease. The acute manifestations of type 1 diabetes are associated with short-term fluctuations in blood glucose levels and include hypoglycemia and DKA, which is a severe form of hyperglycemia.

- Hypoglycemia. Hypoglycemia usually results from having too much insulin (**hyperinsulinism**). Hypoglycemia, sometimes called *insulin reaction* or *insulin shock,* is common in type 1 diabetes (although it can occur in type 2 diabetes) and is related to taking too

Table 7.9   HEMOGLOBIN A1C GLYCEMIC INDEX

Percentage	Interpretation
<6%	Normal
<7%	Good control, target for most patients with diabetes
7–10%	Moderate control, physician should be working with the patient to improve
>10%	Poor control, physician should be working with the patient to improve

much insulin, eating too little food, or underestimating the amount of glucose that is needed in specific situations such as strenuous exercise or during extremely stressful events. Unfortunately, individuals who successfully maintain a normal blood glucose level are more frequent victims of this condition than those who do not control their disease as well. This happens because tight control gives little room for miscalculating the amount of insulin needed for the amount of food ingested. Therefore, if the patient's glucose levels have even minor fluctuations, hypoglycemia will result. Symptoms of hypoglycemia occur when glucose levels fall below 60 to 45 mg/dL of blood. If untreated, hypoglycemia may result in altered consciousness, coma, and death. In addition, some individuals with diabetes may experience **hypoglycemic unawareness**. People who have hypoglycemic unawareness may become unconscious before they have any idea that their glucose levels are low. This condition is seen more often in patients who have very tight control of their glucose levels, take certain heart or blood pressure medications such as beta-blockers, or have neuropathy. This condition is very common in young children who lack the cognitive ability to interpret the warning signs of hypoglycemia (NDEP, 2006).

• **Diabetic ketoacidosis.** DKA is a result of excessive hyperglycemia. Ketoacidosis occurs when the body must break down fat to use as an energy source instead of glucose. Fat metabolism results in increased levels of circulating fatty acids, which stimulate the liver to produce ketones that build up in the blood and cause **acidosis** (a decrease in the pH of the blood). Acidosis causes altered consciousness, coma, and eventual death if not treated.

Table 7.10 compares these manifestations with **hyperglycemic hyperosmolar nonketotic syndrome**, the acute manifestation associated with type 2 diabetes.

Diabetes affects every organ in the body, and the chronic complications associated with it occur slowly over many years. A direct relationship exists between the incidence of complications and the level of glycemic control. The American Diabetes Association reports that less than 10% of patients with diabetes achieve all three of the following treatment goals (ADA, January 2006):

• HbA1c level less than 7%
• Blood pressure less than 130/80
• Cholesterol levels less than 200 mg/dL

Therefore, it is a matter of when, not if, these complications will occur. Given the preventive health philosophy of dental practices, dental professionals should be aware of these complications and be able to recognize the need for a prompt medical referral. Complications are not reversible but can be prevented. A listing and brief description of the complications are provided below.

Table 7.10	COMPARISON OF HYPOGLYCEMIA, KETOACIDOSIS, AND HYPERGLYCEMIC HYPEROSMOLAR NONKETOTIC SYNDROME (HHNKS)		
		Hyperglycemia	
	Hypoglycemia	**Diabetic Ketoacidosis (DKA)**	**HHNKS**
Associated with	Type 1	Type 1	Type 2
Blood glucose levels	Less than 60 mg/dL	Greater than 250 mg/dL	Greater than 600 mg/dL
Speed of onset	Very fast	Gradual, many hours to several days	Occurs more gradually than ketoacidosis but the manifestations often have a fast onset
Symptoms	• Altered behavior • Altered consciousness • Anxiety • Coma • Cool, clammy skin • Headache • Hunger • Impaired mental ability • Polydipsia • Sweating • Tachycardia	• Acetone or fruity breath odor • Coma • Dry mouth • Fatigue • Headache • Hypotension • Increased rate and depth of respirations • Nausea • Polydipsia • Polyuria • Tachycardia • Vomiting	• Aphasia (impaired communication capabilities) • Coma • Dehydration • Hyperthermia • Hypotension • Nausea • Polydipsia • Seizures • Tachycardia • Unilateral paralysis • Vision blurring • Vomiting • Weakness • Weight loss
Emergency Care	• Oral or intravenous glucose	• Call EMS	• Call EMS

- **Neuropathy.** Approximately 60 to 70% of diabetics will experience neuropathy (nervous system damage), which presents most commonly as **peripheral neuropathy.** Peripheral neuropathy may manifest as a loss of sensation or pain in the lower legs, feet, or hands. **Autonomic neuropathy** affects the autonomic nervous system and results in gastrointestinal problems such as delayed emptying of the stomach, causing slow digestion of food in type 1 diabetes, and gastroesophageal reflux disease (Chapter 10) in type 2 diabetes. Neuropathy can also be associated with symptoms normally related to repetitive stress injuries such as carpal tunnel syndrome (CDC, 2005). Fluctuations in blood glucose levels have been linked to cognitive impairment such as confusion and delayed decision making. In addition, Alzheimer's disease occurs in up to 65% of patients with diabetes. Recently, after finding that nerve tissue in the brain produces small amounts of insulin, it was proposed that Alzheimer's disease may be associated with diabetes (Odetti et al., 2005; Rivera et al., 2005).

- **Microangiopathy.** Microvascular changes include thickening of the capillary basement membranes, hyperplasia of the endothelium, and thrombosis or blood clots. These changes cause **retinopathy** (retinal disease), **nephropathy** (kidney disease), and skin and joint problems. Microangiopathy has also been implicated in the initiation and progression of periodontal infections (see the section on infections and the application below). Diabetic retinopathy is the leading cause of blindness in all individuals between the ages of 20 and 74 in the United States (CDC, 2005). Diabetic retinopathy results when the capillaries in the retina hemorrhage and the cells in the retina become hypoxic. Blindness develops as fibrous tissue replaces the normal tissues in the retina and optic disk. Nephropathy is the result of tissue damage caused by hyperglycemia and the creation of abnormal substances (i.e., proteins) during glycosylation, among other events. The exact mechanism is unknown, but the end result is sclerosis (hardening) of the glomeruli and kidney failure. Diabetes is the leading cause of kidney failure and end-stage kidney disease in the United States (CDC, 2005). Skin problems associated with diabetes are common. They include the following:
  - Thickening and hyperpigmentation of the skin (**acanthosis nigricans**) on the neck, axillae, and groin areas is associated with diabetes and other endocrine disorders (Fig. 7.15). This condition may present prior to any other overt signs of the disorder, thus making recognition of this entity during the extraoral examination important to making a prompt medical referral.
  - Hardening of the skin
  - **Diabetic dermopathy,** a condition that manifests as chronic oval lesions that are red, hyperpigmented,

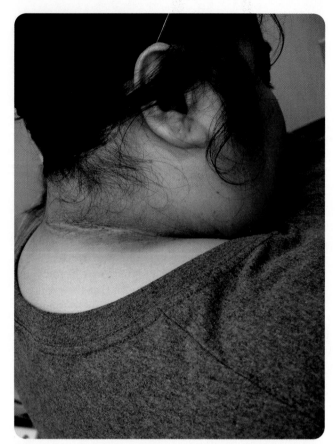

Figure 7.15. Acanthosis nigricans. Hyperpigmentation and thickening of the skin at the nape of the neck is characteristic of this manifestation. (Courtesy of Dr. Frank Varon.)

  papular, and well circumscribed. These are usually found on the shins but may be found on the thighs and forearms (Fig. 7.16).

- Macrovascular disease. Macrovascular disease presents as coronary artery disease, peripheral vascular disease, and/or stroke. Atherosclerosis is the major cause of these disorders and may be directly associated with chronic hyperglycemia, glycosylated proteins and lipids or other AGE, and elevated triglyceride and cholesterol levels often seen in diabetes. Coronary heart disease occurs two to four times more often in diabetics than in the general population and accounts for about 65% of deaths related to diabetes (CDC, 2005). Peripheral vascular disease is also related to high blood pressure, atherosclerosis, and resulting occlusion of the small vessels of the lower extremities. Peripheral vascular disease often results in gangrene (necrosis due to loss of blood supply) and amputation. Diabetes is a major cause (60%) of lower extremity amputations not due to trauma (CDC, 2005). Those with diabetes are two to four times more likely to have a stroke than the general population (CDC, 2005). Strokes, or cerebrovascular accidents, are associated with hypertension, atherosclerosis, and thrombosis, all of which are related to diabetes.

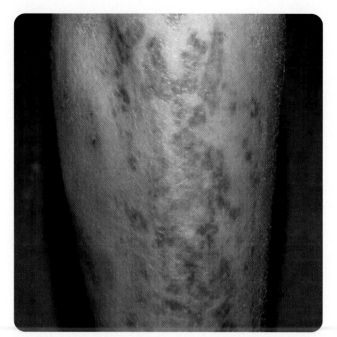

Figure 7.16. Diabetic dermatopathy. Small, brownish, atrophic, scarred, hyperpigmented plaques are seen on the shins. (From Goodheart HP. Goodheart's photoguide of common skin disorders. 2nd ed. Philadelphia: Lippincott Williams & Wilkins, 2003.)

- Infection. Chronic and recurring infections and impaired wound healing are other complications of diabetes. The higher risk of infection in diabetics is associated with a decreased host response thought to be due to the following factors among others:
  - Decreased blood supply because of microangiopathy, resulting in a decrease in the number of white blood cells and nutrients (including oxygen) that are brought to the areas at risk of infection
  - Impaired white blood cell function (WBCs fail to function at glucose levels over 200 mg/dL) resulting in decreased chemotaxic and phagocytic functions
  - Increased bacterial and fungal growth supported by a hyperglycemic environment
  - Decreased vision and sense of touch increase the risk of trauma to the extremities

Specific infections have a tendency to occur more often in diabetics. These include skin infections (bacterial and fungal), oral infections (bacterial and fungal), osteomyelitis (bone infection), urinary tract infection, kidney infection, and tuberculosis (CDC, 2005). Infection in any area of the body makes it hard for individuals to control their glucose levels. Any infection or illness usually requires that individuals increase the amount of insulin that they take to maintain a normal glucose level in the blood. Chronic infections can make maintaining a consistently normal blood glucose level almost impossible.

- Musculoskeletal problems. Research supports a relationship between diabetes and musculoskeletal prob-

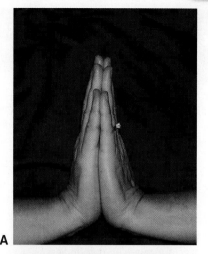

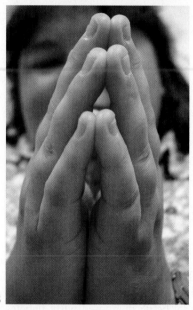

Figure 7.17. Prayer sign. **A.** Normal contact attained between the palms of hands and fingers. **B.** This individual with diabetes is unable to achieve normal contact. (Courtesy of © Chris Ha, M. D., Dermatlas; http://www.dermatlas.org.)

lems, specifically joint and mobility problems. Individuals with diabetes present with limited joint mobility at a young age. Nearly 30% of patients under the age of 28 with type 1 diabetes have limited mobility of the small and large joints, which is exacerbated by thickened skin overlying the joints (Kim et al., 2001). A simple test to determine the presence of this problem is called the **prayer sign**. This involves having the patient place his or her hands in the position seen in Figure 7.17 and observing how much contact the patient can obtain between the opposing fingers as shown. Patients who have limited joint mobility will not be able to obtain good contact. This type of joint mobility problem may affect how well the patient can perform home care procedures, thus affecting the patient's ability to control oral infections. In addition to

Box 7.4   CHRONIC COMPLICATIONS ASSOCIATED WITH DIABETES

Neuropathy	Peripheral neuropathy
	Autonomic neuropathy
Microvascular changes	Retinopathy
	Blindness
	Nephropathy
	Kidney failure
	Foot problems
	Ulcerations
	Charcot's foot (bone deformities)
	Periodontal disease
Macrovascular changes	Atherosclerosis
	Coronary artery disease
	Thrombus formation
	Peripheral vascular disease
	Amputation of lower extremities
	Stroke
	Hypertension
Altered host response	Infection
	Periodontal disease
	Skin
	Urinary tract

joint problems, bone metabolism appears to be affected, especially in type 1 diabetes. Recent studies show that almost 40% of women studied developed **osteopenia** (decreased bone density, Chapter 10) within 2 years of being diagnosed with diabetes (Brown and Sharpless, 2004). Decreased bone density is a predisposing factor for periodontal bone loss.

• Psychosocial Issues. Depression and anxiety have been reported in nearly 40% of patients with diabetes. Eating disorders are also found in about 40% of patients with type 1 and type 2 diabetes.

Box 7.4 lists the long-term complications of diabetes.

Perioral and Intraoral Characteristics: Several oral conditions have been associated with diabetes. Most often these conditions are seen in individuals who are unable to maintain consistently good control of their blood glucose levels. The most destructive of these manifestations is periodontal disease (Fig. 7.18). The diabetic is two to three times more likely to have periodontal infections than nondiabetics, and those who do have periodontal infections also have a much higher rate of severe periodontal disease (CDC, 2005; Mealey, 2004; Faria-Almeida et al., 2006). Refer to the following application for more information on periodontal disease and diabetes. Other oral changes often seen in diabetes include parotid gland enlargement (Fig.

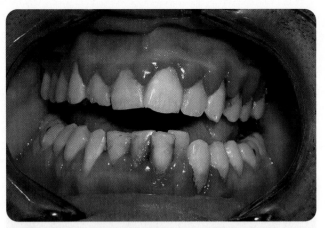

Figure 7.18. Periodontal involvement. Periodontal disease associated with uncontrolled diabetes and local factors.

7.19) with possible xerostomia, burning mouth syndrome (Chapter 10), increased risk for multiple periodontal abscesses, and an increased incidence of fungal (*Candida albicans*) infections (Chapter 14). Not surprisingly, patients who have poor control of their diabetes may exhibit a higher rate of caries than those who have better control.

Distinguishing Characteristics: Not applicable

Significant Microscopic Features: Not applicable

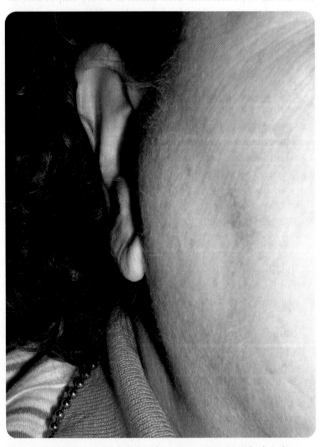

Figure 7.19. Parotid gland enlargement. Parotid gland enlargement and xerostomia are often associated with diabetes. (Courtesy of Dr. Frank Varon)

Dental Implications: A medical referral to evaluate a patient who presents with oral signs of periodontal infection, fungal infections, and/or multiple periodontal abscesses in addition to a suspicious medical history, advancing age, and obesity would be appropriate. This is especially true for patients who have been in the practice for a length of time and have never had such manifestations. Suspicion of diabetes is not unreasonable under these circumstances because of the large number of undiagnosed diabetics, especially of type 2. The patient's glucose level should be determined prior to dental care by either self-reporting or use of a glucometer in the office. Glucose levels of 70 to 80 mg/dL or below should be corrected before continuing with the appointment, to avoid hypoglycemia. A glucose source should be kept close at hand during the appointment in case glucose levels drop suddenly. One source recently suggested that 200 mg/dL glucose was the highest blood glucose level at which dental procedures could be safely performed. Patients who have high glucose levels should be referred to their physician for medical management to achieve levels that range under 140 mg/dL (Stegeman, 2005). The results of the patient's most recent hemoglobin A1c test should also be noted. The HbA1c glycemic index indicates whether a patient has had control of his or her diabetes over time and not just at the time of the dental appointment. This index is a very important indicator of the patient's risk of periodontal disease and treatment outcome after periodontal therapy. Refer to Clinical Protocol 16 for more dental implications.

Differential Diagnosis: Not applicable

Treatment and Prognosis: Treatment for diabetes includes insulin, oral medications, diet control, and exercise programs. Initially after diagnosis, patients undergo diabetes education by a *certified diabetes educator* (either an RN or dietitian), and a diabetes care plan is prepared for the patient. Insulin is absolutely necessary in the treatment of type 1 diabetes. Individuals with either type are very often on medications to control cholesterol levels and high blood pressure as well. All patients with diabetes should be under strict diet constraints, but this is usually the aspect of diabetes that is the most difficult for patient compliance. The age of the individual, lifestyle, and individual personality factors have much to do with how well he or she will adhere to a strict diet. The dental professional has an opportunity to reinforce the dietary plan developed by the diabetes educator and enhance the patient's motivation to stay with a diet program by pointing out all of the oral benefits of maintaining good glucose control. Type 1 diabetes patients should be checking blood glucose levels at least four times per day and should visit a physician two to four times a year to have their HbA1c, blood pressure, and cholesterol assessed. In addition, it is extremely important for these individuals to have annual dilated eye examinations. If the individual is pregnant, a dilated eye examination should be done in the third trimester. Regular foot examinations should be done by a physician or a podiatrist. The core diabetes care team includes the physician (endocrinologist, family practitioner, internal medicine) and the diabetes educator with consulting healthcare specialties including dentistry, podiatry, cardiology, physical therapy, occupational therapy, pharmacology, neurology, and gastroenterology to name a few. Patients who use their diabetes care team will possess the tools to control their disease. However, many patients do not take advantage of this resource. The dental professional has the opportunity to ask patients about their medical care and about how they manage their diabetes. Refer to Clinical Protocol 16.

Oral problems that are treated without first addressing overall diabetes management issues usually have less than optimal treatment outcomes. Dental hygiene treatment should stress thorough periodontal debridement with as little trauma as possible. Patients who have diabetes have a high risk of developing periodontal abscesses; therefore, complete periodontal debridement should be accomplished in one area before moving on to another area or tooth. Treatment of xerostomia, burning mouth syndrome, and fungal infections should be aggressive, with steps to prevent recurrence or long-term effects undertaken. Oral infections can have a severe impact on diabetes control for several reasons, including an inability to follow a proper diet because of oral pain and fluctuating levels of blood glucose caused by the body's need for additional insulin.

Over 200,000 people with diabetes die each year from diabetes-related complications, making diabetes the sixth leading cause of death in America (CDC, 2005). Research is providing hope for preventing diabetes someday. Recent studies on rats have found mechanisms that interfere with the autoimmune destruction of the islet cells in the pancreas, thereby allowing the islet cells to regenerate. If this can be replicated in humans, islet cell destruction could be stopped (Bresson et al., 2006).

Name: Diabetes mellitus type 2

Etiology: Type 2 diabetes has no recognized cause but does have many recognized risk factors with which it is associated. These risk factors include obesity, family history of diabetes, prior gestational diabetes, impaired glucose metabolism, hypertension, physical inactivity, race or ethnicity, and older age (CDC, 2005). Data suggest that type 2 diabetes may be prevented by eliminating as many of these risk factors as possible.

Method of Transmission: Type 2 diabetes is associated with a strong genetic predisposition (Porth, 2004; CDC, 2005).

Epidemiology: As stated above, 90 to 95% of those with diabetes have type 2 diabetes. In addition, most of the people who are unaware that they have diabetes have

APPLICATION

The dental hygiene profession has a special interest in how diabetes affects the periodontal health of an individual. There is strong evidence that diabetes is a risk factor for gingival and periodontal disease. Research also supports findings that uncontrolled diabetes plays an important role in the development and progression of periodontal disease. The data suggest that periodontal disease in those with diabetes is not only related to the impaired host response noted in the previous section but also with the same biologic mechanisms that cause other classic diabetic complications, such as the microvascular changes that are associated with retinopathy and kidney disease (Mealey, Oates, 2006).

The body normally mounts a defense when gingival tissues are challenged by the organisms found in dental biofilm. This defense is impaired in those with diabetes. Defective polymorphonuclear neutrophils (PMNs) are slow to respond to chemotactic factors or they do not respond at all. They also do not recognize the pathogens and are often unable to phagocytize them. In addition, macrophages and monocytes appear to be hyperresponsive in individuals with diabetes, because advanced glycation end products (AGEs), which are present in the periodontal tissues, are able to recruit more of these cells into the area and activate them, increasing their ability to cause extensive destruction of both normal and diseased tissues (Mealey and Oates, 2006). In addition, AGEs can stimulate the production of excessive amounts of chemical mediators such as interleukin (Il-1), prostaglandin E_2, and tumor necrosis factor-α.

These substances accumulate in the soft tissues, causing additional tissue destruction and increased inflammation (Lyle, 2003; Mealey, 2004; Mealey and Oates, 2006). Increased tissue destruction and decreased ability of the body to repair periodontal tissues is also linked to altered collagen production. Collagen production is altered for several reasons including (1) a decrease in the growth of fibroblasts, (2) a decrease in their ability to produce collagen, and (3) an increase in collagenase activity. In addition, osteoblasts exhibit a decreased ability to produce bone matrix, which also leads to increased amounts of periodontal bone loss. Microangiopathy occurs when AGE-modified collagen accumulates in the endothelial cells of the small vessels, causing thickening of the basement membranes, which leads to impaired nutrient supply, and endothelial cell changes, which are linked to clot formation (Mealey and Oates, 2006). These microvascular changes further compromise the periodontal tissues and exacerbate the destructive process (Table 7.11).

The hygienist must be aware that individuals with diabetes do not have to suffer from periodontal disease. Those who have good control of their diabetes have no more risk of developing the disease than those who do not have diabetes. In addition, healthy periodontal tissues are possible, even in those with uncontrolled diabetes if they establish and maintain strict oral infection control and prevention measures. It is in the area of oral health education that the hygienist can make the greatest difference.

---

type 2 diabetes. Type 2 diabetes occurs more frequently in Hispanics, Native Americans, African Americans, and Asian/Pacific Islanders than in non-Hispanic Caucasians. It also occurs more often after the age of 40, with the incidence of type 2 diabetes in people over the age of 60 approaching 20% (CDC, 2005). However, type 2 diabetes is also being seen more frequently in young people, especially in the ethnic groups listed above, because of the alarming rise in childhood obesity that crosses all racial and ethnic boundaries (CDC, 2005).

Pathogenesis: Type 2 diabetes initially occurs because of decreased sensitivity or increased resistance to insulin in the target cells, which are located in the liver, skeletal muscle, and adipose tissues. Obesity, diet, and lack of exercise are the main causes of insulin resistance. Persistent hyperglycemia, caused by poor glycemic control, stimulates the pancreas to produce ever-increasing amounts of insulin. Eventually, the β cells are literally worn out and undergo apoptosis (natural cell death). The pathogenesis of the complications associated with hyperglycemia in type 2 diabetes is essentially the same as for type 1, and the reader is referred to that section for review.

Many individuals with type 2 diabetes can decrease the severity of their disease or eliminate it altogether by losing weight and significantly increasing their activity level.

Extraoral Characteristics: Eighty percent of individuals who have type 2 diabetes are overweight or obese. The classic signs of polydipsia, polyuria, and polyphagia may not be present in this form of diabetes. The symptoms associated with type 2 diabetes are often vague, and since they progress slowly from mild to more severe over time, it is possible that they might go unnoticed by the patient and healthcare providers. Recurrent infections, nonhealing sores, visual changes, and numbness in the extremities are significant findings suggesting type 2 diabetes. The complications of type 2 diabetes can also be described as either acute or chronic. The acute manifestations of type 2 diabetes are hypoglycemia and hyperglycemic hyperosmolar nonketotic syndrome (HHNK), discussed below:

• Hypoglycemia. The manifestation of hypoglycemia in this type of diabetes is much more subtle than that seen in type 1 diabetes, and it is usually due to not eating enough or excessive activity. The patients usually ex-

Table 7.11	DIABETES RELATED CHANGES BELIEVED TO BE ASSOCIATED WITH THE DEVELOPMENT AND PROGRESSION OF PERIODONTAL DISEASE	
Diabetes Complication	**Specific Action**	**Affect on Periodontium**
Impaired PMN function	• Decreased chemotaxis • Decreased adherence • Decreased phagocytosis	Decreased host response
Impaired collagen production	• Decreased growth of fibroblasts • Decreased production of collagen by fibroblasts	Decreased healing/repair and impaired ability to maintain periodontal tissues
Increased collagenase production	• Increased collagen destruction	Increased tissue destruction and decreased healing/repair
Impaired bone formation	• Decreased production of bone matrix by osteoblasts	Decreased ability to maintain periodontal bone levels
Presence of advanced glycation end products	• Increases recruitment of macrophages and monocytes to the area • Activates macrophages and monocytes • Increases production of IL-1 and TNF-α • Associated with microangiopathy	Enhanced destruction of periodontal tissues
Microangiopathy (pathological changes in the small vessels)	• Increased likelihood of blood clot formation • Increased thickness of the capillary basement membrane	Impedes blood flow to the periodontium and compromises the transfer of nutrients necessary to maintain tissue health

hibit a mild behavior or mood change; they may feel lightheaded and hungry.

• **Hyperglycemic hyperosmolar nonketotic (HHNK) syndrome.** HHNK syndrome, although uncommon, is seen in patients with type 2 diabetes. HHNK syndrome is associated with high levels of blood glucose that cause severe dehydration, low blood volume, and low blood flow to vital organs. Severe dehydration leads to coma and death if not reversed. This is seen more often in older persons who have one or more of the chronic complications associated with diabetes, such as heart and/or vascular disease.

Table 7.10 summarizes and compares the acute complications associated with type 1 and type 2 diabetes. The chronic complications of type 2 diabetes are essentially the same as those associated with type 1 diabetes (see Box 7.4).

Perioral and Intraoral Characteristics: Perioral and oral characteristics are the same for both type 1 and type 2 diabetes. Refer to this section under type 1 diabetes.

Distinguishing Characteristics: Not applicable

Significant Microscopic Features: Not applicable

Dental Implications: Refer to dental implications under type 1 diabetes and to Clinical Protocol 16.

Differential Diagnosis: Not applicable

Treatment and Prognosis: Type 2 diabetes is normally treated with medications that increase the amount of insulin that the pancreas produces, decrease the resistance of the cells to the action of insulin, or increase insulin sensitivity within the cells. Insulin is not used frequently to treat type 2 diabetes. Patients with type 2 diabetes should check their blood glucose levels at least twice a day. Otherwise, the management of type 2 diabetes is essentially the same as management of type 1 diabetes.

Name: Prediabetes

Prediabetes, in which blood glucose levels are higher than normal but not yet high enough to be diagnosed as diabetes, always precedes the development of type 2 diabetes.

Etiology: Genetic and environmental factors have a strong influence on the development of type 2 diabetes; therefore, these same factors will influence the development of prediabetes.

Method of Transmission: Type 2 diabetes is associated with a strong genetic predisposition.

Epidemiology: In the United States there are 41 million people, ages 40 to 74, who have prediabetes (CDC,

2005). The ethnic groups that have the highest risk for type 2 diabetes are also at high risk for prediabetes.

Pathogenesis: The pathogenesis of prediabetes is identical to that of type 2 diabetes. Prediabetes may be present for 4 to 7 years or more before it is diagnosed. Recent research has shown that long-term damage to the body, especially the heart and circulatory system, may occur during prediabetes (American Diabetes Association, 2006). In addition, research has shown that early intervention to manage blood glucose levels during the period of prediabetes may delay or prevent the development of type 2 diabetes.

Extraoral Characteristics: Identical to those of type 2 diabetes

Perioral and Intraoral Characteristics: Identical to those of types 1 and 2 diabetes

Distinguishing Characteristics: Patients will have a blood glucose level that is higher than normal but not yet high enough to be considered type 2 diabetes.

Significant Microscopic Features: Not applicable

Dental Implications: All of the oral problems that are associated with type 1 or 2 diabetes may manifest in these patients. Recognition of an individual at risk of having prediabetes and prompt referral may prevent chronic complications from developing.

Differential Diagnosis: Not applicable

Treatment and Prognosis: Treatment usually consists of dietary and lifestyle changes. These individuals have a substantial risk of developing type 2 diabetes and the long-term complications associated with it. Losing weight and starting an exercise program that includes moderate-intensity physical activity is an essential element of preventing type 2 diabetes (CDC, 2005).

Gestational Diabetes Mellitus

Gestational diabetes mellitus (GDM) is glucose intolerance that is first detected during pregnancy. GDM is seen in about 4% of all pregnancies in the United States (CDC, 2005). Those at highest risk include women with a family history of diabetes and those who have had unsuccessful pregnancies or have delivered large or heavy babies or have had five or more pregnancies. In addition, older maternal age and obesity are related to a higher risk of developing gestational diabetes, as is being of an ethnic origin associated with a higher risk for type 2 diabetes. GDM usually manifests after the major fetal morphogenic events have occurred; therefore, the effects of gestational diabetes on the fetus differ from those seen in pregnancies in which the mother has type 1 or type 2 diabetes. In GDM, glucose in the blood crosses the placenta and enters the fetal circulation. If there is too much glucose, a state of hyperglycemia is produced, and in response, the fetal pancreas starts producing more insulin to lower the glucose level. However, the fetus does not need that much energy for its metabolic functions, and the excess glucose is stored as fat. This is the reason for the exceptionally large babies that are born to these mothers. In addition, babies born with excess insulin have a higher risk of being obese children and of developing type 2 diabetes as adults (American Diabetes Association, 2006). Treatment for GDM focuses on nutritional management and physical activity. The goal is to reach a fasting blood glucose level under 106 mg/dL (Porth, 2004). If this cannot be accomplished by diet and exercise, insulin injections will be prescribed. Oral antidiabetes agents are not used during pregnancy because they may be teratogenic. GDM will subside with declining pregnancy hormone levels. However, approximately 5 to 10% of women who have GDM will present with type 2 diabetes after their pregnancy has ended. In addition, women who have had GDM have a 20 to 50% chance of developing type 2 diabetes within 5 to 10 years. GDM patients require medical follow-up for 2 years postpartum.

SUMMARY

- The nervous and endocrine systems are responsible for regulating the many functions of the body. The nervous system is responsible for immediate actions; the endocrine system is responsible for slower processes.
- The endocrine system is composed of glands that secrete hormones or chemical messengers directly into the blood or lymph systems without using any ducts.
- Hormones are received by target cells that have receptors for the hormones on their cell membranes.
- The hypothalamus receives information from the nervous system and the body and directs the pituitary to release the proper hormones to maintain body functions.
- Oral infections may cause the level of prostaglandin to rise, stimulating the release of oxytocin from the posterior pituitary gland, which may result in premature labor.
- The endocrine system is regulated by a negative or positive feedback system. The negative feedback system stops the release of a specific hormone when it senses that there is an adequate level of that hor-

(continued)

SUMMARY *(continued)*

mone in the circulation. The positive feedback system releases one hormone based on the rising level of another hormone and stops releasing that one hormone when the level of the other hormone drops.

- Endocrine disorders take many forms, but the symptoms associated with them are usually linked to either hyposecretion or hypersecretion of the specific hormones associated with that gland.

- Diabetes insipidus is caused by a lower-than-normal level of antidiuretic hormone and is not associated with hyperglycemia. Polydipsia and polyuria are characteristic features of this disorder, as is the potential for severe life-threatening dehydration.

- Hypopituitarism or hyposecretion of any of the pituitary hormones will cause hypofunctioning of the gland that is associated with that particular pituitary hormone. The clinical characteristics would be identical to those caused by hypofunction of the specific gland without any associated pituitary hypofunction.

- Hypopituitarism is more severe in children because the hormones are needed for proper physical and mental development. Hypopituitarism in adults manifests as premature aging and may result in an acute adrenal crisis.

- Hypersecretion of growth hormone by the pituitary will result in gigantism, if it occurs prior to the end of puberty, or acromegaly, if it occurs after the end of puberty.

- The thyroid gland regulates the body's basal metabolic rate (BMR) among other functions. Hyposecretion of the gland causes symptoms associated with a decrease in the BMR in an adult and severe growth and mental deficiencies in children. Hypersecretion causes symptoms associated with a rise in BMR in both adults and children. Uncontrolled hyperthyroidism can lead to a life-threatening condition known as a thyroid storm.

- Goiters are caused by hypertrophy or hyperplasia of the thyroid gland, not neoplastic growth.

- The parathyroid glands regulate the level of calcium in the blood. Hypoparathyroidism causes hyperreflexia and possible hypoplasia of developing teeth. Hyperparathyroidism is associated with musculoskeletal problems, kidney stones, and generalized bone demineralization.

- The adrenal glands produce steroid hormones. Primary adrenal cortical insufficiency, or Addison's disease, may present with bronzing of the skin over high-use areas such as the joints and hyperpigmentation of the oral mucosa. Secondary adrenal insufficiency may result from the sudden withdrawal of corticosteroid medications. Hyperpigmentation is not seen in secondary adrenal insufficiency because there is no rise in ACTH. Hypoglycemia is common, and there is a potential for adrenal crisis.

- Hyperadrenalism causes Cushing disease (hyperfunctioning gland) or Cushing syndrome (medical use of steroids). The most common manifestation is Cushing syndrome. Hyperglycemia is common in hyperadrenalism as are the classic cushingoid features. Adrenal crisis should be anticipated when treating individuals who have a history of corticosteroid use.

- The pancreas has both endocrine and exocrine functions. The endocrine pancreas secretes insulin, which regulates carbohydrate, protein, and fat metabolism. Diabetes mellitus is the most common disorder associated with the pancreas.

- Hypofunctioning of the pancreas due to destruction of the β cells is known as type 1 diabetes. Type 2 diabetes is caused by a decrease in the amount of insulin produced and/or by increased resistance of the target cells to insulin. Diabetes presents with both acute and chronic manifestations. The chronic manifestations of diabetes cause significant morbidity and mortality, making diabetes the sixth leading cause of death in the United States.

- Prediabetes (type 2 only) is associated with an increased risk of developing both diabetes and the long-term complications associated with diabetes.

- Gestational diabetes increases a woman's risk of developing type 2 diabetes after the birth of her child.

- Diabetes is associated with a significant risk of developing dental infections including periodontal disease. An inadequate host response coupled with microangiopathy is considered to be the most likely pathogenesis.

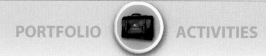

PORTFOLIO ACTIVITIES

1. Go online and find some web sites to which you can refer diabetic patients for assistance with oral health, meal planning, exercise programs, and other topics that you find interesting. Try to find a variety that enables you to separate them into a list of web sites for general information, those that might appeal to children or teens, ones appropriate for women or men, or some that are specific for type 1 or type 2 diabetes. Prepare a patient reference sheet with these sites listed, along with a brief description of the information at the site and the appropriate audience. Distribute these sheets to your patients in your school dental hygiene clinic. You can also use this as a handout when performing community service at health fairs, etc.

Critical Thinking Activities

1. Determine your risk factors for type 2 diabetes including sex, age, weight, ethnicity, diet, relatives who have diabetes, activity levels, and any other individual factors that might be related to your risk of diabetes. Answer the following questions and discuss them with your classmates.
   A. What are some measures that you can take to decrease your risk of becoming diabetic?
   B. What are the risk factors that you cannot change?
2. Imagine that you have just been told that you have type 1 diabetes, what are your first thoughts? What changes do you feel you will have to make to control your diabetes?
3. Are there cultural differences in how a person would react to having and managing diabetes? If you or any of your classmates have culturally diverse backgrounds, discuss how this diagnosis would be handled from that perspective.

Case Study

1. A 36-year-old female patient of record presents for a regularly scheduled preventive dental hygiene appointment. As you update her medical history, she tells you that she has gained about 20 pounds in the last 6 months for no reason that she can determine and that she has continued her level of activity even though she has been extremely tired. During her extraoral examination you observe what you think is a slight thickening of her neck in the area of the thyroid gland.
   A. If you assume that this is evidence of a goiter, what type of thyroid dysfunction would you suspect?
   B. What other history questions could be asked to help determine the type of disorder?
   C. What are the physical symptoms that would accompany this dysfunction?
   D. What are the dental abnormalities that are associated with this type of dysfunction?
   E. What is the prognosis of this disorder if treated? If untreated?
   F. What is your responsibility as a healthcare professional in this instance?

INTERNET RESOURCES

- American Diabetes Association
  http://www.diabetes.org
- The Nephrogenic Diabetes Insipidus Foundation
  http://www.ndif.org
- The Diabetes Insipidus Foundation
  http://www.diabetesinsipidus.org
- Endocrine and Metabolic Diseases Information
  Services: A Service of the National Institute of
  Diabetes and Digestive and Kidney Diseases
  http://www.endocrine.niddk.nih.gov

- National Diabetes Clearing House: A Service of the
  National Institute of Diabetes and Digestive and
  Kidney Diseases
  http://diabetes.niddk.nih.gov
  Addison's Disease Self Help Group
  http://www.adshg.org.uk

REFERENCES

Adler G. Cushing syndrome. Last updated March 15, 2006. e medicine: Instant Access to the Minds of Medicine. Available at: *http://www.emedicine.com/emerg/topic117.htm*. Accessed July 1, 2006.

American Diabetes Association. Diagnosis and classification of diabetes mellitus. Diabetes Care 2005; 28, Supplement 1: S37−S42.

American Diabetes Association. Standards of medical care in diabetes − 2006. Diabetes Care 2006; 29(S1): S4-S42.

Anderson DM, Keith J, Novak PD, Elliot MA. Mosby's medical, nursing & allied health dictionary. 6th ed. Philadelphia: Mosby, 2002.

Bresson D, Togher L, Rodrigo E, et al. Anti-CD3 and nasal proinsulin combination therapy enhances remission from recent-onset autoimmune diabetes by inducing Tregs. J Clin Invest 2006;116:1371–1381.

Brown SA, Sharpless JL. Osteoporosis: an under-appreciated complication of diabetes. Clin Diabetes 2004;22(1):10–20.

Carter WB, Carron JD. Parathyroid physiology. Last updated November 1, 2005. e medicine: Instant Access to the Minds of Medicine. Available at: *http://www.emedicine.com/ped/topic660.htm*. Accessed July 1, 2006.

Centers for Disease Control and Prevention. National diabetes fact sheet: general information and national estimates on diabetes in the United States, 2005. Atlanta, GA: U. S. Department of Health and Human Services, Centers for Disease Control and Prevention, 2005.

Chrousos GP, Lafferty A. Glucocorticoid therapy and Cushing syndrome. Last updated June 23, 2006. e medicine: Instant Access to the Minds of Medicine. Available at: *http://www.emedicine.com/ped/topic1068.htm*. Accessed July 1, 2006.

The Diabetes Insipidus Foundation, Inc. available at: *http://www.diabetesinsipidus.org/index.htm*. Accessed June 28, 2006.

Donatelle RJ. Health: the basics. 7th ed. San Francisco: Pearson Education, Benjamin Cummings, 2007.

Drug Enforcement Administration. Steroid abuse in today's society. Office of Diversion Control, U. S. Department of Justice, Drug Enforcement Administration. Available at: *http://www.deadiversion.usdoj.gov/pubs/brochures/steroids/professionals/*. Accessed July 1, 2006.

Faria-Almeida R, Navarro A, Bascones A. Clinical and metabolic changes after conventional treatment of type 2 diabetic patients with chronic periodontitis. J Periodontol 2006:77:591–598.

Gonzalez-Campoy JM. Hyperosmolar coma. Last updated January 17, 2006. e medicine: Instant Access to the Minds of Medicine. Available at. *http://www.emedicine.com/med/topic1091.htm*. Accessed July 1, 2006.

Halpern J, Wang NE. Hypoparathyroidism. Last updated August 24, 2006. e medicine: Instant Access to the Minds of Medicine. Available at: *http://www.emedicine.com/emerg/topic276.htm*. Accessed July 1, 2006.

Hirsch IB, Parkin CG. Is A1c the best measure of glycemic control? US Endocr Rev September 2005. Available at: http://www.touchbriefings.com/cdps/cditem.cfm?nid=1479&cid=5 Accessed July 14, 2006.

Hoffman R. Panhypopituitarism. April 20, 2006. e medicine: Instant Access to the Minds of Medicine. Available at: *http://www.emedicine.com/ped/topic1812.htm*. Accessed July 1, 2006.

Hopkins RL, Leinung MC. Exogenous Cushing's syndrome and glucocorticoid withdrawal. Endocr Metabol Clin North Am 2005;34(2): 371–384.

Huether SE, McCance KL. Understanding pathophysiology. 3rd ed. St. Louis: Mosby, 2004:449–506.

Ibsen OAC, Phelan JA. Oral pathology for the dental hygienist. 4th ed. St. Louis: WB Saunders, 2004:216–253.

Jabbour SA. Conn syndrome. Last updated April 19, 2005. e medicine: Instant Access to the Minds of Medicine. Available at: *http://www.emedicine.com/med/topic432.htm*. Accessed July 1, 2006.

Khandwala HM. Acromegaly. Last updated May 21, 2005. e medicine: Instant Access to the Minds of Medicine. Available at: *http://www.emedicine.com/med/topic27.htm*. Accessed July 1, 2006.

Kim RP, Edelman SV, Kim DD. Musculoskeletal complications of diabetes mellitus. Clin Diabetes 2001;19(3):132–135.

Klauer K. Adrenal insufficiency and adrenal crisis. Last updated April 18, 2005. e medicine: Instant Access to the Minds of Medicine. Available at: *http://www.emedicine.com/emerg/topic16.htm*. Accessed July 1, 2006.

LaBagnara J. Hyperparathyroidism. Last updated December 9, 2005. e medicine: Instant Access to the Minds of Medicine. Available at: *http://www.emedicine.com/ent/topic299.htm*. Accessed July 1, 2006.

Lee SL. Hyperthyroidism. Last updated July 20, 2005. e medicine: Instant Access to the Minds of Medicine. Available at: *http://www.emedicine.com/med/topic1109.htm*. Accessed July 1, 2006.

Lin L, Achermann JC. Inherited adrenal hypoplasia: not just for kids! Clin Endocrinol 2004;60:529–537.

Lyle DM. Diabetes mellitus. RDH 2003; 23(3):54–56, 88.

Mann NK. Cushing's syndrome. Access 2003; 17(7): 25-29.

Marzotti S, Falorni A. Addison's disease. Autoimmunity 2004;37(4): 333–336.

Mealey BL. Clinical considerations in dental treatment of the diabetic patient. J Pract Hyg 2004;13(6):12–18.

Mealey BL, Oates TW. AAP-Commissioned review: diabetes mellitus and periodontal diseases. J Periodontol 2006;77:1289–1303.

Mulinda JR. Hypopituitarism (panhypopituitarism). Last updated January 17, 2006. e medicine: Instant Access to the Minds of Medicine. Available at: *http://www.emedicine.com/med/topic1137.htm*. Accessed July 1, 2006.

Narayan KM, Boyle JP, Thompson TJ, et al. Lifetime risk of diabetes mellitus in the United States. JAMA 2003;290(14):1884–1890.

National Diabetes Education Program. Overview of diabetes in children and adolescents. National Diabetes Education Program 2006. Available at: http://ndep.nih.gov/diabetes/pubs/Youth_FactSheet.pdf Accessed July 14, 2006.

National Institute on Drug Abuse. Steroids (Anabolic-Androgenic). NIDA InfoFacts, March 2005. Available at: *http://www.drugabuse.gov.* Accessed December 15, 2005.

Nephrogenic Diabetes Insipidus Foundation. Available at: *http://www.ndif.org/.* Accessed December 21, 2005.

Odeke S, Nagelberg SB. Hashimoto thyroiditis. Last updated May 30, 2006. e medicine: Instant Access to the Minds of Medicine. Available at: *http://www.emedicine.com/med/topic949.htm.* Accessed July 1, 2006.

Odetti P, Piccini A, Giliberto L, et al. Plasma levels of insulin and amyloid β 42 are correlated in patients with amnestic mild cognitive impairment. J Alzheimer's Dis 2005;8(3):243–245.

Omori K, Nomura K, Shimizu S, et al. Risk factors for adrenal crisis in patients with adrenal insufficiency. Endocr J 2003;50(6):745–752.

Orlander PR, Woodhouse WR, Davis AB. Hypothyroidism. Last updated September 23, 2005. e medicine: Instant Access to the Minds of Medicine. Available at: *http://www.emedicine.com/med/topic1145.htm.* Accessed July 1, 2006.

Porth CM. Essentials of Pathophysiology: concepts of altered health states, Philadelphia: Lippincott Williams & Wilkins, 2004:529–579.

Postellon D, Bourgeois MJ, Varma S. Congenital hypothyroidism. Last updated June 8, 2006. e medicine: Instant Access to the Minds of Medicine. Available at: *http://www.emedicine.com/ped/topic501.htm.* Accessed July 1, 2006.

Regezi JA, Sciubba JJ, Jordan RCK. Oral pathology: clinical pathologic correlations, 4th ed. St. Louis: WB Saunders, 2003.

Rivera EJ, Goldin A, Fulmer N, et al. Insulin and insulin-like growth factor expression and function deteriorate with progression of Alzheimer's disease: link to brain reductions in acetylcholine. J Alzheimer's Dis 2005;8(3):247–268.

Rubin E, Gorstein F, Rubin R, et al. Rubin's pathology: clinicopathologic foundations of medicine. 4th ed. Baltimore: Lippincott Williams & Wilkins, 2005:1125–1184.

Schraga ED, Kulkarni R, Manifold CA. Hypothyroidism and myxedema coma. Last updated May 25, 2006. e medicine: Instant Access to the Minds of Medicine. Available at: *http://www.emedicine.com/emerg/topic280.htm.* Accessed July 1, 2006.

Shim M, Cohen P. Gigantism and acromegaly. Last updated July 29, 2004. e medicine: Instant Access to the Minds of Medicine. Available at: *http://www.emedicine.com/ped/topic2634.htm.* Accessed July 1, 2006.

Simm PJ, McDonnell CM, Zacharin MR. Primary adrenal insufficiency in childhood and adolescence: advances in diagnosis and management. J. Paediatr. Child Health 2004;40:596–599.

Stedman's medical dictionary for the health professions and nursing. 5th ed. Baltimore: Lippincott Williams & Wilkins, 2005.

Stegeman C. Blood glucose monitoring: a paradigm shift. Abstract presented at the DCE Diabetes Translation Conference, May 5, 2005, Miami, Fl.

Tfelt-Hansen J, Brown EM. The calcium-sensing receptor in normal physiology and pathophysiology: a review. Crit Rev Clin Lab Sci 2005;42(1):35–70.

Votey SR, Peters AL. Diabetes mellitus, type 2—a review. Last updated July 14, 2005. e medicine: Instant Access to the Minds of Medicine. Available at: *http://www.emedicine.com/emerg/topic134.htm.* Accessed July 1, 2006.

Votey SR, Peters AL. Diabetes mellitus, type 1—a review. Last updated February 2, 2006. e medicine: Instant Access to the Minds of Medicine. Available at: *http://www.emedicine.com/emerg/topic133.htm.* Accessed July 1, 2006.

Wong V, Yan T, Donald A, McLean M. Saliva and bloodspot cortisol: novel sampling methods to assess hydrocortisone replacement therapy in hypoadrenal patients. Clin Endocrinol 2004;61:131–137.

8 Cardiovascular Disorders

Key terms

- **Aneurysm**
- **Angina**
- **Arteritis**
- **Autonomic neuropathy**
- **Carditis**
- **Distal**
- **Dysrhythmia**
- **Embolus/emboli**
- **Endocardium**
- **Epistaxis**
- **Exsanguination**
- **Heart murmur**
  Physiologic murmur
  Pathologic murmur
- **Hypercholesterolemia**
- **Infarction**
- **Ischemia**
- **Laminar**
- **Nocturia**
- **Orthopnea**
- **Paroxysmal nocturnal dyspnea**
- **Petechiae**
- **Polycythemia**
- **Pulmonary hypertension**
- **Regurgitate**
- **Shunt**
- **Thrombus**
- **Transient ischemic attack (TIA)**
- **Unstable angina**
- **Ventricular fibrillation**

Objectives

1. Define terminology used in discussing cardiovascular disorders and state the etiology of the disorders discussed in this chapter.

2. Recognize the epidemiologic characteristics, the method of transmission, and the pathogenesis of the disorders discussed.

3. Describe the characteristics and distinguishing features of vascular and heart disorders.

4. Briefly describe possible therapies and prognoses for individuals with cardiovascular disorders.

5. State the significance of turbulent blood flow and describe ways in which normal laminar blood flow may become turbulent.

6. Describe the possible connection between oral infections and atherosclerosis.

7. Describe the dental implications and therapy with the use of anticoagulant therapy and patients with hypertension.

8. List behavior and lifestyle changes that could be suggested to help control hypertension.

9. List oral problems associated with stroke.

10. List heart disorders that are associated with an increased risk of infective endocarditis.

11. Describe the rationale for giving prophylactic antibiotics to patients with certain heart disorders prior to some dental procedures.

12. Identify the most common congenital heart defects.

13. Compare the characteristics associated with "left to right" and "right to left" heart shunts.

14. Compare physiologic and pathologic heart murmurs.

15. Identify the most common heart valve defect.

16. List diseases and disorders that may result in the development of congestive heart failure.

17. Describe dental treatment modifications for patients who have chronic ischemic heart disease and acute coronary syndromes.

18. Describe the significance of a cardiac dysrhythmia.

Chapter Outline

THE CARDIOVASCULAR SYSTEM

The cardiovascular system is comprised of the heart and two distinct circulatory systems: (1) pulmonary circulation, right side of the heart, which carries blood from the heart to the lungs and back to the heart, and (2) systemic circulation, left side of the heart, which carries blood from the heart to the rest of the body and then back to the heart. Within the circulatory systems, arteries take blood away from the heart in progressively smaller vessels until the blood reaches a capillary bed, where nutrient exchange occurs. At this point the venous system takes over, and the blood flows through progressively larger veins until it is returned to the heart.

The Heart

The heart receives blood from the vena cava into the right atrium. The blood travels through the tricuspid valve into the right ventricle, at which time it enters the pulmonary circulation and is pumped through the pulmonary valve (semilunar) into the pulmonary artery (the only artery carrying nonoxygenated blood), and then into the lungs. The oxygenated blood travels through the pulmonary vein (the only vein to carry oxygenated blood) into the left atrium. The blood is now in the systemic circulatory system. Once the blood is in the left atrium, it is pumped through the bicuspid or mitral valve into the left ventricle. The blood is then pumped through the aortic valve (semilunar) into the aorta and then to the rest of the body (Fig. 8.1). All of the valves are continuous with the **endocardium** (the innermost lining of the heart) and function to prevent back flow. The endocardium is continuous with the lining of the blood vessels. The electrical stimulation of the heart is regulated by the autonomic nervous system. The impulses begin in the sinoatrial (SA) node in the right atrium and travel to the atrioventricular (AV) node, which lies in the right atrial wall just superior to the tricuspid valve. At this point the impulses travel through fibers from the AV node to the bundle of His, located in the inferior portion of the ventricular septum, where the fibers split and carry the impulses to the right and left ventricles, terminating in the Purkinje fibers. The heart muscle is provided with oxygen and nutrients through the coronary arteries.

The Vessels

All vessels except the capillaries are comprised of three distinct layers: the tunica externa, tunica media, and tunica intima. The tunica externa is comprised of fibrous tissue that supports the vessel. The tunica media is comprised mostly of smooth muscle that causes the vessels to constrict or dilate, regulating the amount of blood that is flowing through the vessel and the pressure within the vessel. The tunica intima is the innermost layer, which is comprised of an elastic layer that connects the intima with the media and a thin layer of endothelial cells that provide a smooth, slick surface over which the blood flows (Fig. 8.2). Normal blood flow is **laminar**, or layered, with the slower plasma flowing closest to the endothelial layer and the cellular components flowing more quickly within the innermost portion of the vessel. Turbulent blood flow occurs when there is a defect or injury to the vessel or endothelial surface or a change in the amount of pressure within the vessel. Turbulent blood flow allows the blood components to become more mixed with the plasma and increases the chance that platelets and other factors that encourage clotting can come in contact with the endothelium and create a clot, or **thrombus** (Fig. 8.3A and B). Blood flows through the vascular system under a certain amount of pressure. The blood pressure within the pulmonary circulation is low compared with the higher pressure that is required to move the blood through the systemic circulation. Abnormal variations in blood pressure in either the pulmonary or the systemic circulation can have serious effects, such as cardiac enlargement, valve disorders, and stroke, among others.

Arteries are thick-walled vessels that can handle the high pressure needed to move blood through them to the outermost parts of the body. Veins are thinner-walled vessels that do not have to contend with the high pressure associated with arteries. However, veins must work against gravity to bring blood back from the extremities to the heart. Therefore, unlike arteries, veins are equipped with valves that prevent the backflow of blood that has already passed through them (see Fig. 8.2).

If any of the parts of these systems are compromised by disease or defect, blood will not move efficiently through them, and tissues and organs will not receive the nutrients that are necessary to maintain health. Vascular system disorders are discussed before disorders of the heart because

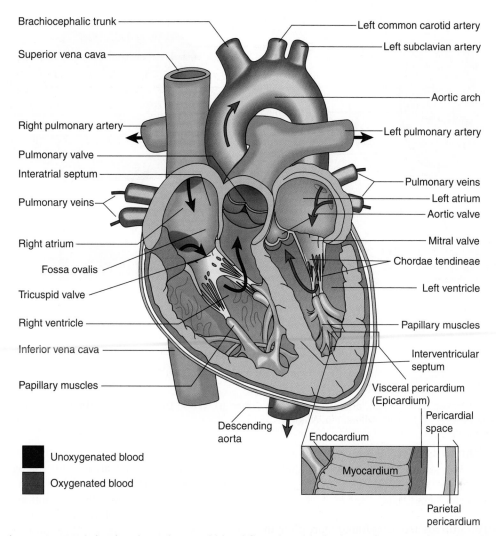

Brachiocephalic trunk

Superior vena cava

Right pulmonary artery

Pulmonary valve

Interatrial septum

Pulmonary veins

Right atrium

Fossa ovalis

Tricuspid valve

Right ventricle

Inferior vena cava

Papillary muscles

Left common carotid artery

Left subclavian artery

Aortic arch

Left pulmonary artery

Pulmonary veins

Left atrium

Aortic valve

Mitral valve

Chordae tendineae

Left ventricle

Papillary muscles

Interventricular septum

Visceral pericardium (Epicardium)

Pericardial space

Descending aorta

Endocardium

Myocardium

Parietal pericardium

Unoxygenated blood

Oxygenated blood

Figure 8.1. The heart. Anatomic landmarks and normal blood flow through the heart. (From Smeltzer SCO, Bare BG. Brunner and Suddarth's Textbook of medical-surgical nursing. 9th ed. Philadelphia: Lippincott Williams & Wilkins, 2002.)

vascular pathology is involved in the etiology of many heart disorders. In addition, vascular pathology is often caused by heart disorders, making it essential to have an understanding of vascular pathology first.

VASCULAR DISORDERS

Abnormalities of the vascular system can be congenital, hereditary, or acquired. Most often they are caused by a combination of genetic and environmental factors. The following sections focus on diseases or disorders of the arteries and veins and abnormal blood pressure.

Name: Atherosclerosis

Etiology: Atherosclerosis is a disease of the arteries in which inflammatory cells, smooth muscle cells, lipids, and connective tissues accumulate within the tunica intima. The exact cause of atherosclerosis is not clearly understood. It is not known why some individuals live their entire lives

without vascular pathology due to atherosclerosis while others have pathology at a very early age. There are specific risk factors associated with the development of this disease. Risk factors such as increasing age and being male as well as having a family history of atherosclerosis cannot be altered. However, other risk factors that have been strongly associated with this disease such as: hypertension, **hypercholesterolemia** (high cholesterol), cigarette smoking, physical inactivity, and high stress levels can be modified by the individual. Familial hypercholesterolemia is an autosomal dominant genetic disorder that is due to a defect or absence of a specific cellular receptor that removes or transports cholesterol out of the blood. Without these receptors, the blood cholesterol level is markedly elevated, and the individual's risk for atherosclerosis is likewise increased. Diabetes is also a risk factor for atherosclerosis. While type 1 diabetes cannot be prevented at this time, type 2 diabetes can be prevented or its severity lessened in most cases by maintaining a healthy weight, staying active, and following a healthy diet.

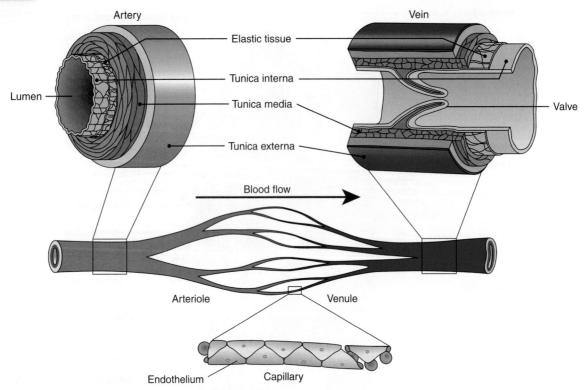

Figure 8.2. Anatomy of capillaries, veins, and arteries. (From Cohen BJ, Wood DL. Memmler's the human body in health and disease. 9th ed. Baltimore: Lippincott Williams & Wilkins, 1999.)

Method of Transmission: Atherosclerosis is not transmissible. However, several risk factors for it including hypertension, type 2 diabetes, and hypercholesterolemia have a strong genetic base.

Epidemiology: Atherosclerosis is found more often in men than in women and is usually diagnosed between the ages of 40 and 70 (Orford and Selwyn, November 2005). It is difficult to determine the number of people affected by this disease because most of the morbidity and mortality statistics are associated with coronary heart disease, stroke, heart attack, aneurysm, and peripheral vascular disease, all of which are major sequelae, or complications, of atherosclerosis. Some 75% of all deaths from cardiovascular diseases are ultimately caused by atherosclerosis (AHA, 2005).

Pathogenesis: Atherosclerotic lesions do not form on the inside of arteries but within the tunica intima layer. The exact mechanism behind the development of the lesions is not known. The lesions or plaques contain inflammatory cells, smooth muscle cells, lipids (mostly cholesterol), and connective tissues. They start out as flat or slightly elevated fatty streaks in the intima. As the disease progresses, the accumulation of cells and lipids increases, and the intima layer gets thicker, bulging into the artery and decreasing in the diameter of the lumen (Fig. 8.4). As the lesions get progressively thicker, they change the geography of the inner vessel from slick and smooth to rough and bumpy. Blood pressure also changes because of

atherosclerosis, since it takes more pressure to force blood through the narrowed areas. This changes the laminar blood flow to turbulent blood flow that not only has a higher chance of creating thrombi but also increases the chance that the endothelium will become injured or that the atherosclerotic plaques will rupture. Injured endothelial surfaces increase the chance of thrombus formation because they are rough, and the substances that the injured cells secrete attract blood products that encourage clot formation. Ruptured plaques expose the blood to the contents of the plaque, much of which will also encourage the formation of a thrombus. Most often it is a thrombus that eventually causes occlusion of the artery and necrosis or **infarction** of the area that is supplied by blood from that vessel. Continued injury can weaken the walls of the vessel and lead to **aneurysm**, or a bulging and thinning of the vessel wall, and eventually to rupture of the artery.

Extraoral Characteristics: Clinical manifestations of atherosclerosis are only seen as they relate to the major complications of the disease, which is discussed throughout this chapter.

Perioral and Intraoral Characteristics: Not applicable

Distinguishing Characteristics: Not applicable

Significant Microscopic Features: Not applicable

Dental Implications: Atherosclerosis is considered a contributing or etiologic factor for many of the cardiac

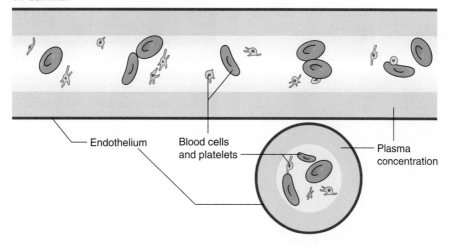

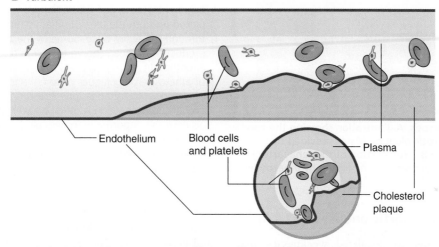

Figure 8.3. Laminar vs. turbulent blood flow. **A.** Laminar flow. In laminar flow the plasma is concentrated around the periphery of the vessel, allowing the solid blood components to flow through the center of the vessel. This maximizes flow rate and minimizes the chances for platelets and other solid components to initiate clot formation. **B.** Turbulent flow. Rough cholesterol plaques have formed within the intima of this vessel, causing the plasma to be deflected from the periphery of the vessel. When this occurs, the blood cells and other solid components of the blood are bounced off the endothelial walls, and the smooth flow of blood is interrupted. Clot formation is enhanced when platelets and other clotting factors come in contact with endothelial cells.

and vascular disorders that are discussed in this chapter; therefore, dental implications are specific for these conditions. In addition, current research may support a link between oral infections and the formation of atherosclerotic plaques. Refer to the application following this section.

Differential Diagnosis: Not applicable

Treatment and Prognosis: Treatment focuses on two areas: (1) eliminating or managing the risk factors and (2) managing the complications of the disease. Individuals at risk of, or affected by, atherosclerosis must make critical choices that may ultimately determine the length and quality of their lives. Risky behaviors such as smoking and physical inactivity need to be addressed and altered. Dietary changes that lower blood pressure, cho-

lesterol, and lipid levels and those that help to prevent or manage type 2 diabetes are very important in reducing not only the risk of atherosclerosis but in decreasing the risk of complications from disease that is already present. Maintaining tight glycemic control over both types of diabetes has been shown to decrease all of the complications associated with that disease, including atherosclerosis. Medications can be used to assist the individual in achieving lower blood pressure and lipid and cholesterol levels if dietary changes alone are not sufficient. Treatment that focuses on managing the complications of atherosclerosis is discussed as the complications are described throughout the rest of this chapter. The prognosis is determined by the complications that are present, which is also discussed with each specific complication listed.

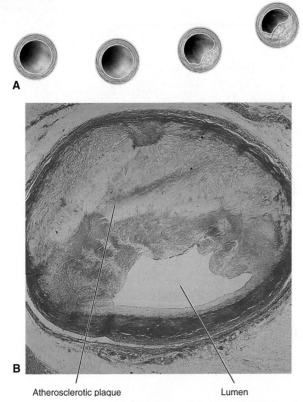

Figure 8.4. Atherosclerosis. **A.** Illustration showing the formation of atherosclerotic plaques. (Asset provided by Anatomical Chart Co.) **B.** Cross-section of the renal artery showing significant narrowing of the lumen by atherosclerosis.

Atherosclerotic plaque   Lumen

APPLICATION

The oral-systemic connection has been the topic of much research lately, and oral health has been shown to be an important aspect of total health. Not too many years ago it was hypothesized that oral infections played a part in the development of atherosclerotic disease and therefore played a part in the development of coronary artery disease, stroke, hypertension, and other cardiovascular diseases. As studies are published, the connection seems to vacillate among stronger and weaker links between periodontal infections and the development of atherosclerosis. At the present time most dental and medical professionals agree that what goes on in the mouth is important to the health of the rest of the body. The current theory is that substances that are produced by the inflammatory process in response to infections, such as interleukin-1, tumor necrosis factor-α, and prostaglandin E_2, are eventually picked up from the area of inflammation and circulated through the entire body. Some of these inflammatory products have been shown to elicit a response within the endothelial cells that appears to encourage the formation of atherosclerotic plaques or to enhance the progression of already established lesions. If this is indeed the case and even if the connection is much weaker, dental professionals have the opportunity to help people prevent or slow the progression of atherosclerosis and thus help to prevent or limit the severity of the many cardiovascular problems associated with it.

Name: Abdominal aortic aneurysm (AAA)

Etiology: Aneurysms are localized weaknesses that manifest as bulges or bubbles in the wall of an artery. The abdominal aortic aneurysm is an aneurysm located in the abdominal aorta. While most AAAs are caused by atherosclerosis and related hypertension, they can also be caused by congenital defects, trauma, or infection.

Method of Transmission: Genetic influences appear to play a part in the development of AAAs. The tendency to form AAAs is a component of many inherited connective tissue disorders, such as Marfan and Ehlers-Danlos syndromes. There is also evidence that a single dominant gene may be involved in some cases. AAAs that are caused by an infectious process are associated with syphilis, tuberculosis, and, more often, infective endocarditis. Preventing and treating these infections would effectively eliminate the chance of transmitting the responsible organisms.

Epidemiology: It is estimated that 0.5 to 9% of the population has an AAA (Porth, 2004; Pearce and Peterson, May 2005). Most of these cases will be asymptomatic and diagnosed at autopsy. AAA is uncommon in African Americans, Asians, and Hispanics. It is more common in men than in women and probably starts developing at age 50, with a peak incidence in men at age 80. About 5 of every 100,000 aneurysms will rupture (Pearce and Peterson, May 2005).

Pathogenesis: The pathogenesis of an AAA is essentially the same regardless of the actual cause. Most AAAs are located just inferior to where the renal arteries branch off the aorta and prior to the bifurcation of the aorta into the iliac arteries, but they can affect any or all of these arteries (Fig. 8.5). Once the vessel wall is weakened, it begins to expand under the constant pressure from cardiac systole (contraction). As it expands, there is increased risk of rupture and thrombus formation. Thrombi may form because of the turbulent blood flow through the aneurysm, but rupture is more common.

Extraoral Characteristics: Most AAAs are asymptomatic and are often found by mistake when looking for something else. As the aneurysm enlarges, there may be pain focused in the lower back or in the groin area, and the individual may experience dysphagia (difficulty swallowing). A pulsating mass in the belly around the area of the umbilicus may be observed. A thrombus that forms in the aneurysm may become detached from the vessel wall and move through the circulation with the flow of blood. When this occurs, the blood clot is known as an **embolus.** An embolus may lodge in another area, blocking the flow

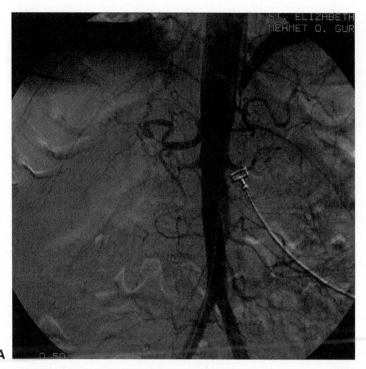
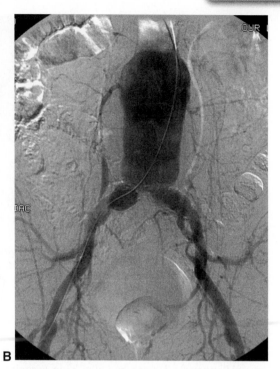

Figure 8.5. Abdominal aortic aneurysm. **A.** Normal aorta and iliac arteries. **B.** Abdominal aneurysm 8 cm in diameter affecting the aorta and the iliac arteries.

of blood, causing **ischemia** (lack of oxygen) in that area. Ischemia can cause permanent cellular damage or necrosis.

Perioral and Intraoral Characteristics: Not applicable

Distinguishing Characteristics: Not applicable

Significant Microscopic Features: Not applicable

Dental Implications: Patients who have been diagnosed with an abdominal aneurysm may be taking medications such as beta-blockers to prevent enlargement of the aneurysm. Xerostomia is often a side effect of this type of medication. In addition, identification of an individual who is at risk and knowledge of the warning signs, such as back pain or dysphagia, may prompt a medical referral that could save a life.

Differential Diagnosis: Not applicable

Treatment and Prognosis: Since atherosclerosis is associated with many AAAs, much of the medical treatment focuses on reducing the risk factors associated with progression of the atherosclerosis. This includes managing hypertension, hypercholesterolemia, and diabetes. In addition, most of the small aneurysms are monitored for signs of progression. Large aneurysms, such as the one in Figure 8.5, need to be surgically corrected. The most common treatment is to replace the damaged part of the aorta with a synthetic Dacron graft. Even the renal and iliac arteries can be attached to this graft if necessary, depending on the extent of aortic involvement. The prognosis is very poor for an untreated or undiagnosed large AAA. AAAs of

4 cm or less have a 2% chance of rupture, those over 5 cm have a 25–40% chance of rupture within 5 years after diagnosis. A ruptured AAA is a life-threatening emergency, with over 50% causing immediate death from **exsanguination**, or bleeding out (Rubin et al., 2005). The prognosis for those with successful graft replacements is just about equal to that for those of the same age who have never had an AAA (Pearce and Peterson, May 2005).

Name: Raynaud's disease or phenomenon

Etiology: Primary Raynaud's or Raynaud's disease appears to have no specific cause. Secondary Raynaud's or Raynaud's phenomenon is associated with other diseases, including scleroderma and lupus erythematosus. It is also linked to previous trauma such as frostbite or occupational trauma such as carpal tunnel syndrome and other repetitive stress disorders.

Method of Transmission: None

Epidemiology: Raynaud's disease is estimated to be found in 3–4% of the population. There is no race predilection, but it appears that more women are affected than men. The usual age at diagnosis is between 10 and 20 (Lisse and Oberto-Medena, April 2006). The incidence of Raynaud's phenomenon is related to the incidence of the disease with which it is associated.

Pathogenesis: The symptoms of this disorder are caused by ischemia of the cells in the fingers, toes, and sometimes the ears and nose. The ischemia is the result of episodes of vasospasms in the small arteries of the

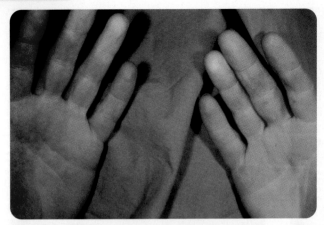

Figure 8.6. Raynaud's disease or phenomenon. Characteristic pallor of the finger tips associated with vasospasms characteristic of Raynaud's disease or phenomenon. (From Rubin E, Farber JL. Pathology, 3rd ed. Philadelphia: Lippincott Williams & Wilkins, 1999.)

skin that are brought on by cold and/or emotional stress. Raynaud's disease has also been associated with smoking.

Extraoral Characteristics: The first sign of an episode is a color change in the affected tissues from normal to pale and then cyanotic (Fig. 8.6). The color change is accompanied by numbness and tingling. The end of an episode is characterized by increased redness, pain, throbbing, and altered sensations. The finger tips are affected more often then the toes, nose, and ears.

Perioral and Intraoral Characteristics: Not applicable

Distinguishing Characteristics: Numbness and color change in the fingers is characteristic of this disorder.

Significant Microscopic Features: Not applicable

Dental Implications: Since Raynaud's phenomenon may have an underlying cause, it would be appropriate to refer an individual complaining of these symptoms for a medical evaluation.

Differential Diagnosis: Not applicable

Treatment and Prognosis: Most cases of Raynaud's disease do not need treatment other than trying to avoid such precipitating factors as cold and stress and protecting the areas during an episode. The most severe cases may be treated with medications, such as calcium channel blockers, which support vasodilation, or a surgical procedure that cuts the sympathetic nerve supply to the area, thereby reducing the occurrence of vasospasms. In rare cases, severe disease can result in necrosis of the tips of the fingers or other affected tissues.

Name: Thromboembolic venous disorders

Etiology: Although not completely understood, thrombus formation is known to be associated with endothelial injury, blood stasis or slow flow, and hypercoagulability.

Method of Transmission: None

Epidemiology: The American Heart Association estimates that 100 of every 100,000 persons in the United States will experience an initial venous thrombosis every year. Deep venous thrombosis (DVT) will account for two thirds of this number, and pulmonary embolism (PE) will account for the other one-third. Men have a higher incidence of this disease than women, and the overall incidence increases with age. Caucasians and African Americans are more likely to experience venous thrombosis than Hispanics or Asians (AHA, 2005).

Pathogenesis: Box 8.1 lists risk factors associated with the development of venous thromboembolisms. Although thrombi can form in any area, the most common site is in the deep veins of the leg, where it is called deep venous thrombosis (DVT). When a thrombus breaks away from the endothelium and becomes an embolus, it can travel through the circulatory system and end up anywhere. However, one of the more common scenarios is that it finds its way into the pulmonary circulation and lodges in the lung as a PE.

Extraoral Characteristics: Individuals with DVT may be asymptomatic and may never have any complica-

---

Box 8.1   FACTORS ASSOCIATED WITH THE DEVELOPMENT OF DEEP VENOUS THROMBOSIS

STASIS

- Heart failure
- Venous obstructions
- Immobility due to bed rest, paralysis, or inactivity
- Myocardial infarction

HYPERCOAGULATION

- Oral contraceptive use
- Pregnancy
- Childbirth
- Stress
- Cancer

VASCULAR TRAUMA

- Severe accidental trauma
- Surgical trauma
- Severe infections

tions from their disease. The symptoms associated with DVT are deep muscle pain and swelling in the area **distal** to the clot or away from the trunk. There is a potential for fever, malaise, and other general signs of inflammation as well.

The symptoms associated with a pulmonary embolism are directly related to the size of the embolus and the health of the individual. A small PE may be asymptomatic or may present with transient dyspnea and tachypnea. Areas that are distal to the embolus undergo ischemia and have the potential for becoming necrotic. Areas of necrosis heal with a scar that can impair lung function if the scar is large enough. Emboli may also resolve and leave little if any evidence of their presence. Large emboli may lodge in the bifurcation of the pulmonary artery and obstruct blood flow to both lungs, causing severe hypotension and sudden death. Smaller emboli that obstruct 50% or more of the lungs also have a high risk of causing death.

Perioral and Intraoral Characteristics: Not applicable

Distinguishing Characteristics: Not applicable

Significant Microscopic Features: Not applicable

Dental Implications: Individuals who have a thromboembolic venous disorder will be taking anticoagulant medications. Anticoagulant therapy increases the risk of uncontrolled bleeding. Anticoagulant therapy is prescribed for many cardiovascular disorders, and the dental implications associated with it are referred to numerous times; therefore, this vital information is presented in Box 8.2. Sudden symptoms of difficult breathing or unconsciousness, which might indicate that a clot is obstructing vital circulation, should prompt the dental healthcare worker to activate emergency medical services (EMS).

Differential Diagnosis: Not applicable

Box 8.2 DENTAL IMPLICATIONS OF ANTICOAGULANT THERAPY

The reason for anticoagulant therapy should be established, and the patient's coagulation status determined prior to dental treatment during which bleeding is anticipated. A medical consultation may be indicated to make sure that all of the important information about the patient is known by the dental healthcare workers. Patients who are on low-dose anticoagulant therapy (including aspirin) do not have a high risk of major blood loss during routine dental procedures. However, it remains a good policy to consult with the physician and determine the current clotting status of the individual. Data indicate that interrupting or reducing anticoagulant therapy prior to dental surgery may not only be unnecessary but may actually cause the formation of thrombi that may result in death of the patient (Wahl, 2000; Rose et al., 2002; Pickett and Gurenlian, 2005).

Prothrombin time (PT) is the most relied upon test for coagulation status, and PT times that are 1.5 to 2.0 times normal are considered safe for most dental procedures. However, the results of this test vary between laboratories and materials used, setting the stage for inaccurate interpretation of the results. The International Normalized Ratio or INR corrects these differences mathematically, creating a standardized measure of clotting time expressed in values from 1.0 to 10 or more. INR levels of 3 or less are not usually associated with uncontrolled bleeding, and it is believed that most dental procedures that might involve bleeding can be safely performed at these levels (Rose et al., 2002). Local hemostatic measures should be used to control bleeding in these patients. The following local hemostatic measures should result in the formation of a clot and cessation

of bleeding for most patients being treated with anticoagulant therapy (AAP, 2002).
- Applying direct pressure
  o Biting on a moistened tea bag (tea contains a hemostatic agent, tannic acid)
- Rinsing with tranexamic acid (a hemostatic agent)
- Placing Gelfoam (an absorbable gelatin substance that provides a framework for clot formation) within a wound such as an extraction site
- Using sutures

Several medications that are commonly prescribed in dentistry can interfere with clot formation and should be avoided when treating the anticoagulated patient. The following medications are contraindicated for patients taking anticoagulant therapy.

INCREASE PROTHROMBIN TIME (DECREASE CLOT FORMATION)

- Aspirin
- Other nonsteroidal antiinflammatory medications
- Tetracycline
- Erythromycin
- Clarithromycin
- Metronidazole

DECREASE PROTHROMBIN TIME (INCREASE RISK OF CLOT FORMATION)

- Penicillins

Treatment and Prognosis: Treatment for DVT consists of anticoagulant therapy to stop further thrombus formation or enlargement and fibrinolytic therapy to dissolve the thrombus. Surgery may be necessary to remove thrombi that are not responding to medical interventions. Individuals who have had one episode of DVT are at very high risk of experiencing more. Prevention is a very important aspect of treatment for the individual at risk for DVT or who has already experienced DVT. Prevention focuses on anticoagulant therapy and using physical and mechanical means to help move blood more quickly through the venous system in the lower extremities. Physical means include early walking or other physical activity following surgery. Mechanical means include wearing support stockings or using air compression devices that put pressure on the legs, thereby forcing blood up toward the trunk of the body.

Name: Hypertension

Etiology: There are two forms of hypertension: primary, or essential, and secondary. Secondary hypertension is a sequela of another disease process such as renal disease or hyperthyroidism and will be eliminated if the disease causing it is eliminated or adequately treated. This section focuses on primary hypertension because 95% or more of the cases of hypertension are considered primary. Primary, or essential, hypertension has a multifactorial etiology that includes numerous genetic and environmental factors. Research has shown that multiple genes are involved in determining a predisposition to hypertension. The exact genetic mechanism that triggers hypertension is unknown, as is the exact impact that environmental factors have on the establishment and progression of the disease. See Table 8.1 for a summary of the classifications of adult blood pressure measurements.

Method of Transmission: Evidence points to a certain amount of genetic predisposition to hypertension, but the inheritance pattern is not understood and appears to be very complex. Otherwise, hypertension is a nontransmissible disease.

Epidemiology: The statistics related to hypertension are ominous; 1 of every 3 adult Americans is hypertensive. Overall, 39% of the population is normotensive or normal, 31% is prehypertensive, and 29% is hypertensive. Approximately 30% of those with hypertension are unaware of it. More men than women are hypertensive until the age of 55, when the trend reverses, and more women are hypertensive than men. African Americans have a much higher rate of hypertension than Caucasians. In addition, their hypertension is more severe and begins at an earlier age (AHA, 2005).

Pathogenesis: The pathological basis of hypertension can be seen in several areas including: the kidney, where blood volume is controlled by regulation of the salt and water balance, in hormones such as aldosterone that affect vascular muscle tone and regulate renal blood flow and salt metabolism, and in the sympathetic nervous system that stimulates the vessels to contract or to dilate. A change in the delicate balance among these systems can result in hypertension. Atherosclerosis, if present, narrows the lumen of blood vessels, increasing the amount of pressure needed to force blood through them. It also interferes with the ability of the vessel to dilate and lower blood pressure. Other risk factors that are associated with hypertension are smoking, high cholesterol, physical inactivity, and being overweight. Being older, having diabetes, being a male, and/or being an African American are also considered risk factors. The major problem associated with hypertension is not the high blood pressure itself, but the effect that the high blood pressure has on al-

Table 8.1	**CLASSIFICATION OF BLOOD PRESSURE MEASUREMENTS FOR ADULTS OVER 18 YEARS OF AGE**			
	Blood Pressure Range			
Stage	**Systolic (mm Hg)**		**Diastolic (mm Hg)**	**Follow-Up Recommendation[a,b]**
Normal	<120	and	<80	Recheck in 2 years
Prehypertension[c]	120–139	and	80–89	Recheck in 1 year
Hypertension[c]				
Stage 1	140–159	or	90–99	Recheck in 2 months
Stage 2	>160	or	>100	Refer for evaluation within 1 month
	>180	or	>110	Refer for immediate evaluation

[a] If systolic and diastolic categories differ, follow recommendations for shorter-time follow-up (e.g., 160/86 mm Hg should be evaluated or referred to source of care within 1 month).

[b] Modify the scheduling of follow-up according to reliable information about past BP measurements, other cardiovascular risk factors, or target organ disease.

[c] The classification is based on the average of two or more properly measured, seated BP readings on each of two or more office visits.

Adapted with permission from Chobanian AV, et al. The seventh report of the Joint National Committee on Prevention, Detection, Evaluation, and Treatment of High Blood Pressure. Hypertension, December 2003;42:1206–1252 Tables 3 and 4.

most every system in the body. Hypertension is a risk factor for the development of almost all cardiovascular diseases and disorders, kidney disease, stroke, and thrombohemolytic disorders.

Extraoral Characteristics: Hypertension is usually asymptomatic. However, severe hypertension has occasionally been associated with headaches, dizziness, **epistaxis** (nose bleeds), and visual disturbances.

Perioral and Intraoral Characteristics: Not applicable

Distinguishing Characteristics: Not applicable

Significant Microscopic Features: None

Dental Implications: Each practice should establish guidelines for when to refer patients for medical evaluation and when to postpone dental procedures, based on current evidence. Table 8.1 lists blood pressure categories and follow-up recommendations for medical referral suggested by the *Seventh Report of the Joint National Committee on Prevention, Detection, Evaluation, and Treatment of High Blood Pressure.* Dental professionals should always inform their patients of their blood pressure measurements. Stress reduction protocols should be considered for all dental patients, especially for those with cardiovascular problems, including high blood pressure. Elective dental care should be postponed and a medical release obtained if the patient's systolic blood pressure is 180 or more and/or the diastolic pressure is 110 or more (Pickett and Gurenlian, 2005). When the patient's blood pressure is observed at these high levels, emergency dental care should be performed in facilities that have access to the necessary emergency equipment and personnel. In addition, dental professionals must be aware of the side effects of medications that the patient is taking to control hypertension. Most will cause xerostomia, and protocols to prevent caries should be started as soon as possible. Most of these medications also cause orthostatic hypotension (decrease in blood pressure upon rising from a supine position) and measures to prevent this, such as keeping the patient in the chair for a few minutes prior to dismissal, are appropriate. The use of local anesthetics that contain epinephrine (1:100,000) should be limited or avoided if possible because of their potential to increase blood pressure.

Differential Diagnosis: Not applicable

Treatment and Prognosis: The blood pressure treatment goal for patients who do not have diabetes is <140/90. If the patient has diabetes in addition to hypertension, the treatment goal is <130/80 (Chobanian et al., 2003). The lower treatment goal for those with diabetes is based on the strong association between diabetes and an increase in the incidence of all forms of cardiovascular diseases, stroke, renal disease, and blindness (Chobanian et al., 2003). Blood pressure can be reduced by pharmacologic means and by changes in behaviors and/or lifestyles. The drugs most often prescribed regulate heart rate, decrease cardiac output, reduce vasoconstriction, and reduce levels of substances that would act to increase blood pressure, such as aldosterone and angiotensin. Diuretics have been returned to most basic treatment regimens because of their ability to lower blood volume initially and eventually to decrease peripheral resistance throughout the vascular system. Behavioral and lifestyle changes include losing weight; limiting alcohol consumption; decreasing sodium, saturated fat, and cholesterol intake; increasing aerobic activity; smoking cessation; and maintaining adequate dietary levels of potassium, calcium, and magnesium (Chobanian, 2003). The prognosis for those with hypertension obviously varies greatly with each individual, but when considered as part of a group, hypertensive individuals will become more hypertensive as they age. Untreated hypertension drastically increases an individual's risk for early death. Even mild-to-moderate untreated hypertension is associated with a 30% increased risk of atherosclerosis and a 50% increased risk of organ damage after only 8 to 10 years (Sharma and Kortas, 2005).

Hypertensive Heart Disease

Hypertensive heart disease is caused by chronic hypertension and is characterized by hypertrophy of the left ventricle due to the heart working so much harder than normal to pump blood through arteries and veins that have become narrowed by atherosclerosis or hardened by the persistent vascular trauma associated with hypertension. See Chapter 2, Figure 2.4 for an example of left ventricular hypertrophy due to hypertensive heart disease. Eventually the heart can no longer compensate for the added work, and it begins to fail. Congestive heart failure is the most common cause of death in hypertensive individuals who have not received treatment (Rubin et al., 2005).

Name: Stroke (Cerebral Vascular Accident)

Etiology: A stroke is caused by partial or total obstruction of blood flow to the brain. There are two forms of stroke, cerebral ischemia (infarction) and intracranial hemorrhage. Cerebral ischemia is caused by occlusion of the cerebral arteries by a thrombus or an embolus. Intracranial hemorrhage can occur in any of the layers of tissues surrounding the brain or in the brain itself. The most common causes of intracranial hemorrhage are trauma, hypertension, and aneurysm, specifically "berry" aneurysm. Berry aneurysms are small saclike bulges in the bifurcations or junctions of vessels in the brain. The most common area for berry aneurysm formation is in the circle of Willis (Fig. 8.7).

Method of Transmission: Genetic predisposition associated with both atherosclerosis and hypertension plays a role in stroke occurrence. Otherwise, stroke is not a transmissible disorder.

Epidemiology: Approximately 700,000 new or recurrent strokes occur annually in the United States; essen-

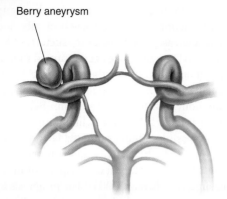

Berry aneyrysm

Figure 8.7. Berry aneurysm. The major blood vessels supplying the brain branch off the circle of Willis, located in the floor of the cranial cavity. The circle of Willis is a common area for the development of berry aneurysms. (Reprinted with permission from Porth CM. Pathophysiology. 6th ed. Philadelphia: Lippincott Williams & Wilkins, 2002:443.)

tially, someone has a stroke every 45 seconds. The incidence of stroke is higher in men than in women and almost twice as high in African Americans as in Caucasians. The incidence of stroke increases as the age of the individual increases (AHA, 2005).

Pathogenesis: Ischemic type strokes account for about 90% of all strokes (AHA, 2005). In ischemic stroke, blood flow is either gradually decreased by a growing thrombus or suddenly obstructed by an embolus. In either case, the brain cells located distal to the obstruction will become necrotic. The typical lesion shows a central area of necrosis and a larger surrounding area that has the potential to recover. Initial emergency treatment of the ischemic stroke focuses on restoring blood flow to this area, thereby limiting the extent of the permanent damage.

Often, individuals who are at risk of ischemic strokes have a temporary obstruction of a cerebral artery, or a **transient ischemic attack (TIA)**, that results in temporary neurologic signs and symptoms. There is overwhelming evidence that these TIAs are warning signs that signify a sharp increase in an individual's risk for a stroke, as 30% or more of strokes are preceded by TIAs.

Hemorrhagic strokes are less common than ischemic strokes but are more frequently fatal. Rupture of the blood vessels in the brain will result in increased pressure in the brain and may cause the brain to push into the foramen magnum causing further damage to the tissues. The increased pressure also compresses other blood vessels and causes ischemia within the tissues that they supply. Interruption of the blood supply to the brain cells distal to the rupture will result in necrosis of these tissues as well.

Extraoral Characteristics: Common symptoms of stroke include full or partial paralysis involving one side of the body, visual disturbances including double and blurred vision, inability to speak or slurred speech, dizziness, and a change in the level of consciousness.

Hemorrhagic strokes may also present with nausea, vomiting, severe headache, loss of consciousness, and coma.

Perioral and Intraoral Characteristics: It is common for stroke symptoms to be observed in the oral area. Unilateral weakness may affect chewing, swallowing, and the ability to clear the mouth of residual food. The patient may appear to drool uncontrollably, not due to excessive salivation but to a decrease in the ability to swallow or to know when to swallow. Patients will favor chewing on the unaffected side of their mouths, so that the natural cleansing mechanism of the oral cavity is impaired. Food pocketing is also a problem with some stroke patients because they cannot feel the location of the food, and it stays in the mucobuccal fold area and in other nooks and crannies within the oral cavity. There is usually at least some motor impairment that makes oral hygiene quite difficult for many stroke patients.

Distinguishing Characteristics: Not applicable

Significant Microscopic Features: Not applicable

Dental Implications: The dental implications associated with stroke fall into four categories as follows:

1. Managing the side effects of medications taken to prevent thrombus formation (see Box 8.2).
2. Management of poststroke physical effects. The severity of physical impairment ranges from insignificant to total incapacitation. The dental professional must evaluate the impact that general physical as well as oral and perioral impairments will have on the physical, mental, and oral health of the individual. Dysphagia, food pocketing, speech impediments, drooling, and other manifestations of neurologic damage can adversely affect all aspects of the person's well-being. Dental professionals will want to work in cooperation with other healthcare professionals to develop a plan to maximize the patient's recovery potential.
3. Home care modifications. The dental hygienist is the ideal person to evaluate the patient's ability to perform home care procedures. Home care modifications should be based on the individual's level of function. Every effort should be made to help the patient achieve as much autonomy as possible through modification of home care implements, such as toothbrushes, and practices, such as using supplemental fluorides. If the patient must have help from a caregiver, the dental hygienist should be able to provide instruction to make oral health maintenance effective and as easy as possible.
4. Emergency management of stroke. If the dental professional suspects that a patient is having a stroke, emergency medical services should be summoned immediately. Aside from reassuring the patient and keeping them comfortable, there is little that can be done in the dental office other than positioning the patient in an upright or semisupine position to limit blood flow to the brain, pro-

viding supplemental oxygen, and monitoring vital signs. The symptoms that are present may be vague, and the patient may not want to attend to them immediately. Therefore, the most important contribution that the dental professional can make is to recognize the symptoms associated with stroke and act appropriately, even if in doubt, because time is of the essence. Quick administration of medical treatment may prevent extensive permanent damage. Thrombolytic drugs (also know as "clot busters") are highly effective but must be given within 3 hours of the onset of stroke symptoms or not at all.

Differential Diagnosis: Not applicable

Treatment and Prognosis: Treatment protocols for ischemic and hemorrhagic strokes differ. With ischemic strokes the emphasis is to treat rapidly, within 3 hours of the onset of symptoms, and to try to preserve as much brain tissue as possible (Arnold and March, 2005). Thrombolytic drugs that dissolve blood clots are used to reestablish circulation to the area of the brain that still has the potential to recover. Hemorrhagic strokes have no specific therapy except to monitor the patient and provide basic and advanced life support. Surgical removal of the intracranial hematoma is one treatment that may be successful in limiting the mortality and disability associated with hemorrhagic strokes.

Stroke is considered to be the third leading cause of death (heart disease and cancer are first and second) in the United States, with approximately 1 death occurring every 3 minutes. In addition, stroke is the leading cause of long-term disability, causing permanent disability in up to 30% of those affected (AHA, 2005).

HEART DISORDERS

Although the heart has a very romantic history, it is in reality a muscular pump that has the capacity to work nonstop for the life of the individual, or approximately 70 to 80 years. When the heart stops pumping, life as we know it ceases. Many of the medical problems of dental patients involve the heart, and many of the procedures that dental professionals perform have an impact on the heart. The dental professional must have a basic understanding of how the heart works and how diseases of the heart impair its function. This knowledge will enable the dental professional to recognize potential problems and modify planned treatment to protect the patient and provide the safest and most appropriate therapy possible. Refer to Clinical Protocol 17 for additional information.

Cardiac abnormalities include both congenital and acquired disorders that affect the form and function of the heart muscle, valves, blood supply, and conduction of electrical impulses. The following sections focus on these abnormalities.

Name: Congenital heart defects

Etiology: The exact etiology of most congenital heart defects is not known. However, there is growing evidence that implicates a combination of genetic and environmental factors in the development of most congenital heart defects. Table 8.2 lists many of the known environmental causes of congenital heart defects. Genetic factors are also known to be involved in the development of congenital heart defects. Many of the more common genetic syndromes include congenital heart defects as one of their elements; some of these syndromes are listed in Box 8.3. Genetic research has uncovered several single-gene abnormalities that appear to be involved in creating heart defects. The cardiac regulatory gene *NKX2.5* has been associated with atrial septal defects and with conduction disorders in the heart (Winlaw et al., 2005). As the role of genes in the development of heart defects continues to be uncovered, there will be many opportunities to find ways to intervene and possibly prevent heart defects (MOD, 2006).

Table 8.2	ENVIRONMENTAL FACTORS ASSOCIATED WITH CONGENITAL HEART DEFECTS.
Maternal infections	Rubella TORCH syndrome agents
Maternal illness	Diabetes Phenylketonuria (PKU)
Maternal medications/drugs	Retinoids (Accutane) Lithium Alcohol Cocaine Phenytoin Dextroamphetamine Vitamin D Thalidomide Estrogenic steroids
Higher maternal age	

Box 8.3 — GENETIC SYNDROMES AND DISORDERS ASSOCIATED WITH CONGENITAL HEART DEFECTS

Trisomy 21
Trisomy 18
Trisomy 13
Cri du chat syndrome
Turner syndrome
Klinefelter syndrome
Marfan syndrome
22q11 Deletion syndromes
• DiGeorge syndrome
• Velocardiofacial syndrome (VCFS)
Noonan syndrome
Ehlers-Danlos syndrome
Osler-Weber-Rendu syndrome
Treacher Collins syndrome

Method of Transmission: Congenital heart defects are not transmitted from one person to the next except in the case of maternal infections and through inheritance.

Epidemiology: The American Heart Association estimates that 9 congenital heart defects per 1000 live births occur in the United States annually (about 36,000 defects). Approximately 2.3 per 1000 or 9200 babies born with these defects will need surgical intervention to correct or manage the defects. Males, females, and different ethnic groups seem to be affected equally (AHA, 2005). The most common types of heart defects are noted in Box 8.4.

Pathogenesis: Errors in morphogenesis that affect the heart and much of the vascular system occur between weeks 2 and 6 in utero. The errors can range from faulty production of a crucial protein to skipping a step in the development process. These errors can result in incomplete formation of structures or development of defective components of the structures, such as the excessive elasticity

Box 8.4 — COMMON HEART DEFECTS

• Ventricular septal defects
• Atrial septal defects
• Patent ductus arteriosus
• Tetralogy of Fallot
• Pulmonary stenosis
• Coarctation of the aorta
• Transposition of the great arteries/vessels

of blood vessels seen in Marfan syndrome. Regardless of the cause, these defects range in severity from innocuous anomalies that are only discovered by accident and have no effect on the individual to major defects that cause the death of a newborn child or the fetus in utero. Heart defects can initiate a series of events that can change the ability of the heart to function over the life span of the individual and can eventually cause premature death. Some of the most common defects allow a mixing of oxygenated blood from the lungs with deoxygenated blood coming from the systemic circulation. This abnormality is called a **shunt**. There are two types of shunts, right-to-left and left-to-right. The right-to-left shunt moves blood from the right side of the heart into the left side of the heart, mixing blood that has not yet been oxygenated into oxygenated blood that is about to be pumped to the rest of the body. This type of shunt can cause cyanosis and cellular hypoxia in all of the body's tissues and is considered more serious than the second type of shunt. The left-to-right shunt moves blood from the left side of the heart to the right side of the heart, mixing blood that has already been oxygenated with blood that is about to be pumped to the lungs to be oxygenated, the resulting mixture is sent to the lungs to be oxygenated (some for the second time), and from there it returns to the heart to be pumped to the rest of the body. This type of shunt results in the heart overworking, but the tissues receive adequate oxygen, making this a less serious condition. One way to remember which one of the two is the "better" shunt is to think of this as one situation in which it is "easier" to be left (handed) than right (handed). More detailed information is presented with each specific defect.

Extraoral Characteristics: Each of the most common heart defects is described in this section along with any information on pathogenesis that is important to understanding the impact of the defect on the function of the system or well-being of the individual.

• The ventricular septal defect (VSD) is a hole in the septal wall between the left and right ventricles. VSD is the most common congenital heart defect, occurring alone or in combination with other defects in about 25–30% of cases (Rubin et al., 2005). Initially, this is a left-to-right shunt with no symptoms of cyanosis. However, if the hole is large enough and is not corrected, the pulmonary arteries can become damaged from the excess pressure of having to carry a greater-than-normal blood flow. The damage results in thickened vessel walls that do not expand as much as they should, which causes the blood pressure within them to increase. The increased blood pressure going to the lungs creates resistance, causing the pressure in the right ventricle to become greater than the pressure in the left ventricle and shifting the shunt from a left-to-right shunt to a right-to-left shunt following the pressure gradient. Symptoms range from none to generalized cyanosis that occurs when the shunt shifts direction. Cyanosis is a sign that the tissues are hypoxic, and symptoms of fatigue, shortness of breath, and tachycardia will be present to some degree. Individuals with chronic hypoxia for any reason tend to present with a characteristic clubbing of the finger tips (Fig. 8.8). Eventually the right ventricle will hypertrophy to try and compensate for the increased workload, and when it can no longer adapt, right-sided congestive heart failure will occur. Congestive heart failure is discussed below in this chapter. Ventricular septal defects leave the affected individual at a higher risk for infective endocarditis, aortic valve prolapse, and blood clots in the circulation or emboli.

• The atrial septal defect (ASD) is a hole in the wall between the right and left atria. ASDs account for about 10 to 15% of congenital heart defects (Rubin et al., 2005). Most of these defects are left-to-right shunts and are asymptomatic unless they are large. If they are large, the initial left-to-right shunt can shift to a right-to-left shunt as with ventricular septal defects. Cyanosis and hypoxia along with right-sided congestive heart failure can result from a large untreated ASD. Symptoms include fatigue, shortness of breath, **dysrhythmias** (abnormal heart beats), and clubbing of the fingers. These individuals are at a higher risk for infective endocarditis and emboli.

• Patent ductus arteriosus (PDA) occurs when the ductus arteriosus, which bypasses the lungs and allows blood from the right side of the heart to go directly into the circulation during fetal development, does not close within a few days after birth (Fig. 8.9). Delayed closure of the ductus arteriosus (sometimes taking several weeks or months) often occurs in premature infants, but full-term infants with PDA rarely have closure of the defect after the first several days. PDA causes a left-to-right shunt between the aortic artery and the pulmonary circulation. Symptoms include a **heart murmur** or abnormal heart sound and, later in life, the possibility of developing **pulmonary hypertension**

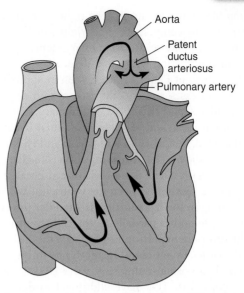

Figure 8.9. Patent ductus arteriosus. (From Pillitteri A. Maternal and child nursing. 4th ed. Philadelphia: Lippincott Williams & Wilkins, 2003.)

(high blood pressure within the lungs) due to excessive blood flow to the lungs. Individuals with untreated PDA are at a higher risk for infective endocarditis and **arteritis** (infection of an artery).

• Pulmonary stenosis (PS) accounts for 5 to 7% of congenital heart defects (Rubin et al., 2005). PS is a narrowing of the pulmonary valve at the entrance of the pulmonary artery coming from the right ventricle (Fig. 8.10). PS is often caused by a fusion of the valve leaflets or cusps so that they form a sort of funnel when the valve opens instead of the wide opening that should be there. Symptoms depend on the extent of the defect. If the stenosis is severe, it will be difficult for the heart to

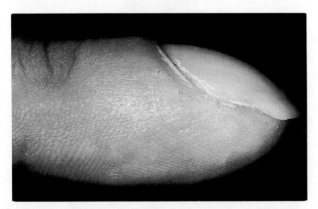

Figure 8.8. Clubbing of the finger tips. Clubbing of the finger tips is associated with chronic tissue hypoxia. (From Bickley LS, Szilagyi PG. Bates' Guide to Physical Examination and History Taking, 7th ed. Baltimore: Lippincott Williams & Wilkins, 1999.)

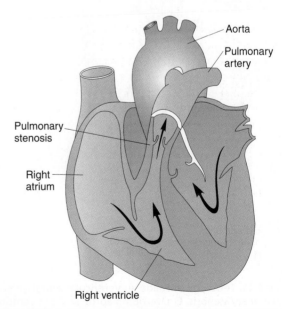

Figure 8.10. Pulmonary stenosis. (From Pillitteri A. Maternal and child nursing. 4th ed. Philadelphia: Lippincott Williams & Wilkins, 2003.)

pump blood into the lungs. The right ventricle will hypertrophy to compensate, and right-sided congestive heart failure may result. Pulmonary stenosis often occurs in conjunction with other defects.

• The tetralogy of Fallot (TOF) is seen in approximately 4 to 9% of cases and is comprised of four defects: (1) ventricular septal defect, (2) pulmonary stenosis, (3) overriding aorta, and (4) right ventricular hypertrophy (Rubin et al., 2005) (Fig. 8.11). VSD and PS have been described above. The overriding aorta is the hardest defect to visualize. The aorta is displaced because of the hole in the septum between the ventricles, and instead of opening in the left ventricle it straddles the break in the septum and is partially in the right ventricle. The right ventricle hypertrophies because the heart has to work harder to get blood to the lungs through a narrower-than-normal pulmonary valve (PS). Often children born with TOF have additional cardiac defects. The symptoms of this disorder depend on the severity of the stenosis and the size of the VSD. Larger VSDs are associated with right-to-left shunting of blood, cyanosis, and hypoxia. Individuals with this disorder have shortness of breath, especially on exertion, poor growth, and clubbing of the fingers. Because they have chronic hypoxia, they also have a tendency to have **polycythemia** (an abnormal increase in the number of red blood cells). Polycythemia and its complications are discussed in Chapter 9. TOF increases the risk of

infective endocarditis, emboli, brain abscesses due to embolization of bacterial vegetations formed in endocarditis, and acute episodes of cyanosis during which seizures, loss of consciousness, and sudden death are possible.

• Coarctation of the aorta (COA) is a constriction of the aorta near the ductus arteriosus after the left subclavian artery branches off the aorta (Fig. 8.12). COA occurs in about 5 to 7% of congenital heart defects; this defect is seen more frequently in males and often in conjunction with other defects (Rubin et al., 2005). COA presents with a discrepancy in blood pressure and pulses in the upper body compared with those in the lower extremities. The heart must pump excessively hard to move blood through the constricted area. Pressure in the upper body is increased because the arteries that supply the upper body branch off the aorta before the area of constriction; the blood flow follows the path of least resistance and overflows into the upper body. The blood pressure in the lower extremities is diminished because a lower volume of blood is able to get past the constricted area. Pulses in the arms and neck appear to be bounding, compared with the weak pulses found in the lower extremities. Signs and symptoms in the upper body include left ventricular hypertrophy, dizziness, headache, and epistaxis. Weakness, pain, pallor, and coldness are found in the lower extremities. Untreated COA is associated with an increased risk of stroke, ruptured aortic and cerebral aneurysms, arteritis at the site of the constriction, or infective endocarditis at the aortic valve.

• Transposition of the great arteries (TGA) occurs in 4 to 10% of heart defects. It is seen more often in males and in those born to diabetic mothers. It is responsible for more than 50% of infant mortality due to heart defects

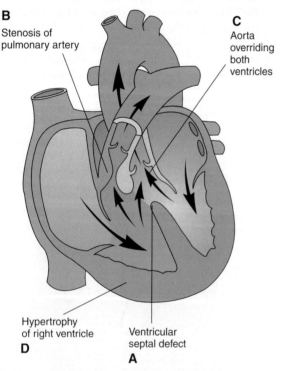

Figure 8.11. Tetralogy of Fallot. *A.* Ventricular septal defect. *B.* Pulmonary stenosis. *C.* Overriding aorta. *D.* Right ventricular hypertrophy. (From Pillitteri A. Maternal and child nursing. 4th ed. Philadelphia: Lippincott Williams & Wilkins, 2003.)

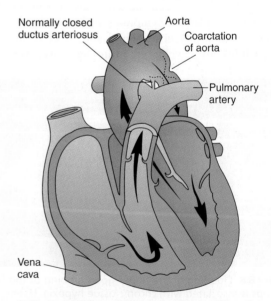

Figure 8.12. Coarctation of the aorta. (From Pillitteri A. Maternal and child nursing. 4th ed. Philadelphia: Lippincott Williams & Wilkins, 2003.)

that cause cyanosis (Rubin et al., 2005). TGA is exactly what its name implies, a complete reversal of normal anatomy. The aorta exits from the right ventricle, and the pulmonary artery exits from the left ventricle (Fig. 8.13). Most of the time there is an associated septal defect that allows mixing of blood from the lungs and from the rest of the body; if there is no associated VSD or ASD, this defect is lethal. The major presenting symptom in a newborn with this disorder is cyanosis and hypoxia.

Perioral and Intraoral Characteristics: Any of the congenital heart defects that cause cyanosis will cause cyanosis in the soft tissues of the oral cavity, including the lips.

Distinguishing Characteristics: Not applicable

Significant Microscopic Features: Not applicable

Dental Implications: The presence of cyanosis in any individual should alert the dental professional to the possibility of the presence of a significant heart defect or disorder and should be investigated thoroughly prior to any treatment. Dental treatment modifications that should be considered include prophylactic antibiotic medication to prevent infective endocarditis (discussed below in this chapter) or arteritis, supplemental oxygen, stress reduction protocols, and caution in selecting local anesthetics. The American Heart Association's recommendations for prophylactic antibiotic regimens should be followed whenever indicated by the individual's medical history. Box 8.5 identifies cardiac conditions that are associated with an increased risk of endocarditis. Box 8.6 lists common dental procedures that might require prophylactic antibiotics. Table 8.3 lists the medications recommended by the American Heart Association for prophylactic antibiotic regimens.

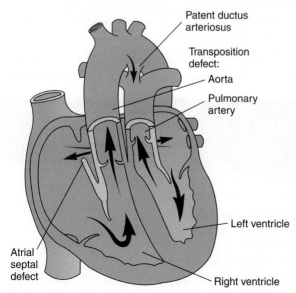

Figure 8.13. Transposition of the great arteries. (From Pillitteri A. Maternal and child nursing. 4th ed. Philadelphia: Lippincott Williams & Wilkins, 2003.)

Box 8.5 CARDIAC CONDITIONS ASSOCIATED WITH THE HIGHEST RISK OF ADVERSE OUTCOME FROM

ENDOCARDITIS FOR WHICH PROPHYLAXIS WITH DENTAL PROCEDURES ARE RECOMMENDED

- Prosthetic cardiac valve
- Previous infective endocarditis
- Congenital heart disease (CHD)[1]
  - o Unrepaired cyanotic CHD, including palliative shunts and conduits
  - o Completely repaired congenital heart defect with prosthetic material or device, whether placed by surgery or by catheter intervention, during the first 6 months after the procedure[2]
  - o Repaired CHD with residual defects at the site or adjacent to the site of a prosthetic patch or prosthetic device (which inhibit endothelialization)
- Cardiac transplantation recipients who develop cardiac valvuloplasty

[1]Except for the conditions listed above, antibiotic prophylaxis is no longer recommended for any other form of CHD.

[2]Prophylaxis is recommended because endothelialization of prosthetic material occurs within 6 months after the procedure.

From Wilson W, Taubert KA, Gewitz M, et al. Prevention of Infective Endocarditis. Guidelines From the American Heart Association. A Guideline From the American Heart Association Rheumatic Fever, Endocarditis, and Kawasaki Disease Committee, Council on Cardiovascular Disease in the Young, and the Council on Clinical Cardiology, Council on Cardiovascular Surgery and Anesthesia, and the Quality of Care and Outcomes Research Interdcisciplinary Working Group. Circulation. 2007 Apr 19; [Epub ahead of print]

Box 8.6 DENTAL PROCEDURES FOR WHICH ENDOCARDITIS PROPHYLAXIS IS RECOMMENDED FOR PATIENTS IN BOX 8.5

All dental procedures that involve manipulation of gingival tissue or the periapical region of teeth or perforation of the oral mucosa*

*The following procedures and events do not need prophylaxis: routine anesthetic injections through noninfected tissue, taking dental radiographs, placement of removable prosthodontic or orthodontic appliances, adjustment of orthodontic appliances, placement of orthodontic brackets, shedding of deciduous teeth, and bleeding from trauma to the lips or oral mucosa.

From Wilson W, Taubert KA, Gewitz M, et al. Prevention of Infective Endocarditis. Guidelines From the American Heart Association. A Guideline From the American Heart Association Rheumatic Fever, Endocarditis, and Kawasaki Disease Committee, Council on Cardiovascular Disease in the Young, and the Council on Clinical Cardiology, Council on Cardiovascular Surgery and Anesthesia, and the Quality of Care and Outcomes Research Interdcisciplinary Working Group. Circulation. 2007 Apr 19; [Epub ahead of print]

Table 8.3   PROPHYLACTIC REGIMENS FOR A DENTAL PROCEDURE

Situation	Agent	Regimen: Single Dose 30 to 60 Minutes Before Procedure
Oral	Amoxicillin	Adults: 2.0g Children: 50mg/kg
Unable to take oral medications	Ampicillin or Cefazolin or Ceftriaxone	Adults: 2.0g IM or IV Children: 50mg/kg IM or IV Adults: 1.0g IM or IV Children: 50mg/kg IM or IV
Allergic to penicillin or ampicillin – oral	Cephalexin[1] or Clindamycin or Azithromycin or Clarithromycin	Adults: 2.0g Children: 50mg/kg Adults: 600mg Children: 20mg/kg Adults: 500mg Children: 15mg/kg
Allergic to penicillin or ampicillin and unable to take oral medications	Cefazolin or Ceftriaxone[2] or Clindamycin	Adults: 1.0g IM or IV Children: 25mg/kg IM or IV Adults: 600mg IM or IV Children: 20mg/kg IM or IV

IM indicates intramuscular; and IV, intravenous.

[1]Or other first- or second-generation oral cephalosporin in equivalent adult of pediatric dosage.

[2]Cephalosporins should not be used in an individual with a history of anaphylaxis, angioedema, or urticaria with penicillins or ampicillin.

From Wilson W, Taubert KA, Gewitz M, et al. Prevention of Infective Endocarditis. Guidelines From the American Heart Association. A Guideline From the American Heart Association Rheumatic Fever, Endocarditis, and Kawasaki Disease Committee, Council on Cardiovascular Disease in the Young, and the Council on Clinical Cardiology, Council on Cardiovascular Surgery and Anesthesia, and the Quality of Care and Outcomes Research Interdisciplinary Working Group. Circulation. 2007 Apr 19; [Epub ahead of print]

The patient should be educated about the relationship between oral bacteria/oral infections and infective endocarditis and how adequate home care regimens can decrease the risk of an autogenous (caused by the patient's own bacteria) endocardial infection. Refer to Clinical Protocol 17.

Differential Diagnosis: Not applicable

Treatment and Prognosis: Most congenital heart defects can be corrected with surgery, and most individuals have an excellent prognosis after successful correction of the defects. The prognosis for individuals with an untreated or undiagnosed congenital heart defect depends on the type and severity of the defect. An unknown number of individuals may be living happily with slight congenital defects; on the other hand, it is not unusual for a premature death to be caused by an undiagnosed heart defect that is initially discovered at autopsy. The overall death rate from congenital cardiovascular defects was 1.5 per 1000 babies in 2001. This is the leading cause of death in infants under the age of 1 year (AHA, 2005).

Name: Heart valve defects

Etiology: While heart valve defects can affect any of the heart valves, our discussion of valve disorders will be limited to disorders of the mitral and aortic valves because they are much more common than disorders of the pul-

monary and/or tricuspid valves. Disorders of the heart valves can be caused by a variety of factors. The most common causes are listed in Box 8.7.

Method of Transmission: Heart valve defects cannot be passed from person to person unless they are inherited. Some infectious agents such as syphilis, associated with the development of heart valve defects, may be passed between people.

Epidemiology: Specific incidence data is not available for most valve defects; however, in 2002 approximately

Box 8.7   COMMON CAUSES ASSOCIATED WITH HEART VALVE DISORDERS

- Rheumatic fever
- Congenital defects
- Infective endocarditis
- Syphilis
- Marfan syndrome
- Select pharmacologic weight loss aids (fenfluramine and dexfenfluramine)
- Degenerative changes that occur with age

93,000 valve procedures, ranging from minor repairs to total replacement, were performed in hospitals in the United States (AHA, 2005).

Pathogenesis: Defective heart valves are either stenotic, insufficient, or both (Fig. 8.14). Stenotic heart valves do not open wide enough to let the normal amount of blood flow through them. Two things happen when a heart valve becomes stenotic. The muscles of the chamber behind the valve must hypertrophy so that they can work harder to get blood through the narrow opening; when the muscles can get no larger, they relax, and the chamber becomes larger or dilates so that it can hold more of the blood that it can no longer force through the stenotic valve. Insufficient heart valves do not close completely. When a valve does not close completely it allows blood to **regurgitate** (flow back) into the chamber that it just came from. The chamber behind the valve will again hypertrophy to work harder to force more blood through the valve to make up for the backflow. When it can not enlarge any more, the chamber will dilate so that it can hold the backflow of blood that it can no longer efficiently move through the valve. In both cases, blood flow through the valves is turbulent or rough instead of smooth and, as such, causes even more damage to the valves. As time passes, the heart weakens even more, and congestive heart failure will result.

Extraoral Characteristics: Most valve defects present with an audible murmur. Benign or **physiologic murmurs** represent the normal functioning of the heart and are heard most often in young children because their chest walls are very thin. Physiologic murmurs are the type that individuals "grow out of" as they get older. Physiologic murmurs do not need any type of treatment and are not associated with an increased risk for endocarditis. Murmurs that are caused by a valve defect are called **pathologic murmurs**, and each defect has a characteristic sound with which it is associated. The sounds are made by the noise that the valve produces while it is working and by the turbulent blood flow through the valve. Symptoms are varied and depend on the type and severity of the defect. In general, stenotic valves will cause symptoms to manifest when

the heart is put under stress because there is less time for the affected chamber to fill before the blood is pumped to the next chamber or out to the rest of the body. This will result in less-oxygenated blood getting to the tissues. The person experiences shortness of breath and possibly chest pains. Insufficient valves are usually better tolerated by the individual and may be asymptomatic for many years. Defective valves also have a tendency to put the heart at a high risk for dysrhythmia or abnormal heart rhythm, and many affected individuals present with an irregular heart beat. In addition, the possibility of having areas within the heart where blood can pool for even short times increases the person's risk of developing a blood clot or thrombus that can break free to travel to the lungs or to other parts of the body as an embolus.

Perioral and Intraoral Characteristics: None

Distinguishing Characteristics: Not applicable

Significant Microscopic Features: Not applicable

Dental Implications: The major significance of a heart valve defect involves the potential for developing infective endocarditis when a bacteremia is created while manipulating oral tissues. The operative word in the last sentence is "when," not "if." Research has shown that even daily home care can cause a bacteremia, especially in the presence of oral infections. Individuals with normal cardiac function have no problem eliminating transient bacteremia. However, individuals who have abnormal blood flow through their hearts may have an area in their heart where some blood can stay out of the main flow for a period of time, allowing any bacteria within that blood to attach to the endocardium. Or the turbulent blood flow can cause surface damage to the tissues of the valves, providing a rough spot that can facilitate adherence of the bacteria, which can then start reproducing. The American Heart Association no longer recommends prophylactic antibiotic medication prior to dental procedures for patients who have heart murmurs (Wilson et al., 2007). Individuals who have had valve replacements are at a very high risk of infective endocarditis and thrombus formation. These individuals may be on daily prophylactic antibiotics, which will need to be augmented with a different antibiotic prior to dental procedures and will require consultation with the patient's physician. In addition, they may be taking anticoagulants to decrease the chance of thrombus formation. Anticoagulant therapy may indicate the need for tests to determine whether the patient can safely undergo certain dental procedures without the risk of severe hemorrhage (Box 8.2). Refer to Clinical Protocol 17.

Differential Diagnosis: None

Treatment and Prognosis: The treatment for a valve defect depends on the type and severity of the defect. Minor defects may need no treatment at all, while major defects might require surgical replacement of the valve. Medical treatment of valve disorders focuses on

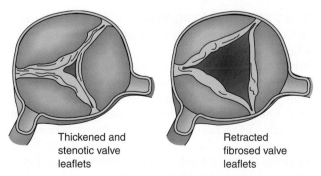

Thickened and stenotic valve leaflets

Retracted fibrosed valve leaflets

Figure 8.14. Valvular disease. Illustration showing a stenotic valve *(left)* that is thickened and narrowed and a valve that is insufficient *(right)* and unable to close completely.

maintaining a normal heart rhythm, preventing the formation of blood clots or infection, and preventing congestive heart failure. These conditions are discussed below in this chapter. The prognosis for this type of disorder is determined by the specific valve involved, the severity of the defect, and whether the individual is treated or not. In most cases of moderate-to-severe defects, an untreated individual will experience a progression of the disorder into congestive heart failure and eventual death from the heart failure or other complications. In 2002 about 19,700 people died from valve defects (AHA, 2005).

Name: Mitral valve prolapse (MVP, floppy mitral valve)

MVP deserves individual attention in this discussion because it is the most common valve defect that will be encountered in a dental care setting.

Etiology: Although some cases of MVP may be due to random errors in morphogenesis, inheritance appears to play a strong role in the development of mitral valve prolapse. The major cause of the defect is an abnormal connective tissue component of the valve leaflets, which results in stretching and ballooning of the valve back into the left atrium during ventricular contraction or systole.

Method of Transmission: MVP is thought to have an autosomal dominant pattern of inheritance. MVP can occur alone or in conjunction with other cardiac defects, and it is associated with many connective tissue disorders such as Marfan syndrome (Chapter 6), Ehlers-Danlos syndrome (Chapter 6), and osteogenesis imperfecta (Chapter 21).

Epidemiology: MVP occurs in up to 6% of the United States population (Huether, 2004; MOD, 2006; AHA, 2005). It appears equally among the different races, but females are affected three times more often than men. However, men seem to have more risk of severe complications than women. MVP is usually diagnosed after adolescence.

Pathogenesis: MVP is seldom if ever diagnosed in the neonate or even in early childhood. The disorder usually takes time to manifest and is normally diagnosed in the late teens or in early adulthood as stated above. Because the connective tissue of the valve leaflets is defective, they stretch and enlarge so that they eventually balloon into the left atrium during systole (Fig. 8.15). This puts added pressure on the valve and, over time, increases the amount of deformity. Constant injury causes the tissues to undergo fibrotic changes that further impair the function of the valve. MVP may present initially with or without regurgitation of blood back into the left atrium. If there is no initial regurgitation it may become evident after many years or it may never occur. Regurgitation due to MVP is the most frequent reason for surgical replacement of the mitral valve (Rubin et al., 2005).

Extraoral Characteristics: MVP has been associated with a thin body type, thoracic deformities, and other

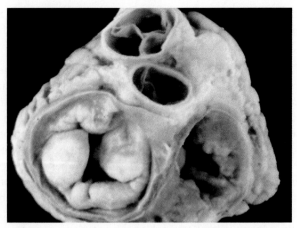

Figure 8.15. Mitral valve prolapse. A view of the mitral valve *(left)* from the left atrium shows stretched and deformed leaflets, which billow into the left atrial cavity. (From Rubin E, Farber JL. Pathology. 3rd ed. Philadelphia: Lippincott Williams & Wilkins, 1999.)

connective tissue disorders. In most cases, this disorder is asymptomatic. However, a myriad of symptoms have been associated with MVP over the years, and there is much controversy about whether the symptoms are related to MVP or not and exactly what impact MVP has on the health of an individual. Some of the symptoms that have been associated with MVP are angina-like chest pain, palpitations, tachycardia, lightheadedness, dyspnea (difficult breathing, shortness of breath), and fatigue.

Perioral and Intraoral Characteristics: None

Distinguishing Characteristics: Not applicable

Significant Microscopic Features: Not applicable

Dental Implications: The American Heart Association no longer recommends prescribing prophylactic antibiotic medication for patients with MVP with or without regurgitation (Wilson et al., 2007). The dental hygienist has an opportunity to educate this patient about the importance of maintaining a disease-free oral environment to decrease the risk of creating a bacteremia that can result in infective endocarditis. Refer to Clinical Protocol 17.

Differential Diagnosis: Not applicable

Treatment and Prognosis: No treatment is necessary for MVP that is not regurgitant or symptomatic. This patient is usually seen by a physician as necessary to make sure that the prolapse is not presenting with any regurgitation. Medical treatment for MVP associated with symptoms is directed toward relieving or eliminating the symptoms. Often, reducing or eliminating dietary stimulants such as caffeine and alcohol are all that is necessary to control the symptoms. In addition, beta-adrenergic-blocking drugs that target palpitations, tachycardia, and chest pain may be prescribed if dietary restrictions alone do not suffice. MVP with regurgitation needs to be followed more closely because of its association with increased risks for infective endocarditis, thrombus formation, and congestive heart failure. Approximately 15% of those with MVP may develop damage that is severe enough to indicate replacing the mitral valve (Rubin et al., 2005).

Name: Rheumatic heart disease

Etiology: Rheumatic heart disease is a sequela of rheumatic fever. Rheumatic fever is thought to be an autoimmune reaction that follows a throat infection caused by group A (beta-hemolytic) streptococcus.

Method of Transmission: Rheumatic heart disease is not transmitted from person to person; however, the triggering infection is caused by streptococci that can be transmitted between persons.

Epidemiology: The incidence of rheumatic fever (and thus rheumatic heart disease) has declined in the United States. Death rates from rheumatic fever/heart disease were 14.5 per 100,000 in 1950, 6.8 per 100,000 in 1972 (Rubin et al., 2005), and 1.2 per 100,000 in 2002 (AHA, 2005). Rheumatic fever is a childhood disease usually occurring between the ages of 5 and 15. This disease is still a significant cause of death in less-developed countries. Rheumatic fever only follows 0.3–5% of untreated streptococcal throat infections, and rheumatic heart disease occurs in about 39% of those who have rheumatic fever (Rubin et al., 2005; Chin and Siddiqui, October 2004). Rheumatic heart disease may not manifest for months or years after the initial rheumatic fever (Rubin et al., 2005).

Pathogenesis: Although there is an association between a particular streptococcal infection and rheumatic fever, it is not known exactly how the disease develops. The most widely accepted theory at this time is that antibodies that form against the bacteria end up attacking the cells of the host after the bacterial challenge is eradicated in a type II cytotoxic hypersensitivity reaction. The specific cells that are affected contain elements that are very close to elements found in the bacteria, thus causing a cross-reaction between the antibodies and normal cells. The cells most likely to be affected are cardiac and smooth muscle cells. The end result is a systemic, immune-mediated inflammatory disease, or rheumatic fever. Rheumatic fever presents about 1 to 4 weeks after a streptococcal throat infection with a high fever; pain in the large joints; rash; subcutaneous nodules over the muscles of the wrist, elbow, ankle, and knee joints; and **carditis**, or inflammation of the heart. All of these manifestations, except the carditis, usually resolve within 3 months. Carditis can affect all of the layers of the heart muscle; however, it is the endocardium, especially of the valve structures, that appears to acquire the most severe and possibly permanent damage. Rheumatic heart disease is the chronic sequela of acute carditis and usually manifests as mitral or aortic valve damage that is often observed clinically as a heart murmur.

During the acute stage of carditis, the valves of the heart become swollen and inflamed, and small nodules form on the edges of the leaflets. This is seen in all of the heart valves but is usually more severe in the valves of the left side of the heart because the blood being pumped though these valves is under higher pressure than those on the right side, causing even more inflammation. As the disease progresses and then begins to resolve, the nodules are replaced by fibrous scar tissue that tends to change the anatomy of the valve, thereby causing the leaflets to thicken, contract, and fuse together, resulting in a stenotic and incompetent valve. Figure 8.16 illustrates the damage done to the mitral valve in rheumatic heart disease. As time passes, the damage becomes more extensive because of the continuing trauma from blood moving through the already damaged valve.

Extraoral Characteristics: Not applicable

Perioral and Intraoral Characteristics: Not applicable

Distinguishing Characteristics: None

Significant Microscopic Features: The heart muscle develops a specific lesion in rheumatic fever, called an Aschoff body. The Aschoff body is a localized area of tissue necrosis surrounded by lymphocytes. This lesion is replaced with fibrous scar tissue as the disease resolves (Rubin et al., 2005).

Dental Implications: Rheumatic heart disease should be suspected whenever a patient reports a history of rheumatic fever. These individuals are sometimes given daily prophylactic antibiotics to prevent streptococcal infections that could lead to a recurrence of rheumatic fever. In addition, the patient may be receiving anticoagulation therapy, indicating the need to determine the coagulation status. Refer to Clinical Protocol 17.

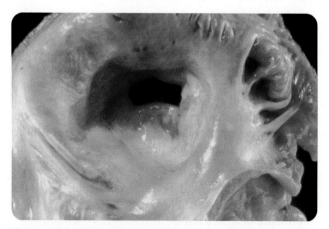

Figure 8.16. Rheumatic heart disease. A view of the mitral valve from the left atrium shows rigid, thickened, and fused leaflets with a narrow orifice, creating the characteristic "fish mouth" appearance of rheumatic mitral stenosis. (From Rubin E, Farber JL. Pathology. 3rd ed. Philadelphia: Lippincott Williams & Wilkins, 1999.)

Differential Diagnosis: Not applicable

Treatment and Prognosis: Preventing rheumatic fever is the best strategy for preventing rheumatic heart disease. Prompt diagnosis of any sore throat especially those with accompanying fever, headache, and malaise will optimize treatment of streptococcal infections and help prevent most cases of rheumatic fever. Prompt diagnosis and treatment of rheumatic fever can limit the severity of symptoms and decrease the potential for severe permanent heart damage. An individual who has once had rheumatic fever is at a considerably higher risk of a recurrence, which would lead to even more heart damage.

Name: Infective endocarditis

Etiology: Bacteria, especially *Staphylococcus* and *Streptococcus*, are the most common causative agents associated with infective endocarditis. Gram-negative bacilli, yeasts, and fungi have also been found, generally associated with the disease found in intravenous drug abusers (Rubin et al., 2005; Porth, 2004).

Method of Transmission: Infective endocarditis is considered an autogenous infection; therefore it is not transmissible from person to person. Individuals must have bacteria in their bloodstream (bacteremia) before they can develop infective endocarditis. In most cases, these are transient or short lived bacteremias, which are eliminated by the body in the natural course of immune system and bodily functions. The infective agents are introduced into the bloodstream of the patient in a variety of ways ranging from illegal intravenous drug use with dirty needles to brushing and flossing at home to remove dental biofilm. Endocarditis can occur in a healthy heart, but the chances of occurrence are much higher in a heart that has been compromised by congenital or acquired heart defects, especially valve defects.

Epidemiology: The incidence of infective endocarditis in the United States is about 2 to 4 cases per 100,000 people. The disease occurs two to three times more frequently in males than in females, and the frequency of infections occurring in those over 60 years of age accounts for up to 50% of all cases (Brusch, August 2005). Rates of infective endocarditis are highest in those with congenital heart defects, mitral valve prolapse, or prosthetic heart valves and in intravenous drug abusers (Rubin et al., 2005; Porth, 2004).

Pathogenesis: The development of infective endocarditis depends on the following factors:

- Presence of a bacteremia
- An underlying cardiac defect in almost all cases (except those associated with intravenous drug abuse)
- Adherence of the bacteria or other causative agent to the endocardial surface (usually the valve leaflets)
- Invasion of that surface by the organism

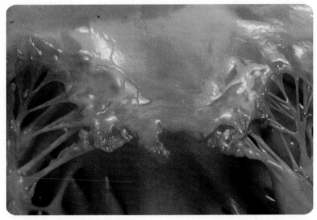

Figure 8.17. Infective endocarditis. The mitral valve shows destructive bacterial vegetations that have eroded through the free margins of the valve leaflets. (From Rubin E, Farber JL. Pathology. 3rd ed. Philadelphia: Lippincott Williams & Wilkins, 1999.)

Vegetative growths or clumps of organisms, cellular debris, and clotted blood appear on the valve leaflets after the organism establishes itself (Fig. 8.17). These vegetations destroy the connective tissues of the valve leaflets. The vegetations adhere loosely to the endocardial surfaces and frequently break free, becoming emboli. The emboli travel to distant parts of the body and may cause infarcts (areas that become necrotic because the blood supply is obstructed by a clot or in this case a mass of bacteria). Abscesses may occur in many organs including the brain, lungs, and kidneys.

Extraoral Characteristics: The disease can manifest as an acute or subacute infection. The acute manifestation presents with high fever, chills, severe shortness of breath, and fatigue associated with congestive heart failure (discussed below in this chapter). Asymmetrical joint pain, a red macular rash, and petechiae on the hands, feet, chest, and abdomen may also be observed.

The subacute infection has a less dramatic course characterized by low-grade fever, flulike symptoms, anorexia, and weight loss. A detectable heart murmur is present in about 99% of cases (Brusch, August 2005). Chest pain, joint pain, and back pain are frequently reported. Neurologic symptoms similar to those associated with a stroke are often present. Congestive heart failure occurs more gradually with the subacute form of the infection.

Perioral and Intraoral Characteristics: Petechiae (minute hemorrhagic spots) may be found on any of the oral mucosal surfaces, especially the soft palate and buccal mucosa (Brusch, August 2005).

Distinguishing Characteristics: Not applicable

Significant Microscopic Features: The causative organism can be cultured from the blood of the individual. Treatment is not successful until all signs of the organism are eliminated from the blood and from any thrombi or emboli in the body.

Dental Implications: The American Heart Association recommends that individuals with a history of infective endocarditis receive prophylactic antibiotic coverage prior to many dental procedures (Table 8.3). Gingival and periodontal infections are the most common source of transient bacteremias. Even more interesting is the fact that surveys have shown that few individuals who are at risk for infective endocarditis are aware of the importance of maintaining good oral health as a method of preventing this terrible disease (Brusch, August 2005). Dental professionals can make a significant impact in this area by identifying those individuals at risk for infective endocarditis and stressing the importance of maintaining oral health to prevent the likelihood of a significant bacteremia being produced.

Differential Diagnosis: Not applicable

Treatment and Prognosis: Treatment focuses on two areas: (1) identifying and eliminating the causative organism and (2) managing complications due to valve damage. Antibiotic therapy is the treatment of choice to destroy bacterial organisms. Other causative organisms are treated with drugs that target those specific organisms. Surgery may be necessary to eliminate abscesses that develop in other areas of the body. Heart valve damage may be so severe that one or more valves must be replaced to manage the congestive heart failure that occurs.

The prognosis for infective endocarditis varies; untreated disease is invariably fatal. The American Heart Association estimated that 2420 individuals died from infective endocarditis in the United States in 2001. In addition, there were 17,000 hospital discharges that listed infective endocarditis as a primary or secondary diagnosis (AHA, 2005). Relapses are common and are highest among those who abuse intravenous drugs, have congenital heart defects or prosthetic heart valves, or have had a previous episode of infective endocarditis (Brusch, August 2005).

Name: Congestive heart failure (CHF)

Etiology: Congestive heart failure occurs when the heart is no longer able to move an adequate amount of blood throughout the body, allowing body tissues to become congested with retained fluids. This can be caused by ischemic heart disease, congenital heart defects, defective heart valves, hypertension, chronic obstructive pulmonary disorders, and anything else that causes the heart to overwork or impairs its function (Rubin et al., 2005; Porth, 2004; Singh, April 2006). Diabetes appears to be a major risk factor, especially among women (AHA, 2005).

Method of Transmission: Not applicable

Epidemiology: In 2002 approximately 4,900,000 individuals in the United States were living with CHF (AHA, 2005). The disorder affects women and men equally, but men have a lower survival rate once they are diagnosed (Singh, April 2006). The risk of developing CHF increases with age; 10 of every 1000 individuals over the age of 65 are affected (AHA, 2005). The available data did not portray any striking differences in incidence among different ethnic groups. Approximately 75% of all cases of CHF occur in conjunction with chronic hypertension (AHA, 2005).

Pathogenesis: CHF is the end result of many chronic and some acute conditions that cause progressive weakening of the heart muscle. CHF manifests as an inability of the heart to pump enough blood to all of the tissues of the body. The edema that results is caused by the decreased cardiac output, which in turn, causes a decrease in the volume of blood that the kidneys can filter. Any decrease in the rate of filtration by the kidney eventually triggers the release of higher-than-normal levels of aldosterone from the adrenal glands. High levels of aldosterone cause sodium reabsorption by the kidneys and fluid retention. As this disease progresses, individuals become more and more incapacitated as less and less blood reaches their tissues. There are several ways to classify heart failure; however, left- and right-sided heart failure will suffice for the purposes of this text.

Left-sided heart failure reflects the inability of the heart to move adequate blood from the pulmonary circulatory system into the systemic circulatory system. Symptoms associated with pulmonary edema (listed below) result from left-sided heart failure. Right-sided heart failure reflects the inability of the heart to move the blood returning from the venous circulation into the pulmonary circulation for oxygenation. Symptoms associated with peripheral edema and edema of central organs (listed below) result from right-sided heart failure. One way to remember what side is associated with which symptoms, is to associate "left" with "lungs" then right must be associated with return of the venous circulation.

Extraoral Characteristics: Symptoms associated with heart failure are initially confined to one or the other side of the heart. However, as the disease progresses both sides of the heart are eventually involved.

Left-sided heart failure results in pulmonary edema. Symptoms of this include impaired gas exchange that causes an inability to perform normal activities, cyanosis, **paroxysmal nocturnal dyspnea** (acute episodes of shortness-of-breath and coughing that occur during the night), and **orthopnea** (an inability to breathe comfortably in a supine position).

Right-sided heart failure results in peripheral edema, which most notably occurs in the lower extremities during the initial stages of the disease (Fig. 8.18). Slowing of the venous blood flow back to the heart causes blood and fluid buildup in the abdominal organs as well. Liver failure, enlargement of the spleen, and gastrointestinal symptoms of anorexia, weight loss, and severe anemia will manifest later in the disease progression. Increased urine

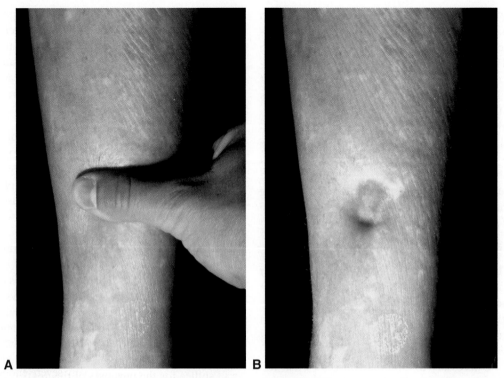

Figure 8.18. Pitting edema of the leg. **A.** In a patient with congestive heart failure, severe edema of the leg is demonstrated by applying pressure with a finger. **B.** The resulting "pitting" reflects the inelasticity of the fluid-filled tissue. (From Rubin E, Farber JL. Pathology. 3rd ed. Philadelphia: Lippincott Williams & Wilkins, 1999.)

output at night (**nocturia**) occurs because the effects of gravity are removed when in the supine position and the fluid can flow more easily back to the heart and through the kidney.

Perioral and Intraoral Characteristics: Cyanosis of the lips and oral mucosal surfaces is possible in both right or left heart failure and would be associated with any severe or end-stage disease. In severe right-sided heart failure the jugular veins become distended and can be observed when the individual is in an upright position, as when an extraoral examination is done. Although not associated with CHF, xerostomia caused by medication taken to manage the disease is a consistent finding.

Distinguishing Characteristics: Not applicable

Significant Microscopic Features: Not applicable

Dental Implications: Modifications in dental care would depend on the stage of the disease and the symptoms present in the individual. Modifying the patient's chair position to semiupright or upright might be indicated as well as providing supplemental oxygen to aid in breathing.

Differential Diagnosis: Not applicable

Treatment and Prognosis: Treatment focuses on removing the cause of the heart failure if possible; for example, repairing a defective heart valve or replacing it, repairing a septal defect, managing hypertension, or treating

a pulmonary disorder. Medical management focuses on relieving the symptoms and maintaining quality of life for the individual. Drugs can help to decrease the levels of aldosterone, remove excess fluid from the body, and increase the force of the heart's contractions.

Approximately 52,828 individuals died from CHF in 2001. Congestive heart failure was listed as the cause of death or contributing to the cause of death on approximately 264,900 death certificates across the United States in 2001 (AHA, 2005). Data gathered from following participants in the Framingham Study suggests that 70% of women and 80% of men who have CHF will die within 8 years of the diagnosis; both sexes have 6 to 9 times more sudden cardiac deaths then the general population and 1 of 5 will die within one year (AHA, 2005).

Name: Coronary heart disease (CHD)

Etiology: Coronary heart disease occurs when the oxygen demands of the heart muscle are not met because blood flow to the heart muscle through the coronary arteries is inadequate. The most common cause of CHD is atherosclerosis. Anything that causes development of atherosclerosis will contribute to the risk of developing CHD. High cholesterol, poor dietary habits, inactive lifestyles, smoking, diabetes, hypertension, age, and genetics all play a role in determining an individual's risk of developing atherosclerosis and, subsequently, CHD.

Method of Transmission: Coronary heart disease is not passed from person to person; however, a family history of CHD can sometimes be linked to a common genetic abnormality called familial hypercholesterolemia. This condition is transmitted in an autosomal dominant inheritance pattern.

Epidemiology: In 2002, 13,000,000 Americans, or 6.9% of the population (Census, 2000), had coronary heart disease (AHA, 2005). Men have a higher prevalence of CHD than women, but only until women experience menopause, when the prevalence of CHD in women steadily increases until it is about equal to that of men of the same age. African Americans of either sex have a higher mortality rate than Caucasians (Singh, August 2005). The incidence of CHD increases with advancing age no matter what additional risk factors are present (AHA, 2005; Singh, August 2005).

Pathogenesis: There are two basic types of CHD: chronic ischemic heart disease and acute coronary syndromes. Chronic ischemic heart disease includes stable angina and silent myocardial ischemia and occurs when the blood supplied to the heart by the coronary arteries is not adequate to meet the demands of the heart muscle. This does not normally occur until one or more of the coronary vessels are 75% or more occluded. Usually the ischemia is not noticeable until the heart is exposed to stress that increases the heart rate, such as: physical exercise, emotional stress, cold temperatures, and large meals. The normal amount of blood that is able to flow through the obstructed arteries is not sufficient to supply the needs of the heart muscle when it is stressed, and ischemia occurs. Ischemia can manifest with or without symptoms. Ischemia that presents with symptoms is called **angina**, or angina pectoris. Silent myocardial ischemia occurs without symptoms of pain. The reason for this is not clearly understood, and it is not known how many people suffer from this form of CHD. Individuals with diabetes suffer from the silent form more often than the symptomatic form. In this case, the lack of pain is thought to be caused by impaired sensory nerve transmission within the autonomic system, or **autonomic neuropathy.**

Acute coronary syndromes include unstable angina, myocardial infarction, and sudden death. **Unstable angina** describes a worsening of the symptoms of angina that usually culminates in a myocardial infarction. Angina pain that occurs when the individual is at rest is the most common sign indicating a progression to unstable angina. Myocardial infarction is the actual death of myocardial cells due to prolonged lack of oxygen. The severity of the infarction depends on the amount of heart tissue that is affected, the location of the infarct, and the length of time that the heart cells are without oxygen. If blood flow is restored to the affected area within 15 to 20 minutes, permanent damage may be avoided. On the other hand, heart cells stop functioning correctly minutes after the onset of ischemia, long before cell death occurs, so that even if blood flow is restored quickly, the myocardial cells may

be unable to begin functioning well enough to sustain life without outside intervention. Dysrhythmias, specifically **ventricular fibrillation,** in which the heart quivers but does not produce a functional beat, are often caused by the malfunction of the ischemic myocardial cells. In these cases, death may be related more to the dysrhythmia than to the actual amount of permanent damage done to the heart. If blood flow is not restored, the myocardial cells undergo coagulative necrosis and then fibrous scar formation. Scar formation takes between 6 and 8 weeks and leaves the heart muscle compromised because the scar tissue does not function like cardiac muscle. How badly the heart is compromised depends on the number and location of the cells that were destroyed. Sudden death is also considered an element of acute coronary syndromes. When an individual dies within 1 hour of the onset of symptoms of a myocardial infarction, it is called sudden death. Sudden death is most often associated with severe dysrhythmia, usually ventricular fibrillation.

Extraoral Characteristics: Angina pain usually centers in the substernal area of the chest and is described as crushing, suffocating, or "like having an elephant stand on your chest." The pain is normally severe enough to stop the individual from doing whatever he or she is doing. The pain may stay in the chest area or may radiate up into the left jaw or into the left arm; the right arm may also be affected. If the pain is not severe, the chest pain can be easily confused with indigestion or the arm and shoulder pain with arthritis. Symptoms associated with an acute myocardial infarction are varied, and many people who have had myocardial infarctions are not aware that they have had them. In fact, 25 to 50% of nonfatal myocardial infarctions are not symptomatic and are identified only later by electrocardiogram or at autopsy (Rubin et al., 2005). The patient may feel severe angina pain that may radiate to the jaw or arms accompanied by nausea, vomiting, shortness of breath, and copious sweating; or the patient may only experience one or two symptoms or a lesser degree of all of the symptoms.

Perioral and Intraoral Characteristics: Not applicable

Distinguishing Characteristics: Not applicable

Significant Microscopic Features: Not applicable

Dental Implications: Elective dental/dental hygiene care should be avoided until 6 months after an acute myocardial infarction, and care should not be rendered to someone with unstable angina except in a setting where appropriate life support is immediately available. Stress reduction techniques should be used to limit anxiety during dental appointments, and supplemental oxygen should be considered if appropriate. Drugs that are used to manage coronary heart disease have many oral side effects, and the professional should be aware of the specific side effects associated with each type of drug. For example, calcium channel blockers are associated with gingival hyperplasia. When gingival hyperplasia is identified, the dental professional may consult with the patient and the patient's physician to develop a plan to try to prevent any further hyperplastic growth. Each patient should be evaluated for the presence of xerostomia because most of the drugs prescribed for treating coronary heart disease will cause xerostomia in most individuals. Above all, each patient should be encouraged to maintain as healthy an oral environment as possible to limit the systemic effects of oral infections. Refer to Clinical Protocol 17.

Differential Diagnosis: Not applicable

Treatment and Prognosis: Treatment for coronary heart disease depends on the specific type that is present. Treatment for chronic ischemic heart disease focuses on relieving symptoms and preventing acute coronary syndromes. Current treatment is aggressive and aimed at not only medical and surgical therapies but also on eliminating preventable risk factors such as smoking, and managing disorders that are associated with progression of this disease such as hypertension, diabetes, and high cholesterol. Medications such as nitroglycerin are used to treat the symptoms of angina by relaxing systemic blood vessels and thereby decreasing cardiac workload and lessening the oxygen requirements of the heart muscle. Drugs that decrease the heart rate, decrease cholesterol levels, and reduce the potential for thrombus formation in atherosclerotic arteries are considered life prolonging and are a mainstay of therapy for coronary heart disease. Surgical treatment is often necessary to reestablish adequate blood flow to the heart muscle. These interventions include coronary angioplasty, the placing of stents or wire tubes that hold the arteries open, and coronary artery bypass procedures. In coronary angioplasty, a collapsed balloon is threaded through arteries in the groin to the coronary artery that is blocked. The balloon is placed in the narrowed area and then inflated, causing the matter within the intima and in the lumen of the vessel to be compressed and resulting in a larger lumen. A stent may be placed in the artery to maintain the open position (Fig. 8.19). Coronary bypass surgery uses a vein graft from the leg to go around, or bypass, a blockage in one or more of the coronary arteries, thus reestablishing blood flow to the area.

Treatment of acute coronary syndromes focuses on reestablishing blood flow to the area of infarction as soon as possible to limit the extent of permanent damage. The ideal intervention occurs within 60 to 90 minutes of the onset of symptoms. Drugs that dissolve blood clots. or thrombolytic drugs, are known to reduce death incidence and limit the extent of damage. Aspirin is a strong antiplatelet drug that can be given to someone who is experiencing a myocardial infarction, even before medical help is obtained. Aspirin has been shown to increase survival chances by decreasing the chance of new or larger clot formation. Definitive therapy for acute coronary syndromes is basically the same as for chronic ischemic heart disease, only performed under emergency conditions.

Individuals who have had experience with these diseases should take part in a cardiac rehabilitation program

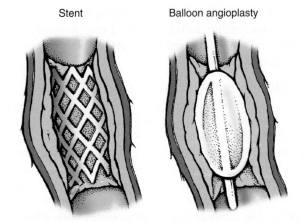

Figure 8.19. Balloon angioplasty. Atherosclerosis treatment. Close-up views of coronary arteries showing balloon angiography and stent placement, both of which are intended to increase blood flow to the heart. LifeART image 6 2007. Lippincott Williams & Wilkins. All rights reserved.

designed specifically to meet their needs. The rehabilitation programs are meant to safely return a person with coronary heart disease to as normal a routine as possible and to address changes that need to be made such as diet and tobacco use.

Dysrhythmias

Dysrhythmias are abnormal heart rhythms or beats. Cardiac dysrhythmias occur in a high percentage of the population. These abnormalities are associated with the conduction of abnormal or inappropriate electrical impulses through the heart muscle and can be caused by scar tissue from myocardial infarctions, valve dysfunction, or other cardiac disorders. Examples of irregular heart beats include tachycardia (fast heart beat), bradycardia (slow heart beat), and ventricular and atrial fibrillation. Tachycardia and bradycardia can occur occasionally or frequently, and the symptoms can range from insignificant to life threatening. If symptoms such as shortness of breath or chest pain occur, then the individual should receive treatment. Ventricular fibrillation occurs when there is an irregular spread of impulses through the bundle of His up to the Purkinje fibers. This leads to twitching of the heart muscle and little or no blood being pumped through the circulatory system. Cardiac arrest will occur if ventricular fibrillation is not stopped. Atrial fibrillation is caused by erratic conduction of impulses from the SA node, which results in uncoordinated atrial contractions. Atrial fibrillation is associated with an increased risk of stroke. Medications such as digoxin or beta-blockers may be used to manage abnormal heart rhythms. Serious disorders are treated with cardiac pacemakers and implanted defibrillators that normalize the beat and, if necessary, shock the heart to stop fibrillation.

The dental professional has the opportunity to identify abnormal heart rhythms while obtaining vital signs and through discussion of the patient's medical history. Because many dysrhythmias are caused by an underlying cardiac condition, it is important to refer these patients to their physician for evaluation. The presence of an implanted pacemaker or defibrillator does not indicate the need for prophylactic antibiotic coverage unless warranted by the underlying cardiac condition. Refer to Clinical Protocol 17 for more dental implications.

SUMMARY

- The cardiovascular system is composed of the heart and the vessels that carry blood throughout the body.
- Cardiovascular abnormalities can be genetic or they may be acquired during morphogenesis or at some other time during life.
- Turbulent, as opposed to laminar, blood flow contributes to atherosclerosis and other forms of cardiovascular injury, infection, or disease.
- Atherosclerosis is a major risk factor for most acquired chronic cardiovascular disorders.
- Oral infections increase the amount of circulating inflammatory products, which may contribute to endothelial injury and encourage the development of atherosclerosis.
- Abdominal aortic aneurysm is a sequela of atherosclerosis that involves the weakening and bulging of the arterial wall. The most significant complications of AAA are rupture and thrombus formation.
- Raynaud's disease/phenomenon is caused by vasospasms in the small vessels of the skin of the fingers and toes and, less often, the nose and ears.
- Deep venous thrombus is characterized by the formation of thrombi in the deep veins of the legs. Aside from pain, inflammation, and swelling of the lower extremities, DVT can result in the creation of emboli that can travel to the lungs as pulmonary emboli.
- Hypertension affects 1 of every 3 American adults. The etiology and pathogenesis are complex, but there are known risk factors that can be altered to prevent or limit the extent of the disease and its complications or sequela.
- Stroke is a sequela of hypertension and atherosclerosis. Strokes occur when there is ischemia to an area of the brain either because of a thrombus, embolus, or intracranial hemorrhage. Blood flow to the area must be restored quickly to reduce the amount of permanent damage.
- Transient ischemic attacks are temporary episodes of ischemia that often warn of, or precede, a stroke.
- Congenital heart defects can be very slight or they can be so severe that they cause death in utero or during the neonatal period. The most common congenital heart defect is the ventricular septal defect.
- Cyanosis is associated with some congenital heart defects and is a sign that there is mixing of blood returning from general circulation with blood from the pulmonary circulation. The heart must work harder to get oxygen to all of the body's tissues. Congestive heart failure is a possible result of these conditions.
- Heart valve disorders can cause valvular stenosis, insufficiency, or both. The most common disorder is mitral valve prolapse, which can occur with or without regurgitation.
- Infective endocarditis is the result of a bacteremia. Often, bacteria enter the blood by way of the oral cavity through trauma or everyday oral hygiene care. Oral infections, particularly periodontal infections, increase the risk of creating bacteremia during everyday oral care and eating.
- Rheumatic heart disease is the result of an aberrant immune system response that causes antibodies that have formed against streptococcal bacteria from a throat infection to attack and damage the tissues of the heart, causing carditis. While the carditis usually resolves, there may be permanent damage to the heart valves.
- Congestive heart failure is the end result of many cardiovascular disorders that cause the heart to overwork to move blood throughout the body. Eventually the heart cannot compensate for the added work by hypertrophy or other means, the contractions begin to weaken, fluids build up in either the lungs, extremities, or both, and the heart fails.
- Coronary heart disease occurs when the heart muscle is not supplied with enough oxygen to meet its needs. The two basic types of CHD are chronic ischemic heart disease and acute coronary syndromes.
- Dysrhythmias or abnormal heart beats result from the abnormal conduction of electrical impulses through the heart muscle. A history of dysrhythmia can be associated with many types of heart defects or damage and should be thoroughly investigated prior to performing dental treatment.
- Dental professionals must prepare accurate health information regarding cardiovascular disorders because some of the disorders increase an individual's risk for infective endocarditis and would thus indicate following the AHA's prophylactic antibiotic premedication regimen.

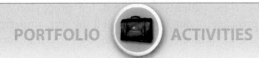

PORTFOLIO ACTIVITIES

1. Develop a patient centered fact sheet dealing with why it is important for an individual who is at risk for infective endocarditis to have excellent oral health.

This can be made available to the dental hygiene clinic patients and can be used as a handout at health fairs and other community events.

Critical Thinking Activities

1. Find information that either supports or negates a connection between periodontal infections and atherosclerosis. Combine your findings with the information found by other classmates and create a class opinion of how strong or weak the connection may be, or if you think that there is one at all. Make sure that you reference the material that you found so that others can refer to the original studies.

2. What do you think the role of a dental hygienist should be in regard to educating patients about cardiovascular diseases? Do you feel that the hygienist should only relate information that is germane to the link between oral and cardiovascular health or do you think that the hygienist should be able to discuss other aspects of cardiovascular health such as diet and exercise?

Case Study

Your first appointment for the day is with a 7-year-old boy named Ben. You have not met Ben before, but you know his father and mother. Ben presents as a healthy-looking young boy who appears rather tall for his age. You are aware that his father has Marfan syndrome but neither his father nor his mother have said that Ben has Marfan syndrome. As you are going over the medical and dental history with Ben's mother you are trying to think of how to ask the questions that you think are necessary.

1. What questions do you think you need to ask Ben's mother?
2. What specific heart or circulatory disorders are associated with Marfan syndrome?
3. What are the possible health implications if you provide dental hygiene therapy for Ben and he has undiagnosed Marfan syndrome?
4. What type of treatment modifications would be necessary to treat Ben if he has the heart disorder associated with this syndrome?

REFERENCES

American Academy of Periodontology (AAP). Academy reports: periodontal management of patients with cardiovascular diseases. J Periodontol 2002;73:954–968.

American Heart Association. Heart disease and stroke statistics—2005 update. American Heart Association, 2005.

Arnold JL. Stroke, ischemic. Last update March 2005. e medicine: Instant Access to the Minds of Medicine. Available at: http://www.emedicine.com/emerg/topic558.htm. Accessed July 12, 2006.

Brusch JL. Infective endocarditis. Last update August 2005. e medicine: Instant Access to the Minds of Medicine. Available at: http://www.emedicine.com/med/topic671.htm. Accessed July 12, 2006.

Chin TK, Chinn E, Siddiqui T, et al. Rheumatic heart disease. Last update May 2006. e medicine: Instant Access to the Minds of Medicine. Available at: http://www.emedicine.com/ped/topic2007.htm. Accessed July 12, 2006.

Chobanian AV, Bakris GL, Black HR, et al. and the National High Blood Pressure Education Program Coordinating Committee. Hypertension December 2003;42:1206–1252.

Feied C. Deep venous thrombosis. Last update March 2005. e medicine: Instant Access to the Minds of Medicine. Available at: http://www.emedicine.com/med/topic2785.htm. Accessed July 12, 2006.

Foster E. Congenital heart disease in adults. West J Med 1995;163:492–498.

Horenstein MS, Pettersen M, Walters HL. Mitral stenosis, acquired. Last update July 2006. e medicine: Instant Access to the Minds of Medicine. Available at: http://www.emedicine.com/ped/topic2868.htm. Accessed July 12, 2006.

Huether SE, McCance KL. Understanding pathophysiology. 3rd ed. St. Louis: Mosby, 2004:639–727.

Lisse JR, Oberto-Medena M. Raynaud phenomenon. Last update April 2006. e medicine: Instant Access to the Minds of Medicine. Available at: http://www.emedicine.com/med/topic1993.htm. Accessed July 12, 2006.

March of Dimes (MOD). Birth defects and genetics: congenital heart defects. March of Dimes. Available at: *http://wwwmarchofdimes.com/printableArticles/4439_1212.asp.* Accessed July 5, 2006.

Nassisi D. Stroke, hemorrhagic. Last update November 2005. e medicine: Instant Access to the Minds of Medicine. Available at: *http://www.emedicine.com/emerg/topic557.htm.* Accessed June 24, 2006.

Orford JL, Selwyn AP. Atherosclerosis. Last update November 2005. e medicine: Instant Access to the Minds of Medicine. Available at: http://www.emedicine.com/med/topic182.htm. Accessed June 24, 2006.

Parrillo SJ, Parrillo CV. Rheumatic fever. Last update May 2006. e medicine: Instant Access to the Minds of Medicine. Available at: http://www.emedicine.com/emerg/topic509.htm. Accessed July 12, 2006.

Pearce W, Peterson BG. Abdominal aortic aneurysm. Last update May 2005. e medicine: Instant Access to the Minds of Medicine. Available at: http://www.emedicine.com/med/topic3443.htm. Accessed June 24, 2006.

Pickett FA, Gurenlian JR. The medical history: clinical implications and emergency prevention in dental settings. Baltimore: Lippincott Williams & Wilkins, 2005.

Plewa MC, Worthington R. Mitral valve prolapse. Last update June 2006. e medicine: Instant Access to the Minds of Medicine. Available at: http://www.emedicine.com/emerg/topic316.htm . Accessed July 10, 2006.

Porth CM. Essentials of pathophysiology: concepts of altered health states. Philadelphia: Lippincott Williams & Wilkins, 2004:231–338.

Rose LF, Mealey B, Minsk L, Cohen DW. Oral care for patients with cardiovascular disease and stroke. JADA 2002;133:375, 385, 395, 405, 415, 425, 435, 445.

Rubin E, Gorstein F, Rubin R, et al. Rubin's pathology: clinicopathologic foundations of medicine. 4th ed. Baltimore: Lippincott Williams & Wilkins, 2005:473–580.

Sharma S, Kortas C. Hypertension. Last update May 2005. e medicine: Instant Access to the Minds of Medicine. Available at: http://www.emedicine.com/med/topic1106.htm. Accessed June 13, 2006.

Singh VN, Deedwanja P. Coronary artery atherosclerosis. Last update August 2005. e medicine: Instant Access to the Minds of Medicine. Available at: http://www.emedicine.com/med/topic446.htm. Accessed June 13, 2006.

Singh VN. Congestive heart failure. Last update April 2006. e medicine: Instant Access to the Minds of Medicine. Available at: http://www.emedicine.com/radio/topic189.htm. Accessed July 12, 2006.

Stephens E. Peripheral vascular disease. Last update October 2005. e medicine: Instant Access to the Minds of Medicine. Available at: http://www.emedicine.com/emerg/topic862.htm. Accessed June 14, 2006.

Wahl MJ. Myths of dental surgery in patients receiving anticoagulant therapy. JADA 2000;131:77–81.

Wilson W, Taubert KA, Gewitz M, et al. Prevention of Infective Endocarditis. Guidelines From the American Heart Association. A Guideline From the American Heart Association Rheumatic Fever, Endocarditis, and Kawasaki Disease Committee, Council on Cardiovascular Disease in the Young, and the Council on Clinical Cardiology, Council on Cardiovascular Surgery and Anesthesia, and the Quality of Care and Outcomes Research Interdisciplinary Working Group. Circulation published April 19, 2007, doi:10.1161/CIRCULATIONAHA.106.183095 Accessed July 6, 2007.

Winlaw DS, Sholler GF, Harvey RP. Progress and challenges in the genetics of congenital heart disease. Med J Aust 2005;182(3):100–101.

Zevitz ME, Singh VN. Myocardial ischemia. Last update June 2006. e medicine: Instant Access to the Minds of Medicine. Available at: http://www.emedicine.com/med/topic1568.htm. Accessed July 12, 2006.

9

Blood Disorders

Key Terms

- **Anemia**
- **Ataxia**
- **Blastic cells**
- **Erythrocytes**
- **Erythropoiesis**
- **Glossitis**
- **Hemarthrosis**
- **Hematocrit**
- **Hematopoiesis**
- **Hematopoietic system**
- **Hematuria**
- **Hemolytic/hemolysis**
- **Hemostasis**
- **Hypercoagulation**
- **Jaundice**
- **Pernicious anemia**
- **Phlebotomy**
- **Plummer-Vinson syndrome**
- **Pluripotential stem cells**
- **Proprioceptive**

Objectives

1. Define and use the key terms listed in this chapter.
2. Briefly describe how blood cells are produced and what regulates their production.
3. Discuss how the body achieves hemostasis.
4. Describe the general oral signs and symptoms that could indicate a systemic condition such as a blood disorder.
5. State the etiology, method of transmission, and pathogenesis of the blood disorders discussed in this chapter.
6. Describe the extraoral, perioral, and intraoral characteristics of disorders involving erythrocytes, leukocytes, and the hemostatic (coagulation) process.
7. Describe the dental implications of disorders involving erythrocytes, leukocytes, and the hemostatic (coagulation) process and discuss possible dental/dental hygiene treatment modifications.
8. Identify the type of anemia that is associated with an increased risk of gastrointestinal, esophageal, and oropharyngeal cancers.
9. Identify the disorders that can cause abnormal vital signs and describe why those changes take place.
10. Differentiate between pernicious anemia and folic acid deficiency.
11. Describe what happens during a sickle cell crisis.
12. Define and differentiate the four major types of leukemia.

Chapter Outline

THE HEMATOPOIETIC SYSTEM

The **hematopoietic system** (blood cell-forming system) comprises lymph tissue, bone marrow, and circulating blood. Lymph tissues are scattered throughout the body. The thymus and bone marrow are considered to be the primary lymph organs. The spleen, lymph nodes, and other lymphoid tissues, such as the tonsils, appendix, and Peyer's patches (organized aggregates of lymphoid tissue found in the intestine) are considered secondary lymph organs. The thymus is the organ in which precursor immune system T cells mature into T cells that can recognize foreign antigens. The thymus attains its largest size about 1 year after birth. This size is maintained until just after puberty, when the gland starts to shrink. At this time the peripheral T cells have become established in lymph tissues throughout the body, and although the thymus continues to function, the gland begins to shrink in size. By the age of 50, the thymus consists largely of fatty tissue and may be only 15% of the size that it once was.

Red and white blood cells are produced during a process known as **hematopoiesis**, which takes place in the red bone marrow. From birth until about the age of 4 years, all of the skeletal bones are packed with red marrow. After the age of 4, the growing size of the bones can accommodate far more red marrow than is necessary for replenishing the body's red and white blood cells; therefore, some of the red marrow is replaced with fatty tissues called yellow marrow. By adulthood, the red marrow is only found in the vertebrae, ribs, sternum, and ilia (hip bones). Yellow marrow can be reactivated to produce red and white blood cells if necessary. Reactivation of yellow marrow may occur in disease states in which there is an increased need for red or white blood cells, such as anemia or leukemia, both of which are discussed below in this chapter.

The spleen is composed of two functional areas and has two main functions. The red pulp is vascular and is responsible for trapping, destroying, and removing injured or senescent (old) red blood cells. The white pulp is packed with T cells, B cells, macrophages, and dendritic cells that filter and remove antigens from the body. Lymph nodes and other lymphoid tissues are found throughout the body. Their functions are to remove foreign matter from the lymph before it enters the lymph vessels and to act as centers for the proliferation of immune system cells. See Chapter 4 for information on the function of the immune system.

The cells of the hematopoietic system are the red and white blood cells and the interstitial space is the plasma. Blood distributes oxygen, nutrients, salts, and hormones to the cells of the body and carries away the wastes from normal cellular metabolism. Blood also provides a line of defense against infection, toxic substances, and foreign antigens. **Erythrocytes,** or red blood cells and platelets, are made in the red bone marrow. Leukocytes, or white blood cells, are made in the red marrow and lymph tissues. Erythrocytes, leukocytes, and platelets make up 45% of the blood, with plasma making up the remaining 55%. See Figure 9.1 for an illustration of hematopoiesis.

As seen in other types of systemic disorders, the first sign of a blood disorder may present in the oral cavity. Any unexplained change in the oral health of an individual should spark the interest of the dental professional. Some of the signs that could indicate a systemic condition, including blood disorders, are as follows:

- Excessive or uncontrolled gingival bleeding
- Spontaneous gingival bleeding
- Unexplained petechiae, ecchymoses, or the tendency to bruise easily
- Pale mucosal tissues
- Glossitis and/or glossodynia (painful tongue)
- Nonhealing mucosal ulcers, recurrent fungal infections
- Exaggerated gingival response to local irritants such as dental biofilm (Wilkins, 2005)

Disorders of the hematopoietic system can be separated into three major groups: (1) diseases of erythrocytes (red blood cells), (2) diseases of leukocytes (white blood cells), and (3) diseases of platelets.

ERYTHROCYTES

Red blood cells are formed in a process called **erythropoiesis.** Approximately 1% of the body's red blood cells are replaced each day, and each normal red blood cell has a life span of about 4 months, or 120 days. Erythropoiesis is regulated by the kidney through release of the hormone erythropoietin. Cells in the kidney are able to sense when there is a low level of oxygen in the circulating blood, which stimulates the production and release of erythropoietin. Erythropoietin, in turn, stimulates the bone marrow to produce red blood cells. Red blood cell develop-

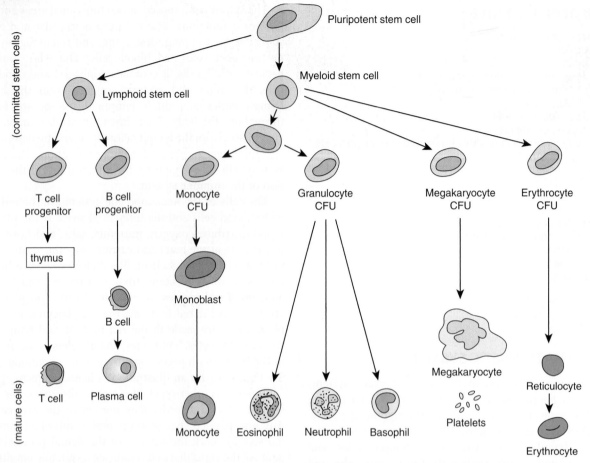

Figure 9.1. Hematopoiesis. Major developmental stages of blood cells in the process of hematopoiesis. (From Porth CM. Essentials of pathophysiology: concepts of altered health states. Philadelphia: Lippincott Williams & Wilkins, 2006.)

ment occurs in the marrow of the flat and long bones of children, but only in the flat bones of the adult. See Figure 9.1 for an illustration of the process of red blood cell development. Red blood cells form from **pluripotential stem cells** (cells that have the ability or potential to produce many different types of cells). Red blood cells are released from the bone marrow as immature cells called reticulocytes, in which the nucleus is absorbed but the endoplasmic reticulum is still present. The reticulocyte takes about 24 hours to become a mature erythrocyte (Fig. 9.2). The presence of blood disorders that cause the red marrow to create excessive numbers of red blood cells can be detected by an increased number of circulating reticulocytes in an individual's blood.

Approximately 1% of the body's red blood cells are destroyed each day. This coincides nicely with the number of red blood cells that are normally produced every day. As red cells age, they become more fragile and have a tendency to rupture when traveling through the tiny vessels of tissues and organs. The spleen will trap most of these red cells, where they will be phagocytized by large mononuclear macrophages. The body salvages and reuses most of the iron and amino acids from the destroyed cells, and the remaining waste is converted to bilirubin (a yellow substance). Bilirubin is transported to the liver and

excreted in bile. **Jaundice** occurs when the liver is unable to remove bilirubin from the blood, either because of liver dysfunction or because of a condition that causes excessive destruction of red blood cells. The yellow substance builds up in the tissues of the body, causing yellowing of the person's skin and mucous membranes (Fig. 9.3).

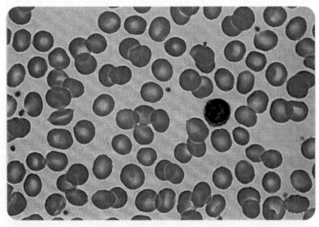

Figure 9.2. Erythrocyte. Scanning micrograph of normal red blood cells shows their characteristic concave appearance. (From Porth CM. Essentials of pathophysiology: concepts of altered health states. Philadelphia: Lippincott Williams & Wilkins, 2006.)

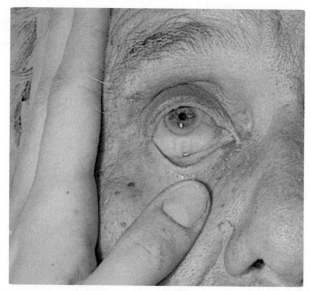

Figure 9.3. Jaundice. The yellow color of this individual's facial skin is compared with the normal skin color of another person's hand. Note also that the sclera of the eye is yellow. (From Smeltzer SC, Bare BG. Textbook of medical-surgical nursing, 9th ed. Philadelphia: Lippincott Williams & Wilkins, 2000.)

Diseases associated with red blood cells can be separated into two categories: (1) those that produce anemia and (2) those that create polycythemia.

Anemia

Anemia can be defined as a decrease in erythrocytes or in the amount, structure, or function of hemoglobin, the substance that carries oxygen to all the cells of the body. A decrease in the number of red cells can be due to excessive loss of blood, destruction of red cells, or decreased production of red cells by the bone marrow. An inadequate amount of hemoglobin is associated with insufficient dietary intake of iron and/or various genetic and acquired conditions that affect the production, function, or structure of hemoglobin.

The result of anemia, whatever its cause, is generalized tissue hypoxia that can be very minor and hardly noticeable or can cause severe dysfunction throughout the body. All forms of anemia share clinical manifestations that are associated with the body's attempt to compensate for the inadequate level of oxygen in the tissues. The severity of the manifestations depends on the severity of the anemia. The individual experiences tachycardia and palpitations because the cardiovascular system compensates for anemia by increasing the heart rate in an attempt to get more blood, thus oxygen, to the tissues. The respiratory system responds by increasing the rate and depth of respirations to bring more oxygen into the circulatory system, which can result in dyspnea (shortness of breath). The individual with anemia will experience dizziness and weakness and will fatigue easily. **Glossitis**, an inflamed sore tongue,

is a common oral finding that is associated with many forms of anemia. Other clinical manifestations are specific for the type or cause of the anemia and are discussed in the following sections.

Name: Hypochromic or iron deficiency anemia

Etiology: Iron deficiency due to insufficient dietary intake or chronic blood loss causes hypochromic, or iron deficiency, anemia. Often the deficiency is not related to a decreased intake of iron but to an increased demand for iron, such as would occur during childhood or during pregnancy when there is a high rate of physical growth. Heavy menstruation, gastrointestinal ulcers, intestinal polyps, or hemorrhoids can cause chronic blood loss that suffices to deplete the body's iron stores and cause iron deficiency anemia.

Method of Transmission: Not applicable

Epidemiology: Iron deficiency anemia is the most common form of anemia found throughout the world. In the United States, it occurs more often in women of childbearing age than in any other age group.

Pathogenesis: Iron deficiency causes the production of red blood cells that are microcytic (small) and hypochromic (pale) and that do not carry the normal amount of oxygen to the cells. This creates a state of chronic hypoxia in which the body tries to increase the level of oxygen and to compensate for a low level of oxygen at the same time. In addition to the cardiac and respiratory compensatory mechanisms, the kidney releases increased levels of erythropoietin, causing an increase in the production of red blood cells. Of course, the new red blood cells will also be deficient in iron and incapable of carrying sufficient oxygen. Thus the kidneys will continue to stimulate the marrow to produce red blood cells. Eventually more and more of the circulating red cells will be immature reticulocytes. Most of the symptoms of iron deficiency anemia begin to manifest at this point.

Extraoral Characteristics: All of the general signs of hypoxia including tachycardia, dyspnea, weakness, dizziness, and fatigue are present. The conjunctiva and exposed skin may appear pale. Long term or chronic anemia may cause the hair to be brittle and fingernails to become brittle, ridged, and concave or spoon shaped. The patient's **hematocrit** (blood test determining the percentage of whole blood that is composed of red blood cells) is lower than normal because of the small size of the erythrocytes. Table 9.1 summarizes the most common blood tests and normal values.

Perioral and Intraoral Characteristics: The mucosal membranes are pale. The growth rate of epithelial

Table 9.1   COMMON BLOOD TESTS AND NORMAL VALUES

Name of Test	Explanation	Normal Range of Values
Hematocrit	Measures the red cell volume as a percentage of total blood volume	Male 42–52 % Female 37–47%
Red blood cell count	Measures the total number of red blood cells/mm^3 of whole blood	Male 4.6–6.2 million/mm^3 Female 4.2–5.4 million/mm^3
Hemoglobin	Measures the total amount of hemoglobin in the blood, which reflects the number of erythrocytes	Male 13.0–18.0 g/dL Female 12.0–16.0 g/dL
Reticulocytes	Measures the total number of reticulocytes in the peripheral blood	25,000–75,000/mm^3 0.5%–1.5% of erythrocytes
Leukocytes, total	Combined total of all types of white blood cells	4,500–11,000/mm^3
Neutrophils	Differential count, percentage of total	60–75%
Lymphocytes	Differential count, percentage of total	25–33%
Monocytes	Differential count, percentage of total	3–7%
Eosinophils	Differential count, percentage of total	1–3%
Basophils	Differential count, percentage of total	0–1%
Iron		75–175 µg/dL

dL, deciliter; mm^3, cubic millimeter; µg, microgram.

cells diminishes because of the generalized hypoxia. This results in the atrophy of oral soft tissues, causing glossitis (Fig. 9.4), angular cheilitis, and a tendency to form ulcers and other mucosal lesions. The patient may report burning sensations in the tongue and oral mucous membranes. Severe cases may present with difficulty swallowing, or dysphagia, due to the formation of a web of mucous and inflammatory cells in the oropharynx.

Distinguishing Characteristics: Glossitis, angular cheilitis, pale mucous membranes, and burning sensa-

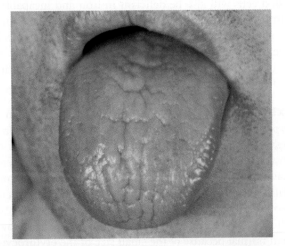

Figure 9.4. Glossitis. Glossitis is a common oral finding in most types of anemia. Atrophy of the dorsal surface and loss of papillae produces a smooth, red and often sore tongue. (Courtesy of Dr. RA Cawson. From Cawson RA. Oral pathology 1st ed. London, UK: Gower Medical Publishing, 1987.)

tions in the tongue or other mucosal tissues might alert the dental professional to a possible systemic disorder.

Significant Microscopic Features: The red cells in hypochromic anemia are microcytic and pale as seen in Figure 9.5.

Dental Implications: The patient who is anemic may exhibit abnormal pulse and respiration rates when vital signs are obtained prior to dental treatment. Review of the medical history may give some indication of the cause of symptoms associated with blood disorders. For example, the patient who is undergoing treatment for bleeding ulcers will have had chronic blood loss that could present as iron deficiency anemia. Patients that exhibit signs of anemia should be referred to their physician for a definitive diagnosis. Patients who are anemic may become very fatigued during dental treatment and may not be able to withstand long dental appointments. Individuals with untreated chronic iron deficiency anemia who exhibit dysphagia may have **Plummer-Vinson syndrome** (discussed below), which is associated with atrophy of the gastric mucosa and an increased risk of developing esophageal and oropharyngeal cancer.

Differential Diagnosis: Since types of anemias share some common characteristics, all of the different forms of this condition need to be ruled out. In addition, the following conditions need to be investigated and ruled out:

1. Burning mouth syndrome, Chapter 10
2. Xerostomia associated with many different conditions
3. Oral candidiasis, Chapters 13 and 14

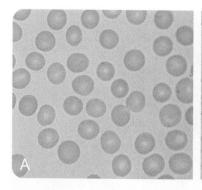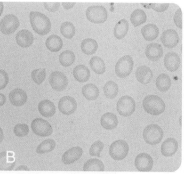

Figure 9.5. Hypochromic (iron deficiency) anemia. **A.** Normal erythrocytes with proper color, shape, and size. **B.** Microcytic-hypochromic (small, pale) erythrocytes in a patient with iron deficiency anemia. (From Willis MC. Medical terminology: a programmed learning approach to the language of health care. Baltimore: Lippincott Williams & Wilkins, 2002.)

Treatment and Prognosis: Treatment for iron deficiency anemia focuses on providing adequate dietary iron and/or determining the source of chronic blood loss and eliminating it. Symptoms associated with iron deficiency anemia will begin to dissipate after about 1 to 2 weeks of oral iron supplementation and/or treatment or correction of disorders that cause chronic blood loss. However, supplementation is usually continued for 6 to 12 months. Untreated chronic iron deficiency anemia is associated with progressive worsening of cardiac dysfunction and increased potential for heart valve problems and congestive heart failure.

PLUMMER VINSON SYNDROME

The characteristic findings of Plummer-Vinson syndrome are iron deficiency anemia and dysphagia, due to the presence of thin mucous membrane webs located in the upper esophagus. The esophageal webs partially obstruct the esophagus, causing difficult swallowing. At present, this is a rare condition because of the improvement in nutritional status and decrease in iron deficiency in the world's population. Plummer-Vinson syndrome is notable because it is associated with an increased risk of esophageal and oropharyngeal squamous cell carcinoma. Other manifestations indicating iron deficiency anemia may also be present, including pale mucous membranes, glossitis, angular cheilitis, and nail abnormalities (Novacek, 2005).

Name: Thalassemia

Etiology: Thalassemia is caused by a genetically determined defect in the production of the hemoglobin molecule. There are several forms of hemoglobin, and each is comprised of several different types of polypeptide chains. Hemoglobin A, the most common adult hemoglobin, is composed of 2 alpha (α)-polypeptide chains and 2 beta (β)-polypeptide chains. Figure 9.6 illustrates the structure of the hemoglobin A molecule. Other forms of hemoglobin are made up of these and other polypeptide chains. The two main types of this disorder are α thalassemia, which is associated with a defect in the α chain, and β thalassemia, which is associated with a defect in the β chain.

There are many other types and subtypes in addition to the two main forms.

Method of Transmission: The thalassemias are caused by mutation or deletion of genetic material on the short arm (p) of chromosome 16 (α thalassemia) and chromosome 11p (β thalassemia). The amount and location of the material that is deleted or changed is what determines the type and severity of the disorder.

Epidemiology: The different forms of thalassemia as a group are the most common inherited disorders in the world. They are found in all ethnic groups and in every geographic area. The α thalassemias are found more often in Southeast Asia, India, the Middle East, and Africa, and the β thalassemias are found more often in the Mediterranean countries of Greece, Italy, and Spain. The most severe forms of thalassemia are not common in the United States; however, the incidence of the types of thalassemia common in Asian populations is increasing rapidly in California and other West Coast states because of high numbers of Asian immigrants (Yaish, December 2005).

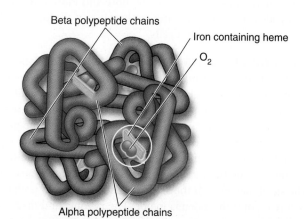

Figure 9.6. Hemoglobin A molecule. Each polypeptide chain is attached to a heme unit that contains an atom of iron. Each atom of iron can carry one molecule of oxygen; therefore, each molecule of hemoglobin can carry four molecules of oxygen (O_2) to the tissues of the body. (From McArdle WD, Katch FI, Katch VL. Essentials of exercise physiology. 2nd ed. Baltimore: Lippincott Williams and Wilkins, 2000.)

Pathogenesis: The α thalassemia defects in the α chain produce hemoglobin that has such a high affinity for oxygen that it will not release it to the cells, thereby causing severe hypoxia. In β thalassemia, defective production of the β chain causes an inadequate production of hemoglobin and leads to an imbalance between the α chains and the β chains that interferes with the normal maturation of the red cell and contributes to its early destruction.

Extraoral Characteristics: Two pairs of genes are associated with α thalassemia, and the clinical manifestations vary with the number of genes that are affected. The most severe manifestation, α thalassemia major, is incompatible with life and occurs when all four genes associated with the production of the α chain of hemoglobin are affected. The deletion of one (silent carrier α thalassemia), two (α thalassemia trait), or even three (Hb H disease) of the associated genes results in a full range of symptoms from none to mild or moderate signs of anemia, respectively.

β thalassemia occurs in three clinical forms: β thalassemia minor, β thalassemia intermedia, and β thalassemia major. Most individuals with the minor form of the disorder do not have symptoms of anemia unless they have a contributing factor, such as inadequate dietary intake of iron or chronic blood loss due to an ulcer, for example. In these instances, the person with β thalassemia minor would be less able to compensate for these factors and would develop signs and symptoms of anemia sooner than someone without the disorder. Individuals with β thalassemia intermedia have mild-to-moderate signs of anemia, and individuals with β thalassemia major have severe anemia that must be treated with transfusions. Those affected by β thalassemia major also exhibit bony malformations and stunted growth due to the expansion of the bone marrow as it tries to create more and more red cells. They also present with jaundice because of the increased destruction of red blood cells.

Perioral and Intraoral Characteristics: Patients with β thalassemia minor and intermedia and the lesser forms of α thalassemia may exhibit no oral abnormalities other than possible pallor of the oral soft tissues. β thalassemia major may cause changes in the trabecular pattern of the oral and cranial bones. The jaw bones may appear more radiolucent and have a honeycomb trabecular pattern, while the radiologic appearance of the surface of the skull may exhibit the "hair-on-end" effect that is characteristic of β thalassemia major. The zygoma and maxilla will be more prominent (Fig. 9.7), and there may be abnormal spacing and flaring of the maxillary incisors. The laminar dura may be thin or absent in some areas. Bossing (protuberance) of the frontal bone is likely.

Distinguishing Characteristics: The craniofacial abnormalities seen in β thalassemia major along with ap-

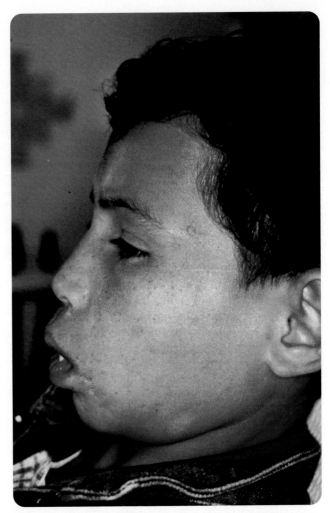

Figure 9.7. β thalassemia major. A patient with β thalassemia major demonstrates the characteristic facial appearance of a prominent maxilla with flaring of the anterior teeth. (Courtesy of Dr. Faiez N. Hattab.)

propriate laboratory test results distinguish this from other forms of this disorder and from other anemias.

Significant Microscopic Features: The red cells produced in thalassemia are microcytic and hypochromic.

Dental Implications: Individuals with thalassemia who have had their spleens removed because of severe enlargement need to be evaluated for prophylactic antibiotics prior to dental/dental hygiene care. In addition, these individuals may be on anticoagulant therapy, and their clotting status should be determined prior to therapy. Annual orthodontic evaluations should be done during childhood because of the tendency for occlusion problems associated with an increased overjet, spacing of maxillary teeth, and delayed eruption of primary and permanent teeth (Hazza'a and Al-Jamal, 2006).

Differential Diagnosis: Not applicable

Treatment and Prognosis: There is no definitive treatment for the thalassemias because of the genetic etiology; however, genetic engineering may hold some promise for the future. Individuals with minor forms of thalassemia usually require little, if any, treatment. β thalassemia major requires routine transfusions to manage the symptoms of the disease. The average life expectancy for those with β thalassemia major is only about 35 years of age because of complications associated with chronic anemia such as heart failure and the chronic iron overload that is associated with frequent transfusions. Untreated individuals do not survive past age 5.

Name: Megaloblastic anemia

Etiology: Megaloblastic anemia is characterized by abnormally large erythrocytes that are the result of defective DNA and RNA synthesis. The most common causes of megaloblastic anemia are vitamin B_{12} deficiency and folic acid deficiency.

One of the major causes of vitamin B_{12} deficiency is **pernicious anemia**, an autoimmune condition that is characterized by the inability of the gastric mucosa to produce intrinsic factor (IF). Intrinsic factor is necessary for the transportation of vitamin B_{12} across the intestinal mucosa. If there is no intrinsic factor, there is no absorption of vitamin B_{12}. Vitamin B_{12} deficiency can also result from inadequate dietary intake, malabsorption syndromes (Chapter 10), alcoholism, and pancreatic disorders, and rarely, it is seen in strict vegetarians.

Folic acid deficiency is usually due to inadequate intake or an increased requirement resulting in inadequate intake of folic acid. However, it can also be due to impaired absorption associated with malabsorption syndromes (Chapter 10), impaired metabolism associated with alcoholism, or the existence of neoplastic disease, which increases the need for folic acid because of the uncontrolled growth of these cells.

Method of Transmission: The deficiency states are not transmissible. However, the inability of the stomach to produce intrinsic factor seen in pernicious anemia appears to have a genetic component.

Epidemiology: In the United States, pernicious anemia occurs in about 10 to 20 of 100,000 individuals. It usually occurs in those over the age of 60. It is more common in people of northern European descent but is found in all races (Conrad, October 4, 2006).

Children and adolescents have a higher requirement for folic acid because of the demands growth places on the body. Pregnant women also require higher levels of folic acid and thus are more apt to be deficient. The elderly are also at a higher risk of folic acid deficiency, not because of growth requirements, but because of dietary choices and socioeconomic status. Women between the ages of 20 and 40 are the most likely to be deficient in folic acid, which, of course, parallels the reproductive years (Gentili et al., May 2006).

Pathogenesis: Vitamin B_{12} and folic acid are both essential for the synthesis of DNA and RNA. Defective DNA and RNA synthesis causes delayed maturation of the nucleus, while the cytoplasm matures normally, producing the large cells seen in this type of anemia. In addition to the large size of the erythrocytes, they are more oval in shape and have a thinner-than-normal cell membrane, which increases the likelihood of rupture. Therefore, these cells have a short life span of several weeks as opposed to the norm of several months. This requires the individual to produce more red cells than normal, which results in anemia. Vitamin B_{12} is also necessary for the maintenance of the myelin sheaths of the nervous system. Without vitamin B_{12} there is a tendency for the myelin sheaths to break down, resulting in central and peripheral nervous system dysfunction.

Extraoral Characteristics: The symptoms associated with red blood cell abnormalities are the same for both vitamin B_{12} and folic acid deficiency. The generic symptoms of anemia are present, including fatigue, dyspnea, and tachycardia. Darker-skinned individuals may present with blotchy skin pigmentation, and lighter-skinned individuals may have a lemon yellow, jaundiced appearance. In addition, chronic vitamin B_{12} deficiency will cause neurologic symptoms such as paresthesia of the hands and feet, loss of **proprioceptive** ability (the ability of a person to be aware of the position of their body), and **ataxia** (jerky uncoordinated movements). Neural tube birth defects have been linked to folic acid deficiency. Recent studies have shown that 50% and more of neural tube defects, such as spina bifida, may be prevented by an adequate dietary intake of folic acid by the mother prior to, and during, pregnancy (Blom et al., 2006).

Perioral and Intraoral Characteristics: Oral mucous membranes may be pale and ulcerated, with the tongue appearing smooth, "beefy red," and sore, due to atrophy of the papillae. Along with neural tube defects, there is evidence to support a link between folic acid deficiency and the development of cleft lip and/or palate.

Distinguishing Characteristics: Vitamin B_{12} deficiency can be differentiated from folic acid deficiency in severe cases because of the additional manifestation of neurologic symptoms; otherwise, there is no difference between the two entities.

Significant Microscopic Features: Megaloblastic erythrocytes are abnormally shaped but have normal hemoglobin concentrations (Fig. 9.8).

Dental Implications: As in iron deficiency anemia, vital signs may be abnormal, and the patient may fatigue easily. These patients should be referred to their physician for evaluation.

Differential Diagnosis: Any of the following could cause similar symptoms and need to be ruled out.

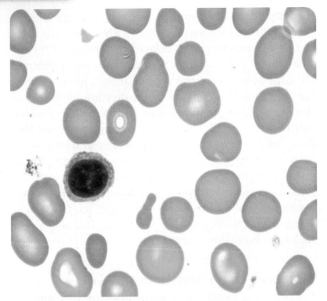

Figure 9.8. Megaloblastic anemia. In this smear of blood from a patient with folic acid deficiency, the erythrocytes are large and often oval as compared with normal erythrocytes as shown in Figure 9.5A. (From Anderson SC. Anderson's atlas of hematology. Wolters Kluwer Health/Lippincott Williams & Wilkins, 2003.)

1. Iron deficiency anemia, Chapter 9
2. Burning mouth syndrome, Chapter 10
3. Oral candidiasis, Chapter 14
4. Xerostomia associated with various disorders.

Treatment and Prognosis: Treatment for folic acid deficiency anemia focuses on replacing folic acid in the individual's diet. The prognosis for treated individuals is excellent because dietary folic acid replacements rapidly eliminate the symptoms of this disorder.

Vitamin B_{12} deficiency is slightly more complex to treat because the reason for the deficiency must first be determined. If the deficiency is due to an inadequate intake of vitamin B_{12} in the diet, the treatment is to increase the intake until normal blood levels are achieved. If the cause of the deficiency is unknown, it must be determined before the deficiency can be treated effectively. Pernicious anemia is treated with lifelong administration of intramuscular injections of vitamin B_{12}, since dietary B_{12} cannot pass across the gastric mucosa. The prognosis is excellent when individuals who have vitamin B_{12} deficiency are treated adequately. However, if left untreated, neurologic symptoms associated with the deficiency may become permanent.

Name: Sickle cell anemia

Etiology: Sickle cell anemia is one disease in a group of inherited disorders that result in the creation of abnormal hemoglobin. The abnormality is caused by the substitution of the amino acid valine for glutamic acid at the sixth position in the hemoglobin β chain. Sickle cell anemia is considered a **hemolytic** anemia because the anemia is caused by the destruction or lysis of the abnormal red blood cells.

Method of Transmission: Sickle cell anemia follows an autosomal recessive inheritance pattern. Heterozygous individuals (with one normal and one defective gene) are said to have sickle cell trait, while those who are homozygous (with two defective recessive genes) are considered to have sickle cell anemia. The genetic abnormality is found on the short arm of chromosome 11 and involves the same genetic material that is associated with β thalassemia.

Epidemiology: Sickle cell anemia occurs in about 0.8% of African-American newborns. Approximately 8% of African Americans carry the sickle cell trait. Sickle cell anemia is also seen in Mediterranean, Middle Eastern, and Indian population groups. Males and females are equally affected (Taher and Kazzi, January 5, 2005).

Pathogenesis: The hemoglobin that forms as a result of the genetic mutation is called hemoglobin S, or Hb S. Hb S reacts to low levels of oxygen or dehydration by combining with adjacent Hb S molecules and forming a larger solidified mass, which causes the erythrocyte to stretch into the long sickle shape that is characteristic of red blood cells in this disease (Fig. 9.9). These abnormally shaped cells tend to get caught in the microvasculature or capillaries because they are not as flexible as the normal red blood cells, which are able to deform and squeeze through tight areas. As more and more cells are trapped in an area, they form aggregates or clots within the microvasculature, causing ischemia or infarcts in the areas

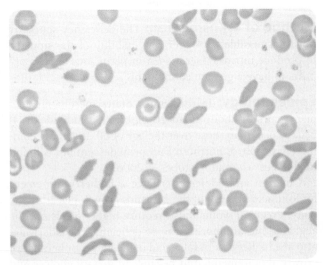

Figure 9.9. Sickle cell anemia. Note the sickled shape of some of the cells in this blood smear. Red blood cells can become permanently sickled after repeated events. (From McKenzie SB, Clare N, Burns C, et al. Textbook of hematology, 2nd ed. Baltimore: Williams & Wilkins, 1996.)

distal to them. These thrombi can form in any tissue or organ, causing severe pain and possible necrosis of the tissues.

Sickle cell crises are episodic exacerbations brought on by cold, stress, physical exertion, dehydration, acidosis, infectious agents, and above all hypoxia or a low level of oxygen. During a crisis there is sickling of many red blood cells, which occlude the microvasculature in many areas, such as the chest, abdomen, and bones, causing extreme pain.

Extraoral Characteristics: Individuals with sickle cell anemia exhibit all of the symptoms of chronic severe anemia. Jaundice may also be present, since this is a hemolytic condition. Sickle cell anemia causes damage in almost every organ in the body. See Table 9.2 for a description of the most common complications related to this disease.

Perioral and Intraoral Characteristics: There are no specific oral manifestations of the disease other than possible bone pattern changes noted in radiographs. "Hair-on-end" spicules may be seen on the surface of the skull, and a "step-ladder" trabecular pattern may be observed between adjacent posterior teeth (Fig. 9.10).

Distinguishing Characteristics: Not applicable

Dental Implications: Dental care focuses on preventing any dental infections that might trigger a crisis.

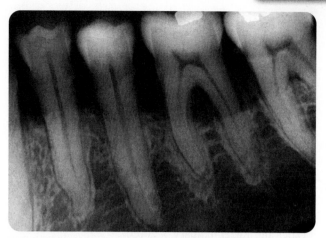

Figure 9.10. Sickle cell anemia. Periapical radiograph showing widely spaced, "step ladder" trabecular pattern. (Courtesy of Dr. Mel Mupparapu.)

Education is extremely important for the individual or family and should be the anchor for a consistent oral care provider relationship with the patient. Short appointments, stress reduction, and the use of local anesthetics with little or no vasoconstrictors should be considered when treating these patients. Poor wound healing can be expected because of the severe chronic anemia. Thus, unnecessary oral trauma during treatment should be avoided. Supplemental oxygen might be used to control the blood oxygen level and avoid the hypoxia that could trigger a crisis.

Table 9.2   COMPLICATIONS OF SICKLE CELL ANEMIA

Organ	Disorder	Causes
Heart	Enlarged heart	Increased work necessary in any chronic anemia
	Congestive heart failure	Due to constant cardiac overload
	Coronary artery obstructions	Thrombus formation from aggregated or clotted sickled cells
Lungs	Acute chest syndrome	Pneumonia associated with lung infarcts
Spleen	Enlarged spleen	Due to the removal of excessive numbers of sickled cells from the circulation
	Fibrosis of the spleen	Chronic damage due to slow blood flow
Brain	Transient ischemic attacks	Thrombus formation from aggregated or clotted sickled cells
	Stroke	Thrombus formation from aggregated or clotted sickled cells
	Hemorrhage	Thrombus formation from aggregated or clotted sickled cells
Kidney	Renal infarcts	Thrombus formation from aggregated or clotted sickled cells
Gall bladder	Gallstones	High levels of bilirubin
	Cholecystitis	Inflammation of the gall bladder due to gallstones
Skin	Ulcers	Obstruction of the cutaneous capillaries resulting in ischemia and necrosis of the tissues
Bones	Aseptic necrosis, especially of the femoral head	Thrombus formation from aggregated or clotted sickled cells
	Osteomyelitis	Infection of the bones in areas of ischemia
Eyes	Retinal hemorrhage	Thrombus formation from aggregated or clotted sickled cells
	Retinal detachment	Thrombus formation from aggregated or clotted sickled cells
	Blindness	Thrombus formation from aggregated or clotted sickled cells

Differential Diagnosis: Not applicable

Treatment and Prognosis: There is no definitive
treatment for sickle cell anemia because it is an inherited
disorder; however, there are ways to manage the disease.
Treatment includes pain control, maintaining adequate
hydration and oxygenation, and managing the complications of the disease. Affected individuals need to avoid situations that expose them to cold, stress, physical exertion,
dehydration, acidosis, and infectious agents. Transfusions
may be necessary in cases of severe disease or crisis.

Fifty percent of individuals with sickle cell anemia succumb to the disease and its complications by the age of 20,
and few of those who survive beyond that age reach age 50
(Taher and Kazzi, January 5, 2005).

Individuals with sickle cell trait very rarely suffer any
symptoms of the disease and then only under conditions
of extreme hypoxia or dehydration. These individuals
have a normal life expectancy. It is well known that individuals with sickle cell trait are less susceptible to malaria
than individuals who do not carry the trait. This can be
explained by the fact that when the malaria organism enters a red blood cell, it actually triggers the cell to become
sickled. The sickled cell is then trapped in the spleen and
destroyed, along with the malaria organism living within
it, making it unable to cause malaria.

ANEMIA ASSOCIATED WITH CHRONIC DISEASES OR DISORDERS

Anemia is often seen as a complication of other conditions.
Treatment of these conditions may eliminate the anemia; if
not, supportive measures to increase the production of red
cells is indicated to manage the disorder. Refer to Table 9.3
for a listing of conditions that may present with anemia as a
comorbid (coexisting but unrelated) condition.

APLASTIC ANEMIA

Aplastic anemia occurs when the bone marrow fails to
produce any of the three types of blood cells. The underlying cause is destruction or injury to the pluripotential
stem cells from which all cellular elements of the blood
originate. Two thirds of all cases are idiopathic; the other
one third can be linked to various chemical and environmental agents (See Box 9.1), and to a rare inherited form
of the disorder.

Whatever the cause, the bone marrow stops, or drastically reduces, production of all of the cellular components
of blood. As the disease progresses, the bone marrow is replaced with fatty tissue. The general symptoms of anemia
are accompanied by increased bleeding tendencies, due to
decreased platelet levels, and an increased chance of infection, due to the decreased white blood cell level. Severe
periodontal and gingival infections may be present, along
with severe and/or spontaneous gingival bleeding. Oral
mucosal tissues may exhibit multiple petechiae and ecchymoses due to bleeding within the oral epithelium.
Epistaxis is also common.

Treatment focuses on identifying and removing the
cause of the anemia when possible. Otherwise, therapy includes bone marrow transplantation and immunosuppressive therapy for those who are not candidates for bone
marrow transplant. Untreated aplastic anemia is fatal.

Polycythemia

Polycythemia is the opposite of anemia. Polycythemia
refers to an excess of red blood cells in relationship to
plasma or a hematocrit over 55%. The increase in volume
of blood cells causes an increase in the viscosity of the
blood, which can impair blood flow to the extremities and
increase the tendency to form thrombi. Polycythemia can

Table 9.3	CHRONIC CONDITIONS THAT MAY PRESENT WITH A SECONDARY ANEMIA	
Primary Condition	**Type of Anemia**	**Cause**
Cancer	Iron deficiency	Rapidly reproducing neoplastic cells compete for the available iron
Chronic inflammatory diseases (rheumatoid arthritis, systemic lupus)	Iron deficiency	Inflammatory mediators are believed to interfere with the metabolism of iron
Renal disease	Low RBC count	Decreased release of erythropoietin by the kidneys
Hypertension	Hemolytic	Mechanical destruction of the cells due to the high pressure under which they are moved through the vessels
Prosthetic heart valves	Hemolytic	Mechanical destruction as they move through the replaced valve
Turbulent blood flow	Hemolytic	Mechanical destruction caused by trauma to the red cells as they move through areas of turbulent blood flow

Box 9.1	ETIOLOGIC AGENTS ASSOCIATED WITH APLASTIC ANEMIA
Chemicals/Drugs	Chloramphenicol
	Phenylbutazone
	Gold
	Antineoplastic chemotherapeutic agents
	Benzene
Environment	Ionizing radiation
Microbes	Hepatitis viruses
	Epstein-Barr
	Parvovirus
	HIV
	Mycobacterium
Conditions	Graft-versus-host disease associated with transfusions
	Pregnancy
	Malignancies

be further defined by the following categories: relative, primary, and secondary.

Relative polycythemia occurs when a decrease in plasma fluid is the cause of the increased ratio of red blood cells to plasma. The most common cause of relative polycythemia is dehydration, resulting from inadequate water intake or excessive output, as occurs in diarrhea or the use of diuretics. Treatment for relative polycythemia focuses on replacing the fluid volume, determining the cause of the dehydration, and treating the underlying problem.

Primary polycythemia, or polycythemia vera, occurs when there is an increase in all types of formed blood products, caused by a proliferative neoplastic disease. This rare disorder usually occurs between 55 and 80 years of age. The clinical manifestations are due to the increase in blood volume associated with this disease and include intense reddening of the skin and mucous membranes, increased blood pressure, headaches, visual disturbances, Raynaud's phenomenon, intense pruritus, and **hypercoagulation** (overproduction of clots). Complications from this disorder include thrombus and embolus formation and the resultant infarcts and hemorrhage that they produce. Polycythemia vera is treated with regular **phlebotomies** (blood letting) to decrease the absolute amount of circulating blood. Other treatments include radioactive destruction of some of the bone marrow and myelosuppressive drug therapy, which decrease the production of cells within the bone marrow. Fifty percent of untreated individuals will succumb to the disorder within 18 months of the onset of symptoms (Huether, 2004). Remission of the disease and prevention of the complications have increased the survival time of those affected to about 10 to 15 years after the onset of symptoms.

Secondary polycythemia, sometimes called erythrocytosis, refers to a condition in which only the red cells are increased. Secondary polycythemia occurs in response to chronic tissue hypoxia due to pulmonary disorders, cardiovascular disorders, smoking, living at high altitudes where ambient oxygen levels are low, and sports that require constant strenuous activity, such as marathon running. Tissue hypoxia stimulates the kidney to release erythropoietin, which in turn stimulates the bone marrow to produce more red cells. When there are enough red cells to eliminate the tissue hypoxia, release of erythropoietin will cease and so will production of red cells.

WHITE BLOOD CELLS

Like the other cellular components of blood, white blood cells or leukocytes are formed within the bone marrow from the same pluripotential stem cells that form erythrocytes. Differentiation results in the formation of a lymphoid stem cell that develops into lymphocytes and a myeloid stem cell that develops into monocytes, granulocytes, platelets, and erythrocytes. Figure 3.5 in Chapter 3 illustrates the major types of white blood cells. The following sections focus on disorders of the granulocytes, monocytes, and lymphocytes. See Figure 9.1 for an illustration of hematopoiesis.

Name: Neutropenia or agranulocytosis

Etiology: Neutropenia is defined as a low neutrophil count, less than 1500 cells per microliter (μL) of blood (Porth, 2004). Agranulocytosis usually refers to severe neutropenia with neutrophil counts less than 200 cells/μL of blood. For the purpose of this discussion, all inadequate neutrophil levels are called neutropenia. The most

---

APPLICATION

A simple experiment can illustrate the phenomenon that occurs at high altitudes. The next time you take a trip from sea level to a higher altitude, be aware of the length of time it takes you to become accustomed to the high altitude and lower oxygen level. The experimental aspect begins when you return home or at least to a much lower altitude and try to jog a few miles. You will find that you have more energy and stamina than you ever thought possible. In fact, you will probably be motivated to attempt it again the next day. However, it is very likely that your next day's experience will not be anywhere near as satisfying as the previous day's because the effects of erythrocytosis have already dissipated. This occurs because of the normal daily destruction of red cells and the fact that tissue hypoxia is not present to stimulate the production of more red cells.

common cause of neutropenia is either an idiosyncratic or adverse reaction to a drug. Other causes include inherited syndromes, overwhelming viral or bacterial infections, autoimmune destruction of the neutrophils, bone marrow neoplasms, or anemia. Transient neutropenia is an expected side effect of almost all of the chemotherapeutic agents used to treat cancer.

Method of Transmission: Not applicable

Epidemiology: The exact frequency of neutropenia is unknown. It occurs more frequently in women than in men, and it occurs in all age groups (Distenfeld, January 2006).

Pathogenesis: The absolute number of circulating neutrophils is decreased in this disorder because of decreased production, production of defective cells, increased destruction, or removal of the cells from the circulation. The major effect of this condition is an increased susceptibility to infections. Individuals are usually asymptomatic until the neutrophil count approaches about 500 cells/μL. One specific form of inherited neutropenia is associated with drops in neutrophil numbers that occur on a regular basis of every 21 to 30 days and last for about 3 to 6 days (Porth, 2004). This type of disorder is appropriately called cyclic neutropenia. Cyclic neutropenia is inherited as an autosomal dominant disorder.

Extraoral Characteristics: Individuals with neutropenia present with fatigue, fever, malaise, and extreme weakness. Vital signs may show a rapid pulse, increased respirations, and hypotension due to septic shock (a condition that causes dilation of the peripheral blood vessels). They may have obvious signs of skin infections, but without the purulent exudate and erythema that would accompany a cellular immune response. Upper respiratory and genitourinary tract infections are very common and are usually caused by microorganisms that inhabit the body and are not normally pathogenic.

Perioral and Intraoral Characteristics: Oral infections are common and very severe. Periodontal disease in these individuals is very aggressive and painful. Chronic neutropenia and the cyclic form of neutropenia invariably lead to premature loss of the dentition. Oral ulcers are common with this condition and can impair the individual's ability to maintain adequate nutrition and hydration (Fig. 9.11).

Distinguishing Characteristics: Rapid, progressive loss of periodontal attachment indicates this disorder as well as other disorders that affect the number of white blood cells that are available to fight infection. Cyclic neutropenia is distinguished by recurrent decreases in white blood cells followed by a return to normal levels.

Dental Implications: Dental care for individuals with neutropenia focuses on preventing infections and preserv-

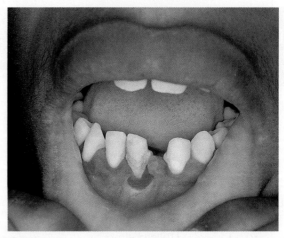

Figure 9.11. Neutropenia. Transient neutropenia caused by chemotherapy can cause gingival infections and ulceration as seen in this photo. (From Fleisher GR, Ludwig S, Baskin MN. Atlas of pediatric emergency medicine. Philadelphia: Lippincott Williams & Wilkins, 2004.)

ing the dentition. Patient education related to oral infection control and biofilm removal is very important. Preventing oral infections is not only crucial in preserving the dentition, but it plays a key role in decreasing the chance of a systemic infection as well. Appropriate medical consultation and laboratory tests should be obtained, since dental treatment should not be performed when neutrophil levels are below 1000 cells/μL (Pickett, 2005).

Differential Diagnosis: Any disorder that presents with severe periodontal infections needs to be ruled out, including the following:

1. Papillon-Lefèvre syndrome, Chapter 6
2. Leukemia, Chapter 9
3. Diabetes associated periodontal disease, Chapter 7

Treatment and Prognosis: Treatment focuses on using antibiotics to prevent infections and boosting the production of neutrophils by administering drugs that contain *colony-stimulating factor*. This factor stimulates the precursor cells in the bone marrow to produce more neutrophils, thereby accelerating their maturation and releasing them into the circulation. The prognosis for neutropenia depends on the type, cause, and severity of the disorder. Untreated neutropenia usually results in death from infection. Most forms of neutropenia have an excellent prognosis once the condition is identified and the etiologic agent removed; recovery may be complete. Neutropenia caused by cancer chemotherapy is eliminated once the treatments are completed.

Lymphoma

The term "lymphoma" represents a heterogeneous group of malignancies involving the lymphocyte. Hodgkin's lymphoma, a malignancy involving an atypical form of B cell, is discussed separately from the other forms of lymphoma (non-Hodgkin's lymphomas), because of its distinctive cellular morphology and disease manifestations. Non-Hodgkin's lymphomas include neoplasms associated with B cells, T cells, and natural killer cells.

Name: Hodgkin's Lymphoma (Hodgkin Disease, Hodgkin's Disease, Hodgkin Lymphoma)

Etiology: The etiology of Hodgkin's lymphoma is unknown, but several risk factors exist. Infection with the Epstein-Barr virus, conditions that cause immunosuppression, such as infection with human immunodeficiency virus (HIV), and genetic factors have been tentatively identified by researchers (ACS, 2006). Almost 100% of Hodgkin's lymphoma cases seen in individuals infected with HIV have Epstein-Barr virus within the tumor cells (Dessain et al., July 2006). Genetic predisposition is suggested by the fact that siblings of an affected individual have a three to seven times greater risk for developing the disease during their lifetimes than those without this connection (Dessain et al., July 2006).

Method of Transmission: There is little direct evidence that Hodgkin's lymphoma is transmissible. However, its association with Epstein-Barr virus indicates a need for further research in this area. In addition, there may be a genetic predisposition to the malignancy.

Epidemiology: The American Cancer Society estimates that about 7800 new cases of Hodgkin's lymphoma will be diagnosed in 2006; of these about 3600 will occur in women and 4200 in men. About 85 to 90% of cases are seen in adults between the ages of 25 and 30 and those older than 55 years. Only 10 to 15% of cases are seen in children between the ages of 5 and 16. Hodgkin's lymphoma occurs more frequently in Caucasians than in African Americans (ACS, 2006).

Pathogenesis: Hodgkin's lymphoma is characterized by the presence of an abnormal cell within the tumors called a *Reed-Sternberg* cell. This cell is thought to result from malignant transformation of a B lymphocyte. Hodgkin's lymphoma usually starts in a single lymph node in the upper body and then spreads to the adjacent nodes. The nodes most commonly affected are the cervical, supraclavicular, axillary, inguinal, and retroperitoneal. Spread of Hodgkin's lymphoma usually progresses in a systematic manner, moving from the original node to the next in the chain. Advanced Hodgkin's lymphoma can spread to any organ of the body, but the spleen, bone marrow, lungs, digestive tract, and liver are the most common sites. As the disease progresses, the individual becomes highly susceptible to infections because of the immune system dysfunction. Eventually, organs begin to shut down due to the increasing numbers of cancer cells that block their normal function and death occurs.

Extraoral Characteristics: Asymmetric enlargement of one or more lymph nodes without reason is the first sign of this disease. The disease normally begins in the upper part of the body, specifically, the chest, neck, or under the arms. Aside from the swollen lymph nodes, other symptoms are significant weight loss, fever, extreme night sweats, pruritus (itchiness), and fatigue.

Perioral and Intraoral Characteristics: Intraoral growth of a tumor in Hodgkin's lymphoma is highly unlikely and only occurs in very advanced metastatic cases.

Distinguishing Characteristics: See Significant Microscopic Findings

Significant Microscopic Features: Presence of the Reed-Sternberg cell in biopsy specimens from affected lymph nodes is diagnostic of this disease (Fig. 9.12).

Dental Implications: The dental professional may well be the first person to detect the enlarged lymph nodes associated with this disease because the cervical and supraclavicular nodes are commonly involved. Any suspicious finding should prompt the dental professional to refer the individual for a definitive diagnosis.

Differential Diagnosis: Infectious diseases that present with lymph node enlargement, such as mononucleosis and tuberculosis should be ruled out, as well as other forms of lymphoma, discussed in the following sections.

Treatment and Prognosis: Treatment depends on the severity of the disease and the specific microscopic appearance of the malignant tissues. The most common treatment is a combination of chemotherapy and radiation therapy. Chemotherapy usually consists of a regimen combining multiple drugs administered over a specific period of time. Radiation of the involved nodes is accomplished after the completion of chemotherapy. Other

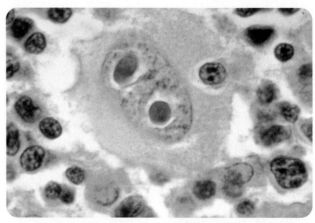

Figure 9.12. Reed-Sternberg cell. Mirror image nuclei are characteristic of the Reed-Sternberg cell which is diagnostic of Hodgkin lymphoma. (From Rubin E, Farber JL. Pathology. 3rd ed. Philadelphia: Lippincott Williams & Wilkins, 1999.)

treatments that are being tested involve bone marrow and stem cell transplants.

The American Cancer Society estimates that 1500 people will die from Hodgkin's lymphoma in 2006. Death rates have dropped more than 60% since 1970 because of improved therapies. The survival rates for patients are 1 year, 93%; 5 years, 85%; and 10 years, 80% (ACS, 2006).

Name: Non-Hodgkin's lymphoma

Non-Hodgkin's lymphoma is a generic term used to describe a group of malignant neoplasms that arise from B lymphocytes and T lymphocytes. Approximately 85% of non-Hodgkin's lymphomas are B cell neoplasms, and the remaining 15% are T cell neoplasms (ACS, 2006). See Box 9.2 for a listing of the most common forms of non-Hodgkin's lymphoma. Note that acute and chronic lymphocytic leukemia are considered forms of lymphoma. These are discussed along with myelogenous leukemia in the next section.

Etiology: The etiology of most forms of non-Hodgkin's lymphoma is unknown; however, risk factors that seem to be related to an increase in their occurrence have been identified. The presence of chromosomal mutations including translocation of genetic material plays an important role in predisposing an individual to the development of non-Hodgkin's lymphoma. Advancing age also appears to be a major risk factor, since most of these cancers oc-cur in individuals over the age of 60. Celiac diseases that are characterized by sensitivity to gluten and associated with inflammation of the mucosa of the small intestine are associated with a higher risk of lymphoma development. Previous experience with radiation or chemotherapy for another malignancy or due to accidental environmental exposure (such as a nuclear accident) increases the individual's risk for developing a lymphoma, as does chronic immunosuppression due to either drug therapy or acquired or congenital disorders. Sjögren syndrome and Hashimoto thyroiditis, both autoimmune disorders, are associated with a higher-than-normal risk of developing lymphomas. *Helicobacter pylori,* the microorganism that causes stomach ulcers, is specifically associated with mucosa-associated lymphoid tissue lymphomas that occur almost exclusively in the gastric mucosa. HIV infection is considered to carry a very high risk of non-Hodgkin's lymphoma development because it causes severe long-term immunosuppression. Recent studies have also included hepatitis B and C, human herpesvirus-8 (HHV-8), Epstein-Barr virus, and human T cell lymphoma virus (HTLV-1) as possible etiologic agents for some forms of lymphoma (ACS, 2006).

Method of Transmission: Both bacterial and viral agents have been implicated in the development of non-Hodgkin's lymphoma.

Epidemiology: The American Cancer Association estimates that 58,870 men and women will be diagnosed with non-Hodgkin's lymphoma in the United States during 2006. This form of cancer is slightly more common in men than in women, and 95% of cases develop in adults. A person's risk of developing non-Hodgkin's lymphoma during his or her lifetime is about 1 in 50 (ACS, 2006).

Pathogenesis: Whatever the cause, somewhere in the development of the lymphocyte a genetic mutation occurs that is not repaired by any of the mechanisms (such as caretaker genes) that are in place to repair this type of genetic damage (see Chapter 5). In addition, for some reason, the cell is not destroyed by the body's defenses against neoplastic growth, as it should be. This may be due to the activation of oncogenes or the inactivation of tumor suppressor genes as well as others. Uncontrolled replication of the defective cell ensues, and lymphoma develops. The organs associated with the lymphatic system are affected first, with eventual spread to any body tissue or organ.

Extraoral Characteristics: The most common clinical manifestation of the disease is superficial lymphadenopathy that is nontender and very likely fixed to the surrounding tissues. The cervical, axial, and inguinal nodes are commonly the first to be affected or noticed (Fig. 9.13). Spread can be contained within contiguous nodes or the disease can spread to noncontiguous nodes and tissues. In addition to soft tissues, the bones may be

---

Box 9.2 TYPES OF NON-HODGKIN'S LYMPHOMA

B CELL LYMPHOMA	PERCENTAGE
Diffuse large B cell lymphoma	31%
Follicular lymphoma	22%
Small cell lymphocytic lymphoma/ chronic lymphocytic leukemia	7%
Mantle cell lymphoma	6%
Mucosa-associated lymphoid tissue lymphoma	8%
Nodal marginal zone B cell lymphoma	2%
Primary mediastinal B cell lymphoma	2%
Burkitt lymphoma	2%

T CELL LYMPHOMA	
Precursor T lymphoblastic lymphoma/leukemia	2%
Peripheral T cell lymphomas	7%

affected by tumors. Systemic symptoms of fever, night sweats, and weight loss are not as common as in Hodgkin's lymphoma, and their presence usually indicates a poor prognosis.

Perioral and Intraoral Characteristics: Oral manifestations of lymphoma are uncommon but when present usually appear as a soft tissue mass in the Waldeyer's ring area, in the lymphoid tissues found at the base of the tongue, or in the major and minor salivary glands. The lesions may, or may not, be ulcerated. When bone is involved, the most common intraoral site is the hard palate (Fig. 9.14). Tumors within bone, or central tumors, may present as an ill-defined radiolucency that can progress to expansion of the bone and perforation of the cortical plate, resulting in a soft tissue swelling at the site of the tumor. These tumors can cause loss of alveolar bone, tooth mobility, swelling, pain, paresthesia, and pathologic bone fractures. Figure 9.15 illustrates a non-Hodgkin's lymphoma of the gingiva.

Lymphomas that are associated with HIV infection manifest in the oral cavity more often than those associated with other causes and account for about 3% of intraoral tumors seen in AIDS affected individuals (Regezi et al., 2003).

Significant Microscopic Features: The microscopic appearance of the tumor cells varies with each type of lymphoma.

Dental Implications: Extraoral examination for signs of lymphadenopathy should be performed for every patient when they present for their preventive appointments or for any new or emergency patient. Any patient who

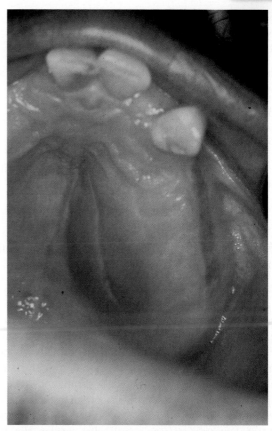

Figure 9.14. Oral non-Hodgkin's lymphoma. Posterior palatal enlargement caused by non-Hodgkin's lymphoma. (Courtesy of the United States Department of Veteran's Affairs.)

presents with indurated, nontender, fixed nodes should be referred immediately to a physician for further diagnosis. Intraoral swelling with or without associated radiolucencies should be definitively diagnosed.

Differential Diagnosis: The differential diagnosis for non-Hodgkin's lymphoma is extensive and includes such other neoplasms as

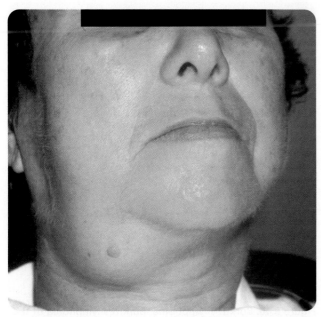

Figure 9.13. Lymphadenopathy. Enlarged submandibular lymph node caused by a non-Hodgkin's lymphoma. (Courtesy of Dr. Michael Brennan.)

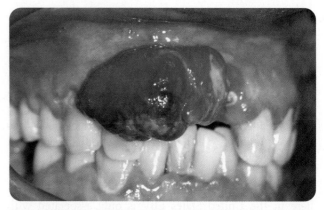

Figure 9.15. Non-Hodgkin's lymphoma. This exophytic mass is an example of a non-Hodgkin's lymphoma found in the attached gingiva. From Neville BW, Damm DD, White DK. Color Atlas of Clinical Oral Pathology; 2nd Edition. Ontario, Canada: BC Dekker Inc., 1999. (Courtesy of Brad Neville.)

1. Squamous cell carcinoma
2. Nasopharyngeal carcinoma
3. Thyroid carcinoma

Lymphadenopathy from infectious etiologies would also be included in the differential diagnosis, including

1. Bacterial (tuberculosis)
2. Viral (mononucleosis, cytomegalovirus, HIV)
3. Parasites (toxoplasmosis)

The differential diagnosis for a central presentation of lymphoma include

1. Metastatic neoplasms
2. Osteogenic sarcoma

These lesions need to be distinguished from one another by biopsy.

Treatment and Prognosis: Treatment depends on the type of non-Hodgkin's lymphoma and the stage of the disease. Lymphomas are usually very radiosensitive; therefore, radiation therapy is used aggressively in many cases. Chemotherapy is also effective and is normally given in combinations of two or more drugs taken every 2 to 4 weeks for variable lengths of time. Resistant and recurrent lymphomas may be treated with a stem cell or bone marrow transplant after high doses of chemotherapy or radiation. Additional treatments using antibodies against the lymphoma cells or monoclonal antibodies and interferon are starting to be used with some success in specific cases.

The prognosis also depends on the type of lymphoma and the stage of the disease when treatment is started. The American Cancer Society estimates that 18,840 men and women will die from non-Hodgkin's lymphoma in 2006. The overall 5-year relative survival rate for non-Hodgkin's lymphoma is about 60%, and the 10-year relative survival rate is about 49%. The relative survival rates only take into account those individuals who die from the non-Hodgkin's lymphoma and not from other related causes, such as heart disease (ACS, 2006).

BURKITT'S LYMPHOMA

Burkitt's lymphoma is a very aggressive form of non-Hodgkin's lymphoma and is thought to be the most rapidly growing cancer known. There are three forms of the disease: (1) an endemic form found in Africa, (2) a more sporadic form seen in North America and Europe, and (3) a form that is associated with immunodeficiency. Burkitt's lymphoma affects children and young adults more often than older adults, and 90% of its victims are male (ACS, 2006). In parts of Africa, Burkitt's lymphoma is associated with the Epstein-Barr virus in about 95% of cases, while here in the United States EBV is only associated with about 20% of cases (Huang, November 2005). The endemic form often manifests in the maxilla or the mandible, while the sporadic form seen in the United States presents as a mass in the abdomen, with our with-

out bone marrow involvement, or it may only affect the bone marrow (Regezi et al., 2004). Oral manifestations of the endemic form consist of rapidly expanding bone lesions that quickly deform the face (Fig. 9.16) and loosening of the affected teeth; the sporadic form does not usually manifest with oral lesions. Treatment consists of intense chemotherapy with multiple drugs. In spite of the aggressive nature of this disease, the American Cancer Society estimates that 50% or more of persons with this form of lymphoma are cured (ACS, 2006).

Burkitt's lymphoma associated with immunodeficiency disorders, specifically AIDS, is usually diagnosed at an advanced stage (Huang, November 2005). Figure 9.17 depicts Burkitt's lymphoma in the oral cavity of an HIV-positive male. The prognosis for these individuals is dismal because of their already compromised immune status and the individual's inability to withstand any type of aggressive therapy. Death normally occurs shortly after the diagnosis (Huang, November 2005).

Name: Leukemia

The term "leukemia" describes a group of malignant neoplasms involving leukocytes. Two basic classifications denote whether the disorder involves cells that are derived from a lymphoid stem cell, B and T lymphocytes, or cells that are derived from a myeloid progenitor cell, granulocytes and monocytes. (Refer to Figure 9.1 for a review of the process of hematopoiesis). Further classification identifies whether the disease is acute or chronic. There are four main types of acute and chronic leukemia, listed below:

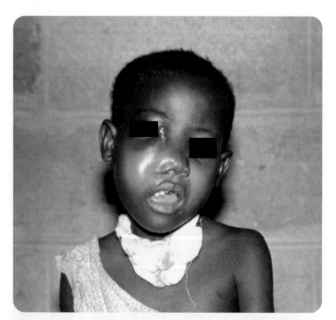

Figure 9.16. Burkitt's lymphoma. Burkitt's lymphoma of the jaw is distorting the facial features of this African child. (From Rubin E, Farber JL. Pathology. 3rd ed. Philadelphia: Lippincott Williams & Wilkins, 1999.)

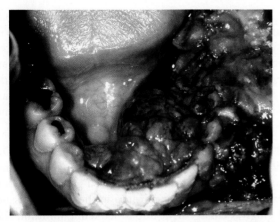

Figure 9.17. Burkitt's lymphoma. This Burkitt's lymphoma tumor was discovered in an HIV positive male patient. (Courtesy of Dr. Douglas Damm.)

- Acute lymphoblastic leukemia (ALL)
- Chronic lymphocytic leukemia (CLL)
- Acute myeloblastic leukemia (AML)
- Chronic myelogenous leukemia (CML)

Etiology: In most cases of leukemia, the cause is unknown. Some risk factors have been identified and include environmental exposure to radiation and certain chemicals, previous exposure to chemotherapeutic drugs, and some genetic syndromes. Table 9.4 provides more specific information regarding the etiology, epidemiology, and prognosis for leukemia.

Method of Transmission: Not applicable

Epidemiology: Refer to Table 9.4 for epidemiologic information related to the four types of leukemia.

Pathogenesis: The acute forms of leukemia usually present with symptoms within days to several weeks of the start of disease activity. The chronic forms exhibit a more insidious or gradual progression of the disease and are sometimes in advanced stages at the time of diagnosis.

In acute leukemia there is an overgrowth of **blastic cells** (cells that fail to mature). Chronic leukemias produce stem cells that do not respond to the body's attempts to regulate their proliferation. In both instances, extremely high numbers of the specific white cells are pro-

Table 9.4   LEUKEMIA

Type of Leukemia	Etiology	Epidemiology	Prognosis
Acute lymphoblastic leukemia (ALL)	• Mostly unknown	• Found more often in children, 66%, than in adults, 33% • Peak age 2–5 • Slightly more in males • More in Caucasians than in African Americans	• Cure rate for children 1 to 10 years of age is 80% • Survival rate for infants under 1 year of age is 30% • Adults experience a 20–30% long-term remission or cure rate
Chronic lymphocytic leukemia (CLL)	• Mostly unknown • Agent Orange (herbicide used in the Vietnam War) • High doses of radiation such as in a nuclear accident	• 50% of cases occur over the age of 70, very rare at ages under 40 • Slightly more in males • More in Caucasians than in African Americans	• Survival time varies from 1 year to 10–20 years or more depending on the course of the disease
Acute myeloblastic leukemia (AML)	• Mostly unknown • Inherited syndromes (trisomy 21, von Recklinghausen's disease, Chapter 17) • Prior chemotherapy for another malignancy • Irradiation (accidental or therapeutic) • Slightly increased risk associated with smoking	• Average age 65 • 90% in adults • Slightly more males • More in Caucasians than in African Americans	5-year survival rate for individuals under the age of 65 is 33%; over the age of 65 is 4%
Chronic myelogenous leukemia (CML)	• Mostly unknown • Radiation exposure • Slightly higher in smokers	• Average age 66 • 2% in children	• 5-year survival rate of 50–60%

duced, increasing the viscosity (thickness) of the blood and causing an infiltration or overflow of the excess white blood cells into the organs and tissues that normally contain leukocytes. In addition, the cells that are produced are malignant cells that do not function normally and therefore do not fulfill their role in protecting the body against infection.

Increased production of the affected leukocyte causes an increase in the amount of marrow associated with that leukocyte, which eventually overwhelms the rest of the bone marrow. This event causes a decrease in the production of red blood cells, platelets, and other nonaffected white blood cells. The symptoms of leukemia are associated with the disorders produced by the decrease in the numbers of these cells, specifically, anemia, neutropenia, and thrombocytopenia (low blood platelets).

Extraoral Characteristics: The initial symptoms of ALL and AML are similar. Patients normally exhibit symptoms associated with anemia (fatigue, pallor, etc.), infection (fever, night sweats), thrombocytopenia (epistaxis, petechiae, bruising), increased metabolism of the cancer cells (weight loss), bone marrow expansion (bone pain), and the infiltration of the liver, spleen, and lymph nodes by leukemic cells, causing enlargement of these organs. Leukemic infiltration of the skin can cause pruritus. Infiltration of the central nervous system is more common in ALL than in AML and can cause headache, nerve dysfunction, nausea, vomiting, and sometimes seizures. Hyperviscosity of the blood caused by leukocytosis (leukocyte levels of 100,000 cells/mm^3), can effectively plug up the microvasculature, causing infarcts and vessel rupture in the lungs, brain, and other organs.

Chronic leukemia may be present for years without being noticed and may only be discovered while performing routine blood work. Symptoms of CLL are usually not apparent at diagnosis but appear slowly as the bone marrow is gradually overtaken by the production of lymphocytes. Symptoms include those associated with anemia, neutropenia, and thrombocytopenia. Repeated infections, increasing fatigue, enlargement of the lymph nodes, increased bleeding tendencies, and bone pain signal progression of the disease. The course of CML differs from that of CLL because it progresses through three distinct phases:

1. The first, or chronic, phase is characterized by leukocytosis that is well controlled by medication and can last for 2 to 10 years or more. During this phase the symptoms associated with anemia, neutropenia, and thrombocytopenia are minor or not noticed by the patient.
2. The second, or accelerated, phase is associated with loss of medical control of the disease and is characterized by increasing numbers of leukemic cells and the appearance of more severe symptoms associated with anemia, neutropenia, and thrombocytopenia. Weight loss can be expected due to the high nutritional needs of the proliferating malignant cells.
3. The last phase is called the acute phase, or blast crisis, and is preceded by bone pain and fever. More severe symptoms are seen in this stage, and the leukemic cells tend to infiltrate the skin, bones, lymph nodes, and central nervous system. Infarcts and hemorrhage due to leukocytosis are more common in this phase. Survival after the initiation of a blast crisis is counted in months.

Perioral and Intraoral Characteristics: Oral findings in all types of leukemia include increased gingival or periodontal infections, increased gingival bleeding, unexplained petechiae or purpura in the oral soft tissues, and gingival enlargement due to leukemic infiltrate (Fig. 9.18). Gingival enlargement is seen most often in AML and CML. Many patients seek dental care prior to medical care because of the rapid decline in oral health and appearance of the tissues.

Distinguishing Characteristics: The presence of a specific genetic abnormality involving translocation of genetic material from the long arm of chromosome 9 to the long arm of chromosome 22 indicates CML. The enlarged chromosome 22 is called the *Philadelphia chromosome,* and it is present in approximately 85% of CML and about 5% of ALL cases. The presence of this chromosomal aberration is being used by researchers to develop new treatment methods that target cells with this abnormality and not normal cells, resulting in less untoward effects from treatment (ACS, 2006).

Significant Microscopic Features: Microscopic features vary according to the type of leukemia.

Dental Implications: The clinician must investigate any case of gingival or periodontal inflammation or infection that does not respond to normal interventions, especially if other systemic manifestations, such as fever, weight loss, or night sweats are present. Patients should be referred to their physician for further evaluation. Elective dental care would not be appropriate during periods when bleeding is excessive or white cell counts are low. Consultation with the oncologist to determine adequate levels of white blood cells and the International

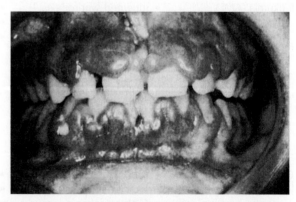

Figure 9.18. Gingival enlargement. The gingival enlargement seen in this picture is caused by leukemic infiltrate.

Normalized Ratio (INR) should precede any dental or dental hygiene care.

Differential Diagnosis: The gingival enlargement associated with leukemia could be caused by hormonal influences in puberty or pregnancy or it could be drug induced by calcium channel blockers (antihypertensives), phenytoin (antiseizure), and cyclosporine (immunosuppressive).

Treatment and Prognosis: The traditional treatment for acute leukemia of either type is aggressive chemotherapy. This may be augmented by treatment with *monoclonal antibodies.* Monoclonal antibodies are produced by engineered cells that are made in the laboratory by fusing tumor cells that grow continuously with mammalian cells that can produce antibodies. The resulting engineered cells replicate continuously and produce large amounts of antibody against the tumor cells. The antibody that is produced can be engineered to target just about any cell or portion thereof, such as a particular protein or enzyme. Several monoclonal antibodies are being used to treat the different forms of leukemia. Another type of drug, *imatinib mesylate,* or Gleevec, has been developed to target and destroy cells that contain the Philadelphia chromosome. This oral drug is being used successfully as the primary treatment for most cases of CML and some cases of ALL. Both monoclonal antibodies and *imatinib mesylate* target only abnormal cells and not the normal cells of the body, which results in fewer side effects and a better quality of life.

Bone marrow and peripheral blood stem cell transplants are an option for treating ALL, AML, and CML. Both of these procedures require that the individual's bone marrow cells be destroyed by high doses of chemotherapy, radiation, or both. After the cells are destroyed, the transplant cells are infused into the bloodstream, where they will go to the bone marrow and, one hopes, begin to produce new normal blood cells. Neither bone marrow transplants nor stem cell transplantation is indicated for the treatment of CLL.

Supportive treatment includes using antibiotics, antifungals, and antivirals to control or prevent infections. Low platelet counts might require a transfusion of platelets to control bleeding. Anemia is often treated with drugs that stimulate the production of red cells or red cell transfusions. Neutropenia caused by the disease and the treatments can be treated with drugs that increase the production of these cells. Refer to Table 9.4 for the prognoses for the different types of leukemia.

Name: Multiple myeloma

Etiology: Multiple myeloma is a B cell cancer that results in the overproduction of malignant plasma cells. Plasma cells are the cells that are responsible for producing all of the body's immunoglobulins. The most common cause of the disease is acquired genetic abnormalities involving translocation of genetic material from a number of different chromosomes to chromosome 14, which regulates the formation of most immunoglobins. The genetic abnormalities have been linked to environmental radiation, such as nuclear accidents, and with the accumulation of genetic errors that occur within our cells as we age. The deletion of pieces of chromosome 13 has been associated with a very aggressive form of the disease.

Method of Transmission: There may be a slight genetic tendency because there is a higher rate of disease within first-degree relatives (mother, father, sisters, and brothers) and because of the significantly higher rate in African Americans.

Epidemiology: The American Cancer Society estimates that 16,570 Americans (9,250 men and 7,320 women) will be diagnosed with this disease in 2006. African Americans develop this disease two times more often than Caucasians, and men are affected more often than women. The average age at diagnosis is 68 years for men and 70 years for women (Grethlein, June 2006).

Pathogenesis: The manifestations of this disease are caused by excessive production of an abnormal immunoglobin called M-protein, increased activation of osteoclasts, and the production of abnormal proteins that are excreted in the urine. The malignant cells produce excessive amounts of M-protein, which causes a decreased production of all other immunoglobulins, and results in immunosuppression. The malignant plasma cells also stimulate osteoclastic activity with resultant bone resorption. Normally the body does not eliminate protein through the kidneys. In multiple myeloma an abnormal protein called *Bence Jones protein* is eliminated through the kidney. Bence Jones protein is toxic to the kidney and accumulates in the tubules, eventually causing renal failure.

Extraoral Characteristics: The most common presenting feature of multiple myeloma is related to infiltration of the bone by the plasma cells and the activation of osteoclasts, resulting in bone resorption, pathological fractures, and bone pain. The vertebrae, ribs, skull, pelvis, and femur are most frequently affected. Localized and generalized infections, especially bacterial infections, are caused by the lack of normal immunoglobulins, excessive M-protein, and suppression of leukocyte production in affected bone marrow. Renal failure results from high calcium levels in the blood (hypercalcemia) and damage done by the Bence Jones protein. The most common causes of death are severe infection or renal failure. There are two other forms of the disease: (1) solitary plasmacytoma and (2) extramedullary plasmacytoma.

The solitary plasmacytoma is seen as a single area of bone destruction, usually in the vertebrae, ribs, or pelvis.

It is rarely seen in the oral cavity. Some 30 to 75% of these cases progress to multiple myeloma.

Plasma cell tumors that are found in soft tissues are called extramedullary plasmacytomas. Most of these tumors (80%) are found in the upper respiratory tract and the oral environment (Regezi et al., 2003). These tumors present as exophytic red masses that may or may not eventually ulcerate. Progression to multiple myeloma is rare in these individuals.

Perioral and Intraoral Characteristics: Bone lesions in the skull are common and manifest as multiple, well-defined, radiolucent areas that appear "punched out" from the surrounding bone (Fig. 9.19). Jaw lesions are seen more in the mandible than in the maxilla, and they are found more often in the posterior areas. Some of the abnormal immunoglobulins created by this disease combine to form what is called *amyloid*. Amyloid is an abnormal protein that is deposited in tissues throughout the body such as in the heart, lungs, or kidneys, where it interferes with normal functioning and causes tissue enlargement. It is very common to see amyloid accumulation in the tongue, where it results in macroglossia (Fig. 9.20). The immunosuppressive nature of this disease increases the risk that these individuals will have some form of periodontal infection.

Distinguishing Characteristics: The "punched-out" radiographic lesions are characteristic of this disease.

Significant Microscopic Features: Bone marrow samples that contain over 30% plasma cells indicate this disease.

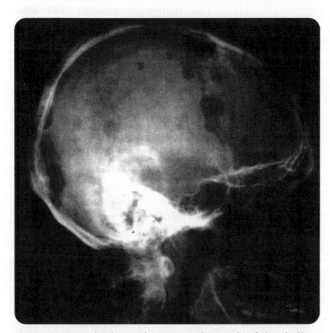

Figure 9.19. Multiple myeloma. A radiograph of the skull shows the "punched-out" radiolucent lesions that are characteristic of multiple myeloma. (From Rubin E, Farber JL. Pathology. 3rd ed. Philadelphia: Lippincott Williams & Wilkins, 1999.)

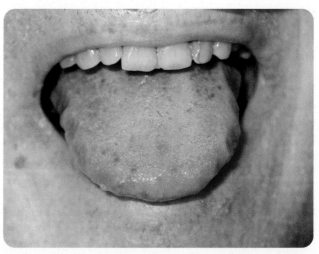

Figure 9.20. Macroglossia. This is an example of macroglossia that was caused by the deposition of amyloid proteins within the tongue. Note the scalloping from pressure on the lingual surfaces of the teeth. (From Stedman's medical dictionary for the health professions and nursing, 5th ed. Baltimore: Lippincott Williams & Wilkins, 2005.)

Dental Implications: Dental hygiene/dental care should focus on controlling infections associated with a compromised immune system. Tests to determine white cell levels and clotting times or the International Normalized Ratio (INR) should be performed if indicated.

Differential Diagnosis: The presence of only intraoral manifestations necessitates ruling out any disorder that causes well-defined radiolucent bone lesions. These include

1. Traumatic bone cyst, Chapter 20
2. Langerhans cell disease, Chapter 20
3. Metastatic cancer, Chapter 5

Macroglossia could be the result of the following:

1. Acromegaly, Chapter 7
2. Trisomy 21, Chapter 6
3. Lymphangioma, Chapter 17
4. Vascular malformation, Chapter 13
5. Neurofibroma, Chapter 17
6. Amyloid accumulation as a result of another chronic illness

Exophytic red soft tissue masses that are found in the oral cavity include

1. Pyogenic granuloma, Chapter 13
2. Peripheral giant cell granuloma, Chapter 13
3. Kaposi's sarcoma, Chapters 13 and 22
4. Squamous cell carcinoma, Chapters 5 and 12

Treatment and Prognosis: Both treatment and prognosis vary, depending on the specific type of abnormality that is present. Not all of the abnormal immunoglobulins that are produced are the same. One person may have abnormal IgG while another may have abnormal IgD; the disorder is still multiple myeloma, but the course and outcome of the disease may differ. In general, multiple myeloma is treated with chemotherapy. Combinations of different drugs have been shown to have the best results. Solitary or painful bone lesions that are not responding to chemotherapy can be treated with radiation. Because this disease causes destruction of bone, it is important to try to strengthen the bone during or directly after therapy. Drugs that are used to treat osteoporosis such as bisphosphonates that interfere with osteoclast activity are indicated to help prevent further damage and permit osteoblasts to strengthen weakened areas. Individuals with this disorder may go into remission for many years or may not be able to control the disease from the outset. The mean survival rate for treated multiple myeloma is 3 years, untreated it is 6 months (Rubin et al., 2005).

HEMOSTASIS

Hemostasis is the process by which the body prevents blood loss from injury. Platelets and circulating coagulation factors are the major participants in the maintenance of hemostasis.

Platelets are created from a cell called a megakaryocyte, which is derived from the same pluripotential stem cells from which the red and white blood cells are created. The nuclear material in the megakaryocyte undergoes division; however, the cytoplasm does not. The cell expands to hold the extra DNA, but it is unsuccessful and breaks up into small pieces called platelets (see Fig. 9.1).

There are 12 numbered coagulation factors found in the blood plasma. The numbers indicate the order in which factors were discovered, not the order in which they work. In addition, the number 6 was never used. The coagulation factors are produced by the liver. Refer to Box 9.3 for a list of the coagulation factors. Vitamin K is necessary for the production of most of the factors, and calcium (factor IV) is necessary for almost all of the reactions that take place in the cascade. Cascade systems, such as the coagulation cascade, consist of a series of inactive enzymes. Once the first enzyme (coagulation factor) in the series is activated, it initiates the next in a series of reactions in which the product of the last reaction is the initiator of the next reaction. The coagulation cascade is illustrated in Figure 9.21. The end result of the coagulation cascade is that thrombin converts fibrinogen into fibrin. Fibrin forms the substance of a blood clot. It is not important to remember the specific names of the factors, but it is important to realize that a defect at any point in the cascade or in the substances that initiate the cascade can result in malfunction of the clotting system and uncontrolled blood loss.

There are specific events that must occur in sequence to achieve hemostasis in the face of vascular injury. The initiating event causes damage to the body and bleeding.

Box 9.3 COAGULATION FACTORS

Factor I	Fibrinogen
Factor II	Prothrombin
Factor III	Tissue factor
Factor IV	Calcium
Factor V	Proaccelerin
Factor VII	Proconvertin
Factor VIII	Antihemophilic factor
Factor IX	Plasma thromboplastin
Factor X	Stuart-Prower factor
Factor XI	Plasma thromboplastin antecedent
Factor XII	Hageman factor
Factor XIII	Fibrin-stabilizing factor

The involved vessels immediately constrict to limit the loss of blood. The damaged endothelial cells release von Willebrand factor, which literally grabs the circulating platelets and causes them to adhere to the injured vessel wall. Other substances released by the platelets cause the adherence of more platelets, creating a "platelet plug." As the platelet plug is forming, the coagulation cascade is being activated, and fibrin strands are being created to reinforce the platelet plug, making it stable and insoluble (Fig. 9.22).

Hemostasis can be compromised by an insufficient number of platelets, dysfunction of the platelets, or defective coagulation factors. The end result of compromised hemostasis is either hypercoagulation (overproduction of clots) or bleeding disorders. Hypercoagulation is discussed briefly above in this chapter under "Polycythemia" and in Chapter 8 regarding thrombus formation associated with atherosclerosis. Table 9.5 lists common blood tests used to evaluate hemostasis.

Name: Bleeding disorders

Etiology: The etiology and method of transmission of various bleeding disorders are listed in Table 9.6.

Method of Transmission: See Table 9.6.

Epidemiology: The National Hemophilia Foundation estimates that hemophilia A affects 1 in every 5,000 to 10,000 male births, hemophilia B affects 1 of every 34,500 male births, and hemophilia C affects 1 of every 100,000 male/female live births. von Willebrand disease is the most common inherited platelet disorder, affecting 1 to 2% of the United States population both male and female (NHF, 2006).

Pathogenesis: All of the hemophilias are associated with a deficiency or defect in one of the factors in the co-

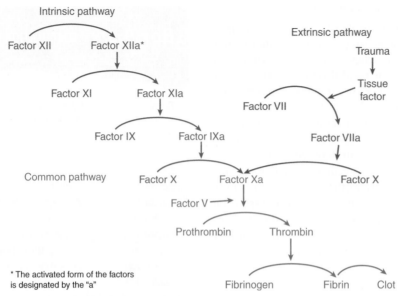

Figure 9.21. Coagulation cascade. The coagulation cascade is initiated when factor XII (Hageman factor) contacts an injured endothelial surface (intrinsic pathway), or when tissue factor (released by damaged endothelial cells) comes in contact with factor VII in the plasma (extrinsic pathway). Intrinsic and extrinsic pathways converge at the activation of factor X (Xa) and follow a common pathway that results in clot formation.

agulation cascade, which results in defective or inadequate clot formation. von Willebrand disease is associated with defective or inadequate levels of von Willebrand factor. This causes defective or inadequate platelet adhesion to sites of injury. In addition, since von Willebrand factor

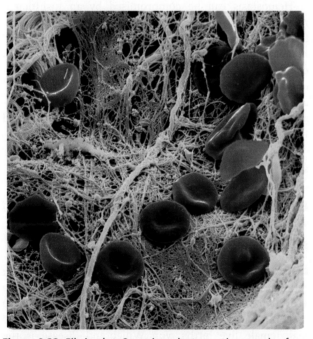

Figure 9.22. Fibrin clot. Scanning electron micrograph of a blood clot (3 × 600). The filaments that form a meshwork between the red blood cells are fibrin fibers that have formed as an end product of the coagulation cascade. (From Porth CM. Essentials of pathophysiology: concepts of altered health states. Philadelphia: Lippincott Williams & Wilkins, 2006.)

carries factor VIII, there may be a concomitant deficiency of this factor, which would add defective clot formation to the platelet disorder. Acquired bleeding disorders (bleeding disorders that are not genetic, but develop during life) are often associated with liver disease, because almost all of the coagulation factors are manufactured in the liver. If the liver is not functioning correctly, then the coagulation factors will not be produced effectively. Vitamin K is essential for appropriate clotting to take place. Normally, vitamin K is produced by the bacteria living in our intestines, so that it is almost impossible to have a deficiency. However, anything that disrupts or destroys the normal intestinal flora (bacteria), such as long-term use of broad-spectrum antibiotics, might cause a deficiency of vitamin K and produce an acquired bleeding disorder.

It might be thought that bleeding disorders would be a problem only when there is traumatic injury to the body. However, the human body is a very complex machine, and there are many opportunities for this machine to malfunction and produce minor, even microscopic, injuries on a daily basis. These are the injuries that someone with a bleeding disorder needs to be concerned about, since there is no way to avoid them and no way to know when they have occurred until it is too late. The major clinical manifestations of bleeding disorders are all associated with either excessive bleeding or reactions to the products given to treat the condition.

Extraoral Characteristics: All of the disorders exhibit a full range of severity of bleeding from unnoticed and undiagnosed, to severe and spontaneous hemorrhages. The severity depends on the amount and activity of the associated coagulation factor or platelet defect.

Table 9.5   BLOOD TESTS THAT EVALUATE HEMOSTASIS

Test	Normal Values	Etiology of Abnormal Findings
Platelet count determines if there is an adequate number of platelets	150,000–400,000/mm^{3a}	Increased—polycythemia, CML, sickle cell anemia and other hemolytic anemias Decreased—ALL, AML, liver disease, thrombocytopenia, pernicious and aplastic anemia
Bleeding time Evaluates the function of platelets	0–9.5 minutes^a	Increased (prolonged)—platelet disorders, thrombocytopenia, leukemia, von Willebrand's disease, antiplatelet drug therapy (aspirin)
Partial thromboplastin time, activated (aPTT) Evaluates the time it takes to form a fibrin clot when calcium and tissue factor are added to the plasma (intrinsic pathway)	<35 seconds^a	Increased (prolonged)—hemophilia, von Willebrand's disease, anticoagulant therapy
Prothrombin time (PT) Evaluates the time it takes to form a fibrin clot when a platelet factor and a surface activating factor are added to the plasma (extrinsic pathway)	11–14 seconds^a	Increased (prolonged)—anticoagulant therapy, prothrombin deficiency, vitamin K deficiency, liver disease, polycythemia, antiplatelet drugs
Clotting Time Measures the time it takes for a clot to form in a glass tube	4–8 minutes	Increased (prolonged)—anticoagulant therapy, vitamin K deficiency, hemophilia, liver disease
International Normalized Ratio (INR) Expresses prothrombin time as a ratio to thromboplastin activity	<1.5	

^{a}Normal values may differ among individual laboratories.

Excessive bleeding in response to minor trauma is consistent throughout all of the disorders. Bleeding into the joint spaces (**hemarthrosis**) is a sign of moderate or severe dysfunction. The bleeding causes joint deformity and severe pain and usually occurs in the weightbearing joints. Bleeding into the muscles of the arms and legs and into the gastrointestinal tract is also common. Ninety percent of patients will have bleeding within the urinary tract, leading to blood in the urine, or **hematuria**. Women with bleeding disorders usually have heavy menstrual flow and

Table 9.6   BLEEDING DISORDERS

Name	Etiology	Method of Transmission
von Willebrand disease	Inadequate or defective von Willebrand factor	• Autosomal dominant or recessive, dominant is less severe • Acquired, damage due to aortic valve stenosis
Hemophilia A (classic hemophilia)	Factor VIII deficiency	• X-linked recessive disorder
Hemophilia B (Christmas disease)	Factor IX or Christmas factor deficiency	• X-linked recessive disorder
Hemophilia C	Factor IX deficiency	• Autosomal recessive disorder
Acquired deficiency of coagulation factors	• Liver disease • Vitamin K deficiency	Not applicable

may have excessive loss of blood during the birth of a child. Childbirth can be life threatening to a woman with a severe bleeding disorder. The most serious form of bleeding is intracranial hemorrhage, or bleeding into the brain. Patients with the severe forms of bleeding disorders have a 10% lifetime chance of having intracranial hemorrhage (Agaliotis and Ozturk, January 2006). The symptoms and sequela of these hemorrhages are mostly identical to those seen with strokes. Most of these patients exhibit easy bruising and many exhibit petechiae on the skin and mucous membranes. In addition, prior to mid 1980, the supply of blood, factors, and other products that are derived from blood were not safe from viral contamination. By 1983, over 50% of those with hemophilia were HIV positive. The most common cause of death in patients who have severe hemophilia is still AIDS (Agaliotis and Ozturk, January 2006). Advances made since then ensure that the blood supply is free of contaminants. The hepatitis viruses were also frequent contaminants of the blood supply, and many with hemophilia are positive for hepatitis B and C.

Perioral and Intraoral Characteristics: The severity of the oral manifestations depends on the severity of the defect or deficiency. Many of the less severe disorders will be asymptomatic or will present with minor gingival bleeding and petechiae on the oral mucous membranes or around the lips. Spontaneous gingival hemorrhage or bleeding after minor trauma occurs frequently in those with severe bleeding disorders. The tendency for hemorrhage will be exacerbated by the presence of gingival or periodontal infections. Significant bleeding will occur after periodontal surgery or therapy, tooth extraction, or oral trauma of any type. In fact, excessive bleeding after dental extractions may be the first indication of a minor bleeding disorder.

Distinguishing Characteristics: Not applicable

Significant Microscopic Features: Not applicable

Dental Implications: The clinician should be curious when there is unexplained bleeding, especially in the absence of trauma or periodontal infection. Referral to a physician should be made based on the presenting oral conditions; the concomitant presence of systemic symptoms such as lymphadenopathy, fever, or weight loss; and the previous medical/dental history. Dental care is very important for these individuals; however, many are afraid to seek dental care, and regrettably, many dental professionals are reluctant to provide treatment for them. Treatment can be accomplished safely in a normal dental environment for all but the most severely affected patients. Consult with the patient's hematologist prior to treatment to discuss the type and severity of the factor deficiency, the need for antibiotic premedication because of a joint replacement or central venous line, the nature of the planned dental procedure, and

the recommendations for hemostatic control before, during, and after the procedure. The hematologist will request appropriate laboratory tests to determine the patient's current factor levels and clotting capabilities. Some surgical procedures will require daily factor infusion starting several days prior to the procedure. Others will only require infusion on the day of the procedure. Local anesthesia is not contraindicated in persons with hemophilia, but the factor level should be raised to at least 50% of normal before giving a mandibular block injection, because the mandibular block can cause major bleeding in the area of the neck. In most cases, buccal infiltration and intrapapillary and intraligamentary injections require only local hemostatic measures and are preferable to the mandibular block (Brewer and Correa, 2006). Oral rinses with fibrin and/or tranexamic acid (a preparation that enhances clot formation) and oral administration of aminocaproic acid (a substance that prevents destruction of a clot), can help to maintain hemostasis until any sutures placed during treatment have been removed and healing has occurred. Gel foam, an absorbable gelatin sponge that provides a framework for clot formation, can be soaked in a thrombin solution and then used in an extraction site to help to control bleeding. Dental care that stresses prevention and anticipates problems is essential for the maintenance of oral health in those with hemophilia (Brewer and Correa, 2006). The infusion treatments are extremely expensive; therefore, measures should be taken to decrease the frequency of performing them. Everyday occurrences, such as the exfoliation of primary teeth, while bothersome to the normal child, can cause a severe loss of blood in the child with hemophilia. Spontaneous bleeding is often associated with severe periodontal infections in normal individuals. Even slight gingival infections could cause severe bleeding for someone with hemophilia. Chlorhexidine gluconate can help minimize gingival inflammation prior to periodontal therapy. Education should stress the importance of maintaining healthy tissues, which could possibly eliminate the need for factor replacement therapy before routine dental care (Brewer and Correa, 2006).

Differential Diagnosis: Any condition that can cause decreased clotting or excessive bleeding should be ruled out. Some of these are

1. Leukemia, Chapter 9
2. Thrombocytopenia, Chapter 9
3. Agranulocytosis or cyclic neutropenia, Chapter 9
4. Anticoagulant therapy, Chapter 8
5. Hereditary hemorrhage telangiectasia, Chapter 13
6. Vitamin C deficiency

Treatment and Prognosis: All of the bleeding disorders are treated with replacement of the specific factor that is missing or defective. Thus hemophilia A requires infusion with concentrated factor VIII, and hemophilia B requires infusion with factor IX. von Willebrand's disease requires replacement of von Willebrand factor (vWF). Because factor

VIII depends on the presence of vWF to function correctly, both substances are usually given at the same time. Factor infusion is normally done prophylactically to maintain an adequate level of factor in the blood to prevent bleeding. It can also be done on demand to stop bleeding.

Desmopressin acetate, a hormone that mimics the action of vasopressin to release factor VIII from endothelial cells, is used in some cases of von Willebrand's disease and mild hemophilia. Desmopressin acetate comes in an injectable form or as a nasal spray. Both forms are used to stop bleeding in progress or as a prophylactic and are administered no more than once daily. Individuals with hemophilia must be careful about the kind of drugs that they take; nothing with aspirin should be taken, nor should any of the nonsteroidal antiinflammatory drugs. Even some over-the-counter herbal preparations are dangerous for someone with a bleeding disorder, for example, garlic, ginger, ginkgo, and ginseng, among others.

Mild and moderate forms of hemophilia and von Willebrand's disease have an excellent prognosis for a normal life expectancy at this time. Severely affected individuals have a life expectancy of 50 to 60 years, compared with 11 years in the 1960s. The supply of factor and blood products is safer than it has ever been, and new developments in treatment and prevention are occurring regularly.

Name: Thrombocytopenia

Etiology:
When the platelet count drops below $100,000/mm^3$ of blood, there is increased risk of excessive blood loss associated with minor trauma. This condition is called thrombocytopenia. Thrombocytopenia usually occurs as a sequela of another condition or therapeutic regimen. Any disorder that suppresses the function of the bone marrow will affect the number of platelets. Aplastic anemia, chemotherapy, radiation therapy, and some types of drugs all have the potential to produce this disorder. Some of the more common drugs in addition to cytotoxic drugs used in chemotherapy include: thiazide diuretics, ibuprofen, tamoxifen, phenytoin, and ranitidine. Individuals who abuse alcohol are at risk for this disorder because alcohol has the potential to suppress platelet production. Several forms of rare inherited disorders also suppress the production of platelets. In addition, idiopathic or immune thrombocytopenia purpura (ITP) is caused by the destruction of platelets by antibodies that the immune system creates. Most often, ITP is associated with leukemia, HIV infection, and collagen disorders such as systemic lupus. Children may present with temporary ITP after a viral illness.

Method of Transmission: Not applicable

Epidemiology:
ITP is seen in about 66 of 1,000,000 adults and 50 of 1,000,000 children. More adult females than males are affected, but both sexes are equally affected in children. The peak age at diagnosis is 2–4 years in children and 20–50 years in adults (Silverman, March 2005). No statistics are available for thrombocytopenia that is secondary to another disorder.

Pathogenesis:
No matter what causes this disorder, the results are the same; there is a severe decrease in the numbers of circulating platelets. Since the platelets are essential for proper hemostasis, most of the clinical manifestations are related to impaired clot formation.

Extraoral Characteristics:
Petechial hemorrhages in the skin of the lower extremities, easy bruising, purpura, epistaxis, heavy menstrual flow, gastrointestinal bleeding, and retinal hemorrhages are characteristic of platelet deficiency.

Perioral and Intraoral Characteristics:
Gingival bleeding is one of the most common presenting features of thrombocytopenia. Petechiae and hemorrhagic bullae within the oral mucosa and lips are also common (Fig. 9.23A and B).

Distinguishing Characteristics: Not applicable

Significant Microscopic Features:
The bone marrow will show increased numbers of megakaryocytes being created to increase the number of platelets.

Dental Implications:
Any unexplained excessive oral bleeding should prompt the clinician to refer the patient to a physician for further evaluation. If excessive bleeding occurs during dental treatment, the same type of local hemostatic measures used in other bleeding disorders should be used. In addition, platelet levels should be determined by blood tests prior to dental/dental hygiene therapy.

Differential Diagnosis:
Any condition that can cause decreased clotting or excessive bleeding should be ruled out. Some of these include

1. Leukemia, Chapter 9
2. Hemophilia, Chapter 9
3. von Willebrand's disease, Chapter 9
4. Agranulocytosis or cyclic neutropenia, Chapter 9
5. Anticoagulant therapy, Chapter 8
6. Hereditary hemorrhage telangiectasia, Chapter 13
7. Vitamin C deficiency

Treatment and Prognosis:
The treatment for these disorders depends on the cause or suspected cause. Thrombocytopenia associated with the use of drugs can usually be reversed by eliminating the drug. Thrombocytopenia caused by cancer treatments usually resolves with the termination of treatment. ITP is treated with transfusions of platelets, steroids to inhibit the production of antibodies, and intravenous immunoglobulin infusions.

Children usually recover within 6 to 8 weeks, with 89% eventually achieving full recovery. Only about 64% of adults recover fully; 30% have chronic dysfunction. Mortality rates for children and adults are 2% and 5%, respectively.

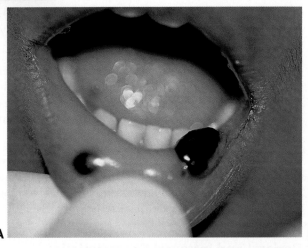
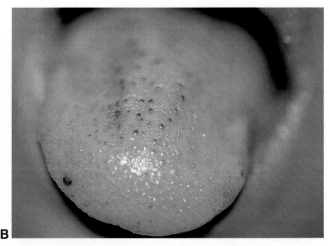

Figure 9.23. Idiopathic thrombocytopenic purpura. This child presents with areas of hemorrhage in the tissues of the lip **(A)** and petechiae on the tongue **(B)** that are characteristic of this disorder. (From Fleisher GR, Ludwig W, Baskin MN. Atlas of pediatric emergency medicine. Philadelphia: Lippincott Williams & Wilkins, 2004.)

SUMMARY

- Lymph tissue, bone marrow, and the circulating blood form the hematopoietic system. Hematopoiesis, the process of red and white blood cell production, occurs in the bone marrow.
- The pluripotential stem cells that reside in the marrow differentiate into the three types of blood cells: red, white, and platelets.
- The normal life span of an erythrocyte (red blood cell) is about 120 days. The kidney regulates the process of erythropoiesis by secreting erythropoietin when a low blood oxygen level is sensed. Old or damaged erythrocytes are removed from the circulation by the spleen.
- Anemia manifests as a decreased level of oxygen in the blood and can be caused by a decrease in the number of cells or amount of hemoglobin or a defect in the structure or function of hemoglobin.
- The symptoms associated with anemia include tachycardia, palpitations, dyspnea, dizziness, weakness, and fatigue. Glossitis is a common oral manifestation that occurs with many forms of anemia.
- Hypochromic or iron deficiency anemia can be due to inadequate dietary intake of iron or chronic blood loss as seen in gastrointestinal ulcers or heavy menstruation. Physical manifestations range from mild to severe, depending on the severity of the deficiency. Oral manifestations include pale mucous membranes, glossitis, oral ulcers, and angular cheilitis.
- Plummer-Vinson syndrome, a form of severe long-standing iron deficiency anemia, is associated with

increased risk of developing esophageal and oropharyngeal cancers.
- Thalassemia is a genetic disorder that causes the formation of a defective hemoglobin molecule. The different forms of thalassemia make up the most common inherited disorders in the world.
- Megaloblastic anemia occurs when defective RNA or DNA synthesis results in the production of abnormally large red cells. Vitamin B_{12} and folic acid deficiencies are the most common cause of megaloblastic anemia.
- Pernicious anemia is an autoimmune condition that inhibits the production of intrinsic factor, which is necessary for the transportation of vitamin B_{12} across the gastrointestinal mucous membranes. Pernicious anemia presents with the general and oral symptoms of anemia plus neurologic problems such as paraesthesia, loss of proprioception, and ataxia.
- Folic acid deficiency presents with all of the symptoms of pernicious anemia except the neurologic symptoms. Folic acid deficiency has been linked to an increased risk for neural tube defects, such as spina bifida, and oral clefting.
- Sickle cell anemia, a form of hemolytic anemia, is an autosomal recessive genetic disorder that results in the production of defective hemoglobin molecules that become misshapen (sickled) when exposed to specific conditions, such as hypoxia and dehydra-

(continued)

SUMMARY *(continued)*

tion. Sickled cells tend to get trapped in the microvasculature and cause tissue infarcts.

- Anemia can be a secondary complication of many chronic disorders.
- Aplastic anemia occurs when disruption of the bone marrow causes it to limit or stop producing all three types of blood cells.
- Polycythemia refers to an increase in blood cells in relationship to blood plasma. Relative polycythemia occurs when there is a decrease in plasma fluid related to dehydration. Primary polycythemia occurs when there is an increase in all types of cells, usually resulting from a neoplastic disease. In secondary polycythemia, only red blood cells increase.
- Neutropenia (agranulocytosis) refers to an abnormal decrease in the numbers of neutrophils. The most common cause of neutropenia is an adverse reaction to a drug. Severe periodontal disease resulting in tooth loss is associated with the chronic forms of neutropenia.
- Hodgkin's lymphoma often presents in the head and neck area as cervical lymphadenopathy. The Reed-Sternberg cell differentiates this lymphoma from other types of lymphoma.
- Non-Hodgkin's lymphoma refers to a diverse group of neoplasms that arise from T and B lymphocytes. Patients who are HIV positive have a higher risk of developing non-Hodgkin's lymphoma than the general population. Intraoral non-Hodgkin's lymphoma may present as a soft tissue swelling in the area of Waldeyer's ring, at the base of the tongue or in the salivary glands. The hard palate is the most common area for the development of a bone lesion.
- The most aggressive form of lymphoma is Burkitt's lymphoma. The African form presents as a neoplastic growth in the head and neck area and is associated with the Epstein-Barr virus. The sporadic form usually presents as a mass in the abdomen and is less often associated with Epstein-Barr virus.
- Leukemia refers to a diverse group of neoplastic disorders involving leukocytes. The acute forms of the disease exhibit symptoms very early in the disease process; the chronic forms progress more slowly.
- Immune suppression is a characteristic feature of all forms of leukemia because the white cells that are produced do not function correctly. Often the first sign of a problem is an unexplained gingival infection accompanied by excessive gingival bleeding and gingival enlargement.
- The Philadelphia chromosome is present in most cases of chronic myelogenous leukemia (CML).
- Multiple myeloma is a malignant neoplasm of B lymphocytes, usually caused by an accumulation of genetic defects within the cells. The disease is associated with severe immunosuppression, bone resorption, and kidney failure.
- Extramedullary plasmacytomas are found in the soft tissues and may frequently be found in the oral cavity.
- Severe loss of blood from injuries is prevented by the process of hemostasis (coagulation). Platelets and the coagulation factors (produced in the liver) act together to maintain hemostasis. The process of coagulation centers on the coagulation cascade.
- Bleeding disorders are seen when there are too few or defective platelets or inadequate or defective coagulation factors.
- Severe hemophilia presents with hemarthrosis, hematuria, and bleeding into the muscles and gastrointestinal tract. Cerebral hemorrhage is also common in more severe cases. Intraoral findings include spontaneous gingival hemorrhage, petechiae, and ecchymoses.
- Dental management of a bleeding disorder focuses on preventing excessive blood loss and maintaining healthy oral tissues to decrease inflammation.
- An inadequate number of platelets or defective platelets presents as thrombocytopenia. Idiopathic thrombocytopenia purpura is caused by an autoimmune reaction that destroys the platelets.

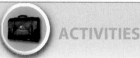

PORTFOLIO ACTIVITIES

1. Contact a community group in your area that provides education and support for patients who have hemophilia, sickle cell anemia, or thalassemia. Tell them that you are a dental hygiene student and ask if you can present a short oral health program focused on maintaining healthy oral tissues and addressing the dental problems associated with that particular condition to some of their members. You might be able to survey some members to see if they have any specific oral health questions that you could help them find answers to. When you present your program, make sure that you ask questions about the participant's dental experiences, both good and bad. After your visit, write a summary of your experience with reflections on the information that you received from the individuals with whom you spoke. Include how some of their bad experiences might have been changed into good experiences and how the good experiences might have been made even better. The following are good places to start looking for a community group:
   - National Hemophilia Foundation *http://www.hemophilia.org* go to the Chapter Center
   - Sickle Cell Disease Association of America *http://www.sicklecelldisease.org* go to Member Organizations
   - Cooley's Anemia Foundation *http://www.thalassemia.org* go to local chapters

Critical Thinking Activities

1. List several obstacles that you think might cause someone with a bleeding disorder to avoid receiving routine dental care. Look at your list, and using information from any available source and your imagination, develop strategies to overcome these obstacles. Share these with your classmates.

2. Examine your school's medical/dental history form and identify the items that pertain to blood or bleeding disorders. Write down questions that you would want to ask to get the most complete information from your patients.

Case Study

One of your favorite patients has brought his wife along with him to your dental hygiene clinic for an oral cancer examination while he is having periodontal debridement. She is 69 years old, edentulous, and wears full upper and lower dentures. Her main complaint is that her dentures have been difficult to wear lately. Her medical history is unremarkable except for stage 1 hypertension, treated with a diuretic, and a recent history of heart palpitations. Figure 9.24 shows what you see before you even start your intraoral examination.

1. What is the most striking observation?
2. What else do you see?
3. What types of follow-up questions would you want to ask?
4. What conditions would you want to include in a differential diagnosis?

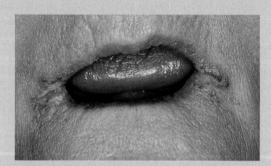

Figure 9.24. Case study for text. (From Neville B, et al: Color atlas of clinical oral pathology. Philadelphia: Lea & Febiger, 1991, with permission.)

5. Can you determine what the cause of this clinical presentation is without any other information? What other information would you want to have?
6. What would be the outcome of this visit?

INTERNET RESOURCES

American Cancer Society
http://www.cancer.org
National Anemia Action Council
http://www.anemia.org
American Sickle Cell Anemia Association
http://www.ascaa.org
Sickle Cell Disease Association of America
http://www.sicklecelldisease.org
Sickle Cell Information Center
http://www.scinfo.org
Cooley's Anemia Foundation
http://www.thalassemia.org
Lymphoma Research Foundation
http://www.lymphoma.org

The Leukemia and Lymphoma Society
http://www.leukemia-lymphoma.org
Lymphoma Association
http://www.lymphoma.org.uk
National Cancer Institute
http://www.cancer.gov
National Hemophilia Association
http://www.hemophilia.org
World Federation of Hemophilia
http://www.wfh.org
Hemophilia Galaxy
http://www.hemophiliagalaxy.com

REFERENCES

Agaliotis DP, Ozturk S. Hemophilia, overview. Last update January 6, 2006. e medicine: Instant Access to the Minds of Medicine. Available at: *http://www.emedicine.com/med/topic3528.htm*. Accessed October 7, 2006.

American Cancer Society. Available at: http://www.cancer.org. Accessed October 7, 2006.

Besa EC, Woermann U. Chronic myelogenous leukemia. Last update July 12, 2006. e medicine: Instant Access to the Minds of Medicine. Available at: *http://www.emedicine.com/med/topic371.htm*. Accessed October 7, 2006.

Blom HJ, Shaw GM, den Heijer M, Finnell RH. Neural tube defects and folate: case far from closed. Nature Rev Neurosci Sep 2006;7(9): 724–731.

Brewer A, Correa ME. Guidelines for dental treatment of patients with inherited bleeding disorders ©World Federation of Hemophilia, 2006. Available at: http://www.wfh.org/2/docs/Publications/Dental_Care/TOH-40_Dental_treatment.pdf . Accessed October 15, 2006.

Conrad M. Iron deficiency anemia. Last update October 4, 2006. e medicine: Instant Access to the Minds of Medicine. Available at: *http://www.emedicine.com/med/topic1188.htm*. Accessed October 7, 2006.

Conrad M. Pernicious anemia. Last update October 4, 2006. e medicine: Instant Access to the Minds of Medicine. Available at: *http://www.emedicine.com/med/topic1799.htm*. Accessed October 7, 2006.

Cotran RS, Kumar V, Collins T. Robbins: pathologic basis of disease. 6th ed. Philadelphia: WB Saunders, 1999:139–187.

Dessain SK, Wasilewski C, Argiris A, Kaklamani V. Hodgkin disease. Last update July 21, 2006. e medicine: Instant Access to the Minds of Medicine. Available at: *http://www.emedicine.com/med/topic1022.htm*. Accessed September 12, 2006.

Distenfeld A. Agranulocytosis. Last update January 10, 2006. e medicine: Instant Access to the Minds of Medicine. Available at: *http://www.emedicine.com/med/topic82.htm*. Accessed October 7, 2006.

Gentili A, Vohra M, Subir V, et al. Folic acid deficiency. Last update May 2006. e medicine: Instant Access to the Minds of Medicine. Available at: *http://www.emedicine.com/med/topic802.htm*. Accessed October 3, 2006.

Grethlein S. Multiple myeloma. Last update June 16, 2006. e medicine: Instant Access to the Minds of Medicine. Available at: *http://www.emedicine.com/med/topic1521.htm*. Accessed October 7, 2006.

Harper JL. Anemia, megaloblastic. Last update June 2005. e medicine:

Instant Access to the Minds of Medicine. Available at: *http://www.emedicine.com/ped/topic2575.htm*. Accessed October 1, 2006.

Hazza'a AM, Al-Jamal G. Dental development in subjects with thalassemia major. J Contemp Dent Pract @ www.thejcdp.com, September 1, 2006;7(4):063–070.

Huether SE, McCance KL. Understanding pathophysiology. 3re ed. St. Louis: Mosby, 2004:507–596.

Ibsen OAC, Phelan JA. Oral pathology for the dental hygienist. 4th ed. St. Louis: WB Saunders, 2004:216–253.

National Hemophilia Foundation. Available at: http://www.hemophilia.org/NHFWeb/MainPgs/MainNHF.aspx?menuid=0&contentid=1. Accessed September 29, 2006.

Novacek G. Plummer-Vinson syndrome. Orphanet encyclopedia, July 2005. Available at: http://www.orpha.net/data/patho/GB/uk-Plummer-VinsonSyndrome2005.pdf. Accessed October 4, 2006.

Perry M, Rasool H. Chronic lymphocytic leukemia. Last update July 11, 2005. e medicine: Instant Access to the Minds of Medicine. Available at: http://www.emedicine.com/med/topic370.htm. Accessed October 2, 2006.

Pollak ES, Stein S. von Willebrand's disease. Last update July 5, 2006. e medicine: Instant Access to the Minds of Medicine. Available at: http://www.emedicine.com/med/topic2392.htm. Accessed October 5, 2006.

Porth CM. Essentials of pathophysiology: concepts of altered health states. Philadelphia: Lippincott Williams & Wilkins, 2004:191–230.

Prchal JT, Chen G. Polycythemia vera. Last update June 15, 2005. e medicine: Instant Access to the Minds of Medicine. Available at: *http://www.emedicine.com/ped/topic1850.htm*. Accessed September 29, 2006.

Regezi JA, Sciubba JJ, Jordan RCK. Oral pathology: clinical pathologic correlations. 4th ed. St. Louis: WB Saunders, 2003:122–125, 51, 223–239.

Rick ME, Walsh CE, Key NS. Congenital bleeding disorders. Hematology Jan 2003;559–574.

Rubin E, Gorstein F, Rubin R, et al. Rubin's pathology: clinicopathologic foundations of medicine. 4th ed. Baltimore: Lippincott Williams & Wilkins, 2005:1019–1123.

Satake N, Sakamoto K. Acute lymphoblastic leukemia. Last update July 11, 2006. e medicine: Instant Access to the Minds of Medicine. Available at: *http://www.emedicine.com/ped/topic2587.htm*. Accessed October 7, 2006.

Seiter K. Acute myelogenous leukemia. Last update January 24, 2006. e medicine: Instant Access to the Minds of Medicine. Available at: http://www.emedicine.com/med/topic34.htm. Accessed October 7, 2006.

Stedman's medical dictionary for the health professions and nursing, 5th ed. Baltimore: Lippincott Williams & Wilkins, 2005.

Wilkins EM. Clinical practice of the dental hygienist. 9th ed. Baltimore: Lippincott Williams & Wilkins, 2005:1059.

Yaish HM. Thalassemia. Last update December 19, 2005. e medicine: Instant Access to the Minds of Medicine. Available at: http://www.emedicine.com/ped/topic2229.htm. Accessed October 8, 2006.

Chapter 1

Respiratory, Gastrointestinal, Neurologic, and Skeletal Disorders

Key Terms

- **Abfraction**
- **Atelectasis**
- **Aura**
- **Bradykinesia**
- **Demyelination**
- **Diverticula**
- **Droplet nuclei**
- **Dyskinesia**
- **Emulsifier**
- **Febrile**
- **Hemoptysis**
- **Hyperacusis**
- **Hypercementosis**
- **Nosocomial**
- **Osteonecrosis**
- **Osteophyte**
- **Parafunctional**
- **Paroxysm**
- **Peristalsis**

Learning Outcomes

1. Define and use the key terms in this chapter.

2. Describe how to limit the spread of the common cold and influenza within the dental office.

3. Discuss why antibiotics should not be used to treat the common cold or influenza.

4. Identify the medication associated with Reye syndrome and note those at highest risk for the syndrome.

5. Describe how dental biofilm may be associated with nosocomial pneumonia.

6. Discuss why the long incubation period associated with SARS facilitates widespread transmission of the disease.

7. Describe the dental management of an individual suspected of having tuberculosis.

8. Identify the type of personal protective equipment and environmental controls that need to be available for the dental professional to safely treat an individual with active tuberculosis.

9. Compare and contrast the clinical characteristics of emphysema and chronic obstructive bronchitis.

10. Discuss the myriad of difficulties associated with dysphagia.

11. Identify the gastrointestinal disorders that are associated with an increased risk of cancer within that system.

12. Identify one special population group that is at high risk for meningococcal disease.

13. Discuss the distinguishing feature of burning mouth syndrome.

14. Compare and contrast osteoarthritis and rheumatoid arthritis.

15. Describe bisphosphonate-associated osteonecrosis and the factors associated with an increased risk of BON.

16. Describe methods to identify and manage the patient with a temporomandibular joint disorder.

Chapter Outline

The most important aspects of general pathology are covered in this text up to this point. However, some additional medical disorders should be reviewed to help prepare the student to safely provide appropriate patient treatment. This chapter discusses the pertinent information and dental implications related to these conditions.

THE RESPIRATORY SYSTEM

The respiratory system comprises several different types of structures: (1) structures that bring air into the lungs, (2) structures that transfer oxygen into the bloodstream, and (3) structures that allow the lungs to expand and contract. The nasal cavity, oral cavity, larynx, pharynx, trachea, bronchi, and bronchioles bring air from the environment into the lungs. Oxygen is exchanged for carbon dioxide in the alveoli. The diaphragm and the external intercostals are the muscles of inspiration. When these muscles contract, the volume of the chest cavity increases, and outside air enters the lung. The rate of contraction of these muscles is regulated by the respiratory center in the medulla of the brain. This center senses the carbon dioxide level in the blood and stimulates the muscles of inspiration to contract. Air leaves the lungs when these muscles relax. The abdominal and internal intercostal muscles assist with expiration, if necessary, an example being the compensation that may occur in emphysema. The lungs are enclosed by a double membrane called the pleura. The area between these layers is called the pleural cavity and is filled with a special fluid that lubricates the lungs as they expand and contract. The respiratory tract is lined with specialized respiratory epithelium that contains cilia. The cilia help to prevent foreign objects or substances from entering the lungs. The respiratory system is divided into the upper respiratory tract, which is composed of the structures of the nose and throat, and the lower respiratory tract, which is composed of the trachea, bronchi, and lungs.

Upper Respiratory Diseases

Upper respiratory diseases are among the most common infections known to man and cause significant amounts of time away from school and work each year. The common cold and influenza are examples of these types of diseases.

Name: Common cold

Etiology: The common cold is an acute inflammation of the mucous membrane lining of the upper respiratory tract. The virus most often associated with the common cold is the rhinovirus, of which there are more than 100 different types.

Method of Transmission: Although these viruses can be transmitted through the air and inhaled, transmission by hands and fingers that have touched objects contaminated with the viruses is more likely to occur. As few as 1 or as many as 30 viral particles have been known to cause an infection.

Epidemiology: About 61 million of these infections occur every year in the United States alone. Adults average about two infections per year, while children may have up to six or more infections per year (DePaola, 2005).

Pathogenesis: Symptoms of the infection can occur within 10 to 12 hours after the virus is introduced to the nasal mucosa (DePaola, 2005). The first symptom is usually a sore throat, followed by congestion and nasal discharge. The initial congestion is due to the swelling of the mucous membranes, which narrows the nasal passageways. The discharge that comes next is caused by the secretion of copious amounts of mucus by the inflamed glands. Viral-induced mucosal secretions are clear and watery. The altered environment of the nasal passages and the compromised immune status of the affected individual predispose him or her to infection by bacterial organisms.

Thick, yellow or green mucous secretions caused by pyogenic bacteria are evidence of a bacterial infection superimposed on the original viral infection. The offending bacterial organisms are usually streptococci, staphylococci, or pneumococci.

Treatment and Prognosis: There is no cure for the common cold, which resolves on its own in 7 to 10 days, and there is no need for the use of antibiotic medications unless there is a concomitant bacterial infection. In the past it was common medical practice to prescribe antibiotics for the individual with a cold. This was not to treat the cold, which is viral, but to prevent a bacterial coinfection. This practice is no longer considered appropriate because of the risk of creating antibiotic-resistant organisms. Medications that alleviate the symptoms associated with colds include decongestants, cough suppressants or antitussives, and expectorants, which help to remove mucus from the respiratory tract.

Name: Influenza

Etiology: Influenza can affect both the upper and lower respiratory tracts and is caused by influenza virus types A, B, and C.

Method of Transmission: The virus is transmitted to an uninfected host's oral or nasal mucous membranes through inhalation of aerosols that contain the organism (created when an infected person coughs, sneezes, or speaks) or through contact with contaminated objects.

Epidemiology: Influenza occurs in epidemic or pandemic (worldwide) proportions causing approximately 500,000 deaths every year (DePaola, 2005). Influenza is a known killer, usually affecting the elderly and the very young.

Pathogenesis: There is a short incubation period of up to 4 days, and the affected individual is capable of spreading the virus from a day or two before the symptoms arise to about 5 days after symptoms appear. Children and severely immunocompromised individuals may shed the virus for weeks or months (DePaola, 2005). Early symptoms of influenza include fever, headache, and malaise. These are followed closely by sore throat, cough, and copious nasal discharge. The infection causes necrosis and shedding of the serous and ciliated cells lining the respiratory tract, allowing extracellular fluid to leak out and produce the nasal discharge. In addition, the serous cells are among the first to recover, allowing the renewed production of mucus. However, without the ciliated cells, the body has difficulty moving the mucus, which results in the coughing and nose blowing characteristic of the flu (Porth, 2004).

Treatment and Prognosis: The influenza viruses are known for their ability to mutate into new and often more virulent strains. Every mutation requires the development of a new vaccine to stop the spread of the disease. Consequently, new vaccines need to be produced every year to combat the newest forms of the virus. This also explains why people who have the flu one year are not immune to the flu the next year. The infection is normally self-limiting, with symptoms resolving in 7 to 10 days. However, the greatest danger associated with influenza is its ability to cause more severe infections in high-risk individuals, such as the very young, the elderly, those with preexisting cardiac or pulmonary disorders, and the immunocompromised. Viral pneumonia and/or a bacterial coinfection can cause death from respiratory failure in just days. Antiviral medications are available to help prevent the flu and also to treat the infection. When given within 2 days of the onset of flu symptoms, these drugs can shorten the length of time that the individual is affected by symptoms of the infection by 1 or 2 days. The drugs can also decrease the potential for transmitting the virus and decrease the severity of the symptoms associated with the infection. The use of these drugs should be considered carefully, because severe side effects have been associated with them. For example, there have been reports of an increase in seizure events in those with a seizure disorder, an increase in the level of renal dysfunction in those with preexisting renal disease, and an increase in respiratory dysfunction in those with an underlying respiratory condition (Smith et al., July 2006).

REYE SYNDROME

In the early 1960s, several physicians observed a distinct set of symptoms that seemed to occur following a viral illness that had been treated with aspirin. Reye syndrome was named after the Australian physician who first recognized it. The etiology and pathogenesis of Reye syndrome are obscure. However, Reye syndrome is associated with the use of aspirin or aspirin-containing products to treat the symptoms of influenza and several other **febrile** (fever producing) diseases of viral etiology in young children. Reye syndrome consists of liver damage and brain pathology, usually associated with edema from inflammatory exudates, which can lead to brain damage, coma, and death. Because of the potential for this syndrome, it has become standard practice to never prescribe or give aspirin or aspirin-containing products to children, especially those who have colds or other febrile illnesses (Weiner, November 2005).

Lower Respiratory Diseases

Lower respiratory tract diseases are usually more severe and are often chronic, unlike upper respiratory diseases. Disorders of the lower respiratory tract include pneumonia, tuberculosis, and obstructive airway disorders, specifically, asthma, chronic obstructive pulmonary disease, and cystic fibrosis, as well as others.

APPLICATION: PREVENTING COLDS/FLU

The best treatment for colds and flu is to try to prevent them. While exposure to infectious organisms cannot be eliminated, there are many ways to limit exposure to these organisms. The following are some strategies that can be implemented in the dental office that may help in preventing the spread of both colds and flu.

- Perform frequent hand hygiene (washing). This is probably the most effective weapon available for preventing the spread of these and other infections. Hand hygiene should be performed after any patient contact or contact with surfaces that are potentially contaminated with respiratory secretions.
- Use a preoperative antimicrobial mouth rinse to limit the microorganisms that could be aerosolized during a dental procedure.
- Place dispensers of alcohol-based hand rub or towelettes for patient use where sinks are not available, such as in the reception room.
- Encourage dental healthcare workers to remain at home if they have flu or cold symptoms.
- Make sure all dental healthcare workers receive a flu vaccination if appropriate and available.
- Disinfect as much of the reception room furniture as possible. Disinfect toys and discard any toy that cannot be disinfected.
- Encourage everyone to cover their nose and mouth with tissues when coughing or sneezing. Tissues and receptacles for contaminated tissues should be placed throughout the office.
- Keep a mask on when working with a patient who may have a cold or the flu and leave it on after the patient has left the room and during cleanup.
- Avoid close contact with sick people. Reschedule sick patients.
- Perform hand hygiene prior to eating or touching your mouth, nose, or eyes.

Name: Pneumonia

Etiology: Pneumonia can be defined as an inflammation of the bronchioles and the alveoli within the lungs. Most cases of pneumonia are caused by bacteria or viruses. However, pneumonia can also result from a fungal infection, inhalation of toxic fumes, or aspiration of chemical substances into the lungs. These substances include vomitus or bacterial organisms, such as those associated with dental biofilm. Dental biofilm has been associated with **nosocomial** or hospital-acquired pneumonia, especially in the elderly population (Mojon, 2002).

Method of Transmission: Bacterial and viral pneumonia are transmitted through inhalation of contaminated aerosols or through inoculation of the respiratory mucosa by contaminated hands, fingers, or other objects. The method of transmission of pneumonia is categorized into the following two types, depending on the setting or circumstances surrounding its occurrence or transmission:

- Community-acquired pneumonia is contracted outside of a hospital or long-term care facility.
- Nosocomial pneumonia is contracted within a hospital or long-term care facility by susceptible individuals.

Some of the conditions that make an individual susceptible to pneumonia include altered levels of consciousness impairing the individual's ability to clear the lungs by coughing, esophageal dysfunction causing the aspiration of matter into the lungs, neurologic disorders such as dementia, and mechanical intrusions into the body such as breathing tubes or endoscopic examination of the esophagus or lungs.

Epidemiology: Approximately 3 million cases of pneumonia occur in the United States each year (Stephen, February 2005). Males are diagnosed with pneumonia more often than females, and the elderly are affected more often than younger individuals. Individuals with preexisting pulmonary conditions, smokers, and those who are immunocompromised are at the highest risk of developing pneumonia.

Pathogenesis: The specific pathogenesis depends on the cause of the pneumonia; however, all cause an inflammatory response within the lung tissues. This inflammation results in the production of an exudate that obstructs the air spaces within the lung, preventing the exchange of gases that normally occurs in these areas. Symptoms of pneumonia include fever, dyspnea, productive cough (cough that brings up sputum), tachycardia, weakness, anorexia, and chest pain.

Dental Implications: Dental professionals have a responsibility to increase awareness of the link between oral pathogens and pneumonia. Oral bacteria in dental biofilm can be aspirated into the lungs and cause pneumonia. Several studies have reported up to a 50% reduction in the rate of pneumonia in hospital patients who have daily mechanical removal of dental biofilm with or without antibacterial rinses (Teng et al., 2002). While most of the studies that explored this relationship were conducted in hospitals or long-term care facilities, the information can be applied to situations in which debilitated patients are being cared for in the home and to anyone with a respiratory disorder. Dental hygienists have an excellent opportunity to provide this information during patient visits and during community education programs.

Treatment and Prognosis: Both the treatment and prognosis depend on the cause of the pneumonia and the immune status of the host. All forms are treated with supportive therapy as needed, including adequate hydration, nutrition, supplemental oxygen, and mechanically assisted ventilation. Bacterial pneumonia, including aspiration pneumonia, is treated with antibiotics. Viral pneumonia is sometimes treated with antivirals, depending on the specific risks involved and the general health of the individual. Chemical aspiration pneumonia is usually treated by removal of the offending agent, if possible, and with supportive oxygen therapy. Most individuals will recover from pneumonia; however, those with preexisting respiratory disorders often see a worsening of the underlying condition and may be subject to frequent recurrences of the pneumonia. Data for mortality rates are specific for the type of pneumonia, but in all cases, the elderly have the highest mortality rates. Prevention is possible through strict adherence to standard precautions and through vaccination for one of the more common bacterial pneumonias, pneumococcal pneumonia. The vaccine is recommended for individuals over the age of 65, those with a compromised immune system, those with chronic illness, and residents of long-term care facilities.

SEVERE ACUTE RESPIRATORY SYNDROME (SARS)

The SARS outbreak that occurred in 2003 is considered to be the first pandemic of the 21st century. Eight thousand individuals in 26 countries on five continents were affected, and 774 deaths were reported (Peiris et al., 2003). An atypical form of a coronavirus, normally associated with the common cold, called SARS-CoV has been identified as the etiologic agent. The virus appears to be transmitted through direct or indirect contact with the oral or respiratory mucous membranes of a susceptible host. Inhalation of the virus in contaminated air is most likely the reason for the many reported cases that occurred to those in close contact while traveling in planes, taxis, and other methods of transportation. Hospital transmission during procedures that created aerosols was also implicated as a cause for the disease (Peiris et al., 2003). Disease transmission was facilitated by the fact that the infection has a longer incubation period, up to 14 days, than others of its type. The longer incubation period enabled transmission over large geographic areas (Peiris et al., 2003).

The pathogenesis of SARS is not well known. The initial symptoms are fever, malaise, muscle pains, chills, and cough. Later symptoms that are characteristic of SARS include dyspnea, tachypnea, and pleurisy (inflammation of the pleural membranes). One third of the affected individuals recovered uneventfully, two thirds had worsening symptoms and required more intense interventions. Admission into intensive care facilities and the use of mechanical ventilation was required for almost 30% of the patients who manifested worsening symptoms (Peiris et al., 2003). There is no vaccine for SARS as of this date. The dental professional who is aware of the potential signs and symptoms of this disease may be able to make a timely medical referral. In addition, cases of highly contagious diseases such as SARS should be reported to the local health department.

Name: Tuberculosis

Etiology: *Mycobacterium tuberculosis* is the etiologic agent associated with tuberculosis. Most of these organisms are susceptible to the drugs that are commonly used to treat an infection with them. However, over time, forms of the bacterium that are not susceptible to these drugs have developed. These organisms are multidrug-resistant (MDR) strains of *M. tuberculosis* that have developed in response to inappropriate drug therapy or as a result of incomplete or early discontinuation of treatment.

Method of Transmission: Tuberculosis is spread through inhalation of **droplet nuclei,** microscopic particles containing the *M. tuberculosis* organism. Transmission depends on the number of bacilli that are inhaled, the environment from which they are inhaled, the duration of the exposure, and the virulence of the organism. *M. tuberculosis* can also be spread by contact with contaminated surfaces.

Epidemiology: In the early to middle 1980s, after years of a steady decline in TB, there was an increase in the number of cases of tuberculosis in the United States. This increase was attributed to the HIV epidemic, the increase in the number of immigrants from areas that had endemic TB, outbreaks in institutional settings, and the emergence of a drug resistant form of bacteria. This increase continued until 1993, when the number of cases again started to drop. The CDC's most current data show that the 2005 TB rate of 14,093 new cases is the lowest reported since national TB data started being collected in 1953 (CDC, MMWR, March 24, 2006). More troubling are the data showing that 13% of new cases in 2004 were considered to be MDR, which was an increase over the number of cases in 2003 (CDC, MMWR, March 24, 2006). Factors that increase an individual's risk of acquiring tuberculosis infection are listed in Box 10.1.

Pathogenesis: After the organisms have been inhaled, they are carried into the alveoli, where they are surrounded by macrophages and ingested.

Most of the bacilli will be destroyed; however, some may survive within the macrophages and begin to multiply. Eventually the bacilli are released when the macrophage dies. The immune system is activated by antigen-presenting macrophages, and a cell-mediated immune response against the organism is mounted. This immune response is usually a localized inflammatory reaction in which the *M. tuberculosis* is surrounded by more macrophages and other white blood cells, creating a granuloma or tubercle. The tissues within the tubercle undergo caseous necrosis (Chapter 2), and the entire area becomes surrounded by fibrous scar tissue, effectively isolating any remaining *M. tuberculosis*. At this point the infection is contained, and the person is said to have latent TB infection. Some 90% of individuals with healthy immune systems who are exposed to *M. tuberculosis* remain in this status for the rest of their lives. They do not have active TB infection, and they are not considered to have a case of TB. They will, however, have positive Mantoux skin test results for the rest of their lives, because of a type 4 delayed hypersensitivity reaction (Chapter 4).

Approximately 10% of individuals with healthy immune systems progress to secondary TB within 2 years of the original infection or possibly many years later. Secondary TB can result from either a reactivation of the original infection or exposure to a second infection. Reactivation of the original infection is most often due to a change in the immune status of the individual, such as: the use of immunosuppressive drugs, infection with HIV, diabetes mellitus, head and neck cancer, end-stage renal disease, malnourishment, and intravenous substance abuse. The secondary infection differs from the primary infection. The immune response causes many tubercles to form, resulting in tissue destruction by both the infection and the hypersensitivity reaction that is caused by the bacteria. Large, cystic areas, or cavities, up to 10 cm in diameter, may form within the lungs (Fig. 10.1). If these cavities compromise or break through into a bronchus, the contents of the cavity will be released into the lungs, and the individual will cough up infected sputum. Lung collapse, **atelectasis**, can result if the formation of tubercles compromises the pleural cavity. **Hemoptysis**, blood in the sputum, results if one of the cavities destroys a pulmonary blood vessel, causing bleeding into the lungs. Blood vessel involvement and involvement of the lymphatic system can result in the circulation of TB throughout the body. Any organ or part of the body can therefore become infected; this diffuse infection is called acute miliary tuberculosis, or disseminated TB. Miliary TB can occur in either primary or secondary infections and most commonly affects the lungs, lymph nodes, kidneys, spleen, and liver.

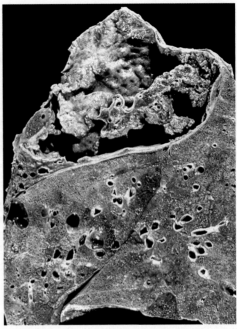

Figure 10.1. Secondary tuberculosis. This example of secondary tuberculosis shows the formation of a necrotic cavity involving the entire upper lobe. Involvement of any of the blood vessels, as was very likely, would have caused bleeding into the lung and hemoptysis. (From Cagle PT, Color atlas and text of pulmonary pathology. Philadelphia: Lippincott Williams & Wilkins, 2005.)

Extraoral Characteristics: Primary TB is usually asymptomatic, with most individuals only becoming aware of its presence when they have a positive Mantoux skin test. A positive test result should be followed by a chest x-ray to determine the presence of lung lesions. The final diagnosis is made by bacteriologic or histologic examination of the sputum, if present. The symptoms associated with secondary TB are afternoon fevers, night sweats, weight loss, weakness, chest pain, a productive cough (sputum), and hemoptysis.

Perioral and Intraoral Characteristics: Oral lesions usually develop secondary to a primary lung infection. Oral lesions are caused by implantation of infected sputum into a break in the mucosal surface during coughing episodes. Oral tuberculosis lesions appear as painful nonhealing ulcers found most often on the tongue, although they can be found on any mucosal surface (Fig. 10.2).

Dental Implications: Dental professionals need to be aware of the potential for the spread of tuberculosis within the dental office environment. There should be prompt detection of suspected cases, isolation of infectious patients, and referral for appropriate treatment. Persons with active TB should not be treated in dental facilities that do not have proper air treatment capabilities. For dental professionals to safely treat TB patients, the facility must have an effective ventilation system containing high-efficiency particulate air (HEPA) filtration and ultra-

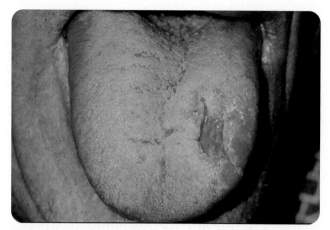

Figure 10.2. Oral tuberculosis ulcer. This oral ulcer is caused by implantation of *M. tuberculosis* from an already present lung infection in compromised oral mucosa. (Courtesy of the U. S. Department of Veteran's Affairs.)

violet germicidal irradiation (UVGI). Healthcare workers should use personal respirators effective at the N-95 particulate level in instances when air filtration and irradiation are not in use. Precautions to prevent the production of airborne particles should also be used, for example, using hand instrumentation instead of ultrasonic instruments during dental hygiene therapy.

Treatment and Prognosis: Individuals who are infected with the organism but who do not have active disease are usually treated with a prophylactic regimen to eliminate the organism and prevent a secondary infection. Active infection is treated with a combination of drugs to which the organism is susceptible in an effort to prevent the development of more resistant strains. The treatment regimen recommended for most individuals contains four drugs: (1) isoniazid, (2) rifampin, (3) pyrazinamide, and (4) either ethambutol or streptomycin. The drugs are usually given for 6 to 9 months. MDR tuberculosis presents extremely difficult treatment problems, and compliance with the treatment regimen should always be stressed, since the major variable in the outcome of drug therapy is patient compliance with the regimen.

Often patient compliance is lacking, usually due to the characteristics of the population that is at highest risk for the disease. Drug abusers, homeless persons, individuals with mental health alterations, and other high-risk individuals are not always the most reliable when it comes to being responsible for taking medications at a specific time. Even in areas where health workers are sent to deliver and watch the patient take the medication in a program called Directly Observed Therapy (DOT), treatment is often interrupted prior to completion. The development of MDR strains of *M. tuberculosis* is directly related to this problem. In the absence of complications, the prognosis for most individuals is good. The immune status of the host and the susceptibility of the organism to the medications currently available are significant factors in the determination of an individual's prognosis. The CDC reported

704 TB related deaths in 2003, or about 0.2 deaths per 100,000 individuals (CDC, September 2005).

Obstructive Pulmonary Diseases

Obstructive pulmonary diseases are associated with airway obstruction that is either chronic or episodic and in which difficult expiration or exhalation of air is the major presenting feature. Asthma, emphysema, chronic obstructive bronchitis, and cystic fibrosis, among others, are considered to be obstructive pulmonary diseases.

Name: Asthma

Etiology: Asthma is caused by an inflammatory reaction that occurs within the bronchial airways. The inflammatory reaction is caused by excessive sensitivity of the mucosal membranes and muscles to any number of triggers. See Box 10.2 for a list of possible triggers.

Epidemiology: Approximately 30 million Americans have been diagnosed with asthma at some time in their lives. Asthma is the number one serious chronic illness in children and the third leading cause of childhood hospitalizations. Women are afflicted with asthma more often than men, but only after puberty; until then, more boys than girls are affected. Asthma rates are significantly higher among African Americans (39%) than Caucasians (ALA, Lung Disease Data: 2006).

Pathogenesis: The inflammatory response is elicited by exposure to one of the triggers. This causes mast cell degranulation (Chapter 3) and the release of multiple chemical mediators, including histamine, prostaglandins, leukotrienes, and interleukins. The release of these substances causes smooth muscle spasm, mucosal edema, and the production of a thick and tenacious mucus. The end result of this process is hyperresponsiveness or hyperexcitability of the airways and airway obstruction. Airway obstruction interferes with the release of air from the areas of the lung that are distal to the obstruction and in-

Box 10.2   SUBSTANCES ASSOCIATED WITH THE INITIATION OF AN ASTHMA ATTACK

- Lung infections
- Tobacco smoke
- Allergies (molds, pollen, animals, etc.)
- Exercise
- Cold air
- Excitement
- Stress
- Drugs
- Air pollution

creases breathing difficulty. Individuals with asthma become cyanotic because they cannot exhale fully; therefore, they cannot inhale enough oxygen-rich air to keep the appropriate level of oxygen in the blood.

Extraoral Characteristics: After exposure to a trigger, the individual with asthma exhibits **paroxysms**, sharp spasms of wheezing, dyspnea, and cough. The wheezing initially appears during exhalation only but may affect inhalation as the attack progresses. Exhalation becomes so difficult that the accessory muscles of expiration must be mobilized. The individual who is having trouble breathing becomes anxious, which only adds to the hyperresponsiveness of the airways. If the attack is not brought under control by initial administration of medication, the individual is said to have status asthmaticus, a life-threatening emergency. Status asthmaticus may continue for hours or even days without remission. The patient should never be discharged from the dental office while still experiencing symptoms of an attack, emergency medical services should be contacted, and treatment in a hospital emergency room is essential (Malamed, 2000).

Perioral and Intraoral Characteristics: Asthma does not cause any specific manifestations in the oral cavity. However, the medications that are taken by individuals with asthma may contribute to several oral conditions. One of the most common oral side effects of inhaled corticosteroids is an increased risk of oral fungal infections (candidiasis, Chapter 14). Many of the medications that are used to treat asthma have the potential to cause xerostomia (dry mouth), which is associated with a higher rate of caries and periodontal or gingival infections. In addition, an increase in gastroesophageal reflux, associated with some asthma medications, can cause a higher than normal oral pH (acidic), which is related to enamel erosion.

Dental Implications: Dental hygienists have the opportunity to help individuals with asthma to maintain healthy oral tissues by educating them about the adverse effects of the drugs they may be taking. In addition, the dental hygienist should make homecare recommendations focused on controlling the oral effects of the medications. A thorough review of the patient's medical/dental history should make the dental professional aware of the patient's risk for having an asthma attack during dental treatment. Steps should be taken to prevent exposing the patient to triggers and to facilitate treatment of the patient should an attack occur. Some preventive measures include stress management, aerosol control to limit the potential of inhaling foreign matter, and avoiding the use of latex-containing gloves and disposables. The patient's medication should be available and readily accessible throughout the entire dental appointment.

Treatment and Prognosis: Medical therapy for asthma consists of the use of bronchodilators to open the airways and antiinflammatory medications to interfere with and/or prevent the inflammatory response, such as leukotriene modifiers that block the action of leukotrienes (Chapter 3) and corticosteroids. Epinephrine (1:1,000 or 1:10,000) may be necessary to control asthma during a severe attack. Emergency medical services should be summoned if the administration of epinephrine appears to be indicated (Malamed, 2000).

The American Lung Association reports that deaths from asthma in the United States have been declining for the last 5 years. The most recent mortality data estimates that 4000 Americans died from asthma in 2002 (ALA, Lung Disease Data: 2006).

Name: Chronic obstructive pulmonary disease (COPD)

Etiology: There are two forms of COPD: (1) emphysema and (2) chronic obstructive bronchitis. Smoking and inhaling secondhand smoke are the most common causes associated with COPD. In addition, air pollution and occupational exposure to toxic inhalants have been linked to cases of COPD.

Epidemiology: In 2003 about 10.7 million Americans had COPD, most having chronic obstructive bronchitis. Most of those affected were over the age of 45, and most were Caucasians. In recent years males and females have been equally affected (ALA, Lung Disease Data: 2006).

Pathogenesis: Emphysema is characterized by decreased elasticity of lung tissue and destruction of alveolar tissue, resulting in enlarged air spaces and increased total lung capacity. Chronic obstructive bronchitis is characterized by obstruction of the small airways by inflamed and hyperplastic mucosal tissues accompanied by excessive production of mucus.

Extraoral Characteristics: Individuals with emphysema have been called "pink puffers" because they are able to maintain normal blood oxygen levels by increasing their rate of breathing. They often present with a "barrel chest," which results from an increase in the size of the chest because of air becoming trapped in the lungs. Exhaustion after minor activity is common because of the amount of energy required to just keep breathing. Eating becomes a problem because the individual cannot stop breathing long enough to swallow, and drastic weight loss is often experienced in advanced disease.

Individuals with chronic obstructive bronchitis have been called "blue bloaters" because they cannot maintain a normal level of oxygen in their blood by simply increasing their respiratory rate. Cyanosis is common in chronic bronchitis and occurs because the airways are blocked by inflamed and hyperplastic tissues and by the presence of excessive mucus and fluids that interfere with oxygen exchange. These individuals have marked shortness of breath and usually present with a productive cough that has worsened over the course of many years.

Dental Implications: Maintaining patient comfort and an adequate oxygen level during dental treatment is imperative. The position of the dental chair may have to be modified so that the patient is in a comfortable position for breathing, and supplemental oxygen may be indicated. Procedures that create aerosols, such as ultrasonic scaling and air abrasion or polishing, should be avoided in most cases. Tobacco cessation interventions may also be appropriate for patients who continue to smoke.

Treatment and Prognosis: Most patients seek medical care when COPD is in an advanced stage. The lung damage is irreversible, but there are treatments that can improve the individual's quality of life. Common medications that are used to control the symptoms and slow the progression of the disease include (1) bronchodilators that open the airways, (2) antiinflammatory medications that inhibit or prevent the inflammatory response, and (3) expectorants that help to clear the excess mucus from the lungs. By far the most important adjunct to treatment is tobacco cessation for those who smoke. In 2002, 120,555 Americans died from COPD. Eighty to 90% of these deaths were related to smoking (ALA, Lung Disease Data: 2006).

Name: Cystic fibrosis (CF)

Etiology: Cystic fibrosis is an inherited disorder resulting from a mutation of the *CF* gene on chromosome 7.

Method of Transmission: Cystic fibrosis follows an autosomal recessive inheritance pattern.

Epidemiology: According to the American Lung Association, 30,000 Americans have cystic fibrosis, and 1,000 new cases are diagnosed each year. It affects males and females equally and is considered the most common lethal autosomal disorder in the Caucasian population (ALA, Lung Disease Data: 2006).

Pathogenesis: The genetic abnormality causes the development of defective epithelial cells, specifically those lining the respiratory system, bile ducts, pancreas, and sweat ducts. The defect causes these cells to produce abnormally thick mucus. All of the pathologic consequences of cystic fibrosis can be attributed to this abnormal mucus obstructing the lumina of the affected organs. Blocked pancreatic ducts decrease fat metabolism, decrease the absorption of fat-soluble vitamins, and decrease body weight. Excessive salt is lost through defective sweat glands causing electrolyte imbalance and leaving the individual susceptible to heat exhaustion. The most serious complications involve the lungs, resulting in chronic pulmonary disease and frequent infections. Death is usually the result of respiratory failure related to damage done by repeated lung infections.

Extraoral Characteristics: The most common symptoms of cystic fibrosis are chronic coughing or wheezing accompanied by recurrent severe lung infections. The individual with CF may be underweight and may have a barrel chest.

Perioral and Intraoral Characteristics: Patients may present with a high caries rate due to frequent ingestion of high-caloric foods necessary to maintain an appropriate weight. Medications may cause xerostomia and/or the quality of the saliva may be altered by the disease, the medications, or both. Inadequate levels of vitamin K may cause excessive gingival bleeding, especially in the presence of oral infections.

Dental Implications: Patients with CF usually take prophylactic antibiotic medications to prevent lung infections (usually from *Staphylococcus aureus* or *Pseudomonas aeruginosa*) for their entire lives. Medical consultation should be obtained to determine any need for additional prophylactic antibiotics to decrease the risk of respiratory infection due to the aspiration of oral bacteria during dental procedures. Any dental procedure that produces aerosols should be avoided. The patient should be positioned in the dental chair in a manner that optimizes respiration and aids in mucus drainage. Patients with CF are not considered candidates for nitrous oxide analgesia. Vitamin K supplements may be needed to enhance blood clot formation prior to procedures in which bleeding is anticipated. Homecare recommendations focus on preventing caries and maintaining healthy oral tissues, which will decrease the number of oral bacteria (DeAngelis, 2001).

Treatment and Prognosis: The mainstays of treatment focus on preventing the respiratory complications associated with cystic fibrosis. Inhaled and oral antibiotics are used to treat and prevent lung infections. Other inhaled drugs are used to thin out the thick mucus in the lungs. Bronchodilators help open the airways, and mechanical chest therapy helps to break up the mucus in the lungs. The patients usually take vitamin supplements, pancreatic enzyme supplements, oral corticosteroids, antigastroesophageal reflux medications, and laxatives to manage the effects of the disease.

The prognosis for those affected by this disease is improving. Only 484 individuals died from this disease in the United States in 2002. About 50% are now expected to live past the age of 20 years (ALA, Lung Disease Data: 2006).

THE GASTROINTESTINAL SYSTEM

The gastrointestinal system is responsible for the ingestion, digestion, and absorption of food, as well as the elimination of wastes from the body. The oral cavity is the starting point for all of the actions of this system. Mastication (chewing) breaks the food into small pieces and mixes it with saliva. Saliva lubricates the bolus of food and contains salivary amylase, which starts the digestion of carbohydrates. The food is swallowed in a complex action that is usually automatic. The motor impulses for swallowing are supplied by the trigeminal, glossopharyngeal, vagus, and hypoglossal cranial nerves. Once the bolus is moved into the esophagus and swallowed, involuntary muscle contractions cause **peristalsis** (rhythmic muscle contractions that propel the food toward the stomach). The lower esophageal sphincter controls the entrance of food into the stomach; therefore, it is the culprit when food and gastric juices back up out of the stomach and into the esophagus during vomiting and in cases of gastric reflux. The stomach is lined by special mucosal cells that secrete digestive enzymes and hydrochloric acid, which activates the enzymes. It also contains copious amounts of thick mucus that protect the lining of the stomach from the acidic environment. The gastric juices mix with the food and create a semidigested mixture called chyme. The chyme is released from the stomach through the pyloric sphincter into the small intestine, where peristalsis moves it along. Most of the digestion of food takes place in the upper part of the small intestine, or duodenum. Here the pancreas secretes enzymes through the pancreatic duct, which aid in the digestion of proteins, lipids, and carbohydrates. It also secretes an alkaline substance that neutralizes the acid from the stomach. Bile, manufactured in the liver, enters the duodenum from its storage area in the gall bladder through the common bile duct. Bile is an **emulsifier** (a substance that allows fat to mix with water) that facilitates the digestion of lipids. The nutrients are absorbed into capillaries and lymph vessels that are found in the surface of the small intestine. The surface area of the small intestine is vast, because it is covered with many tiny projections called villi that increase the surface area of the intestine and thereby help to absorb more nutrients. The substance that is left after digestion passes through the small intestine into the large intestine, where water and minerals are absorbed into the body. The remaining waste is eliminated as feces. Many gastrointestinal disorders have oral manifestations associated with them. This section discusses a few of the more common disorders.

Name: Dysphagia

Etiology: Dysphagia, difficulty swallowing, can result from a physical obstruction or a muscular or neurologic disorder. Tumors (neoplastic growths) and pockets (**diverticula**) that form in the wall of the esophagus can obstruct the flow of food from the mouth to the stomach. Individuals with scleroderma (Chapter 23) may exhibit fibrosis of the muscle layer in the esophagus, causing dysphagia. Strokes can cause damage to the nerves that control the muscles of swallowing and impair a person's ability to safely swallow food.

Perioral and Intraoral Characteristics: Pain occurring during and within 2 to 5 seconds after swallowing usually indicates a problem in the upper esophagus, while pain occurring 10 to 15 seconds later indicates a lower esophageal problem. If the dysphagia is due to diverticula, food may lodge in the pouches and ferment, causing a foul odor and increasing the risk of infections. Swallowing difficulties associated with nerve or muscle dysfunction can cause food to be aspirated into the lungs, resulting in pneumonia. This type of dysphagia can also cause the regurgitation of food and can limit the individual's ability to ingest adequate nutrients, resulting in malnourishment.

Dental Implications: The patient must be properly positioned in the dental chair to decrease the risk of accidental aspiration of oral fluids during dental treatment. Dietary modifications that are necessary to decrease the problems associated with dysphagia may encourage increased caries activity, and preventive strategies should be included in homecare recommendations.

Treatment and Prognosis: Treatment depends on the cause of the dysphagia. Physical therapy to train muscles that control mastication and swallowing has helped in cases of stroke or other neurologic impairments. Eating small meals, eating slowly, and preparing foods in a form that is easier to swallow are important elements for managing dysphagia. The main objectives of treatment are maintaining proper nutrition, eliminating pain, and preventing aspiration of food into the lungs.

Name: Gastroesophageal reflux disease (GERD)

Etiology: GERD is caused by a weak lower esophageal sphincter that allows the flow of gastric contents back into the esophagus.

Epidemiology: About 7% of the United States population experiences symptoms of heartburn daily. It is estimated that 20 to 40% of these people have GERD, while the rest have other problems (Fisichella and Patti, September 2006). Males and females are equally affected, and while the disorder can occur at any age, it occurs more frequently over the age of 40 (Fisichella and Patti, September 2006).

Pathogenesis: Exposure of the esophagus to the acid in the gastric contents causes mucosal erosions that can eventually cause permanent tissue damage. The most severe form of damage is called Barrett esophagitis and is associated with an increased risk of esophageal cancer.

Perioral and Intraoral Characteristics: In addition to cancer of the esophagus, cancer of the pharynx and the tonsils have been found to be associated with GERD. GERD has also been associated with an increased risk of enamel erosion in some individuals (Fig. 10.3).

Dental Implications: Dental appointment modifications include positioning the patient's chair in a more

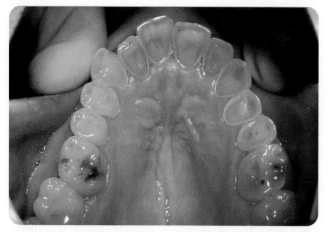

Figure 10.3. Enamel erosion. This extensive enamel erosion was seen in an individual with chronic severe GERD of more than 10 years duration.

semisupine position for the patient's comfort, especially during longer appointments. Specific attention should be given to the pharyngeal and tonsillar areas during the intraoral examination, because of the increased risk of cancer associated with GERD. Education about the oral effects of GERD and recommendation of additional fluoride to counteract increased levels of oral acid are appropriate. Custom trays can be fabricated to provide optimal contact between the teeth and the fluoride.

Treatment and Prognosis: Treatment includes use of medications that decrease the production of acid in the stomach, modifying eating habits, and avoiding foods that cause the lower sphincter to be less effective, such as alcohol, caffeine, chocolate, and fats. Smoking has been associated with an increased risk of GERD; therefore, cessation therapy is advised for those suffering from this disorder. Reflux occurs more easily when the person is in a supine position, and sleeping with the head elevated is advised.

Barrett esophagitis occurs in about 376 of every 100,000 men and women in the United States. It is estimated that 5%, or 18, of these progress to adenocarcinoma every year (Johnston and Eastone, June 2005).

Name: Peptic ulcer

Etiology: Peptic ulcers occur in the duodenum and less frequently in the stomach. The most common cause of peptic ulcer is infection with *Helicobacter pylori (H. pylori)*; the second most common cause is medications containing aspirin or other nonsteroidal antiinflammatory drugs (NSAIDs) (Porth, 2004). Other factors that are associated with peptic ulcers include smoking, alcohol, older age, and some chronic diseases such as emphysema and diabetes (Huether, McCance, 2004).

Pathogenesis: Infection with *H. pylori* causes the creation of ammonia, which destroys mucosal cells. Likewise, NSAIDs interfere with the production of mucus.

Both processes compromise the effectiveness of the mucosal barrier in the stomach or small intestine. Once the barrier is compromised, underlying tissues come in contact with the acidic gastric contents, and ulceration occurs. If left untreated, the ulcers can cause excessive loss of blood, perforation of the stomach or duodenum, obstructions due to swelling associated with inflammation, or scarring associated with repeated injuries.

Extraoral Characteristics: Pain that is relieved by eating is the most common presentation of peptic ulcers. Anorexia, weight loss, and vomiting are more common with ulcers in the stomach than those in the duodenum.

Dental Implications: Frequent eating to alleviate pain may increase caries activity, especially if cariogenic foods are chosen. Vomiting, if present, increases the risk of enamel erosion, and the patient should be advised about not brushing immediately after vomiting. Home fluoride treatments and nutrition counseling should be considered for these patients.

Treatment and Prognosis: Treatment focuses on eliminating the infection and decreasing the acid level in the stomach. The most common therapy is a combination of antibiotics with drugs that lower the amount of acid that is produced (such as proton pump inhibitors). When aspirin and/or NSAIDs are the cause of the ulcers, the most appropriate course of action is to eliminate the drugs. This may not always be possible; therefore, the use of antacids and drugs that lower the acid levels may be helpful. The prognosis for most patients is excellent.

Name: Malabsorption syndromes

Etiology: Malabsorption refers to the body's inability to absorb specific substances from the digestive tract. The substances can be vitamins, minerals, or fats. There are several causes associated with malabsorption syndromes, including: chronic intestinal disease, removal of large sections of the intestine, deficiency of specific digestive enzymes, or deficiency of bile acids.

Pathogenesis: Celiac sprue is an example of a malabsorption syndrome caused by a hypersensitivity reaction to gluten, a substance found in wheat, rye, barley, and oat grains in the diet. Gluten appears to cause an autoimmune reaction in which the intestinal villi are destroyed, leaving large ulcerative lesions, and resulting in poor nutrient absorption across the affected mucosal surfaces (Porth, 2004).

A deficiency in pancreatic enzymes or bile acids causes poor digestion of most nutrients, especially fats and fat-soluble vitamins. Symptoms associated with this condition are related to deficiencies of vitamins A, D, E, and K. Diarrhea, fatty stools, flatulence (passing gas), bloating, pain, and cramping are all associated with ineffective absorption of fats. Vitamin K is essential for proper clot formation, and any deficiency is associated with increased bleeding.

Lactase deficiencies, or the production of a defective lactase enzyme, will produce what is commonly referred to as lactose intolerance. Lactose intolerance leads to the accumulation of undigested lactose in the intestine. Bacteria ferment the lactose, producing gases that cause pain, bloating, and flatulence. Diarrhea is a common symptom due to a change in the rate of water absorption caused by the abundance of lactose.

Extraoral Characteristics: Not applicable

Perioral and Intraoral Characteristics: Occasionally, malabsorption syndromes are associated with oral ulcers, glossitis (Fig. 10.4), and angular cheilitis, all of which are linked to nutrient deficiencies.

Dental Implications: It is important to identify the patient with a malabsorption syndrome to take appropriate measures to manage any oral manifestations. This is especially important since these manifestations can mimic many other oral lesions, such as aphthous ulcers and fungal infections.

Treatment and Prognosis: Once malabsorption syndromes have been identified, most can be controlled by avoiding foods that exacerbate the condition, providing supplements to prevent nutrient deficiencies, and in some cases replacing the enzymes that are deficient.

Name: Crohn's disease

Etiology: The etiology of Crohn's disease is unknown. It is suspected that there may be a genetic component because 10 to 20% of affected individuals have a positive family history of the disease (Huether and McCance, 2004). It is also suspected that immune system dysfunction associated with increased suppressor T cell activity, defective IgA production, and possible interactions with

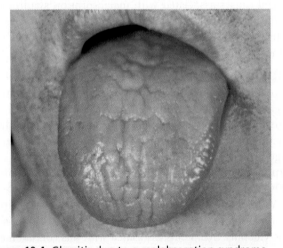

Figure 10.4. Glossitis due to a malabsorption syndrome. Vitamin or iron deficiencies that result from malabsorption syndromes cause atrophy of the papillae and create a smooth, often sore, tongue. (From Weber J, Kelley J. Health assessment in nursing. 2nd ed.. Philadelphia: Lippincott Williams & Wilkins, 2003.)

indigenous gastrointestinal bacteria might contribute to causing the disease.

Pathogenesis: Crohn's disease is a chronic inflammatory disorder of the granulomatous type that affects the gastrointestinal tract at any point from the oral cavity to the anus. The characteristic ulcerative lesion involves all layers of the tissues in the GI tract. The lesions may be found scattered among normal mucosal tissues. The ulcerations usually progress into deep fissures, which may eventually form fistulas that communicate with other parts of the GI tract or with the skin, bladder, or vagina. Fistulas have the potential to become infected, thereby creating abscesses. The chronic nature of the inflammation causes affected tissues to become fibrotic and thickened, leading to malabsorption syndromes. The risk of colon cancer is increased in those with long-term disease (Rowe, June 2006).

Extraoral Characteristics: The most common symptom presentation is an irritable bowel manifesting as either constipation or diarrhea. There is often crampy pain in the lower right abdomen. Vitamin deficiencies associated with malabsorption of nutrients are common, as are weight loss, low energy levels, and low-grade fevers. Children with Crohn's disease are likely to experience growth retardation. Ulcers that perforate the mucosal lining may cause chronic loss of blood, resulting in anemia.

Perioral and Intraoral Characteristics: Compromised mucosal tissues result in aphthouslike ulcers seen on the buccal and labial mucosa and the tongue. These ulcers are sometimes multiple and large, and they are deep, because the lower layers of the mucosa are affected. Other oral manifestations may include diffuse swelling of the buccal and labial mucosa, angular cheilitis, glossitis, and cobblestoning (mild fissuring) of the buccal mucosa. The oral manifestations are usually associated with exacerbation of the intestinal symptoms (constipation or diarrhea and pain). and they tend to resolve when the intestinal disease is under control (Gurenlian, 2003).

Dental Implications: The patient should be educated about the benefits of maintaining a healthy oral environment as a means of helping to prevent the oral complications of Crohn's disease. Pain management should be accomplished without using NSAIDs or aspirin-containing products, since they tend to affect the mucosal tissues of the GI tract.

Treatment and Prognosis: Treatment focuses on controlling the inflammation, eliminating or preventing nutritional deficiencies, preventing complications, and relieving symptoms. Current therapies include medications such as: antiinflammatories, immunosuppressants, antidiarrheal agents or laxatives, and some new drugs that affect certain chemical mediators crucial to the activation of the inflammatory response (tumor necrosis factor). Nutritional supplements are necessary to prevent nutrient deficiencies. If these treatments are unsuccessful or if there are complications such as fistula or abscess formation, surgery to remove the diseased section of the intestine is indicated. Occasionally, patients must have their entire colon removed, after which solid wastes are removed through a colostomy and collected in a colostomy bag. Oral lesions are treated with topical steroids, if necessary.

Crohn's disease is a chronic debilitating disease that is characterized by frequent remissions and exacerbations. The mortality rate of those with Crohn's disease is higher than in the general population because of a higher risk of affected individuals developing gastrointestinal cancer than those without the disease (Chen and Zhou, 2004).

Name: Peutz-Jeghers syndrome

Etiology: Peutz-Jeghers syndrome is an inherited condition that results from a mutation of gene *LKB1* on the short arm (p) of chromosome 19.

Method of Transmission: Peutz-Jeghers syndrome follows an autosomal dominant inheritance pattern.

Extraoral Characteristics: Individuals with this genetic mutation have multiple intestinal polyps that resemble neoplastic growths but are comprised of normal cells and grow at a normal rate. The polyps may also occur in the stomach or the colon. This genetic disorder is associated with an increased risk for developing cancers of the breast, pancreas, testis, and ovary in addition to the increased risk of developing adenocarcinoma of the lining of the GI tract.

Perioral and Intraoral Characteristics: The striking melanin pigmentation that forms on the buccal and labial mucosa and skin of the face, hands, and feet is characteristic of this condition (Fig. 10.5).

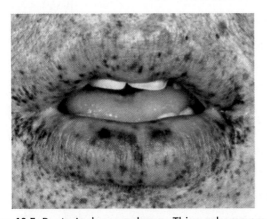

Figure 10.5. Peutz-Jeghers syndrome. This syndrome presents with pigmented spots on the lips that are more prominent than the freckling of the surrounding skin. Pigment in the buccal mucosa helps to confirm the diagnosis. The hands and face may also have scattered pigmented spots. (From Robinson HBG, Miller AS: Colby, Kerr, and Robinson's color atlas of oral pathology. Philadelphia: JB Lippincott, 1990.)

Dental Implications: Dental professionals need to be aware of the characteristic pigmentation to make appropriate referrals when indicated.

Treatment and Prognosis: Treatment consists of identification of the syndrome and careful monitoring of the tissues that are at risk for cancer development. Intestinal polyps are usually removed when discovered during colonoscopy. Approximately 3% of patients develop intestinal adenocarcinoma (Rubin et al., 2005).

NERVOUS SYSTEM

The nervous system is designed to receive sensory information, process it, and determine what actions to take to maintain homeostasis. It also protects the body with little or no conscious thought by the individual. There are two main parts of the nervous system: (1) the central nervous system (CNS), which comprises the brain and the spinal cord, and (2) the peripheral nervous system (PNS), which comprises all nervous tissues found outside the CNS. The neuron is the basic cell of both systems. The neuron is so specialized that other cells must help to provide nutritional and other metabolic support. Schwann cells provide nutritional and metabolic support for the PNS; glial cells, such as the oligodendroglia, provide these functions for the CNS. These cells also produce the myelin sheaths that cover the axons of the neurons. Myelin increases the rate of transmission of a nerve impulse and is necessary for the continued existence of the axon.

Glucose is the major energy source for the nervous system. Since there is no place to store glucose in the neurons, these cells depend on a constant availability of glucose in the blood. Nervous tissue consumes high levels of oxygen, which it also has no place to store. In addition, unlike some other tissues, nervous tissue cannot undergo anaerobic metabolism. Nerve cells become nonfunctional after about 10 seconds without oxygen and begin to die within 4 to 6 minutes. The disorders discussed in this section have their basis in the tissues of the nervous system.

Name: Meningitis and encephalitis

Etiology: Meningitis is an inflammation of the meninges, the membranes that cover the brain and the spinal cord. Encephalitis is an inflammation of the nerve tissues of the brain and/or spinal cord. Both of these conditions can be caused by a variety of organisms. Bacteria such as: *Escherichia coli, Haemophilus influenzae, Streptococcus pneumoniae,* and *Neisseria meningitidis* are the most common cause of bacterial meningitis. Viral meningitis is most often associated with enteroviruses, such as coxsackievirus B; however, mumps, Epstein-Barr, and herpes simplex viruses have all been linked to the infection. Encephalitis can be caused by bacteria, viruses, fungi, or other organisms. Rabies is an example of a virus that specifically targets the nervous tissue of the brain, causing encephalitis. Herpes simplex is one of the more common agents associated with viral encephalitis. Viruses carried by insects such as mosquitoes and ticks may also cause encephalitis. Western and Eastern equine encephalitis are carried by the mosquito that bites an infected animal to the human whom it bites next.

Epidemiology: Approximately 0.5 to 1.1 individuals per 100,000 population, or 1400 to 2800 cases of meningococcal disease occur in the United States every year. Of interest is the fact that college students who reside in dormitories are 9 to 23 times more likely to contract this infection than students who live off campus (MMWR 2005, 54[no. RR-7]).

Pathogenesis: In meningitis, the organisms infect all layers of the covering of the brain and or the spinal cord. Bacterial infection produces purulent exudate that blocks movement of the cerebrospinal fluid and pinches off the capillary blood supply, causing tiny infarcts in the tissues. If not treated, the infection causes edema of the brain, coma, and death. Viral meningitis follows a less severe, self-limiting course, with no production of purulent exudate.

Encephalitis causes generalized edema, hemorrhage, and necrosis of brain and spinal tissues. Most forms of encephalitis target specific areas of the central nervous system.

Extraoral Characteristics: Meningitis and encephalitis exhibit similar symptoms of headache, stiff neck, fever, chills, nausea, vomiting, altered mental status, and pain in the back, abdomen, and extremities. Meningitis symptoms often have an abrupt onset with rapid development of symptoms, sometimes leading to death within 24 hours. Individuals with meningitis may exhibit a petechial rash that covers large portions of the body.

Dental Implications: Dental professionals need to be aware of the signs and symptoms of these infections to make an appropriate medical referral if they are observed in a patient.

Treatment and Prognosis: Treatment depends on the etiologic agent. Antibiotics are given for a bacterial infection. Corticosteroids are often given to offset the inflammatory response to massive bacterial deaths and the subsequent release of endotoxins from the cell walls.

The CDC recommends routine immunization against *N. meningitidis*, the most common cause of bacterial meningitis, for all preadolescents, teenagers, and college-bound students (MMWR 2005; 54[no. RR-7]).

The prognosis depends on the general health and immune status of the individual. The highest mortality rates are associated with individuals who have a compromised immune system, low level of consciousness, and infection with *S. pneumoniae*. In any case, the potential exists for neurologic damage causing seizures and decreased mental capacity after resolution of the infection.

Name: Parkinson's disease

Etiology: Parkinson's disease (PD) is a degenerative disease of the basal ganglia located at the base of the cerebral hemisphere. The exact cause is unknown; however, genetic, viral, and environmental agents have been suggested. Genetic factors may be more involved with PD that occurs early in life, at about 40 years of age.

Epidemiology: The American Parkinson Disease Association estimates that 1.5 million Americans are affected by PD. The disease occurs more often in men and more frequently in those over the age of 60 (APDA, 2006).

Pathogenesis: PD originates within a region in the brainstem called the substantia nigra. Cells within the substantia nigra produce the neurotransmitter dopamine, which enables cells of the CNS to function correctly, thereby controlling movement and balance. In PD, the cells of the substantia nigra are destroyed, and the level of dopamine decreases, causing a syndrome of abnormal movement. This syndrome is characterized by **bradykinesia** (slowed movements), resting tremor (alleviated by voluntary movement), muscle rigidity, and postural abnormalities.

Extraoral Characteristics: See Figure 10.6 for a listing of the physical characteristics of PD. Nonmotor symptoms are associated with autonomic nervous system dysfunction and can include sleep disturbances, depression, dementia, constipation, hyperhydrosis (excessive sweating), and urinary incontinence.

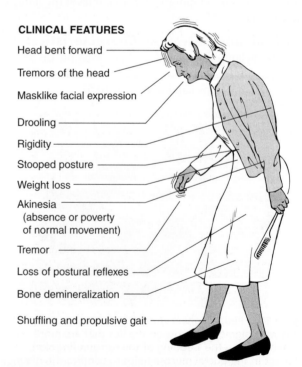

Figure 10.6. Parkinson's disease. Illustration showing the typical physical characteristics of Parkinson's disease. (Reprinted with permission from Rosdahl CB. Book of basic nursing. 7th ed. Philadelphia: Lippincott-Raven; 1999:1063.)

Perioral and Intraoral Characteristics:

Patients with PD often exhibit masklike facial features. Tremors affect the muscles of mastication and facial expression. Constant **parafunctional** (not related to mastication) jaw movements cause an increase in enamel attrition and **abfraction** (loss of tooth structure due to biomechanical forces). As the disease progresses, the muscles of the tongue and throat become more rigid and result in dysphagia and unintelligible speech. Dysphagia may become so severe that the patient is unable to eat and must be fed through a feeding tube. The patient drools because of infrequent swallowing and pooling of the saliva in the anterior of the mouth.

Dental Implications:

Dental healthcare workers need to modify some of their appointment procedures for patients who have PD. All precautions should be taken to avoid patient and operator injuries from sharp instruments that may occur due to the uncontrolled motions that are characteristic of this disease. Mouth props and bite blocks may help to keep the mouth open and stable. Also, the use of a rubber dam may avoid saliva contamination during restorative procedures. Pillows or gentle hand pressure will help to stabilize the patient's head in the headrest during treatment. The patient should be gradually raised from the supine position after dental care, since some medications that are given to control PD may cause postural hypotension. Xerostomia is a side effect of many of the PD medications, and frequent use of fluoride is recommended. It is difficult for some patients with PD to tolerate the normal tray delivery; therefore, fluoride varnish instead of trays is recommended. Supplemental fluoride in the form of a gel, not rinse, should be used daily. The patient with PD should have frequent maintenance appointments to monitor oral health. Every effort should be made to adapt homecare implements to the specific needs and abilities of the patient, to provide independence for as long as possible. Examples of modifications include increasing the width of toothbrush handles and using floss holders. Mechanical toothbrushes may be useful in many instances. Caregivers should be trained to use appropriate homecare procedures to maintain the patient's oral health when necessary (Mitchell, 2006).

Treatment and Prognosis:

Medical treatment is available for the symptoms of PD, but no treatment will reverse the course of the disease. There are drugs available that prevent the degradation of dopamine and thereby increase its availability. Other drugs stimulate the same receptors as dopamine on the neurons, mimicking its action and decreasing the need for dopamine. All patients with PD will eventually take levodopa, a drug that is converted to dopamine by the body, thereby elevating its level. Long-term therapy with levodopa and continued neural degeneration often produces dyskinesias. **Dyskinesias** are uncontrollable movements including writhing, twitching, and shaking. Continued use of levodopa at this time is usually not tolerated by the patient, and other means of controlling the symptoms should be considered. Surgery is one of these options. Irreversible surgical procedures destroy specific portions of the brain that are involved with the creation of movements, while sparing sensory and motor neurons. Deep brain stimulation is a relatively new form of therapy that uses implanted electrodes to produce constant electrical stimulation of areas of the brain that affect unwanted motions. This procedure is promising some hope for patients with PD who have not responded well to medical therapy.

Continued neural degeneration eventually leads to death, often from aspiration pneumonia. In 2003, 0.7% of the total deaths (17,997) in the United States were attributed to PD. PD is considered the 14th leading cause of death in the United States at this time (Hoyert et al., 2006).

Name: Bell's palsy

Etiology:

The herpes simplex virus is considered to be the prime suspect in most cases of Bell's palsy at this time (Shenaq, Kim, August 2005). Box 10.3 lists examples of other suspected etiologic agents associated with facial nerve paralysis, or Bell's palsy.

Epidemiology:

Bell's palsy affects approximately 23 of every 100,000 individuals in the United States. Males and females are affected equally, and most have unilateral paralysis of the right side. The population under the age of 10 has the lowest incidence, while those over 60 years have the highest incidence. Individuals with diabetes and pregnant women in their third trimester have the highest risk of developing this condition (Monnell and Zachariah, June 2005).

Pathogenesis:

The specific pathogenesis depends on the etiology of the paralysis. The paralysis is thought to result from edema and compression of the nerve or **demyelination** (loss of the myelin sheath) and subsequent death of the neurons. The end result, however, is total or partial paralysis of the tissues innervated by the affected facial nerve (Fig. 10.7). The severity of the dysfunction is rated on a scale from mild dysfunction to total paralysis. The functions that are evaluated include forehead wrinkling, eye closure, widely smiling, whistling, and blowing air through puckered lips. The palsy may be temporary, recurrent, or permanent.

Extraoral Characteristics:

The symptoms associated with Bell's palsy depend on the extent of facial nerve involvement and can include keratoconjunctivitis sicca (dry eyes), posterior auricular pain, facial numbness, and **hyperacusis** (increased sensitivity to sound because of relaxed muscles in the ear). Normally, the individual is unable to completely close the eye and will roll the affected eye upward and inward in an attempt to do so (Bell phenomenon).

Box 10.3 — SUSPECTED ETIOLOGIES ASSOCIATED WITH FACIAL NERVE PARALYSIS

- Birth trauma
- Accidental trauma
  - o Brain injuries
  - o Facial injuries
  - o Electrical injuries
- Infections
  - o Herpes simplex and numerous other bacterial and viral organisms
  - o Ramsey-Hunt syndrome
  - o Otitis media
- Diabetes
- Hyperthyroidism
- Hypertension
- Pregnancy
- Neoplastic growths
- Alcoholism
- Iatrogenic
  - o Mandibular block injections
  - o Postimmunization
  - o Parotid or mastoid surgery
  - o Tonsillectomy
  - o Dental surgery
- Idiopathic
  - o Familial
  - o Melkersson-Rosenthal syndrome
  - o Multiple sclerosis
  - o Myasthenia gravis
  - o Sarcoidosis

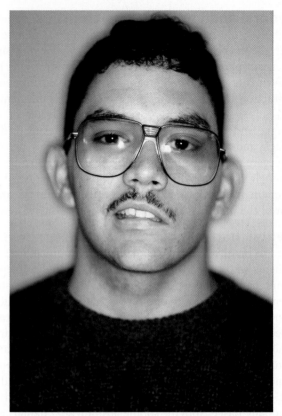

Figure 10.7. Bell's palsy. This patient has paralysis of the left side of his face, affecting the muscles innervated by the facial nerve. (Courtesy of Dr. Carolyn Bentley.)

Perioral and Intraoral Characteristics: Patients are not able to smile and complain of drooling because of lip incompetence. Speech may be slurred, and mastication and swallowing may be impaired. The gag reflex may be inhibited also. Xerostomia may be present because of lack of nerve stimulation of the salivary glands on the affected side and because the mouth is always partially open. Sensory loss may occur in addition to paralysis of the muscles innervated by the facial nerve. Taste disturbances are common, and the individual may consistently traumatize the oral mucosa and not be aware of it.

Dental Implications: While safety glasses should be provided for all patients, it is especially important for patients like the Bell's palsy patients, who can not close their eyes completely. Patients should be given appropriate postoperative instructions after treatment that has included local anesthetic use on the nonaffected side, to avoid accidental trauma. Patients with Bell's palsy should have frequent maintenance appointments to monitor their oral health. Bell's palsy compromises the

natural cleansing mechanisms of the oral environment, resulting in food and debris accumulation in the side of the mouth that is affected. Diminished feelings in the affected area also contribute to food retention. Xerostomia and food retention enhance caries activity, making frequent fluoride use important. Nighttime xerostomia may be severe, and saliva substitutes may be appropriate. Refer to Clinical Protocol 4 for additional suggestions to manage xerostomia.

Treatment and Prognosis: Most patients recover completely from Bell's palsy within 6 weeks to 3 months. Those with a less favorable outcome are usually over the age of 60 and have total paralysis, hyposalivation, and taste disturbances. Medical therapy depends on the suspected etiology of the condition. Most often corticosteroids and acyclovir are used alone or in combination for specified lengths of time. Performing surgical procedures on individuals with less than optimal recoveries has been successful in restoring more normal function to the tissues innervated by the facial nerve. Some of the procedures that are being used involve nerve grafting and relocation and muscle transfer from one area to another. In these cases, the patient has to train the new muscles and nerves to perform the appropriate motions needed to smile or close the eye (Shenaq and Kim, August 2005).

Name: Trigeminal neuralgia

Etiology: Trigeminal neuralgia presents as excruciating pain in the tissues innervated by the trigeminal nerve. There are two forms of this condition: (1) idiopathic and (2) secondary. Idiopathic trigeminal neuralgia has no known cause. Secondary trigeminal neuralgia has been commonly associated with vascular anomalies and, less often, neoplastic growths that impinge, or put pressure, on the nerve, and inflammatory conditions. There is also an association between multiple sclerosis and trigeminal neuralgia, since trigeminal neuralgia occurs more frequently in individuals with multiple sclerosis (Burchiel et al., October 2006).

Epidemiology: Approximately 15,000 cases of trigeminal neuralgia are identified in the United States every year (Lenaerts and Couch, March 2006). Twice as many females are affected than males, and most cases occur over the age of 40 (Lenaerts and Couch, March 2006). Approximately 4% of patients who have multiple sclerosis also have trigeminal neuralgia (Burchiel et al., October 2006).

Pathogenesis: The actual mechanism of producing a pain impulse is altered in this condition. Damage to the small and large nerve fibers is present, and it is thought that demyelination of the axons permits uncontrolled transmission of pain impulses along the nerve fiber. Either the second or third division of the trigeminal nerve is most frequently affected, rarely both are affected, and even more rarely, there is involvement of the first division of the nerve. In most cases the involvement is unilateral. Trigeminal neuralgia is considered a chronic condition, even though there may be intermittent remissions lasting several months at a time.

Perioral and Intraoral Characteristics: The pain that accompanies this condition is described as lightning-like, with the impulses firing so quickly that the patient often thinks that it is constant instead of intermittent. A strange residual sensation may linger in the tissues after each episode. The pain is usually initiated by contact with a particular trigger, such as touching a specific area, having cold or hot touch an area, air blowing on an area, chewing, yawning, and various food stimuli.

Dental Implications: Patients may avoid dental care because they are afraid of initiating pain. All efforts should be made to identify and avoid the triggers during dental treatment. Homecare procedures may also be neglected for fear that they will trigger the painful episodes. Homecare recommendations should be made after careful consideration of the needs of these patients. Patients should be referred to professionals who can help them cope with the full range of dental, medical, and psychologic problems that can accompany this type of chronic pain.

Treatment and Prognosis: Treatment is focused on preventing the pain as opposed to stopping it once it starts, because the pain is of such short duration. Medical therapy consists of drug regimens that include anticonvulsants, antidepressants, BOTOX injections, and drugs that reduce painful nerve impulses. All of the drugs have been used with varying degrees of effectiveness. Surgery has been used to alleviate pressure on the nerve from arteries and growths. Substances have been injected into the ganglion to destroy those fibers associated with painful stimuli with good results. One new therapy that is highly effective involves using high-energy photons aimed at the trigeminal nerve root to destroy specific parts of the nerve, thereby eliminating the pain.

There is no mortality associated with this condition; however, significant morbidity is common. The pain is reported as being severely intense, and its severity may be associated with the higher rate of suicides reported among people with this condition (Lenaerts and Couch, March 2006).

Name: Glossopharyngeal neuralgia

Etiology: Glossopharyngeal neuralgia presents with recurring episodes of severe pain located in the back of the throat at the base of the tongue near the tonsils. Pressure on the glossopharyngeal nerve by an artery that is abnormally close or in the wrong position is the most common cause of this condition.

Perioral and Intraoral Characteristics: Intense shooting pain at the back of the throat is the presenting feature of this disorder. The pain can be triggered by swallowing or it may occur spontaneously. The course of the condition is similar to that of trigeminal neuralgia in that it is a chronic condition with remissions and exacerbations likely.

Treatment and Prognosis: Medical therapy involves the identical drugs used for trigeminal neuralgia and a surgical procedure similar to the one listed above. Most patients are able to function well with only pharmacologic (drug) therapy. Those who are not helped with medications can have surgery to remove pressure from the nerve. Most of those treated surgically have good results (NINDS, 2006).

Name: Temporal arteritis

Etiology: Temporal arteritis is a focal granulomatous inflammation of the temporal arteries. The cause is unknown, but there is evidence of a possible genetic tendency.

Epidemiology: Information regarding the epidemiology of temporal arteritis is incomplete. Temporal arteritis is known to affect more females than males, and it occurs more often in those over the age of 60 (Paget and Leibowitz, February 2006).

Pathogenesis: The granulomatous inflammation causes a general thickening of the vessel walls, resulting in a narrowed lumen, which can be easily blocked by a thrombus. The inflammatory reaction brings massive numbers of inflammatory cells into the area, causing damage to all layers of the vessel walls. Other branches of the external carotid can also be affected. If the ophthalmic artery is involved, sudden and irreversible blindness can occur. Rarely, thrombus formation leads to potentially fatal brain infarcts.

Extraoral Characteristics: The sudden onset of a throbbing headache sometimes accompanied by erythema, edema, and tenderness in the scalp covering the temporal artery is characteristic of this disorder (Fig. 10.8). These specific symptoms may be seen concomitantly with general malaise, fever, night sweats, weight loss, muscle aches, weakness, and stiffness. Changes in visual acuity are ominous and may indicate involvement of the ophthalmic artery, leading to possible permanent blindness.

Perioral and Intraoral Characteristics: Jaw stiffness and pain when chewing are classic signs of this condition, occurring in about 50% of those affected. Ear pain and pain in the parotid gland are also common. If the maxillary or lingual arteries are involved, there is pain in the jaw and in the tongue when talking or eating. Thrombus formation in the lingual artery has been reported to have caused ischemia and subsequent necrosis and gangrene of the tongue in at least one case (Paget and Leibowitz, February 2006).

Dental Implications: An astute dental professional might recognize the signs associated with this disorder

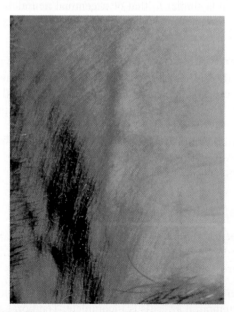

Figure 10.8. Temporal arteritis. A prominent, tender temporal artery found in a patient with temporal arteritis. (From Gold DH, Weingeist TA. Color atlas of the eye in systemic disease. Baltimore: Lippincott Williams & Wilkins, 2001.)

upon obtaining the medical history or during the extraoral examination and should refer the patient for further medical evaluation.

Treatment and Prognosis: Corticosteroids are used to treat this disorder. The symptoms usually decrease dramatically over the course of a few days. Therapy generally continues for 2 to 5 years. Often the side effects of long-term steroid use produce more morbidity and mortality than the disorder itself. Permanent blindness occurs in about 20 to 50% of individuals with ophthalmic artery involvement (Paget and Leibowitz, February 2006).

Name: Migraine headache

Etiology: Migraine or vascular headaches are thought to be caused by a complex interaction between vascular and neural events, culminating in the classic signs of a migraine headache (Sahia-Srivastava and Cowan, August 2005). Some 70% of those who experience migraines report having a first-degree relative (mother, father, sister, or brother) who also has migraines. This may indicate at the very least an inherited predisposition for the disorder.

Epidemiology: An estimated 17% of women and 8% of men in the United States are reported to have migraine headaches (Sahia-Srivastava and Cowan, August 2005).

Extraoral Characteristics: Migraines can occur with or without an **aura** (subjective symptoms that occur prior to the onset of a migraine headache). The headaches are usually unilateral and are described as throbbing or pulsating. Nausea, vomiting, photophobia, noise sensitivity, irritability, and malaise frequently accompany the headaches, which can last from a few hours to several days. Often individuals can identify events or situations that will trigger a headache, such as: certain foods or food additives, hormonal fluctuations, physical exertion, fatigue, stress, or trauma to the head. Migraines with aura are preceded by some type of visual or other sensory disturbance. The usual visual disturbances reported are flashes of light, wavy lines obstructing the visual field, or blurred vision. Individuals experiencing migraines can be severely disabled by the symptoms.

Dental Implications: The dental implications associated with migraine headaches focus on managing the side effects of medications. Most of the medications that are being prescribed have the potential to cause xerostomia. In addition, individuals who have frequent migraines and experience vomiting on a regular basis are at increased risk of dental erosion. Frequent applications of topical fluorides at home and recommendations that will help to alleviate xerostomia are appropriate for these patients. See Clinical Protocol 4.

Treatment and Prognosis: Treatment usually depends on the severity of the symptoms and the amount of disability that they cause. Medications are available that can reduce the pain and limit the severity of any additional symptoms such as nausea and vomiting. In addition, prophylactic medications are given to reduce the frequency of the headaches. The prophylactic medications include antiepileptics, antidepressants, and antihypertensives. Alternative therapies such as biofeedback, relaxation therapy, and stress reduction therapy have been successful in reducing the number of headaches for some individuals. Since each individual is different, the circumstances surrounding the creation of a migraine must be determined on an individual basis; therefore, much time is spent by the physician and the patient trying to identify what triggers that person's headaches.

Name: Burning mouth syndrome

Etiology: A diagnosis of burning mouth syndrome is usually made when all other etiologic possibilities for the symptoms have been ruled out. Refer to Box 10.4 for a list of disorders that may present with symptoms of burning mouth syndrome.

Epidemiology: Approximately 0.7 to 2.6% of the population suffers from symptoms of burning mouth syndrome. Most of those affected are women during and after menopause; men appear to be affected at an older age (Gutkowski, 2004).

Perioral and Intraoral Characteristics: The most important clinical feature of this disorder is that there are no clinically observable abnormalities present. There are no mucosal changes or functional changes, and nothing seems to be out of order, except for the fact that the individual is reporting a burning sensation, often severe, in the oral tissues. The burning occurs most often in the anterior two thirds of the tongue, the anterior hard palate, and the mucosa of the lower lip (Grushka et al., 2002). Typically there is an absence of symptoms during

Box 10.4 — CONDITIONS ASSOCIATED WITH BURNING SENSATIONS IN THE ORAL MUCOSA

- Xerostomia
- Vitamin deficiencies
- Mineral deficiencies
- Gastrointestinal disorders
- Fungal infections
- Hormone deficiencies
- Neurologic problems
- Blood diseases
- Allergic and inflammatory disorders
- Adverse effects of drugs
- Psychologic disorders
- Phantom pain

sleep, and the symptoms are less severe in the morning, but increase as the day progresses. The sensations also disappear when the person is eating (Gutkowski, 2004). Other oral symptoms associated with burning mouth syndrome are intermittent xerostomia and taste perversions (abnormal taste sensations).

Treatment and Prognosis: The most important element in successfully treating this disorder is to identify the cause, if possible, and eliminate it. Complete blood counts, allergy testing, tests to determine nutritional status, and oral cultures or biopsies should be done to try to determine the exact cause of the sensations. In cases in which no causative agent is discovered or nerve damage is suspected, several medications have been prescribed with varying degrees of success. These medications include tricyclic antidepressants, benzodiazepines, and other anticonvulsants. Another substance that has been shown to reduce the burning sensations is capsaicin, which is the substance that is responsible for the "heat" in hot chili peppers. Apparently the topical application of capsaicin blocks one of the neurotransmitters associated with pain impulses and gives the individual temporary relief from the painful sensations (Gutkowski, 2004). The patient should be advised to avoid mouth rinses containing alcohol or cinnamon flavoring as well as tobacco products, since these substances may increase the level of discomfort. Chewing on ice chips and chewing sugar-free gum may alleviate the symptoms for short periods of time. Burning mouth syndrome may persist for years with no relief, become episodic, and then disappear altogether, or it may never resolve.

SKELETAL SYSTEM DISORDERS

Several skeletal disorders should be discussed for the simple reason that they are among the most common chronic diseases known to mankind. Osteoarthritis or rheumatoid arthritis affects almost 100% of the population at some point in their lives. Osteoporosis is a major preventable health problem for women and men. Paget's disease and fibrous dysplasia, even though uncommon, have specific oral implications and manifestations. The dental hygienist will have to manage disorders of the TM joint on a daily basis, not only because of the need to identify patients with symptoms, but also to be able to modify treatment procedures to put as little stress as possible on the joint.

Name: Osteoarthritis

Etiology: Osteoarthritis affects the joints, specifically the articular cartilage and bone directly underneath it. This is a degenerative disease and considered to be idiopathic. It appears to be related to the process of aging and typically appears in older individuals. Many feel that it is due to excessive wear and tear on the joints, but often there is no trauma associated with its occurrence.

Epidemiology: Osteoarthritis is widespread, and it is estimated that 80 to 90% of the United States population over the age of 65 have evidence of this disease (Stacy and Basu, November 2005). It affects all races, and women are more susceptible to some forms of the disease than are men.

Pathogenesis: The underlying pathology in osteoarthritis is the destruction of the cartilage covering the articular surfaces of the bones in synovial joints. Eventually, the opposing bones rub directly on each other because there is so little cartilage. During this process, small pieces of cartilage break away and float freely in the joint space, causing more impairment of joint function. In response to the destructive process, the body forms new bone at the margins of the joint. This new bone takes the form of a bone spur, or **osteophyte**, causing even more impairment of joint function. Eventually the bone underlying the articulating surfaces collapses, causing severe limitation of motion with accompanying pain.

Extraoral Characteristics: The joints of the fingers are affected most often. Some definitions of osteoarthritis limit the disease to the hands; however, other definitions include most of the weightbearing joints such as the knee, hip, and sometimes the cervical and lumbar (lower) regions of the spine. The pain associated with osteoarthritis has been characterized as a deep, achy joint pain that increases as the joint is used. Small pea sized areas of exostosis, or bony outgrowth, are seen in the joints of the fingers. These areas are called Heberden nodes and are seen often in women but seldom in men (Fig. 10.9).

Dental Implications: Treatment modifications might include adapting the patient's position for comfort, keeping appointments short, and scheduling appointments at a time when the patient is feeling best. Methods to manage excessive bleeding during dental/dental hygiene procedures should be planned, since many medications used to treat osteoarthritis have an anticoagulant effect. The dental hygienist may have to recommend modifying homecare implements, making them easier to hold, to enable patients to effectively remove dental biofilm from their teeth.

Treatment and Prognosis: Treatment of osteoarthritis focuses on relieving the symptoms and rehabilitative measures, which attempt to enhance the supporting structures of the joints. Resistance training exercises and exercising with weight partially removed from the joint, as occurs in water aerobics, has been found to be very helpful. Medications that reduce inflammation and pain, such as the NSAIDs and other antiinflammatories, are important. Injection of sodium hyaluronate (a substance that mimics the actions of synovial fluid) directly into the joint space appears to help lubricate the joint and provides temporary comfort for many patients. When all else fails to provide relief, surgery is considered. Some forms of surgery simply remove the floating bodies or spurs around the joints; others actually remodel the bone surfaces. In the case of hip or knee osteoarthritis, the joint may eventually need to be replaced.

Name: Rheumatoid Arthritis (RA)

Etiology: RA is a chronic systemic inflammatory disease. The exact cause is unknown, but it is thought that infectious organisms such as Epstein-Barr virus, autoimmune processes, and genetics may be part of the etiology.

Epidemiology: Approximately 3 of every 10,000 individuals will have RA. RA affects all races and all age groups. Females are 2 to 3 times more likely to have RA, and the peak age at onset is between the ages of 35 and 50 years (Smith and Smolen, January 2006).

Pathogenesis: RA is primarily a disease of the joints, but it can also affect any organ, such as the heart or the skin. The inflammation starts in the synovial membrane that lines the joints. The membrane thickens and extends into the joint cavity, often filling the space. The inflammation also affects the articular cartilage on the ends of the bones, causing the formation of scar tissue between the bones. Calcification of the scar tissue causes ankylosis, or fusion of the bones, resulting in the characteristic crippling of the hands (Fig. 10.10). The hands and the feet are affected most often, but other joints (hip, knee, shoulder, and TM) are usually not spared. The spine often becomes involved as the disease becomes more advanced.

Extraoral Characteristics: Pain is the presenting feature of this disorder. Morning stiffness and soft tissue swelling or accumulation of fluid around the joints are also characteristic. There is no bony overgrowth as in osteoarthritis. The individual may have rubbery nodules under the skin, called rheumatoid nodules, at pressure points such as the elbow; these are granulomatous lesions

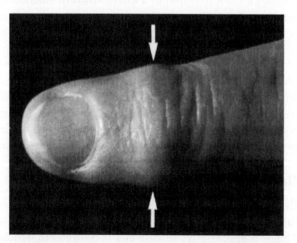

Figure 10.9. Heberden nodes. These are characteristic of the joint deformities (*arrows*) seen in the hands of individuals with osteoarthritis. (From Bickley LS, Szilagyi P. Bates' guide to physical examination and history taking. 8th ed. Philadelphia: Lippincott Williams & Wilkins, 2003.)

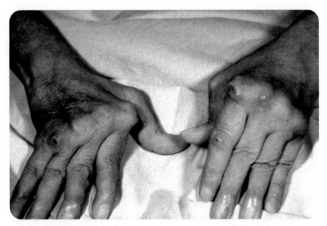

Figure 10.10. Rheumatoid arthritis. The hands of a patient with advanced rheumatoid arthritis show swelling of the joints and the classic ulnar deviation of the fingers. (From Rubin E, Farber JL. Pathology. 3rd ed. Philadelphia: Lippincott Williams & Wilkins, 1999.)

that develop around small blood vessels (Porth, 2004) (Fig. 10.11). Rheumatoid nodules may or may not be painful. Other organ manifestations of the disease include fluid accumulation around the heart and in the lungs, entrapment of nerves in the deformities caused by RA such as carpal tunnel syndrome, and keratoconjunctivitis sicca (dry eyes). RA may be the connective tissue disorder associated with secondary Sjögren syndrome.

Dental Implications: The dental hygienist should pay careful attention to the drug history of the patient with RA because of the possibility of immunosuppression from long-term use of disease-modifying antirheumatic drugs (DMARDs) and corticosteroids (discussed in the next section). Long-term steroid use is also associated with a significant decrease in bone density that can affect the mandible and the maxilla. Blood clotting may be affected by drugs used to treat RA, making it important to determine the individual's bleeding time, especially prior

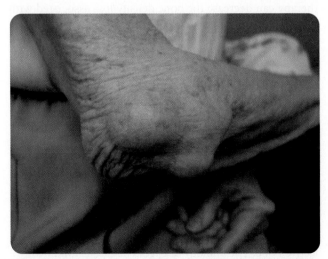

Figure 10.11. Rheumatoid nodule. Several large rheumatoid nodules can be seen on the elbow of this elderly patient. (Image provided by Stedman's.)

to procedures during which bleeding is anticipated. Appointment modifications that might make dental treatment more comfortable include scheduling short appointments, modifying the patient's position in the chair, providing pillows or rolled up towels to support joints, and using bite blocks to assist in keeping the mouth open comfortably. Examination of the TM joint for RA manifestations is important to plan interventions to limit the destruction in this joint. Homecare procedures and instruments might need to be modified to contend with dexterity problems caused by destruction of the joints of the fingers and hands. Finally, many of the drugs given for RA have the potential to cause xerostomia; therefore, preventive strategies for caries and periodontal disease should be initiated early, before any disease can occur.

Treatment and Prognosis: Treatment of RA focuses on slowing the progression of the disease and minimizing the deformities caused by it. Medications, exercise, and rest are all essential components of controlling this disease. Exercises are aimed at strengthening the support system for the joints and maintaining flexibility. Medications that interfere with the disease process, called disease-modifying antirheumatic drugs (DMARDs) are the mainstay of modern drug therapy. Methotrexate, a strong immunosuppressive drug, is the DMARD of choice at this time. Other DMARDs include medications that inhibit the binding of tumor necrosis factor (TNF) to cell surface receptors and those that reduce the infiltration of inflammatory cells into an inflamed area and thus decrease inflammation. These are often combined with anti-inflammatory drugs (corticosteroids and NSAIDs) and analgesic (acetaminophen) drugs to provide the highest level of comfort and function.

The disease usually follows an episodic course with many exacerbations and remissions over the years. Approximately 40% of individuals with RA become significantly disabled after 10 years, and their overall life expectancy is about 5 to 10 years less than someone without RA (Smith and Smolen, January 2006).

Name: Osteoporosis

Etiology: Osteoporosis is a skeletal disorder characterized by low bone density and deterioration of the structure of the bone, leading to an increased risk of fractures. There are two types of osteoporosis: (1) primary and (2) secondary. Primary osteoporosis is seen in postmenopausal women and in the elderly of both sexes. There does not seem to be a clear cause of primary osteoporosis, but there are many risk factors that increase an individual's chance of having osteoporosis. Box 10.5 lists some of these risk factors. Individuals who do not have osteoporosis but have low bone density compared to the norm are said to have osteopenia. Many of those with osteopenia progress to osteoporosis. Secondary osteoporosis is associated with a known cause, which is often an en-

Box 10.5   RISK FACTORS FOR OSTEOPOROSIS

- Female
- Age
- Low body weight
- Family history
- Physically inactive
- Estrogen deficiency
- Caucasian
- Certain medications
- Previous fractures
- Low calcium intake
- Tobacco use
- Alcohol abuse
- Caffeine ingestion

docrine disorder or the use of certain medications, such as corticosteroids, for long periods of time.

Epidemiology: The National Osteoporosis Foundation estimates that 10 million Americans already have osteoporosis, and another 34 million have osteopenia. Eight million women and 2 million men are affected. They also estimate that 1 of every 2 women and 1 of every 4 men will have an osteoporotic fracture in their lifetimes (NOF, 2006).

Pathogenesis: The pathology associated with all forms of osteoporosis is the result of defective bone remodeling. Bone is not a static tissue and is simultaneously undergoing formation and resorption on a continual basis. When the resorption of bone exceeds the formation of bone, the density of the bone decreases as does the quality of the bone. Figure 10.12 compares normal bone structure to osteoporotic bone.

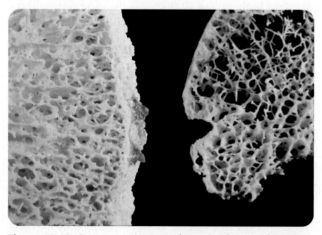

Figure 10.12. Osteoporosis. Bone from the femur of an 82-year-old female with osteoporosis *(right)* compared with a normal bone cut to the same thickness *(left)*. (From Rubin E, Farber JL. Pathology. 4th ed. Philadelphia: Lippincott Williams & Wilkins, 2005.)

Extraoral Characteristics: Some of the clinical findings associated with osteoporosis are a decrease in height of between 10 to 15 cm, dowager's hump (curvature of the upper back), lower back pain, and bone fracture caused by minimal trauma such as coughing. Osteoporosis is considered a "silent" disease. Individuals may not know that they have it until they experience a fracture or one or more of the other signs and symptoms.

Perioral and Intraoral Characteristics: Osteoporosis can be seen in the maxilla and the mandible as loss of trabecular detail and thinning of the cortical bone. Research has suggested a link between osteoporosis and accelerated progression of bone loss due to periodontal infection. The use of bisphosphonates, medications that reduce osteoclast activity, thereby increasing bone density, to treat osteoporosis has been associated with **osteonecrosis** (pathologic death of the bone) of the mandible (AAE, 2006).

Dental Implications: Maintaining periodontal health should be stressed in patients who have been identified as having osteoporosis because of the possibility of accelerated bone loss. In addition, those taking bisphosphonates should be advised to report any pain or swelling in either jaw, infections that produce pus, change of sensation within the jaws, and ulceration of the mucosa covering the jaws that does not heal, all of which may be associated with osteonecrosis of the jaw (AAE, 2006). See the application following this section for more information.

Treatment and Prognosis: Treatment focuses on maintaining the current level of bone density through weightbearing exercises combined with resistance training. Increasing the dietary intake of calcium as well as vitamin D is a crucial element of treatment and prevention. Drug therapy includes medications that increase bone density by reducing the activity of osteoclasts and one that actually increases the formation of bone. Estrogen replacement therapy can decrease the bone density loss associated with menopause. However, estrogen use has been associated with a higher rate of some cancers in women and is very controversial at this time. Prevention is the key to controlling this disease. It is recommended that prevention begin in childhood with the formation of healthy eating habits, maintaining an active lifestyle, and avoiding tobacco use. Prevention should not begin at age 50 when an individual is diagnosed with osteoporosis or osteopenia; however, it is never too late to try to stay healthy and active.

Name: Paget's disease (osteitis deformans)

Etiology: Paget's disease is a skeletal disorder characterized by bone resorption followed by excessive growth of defective bone. The etiology of Paget's disease is unknown.

Epidemiology: Approximately 1 to 3% of the United States population is affected by this disease. More males

APPLICATION

Osteonecrosis is the term that is used to describe a condition in which the bone dies or undergoes necrosis. This condition has long been associated with exposure of the bone to ionizing radiation used to treat malignant growths (osteoradionecrosis). During radiation therapy, the capacity of the bone to repair itself and recover from infections or trauma is permanently altered by the damage done to the bone cells and the structures that supply nutrients to the bone. Similarly, bisphosphonates alter the balance of normal bone turnover by decreasing the number of osteoclasts that are allowed to become active and by causing premature apoptosis (natural death) of already functioning osteoclasts. This causes the inhibition of normal bone formation that could result in a decreased ability of the bone to repair itself. This is thought to be the process associated with the development of bisphosphonate-associated osteonecrosis of the jaw (BON) (ADA, 2006).

Since 2003, cases of BON have been reported among patients who are taking intravenous bisphosphonates to prevent bone loss associated with cancer therapy and with some other chronic conditions, such as Paget's disease (ADA, 2006). In 2006, cases of BON began to be reported among individuals taking oral bisphosphonates (ADA, 2006). In light of the fact that millions of individuals are taking this medication for the prevention of osteoporosis, the dental community has taken steps to address the problem and determine the direction of further research.

Patients who are undergoing IV therapy with bisphosphonates have the highest risk for developing BON (ADA, 2006). Individuals taking oral bisphosphonates have a very low risk of BON. The current data suggest that the incidence (rate at which new cases develop) is less than 1 case per 100,000 person-years of exposure (the risk increases the longer the medication is taken) (ADA, 2006). In addition, since older individuals and those who are taking oral glucocorticoids and/or estrogen in addition to IV bisphosphonates have a higher risk of BON, it is assumed that older age and the use of these drugs also increases the risk for those taking oral bisphosphonates (ADA, 2006).

The American Dental Association has developed several general recommendations for managing patients who are taking oral bisphosphonates (ADA, 2006):

- Performing regular dental examinations beginning prior to the initiation of therapy
- Maintaining healthy oral tissues with good oral hygiene practices
- Telling patients to contact their dentist if any problems arise in the mouth
- Informing patients of the increased risk of developing BON prior to any invasive dental procedures, specifically periodontal therapy or tooth extraction; consulting with an expert in metabolic bone diseases as indicated
- Beginning in a single sextant during invasive therapy and then waiting 2 months to monitor tissue response before completing the other sextants
- Rinsing with chlorhexidine twice daily during the 2-month recovery period, as well as prescribing a 2-week course of oral antibiotics
- Carefully considering the use of any guided bone regeneration, implant placement, and extensive surgical periodontal therapy because the bone repair process may be impaired

BON may appear clinically as a painful soft tissue swelling that may be accompanied by infection, purulent exudate, tooth mobility, and bone exposure. It is more common to see BON at the site of a previous or current infection such as periodontal infection or after trauma such as tooth extraction. However, BON has also occurred spontaneously in an area that is unaffected by infection or trauma. In addition, the lesions may be asymptomatic and only discovered during a regular dental examination (ADA, 2006). The following case is an example of BON.

The area in Figure 10.13 was discovered in a 66-year-old, 5-foot 3-inches tall, 102-lb, Caucasian female patient who presented to the dental hygiene clinic with severe oral pain. Her medical history included severe rheumatoid arthritis of over 10 year's duration, and secondary Sjögren syndrome. Her current medications included methotrexate (an antineoplastic agent used to treat rheumatoid arthritis), an NSAID (for reduction of pain and inflammation), an antimalarial (used to treat rheumatoid arthritis), bisphosphonates (used to treat osteoporosis), thyroid medication (for thyroid disease),

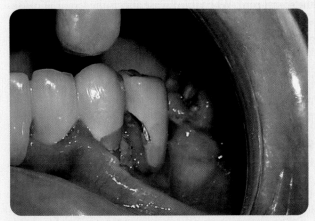

Figure 10.13. Bisphosphonate osteonecrosis of the jaw. An area of necrotic bone is visible in the interproximal area between 21 and 22.

continued

Application, cont.

calcium (for osteoporosis), and a proton pump inhibitor (used to reduce the risk of gastric ulcer development in patients taking NSAIDs).

Clinical examination revealed an area of necrotic bone in the interproximal area between teeth 21 and 22. The surrounding soft tissue was erythematic and swollen and bled easily. There was a corresponding area of necrotic bone on the lingual interproximal surface. The patient was referred to an oral medicine clinic at an area dental school for diagnosis and initial therapy. The initial diagnosis was bisphosphonate-associated osteonecrosis, and the initial therapy consisted of careful debridement of the area, topical alco-

hol-free antibacterial rinses, and a course of systemic antibiotics. The patient was to be monitored closely.

These web sites are recommended to keep abreast of the most current information regarding BON.

American Dental Association
http://www.ada.org/prof/resources/topics/osteonecrosis.asp

National Osteoporosis Foundation
http://www.nof.org

American Society for Bone and Mineral Research
http://www.asbmr.org

---

than females are affected. The disorder rarely occurs under the age of 25, with most cases occurring after the age of 60 (Carbone and Barrow, June 2005).

Pathogenesis: Initially the disease causes excessive resorption of the cancellous bone, which is replaced with a vascular connective tissue. After the initial resorption, new bone is created at a very fast rate, causing enlargement of the affected bones. The new bone is abnormal in structure, causing it to be weaker than normal bone, even though it is highly mineralized. The bones of the spine, skull, sternum, pelvis, and femur are affected most often, but any bone can be affected. In addition to these problems, approximately 1% of affected individuals will develop osteogenic sarcoma within the bone lesions.

Extraoral Characteristics: Involvement of the spine can cause neurologic symptoms ranging in severity from transient pain to complete paralysis due to compression of the spinal cord. When the disease affects the femur, it causes severe bowing and is associated with increased incidences of stress fracture. Radiographs will show enlargement of the bones, with areas of excessive mineralization appearing as radiopaque patches resembling "cotton wool" (Fig. 10.14). Diagnosis of Paget's disease is based on the results of blood tests that show significantly elevated levels of alkaline phosphatase, and radiographic manifestations.

Perioral and Intraoral Characteristics: Involvement of the skull usually results in asymmetric enlargement of the occipital and frontal bones (Fig. 10.15). Depending on the extent of the deformity, neurological symptoms can range from mild headache to dementia. Excessive bone growth around the foramina of the skull can lead to cranial nerve compression and blindness, deafness, constant vertigo, impaired motor function, and more. Maxillary and/or mandibular involvement results in bilateral enlargement of the jaw with increased tooth spacing and malocclusion (Fig. 10.16).

Patients may complain that removable prosthetics no longer fit and that they can no longer close their lips. They may also complain of temporomandibular dysfunction. Loss of the lamina dura and periodontal ligament space as well as **hypercementosis**, or the growth of excessive amounts of cementum, in addition to the cotton

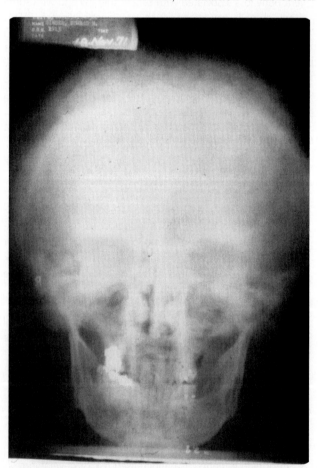

Figure 10.14. Paget's disease. Radiograph showing the cotton wool appearance of the bone in Paget's disease. Note the involvement of the mandible. (Courtesy of Dr. William Carpenter.)

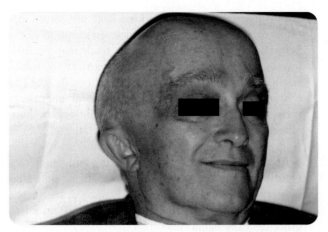

Figure 10.15. Paget's disease. Asymmetric enlargement of the skull bones can cause neurologic problems, and bone growth can encroach on the foramina, putting pressure on the nerves and vessels passing through them. (Courtesy of Dr. William Carpenter.)

wool appearance of the affected bone, may be present in intraoral and panoramic radiographs.

Dental Implications: Dental management of the functional problems associated with malocclusion and temporomandibular joint dysfunction caused by Paget's disease is one challenge presented by these patients. Pain management may become an issue if nerves are impinged upon by thickening bone. In addition, bisphosphonates are used to treat Paget's disease, and patients should be advised about the possibility of osteonecrosis of the jaw.

Treatment and Prognosis: Often the disease is localized, is self-limiting, and requires no treatment. Otherwise, treatment is determined by the severity of the symptoms and the extent of the involvement. Some of the same drugs that are used to treat osteoporosis are used to treat Paget's disease, specifically; the bisphosphonates, which inhibit bone loss by decreasing bone resorption and by slowing the formation of new bone.

The prognosis for individuals with Paget's disease is excellent in cases that are treated appropriately. When osteogenic sarcoma is diagnosed, the prognosis is poor, with most succumbing to the illness within 3 years of diagnosis.

Name: Fibrous dysplasia

Etiology: The etiology of fibrous dysplasia is uncertain. Current thought is that a genetic mutation occurring after birth causes the production of increased levels of a specific protein that enhances the action of certain cells including osteoblasts and fibroblasts.

Method of Transmission: One rare form of the disease, cherubism, is an autosomal dominant genetic disorder.

Pathogenesis: Spongy bone is replaced by fibrous tissue, which precedes the formation of immature woven bone. The woven bone exhibits a characteristic "ground glass" radiographic appearance (Fig. 10.17). Several forms of this disease are discussed below:

• Monostotic fibrous dysplasia occurs in one bone only, usually one of the ribs, femur, tibia, or craniofacial bones. This form of the disease accounts for 70 to 80% of cases and may present with bone pain and pathologic fractures or may be asymptomatic. Diagnosis is usually made between the ages of 10 and 30 years (Anand, 2004).

• Polyostotic fibrous dysplasia occurs in multiple bones and accounts for 20 to 30% of cases (Anand, 2004). The bones most frequently affected include the skull, facial, pelvis, spine, and shoulder girdle. Symptoms of pain, swelling, and spontaneous fracture may be the presenting features of this form of the disease. Over time, the weightbearing bones of the hip, if affected, will become deformed or bowed. More females are affected than males (Rubin et al., 2005).

  • McCune-Albright syndrome consists of polyostotic fibrous dysplasia, cutaneous hyperpigmented areas called café-au-lait macules with characteristic jagged borders (Fig. 10.18), and one or more endocrine ab-

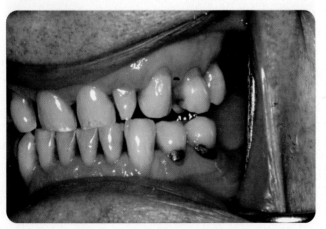

Figure 10.16. Paget's disease. Malocclusion caused by enlargement of the maxilla. Note the normal size of the mandible. (Courtesy of Dr. William Carpenter.)

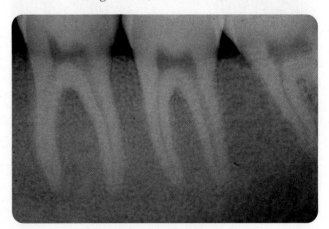

Figure 10.17. Fibrous dysplasia. Radiograph of the mandible showing the characteristic ground-glass appearance of the bone in fibrous dysplasia. (Courtesy of Dr. Charles Dunlap.)

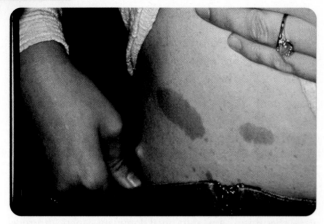

Figure 10.18. Café-au-lait macule. This café-au-lait macule was observed on the abdomen of a patient with McCune-Albright syndrome. Note the jagged border, which is characteristic of the café-au-lait macules seen in fibrous dysplasia. (Courtesy of Dr. Michael Brennan.)

normalities. The most common endocrine abnormality is precocious or very early sexual development. Other abnormalities that may be present include diabetes, hyperthyroidism, hyperparathyroidism, and acromegaly. Oral manifestations including partial anodontia may be present in some cases.

- Jaffe-Lichtenstein syndrome consists of polyostotic fibrous dysplasia and the cutaneous café-au-lait macules without any endocrine abnormalities.
- Cherubism is a rare, painless form of fibrous dysplasia that affects the bones of the face, especially the mandible and, less often, the maxilla. Replacement of spongy bone with fibrous tissues gives the area of the cheeks a very swollen appearance (Fig. 10.19). If the bones of the inferior orbit enlarge, the eyes appear to tilt upward like the eyes of cherubs in religious paintings. Oral problems are encountered with this form of

the disorder. Affected individuals have premature loss of primary teeth and failure or delayed eruption of the permanent teeth. In addition, the teeth may be malformed and out of place or missing (partial anodontia), resulting in severe malocclusion (Fig. 10.20). The characteristic radiographic appearance of cherubism presents as multiple, well-defined, multilocular, radiolucent lesions scattered within the affected bones (Fig. 10.21). The cortical bone thins and may become perforated. The disease is self-limiting and progresses rapidly during childhood, but slows during and after puberty, and normally regresses or resolves by the age of 30, leaving no permanent disability or disfigurement other than the malocclusion.

Treatment and Prognosis: Treatment, other than follow-up and biopsy, is usually unnecessary for small lesions, especially those of the monostotic type. Larger lesions and the multiple lesions of polyostotic fibrous dysplasia are often treated with surgical recontouring after the individual has reached adulthood to decrease the chance for recurrence. Very often hip deformities cause mobility problems and result in the need to use a wheelchair. Individuals with McCune-Albright syndrome need to be treated for their endocrine abnormalities. In addition, there is a very slight chance that the fibrous lesions can undergo a malignant transformation. This has been reported more often in the polyostotic form and in individuals who have a history of radiation treatment for their lesions. Radiation treatment is no longer considered appropriate therapy for this disorder.

Temporomandibular Disorders

The TM joint is comprised of the mandibular condyle, which fits into the mandibular fossa of the temporal bone.

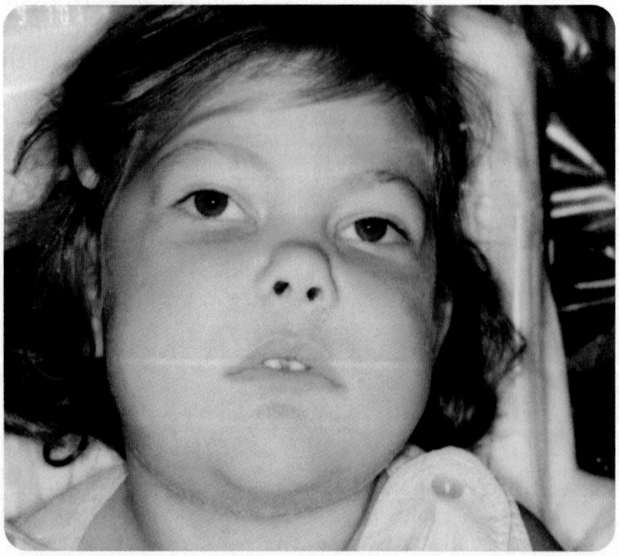

Figure 10.19. Cherubism. This 4-year-old female exhibits the facial features characteristic of cherubism, including the swollen appearance of the cheeks. (Courtesy of Tirza Jo.)

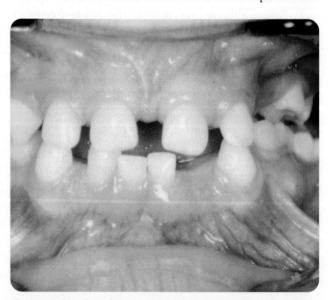

Figure 10.20. Cherubism. Intraoral photograph of the same female shows partial anodontia and malocclusion affecting both the mandible and the maxilla. (Courtesy of Tirza Jo.)

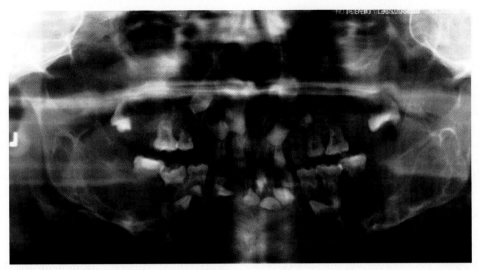

Figure 10.21. Cherubism. Panoramic radiograph of the same female showing partial anodontia, malformed teeth, and multiple well-defined, multilocular, radiolucent lesions scattered throughout the mandible and maxilla. (Courtesy of Tirza Jo.)

These are separated into upper and lower synovial cavities by the articular disk. The joint is surrounded by ligaments that protect the joint and limit motions that could damage it. The muscles of mastication, while not part of the joint, are intimately involved with proper joint function.

Name: Temporomandibular disorder (TMD)

Etiology: TMDs are a group of disorders characterized by functional impairment or pain-related to the temporomandibular joint. These include disorders related to the bone, ligaments, and articular disk of the joint and to the associated muscles of mastication. See Box 10.6 for a classification of TMDs. The most common cause of dysfunc-

tion is acute or chronic trauma. Sudden, forceful trauma such as a blow to the jaw is considered acute, while chronic trauma may take the form of clenching and bruxing. Occlusal conditions that cause deviant or traumatic muscle function such as an anterior open bite, a significant overjet, and five or more nonreplaced missing teeth have been associated with an increase in TMDs (Okeson, 2003). Emotional stress is associated with an increase in muscle tone and unconscious muscle function, which may cause an increase in parafunctional habits (masticatory motions not related to the act of eating such as bruxing or chewing on pens). Patients who complain of chronic mouth, ear, sinus, and, sometimes, cervical neck pain also have a higher risk of developing TMD because the body protects the painful area by limiting its function. Muscles that are in these areas may undergo significant change because of deviant or nonuse.

Epidemiology: Numerous studies have reported TMD signs and/or symptoms in up to 60% of the population. However, only about 10% reported enough pain and/or dysfunction to seek care (Okeson, 2003). Significantly more females than males seek care for TMDs, which occur most frequently between 20 and 40 years of age.

Pathogenesis: The pathogenesis of the condition depends on the specific cause. For example, if an acute traumatic event such as a sharp, forceful blow to the jaw occurs, then the tissues of the joint would show signs of inflammation. There would be swelling and pain; the joint would be tender to touch and might even feel warm. The range of motion or opening would be limited and the individual might notice that his or her teeth did not occlude normally, due to swelling in the joint. With time and proper treatment, the inflammation would resolve and the joint would return to normal with no permanent damage. On the other hand, chronic trauma follows a more insidious or gradual course. For instance, an individual who is missing all of the molars would have to learn how to chew

---

Box 10.6 **CLASSIFICATION OF TEMPOROMANDIBULAR DISORDERS**

- Muscle disorders
- TM joint disorders
  - ○ Articular disk out of place
  - ○ Inflammation of the articular surfaces
    - • Osteoarthritis
    - • Rheumatoid arthritis
- Ankylosis or fixation
- Defective coronoid process
- Growth disorders
  - ○ Bone
    - • Agenesis
    - • Hypoplasia
    - • Hyperplasia
  - ○ Muscles
    - • Hypotrophy
    - • Hypertrophy

on the anterior and premolar teeth. The TM joint is not made to function heavily on these teeth and to do so must attain an abnormal position. In addition, the muscles of mastication will have to function out of their normal range of motion. Over time, the chronic trauma induced by these functional changes will lead to permanent joint damage. Growth disorders can cause either hyperplastic or hypoplastic development of the joint, and the deformity may be unilateral or bilateral. These disorders can affect the condyle, coronoid process, and/or the TM joint itself. Acromegaly is an example of a growth disorder that can result in unbalanced jaw development and TMD.

Perioral and Intraoral Characteristics:
The dental hygienist may be the first professional to identify a possible TMD. A thorough history is very important and will establish the basis for determining the etiology and nature of the dysfunction. Refer to Box 10.7 for examples of questions that might be asked to further investigate a TMD. The most common presenting feature of TMDs is pain, which is usually associated with muscle dysfunction. The pain can be localized to the tissues around the joint or it may be referred to the ear, sinuses, or head. It usually increases in intensity when chewing and as the day progresses into night. When pain involves the joint, it is usually confined to the ligaments and soft tissues surrounding the joint and not the bone itself. Joint dysfunction is the next most common presenting feature. Inappropriate joint sounds indicate dysfunction. When the articular disk is out of place, the condyle will make a sometimes audible click as it bumps over it during opening and closing. Occasionally this is very loud and sounds more like a pop. "Crepitation" is the term used for joint noise that sounds more like grinding or rubbing over a rough surface. Crepitation is felt when the articular surfaces are roughened or if the disk is damaged, allowing the bones of the joint to rub together. This type of sound is heard or felt in cases of osteoarthritis or rheumatoid arthritis. Other signs of dysfunction include deviation (the jaw moves right or left during opening or closing but returns to a normal position when fully opened or fully closed), deflection (the jaw moves to an abnormal right or left position when fully opened), limitation of opening (<40 mm between maxillary and mandibular incisors), occlusion or bite irregularities, locking in the open position, and masseter muscle hypertrophy. Many of the above signs are often seen without any accompanying pain.

Dental Implications:
Joint dysfunction can make dental/dental hygiene care difficult for the operator and very difficult and painful for the patient. The patient might be advised to take antiinflammatory medications prior to the appointment. Appointments should be kept short, and the patient should be given frequent opportunities to close or move the mouth. Alternating hot and cold compresses applied to the joint in addition to the anti-inflammatory pain medications after treatment may help to alleviate posttreatment discomfort.

Treatment and Prognosis:
The goal of treatment is to alleviate pain, restore function, and decrease the potential for permanent joint damage. In many cases, treatment is focused on relieving the symptoms associated with acute trauma. Nonsteroidal antiinflammatory drugs and diet modification may be all that is necessary to allow the joint to recover from the trauma. Dietary modifications include eating softer foods, taking smaller bites, and chewing more slowly. Some patients are bothered by episodic dysfunction and pain separated by long periods of normal functioning; if the causative agent can be identified by careful history and follow-up questions, these episodes might be eliminated.

Trauma from parafunctional habits can be lessened if the patient identifies the habit and consciously tries to eliminate the behavior. Parafunctional habits such as bruxing and clenching that occur at night are more difficult to manage because the patient is not consciously aware of them. Often soft or hard plastic occlusal night guards can help to interfere with the habit or at least decrease the trauma associated with it. In addition, relaxation therapy and massage therapy have been used with some success in alleviating the symptoms of TMD for some individuals.

Chronic trauma from altered masticatory function might necessitate making an appliance that can bring the joint and the muscles of mastication into normal resting positions, thus alleviating the constant stress on them. These appliances are usually worn at night and off and on during the day to relieve symptoms. As the symptoms resolve, the appliance is worn less often, so that the muscles

---

Box 10.7   FOLLOW-UP QUESTIONS IN REFERENCE TO A SUSPECTED TMD

- When were the symptoms first noted?
- Have they been intermittent or constant?
- What type of pain is involved? Where is the focus of the pain?
- When does the pain occur?
- Does your jaw get stuck or lock?
- Are you able to eat what you want to?
- Are you able to open your mouth as wide as you need to without pain?
- Do you have any habits such as bruxing, clenching, chewing on nonfood items, etc.?
- Do you feel stressed?
- Do you have any chronic muscle or bone disorders?
- Have you ever had treatment for TMD such as orthodontia?
- What medications are you taking?

are not locked into any one position for long periods of time. Dental treatment to restore posterior teeth and reestablish proper occlusion may also be necessary to restore proper function.

Surgery may be an option in some cases, if the joint dysfunction is due to bony defects, growth abnormalities, destruction or damage to the disk, or a displaced disk.

SUMMARY

- The common cold is caused by a rhinovirus or other virus. The infection causes swelling of the mucosal tissues and the production of copious amounts of mucus by the inflamed glands.
- The flu is caused by inhalation or mucosal contact with influenza virus. The flu has a short incubation period, and individuals are able to spread the virus about 2 days prior to the appearance of flu symptoms.
- Pneumonia is a lower respiratory tract infection or inflammatory reaction that can be caused by a variety of agents including viruses, bacteria, fungi, chemicals, toxic fumes, or aspirated substances such as vomitus or dental biofilm.
- SARS is caused by an atypical form of a coronavirus. SARS has an unusually long incubation period of up to 14 days, which is associated with a wide geographic range of transmission.
- Tuberculosis is caused by *Mycobacterium tuberculosis*, and it is transmitted through inhalation of droplet nuclei or through contact with the mucous membranes of the respiratory tract.
- Asthma is the most serious chronic illness affecting children. Asthma results from an inflammatory reaction caused by hypersensitivity to one or more numerous triggers, such as infections, allergies, inhaled fumes, exercise, and cold temperatures.
- The most common cause of emphysema and chronic obstructive bronchitis is smoking, followed closely by inhaling second-hand smoke. Emphysema causes destruction of the lung tissue and the formation of large cavities.
- Cystic fibrosis is the most common lethal autosomal disorder in the Caucasian population.
- GERD is a disorder of the lower esophageal sphincter that allows gastric contents to flow back up the esophagus from the stomach. Barrett esophagitis is a severe form of this damage and is associated with the potential for malignant transformation within the damaged epithelial tissues.
- Peptic ulcers are most commonly caused by an infection with *H. pylori* or by use of medications containing aspirin or other NSAIDs.
- Malabsorption syndromes are associated with an inability to absorb specific nutrients. Some of the possible oral manifestations include excessive bleeding, ulcers, glossitis, and angular cheilitis.
- Crohn's disease is a granulomatous inflammatory reaction that has the potential to affect any mucosal surface within the gastrointestinal tract. The risk of colon cancer is increased in those with long-term disease.
- Peutz-Jeghers syndrome is an inherited disorder associated with distinctive perioral and oral pigmentations and an increased risk of cancers of the breast, pancreas, testes, ovaries, and the lining of the gastrointestinal tract.
- Meningitis and encephalitis can be caused by both viral and bacterial organisms. The abrupt onset of symptoms of severe stiff neck, high fever, chills, nausea, and vomiting are characteristic of both of these infections.
- Oral manifestations of Parkinson's disease include dysphagia, abfractions, attrition, speech difficulties, and drooling.
- Bell's palsy is unilateral paralysis of the muscles innervated by the facial nerve.
- Trigeminal neuralgia manifests as sharp intermittent pain impulses located within the tissues innervated by the trigeminal nerve and triggered by touch, movement, or other agents.
- Glossopharyngeal neuralgia is similar to trigeminal neuralgia, but the pain is felt in the back of the throat, base of the tongue, or tonsillar area.
- Temporal arteritis is associated with granulomatous inflammation of the temporal artery that can lead to thrombus formation and ischemia of the tissues distal to the thrombus.
- The most obvious clinical characteristic of burning mouth syndrome is the lack of any clinically observable abnormalities.
- Osteoarthritis is associated with destruction of the articular cartilage and the bones of the joints and appears to be one of the few diseases that are directly related to the aging process. Rheumatoid arthritis is a chronic systemic inflammatory disorder that has no known cause but may be associated with genetics, autoimmunity, or reactions to infectious organisms.

(continued)

SUMMARY *(continued)*

- Osteoporosis is a decrease in bone density that occurs primarily in women after menopause, leading to an increased risk of bone fractures especially of the hip. Osteoporosis of the jaw can accelerate the amount of bone loss associated with a concomitant periodontal infection.

- Paget's disease of bone is associated with initial bone resorption followed by enlargement of the bone with abnormal weak new bone.

- Fibrous dysplasia is thought to have a genetic etiology. There are three forms of the disorder, monostotic, polyostotic, and cherubism.

- The most common presenting feature of temporomandibular disorder is pain, which may be localized in the tissues around the joint or generalized to the surrounding areas of the skull. Treatment focuses on alleviating pain, restoring function, and preventing permanent joint damage.

INTERNET RESOURCES

American Lung Association
  www.lungusa.org
American Parkinson Disease Association
  www.apdaparkinson.org

National Institute of Neurological Disorders and Stroke
  www.ninds.nih.gov
Fibrous Dysplasia Foundation
  www.fibrousdysplasia.org

PORTFOLIO ACTIVITIES

1. Develop an office protocol for identifying and managing a patient who has a productive cough of unknown etiology that is suspicious for TB.

Critical Thinking Activities

1. Observe the operation and physical makeup of your school's dental hygiene clinic and the public areas. What considerations have been made to try to limit the spread of colds and flu? What more could be done to limit the spread of colds and flu? Share your findings and suggestions for improvements with the rest of the class.

Case Study

Patients who have Parkinson's disease can be a challenge to manage in the dental office. You have just been informed that a 70-year-old patient with Parkinson's disease, Mrs. G, has been scheduled for a dental hygiene appointment with you in 1 week. Assume that the patient has moderate symptoms that limit her ability to function independently.

A. What are the extraoral, perioral, and intraoral characteristics of this disease?

B. How can you plan for this appointment? Write a description of the modifications that you might make to ensure that this appointment is successful.
C. What type of homecare suggestions might be appropriate for this patient? Research the internet and other sources to find options that might be able to help this patient care for her teeth independently for as long as possible.

REFERENCES

American Association of Endodontists. Endodontic implications of bisphosphonate-associated osteonecrosis of the jaws. Available at: http://www.aae.org. Accessed June 16, 2006.

American Dental Association (ADA) Council on Scientific Affairs. Dental management of patients receiving oral bisphosphonate therapy, expert panel recommendations. JADA 2006;137:1144–1150.

American Lung Association. Lung Disease Data: 2006: 13. Available at: http://www.lungusa.org/site/pp.asp?c=dvLUK9O0E&b=22542. Accessed June 16, 2006.

American Parkinson Disease Association. Basic information about Parkinson's disease. Available at: http://www.apdaparkinson.org/user/AboutParkinson.asp. Accessed June 17, 2006.

Anand MKN. Fibrous dysplasia. Last updated July 27, 2006. e medicine: Instant Access to the Minds of Medicine. Available at: http://www.emedicine.com/radio/topic284.htm. Accessed October 20, 2006.

Burchiel KJ, Khoromi S, Totah A, Zachariah SB. Trigeminal neuralgia. Last updated October 6, 2006. e medicine: Instant Access to the Minds of Medicine. Available at: http://www.emedicine.com/med/topic2899.htm. Accessed October 21, 2006.

Carbone L, Barrow K. Paget disease. Last updated June 21, 2005. e medicine: Instant Access to the Minds of Medicine. Available at: http://www.emedicine.com/med/topic2998.htm. Accessed October 21, 2006.

Centers for Disease Control and Prevention. Prevention and control of meningococcal diseases: recommendations of the Advisory Committee on Immunization Practices (ACIP). MMWR 2005;54(no. RR-7):1–3.

Centers for Disease Control and Prevention. Trends in tuberculosis—United States, 2005. MMWR 2006;55:305–308.

Centers for Disease Control and Prevention. Reported tuberculosis in the United States, 2004. Atlanta, GA: U.S. Department of Health and Human Services, CDC, September 2005.

Chen YH, Zhou D. Crohn disease. Last updated June 8, 2004. e medicine: Instant Access to the Minds of Medicine. Available at: http://www.emedicine.com/radio/topic197.htm. Accessed September 30, 2006.

DeAngelis S. The patient with cystic fibrosis: a case study. Access 2001;15(8):58–59,65.

DePaola LG. Colds and flu: prevention in the dental office. Infect Control Forum 2005;3(2):1–6.

Fisichella PM, Patti M. Gastroesophageal reflux disease. Last updated September 13, 2006. e medicine: Instant Access to the Minds of Medicine. Available at: http://www.emedicine.com/med/topic857.htm. Accessed October 21, 2006.

Grushka M, Epstein JB, Gorsky M. Burning mouth syndrome. Am Fam Physician 2002;65(4):615–620.

Gurenlian JR. Crohn's disease. Access 2003;17(3):30–32.

Gurenlian JR. Gastroesophageal reflux disease. Access 2004;18(9):30–35.

Gutkowski S. Burning mouth syndrome. Prevent Angle 2004;3(1):1–7.

Hoyert DL, Heron M, Murphy SL, Kung HC. Deaths: final data for 2003. National Center for Health Statistics, Centers for Disease Control and Prevention. Available at: http://www.cdc.gov/nchs/products/pubs/pubd/hestats/finaldeaths03/finaldeaths03.htm. Accessed June 17, 2006.

Huether SE, McCance KL. Understanding pathophysiology. 3rd ed. St. Louis: Mosby, 2004:990–993, 997–999.

Johnston M, Eastone JA. Barrett esophagus and Barrett ulcer. Last updated June 16, 2005. e medicine: Instant Access to the Minds of Medicine. Available at: http://www.emedicine.com/med/topic210.htm. Accessed October 15, 2006.

Kim JYS, Shenaq SM, Niederbichler A, Armenta A. Facial nerve paralysis. Last updated June 14, 2006. e medicine: Instant Access to the Minds of Medicine. Available at: http://www.emedicine.com/plastic/topic522.htm. Accessed September 25, 2006.

Lenaerts ME, Couch JR. Trigeminal Neuralgia. Last updated March 17, 2006. e medicine: Instant Access to the Minds of Medicine. Available at: http://www.emedicine.com/oph/topic512.htm. Accessed October 13, 2006.

Malamed SF. Medical emergencies in the dental office. 5th ed. St. Louis: Mosby, 2000:211.

Mitchell TV. Treating the patient with Parkinson's disease. J Pract Hyg 2006;15(3):17–19.

Mojon P. Oral health and respiratory infection. J Can Dent Assoc 2002;68(6):340–345.

Monnell K, Zachariah SB. Bell palsy. Last updated June 2, 2005. e medicine: Instant Access to the Minds of Medicine. Available at: http://www.emedicine.com/neuro/topic413.htm. Accessed October 21, 2006.

National Institute of Neurological Disorders and Stroke. Glossopharyngeal neuralgia information page. Last updated June 7, 2006. Available at: http://www.ninds.nih.gov/disorders/glossopharyngeal_neuralgia/glossopharyngeal_neuralgia.htm#toc. Accessed June 17, 2006.

National Osteoporosis Foundation. Physician's guide to prevention and treatment of osteoporosis 2003. Available at: http://www.nof.org/physguide/inside_cover.htm. Accessed June 17, 2006.

Okeson JP. Management of temporomandibular disorders and occlusion. 5th ed. St. Louis: Mosby, 2003.

Paget SA, Leibowitz EL. Giant cell arteritis. Last updated February 16, 2006. e medicine: Instant Access to the Minds of Medicine. Available at: http://www.emedicine.com/med/topic2241.htm. Accessed October 20, 2006.

Peiris JSM, Phil D, Yuen KY, et al. The severe acute respiratory syndrome. N Engl J Med 2003;49:2431–2441.

Porth CM. Essentials of pathophysiology: concepts of altered health states. Philadelphia: Lippincott Williams & Wilkins, 2004:359–365, 478–479, 489, 821–824.

Rubin E, Gorstein F, Rubin R, et al. Rubin's Pathology: Clinicopathologic foundations of medicine. 4th ed. Baltimore: Lippincott Williams & Wilkins, 2005:705, 1349–1350.

Rowe WA. Inflammatory bowel disease. Last updated June 27, 2006. e medicine: Instant Access to the Minds of Medicine. Available at: http://www.emedicine.com/med/topic1169.htm. Accessed October 21, 2006.

Sahar-Srivastava S, Cowan R. Pathophysiology and treatment of migraine and related headache. Last updated August 4, 2005. e medicine: Instant Access to the Minds of Medicine. Available at: http://www.emedicine.com/neuro/topic517.htm. Accessed June 17, 2006.

Smith HR, Smolen JS. Rheumatoid arthritis. Last updated May 24, 2006. e medicine: Instant Access to the Minds of Medicine. Available at: http://www.emedicine.com/med/topic2024.htm. Accessed October 12, 2006.

Smith NM, Bresee JS, Shay DK, et al. Prevention and control of influenza: recommendations of the Advisory Committee on Immunization Practice. CDC, MMWR, July 28, 2006/55(RR10);1–42.

Stacy G, Basu AP. Osteoarthritis, primary. Last updated July 19, 2006. e medicine: Instant Access to the Minds of Medicine. Available at: http://www.emedicine.com/radio/topic492.htm. Accessed September 30, 2006.

Stephen J. Pneumonia, bacterial. Last updated September 12, 2006. e medicine: Instant Access to the Minds of Medicine. Available at: http://www.emedicine.com/emerg/topic465.htm. Accessed September 15, 2006.

Teng YTA, Taylor GW, Scannapieco F, et al. Periodontal health and systemic disorders. J Can Dent Assoc 2002;68(3):189.

Weiner DL. Pediatrics, Reye syndrome. Last updated November 28, 2005. e medicine: Instant Access to the Minds of Medicine. Available at: http://www.emedicine.com/emerg/topic399.htm. Accessed October 13, 2006.

11

Lesions That Look Like Vesicles

Key Terms

- **Acantholysis**
- **Ankyloglossia**
- **Antipruritic**
- **Autoinoculation**
- **Bulla**
- **Corticosteroids**
- **Cytotoxic virus**
- **Dysphagia**
- **Erythema**
- **Forchheimer's sign**
- **Herpetic whitlow**
- **Herpesviridae**
- **Immunosuppression**
- **Koplik's spots**
- **Lymphadenopathy**
- **Microstomia**
- **Mucocele**
- **Mucus extravasation phenomenon**
- **Mucus retention cyst**
- **Necrosis**
- **Nikolsky sign**
- **Noncytotoxic virus**
- **Pathognomonic**
- **Perioral skin**
- **Prodrome**
- **Pruritus**
- **Sialolith**
- **Subclinical infections**
- **Tzanck cells**
- **Ulcerations**
- **Vesicular lesions**

Learning Outcomes

1. Define the key terms used in this chapter.

2. Describe the clinical features of the mucocele.

3. State four of the trigger mechanisms that are involved with herpes simplex virus infections.

4. List the sites affected in type 1 and type 2 herpes simplex virus infections.

5. Describe the cycle of varicella-zoster virus infection and the subsequent reactivation resulting in shingles.

6. List the organisms involved in hand-foot-and-mouth disease, rubeola, rubella, herpes labialis, and herpangina.

7. Name the four major types of pemphigus vulgaris.

8. Describe the histologic findings that would differentiate pemphigus vulgaris and mucous membrane pemphigoid.

9. Describe the key factors of the immunofluorescence diagnostic test in the differentiation of pemphigus vulgaris and pemphigoid.

10. List the three types of epidermolysis bullosa.

11. List three diseases to consider in a clinical differential diagnosis involving pemphigoid.

12. Discuss the importance of requesting a thorough eye examination when a diagnosis of mucous membrane pemphigoid or pemphigus vulgaris has been made.

13. Discuss the definition of cytotoxic and noncytotoxic.

14. List at least three sites where a person may self-inoculate with HSV.

Chapter Outline

VESICULOBULLOUS DISORDERS

Vesiculobullous disorders are sometimes grouped as similar in appearance when seen by the clinician. However, with careful evaluation clinically and with the help of diagnostic tests, these lesions can usually be differentiated quite successfully. Based on the patient history, the clinical appearance, and some investigation, the astute clinician can combine the clues observed to solve the mystery. This chapter addresses those lesions in the mouth that have a vesicular appearance. They may be categorized as traumatic or inflammatory lesions, lesions from known infectious agents, immune system disorders, or those that have a genetic or congenital component.

TRAUMATIC OR INFLAMMATORY LESIONS

Traumatic lesions with a vesicle-like appearance may sometimes be ulcerative or they may have a smooth tissue appearance with only slight color differentiation. The lesion may be benign or they may be something more serious and need further evaluation to confirm a diagnosis. A careful evaluation will usually provide the clinician with enough information to sort out the etiology and the course of action related to the lesion.

NAME: Mucocele

The **mucocele** is also known as the **mucus extravasation phenomenon** (lined with granulation tissue), mucous cyst, and **mucous retention cyst** (when lined with epithelium). Figure 11.1A depicts a mucocele in the buccal mucosa. Fig. 11B depicts the histology of a mucocele. The accepted term is "mucus extravasation phenomenon," or "mucous retention cyst." Within the same term, the ranula occurs in the floor of the mouth affecting the ducts of the sublingual and submandibular glands. The ranulas can be very large and are covered in more detail in Chapter 17.

Etiology: Mucoceles are caused by trauma and severance of a salivary excretory duct. The damage to the ductal structure causes mucin to be retained in the surrounding tissue. The lesions related to the mucocele are discussed in more detail in Chapter 17 under salivary gland disorders. The mucocele is mentioned here because the lesion, depending upon the location and whether it is more superficial, may appear vesicle-like. The mucous retention cyst results from a **sialolith**, or salivary gland stone, and sometimes from ductal scar tissue, causing obstruction of the involved salivary gland. Usually found in an older age group, the mucous retention cyst is often found in the floor of the mouth. Figure 11.2 shows a mucous retention cyst in the floor of the mouth).

Method of Transmission: There is no method of transmission of the mucocele because the lesion is caused by trauma.

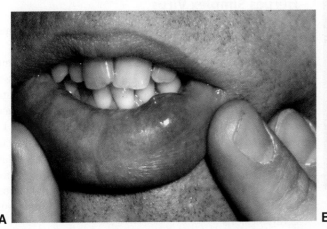
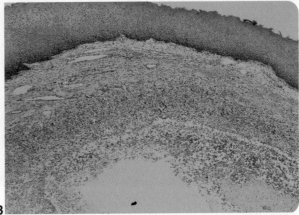

Figure 11.1. A. A mucocele in the buccal mucosa region. (Courtesy of Dr. Harvey Kessler.) **B.** Histology of a mucocele.

Epidemiology: The younger age groups are most often affected, because of the traumatic nature of the lesion. Both sexes are affected equally.

Pathogenesis: The mucocele occurs when a salivary gland duct is severed through trauma and the contents of the duct collect in the tissue, manifested with a raised, seemingly fluid-filled lesion. The more superficial mucoceles will rupture spontaneously, leaving an ulcerlike lesion.

Extraoral Characteristics: None

Perioral and Intraoral Characteristics: Mucoceles may have a blue hue with a somewhat transparent appearance. Most appear slightly elevated and exhibit a smooth appearance. This is especiaally true when they occur in the oral mucosa of the lip area. Mucoceles may also appear in the palate, and they may be in any area where there is salivary gland function.

Distinguishing Characteristics: The clouded blue hue of the mucocele is a distinguishing characteristic and is often used in clinical differentiation. The color variation depends upon how close to the surface the mucin may pool. The patient may be able to confirm that the lesion increases and subsequently decreases in size after trauma because of a rupture in the lesion. Reports of the size vary from millimeters to centimeters.

Significant Microscopic Features: The mucocele is walled off by granulation tissue enclosing the mucin pool. The severed duct shows ductal dilation, and an inflammatory response is initiated. Mucoceles are not true cysts, since they are not epithelial lined. Mucous retention cysts or mucous cysts result because of a salivary gland stone or sialolith composed of calcium carbonate. Additionally, epithelial tissue lining the cyst should be observed microscopically.

Dental Implications: The main dental implication would be tissue trauma to the buccal mucosa or the lip region because of the elevated tissue and tendency for the patient to traumatize the area while eating or chewing.

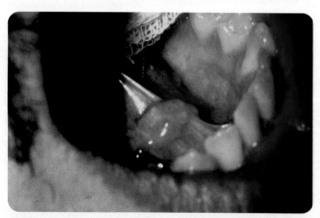

Figure 11.2. Mucous retention cyst in the floor of the mouth. (Courtesy of Dr. Carolyn Bentley.)

Differential Diagnosis: Considerations may be neoplasms, lipomas, vascular malformations, a dermoid cyst (when in the floor of the mouth), and mucoepidermoid carcinoma.

Treatment and Prognosis: When a mucocele is classified as a mucous cyst or blockage of the duct, surgical approaches are warranted. These approaches are discussed in Chapter 17 under salivary gland diseases.

INFECTIOUS VIRAL DISEASES

Viruses may be **cytotoxic** or **noncytotoxic**. Cytotoxic viruses replicate within the host cells and destroy them, releasing new viral particles into adjacent tissues. These particles go on to invade other host cells, allowing progressive cellular destruction to take place. As more host cells are destroyed, more symptoms develop. Humans are exposed to viruses daily, but no symptoms occur if the immune system is healthy. If the body's defenses become weakened, however, through fatigue, stress, injury, or other factors, the person is more susceptible to the cellular destruction.

Noncytotoxic viruses do not cause cellular destruction or they may cause it on an intermittent basis. The virus may lie dormant in an infected cell or take the place of some of the host DNA and become part of the cell. For example, herpesvirus may remain dormant for long periods but become activated when host defenses are altered.

Differentiation between viral and nonviral diseases is important in determining the treatment for a particular lesion. If the disease is viral, the treatment should be started no later than 48 hours after the onset of symptoms to achieve optimal success. If cell destruction and viral replication has occurred before the clinician views the oral lesions, the antiviral medications may be less effective. Antiviral medications are most effective in the **prodromal** stage, when the individual experiences localized tingling, burning, or **pruritic** sensations that signify a pending viral outbreak. The following viral infections are the most common.

Herpes Simplex Virus

Herpes Simplex Virus (HSV) is a member of the human herpesvirus (HHV) family known as Herpesviridae. At least eight human herpesviruses (HHV) have been identified, including those involved in AIDS related illnesses. HHV 1 and HHV 2, however, are commonly associated with disease entities and the simplex virus. The virus may be in either a primary form or a systemic form. HHV 1 is associated with primary herpetic gingivostomatitis, recurrent oral herpes, and herpes labialis; type 2 (HHV-2) is associated with genital herpes. However, it is known that type 2 may be found orally because of oral–genital contact (Lamey et al., 1999), and likewise, HHV type 1 may cause genital lesions.

The two are structurally similar, and their manifestation is identical, but they are antigenically different, in other words, the immune system recognizes as two distinct entities. In this book, the discussion focuses on type I (HHV-1). Additionally, in the same family of the Herpetoviridae, we include the varicella–zoster virus, rubeola, rubella, herpangina and hand-foot-and-mouth disease, which is discussed in this section.

Human Herpesvirus Type 1

As mentioned above, HHV type 1 is commonly associated with the oral conditions that are described in the following sections.

NAME: Primary herpetic gingivostomatitis

Etiology: Primary herpetic gingivostomatitis is caused by human herpesvirus type 1 (herpes simplex). Figure 11.3A demonstrates a primary herpetic infection with vesicles on the lip, tongue, and buccal mucosa.

Method of Transmission: Transmission occurs through physical contact such as kissing, shared utensils, and close contact. It is more readily transmitted in dense and crowded populations. It may be passed through the sharing of eating utensils or through aerosols in close living conditions. Technically, the virus is spread through saliva and has a propensity toward the pharynx, eyes, lips, and oral areas.

Epidemiology: Exposure of one-half of the U.S. population and even up to 85% of populations in crowded living areas has been found. The infection occurs equally among males, females, and young children, and immunocompromised adults or those never exposed to the virus are most commonly affected. Children usually exhibit a subclinical infection.

Pathogenesis: The initial exposure of an individual to the virus is called the primary infection. Recurrent episodes are termed secondary forms. More than 85% of adults in both urban and rural areas have antibodies, showing that they have been exposed to the herpes simplex virus. Many of these individuals are not aware of ever experiencing the primary infection, while others are quite ill. After mucocutaneous contact with an infected individual, there is a 2-day to 2-week incubation period. The disease may present as either a subclinical or a clinical infection. Most primary infections are subclinical. Usually, individuals develop antibodies to herpesvirus during childhood at between 6 months and 6 years of age. However, the primary infection may occur in adulthood in those individuals who were not exposed to the virus as children. Following resolution of the primary infection, antiherpetic antibodies are formed, and the virus may migrate along the trigeminal nerve to the trigeminal ganglion. There it will remain latent until triggered by some future event.

Extraoral Characteristics: Both HHV-1 and 2 may be found in the oral or genital areas. When found in the genital area herpes simplex 1 presents as multiple, painful ulcerations on any mucosal or cutaneous surface. The two are clinically indistinguishable regardless of lesion site.

Perioral and Intraoral Characteristics: The classic feature of this condition is a fiery red, marginal gingivitis that usually affects all areas of the dental arches as shown in the primary severe herpetic lesions in Figure 11.3B and C.

Multiple small vesicular lesions appear on the gingiva, lips, tongue, oral mucosa, and occasionally on perioral skin. The vesicles rupture quickly and appear as ulcerations surrounded by erythema.

Distinguishing Characteristics: The individual experiences extreme pain, elevated temperature, and generalized malaise. Cervical lymphadenopathy and a sore throat commonly occur. Signs and symptoms may be more severe when it occurs in adults. The cycle of primary HSV exposure is represented in Figure 11.3D.

Significant Microscopic Features: HSV exhibits intraepithelial vesicle formation. The clinical characteristics of the disease are readily apparent to the clinician in most cases, but a viral culture can provide a definitive diagnosis when necessary. The cells of HSV are readily apparent in most cases when viewed microscopically. The cells appear as virus-infected epithelial cells with inflammatory cells and a ballooned, degenerating appearance with microscopic inclusions and multi nucleation. Figure 11.4 shows the histology of a HSV infected cell.

A biopsy, cytologic smear, or viral culture can provide a definitive diagnosis when necessary. (See Clinical Protocol Appendix 1 for steps in collecting and processing a smear sample.)

Dental Implications: The clinical appearance and course of the infection are significant factors in determining this diagnosis. Beginning or completing treatment on a patient with herpetic lesions would be detrimental because of spreading the virus. Treatment should be rescheduled until the lesions have healed. Eating is the most significant problem because the course of the disease is 10 to 14 days.

Differential Diagnosis: Diagnosis is based on clinical presentation. Differentiation must be made with other vesicles that occur orally such as the following:

1. *Recurrent aphthae*—elevated temperature may or may not be present with the ulcers, and they usually appear as single lesions rather than coalescing groups. Aphthae appear on freely moveable nonkeratinized mucous membranes such as the labial mucosa, maxillary and mandibular sulci, soft palate, buccal mucosa, and oropharynx. Additionally, the ventral surface of the tongue and the floor of the mouth are often af-

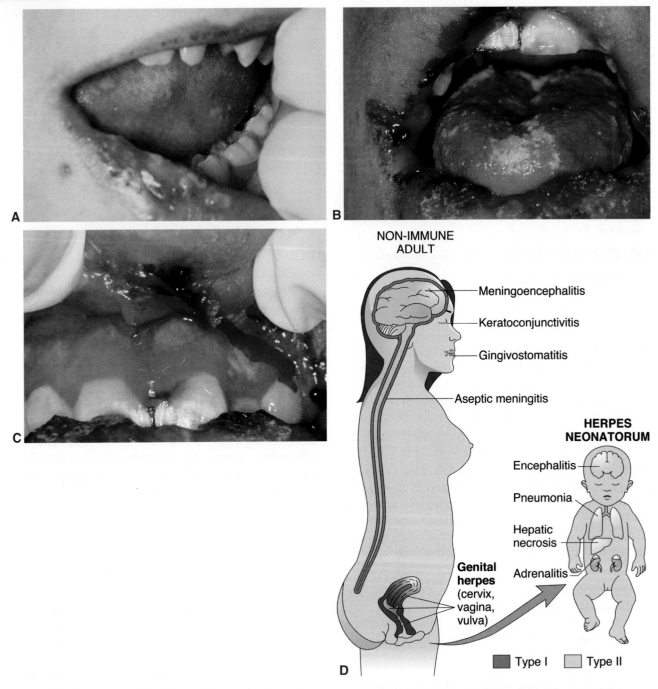

Figure 11.3. A. Primary herpetic gingivostomatitis; lip lesions and tongue lesions. (Courtesy of Dr. Michael Brennan.) **B.** Primary herpetic lesions. (Courtesy of Dr. Terry Rees.) **C.** Primary herpetic lesions. (Courtesy of Dr. Terry Rees.) **D.** Cycle of herpes infections. (From Rubin E, Farber JL. Pathology, 3rd Edition. Philadelphia: Lippincott William & Wilkins, 1999.)

fected. Aphthae appear as ulcerlike lesions, not as vesicles, and are isolated to single lesions without clusters.

2. *Coxsackie virus* might be considered in early differentiation.

3. *Herpes zoster* could be a consideration, but the lesions are unilateral and usually seen in older adults.

A careful health history will assist in differentiating the most likely possibilities.

Treatment and Prognosis: Palliative treatment with a soft diet, liquids that are nonacidic, and noncarbonated beverages are optimal. Cold foods help, such as ice cream or sherbet. Antipyretics, topical application of Benadryl elixir and Kaopectate 50–50% helps to relieve pain to enable eating. Oral antivirals are not helpful once the lesions are present, although their use may prevent viral shedding and make the patient less infectious to others. The lesions

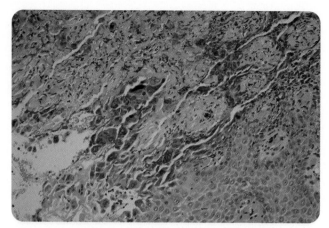

Figure 11.4. Histology of a herpetic lesion (Courtesy of Dr. Yi-Shing Lisa Cheng.)

usually resolve completely within 10 to 14 days. However, herpesviruses often follow a recurring pattern (See Clinical Protocol #8).

NAME: Secondary or recurrent herpes simplex infections

Etiology: Recurrent infections are caused by reactivation of the latent virus. The event that causes the reactivation, or triggering event, is usually one that causes a compromised immune system such as a cold, fever, sunburn, emotional stress, trauma, pregnancy, infection, debilitation, menstruation, systemic disease, and possible allergies. In the oral cavity, activation may be precipitated by manipulation of tissues as in scaling and root planning or periodontal surgery.

Method of Transmission: The virus becomes reactivated and produces a recurrent infection. The virus cannot be considered transmitted in the strict sense of the term; however, the virus particles found in the recurrent lesions are active and can be transmitted to other individuals and to other areas of the affected individual's body.

Epidemiology: Recurrent infections affect 20 to 40% of individuals after the primary infection.

Pathogenesis: This is a latent infection following the primary infection. When the dormant virus in the nerve ganglion is activated, it moves along the trigeminal nerve usually to the place of initial inoculation and infects the epithelial cells of the mucosa, creating vesicular lesions. As a result, the whole cycle begins again.

Extraoral Characteristics: Any extraoral characteristics is evident at the time of an outbreak, and clusters of vesicles would be seen only at this time unless there is some scar formation due to extensive outbreaks.

Perioral and Intraoral Characteristics: These lesions initially appear as clusters of vesicles on the vermilion border, perioral skin, or less commonly on keratinized intraoral surfaces. When occurring on the lip and perioral areas, they are termed **herpes labialis.** Figure. 11.5A depicts early herpetic lesions on the lip.

Intraoral lesions appear unilaterally as very small vesicles on the palatal or attached gingiva. When the lesions occur on the lip, they are often referred to as cold sores or fever blisters, but the correct term is herpes labialis. The vesicles quickly rupture and leave ulcers that crust and usually heal without scarring in 7 to 14 days. Figure 11.5B shows vesicles on the lip in a later stage, beginning to heal and crust.

Distinguishing Characteristics: There are often localized, prodromal symptoms prior to a vesicle appearance such as burning, tingling, or pain before any eruption.

Significant Microscopic Features: Histology of a herpes simplex infection reveals ulceration with fibrin exudates and acantholytic epithelial cells (**Tzanck cells**).

Dental Implications: When lesions are present, routine dental care should be postponed to prevent patient discomfort and spread of the virus. The lesions should be completely healed with no exudates apparent.

Differential Diagnosis: Herpes labialis is usually very distinct in appearance; however, early lesions may not appear as vesicles, but rather as skin irritations or

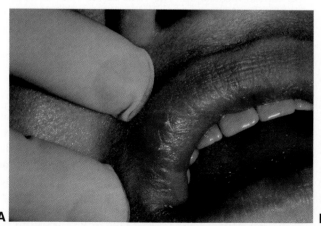
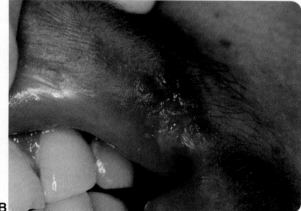

Figure 11.5. A. Early herpes lesions, a beginning herpetic lesion of the lip. **B.** Herpes labialis- lesions at the commissure and upper lip area. (Courtesy of Dr. Michael Brennan.)

raised areas on the lip. Careful questioning of the patient will usually provide the information needed to make a clinical decision. *Impetigo*—no purulent exudates are present in herpes, history of lesions should aid in differentiating the occurrence (see Chapter 23).

Intraorally, *recurrent aphthous stomatitis*—ulcerations tend to be less numerous, single rather than coalescing, and larger. Ulcerations usually occur on nonkeratinized tissues (see Chapter 12) and are single and ulcerlike.

Treatment and Prognosis: (herpes labialis):
Antiviral topical ointments or creams may reduce the duration and may stop some lesions from developing, if applied early, before replication of the virus occurs. Always instruct patients to use a cotton applicator, rubber glove or finger cot to reduce the potential for transmitting the virus to other parts of the body or to other individuals. (See Clinical Protocol 7 for patient education information.) Instruct the patient to avoid sunlight exposure when possible and to use a lip balm of SPF 15 or higher. Unless the topical agent is applied during the prodromal phase before replication is well under way, it is of little benefit. Intraoral lesions—acyclovir 200-mg capsules 5 times daily for 7 days or valacyclovir 2-g orally, 2 times (12 hours apart) for 1 day. Therapy may shorten the duration of lesions, but success is more predictable if treatment is provided in the prodromal stage. There are presently no topical medications recommended for intraoral use. The lesions are self-limiting and will resolve within 7 to 14 days. Using the antiviral medications when prodromal signs first occur is the most effective way to reduce or eliminate the outbreaks. Counseling the patient to use a lip balm sunscreen and to avoid trigger mechanisms may help to limit the frequency of outbreaks (See Clinical Protocol #7).

Other Forms of Herpes Infection

Herpes infection can occur in other areas of the body such as on the fingers, eyes, nose, and skin areas when there is a break in the mucosa or mucosal lining. Safety glasses are mandatory for working in any area where there may be exposure to splash, aerosols, particles from scrubbing any type of instrument, or conducting laboratory work that may be needed. Safety goggles with side shields are a standard in the infection protocol and certainly crucial to avoid any potential contamination of the clinician's eye area.

HERPETIC WHITLOW

Herpetic whitlow is caused by the same HSV type 1 virus as those above; however, the infection occurs on the terminal segment of a finger (Figure 11.6). This can leave the infected individual debilitated for weeks at a time. Herpetic whitlow usually occurs as a primary infection, but cyclic recurrence has been described. Healthcare workers are susceptible, especially when working in the

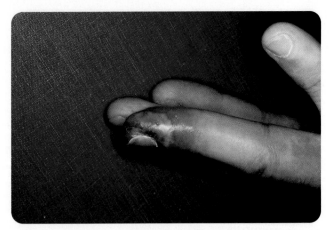

Figure 11.6. Herpetic whitlow. (Courtesy of Dr. Peter Jacobsen.)

mouth. In previous years, before the infection control standards that are currently in place, dental personnel were especially vulnerable. Herpetic whitlow can also cause infection to other areas of the body such as the mouth, nose, and eyes or any other mucosal lining.

OCULAR HERPES

Ocular herpes is a type 1 or type 2 HSV infection, usually caused by autoinoculation. Although relatively rare, it may result from touching a herpetic lesion elsewhere and then touching the eye. There is, of course, a real danger of ocular herpes from any splash that may enter the eye from aerosols or debris that enters the eye during dental procedures. This is very serious and can result in blindness. The child seen in Figure 11.7 has exposed his eye to herpes and exhibits obvious lesions in the mouth and perioral tissues.

Obvious lesions are seen on the mouth and periorally. All individuals who experience herpetic lesions should be warned of the possibility of transferring the virus to the eyes and any mucosal lining. They should use caution not to touch the lesions with unprotected fingers, and they should wash their hands thoroughly after each application of topical medication. The virus can live on surfaces and in droplets for up to 24 hours, and standard infection control procedures must be followed to protect the clinician, patient, and subsequent patients.

HERPES SIMPLEX VIRUS TYPE 2 (GENITAL HERPES)

This form of herpes is transmitted in genital secretions, producing genital ulcerations. The practice of oral sex in the patient population has increased the likelihood of transmission of either type 1 or type 2 to both the oral and genital tissue areas. For the purpose of this book, we mention this fact, although there is no way to differentiate the types without very sophisticated laboratory and histologic tests. Research supports the transmission of type 1 and type 2 transmissions of herpetic viruses through oral sex.

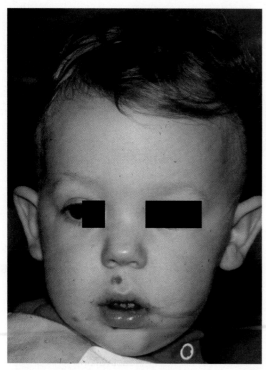

Figure 11.7. Ocular herpes. (Courtesy of Dr. Peter Lockhart.)

Oral sex is also implicated in certain head and neck cancers caused by the human papilloma viruses (See Chapter 16).

NAME: Primary varicella–zoster.
Varicella is the original infection (chickenpox) and zoster (shingles) occurs when the virus is subsequently reactivated. We have discussed the HHV types 1 and type 2, caused by the herpes simplex virus. As discussed earlier in the chapter, there are eight known HHV type categories. The HHV 3 type is known as the varicella–zoster virus. As with types 1 and 2 HHV, type 3 has some oral manifestations and is covered in this section as well.

Etiology: The human herpesvirus type 3, or varicella–zoster virus, is the causative agent of primary varicella infection, or chickenpox.

Method of Transmission: Transmission occurs through air droplets or direct contact with lesions. This is a highly contagious disease when lesions are present.

Epidemiology: Young children are most often affected, but the disease can occur in adults who have never been exposed to the virus. Males and females are affected equally. Figure 11.8A shows a female with a primary varicella infection.

Pathogenesis: The virus normally infects the respiratory tract, and it is carried through the body via the bloodstream into the epidermis. At this point, viral replication begins to destroy the epithelial basal cells. After a 2-week incubation period, symptoms begin to appear. The virus can be transmitted approximately 2 days before the appearance of the rash and until all lesions are crusted, with no detectable drainage. The disease resolves in 2 to 3 weeks. The virus may migrate over sensory nerves to lie dormant in ganglia until triggered later, much like the herpes simplex viruses. If this occurs, the virus remains in a latent stage in ganglia along the sensory nerves and may be reactivated years later to emerge as herpes zoster, or shingles, discussed below.

Extraoral Characteristics: The symptoms usually begin with malaise, sore throat, and upper respiratory congestion. Fever and slight lymphadenopathy usually precede or occur concurrently with a vesicular rash that appears on the trunk, head, and neck. The vesicles form pustules and then ulcers with an erythematous border. Figure 11.8B shows the skin lesions of primary varicella chickenpox. During the peak of the infection, new lesions continue to develop while older lesions are beginning to heal, so that one can observe lesions in all stages of development. The lesions are extremely pruritic, and it is difficult to keep the patient, usually a child, from scratching them. Often scratching will introduce bacteria into the lesions, causing a secondary bacterial infection that usually results in scarring.

Perioral and Intraoral Characteristics: Cutaneous lesions may form anywhere in the head and neck region and appear identical to the lesions found on the trunk and the extremities. Vesicular intraoral lesions are usually found on the lips, hard palate, and the buccal mucosa. The lesions will heal without scarring in most cases. Fig. 11.8C depicts the progression of varicella–zoster (VZV) and, subsequently, shingles or herpes zoster.

APPLICATION

Excellent office protocol is crucial in adhering to good infection control practices for your work environment. Keeping abreast of current standards with methods of safety for both you and the patient is part of good work ethics and practice. As discussed, the HSV virus is easily spread, and any dental procedures must be postponed when infection is active. Infection control issues need to be maintained to protect the health of both practitioner and patient. Adequate safety protection such as goggles with shields; fully protected office wear consisting of long sleeves, fully washable garments, and overgarments; mask and gloves are always mandatory. In some practices, street clothing with open jackets are worn, and this type of office wear does not adequately protect either the patient or the practitioner. The realization that anything worn around a patient or spattered-on clothing worn away from the office will endanger others is key to confining any viral or infectious agents. Contracting ocular herpes or any other form of herpes can be life changing for you, your family, and the patient.

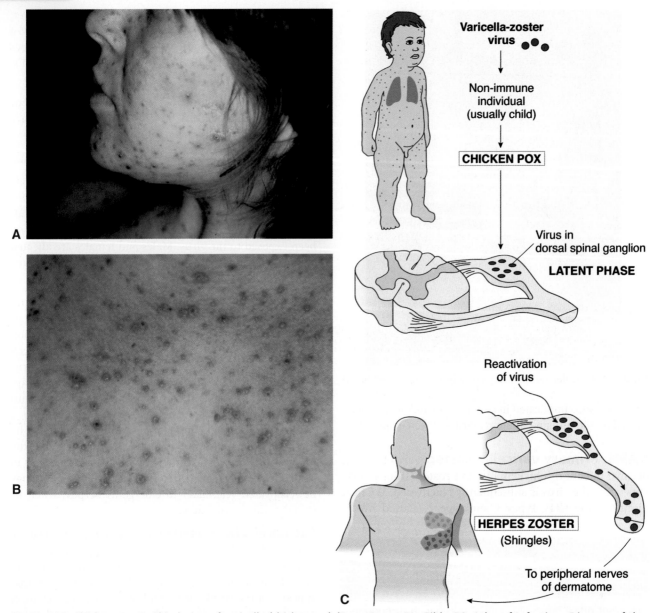

Figure 11.8. Chickenpox. **A.** Skin lesion of varicella (chickenpox) (From Sweet RL, Gibbs RS. Atlas of Infectious Diseases of the Female Genital Tract. Philadelphia: Lippincott Williams & Wilkins, 2005). **B.** Skin lesion of chickenpox (From Sweet RL, Gibbs RS. Atlas of Infectious Diseases of the Female Genital Tract. Philadelphia: Lippincott Williams & Wilkins, 2005). **C.** Progression of varicella and herpes zoster virus—the progression of varicella to shingles (From Rubin E MD and Farber JL MD. Pathology, 3rd Edition. Philadelphia: Lippincott Williams & Wilkins, 1999) .

Distinguishing Characteristics: This disease presents with a wide range of symptoms; and often the infection is subclinical or may be a minor rash of only a few lesions and some upper respiratory symptoms. Occasionally, the disease is so severe that the patient has to be hospitalized to maintain hydration and body temperature. Usually, the disease manifests somewhere between these extremes. The intense pruritus, clinical presentation, and self-limiting course of the disease usually distinguish it from other conditions.

Significant Microscopic Features: Superficial intraepithelial vesicles

Dental Implications: Treatment should not proceed until the person is completely without any visible exudates in any of the lesions, both orally and extraorally.

Differential Diagnosis:

1. HSV type 1—Painful lesions are not present in chickenpox.
2. Pruritus may be present with chickenpox, and hand-foot-and-mouth disease.
3. There are vesicles on the trunk in chickenpox.
4. Aphthae would not be a good differential since the oral lesions are not usually painful in chickenpox.

Treatment and Prognosis: Palliative care is suggested, with topical preparations to relieve pruritus. Nonaspirin antipyretics are recommended for any discomfort. This infection is self-limiting, with complete resolution of the lesions in 2 to 3 weeks. However, complications are occasionally associated with this disease including:

In the adult, encephalitis and pneumonia can occur.

Infection during pregnancy may cause spontaneous abortion or congenital birth defects.

Encephalitis and Reye syndrome may occur in this age group. Vaccines are provided for children and are usually given in the combination MMR, commonly provided as childhood immunizations. Adults may reactivate the virus that leads to herpes zoster (shingles), discussed below. A vaccine recently developed for the prevention of shingles may be used for older adults.

NAME: Secondary varicella–zoster (shingles or herpes zoster)

Etiology: Shingles is caused by reactivation of the latent varicella–zoster virus.

Method of Transmission: Shingles is caused by a latent viral infection, and there is no method of transmission other than that which caused the primary infection. However, the lesions in shingles contain active viral particles, and contact with them by a susceptible person can cause the primary disease, which is chickenpox. The patient should be cautioned to avoid contact with persons at high risk such as immunocompromised persons and pregnant women, since the patient is contagious and may infect other individuals. Anyone in an altered immune state could be at risk.

Epidemiology: Herpes zoster is seen most often in adults, especially the elderly, and slightly more often in males than females.

Pathogenesis: The virus may migrate over sensory nerves to lie dormant in ganglia until triggered later, much like the herpes simplex viruses. Reactivation of latent HZV stems from the dorsal ganglion or the trigeminal ganglion. One of the three branches of the trigeminal nerve may be affected: the ophthalmic branch, the maxillary branch, or the mandibular branch. Figure 11.9A illustrates the nerve areas affected by secondary varicella–zoster. The triggering factors may include stress, compromised immune system, debilitating disease states, etc. Prodromal symptoms of pain or paresthesia are common. The unilateral vesicular lesions develop 2 to 4 days later and may last for 2 to 3 weeks.

Extraoral Characteristics: The disease usually presents unilaterally over the sensory nerves of the head, neck, and trunk as a vesicular rash that is extremely painful. The vesicles rupture and crust in a manner similar to that of chickenpox. Along with the rash, there may be fever, pain, malaise, and lymphadenopathy.

Perioral and Intraoral Characteristics: Intraoral presentation is unilateral and consists of small vesicular eruptions on any mucosal surface or on the palate (Fig. 11.9B).

Distinguishing Characteristics: Shingles may be diagnosed clinically when the unilateral distribution of skin lesions is evident. Additionally, the oral lesions and the distinct halt of the lesions at the midline are very characteristic of the disease. Fig 11.9C illustrates the delineated lesion from the midline to the ramus.

The virus does not migrate far beyond the area of skin or mucous membrane supplied by the infected nerve. Figure 11.9C demonstrates the demarcation of the lesions, which subside at the midline of the face.

Microscopic Features: These are the same as those of a primary infection.

Dental Implications: Shingles is a self-limiting condition and should resolve in 2 to 3 weeks. However, 14% of affected individuals may experience postherpetic neuralgia (persistent and often severe pain) that usually resolves within 2 months but may follow a prolonged course and last for years. Other infrequent complications include Ramsay Hunt syndrome (facial paralysis, diminished hearing, and vertigo) and blindness due to involvement of the ophthalmic division of the trigeminal nerve. One rare and serious complication of herpes zoster is spontaneous tooth exfoliation and necrosis of the mandible.

Differential Diagnosis: The pruritic rash is characteristic of other skin disorders in the early stages such as

1. Herpes simplex
2. Impetigo
3. Rubella
4. Rubeola

Treatment and Prognosis: Routinely, patients are seen by their physicians for treatment; however, dental personnel are often involved initially when oral pain is reported.

Treatment and Prognosis: The recommended therapy includes isolation, local management of the skin lesions, controlling pain, antiviral medications, and treatment of herpetic neuralgia. Palliative procedures are recommended with oral acyclovir 800 mg 5 times a day for 7 to 10 days. This may shorten the duration and decrease the probability of postherpetic neuralgia (see below). Oral lesions should be treated in a palliative way with soothing mouth rinses and/or topical anesthetics. The vaccine for varicella is the prime way of avoiding chickenpox and also shingles later in life. Individuals should talk to their physician about the vaccine. In some cases, the vaccine may not be appropriate, such as in those who are pregnant or have immune system problems, allergy concerns, or cancer, or those receiving treatment for cancer.

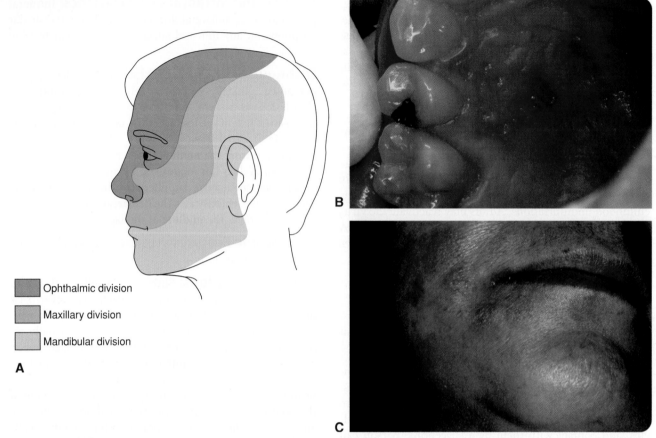

Ophthalmic division

Maxillary division

Mandibular division

A

B

C

Figure 11.9. Varicella–zoster. **A.** Trigeminal nerve branches. **B.** Herpes zoster shingles in the lingual palatal region. (Courtesy of Dr. Michael Brennan.) **C.** Facial shingles from the ramus to the midline.

Coxsackie Virus Infections

Numerous viruses exist in the environment that produce rashes and vesicles. The following section discusses some of the most common that the clinician may see in a dental practice. Picornaviruses are part of the genus Enterovirus. Coxsackie is an enterovirus that causes human herpangina and hand-foot-and-mouth disease.

NAME: Hand-foot-and-mouth disease

Etiology: Hand-foot-and-mouth disease is caused by the coxsackie A-16 virus and other coxsackievirus A and B strains. (Figure 11.10A, 11.10B, and 11.10C depict the lesions associated with hand-foot-and-mouth disease.)

Method of Transmission: The virus is transmitted through airborne and oral/fecal routes. Infection confers immunity against reinfection by that particular strain; however, the person may be infected with other strains later. Hand-foot-and-mouth disease is highly contagious.

Epidemiology: This disease especially affects children under 5, who are vulnerable because of the contact with other children and the numbers who are in schools and daycare centers. Male and females are affected equally.

Pathogenesis: Incubation is 4 to 7 days, and the disease tends to occur in the summer or early fall. Resolution occurs in 1 to 2 weeks.

Extraoral Characteristics: A maculopapular rash occurs on the soles of the feet and the palms of the hands. These lesions develop central vesicles that may or may not rupture and become crusted before healing. Systemic involvement includes fever, sore throat, malaise, and lymphadenopathy.

Perioral and Intraoral Characteristics: Intraoral lesions usually precede the cutaneous rash and may appear on any mucosal surface. The lesions form vesicles that rupture, ulcerate, and become very painful.

Distinguishing Characteristics: Vesicles and ulcers occur on the buccal mucosa, tongue, and palate orally, with external lesions on the soles of the feet, palms of the hands, and fingers and toes. The location of the lesions usually provides a good indication of the disease.

Significant Microscopic Features: Intraepithelial vesicles precede shallow ulcerations.

Dental Implications: The oral lesions cause pain and difficulty with eating and swallowing.

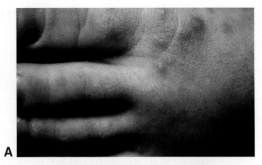

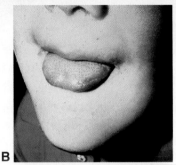

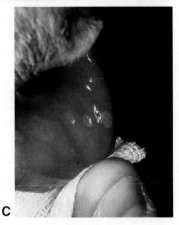

Figure 11.10. Hand-foot-and-mouth disease. **A.** Vesicles on the foot of a young adult. **B.** Vesicles on the tongue of a child. **C.** Vesicles with severe ulceration of the mucosa in an adult. (Courtesy of Dr. Terry Rees.)

Differential Diagnosis: The lesion distribution is usually diagnostic, with the prevalence to the palms of the hands and soles of the feet.

1. Varicella may initially be a consideration.
2. Primary herpetic gingivostomatitis may be considered as well.

Treatment and Prognosis: Treatment is directed toward symptomatic relief. Antipyretic agents and topical medications for sore mouth are the treatments of choice. The prognosis is excellent, and no complications would be expected.

NAME: Herpangina. Herpangina may arise from a number of other types of coxsackievirus A strains. The patient will still be susceptible to other strains of the virus and may contract the disease again. Patients usually complain of a sore throat with fever, loss of appetite, abdomi-

nal pain, and vomiting. Depending upon the length of time and severity of the symptoms, the patient may complain of varying degrees of discomfort.

Etiology: Herpangina is a disease also caused by the coxsackievirus and specifically, the A-16 coxsackievirus. Because of the prevalence of a younger age group, it is often found in schools and daycare centers, and it is easily transmitted. Figure 11.11 depicts lesions in the posterior oropharynx region.

Method of Transmission: Herpangina is easily transmitted via an oral/fecal route.

Epidemiology: Children are most susceptible, with an equal ratio of males and females.

Pathogenesis: Incubation is 4 to 7 days, and the disease tends to occur in the summer or early fall. The onset of symptoms is sudden, with sore throat, dysphagia, fever, headache, and sometimes vomiting. Resolution of the lesions occurs in 1 to 2 weeks; systemic symptoms usually dissipate in 2 to 3 days.

Extraoral Characteristics: Oral lesions are found in the posterior regions of the mouth, soft palate, anterior and posterior pharyngeal pillars, and tonsils. Herpangina presents with a diffuse reddening of the tissues and the appearance of vesicles that rupture and ulcerate.

Perioral and Intraoral Characteristics: Herpangina is characterized by vesicular lesions ranging in size from 1 to 2 mm.

Distinguishing Characteristics: The vesicles of herpangina are small vesicles and ulcerations in the pharyngeal area.

Dental Implications: Dental treatment needs to be postponed until all vesicles and ulcerations are healed.

Microscopic Features: Not applicable

Differential Diagnosis: Diagnosis usually is made from historical and clinical information with little difficulty. Some physicians state that herpangina may appear

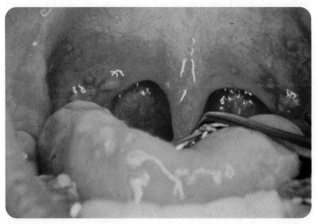

Figure 11.11. Herpangina. (Courtesy of Dr. John Jacoway.)

as strep throat in some cases because of the intense red color.

Treatment and Prognosis: Palliative treatment is recommended and may or may not be required. Excellent prognosis and complications are rare.

ACUTE LYMPHONODULAR PHARYNGITIS

Also caused by the coxsackievirus, ALP is a very rare condition that is also characterized by a sore throat, just as herpangina. The disease is characterized by small nodules in the pharyngeal area and the tonsillar pillars. ALP is caused by a different strain of the coxsackievirus and may vary in appearance from vesicle-like to nodular.

NAME: Paramyxoviridae virus infections: rubeola (measles)

Etiology: The virus originates from the Paramyxoviridae family. Measles has seen a sharp decline, since most children receive the MMR (measles, mumps, rubella) vaccine in early childhood.

Method of Transmission: Measles is airborne and spread through respiratory droplets.

Epidemiology: Children–young adults. There is an equal male to female ratio.

Pathogenesis: Most cases arise in the winter and spring. The incubation period is 10 to 12 days, after which prodromal symptoms occur consisting of fever, malaise, upper respiratory congestion, cough, and conjunctivitis. An erythematous maculopapular rash appears after several days and lasts for 4 to 7 days.

Extraoral Characteristics: The dermal erythematous rash begins on the face and moves downward to cover the trunk and extremities.

Perioral and Intraoral Characteristics: Characteristic lesions called Koplik's spots are found intraorally on the buccal and labial mucosa. These precede the extraoral rash and are considered pathognomonic. The spots are small, bluish white spots on an erythematous background. In severe cases, pitting of the enamel (enamel hypoplasia) in developing teeth may occur.

Distinguishing Characteristics: The intraoral **Koplik's** spots along with the cutaneous rash are usually diagnostic. Figure 11.12 depicts Koplik's spots.

Significant Microscopic Features: Epithelial cells become necrotic. Additional tissue tests may be used to determine the presence of viral antigens.

Dental Implications: All dental work should be postponed until the virus has been eliminated.

Differential Diagnosis: The diagnosis is based on clinical findings both externally and orally.

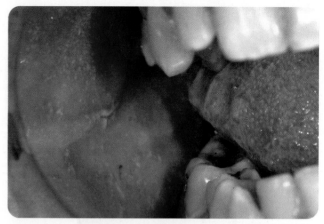

Figure 11.12. Measles (rubeola) Koplik's spots of rubeola. (Courtesy of Dr. James Sciubba.)

Treatment and Prognosis: The treatment is palliative with nonaspirin antipyretics. Complications may include pneumonia and encephalitis. Death may occur in severely immunocompromised individuals.

Togavirus Infections: Rubella (German Measles) Togavirus

NAME: German measles

Etiology: The togavirus and not the paramyxovirus as discussed in rubeola forms of measles cause the German measles, or rubella. The togavirus replicates in the oropharynx and regional lymph nodes and spreads through the bloodstream to skin and distal organs. It can cross the placental barrier, so avoidance of exposure of pregnant women is crucial, since known birth defects have occurred. The birth defect rate is at the highest when the mother is exposed during the first trimester of pregnancy.

Method of Transmission: German measles are highly contagious and spread through respiratory droplets. A vaccine was developed in 1969 reducing the incidence of the virus.

Epidemiology: German measles are most commonly found in children or adults who have not been vaccinated or exposed to the virus. There is an equal predilection. The disease usually occurs in the spring, with a 2- to 3-week incubation period.

Pathogenesis: After an incubation period of 12–24 days, a mild erythematous rash occurs, accompanied by low-grade fever. The rash usually disappears within 3–5 days. Complications during pregnancy include spontaneous abortion or fetal injury causing one or more features of the congenital rubella syndrome (deafness, heart disease, cataracts, encephalopathy, mental retardation, and others). Severe complications are more likely if the mother is infected during the first trimester of pregnancy.

Extraoral Characteristics: Patients usually complain of malaise, fever, nausea, and poor appetite.

Lymphadenopathy is evident, with red and pink papules on the body.

Perioral and Intraoral Characteristics:
Small, discrete, dark-red papules on the soft and hard palate occur in some cases, and these lesions are known as **Forchheimer's signs.**

Distinguishing Characteristics:
Forchheimer's signs may be visible in the soft palate region and are considered an early sign of the infection.

Significant Microscopic Features:
Serologic analysis is required to confirm.

Differential Diagnosis:

1. With rubeola, the signs and symptoms are more severe and much more prolonged.
2. Hand-foot-and-mouth disease may appear more vesicle-like than rubella.
3. Herpangina may appear more vesicle-like than rubella.

Treatment and Prognosis:
Nonaspirin antipyretic medications may be helpful in soothing the discomfort.

NONINFECTIVE VESICULOBULLOUS DISEASES: AUTOIMMUNE DISEASES

This section discusses diseases of an autoimmune nature that have a vesiculobullous intraoral presentation. These diseases are difficult to distinguish on a clinical basis, and microscopic and immunofluorescence features must be determined to obtain a positive diagnosis. However, there are subtle clinical and historical differences that may lead one to suspect one disease over the other possibilities. Multiple lesions that have a gradual onset and a chronic nonhealing course characterize them all. Cutaneous lesions may or may not be present.

NAME: Pemphigus vulgaris

Etiology:
Pemphigus vulgaris is an autoimmune disease.

Method of Transmission:
Since the disease is an autoimmune disease, there is no mode of transmission.

Epidemiology:
There is no sex predilection. Pemphigus vulgaris generally affects patients in the fourth to sixth decades of life; however, the disease may occur in all age groups. Pemphigus is a term used to describe a group of chronic diseases with potential intraoral involvement, including pemphigus vulgaris, pemphigus vegetans, pemphigus foliaceus, pemphigus erythematosus, paraneoplastic pemphigus, and others.

Pemphigus vulgaris is by far the most common form of the disease. Individuals of Jewish or Mediterranean descent may be affected more frequently, and there may be a familial tendency for the disease.

Pathogenesis:
Pemphigus vulgaris is associated with human leukocyte antigens A10, A26, Bw28, and DR4.

Extraoral Characteristics and Clinical Features:
Oral lesions may be the initial sign of pemphigus in over 50% of affected individuals, and virtually 100% of untreated individuals will develop oral lesions. These lesions begin as bullae, usually greater than 1 cm in size, that rupture quickly to form shallow ulcers covered by a gray pseudomembrane. The membrane can be removed to reveal an erythematous surface, as seen in Figure 11.13. The ulcers are painful and can be found on any mucosal surface. If untreated, the lesions persist and enlarge.

Perioral and Intraoral Characteristics:
Lesions may be found on any epithelial surface including the skin, oral cavity, esophagus, larynx, pharynx, vagina, anus, and eyes.

Distinguishing Characteristics:
Nikolsky's sign is usually positive in affected patients. This sign is considered positive when the clinician can initiate bulla formation by stretching or rubbing the mucosa in a clinically unaffected area.

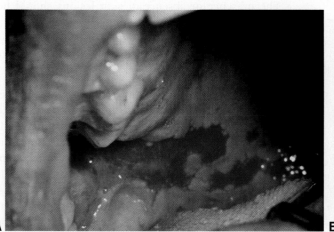
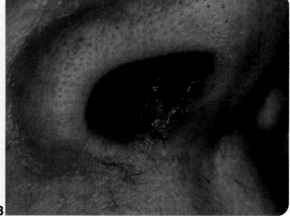

Figure 11.13. Pemphigus vulgaris. **A.** Stripping of the epithelial tissue in the posterior oral region. **B.** Pemphigus of the nose with ulceration and crusting (Both slides courtesy of Dr. Terry Rees.)

Significant Microscopic Features: Microscopically, intraepithelial clefting or acantholysis (cell separation in the stratum spinosum) with freely floating, rounded epithelial cells called **Tzanck cells** are characteristic, as seen in Figure 11.14. Irregularly arranged basal cells may have a tombstonelike appearance. There is also a positive direct and indirect immunofluorescence test (Fig. 11.15). Pemphigus features a separation of epithelial cells (**acantholysis**) caused by autoantibodies that attack a protein component of the desmosomes, which is the adhesion site between two epithelial cells. This protein component binds epithelial cells together (the intercellular cement) in stratified squamous epithelium. This leads to blister formation (bulla) and ulceration of affected tissues.

Dental Implications: An extensive team approach is needed to treat pemphigus, which invariably includes high-dose systemic corticosteroids and immunosuppressive agents. Oral lesions respond to a combination of systemic therapy and high-potency topical steroids such as fluocinonide. Effective oral hygiene is crucial. Alcohol-containing products and abrasive dental products may be harmful; however, use of non-alcohol-containing mouth rinses such as chlorhexidine mixed in water may be beneficial. Although not commercially available, these products can be prepared by compounding pharmacists and tend to be highly effective in treatment. Tooth-whitening agents should not be used because of their abrasive properties and ability to irritate the tissues. Recall appointment guidelines may include gentle debridement with minimal tissue manipulation. This may include multiple appointments to meet the therapeutic goal. Other procedures include taking clinical photographs for optimal monitoring and discontinuing flavoring agents. Hydrogen peroxide and other ingredients of dental hygiene products may be irritating to patients with mucosal disease, and spicy foods should be eliminated.

Clinical Protocol 6 lists the treatment for patients with sensitivity to flavoring agents.

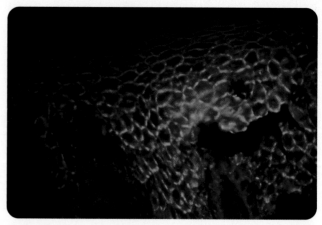

Figure 11.15. Immunofluorescence slide of pemphigus vulgaris. (Courtesy of Dr. Denis Lynch.)

Differential Diagnosis: Any of the bullous conditions need to be considered:

1. Bullous pemphigoid
2. Pemphigus
3. Erosive lichen planus
4. Erythema multiforme
5. Discoid lupus erythematosus

With any nonhealing chronic condition, there is always the possibility that changes have occurred since the last maintenance visit. The clinician should always entertain the possibility that even though a diagnosis was made previously, a patient may have a new disease or the existing disease has taken a different course. This is especially true for any chronic mucosal disease. Chronic inflammation of the tissues may lead to a more serious state, such as carcinoma. Any changes need to be evaluated, and new testing may be warranted. Intraoral photographs that can be compared are crucial in evaluating all mucosal diseases and should be used.

The presence or absence of skin lesions should help with the differential diagnosis; however, definitive diagnosis must be based on microscopic features as well as immunofluorescence results. A biopsy is essential in determination with immunostaining.

Treatment and Prognosis: Pemphigus vulgaris is a potentially life-threatening condition, and it is imperative that the patient receive medical care. Unfortunately, the medications used to treat the condition may induce adverse side effects or systemic complications. For example, complications of chronic steroid therapy may include diabetes mellitus, hypertension, adrenal suppression, weight gain, osteoporosis, peptic ulcers, severe mood swings, and diminished resistance to infectious agents. If left untreated there is a 60 to 80% mortality rate; if treated, the mortality rate is 5 to 10%.

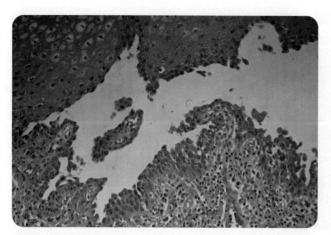

Figure 11.14. Pemphigus photomicrograph with Tzanck cells.

Pemphigoid

Pemphigoid represents a group of chronic, vesiculobullous, pemphigus-like diseases that affect skin and mucous membranes. The oral cavity may be involved in all forms of pemphigoid, and in many instances; it may represent the only site of lesions. On some occasions, pemphigoid lesions may be drug induced by such medications as carbamazepine, clonidine, or penicillamine.

NAME: Mucous membrane pemphigoid (cicatricial pemphigoid, benign mucous membrane pemphigoid)

Etiology: When affecting the gingiva, the term *desquamative gingivitis* is sometimes used.

Method of Transmission: Mucous membrane pemphigoid is idiopathic and classified as an autoimmune disease.

Epidemiology: The disease affects older middle-aged (usually 5th decade) and elderly individuals. Pemphigoid is rare in children. Females are affected more than males in a ratio of 2:1

Pathogenesis: Mucous membrane pemphigoid appears to be caused by antibodies that target the basement membrane and cause weakening of the attachment to the underlying connective tissues. In this disease, bulla formation occurs in the subepithelial area between the connective tissue and the basement membrane. Figure 11.16 shows the histology of this disorder, with separation of the basal cell layer from the underlying connective tissue.

Extraoral Characteristics: Various other mucous membranes may be involved, including the genitalia, and eye and localized skin bulla occasionally occur. Lesions may also be found on the skin, nares, rectum, urethra, and esophagus. The bullae of MMP are short-lived; they break quickly and desquamate, leaving a raw erythematous or ulcerated surface. Scarring rarely occurs in the oral cavity,

but on the skin and ocular mucosa, scarring is a major factor of the disease.

Perioral and Intraoral Characteristics: The oral cavity is the most frequently involved site. Figure 11.17 shows the clinical features of oral mucous membrane pemphigoid, exhibiting erythematous, shiny red gingival tissue. The gingiva is a target site for the oral MMP, and localized or generalized desquamative gingivitis is present more than 90% of the time. The gingiva is highly friable (easily crumbles) and even gentle oral hygiene measures or eating may cause the tissue to slough, leaving a painful, erythematous or ulcerated surface.

Distinguishing Characteristics: The lesions are confined to the gingiva in over 50% of cases. A positive Nikolsky's sign is usually present. (See Clinical Protocol 3 for the mucosal disease maintenance patient.) Eye lesions are more common in MMP. Figure 11.18 shows ocular mucous membrane pemphigoid with scarring of the tissues.

Microscopic Features: Subbasalar separation of the epithelium from the underlying connective tissue is characteristic. The separation occurs within the basal lamina, and the inflammatory infiltrate within the connective tissue is nonspecific. Immunofluorescence is positive, revealing a linear pattern of IgG and complement in the basement membrane. This can be drug induced with patients taking medications such as clonidine and penicillamine, but this is true in few cases.

Differential Diagnosis: Other vesiculobullous diseases need to be considered as well.

1. Other vesiculobullous diseases need to be considered: bullous pemphigoid, pemphigus, erosive lichen planus, erythema multiforme, discoid lupus erythematosus, etc.
2. Generalized desquamative gingivitis is more common in MMP, although localized desquamative gingivitis may be a feature of other vesiculobullous disorders. Extensive skin involvement is rare in MMP in con-

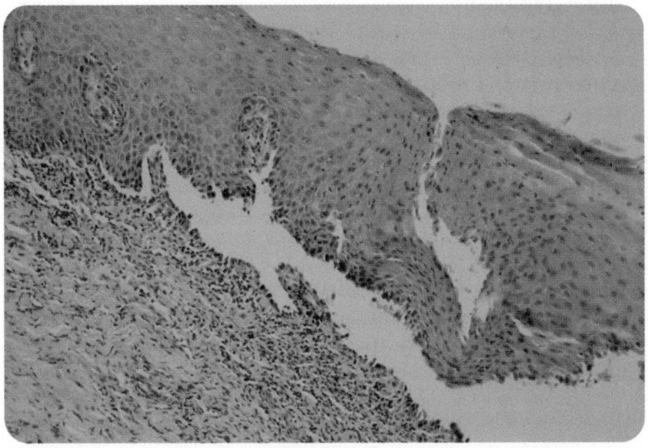

Figure 11.16. Histology of oral mucous membrane pemphigoid.

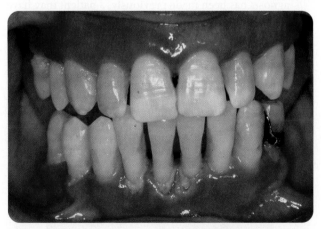

Figure 11.17. Oral mucous membrane pemphigoid demonstrating red, shiny gingival tissue. (Courtesy of Dr. Terry Rees.)

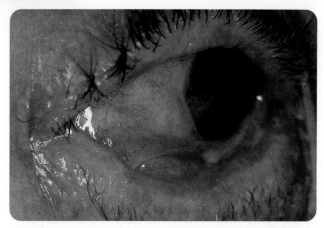

Figure 11.18. Ocular mucous membrane pemphigoid (symblepharon). (Courtesy of Dr. Terry Rees.)

trast with pemphigus, erythema multiforme, lupus erythematosus, and bullous pemphigoid.

3. Contact allergies may be involved. Generalized erythematous gingivitis is a feature of toothpaste allergy, but bullae formation and classic desquamative gingivitis are rare. Cinnamic aldehyde and other flavoring agents are especially common allergens in oral hygiene products and many foods (see Clinical Protocol 6). Since the flavoring agents are used in so many products, the clinical appearance is becoming more common. Generally, the area of tissue that is exposed to the offending products remains inflamed, and areas of tissue not exposed to the product exhibit clearing. This is true for toothpaste and other flavoring agents that the person is using. Figure 11.19 shows a gingival reaction to cinnamon aldehyde, with reddened tissue and clearing in the oral vestibule.

4. MMP lesions are chronic in contrast with the acute onset associated with erythema multiforme.

5. With any nonhealing, chronic-type condition, there is always the possibility that changes have occurred since the last maintenance visit. The clinician should always entertain the possibility that even though a diagnosis has been made previously, a patient may have a new disease or the existing disease has taken a different course. This is especially true for any mucosal disease that is chronic. Chronic inflammation of the tissues may lead to a more serious state, such as carcinoma. Again, intraoral documentation with the use

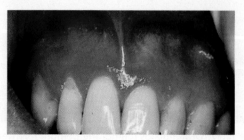

Figure 11.19. Cinnamon aldehyde reaction on gingiva. (Courtesy of Dr. Terry Rees.)

of photography should be used and is a standard part of monitoring chronic disease states.

Treatment and Prognosis: Often, identifying and discontinuing the offending product is all that is needed. Discontinuing the use of oral products that burn, such as alcohol-based mouth washes, spicy foods, cinnamon, and strong flavoring agents, is suggested. This will often help lessen the tissue sloughing that causes erosive lesions. Avoiding toothpaste and mouth rinses on the market that contain sodium laurel sulfate is also helpful. Many hidden flavoring agents are present in foods such as salsa, processed foods, and soft drinks such as colas. Canned goods may also have additives that pose a problem for patients with mucosal disease. A dietary analysis should be performed for patients to assist them in avoiding substances that may cause discomfort or worsen the mucosal condition. Patients who are diagnosed with cinnamon allergy usually exhibit normal tissue within a 2-week period.

The use of corticosteroids may predispose patients to candidal infections and prophylactic prescriptions of an antifungal agent such as nystatin would be considered. (See Clinical Protocols 2 and 5 for diagnosis and treatment.) Individuals afflicted with desquamative gingivitis have difficulty maintaining good oral hygiene and are highly susceptible to dental and/or periodontal disease. Consequently, they should receive frequent maintenance visits, and all treatment procedures should be performed as atraumatically as possible (see Clinical Protocol 3).

NAME: Bullous pemphigoid

Etiology: Bullous pemphigoid is an autoimmune disease.

Epidemiology: Bullous pemphigoid affects a slightly older age group of older adults and elderly, usually in the 7th to 8th decade of life. There is an equal distribution of male and female.

Pathogenesis: The disease is similar to mucous membrane pemphigoid. Bullae are formed because of separation between the basement membrane and the underlying connective tissue.

Perioral and Intraoral Characteristics: Intraoral involvement is relatively rare (10–40%). When present, it affects the gingiva. Cutaneous bullae develop slowly and may last for weeks to months before breaking, thereby creating painful erythematous and ulcerative lesions. Oral lesions are similar in appearance to those of mucous membrane pemphigoid. Lesions usually occur on the gingival, palate, floor of the mouth, tongue, or buccal mucosa. The disease follows a chronic course, although remissions are common. Healing usually occurs without scarring. Unlike mucous membrane pemphigoid, bullous pemphigoid usually affects the skin first.

Microscopic Features: The microscopic features are similar to those of mucous membrane pemphigoid. Figure

11.20 shows a bullous lesion of pemphigoid on the buccal mucosa.

Differential Diagnosis: Microscopic examination and immunofluorescence testing are needed to differentiate this disease from other bullous diseases. The characteristic lack of oral lesions should help separate some cases.

Treatment and Prognosis: Systemic corticosteroids alone or in combination with other immunosuppressive agents are required. Other treatment may include dapsone, cyclosporine, sulfapyridine, and niacinamide. Periodic photographs are helpful in assessing tissue changes in all mucosal diseases (see Clinical Protocol 3). Plaque control is beneficial, with frequent prophylaxis. As discussed above, patients with mucosal disease may have trouble tolerating flavoring agents and abrasive dental products. Alcohol is also an irritant, and alcohol-containing products should be discontinued. Remission is common after 2–3 years. However, bullous pemphigoid can be a chronic disorder for some patients. The disease is rarely fatal.

CONGENITAL OR GENETIC DISEASES

Genetic diseases and disorders affect vital organs and tissues during embryonic development, and congenital disorders may occur at birth. Factors such as exposure to environmental materials, radiation, infections, certain medications, alcohol, and diseases may play a role in congenital disorders. An example would be a woman who is exposed to rubella in the first 3 months of pregnancy is at high risk of producing an offspring with birth defects. Additionally, genetic disorders may be inherited as autosomal dominant and autosomal recessive disorders (see Chapter 6). Certain diseases may occur during cell development and division, while other defects may not be obvious until later in life, and the individual may be affected at certain life stages.

NAME: Epidermolysis bullosa

Etiology: Epidermolysis bullosa (EB) represents a diverse group of inherited and acquired diseases characterized by fragility of the skin and mucosa, with three main categories recognized (simplex, junctional, and dystrophic). Depending upon the specific type of the disease, individuals will exhibit different levels of severity. Epidermolysis bullosa is a disease with several subtypes and varying degrees of debilitation with each type. The disorder is related to genetic defects in basal cells, hemidesmosomes, and anchoring connective tissue filaments.

Method of Transmission: EB is a rare, genetic disease with both autosomal dominant and recessive varieties, and over 20 different forms have been identified. Along with the genetic forms of this disease, there is also a form discussed in the next section, which is an acquired autoimmune form known as **epidermolysis acquisita.**

Epidemiology: Infants are affected with onset at or within a few weeks of birth. The simplex form, which is the least severe, may have a later onset from 0 to 4 years old. The disease affects both males and females equally. The *National Epidermolysis Bullosa Registry Reports* estimate that approximately 12,500 persons have some form of EB. It is estimated that there are 50 EB cases per 1 million births, with more than 92% of these diagnosed as the simplex form discussed below. The numbers of reported cases vary with each country.

Pathogenesis: There are three major subgroup categories: simplex (typically the mildest form), junctional, and dystrophic. The skin and mucosa are fragile and blister following mild trauma. The precise pathogenesis varies in the specific defects in the basement membrane area and the level of tissue cleavage after a traumatic incident.

Extraoral Characteristics: All categories feature bullae formation at birth, but the simplex form is the least severe and may improve at puberty. The dystrophic form may not reach peak severity until puberty, while the junctional form is the most severe and often fatal at birth.

On the skin, exposed surfaces such as the knees and knuckles are most often affected. Crusted erosions, milia, pigmentation, and alopecia, are commonly seen. Digital webbing with mitten-type deformities of the hands and feet may be seen in the severe form of EB. The varying combinations and types of EB that affect various organs such as the musculoskeletal, intestinal tract, eyes, and esophagus produce different degrees of affliction. Additionally, anemia is associated with EB. Ocular disease activity, particularly corneal, is common in some EB subtypes. Figures 11.21A, B, and C show the clinical features of epidermolysis bullosa depicting the mitten-like foot with obvious scarring, the oral enamel hypoplasia, and the oral destruction of tissue, respectively.

Perioral and Intraoral Characteristics: Oral lesions can occur in any subgroup, but individuals who require special dental care are usually those with the dystrophic forms. Their oral erosions can be either mild (usually the dominant form) or severe with scarring (usually the recessive form). Depending upon the type and

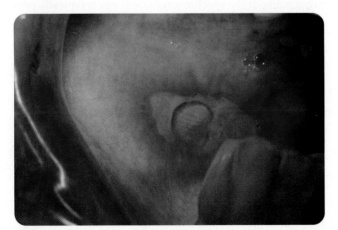

Figure 11.20. Bullous pemphigoid. (Courtesy of Dr. Terry Rees.)

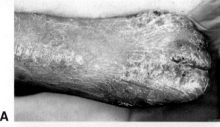

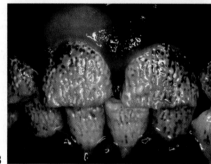

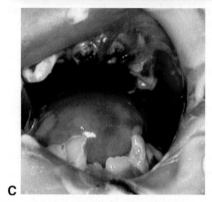

Figure 11.21. Epidermolysis bullosa. **A.** Mittenlike scarring of the foot. **B.** Enamel hypoplasia. **C.** Oral lesions of a child. (Courtesy of Dr. J. Timothy J. Wright.)

severity, oral lesions may be occasional blisters with small discrete vesicles that heal rapidly without scarring or they may be more severe ongoing oral lesions with scar formation. Bullae and painful erythematous or ulcerative lesions may be found on the tongue, buccal mucosa, palate, floor of the mouth, and gingiva. With the more severe types of disease, any food may cause traumatic insult resulting in lesion formation. In fact, the oral and esophageal involvement with scarring and constriction affects eating and swallowing and sometimes makes the passage of food impossible. Many severely affected patients now have G-tubes to assist with nutritional intake.

Distinguishing Characteristics:
All lesions, whether oral or cutaneous, occur as the result of some trauma and can heal with some scarring. Fingernails are often obliterated because of scarring over time. Often the scarring will result in ankyloglossia, and strictures of other oral tissues are common.

Microscopic Features:
Histopathologic features depend on the genetic abnormality that is present. All forms involve separation of the epithelium from the underlying connective tissue. Blistering occurs within the epidermis (simplex type), within the basement membrane (junctional type), or beneath the basement membrane (dystrophic forms) in inherited EB.

Differential Diagnosis:
Occurrence of the disease in infancy rules out the other bullous diseases.

1. Late onset dystrophic epidermolysis bullosa must be differentiated from epidermolyis bullosa acquista (discussed in the next section) by histologic and immunofluorescence studies.
2. Sequencing of the specific causative genes is typically performed to diagnose the different EB subtypes.

Dental Implications:
Enamel hypoplasia can occur in developing teeth in junctional EB types, and there is a high rate of caries in patients with the junctional and dystrophic forms of EB. The ability of the patient to tolerate a dental procedure depends upon the severity of the EB. Patients who have milder forms of the disease can tolerate normal dental procedures without much difficulty. The way that the patient tolerates a dental procedure depends upon the degree of EB. Patients with milder forms may tolerate in-office procedures with a local anesthetic while a patient with a more severe form would usually need hospitalization with general anesthesia. Oral hygiene procedure can be modified to accommodate the various types of EB with limited tissue disruption. Specially formulated rinses without alcohol may help with caries control. Systemic use of fluoride, a soft-bristle brush with a small head, and swabbing the medications on without tissue contact or trauma is optimal. Topical fluorides such as increased-strength dentifrices (e.g., 500 ppm), daily sodium fluoride mouth rinses (0.05%), and fluoride varnishes are very helpful in managing the increased risk for caries in junctional and dystrophic EB patients.

Differential Diagnosis:
Occurrence of the disease in infancy rules out the other bullous diseases. Late onset dystrophic epidermolysis bullosa must be differentiated from epidermolysis bullosa acquista (discussed in next section) by histologic and immunofluorescence studies. Sequencing of the specific causative genes is typically performed to diagnose the different EB subtypes.

Treatment and Prognosis:
Wound care for mild cases, antibiotics to prevent secondary infection, and plastic surgery to correct deformities caused by scarring are all treatments for this disease. Dental care requires nonabrasive, nonirritating chemical substances and avoidance of trauma. Promoting a noncariogenic soft diet helps to reduce future caries. In addition, fluoride applications may assist in reducing carious lesions. Patients should be instructed in gentle home care techniques, and antimicrobial mouth rinses may be required (e.g., 0.12% chlorhexidine). Patients with mild forms of the disease can withstand gentle prophylaxis. Scaling and root planing and the successful use of acellular dermal allografts to gain attached gingiva has been described. Successful osseointegration of endosseous implants has also been reported.

The prognosis depends on the type of genetic defect and can range from good to fatal. Excellent information may be obtained from the following web sites:

www.niams.nih.gov

http://www.niams.nih.gov/hi/topics/epidermolysis_bullosa/epidermol

www.debra.org

EPIDERMOLYSIS BULLOSA ACQUISITA

This unusual autoimmune disease primarily occurs in adults, although it also has been described in children. On occasion onset of EBA correlates with development of a variety of underlying systemic diseases. Other reports correlate onset with the use of specific medications. EBA may have clinical manifestations similar to those of epidermolysis bullosa, but it can usually be differentiated by the age of onset. However, EBA features dermal and mucosal bullae formation as found in other blistering diseases. Fig. 11.22 shows ulcerations in the lower mucosal region of the lip.

Diagnosis may be difficult. For example, clinical features, histologic findings, and immunofluorescence characteristics of EBA may mimic bullous or mucous membrane pemphigoid. Special immunoelectron microscopy evaluation of biopsied tissue is required if the disease is suspected. Treatment most often consists of the use of systemic corticosteroids and immunosuppressive agents.

Because of the similar name, it should not be confused with epidermolysis bullosa. Additionally, because of the bullous and vesicle formations when trauma is induced, the hygienist should use caution in scaling procedures since these patients suffer when ultrasonic devices are used. Harsh or abrasive products cause problems as well.

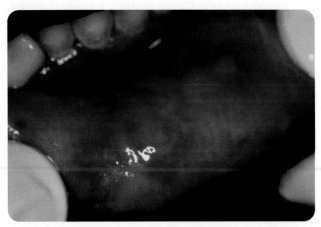

Figure 11.22. Epidermolysis bullosa acquisita. A lesion on the lower oral mucosa. (Courtesy of Dr. Michael Brennan.)

SUMMARY

- Lesions that appear as vesicles can be as innocuous as the mucocele and as extreme and life-threatening as pemphigus vulgaris.
- Viral infections such as herpangina, hand-foot-and-mouth disease, as well as, measles all have vesicle formations but are caused by very different viruses.
- Clues such as clinical features, age, sex of the patient, duration of the symptoms, and the location of lesions begin to play a key part in determining the diseases in question. As the student assesses the vesicle or combinations of lesions, a pattern of factors begin to emmerge in the thought process.
- Further diagnostic testing such as histology, cytology, and immunofluorescence assists in making a definitive diagnosis of lesions.
- The practitioner should be able to account for any lesion in the mouth or any changes that have occurred since a previous visit.
- All lesions have a history, and it is important to account for any tissue change in the mouth by working through the differential process.
- Treatment should be postponed when active herpetic lesions are present.

- Herpetic lesions reoccur and may have prodromal signs prior to the reoccurrence.
- Assisting the patient in containing the spread of herpetic labialis through patient education is crucial.
- Herpes zoster is due to the reactivation of the varicella–zoster that is often contracted during childhood.
- Childhood vaccines not only limit the spread of infectious diseases such as chickenpox and measles, but also eliminate infections such as herpes zoster or shingles.
- Autoimmune diseases may have a vesicle-like appearance such as pemphigus vulgaris, pemphigoid, and other variants of these diseases.
- Specific care and treatment are indicated for each of the mucosal diseases depending upon the severity of the disease.
- Epidermolysis bullosa is found in three major subgroups: simplex, junctional, and dystrophic.
- Epidermolysis bullosa acquisita occurs in later life, resulting from the use of specific medications, and correlates with the development of other systemic diseases.
- Precautions for dental treatment must be taken in both autoimmune and genetic-type diseases that exhibit vesicle formations. Tissue trauma should be minimized.

PORTFOLIO ACTIVITIES

- Construct a patient education sheet for patients with pemphigoid and pemphigus.

  List the facts about the disorders with clear and concise educational information for a newly diagnosed patient. (See the guidelines for Maintenance Appointments in Clinical Protocol 3.) Include dental home care procedures and food products that should be avoided.

- Construct an information sheet for parents of children who may be diagnosed with herpangina, measles, or hand-foot-and-mouth disease. Include phone numbers, contact information and any pertinent information that a parent may find useful.

- Develop a patient diet diary for 1 week. Have the patient list all brands of foods with the amount consumed. This should include any mints, gum, or beverages that the patient may eat for a week. Have the patient bring in the diary, so that you can evaluate the contents. Patients often report more symptoms from their mucosal disease after consuming certain food products. This could be very helpful in the maintenance program for the individual patient.

- The protocol of your practice should be clear to new patients. Your office staff should decide on when a patient should not be seen (unless there is an emergency) and when observed lesions should be biopsied, followed, and evaluated. Consider obvious lesions such as HSV. For example, if the patient has an active lesion, the staff will know that the policy is to give them a reappointment for a later date. Creating a standard information sheet on any shared views, policies, and protocol would alert patients to what standards exist within your practice. Using this sheet when situations arise, ensures that everyone will be aware of the proper office protocol, and there will be no surprises. This information sheet can also be shared with new patients, so that they know from the beginning your office policy.

REFERENCES

Anhalt GJ, Morrison LH. Bullous and cicatricial pemphigoid. J Autoimmun 1991:4:17–35.

Cawson RA, Odell EW. Essentials of oral pathology and oral medicine. 6th ed. London: Churchill Livingstone–Harcourt Brace, 1998.

Crawford EG, Burkes EJ, Briggman RA. Hereditary epidermolysis bullosa: oral manifestations and dental therapy. Oral Surg. 1976:Oct:490–500.

Eisen D. Lynch DP. The mouth—diagnosis and treatment. St. Louis: Mosby 1998.

Langlais R, Miller C. Color atlas of common oral diseases. Baltimore: Lippincott Williams & Wilkins, 2003.

Gazit E, Slomov Y, Goldberg I, et al. HLA-G is associated with pemphigus vulgaris in Jewish patients. Hum Immunol 2004;65(1):39–46.

Greenspan MS. Herpesvirus infections. Dent Clin North Am 1996:40: 359–368.

Lamey P, Hyland PL. Changing epidemiology of herpes simplex virus type 1 infections. HERPES 1999;6:20–24.

Lamey PJ, Rees TD, Binnie WH, et al. Oral presentation of pemphigus vulgaris and its response to systemic steroid therapy. Oral Surg Oral Med Oral Pathol Oral Radiol Endod 1992;74:54–57.

Jordan, RCK, Daniels TE, Greenspan JS, Regezi JA. Advanced diagnostic methods in oral and maxillofacial pathology. Part ll: Immunohistochemical and immunofluorescent methods. Oral Surg Oral Med Oral Pathol Oral Radiol Endod 2002;93:56–74.

Luman ET, Barker LE, Shaw KM, et al. Timeliness of childhood vaccinations in the United States: days under vaccinated and number of vaccines delayed. JAMA 2005;293(10):1204–1211.

Millar EP, Troulis MJ. Herpes zoster of the trigeminal nerve: the dentist's role in diagnosis and management. Scientific 1994;60(5):450–453.

Murray SJ. Herpes zoster: diagnostic and therapeutic considerations. Can J Diagn 1992;91:77–84.

Neville BW, Damm DD, Allen CM, Bouquot JE. Oral & maxillofacial pathology. Philadelphia: WB Saunders, 1995.

Parisi E, Raghavendra S, Werth V, Sollecito TP. Modification to the approach of the diagnosis of mucous membrane pemphigoid: a case report and literature review. Oral Surg Oral Med Oral Pathol Oral Radio Endod 2003;95:182–186.

Plemons JM, Gonzales TS, Burkhart NW. Vesiculobullous diseases of the oral cavity. In: Disorders affecting the periodontium. Periodontology 1999;21:158–175.

Regezi J, Sciubba J, Jordan R. Oral pathology—clinical pathologic correlations. 4th ed. St. Louis: WB Saunders, 2003.

Rivera-Hidalgo F, Stanford TW. Oral mucosal lesions caused by infective microorganisms I. viruses and bacteria. Disorders affecting the periodontium.In Periodontology 1999;21:106–144.

Popovsky JL, Camisa C. New and emerging therapies for disease of the oral cavity. Dermatol Clin 2000;18:1.

Rogers RS, Seehafer JR, Perry HO. Treatment of cicatricial (benign mucous membrane) pemphigoid with dapsone. Am Acad Dermatol 1982; 215–223.

Ruocco V, Ruocco E, Wolf R. Bullous diseases: unapproved treatments or indications. Clin Dermatol 2000;18:191–195.

Scully C. Handbook of oral disease—diagnosis and management. London: Martin Duntz Ltd. Livery House Publishers, 1999.

Seward JF, Watson BM, Peterson CL, Varicella disease after introduction of varicella vaccine in the United States, 1995–2000. JAMA 2002;287(5): 606–611.

Stedman's medical dictionary. Baltimore: Williams & Wilkins. 2000.

Shulman JD. Recurrent herpes labialis in US children and youth. Community Dent Oral Epidemiol 2004;32:402–409.

Tidwell E, Hutson B Burkhart N, et al. Herpes zoster of the trigeminal nerve 3rd branch: review of the literature and case report. Intern Endodontol J 1999;32:61–66.

Wright JT, Fine JD, Johnson L. Hereditary epidermolysis bullosa: oral manifestations and dental management. Pediatr Dent 1993;15:242–247

Wright JT, Fine JD, Johnson L. Oral soft tissues in hereditary epidermolysis bullosa. Oral Surg Oral Med Oral Pathol 1991;71(4):440–446.

Critical Thinking Activities

How would you differentiate benign mucous pemphigoid (BMP) from a toothpaste or dental product allergic response? What factors might lead you toward a toothpaste allergy?

Points to consider:

1. Toothpaste allergy presents with a clearing in the vestibule.

Why does this occur? Try to imagine how the tissue in the vestibule is somewhat protected by the surrounding tissue.

2. Toothpaste allergy does not produce the denuded, friable consistency of the gingiva that can be observed in BMP or other mucosal diseases.
3. Discontinuing the toothpaste and dental products in question will produce a somewhat rapid response and will diminish lesions within a 2-week period.

Case Study

Mr. Anderson, 52, has been seen in your practice every 4 to 6 months for many years. He usually presents with some generalized erythema of the gingival tissues, but you have always attributed this to his lack of compliance with the recommended three month maintenance appointments, and poor oral hygiene when he is out of town or busy. He travels frequently and has missed or rescheduled appointments many times. Today he informs you that he has been told by his family physician that he has ocular pemphigoid. Considering this recent diagnosis, answer the following questions

- Describe the type of oral manifestations that might be associated with this type of vesiculobullous disorder.
- What oral findings in Mr. Anderson's previous dental appointments could be associated with this diagnosis?
- If Mr. Anderson is exhibiting oral manifestations of pemphigoid, what appointment modifications, if any, would need to be made? What information could you give him regarding management of his disorder at home?

Key Terms

- Actinomycosis
- Adenocarcinoma
- Angioedema
- Aphthous ulcers
- Behçet syndrome
- Carcinoma
- Chancre
- Condylomata lata
- Deep fungal infections
- Erosive lesions
- Erythema multiforme
- Erythroleukoplakia
- Erythroplakia
- Factitial injury
- Fibrinous exudate
- Gonorrhea
- Gumma
- Hutchinson's triad
- Keratin pearls
- Libman-Sacks endocarditis
- Lupus erythematosus
- Mucous patches
- Mulberry molars
- Morsicatio buccarum
- Necrotizing sialometaplasia
- Necrotizing ulcerative gingivitis
- Nonpathogen
- PFAPA
- Reiter's syndrome
- Sarcoma
- Speckled erythroleukoplakia
- Squamous cell carcinoma
- Stomatitis medicamentosa
- Stomatitis venenata
- Sutton's disease
- Syphilis
- Traumatic ulcer
- Ulcer
- Urticaria

Chapter Objectives

1. Define three common ways that a patient may develop a traumatic ulcer.

2. Differentiate and define the key words *factitial* and *iatrogenic*.

3. Describe the clinical characteristics and etiology of necrotizing sialometaplasia.

4. Discuss the confusion that may occur related to malignant lesions and necrotizing sialometaplasia.

5. Define each of the key vocabulary terms for this chapter.

6. Describe the clinical characteristics of the major, minor, and herpetiform types of aphthous ulcers.

7. List the lesions associated with each stage of syphilis.

8. Describe the clinical characteristics of gonorrhea.

9. List the organism involved in gonorrhea and the usual oral site that is commonly seen clinically.

10. List the etiology of the following deep fungal infections: mucormycosis, histoplasmosis, blastomycosis, cryptococcosis, and aspergillosis.

11. Describe the triad of signs and symptoms related to Reiter syndrome.

12. Describe the triad of signs and symptoms related to Behçet syndrome.

13. List the etiology and clinical characteristics of Stevens Johnson syndrome.

14. List the key clinical characteristics of squamous cell carcinoma.

15. Define the term "field carcinogenesis."

16. Describe the clinical features of lupus erythematosus.

17. List five characteristics of erythroplakia.

18. What is meant by erythroleukoplakia?

19. List the four most prominent areas of the mouth for oral cancer.

20. List at least four statistical facts related to oral cancer.

21. Describe the clinical characteristics of a hypersensitivity reaction.

22. List the types of erythema multiforme and the clinical significance of each.

Chapter Outline

ULCERS AND INFLAMMATORY LESIONS

An erosive lesion may simply be defined as the loss of the epithelial covering of tissue. The lesion may or may not involve pain and will vary in size. Figure 12.1 depicts an aspirin burn producing an ulcer on the tongue and the buccal mucosa. **Erosive lesions** are denuded areas that occur above the basal cell layer of the epithelium. The term **ulcer** is used when the lesion penetrates the epithelium and extends into the dermis. Ulcers often exhibit a red halo or border with a yellow center. The yellow hue is caused by the thin yellow fibrinous exudate that covers the ulcer. The process of inflammation causes the ulcer to appear red, which accentuates the yellow hue of the exudates.

Ulcers may have multiple causes, but often they are due to **factitial** injury. This is self-induced injury, and an example would be a traumatic lip bite. Figure 12.2 represents a traumatic ulcer that is factitious—this child bit his

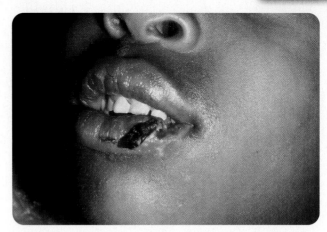

Figure 12.2. The lip was bitten after being anesthetized. (Courtesy of Dr. Terry Rees.)

lip following anesthesia. Figure 12.3 shows a fingernail injury at the gingivae in a 2-year-old child.

The term **traumatic ulcer** is used to denote an injury to the existing tissue. In some cases, a direct chemical injury such as an aspirin burn may occur. Electrical burns have also been reported as the origin of traumatic ulcers. Ulcers may also be **iatrogenic**. Iatrogenic ulcers are caused by the treatment that is rendered. For instance, the patient may have a dental procedure performed and trauma from the actual procedure may induce formation of an ulcer. Perhaps a saliva ejector was pressed down on the tissue in the floor of the mouth for too long or with too much pressure or maybe the patient was injected with anesthesia and an ulcer appeared at the site of the injection. Figure 12.4 shows a traumatic ulcer that is iatrogenic because the tongue was traumatized by an instrument. Figure 12.5 shows a traumatic ulcer caused by multiple carpules of

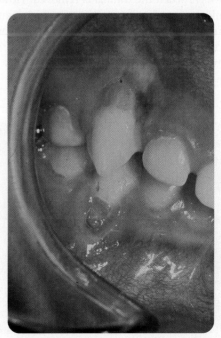

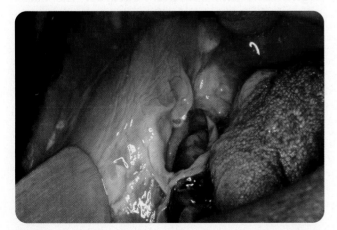

Figure 12.1. Chemical burn (aspirin) to the tongue and buccal mucosa. (Courtesy of Dr. Michael Brennan.)

Figure 12.3. Gingiva has a factitial injury by a young child with a fingernail. (Courtesy of Dr. Terry Rees.)

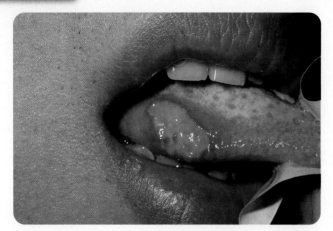

Figure 12.4.   Traumatic ulcer of the tongue due to hand-piece injury. (Courtesy of Dr. Peter Jacobsen.)

anesthetic injected in the site. Sometimes an impression is taken, and the tray scrapes or presses the tissue too forcefully, causing an injury. These examples are considered iatrogenic.

Systemic problems related to medications, diseases, and malignancy may produce ulcerative lesions. It is often a process of elimination and investigation for the practitioner to determine the source of the lesion, based on a good medical history and a thorough clinical evaluation. In the case of factitial injuries (those produced by the patient), removal of the source of likely trauma is the first step in the tissue healing response. For instance, a sharp edge on a tooth may induce an ulcerative response over a period of time, and smoothing the roughness may provide a quick tissue response, or the patient may traumatize an area by biting a lip that is anesthetized. These ulcers usually resolve when the trauma is removed. However, other ulcerlike lesions that have an immunologic component or a bacterial source will take longer to resolve or may continue to be a chronic problem for the patient. This chapter covers many of the ulcerative lesions that the practitioner sees in clinical practice.

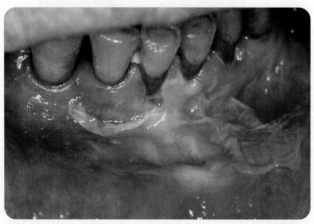

Figure 12.5.   Iatrogenic injury due to multiple carpules of anesthesia. (Courtesy of Dr. Terry Rees.)

Traumatic or Inflammatory Lesions

NAME: Traumatic ulcers

Etiology: Traumatic ulcers may occur at any time and at any location in the mouth. Some patients may traumatize the oral tissue because of improper alignment of the teeth or improper brushing techniques, including brushing aggressively. Dentures that do not fit properly may cause tissue damage, or the patient may traumatize tissue, such as the buccal mucosa or tongue, while chewing.

Method of Transmission: Traumatic ulcers are localized to the area of trauma and are not contagious.

Epidemiology: Traumatic ulcers may occur in any age group, and there is an equal distribution between males and females.

Pathogenesis: External forces are directed toward the tissue causing trauma to the area and subsequently producing the ulcerations.

Extraoral Characteristics: The extraoral characteristics may involve the lip area if traumatized, and this area can appear crusted and sometimes bleeding because of continued trauma.

Perioral and Intraoral Characteristics: Ulcers often have a craterlike appearance with some fibrinous exudate depending upon the degree of trauma.

Distinguishing Characteristics: When repeated trauma occurs, damaging the tissue, the injury may induce scar tissue. The area may be a source of irritation because of the excess tissue and the tendency of continuous injury to the site. Thickened, keratinized tissue in the area of injury often causes the tissue to appear white and may indicate some type of frictional injury to the tissue. An example would be the chronic "cheek chewer," with the technical name of **morsicatio buccarum.**

Significant Microscopic Features: The microscopic findings are nonspecific and not diagnostic, exhibiting an inflammatory process with a loss of the epithelium. Figure 12.6 depicts the histology of an ulcer. The epithelium has been lost in one area of the lesion, and the ulcer is covered by a fibrinous exudate with underlying granulation tissue in the same area. A heavy infiltrate of lymphocytes is present.

Dental Implications: Continued trauma may occur because of more injury to the tissue. Discomfort may be present, and dental work should be postponed until a later date and until the lesions have completely healed. If another injury does not occur in the same region, the traumatic ulcer eventually heals. Scar tissue may form in severely traumatized tissue, and the person may easily traumatize the same area again.

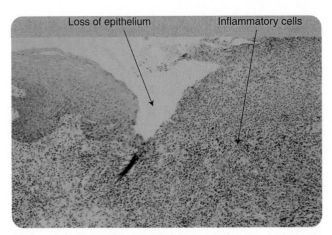

Figure 12.6.   Histology of an ulcer.

Differential Diagnosis: Any ulcerative condition must be considered. Traumatic ulcers may be confused with

1. Ulcers produced by microorganisms, such as those involved with tuberculosis, discussed in Chapter 10
2. Syphilis, discussed in this chapter
3. Gonorrhea, discussed in this chapter
4. Aphthous ulcers, discussed in this chapter

Treatment and Prognosis: Discomfort is usually mild, although in some cases eating may be difficult. The ulcers are usually short-lived and resolve with no problems other than mild discomfort to the patient. Removing the source of injury should allow recovery of the tissue. Of course, any lesion that does not heal within 2 weeks or one in which no possible etiology is found, should be evaluated further.

NAME: Necrotizing sialometaplasia

Etiology: The entity originates from salivary gland ischemia that causes necrosis of the tissue, usually due to trauma in the local area. This may be from trauma due to previous surgery or possibly previous local anesthesia administered in the site. Local blood supply to the area is disrupted, causing ischemia.

Method of Transmission: Necrotizing sialometaplasia is not contagious; it is localized and self-limiting.

Epidemiology: All ages are equally affected and necrotizing sialometaplasia occurs equally in males and females.

Pathogenesis: Necrotizing sialometaplasia is a benign entity that occurs at the juncture of the soft and hard palate, producing disruption of the tissue at this site. Although the lesion is not malignant, it may be confused with malignancies such as mucoepidermoid carcinoma. A careful evaluation and biopsy is needed to produce a definitive diagnosis; however, the lesion will usually heal without complications. Figure 12.7 depicts the palate region with necrotizing sialometaplasia.

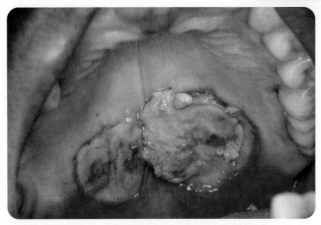

Figure 12.7.   Necrotizing sialometaplasia in the palate region (Courtesy of Dr. Michael Brennan.)

External Characteristics: Not applicable

Perioral and Intraoral Characteristics: The tissue may appear as an elevated mass subsequently becoming ulcerative.

Distinguishing Characteristics: A deep demarcated ulcer is characteristic of necrotizing sialometaplasia. The deep lesion subsequently becomes coated with a thick yellow fibrinous covering.

Significant Microscopic Features: Necrosis of the salivary gland is involved, and there is squamous metaplasia of the salivary duct epithelium. Necrotizing sialometaplasia may resemble malignancies in both clinical and microscopic appearance.

Differential Diagnosis: Considerations would be

1. Syphilitic gummas, discussed later in this chapter
2. Mucoepidermoid carcinoma—Chapter 17
3. Deep fungal infections, discussed later in this chapter
4. Salivary gland neoplasms—Chapter 17
5. Squamous cell carcinoma should be considered. Due to the histologic pattern, necrotizing sialometaplasia is sometimes confused with squamous cell carcinoma. Squamous cell carcinoma is discussed throughout the book.

Treatment and Prognosis: Analgesics may be recommended. There is no surgical intervention, and a biopsy should be taken to confirm the diagnosis. The prognosis is excellent, and healing occurs after several weeks to months.

Infectious Agents

Microorganisms surround us, but most do not cause disease in the host because of the unique properties of the immune system. The natural barriers that provide defense, such as the skin and mucosal surfaces, surround us and help defend us (see Chapters 3 and 4). Some microorganisms are disease causing (pathogens), and many are considered non-disease causing (**nonpathogenic**). Since standard precautions are taken with each patient, the distinction is not an issue in the clinic. The following section focuses on the distinction of common oral disorders that arise from various microorganisms and manifest as oral ulcers or erosions. The chapter is related to the clinical features and treatment of each disorder.

NAME: Syphilis

Etiology: Syphilis is caused by the spirochete *Treponema pallidum* through direct contact with the primary lesion.

Method of Transmission: Syphilis is spread through venereal transmission from sexual contact, from mother to fetus, or by the transfusion of infected blood. Transmission occurs during oral, anal, or vaginal sex. The organism dies quickly on dry surfaces and when it is exposed to air, and this organism is not transmitted through toilet seats, hot tubs, eating utensils, or other casual contact.

Epidemiology: A decline in the incidence of syphilis has occurred since 1900, with a sharp increase during the 1940s and a peak in 1980 primarily because of the increase in AIDS, since unprotected sex is a risk factor in both AIDS and sexually transmitted diseases such as syphilis. A sharp 90% decline occurred from 1990 to 2000. In 2004, the overall incidence was 7353 cases. The South continued to have the highest rates of any region in the United States at 3.6 per 100,000 (CDC & P, 2005 National Report). The disease is more prevalent in African-American men and patients with AIDS and less frequent in Native Americans. Mortality from syphilis occurs in approximately 20% of untreated patients and is most likely due to complications of late disease.

Pathogenesis: Syphilis is transmitted through sexual contact and is classified as a sexually transmitted disease. Although syphilis is a disease spanning decades of persistence, it is a disease that has resurfaced in the last couple of decades and is a concern. Syphilis involves a progression through three stages. Without treatment, the progression continues, with the host experiencing each of the following stages: primary, secondary, and tertiary. There is also a period of latency after the secondary stage that can last for years only to recur as the tertiary stage when the proper treatment has not been given. The infection can also be spread from the mother to her fetus.

Extraoral Characteristics: The features differ depending upon the stage of disease. Skin lesions can be apparent on the extremities. Syphilis lesions appear on the genitals, involving the penis, vulva, and anus. Later-stage syphilis, which has not been treated, can involve the eyes, causing blindness.

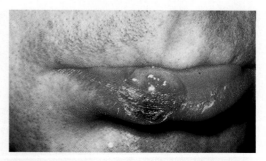

Figure 12.8. Chancre on the lip from syphilis (From Smeltzer SC, Bare BG. Textbook of Medical-Surgical Nursing, 9th Edition. Philadelphia: Lippincott Williams & Wilkins, 2000.

Perioral and Intraoral Characteristics: Syphilis may have various oral appearances that depend on the stage of infection in the individual. Three prime stages occur:

- Primary stage: After direct contact with an infected individual, the person develops a **chancre**. Figure 12.8 shows an ulcerative lesion on the lower lip at the site where the spirochete entered the host within 1 week to 3 months. This usually occurs on the penis, vulva, anus, or mouth. This chancre will heal within several weeks with no other signs of the disease. The most common site for oral lesions is on the lip, but they may be seen on the tongue, tonsils, or other mucosal areas. The lesions are painless, may appear as a firm, indurated lesion with an ulcer-like appearance that rapidly becomes eroded. Lesions at this stage are highly infective, and a diagnosis followed by treatment is crucial.
- Secondary stage: Several weeks after the primary stage, the host develops a secondary stage that manifest with flulike symptoms, fever, swollen lymph nodes that are nontender, skin lesions, and some mucocutaneous lesions. The lesions associated with this stage are called **mucous patches**. Figure 12.9 depicts a mucous patch on the mucosa near the vermillion border of the lip. The patches may be ulcer-like, with a pseudomembranous covering exhibiting yellow, white, or gray coloring. The highly infectious lesions of syphilis are teem-

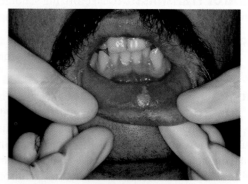

Figure 12.9. Mucous patch on the lip from syphilis. (Courtesy of Dr. E. J. Burkes)

ing with organisms. During this stage, the practitioner may notice papillary lesions known as **condylomata lata**; and there may be a rash on the trunk of the infected person. The saliva is highly infective during this stage (See Chapter 16).

- Tertiary stage: The third stage produces some serious complications that affect multiple organs. A **gumma** may appear initially as an indurated mass; and subsequently, an ulceration that promotes extensive tissue destruction in the localized area of the gumma. Gummas can appear on the face and extremities as well as the genitals. Most frequently, the palate and the tongue are involved. The palatal lesion may be extensive enough to penetrate to the nasal cavity. Gummatous syphilis may affect skin, bone, and mucous membranes, and the lesions often cause local destruction of the affected organ system.

In congenital syphilis (Box 12.1), the organism that infects the mother is passed on to the developing fetus, resulting in numerous clinical malformations. Pregnant women have a high risk of having a stillborn baby. Babies born to infected mothers need to be treated immediately after birth.

Distinguishing Characteristics: As discussed above, some subtle clinical manifestations may go unnoticed or be mistaken for other oral conditions or ulcerlike lesions. With congenital exposure, the teeth are affected, resulting in the molar teeth exhibiting rounded, berry-shaped elevations on the occlusal surfaces, and they are

known as **mulberry molars.** The incisors have a notched appearance due to the spirochetes infecting the enamel organ during formation. The described effects on the teeth are part of a triad of occurrences called **Hutchinson's triad.** See Chapter 21 for a clinical representation of the Hutchinson's triad.

Significant Microscopic Features: Specific stains in a dark-field examination of a smear are used to view the numerous "corkscrew-like" organisms that are diagnostically significant in extraoral syphilis. Specific blood tests are used such as the VDRL and the RPR tests. Results of these tests are positive throughout the first two stages. Serologic tests are also used which include the fluorescent treponemal antibody absorption tests and the *T. pallidum* hemagglutination assays (TPHA). The FTA-ABS is used as a check against test results, and the specific diagnostic tool that is used is determined by the existing stage of the disease.

Dental Implications: Specific to dentistry is what is known as Hutchinson's triad, which involves three factors: (1) inflammation of the cornea, (2) eighth nerve deafness, and (3) dental abnormalities. The abnormalities are related to congenital exposure of the child resulting in the molar teeth being formed with a rounded, cup-shaped appearance and the incisors developing a notched appearance due to the spirochetes infecting the enamel organ during formation. The person who has been exposed may present with external skin lesions, and in some instances,

---

Box 12.1 THE STAGES OF SYPHILIS

Stages of Syphilis	Dental Implications
Primary Incubation: 12–30 days	Chancre—Usually occurs on genitals but can occur orally Lymphadenopathy Patchy alopecia
Latent	The disease appears dormant. This latent stage can occur between the secondary and tertiary stage as well
Secondary	Mucous patch Bilateral cutaneous rash Condylomata lata
Latent	The disease appears dormant. This latent stage can occur between the primary and secondary stage as well. This stage can exist for decades.
Tertiary	Gumma seen orally Syphilis affects the cardiovascular system and the CNS Altered mental state
Congenital	Hutchinson's triad 1. Mulberry molars and notched incisors 2. Inflammation of the cornea 3. Eighth nerve deafness Additional nasal deformity and excessive bone growth may occur—frontal bossing

there may be visible evidence of lesions around the periphery of the lip.

Differential Diagnosis: Since the incidence of syphilis is low, it is sometimes unnoticed and undiagnosed when seen clinically. Syphilis is termed "the great imitator" and rightfully deserves its name because of the multiple clinical manifestations that the disease presents. If oral lesions are not present or are very subtle, the disease could go unnoticed. The ulcerlike lesions make syphilis easily confused with other diseases. The clinician may want to consider the following diseases in a clinical diagnosis:

- Necrotizing sialometaplasia—Chapter 12
- Aphthous ulcers—Chapter 12
- Mucoepidermoid carcinoma—Chapter 17
- Tuberculosis—Chapter 10
- Squamous cell carcinoma—Chapter 12
- Trauma—Chapter 12

Treatment and Prognosis: The standard treatment is penicillin. The outcome of treatment will depend upon the stage of the disease and the amount of the damage that has occurred. The tertiary stage may last for years, and severe damage to organs may have occurred if prior treatment was not initiated.

NAME: Gonorrhea

Etiology: Gonorrhea is sexually transmitted and when treated, can be cured. The bacterium *Neisseria gonorrhoeae,* the gonococcus, infects the genital tract, mouth, and rectum of both men and women.

Method of Transmission: Gonorrhea is transmitted through sexual contact and can be transmitted from mother to child across the placenta and during birth in the birth canal. The oral lesions of gonorrhea result from oral-genital contact. Babies may be infected in the birth canal.

Epidemiology: In 2002, some 351,852 cases of gonorrhea were reported to the Centers for Disease Control and Prevention (CDC). Approximately 200 million new cases of gonorrhea are reported each year internationally. In the United States, approximately 75% of all reported cases of gonorrhea are found in people aged 15 to 29 years. The highest rates of infection are usually found in 15- to 19-year old women and 20- to 24-year-old men. The disease is sexually transmitted. The rate is higher in homosexuals and prostitutes than in the general population. More than a million cases are reported annually in the United States, and this number has risen in the last few years. Approximately 200 million new cases of gonorrhea appear each year. The incubation period is approximately 7 days.

Pathogenesis: Gonorrhea is caused by the organism *N. gonorrhoeae,* the gonococcus. The disease produces inflammation of the reproductive and urinary tracts in the form of urethritis in men and vaginal discharge with in-

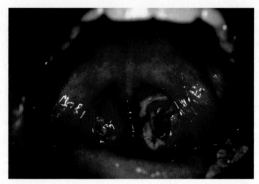

Figure 12.10. Oral gonorrhea. (Courtesy of Dr. Michael Krakow.)

flammation of the cervix in women. In women, the opening to the uterus, the cervix, is the first place of infection. The disease can spread into the uterus and fallopian tubes, resulting in pelvic inflammatory disease (PID), which can cause tubal (ectopic) pregnancy and infertility in as many as 10% of infected women. The disease is mentioned here because oral signs may be present; and although the disease is not common, reported cases have increased in the past few years.

Extraoral Characteristics: The person may appear in poor health and exhibit lymphadenopathy (swollen lymph nodes).

Perioral and Intraoral Characteristics: The most common site is the oral pharynx, with resultant gonococcal pharyngitis. The tonsillar region is often affected, with inflammation and pustular lesions. Figure 12.10 shows the oropharynx with tissue appearing red and swollen. Figure 12.11 shows a heavy coating on the tongue and other tongue lesions associated with gonorrhea. Other common complaints may include halitosis, stinging, and burning. Generalized stomatitis may be seen in some cases.

Distinguishing Characteristics: The presenting features are not diagnostic, and other factors need to be considered such as lifestyle and health history. As noted in the presentation of syphilis, gonorrhea may have a varied clinical appearance.

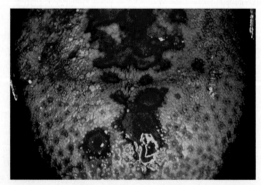

Figure 12.11. Oral gonorrhea. (Courtesy of Dr. Michael Krakow.)

Significant Microscopic Features: Gram stains and serologic tests are used to make a definitive diagnosis. When left untreated, the inflammatory response becomes chronic, with macrophages and lymphocytes predominant.

Dental Implications: When oral lesions are observed, the oropharyngeal areas are the most vulnerable. Because of the usual oral–genital practice involved and the associated trauma to the tissues, the pharyngeal tissues may appear ulcerative and erythremic. Ulcerative lesions may also be observed.

Differential Diagnosis: Other ulcerative conditions should be considered such as
• Aphthous ulcers—Chapter 12
• Herpetic lesions—Chapter 11
• Pemphigus and other mucosal diseases—Chapter 11
• Cancer of the tonsil—Chapter 12

Treatment and Prognosis: Antibiotic therapy is used with combinations of antibiotics, depending on the region of the world. Commonly, the following antibiotics are the drugs of choice and given in a single dose: cefixime, ceftriaxone, ciprofloxacin, ofloxacin, and levofloxacin. This infection results in blindness in some countries where antibiotics are not routinely administered at birth into the conjunctiva. The prognosis is good if discovered early. Urethral stricture is a common complication.

NAME: Actinomycosis

Actinomycosis is a chronic bacterial disease that manifests in the formation of an abscess, sometimes draining externally. The lesion is often observed during the extraoral examination as a draining lesion in the lower facial region.

Etiology: Actinomycosis is caused by *Actinomyces israelii*, an anaerobic or microaerophilic, gram-positive bacterium usually associated with initial tissue trauma. The name of this disease is confusing, since the mycosis suffix would lead one to categorize the name with fungal infections; however, actinomycosis is a bacterial infection. Since these gram-positive bacteria are components of the normal flora, they work in conjunction with other bacteria in the mouth and are kept in check.

Method of Transmission: Since actinomycosis is considered a bacterial infection, it is not a contagious disease. Actinomycosis develops in cases related to trauma such as from surgery, tooth extraction, root canals, tonsil crypts, and carious lesions. These factors predispose the individual to its invasion through mucosal tears and openings, thereby positioning the person for the subsequent development and progression of the bacteria.

Epidemiology: Any age group may be affected, but actinomycosis occurs predominately in adults. The infection occurs in both males and females.

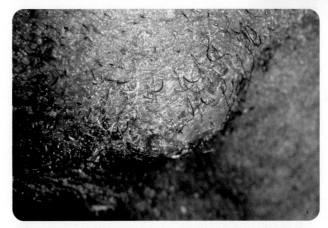

Figure 12.12. Draining fistula of the mandible. (Courtesy of Dr. Michael Brennan.)

Pathogenesis: The primary characteristic of actinomycosis is the abscess formation and the subsequent draining **fistula**. The bacteria do not exist free in nature but are normal inhabitants of the gastrointestinal tract and the oral cavity. The infections have been reported in patients with AIDS.

Extraoral Characteristics: When actinomycosis occurs in the oral region, it may become an indurated, ulcerative lesion developing into a fistula leading out through the skin of the neck or mandible. The extreme exudates that build up eventually develop a tract leading outside of the body. Figure 12.12. shows a draining fistula. Figure 12.13 shows actinomycosis deep within the tissue.

Perioral and Intraoral Characteristics: The site of the lesion is usually ulcerative and may have exudate associated with the ulcer, depending upon the extent of the infection. In the case of extraction sites, the infection would be at the point of the extracted tooth.

Distinguishing Characteristics: The exudate produced is a yellow puslike substance containing what is known as sulfur granules. This is seen seeping from the fistula.

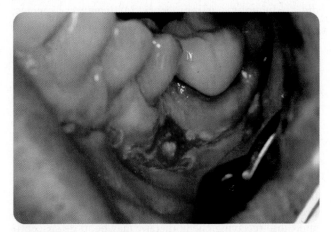

Figure 12.13. Deep fungal infections. (Courtesy of Dr. John Jacoway.)

Significant Microscopic Features: The sulfur granules and the organism are identified through clinical examination, evaluated microscopically, and diagnosed with cultures. See Figure 12.14.

Dental Implications: Other systemic disease states may be present as well, such as AIDS, which has been reported in conjunction with actinomycosis. Often, because of its subtle nature, in many cases, the more serious disease goes unrecognized and not associated.

Differential Diagnosis: Considerations should be given to the following:
- Osteomyelitis—Chapter 20
- Other bacterial and fungal organisms—Chapter 12
- Staphylococcus infections may be considered as well—Chapter 23
- HIV—Chapter 22

Treatment and Prognosis: The prognosis is good upon dissolution of the infection. High-dose penicillin is the required treatment for extensive periods.

NAME: Necrotizing ulcerative gingivitis

Necrotizing ulcerative gingivitis (NUG) is also formally known as acute necrotizing ulcerative gingivitis. Additionally, the older term "trench mouth" was given to soldiers during WW-II. who were diagnosed with NUG. NUG is superimposed on gingivitis or periodontitis (Wilkins, 2005).

Etiology: NUG is an infectious disease primarily of the gingiva, causing gingival bleeding, gingival ulceration, tissue necrosis, and pain. The condition is usually found in young adults. Factors such as stress, lower resistance to disease, poor nutrition, and poor oral hygiene contribute to the disease and predispose the person to the complications of other organisms. The term trench mouth, used for WW II soldiers, evolved because of an inability to maintain adequate oral hygiene along with the living conditions and stress factors that accompany the situations of war. Any of a number of different oral spirochetes is associated with NUG. Organisms such as *Prevotella intermedia*, α-hemolytic streptococci, *Actinomyces* species, *Selenomonas*, *Porphyromonas gingivalis*, *Treponema*, and *Fusobacterium* species are commonly found in NUG.

Method of Transmission: The person has been predisposed by general systemic problems, stress, improper nutrition, and poor oral hygiene practices. Since NUG is an infectious disease, care should be taken to minimize aerosol production during dental procedures.

Epidemiology: NUG is usually found in young adults between the ages of 15 and 30 years, and it is preceded by chronic gingivitis. The NUG is superimposed on gingivitis/periodontitis and usually begins with ulceration and necrosis in the col area. Immunocompromised patients and those receiving chemotherapy may be more susceptible to developing NUG (see Chapter 22 for clinical representation and its relationship to AIDS). An inability to

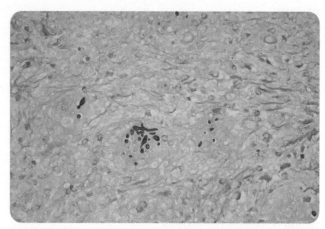

Figure 12.14. Histology of aspergillosis. (Courtesy of Dr. Lisa Chang.)

perform adequate home care is also observed in certain disorders such as Down syndrome, making NUG more likely in these individuals. Smoking is a known predisposing factor as well, since tobacco chemicals affect the tissues. There is an equal distribution of males and females.

Pathogenesis: NUG is has also been known as Vincent's infection because of the description of the lesions in the tonsil and pharynx region by Vincent. The name originates from the spirochete *Borrelia vincentii*, with which it is associated. However, the term Vincent's angina is used incorrectly as a synonym for NUG.

Extraoral Characteristics: The extraoral characteristics may involve the general physical health of the person along with observable characteristics of fever, pain, and swollen lymph nodes.

Perioral and Intraoral Characteristics: NUG presents with sudden, painful swelling of the free gingiva and necrosis with craters in the interdental papillae. (See Chapter 22 on AIDS for clinical representation.) A fiery red gingiva with bleeding is common. A fetid odor is present, and the patient may complain of a metallic taste. The inflammation may extend into the palatal region and the oral pharynx. A clinical slide of NUG is depicted in Chapter 22 (Figures 22.14 and 22.15).

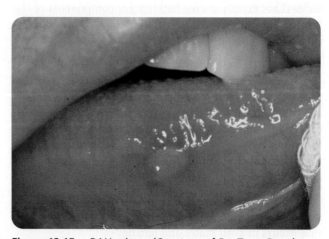

Figure 12.15. RAU minor. (Courtesy of Dr. Terry Rees.)

Distinguishing Characteristics: The fetid odor associated with NUG is a factor in distinguishing the disease from other mucosal disorders. A gray pseudomembrane forms over the necrotic gingiva in NUG and spontaneous bleeding occurs with any tissue manipulation. The pseudomembrane is composed of the necrotic tissue, fibrin, microorganisms, and leukocytes (Wilkins, 2005).

Significant Microscopic Features: A mixed flora of spirochetes (*Treponema* spp.), fusobacteria, *Prevotella intermedia*, *Veillonella* spp., and streptococci has been implicated in the disease.

Dental Implications: Debridement of the teeth and affected soft tissue areas is the recommended treatment, along with a proper diet, rest, and stress reduction. Mouth rinses are sometimes recommended to aid in healing (see Clinical Protocol 3). Instruction in brushing and flossing techniques will help the patient maintain a disease-free state. An oral irrigating device should not be used, since microorganisms can be forced down into the deeper tissues and could produce bacteremia. No ultrasonic devices should be used so that aerosol production is minimized, since NUG is an infectious disease. Encourage the patient to continue treatment because the infection may recur if treatment is prematurely discontinued. The use of salt-water rinses, mixtures of peroxide 3% with equal water or chlorhexidine 0.12% twice daily is suggested (Wilkins, 2005).

Differential Diagnosis: The following disease states may be considered in a differential diagnosis:
- There is a strong connection with HIV and AIDS—Chapter 22
- Confusion may occur with other gingival diseases—Chapter 11
- Herpes simplex infection—Chapter 11
- The severity of the condition and early clinical similarities may cause confusion with other mucosal conditions—Chapter 11

Treatment and Prognosis: The prognosis is excellent once the infection is treated and oral hygiene is maintained. However, the papillae do not return to normal and suffer the damage of the infection.

NAME: Deep fungal infections

Etiology: Fungal infections may arise from soil, bird and bat droppings, or decaying vegetation. Some fungi reside as normal inhabitants on the body, causing problems only when they are able to enter the body through tears or cuts in the skin. The spores or organisms follow specific routes such as the mucous membranes, which allow the organism to enter the body. For instance, the specific organism involved with histoplasmosis is *Histoplasma capsulatum var. capsulatum*, which enters the body through the lungs.

Method of Transmission: (Box 12.2, "Deep Fungal Infections.") The specific route of transmission is stated for various organisms. The organisms involved in deep fungal infections inhabit the soil and are found in the natural environment. Some of the organisms are native to certain geographic locations. For instance, according to the CDC 2005 report, histoplasmosis is especially prevalent in the Ohio and the Mississippi River valleys in the United States, in Central and South America, Africa, India, and Southeast Asia. In most cases, these areas are known to have the organisms within this geographic location. Additionally, of HIV-infected persons in these areas, 10–25% develop histoplasmosis. The fungal infections continue to increase in proportion to the number of HIV-infected patients, transplant patients, diabetic patients, patients with emphysema, cancer patients, and others who are immune-suppressed (Chapter 22).

Epidemiology: Every age group may be affected by fungal infections if the host resistance is lowered. There is

Box 12.2 DEEP FUNGAL INFECTIONS

Disease	Organism	Entry/Source	Clinical Appearance
Histoplasmosis	*H. capsulatum*	Lungs/bat and bird	Ulcers, indurated with rolled borders
Zygomycosis (also called mucormycosis and phycomycosis)	*Absidia, Mucor*	Oral/normal inhabitant	Palatal ulceration with fistulas/necrosis
Aspergillosis	*Aspergillus*	Lungs/soil, water, decaying vegetation	Large necrotic ulcers covered by black coat
Cryptococcosis	*Cryptococcus neoformans*	Lungs/prevalent in AIDS	Nonhealing nodules
Blastomycosis	*B. dermatitidis*	Lungs/immunocompromised	Irregular ulcerations with firm borders
Coccidioidomycosis	*Coccidioides immitis*	Lungs/desert region soil	Large ulcerations

equal susceptibility, depending on the immune defenses of the person. Elderly patients and those who are immunocompromised are at greater risks.

Pathogenesis: Deep fungal infections occur in the internal organs and the submucosal connective tissue. The tissue in the mouth is very vulnerable to tears, scrapes, and normal trauma. This poses a problem for the person who has an immunocompromised state or a lowered state of health and thus a lowered resistance to pathogens and other organisms. Although the diagnosis of such organisms and lesions cannot be made clinically and requires other tests, the clinician should be aware of the possibilities. Delayed treatment for the patient could make the problem worse.

Extraoral Characteristics: The lesions are usually ulcerative, sometimes necrotic depending on the stage, and they are pseudomembranous.

Perioral and Intraoral Characteristics: Some of the specific fungal infections produce an ulcerative lesion with indurated lesions. These fungal infections have some oral manifestations and warrant consideration in a differential diagnosis. Although rare and usually seen in patients who are debilitated, they may be the first clue to the dental hygienist that there may be a more serious disease entity.

Distinguishing Characteristics: The lesions related to fungal infections may mimic other disease states, and they may be in combination with other health conditions. Some chronic infections may persist for long periods.

Microscopic Features: The organism involved is observed through special cultures and staining procedures. Further culture tests would be performed to confirm the diagnosis.

Figure 12.14 depicts a stained slide of aspergillosis.

Differential Diagnosis: Many of the fungal infections mimic lesions such as
- Squamous cell carcinoma
- Mucoepidermoid carcinoma
- Ulcerative conditions such as major aphthae as well as systemic conditions producing ulcerlike lesions

Dental Implications: The correct diagnosis is important to establish a treatment protocol. A referral to the correct facility is important if it is determined that the ulcers may be symptoms of other serious disease states. Identification of the organism is important in successfully treating the lesion or referring the patient for further treatment, depending on the type of lesion involved. Box 12.2 provides some well-known fungal infections that would warrant consideration.

Treatment and Prognosis: The treatment of choice would depend upon the organism. Specific medications are prescribed such as antimicrobial agents including amphotericin B, ketoconazole, and itraconazole. The progress and recovery would depend on the particular organism and the ability of the host to render defenses. Patients who have fungal infections may have lung involvement; a pulmonologist who specializes in lung diseases would be the person who treats this disease.

Immune System Disorders

The function of the immune system is discussed in Chapter 4, with details of the functions in which the body defends itself against disease and pathogens. During evolution the human body has acquired ways in which we defend ourselves from natural predators such as animals, environmental conditions, and organisms. These organisms include pathogens such as viruses, bacteria, parasites, and fungi. Some organisms such as those found in the human intestine actually work in a symbiotic-type relationship. Viruses, which are pathogens, do not assist in our survival and are detrimental to our actual health. The body's natural defenses against microorganisms function in two ways: (1) natural immunity and (2) acquired immunity (Chapter 4). The diseases listed in this section have oral manifestations and involve the immune system.

NAME: Aphthous ulcers

Etiology: The etiology of aphthous ulcers is not fully understood, although some factors associated with aphthous ulcers are stress, trauma, food allergies, genetic predispositions, B_{12} vitamin deficiencies, and hormonal fluctuations. There is also speculation that the initiation is caused by a hypersensitivity reaction, autoimmune response, and trauma, with chemical mediators involved.

Three types of recurrent aphthous ulcers are classified: (1) RAU minor, (2) RAU major, and (3) the herpetiform RAU (not to be confused with the herpes lesions caused by the HSV). The classification is determined by the size of the lesion and the dispersion. The aphthous ulcer is believed to have an immunologic etiology.

Method of Transmission: Aphthous ulcers are not contagious in contrast to the herpetic type lesions, which are spread from person to person, and to other parts of the body on the same person.

Epidemiology: Local factors are sometimes involved such as trauma and may be caused by biting the tissue, consuming hot liquids, dental procedures, or dental hygiene procedures that disrupt the tissues. Aphthous ulcers often begin in childhood and decrease with age. Rivera-Hidalgo, Shulman, and Beach (2004) analyzed the data (as part of NHANES III) from 17,235 adults, reporting a higher annual prevalence in whites, Mexican Americans, and individuals 17–39 years old who were nonsmokers. Blacks were reported to have lower rates of aphthous ulcers. Studies by Tollerud et al., 1991, reported that smoking raises the number of T helper lymphocytes in Caucasians and lowers it in African Americans. Rivera-Hidalgo et al., point out that this may relate to the ethnic differences in why some populations may be more prone to aphthous ulcers. The prevalence in the under 40-year-old age group was almost double that for those over 40 years of age. They have been reported to decrease during pregnancy and increase significantly during stressful events. Females reportedly have a higher rate of occurrence, especially in association with the menstrual cycle and hormonal fluctuations (Ponter and Scully, 2003).

Pathogenesis: Recurrent aphthous ulcers (RAUs), also known as canker sores, or aphthous stomatitis, periadenitis mucosa necrotica recurrens, are the most commonly seen ulcerations in the oral cavity. RAUs appear on unkeratinized tissue such as the buccal mucosa, the labial mucosa, the ventral surface of the tongue, and the floor of the mouth. Additionally, the soft palate and the posterior oropharynx may be involved. The herpetic types (HSV) of lesions appear on keratinized tissue and are preceded by vesicles. The aphthous form of ulcers also has a distinct size, shape, and location. The lesions are reported to occur more frequently in non-tobacco users. This may be due to the effect tobacco has on the mucosa, making it more keratinized and thereby lowering the susceptibility to the ulcers. There is some indication that a substance in nicotine may also play a role in decreasing susceptibility, since patients on nicotine replacement therapy appear to avoid outbreaks. The reported incidence of aphthous ulcers ranges from as low as 5% to 66% of the population.

Ulcerations that appear aphthous have also been reported in disorders such as Sweet syndrome, agranulocytosis, cyclic neutropenia, and periodic fever syndrome. RAU type ulcers are reported in patients who have Crohn's disease, Reiter syndrome, Behçet syndrome, systemic lupus, celiac sprue (caused by gluten sensitivity, and ulcerative colitis, nontropical and tropical) and allergies in general.

THE THREE CATEGORIES OF RAUs

- RAU-Minor. This is the most common of the three types, making up approximately 70 to 87% of all forms of RAU. Those afflicted are usually aware of a prodromal stage in which they report a tingling or burning sensation. The lesion usually develops within 24 to 48 hours and lasts from 7 to 10 days. The ulcer will heal without scar formation. Pain may accompany the lesions for several days, and the craterlike ulcer will develop a fibrinous membrane cover appearing white or yellow. The ulcers are surrounded by an erythematous halo. Lesions usually number from one to five and are less than 1 cm in diameter (Figs. 12.15 and 12.16).
- RAU-Major. This form has the largest lesions of the

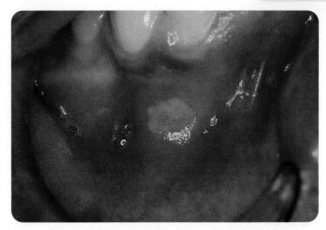

Figure 12.16. RAU Minor. (Courtesy of Dr. Terry Rees.)

three types. Sometimes referred to as **Sutton's disease**, or periadenitis mucosa necrotica recurrens, it is much less common in occurrence. Statistics report that from 7 to 20% of RAUs are classified in this variety. The lesions are much larger, ranging from 1 to 3 cm in diameter and usually number from 1 to 10. They also appear deeper and more craterlike, and have an irregular border. Because of the extensive lesions and the depth, there is scarring of the tissue. The patient may suffer with the chronic disease for 25 years or more (Fig. 12.17).

- RAU Herpetiform (Figure 12.18). These are the smaller of the ulcers, measuring approximately 1 to 3 mm in diameter. They tend to appear in cluster formation of anywhere from 10 to 100 at any time. This form tends to be more predominant in women and occur later in life. The ulcers may coalesce to produce a wide area of lesion. From 7 to 10% (some authors believe this occurs much less frequently) of all cases of aphthous ulcers are of this type. The herpetiform name is not to be confused with the herpetic-type gingivostomatitis lesions found in the primary form of herpes simplex that may occur in children (see Chapter 11). RAU herpetiform is similar in that the vesicles are small and cluster like, but RAU herpetiform is found usually on nonkeratinized tissue and as shown in the figure below, the lesions are found on the ventral surface of the tongue and the floor of the mouth. As shown in the figures be-

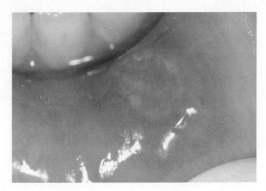

Figure 12.17. RAU major. (Courtesy of Dr. Michael Lewis.)

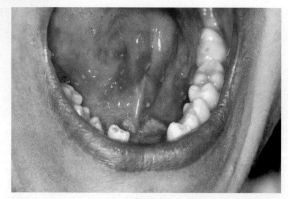

Figure 12.18. RAU Herpetiform. (Courtesy of Dr. Marco Carrozzo.)

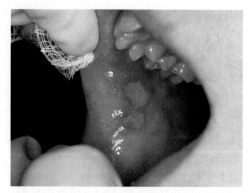

Figure 12.20. Behcet syndrome.

low, herpetic stomatitis HSV is located on the keratinized tissue of the dorsum of the tongue, preceded by vesicles (Fig. 12.19.)

Extraoral Characteristics: There are no oral characteristics related to RAUs unless the lesion is close to the lip and produces edema in that area. The general health and condition of the patient may appear below normal because of pain or fever. Fever is not a noted characteristic; in most cases it is unusual, but it may be evident in some individuals. Syndromes such as **PFAPA** (Marshall et al., 1989) which include periodic fever, aphthous stomatitis, pharyngitis, and adenitis may be a consideration if a fever does occur. Other possible trigger mechanisms are allergic or hypersensitivity reactions. Additionally, gastrointestinal related problems such as Crohn's disease or sprue (gluten sensitivity) are considerations. Further, if the aphthous ulcer is large or has been present for a few days, a secondary infection may produce a systemic infection involving the lymph nodes and a low-grade fever may be produced.

Perioral and Intraoral Characteristics: The appearance and location are important in the clinical diagnosis of all ulcer-type lesions. The ulcer appears as a shallow, and somewhat craterlike lesion with a yellow-to-

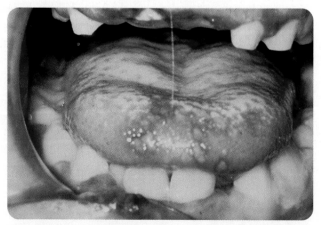

Figure 12.19. Herpes Simplex Virus. (Courtesy of Dr. Peter Jacobsen.)

white pseudomembrane and an erythematous border described as a halo appearance.

Distinguishing Characteristics: The RAUs are found on nonkeratinized tissue. RAUs are not found on the dorsum of the tongue, the attached gingiva, and the hard palate mucosa that are keratinized. This is in contrast to the herpetic lesions that are on attached, keratinized mucosa. However, with the herpetic form of acute herpetic gingivostomatitis, the lesions may be in both attached and movable mucosa (Chapter 11). Aphthous ulcers must be differentiated from trauma ulcerations and from other systemic problems that may cause ulcers.

Significant Microscopic Findings: There are nonspecific findings, and biopsies are usually not needed. The normal findings are lymphocytes, macrophages, and mast cells. Generally, the biopsy specimen is nonspecific, with just an inflammatory composition.

Dental Implications: Pain may make dental procedures difficult. Patients who are susceptible to RAU may have lesions due to any traumatic tissue trauma. Multiple visits may be difficult for dental procedures that require additional appointments. Repairing any sharp teeth or restorations reduce the incidence of trauma. Plaque removal and increasing lubrication of the mouth is beneficial to decrease the bacterial counts and inflammation in the mouth. (See Chapter 22 for the occurrence of aphthous ulcers in relation to AIDS.)

Differential Diagnosis: Some viral infections such as herpangina, gingivostomatitis, and hand-foot-and-mouth disease are part of the differential diagnosis but can usually be eliminated clinically. Some diseases should be considered initially such as

• Erythema multiforme—Chapter 23
• Lichen planus—Chapters 13 and 14
• Mucous membrane pemphigoid—Chapter 11
• Pemphigus vulgaris—Chapter 11
• AIDS/HIV infection—Chapter 22
• Reiter syndrome—Chapter 12
• Behçet syndrome—Chapter 12

- Sprue—Chapter 12
- Crohn's disease—Chapter 12
- Sutton's disease—Chapter 12
- Systemic lupus erythematosus—Chapter 12
- PFAPA syndrome—Chapter 12

Treatment and Prognosis: The use of chlorhexidine gluconate as a rinse is often prescribed. Sometimes topically applied corticosteroid gels such as Kenalog in Orabase are used, depending on the severity and type of ulcerations. (See Clinical Protocol 8). Additionally, tetracycline rinses are sometimes prescribed in addition to corticosteroids. Corticosteroids and over-the-counter medications are sometimes suggested when the patient determines that the first prodromal signs have appeared. For severe problems, further testing and screening may be needed. Depending on the number and severity, the lesions usually subside within 7 to 10 days regardless of treatment. In the major forms, the lesions may remain ulcerative for weeks and eventually heal with evidence of scarring.

NAME: Behçet's syndrome

Etiology: Behçet syndrome is an inflammatory disorder of unknown cause. A viral connection is suspected, with a genetic predisposition.

Method of Transmission: Behçet syndrome is of an unknown origin, but there is no indication of possible transmission from one person to another.

Epidemiology: Behçet syndrome has an onset in the 3rd and 4th decades. It affects men more often, and persons of Mediterranean, Middle Eastern, and Japanese descent in most geographic areas; but in western countries, women are affected most often. Oral lesions are found in over 90% in all types of the disease. Both oral and genital ulcers are found in 65% of Behçet patients with about 80% developing eye lesions as well.

Pathogenesis: The disorder is a rare multisystem disorder noted for a triad of (1) RAU minor,(2) genital ulcers, and (3) ocular lesions. The three factors are required for diagnosis consideration. Other problems may exist also, related to gastrointestinal, vascular, muscular, and hematologic abnormalities. Skin lesions including Behçet are an immune-mediated process leading to vasculitis. Genetic predisposition is suspected, and a viral etiology has been proposed (Fig. 12.20).

Extraoral Characteristics: Cutaneous lesions may be present such as erythema nodosum or acneform skin eruptions, arthritis, CNS lesions, and intestinal ulcerations.

Perioral and Intraoral Characteristics: The ulcerative appearance in Behçet syndrome is very similar to the aphthous ulcer. The lesions may range in size from several millimeters to several centimeters. The lesions are recurrent and painful.

Distinguishing Characteristics: The triad of minor ulcers, genital ulcers, and ocular lesions signal the possibility of Behçet syndrome for a disease consideration. When seen with cutaneous involvement and other symptoms, the characteristics become even more pronounced.

Microscopic Features: Enhanced polymorphonuclear leukocyte chemotaxis and neutrophil/platelet hyperfunction. Vasculitis and perivascular infiltrate ultimately develops.

Dental Implications: Medications used in treatment such as cyclosporine may produce gingival hyperplasia, and other medications may have effects on the tissue as well. Corticosteroids and immunosuppressive agents often produce changes in the tissues, and the patient should be evaluated with each visit. Maintenance can be adjusted for the individual patient as needed.

Differential Diagnosis: Behçet syndrome may be confused with other disorders that also have oral ulcerations such as

- HIV-associated aphthous.(see Chapter 22)
- Confusion may also exist between RAUs and HSV, especially with regard to the herpetiform types (see Chapters 11, 12, and 22)
- Crohn's disease (Chapter 12)
- Reiter syndrome (Chapter 12)
- Lupus (Chapter 12)

Treatment and Prognosis: Topical steroid treatment may be used. Cyclosporine has been shown effective in the treatment of mucocutaneous and ocular lesions. Chlorambucil may be combined with corticosteroids. The lesions can be controlled but recur frequently in most instances.

NAME: Reiter's syndrome

Etiology: Reiter syndrome usually develops after exposure to a venereal disease or a gastrointestinal infection, such as dysentery, and is caused by organisms such as *Salmonella* and *Shigella* (Yates and Stetz, 2006). Males who carry the HLA-B27 are at risk for Reiter's syndrome, which suggests a genetic influence to the disease (Neville et al. 1995, Regezi et al., 2005). Infectious organisms are suspected to be etiologic agents such as *Chlamydia* or *Mycoplasma* spp.

Method of Transmission: Since the syndrome is related to an abnormal immune response, it is not considered contagious. However, an association with HIV-infected individuals has been suggested, and this aspect should be kept under consideration for diagnosis.

Epidemiology: Reiter syndrome usually affects white males in their 30s. Males are affected most often, but females may be affected as well. Although Reiter syndrome has been reported in children, the cases are infrequent. There are no known racial differences.

Pathogenesis: As in Behçet syndrome, this syndrome also comprises a triad of arthritis, urethritis, and conjunctivitis (or iritis, which is inflammation of the iris). See Figure 12.22.

Extraoral Characteristics: The small joints of the patient are affected, which usually involve the lower extremities. The genitals, anus, and rectum may be affected. Thickened hyperkeratotic nodules that resemble pustular psoriasis are characteristic. Conjunctivitis is a component of the triad for Reiter syndrome and occurs early in the disease. Dystrophic nail lesions may also be a dermatologic component. Musculoskeletal problems of the large weightbearing joints and the ankles are frequently involved and may exhibit redness and swelling. The Achilles tendon may be involved, producing tendinitis. The ocular involvement may include cataracts and glaucoma. The eye appears red and swollen in some cases.

Perioral and Intraoral Characteristics: In the mouth, approximately one half of patients have oral ulcerations. They appear sharply demarcated, and a white border often surrounds the lesion. Additionally, some of the lesions may appear aphthous-like. Unlike the painful aphthous ulcers, lesions related to Reiter syndrome are often described as less painful. These lesions may occur anywhere in the mouth.

Distinguishing Characteristics: Reiter syndrome may appear similar to other disease states with common findings such as geographic-like tongue, aphthous ulcers, arthritis, and conjunctivitis (Figs. 12.21 and 12.22).

Significant Microscopic Features: The lesions resemble psoriasis, with parakeratosis and microabscess formation.

Dental Implications: Assisting the patient in diagnosis of the early disease is important, since the oral signs

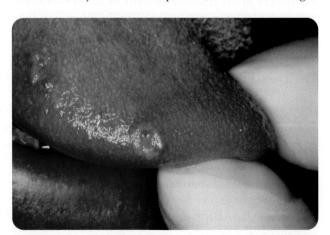

Figure 12.21. Reiter's syndrome (Courtesy of Dr. Terry Rees.)

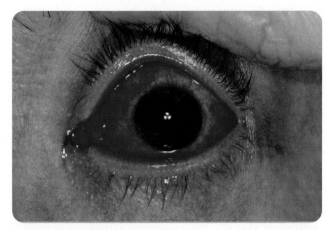

Figure 12.22. Reiter's syndrome with occular inflammation. (Courtesy of Dr. Denis Lynch.)

can mimic other less serious diseases such as common aphthous ulcers. When external symptoms are present along with the intraoral lesions, referral to a medical doctor is indicated.

Differential Diagnosis: The lesions may appear as aphthous-like lesions or geographic tongue, with some lesions appearing as erythematous plaques.
• Aphthous ulcers—Chapter 12
• Behçet syndrome—Chapter 12
• Celiac sprue—Chapter 12
• Crohn's disease—Chapter 12
• Lupus—Chapter 12

Treatment and Prognosis: Nonsteroidal antiinflammatory agents are the medications of choice. The disease may last from weeks to months, and the condition can be chronic with remission and recurrence. In most patients, Reiter syndrome usually remits within a year, but in 15 to 20% of cases, progressive arthritis develops.

NAME: Erythema multiforme

Etiology: Erythema multiforme has been associated with exposure to the herpes simplex virus, tuberculosis, and histoplasmosis, as well as other fungal organisms. Mycoplasma pneumonia and herpes simplex virus infection are often observed within the previous weeks of skin lesion development (Rubin, 2005). The use of certain medications is also associated with erythema multiforme, including sulfonamides, penicillin, barbiturates, phenylbutazone, and phenytoin. Sometimes the cause of the disease is never discovered. As the name implies, the disease can have multiple clinical appearances and forms.

Method of Transmission: Exposure to certain medications, contact with viral, fungal, and bacterial agents are involved in the transmission of erythema multiforme.

Epidemiology: Erythema multiforme affects young adults, and men develop the disease more often than women do. Approximately 25–50% of patients who have

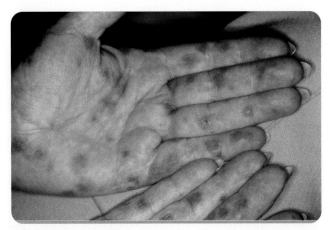

Figure 12.23. Erythema multiforme target lesions. (Courtesy of Dr. Peter Jacobsen.)

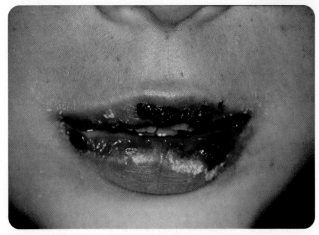

Figure 12.24. Stevens-Johnson syndrome. A 7-year-old with crusting of the lips due to penicillin reaction. (Courtesy of Dr. John Jacoway.)

cutaneous lesions also have oral lesions. The disease can be chronic or may only be seen in an acute form (Plemons et al., 1999).

Pathogenesis: Erythema multiforme is an acute mucocutaneous disease that occurs in two forms. Erythema multiforme minor features distinct skin lesions that are termed *target lesions*. This form may or may not have oral involvement (Fig. 12.23). Figure 12.23 depicts the skin lesions known as "target lesions" or "iris lesions." The lesions resemble a target or the iris with a circular pattern. Both cutaneous lesions and intraoral involvement characterize erythema multiforme major. The second form (more severe form) is also referred to as **Stevens-Johnson syndrome.** The oral cavity, conjunctiva, and genitalia are involved, and a mortality rate of 5–15% is reported (Pont, 2004).

Extraoral Characteristics: The skin lesions present as erythematous papules that enlarge to form central vesicles, or bulla, creating what are referred to as "iris," "target," or "bull's eye" lesions.

Perioral and Intraoral Characteristics: Oral, genital, and ocular lesions may be present, depending upon the type and severity of the disease. The lesions may be bordered by a blanched halo with an erythematous zone at the periphery. Ocular lesions may vary in severity when present. Often, the lips are involved and may be covered by a black hemorrhagic crust; the mucosal lesions are raw and red in appearance. Figure 12.24 demonstrates the hemorrhagic state of Stevens Johnson syndrome in a child.

The oral ulcers may vary from a few aphthous lesions to a large number when the disease is in a major form.

Distinguishing Characteristics: The cutaneous target lesions that are initially seen are the most characteristic sign of erythema multiforme. The lesions appear as concentric rings with a lighter outer edge and a deeper colored core. The major form of EM is known as Stevens Johnson syndrome, and this form is often triggered by

medications, resulting in a heavy crusting of the lips, which become swollen and hemorrhagic. Figure 12.24 depicts the oral tissue lesions in a patient diagnosed with erythema multiforme who had a reaction to penicillin.

Significant Microscopic Features: Histologic findings include epithelial hyperplasia, spongiosis, vesicles, and lymphocytic infiltrate. Necrotic keratinocytes and extensive vesicular changes are seen on histologic diagnosis.

Dental Implications: Dental work may exacerbate the disease and must be postponed until the lesions have completely healed.

Differential Diagnosis: Confusion sometimes occurs with the following disease states:

- Herpes simplex
- Primary herpetic gingivostomatitis
- Other dermatological disorders such as pityriasis, erosive oral lichen planus, pemphigus and pemphigus vulgaris

Treatment and Prognosis: Treatment is usually palliative, but short term. Corticosteroids are used in more extreme cases as well as antiviral medications. The lesions usually subside within a few weeks, but recurrent lesions are possible in about 25% of cases.

NAME: Hypersensitivity Reactions

Etiology: Immunity and hypersensitivity reactions are discussed fully in Chapter 4. The main type of hypersensitivity that occurs in the mouth is a delayed hypersensitivity reaction mediated by sensitized T lymphocytes.

Method of Transmission: Hypersensitivity is caused by a reaction to a medication or contact with a product that produces a tissue reaction.

Epidemiology: Any age may be affected, and an equal distribution of males and females has been reported. With

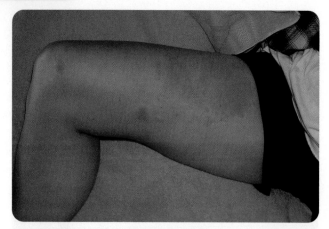

Figure 12.25. Hypersensitivity reactions.

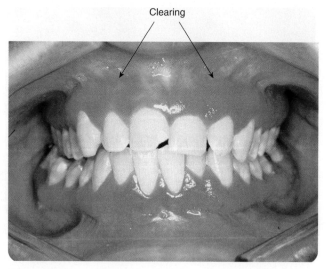

Clearing

Figure 12.26. Toothpaste allergy—cinnamonaldehyde. (Courtesy of Dr. Terry Rees.)

exposure to more chemicals than in previous decades, the numbers of hypersensitivity reactions has increased and is expected to continue to rise.

Pathogenesis: Hypersensitivity is often related to medications and products that the patient may be using at the time. These reactions can occur at any point of exposure but may especially appear when a new medication is being used. The reaction may occur at anytime during use, but is usually after 24 to 48 hours of consuming the medication. Any individual may be susceptible to the effects of a hypersensitivity reaction. **Stomatitis medicamentosa,** or fixed drug reaction occurs with systemic drug usage, and **stomatitis venenata** appears with contact hypersensitivity.

In fixed drug reactions, the lesions can be ulcerative, and the reaction is usually within 24 hours after ingestion of the medication. The result can be what is termed **angioedema** (a diffuse swelling of the tissue) and/or **urticaria** (hives). Figure 12.25 is an example of a hive in an allergic response to a product. Figure 12.25 is an example of contact dermatitis. During angioedema and urticaria, a chemical mediator called histamine is released that is stimulated by IgE antibodies, causing vascular permeability. Antihistamine medications are used to control the effects of the symptoms. Avoidance of the trigger agent is important in the management of future episodes, however, in many cases no specific causative agent may be found.

In contact stomatitis, which is a local reaction, the tissue in contact with the mucosa appears erythematous and may be ulcerated. An example of contact stomatitis is cinnamon aldehyde allergy caused by the use of cinnamon products. When the patient is hypersensitive to cinnamon, the tissues are bathed in the substance, but the area in the vestibule is protected because of the overlapping tissues. When viewed clinically, there will be what is described as a "clearing," in which the product is not coming in contact with the tissue. Figure 12.26 is an example of the erythematous gingiva of contact hypersensitivity. With cinnamon products being used more widely, reported cases of this type of allergy are being documented

(see Clinical Protocol 6). Another compound that may produce a type of contact allergic response is amalgam. Lichenoid type reactions are seen as sensitivity to the restoration material. Toothpaste hypersensitivity is another frequent problem for patients, with sloughing of tissue along with the redness and irritation. Figure 12.27 depicts the sloughing of tissue that is common in patients who experience a toothpaste allergy.

Extraoral Characteristics: Hives are common in severe allergic reactions. The external lesions can vary in size, and pruritus may accompany the lesions.

Perioral and Intraoral Characteristics: Vesicles, erythematous tissue, rash with various sized macules, and ulcers may be seen depending upon the type of reaction and the person's immune system. Angioedema (tissue swelling) and urticaria (hives) may be present.

Distinguishing Characteristics: Angioedema and urticaria are common symptoms in hypersensitivity reactions.

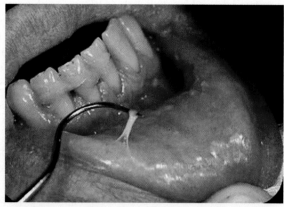

Figure 12.27. Tissue sloughing due to sensitivity reaction. (Courtesy of Dr. Terry Rees.)

Microscopic Features: Nonspecific features are seen such as spongiosis (collections of neutrophils surrounded by clear spaces or halos), apoptotic keratinocytes, lymphoid infiltrates, eosinophils, and ulceration. In addition, mononuclear or polymorphonuclear infiltrations in a subepithelial or perivascular infiltration, basal cell destruction, edema, and keratinocyte necrosis are seen.

Dental Implications: Patients who have hypersensitivity may be predisposed to react to certain dental products or chemicals used in the dental office. An example is latex allergy and flavoring agents that are found in prophy paste, toothpaste, mouth rinses, and even fluoride. Certain restorative products may produce a response in some patients. When obvious allergy-related problems continue after discontinuing the offending products, it will be necessary to refer the patient to someone for a more extensive evaluation of the condition. A skin prick test or a patch test may be used to determine specific products that the patient is not tolerating well.

Differential Diagnosis: A careful health history is crucial, with emphasis on the current use of medications that may be contributing to the reactions. The oral membranes may be affected or there may be more systemic problems and symptoms. Intolerance or an allergy may occur at anytime during life. The following items should be considered: certain foods, central products, and many household products. Clinically, patients may appear with many ulcerative type lesions that may clinically appear as

    RAU—Chapter 12
    Lichen planus—Chapters 13 and 14
    Pemphigus—Chapter 11
    Pemphigoid—Chapter 11
    Lupus erythematosus—Chapter 11
    Cinnamon aldehyde reaction—Chapter 11, Chapter 13

Treatment and Prognosis: Discontinuing the medication or changing to another commonly used medication is considered. In the case of stomatitis venenata, discontinuing the product responsible is the treatment of choice. Withdrawal of the offending source usually produces results within several days to 2 weeks.

Name: Lupus erythematosus

Etiology: Lupus is classified as an autoimmune disease and a type III hypersensitivity reaction (Rubin, 2004). In systemic lupus, although the cause is unknown, there is a breakdown in the normal immune surveillance mechanisms. There does appear to be some genetic predisposition to lupus.

Method of Transmission: Lupus erythematosus is an autoimmune disease and is not contagious.

Epidemiology: Adults are most affected by lupus and predominately women in their 30s. As with most autoimmune-type diseases, females are affected more than males.

The Lupus Foundation of America estimates that approximately 1,500,000 Americans have some form of the disease (2006). Lupus is 10 to 15 times more common in adult females, and more common in Blacks (1:250) and nonwhite groups (1:1000). There is a higher incidence in Europe and Australia than in the United States. In Europe, the highest prevalence was reported in Sweden, Iceland, and Spain (Lupus, 2006).

Pathogenesis: Lupus is a chronic autoimmune disorder that affects the skin surfaces, the organs (mainly the kidneys), joints, serous membranes, and skin, although any organ can be affected. The disorder arises because of an antigen–antibody response that causes inflammation of multiple organs throughout the body as in a type III hypersensitivity reaction. Antibodies (IgG, IgM, and IgA) are formed against exogenous or endogenous antigens, and complement and leukocytes (neutrophils and macrophages) are often involved. This scenario is typical for most lupus erythematosus.

The oral tissues are also affected and the tissues can be extremely erythematic and painful. Certain pharmaceutical agents have been implicated in the pathogenesis of lupus such as hydralazine, lovastatin, penicillamine, recombinant cytokines, L-tryptophan, and procainamide. There is a genetic predisposition to the disease. Lupus is classified into two groups. Discoid lupus erythematosus (chronic form, DLE) accounts for 70% of all cases, and systemic lupus erythematosus (acute form, SLE), accounting for 10% of cases, is a multisystem disorder affecting the kidneys, joints, heart, lungs, central nervous system, and the skin. In SLE, the heart may develop thrombus formation and thrombocytopenia may lead to bleeding with anemia due to suppression of the platelet and red blood cell counts. The kidney is also affected, and renal failure is a problem for these patients. Along with the DLE and SLE forms, drug-induced lupus is found in about 10% of cases, and another 10% have a relationship with other connective tissue diseases such as scleroderma. The oral and cutaneous lesions may be seen in varying degrees with all forms of lupus erythematosus. Small, nonbacterial vegetations may form on the heart valves and are called **Libman-Sacks endocarditis**. As with any severe systemic disease, working together with the physician is important and premedication may be needed for certain procedures.

Extraoral Characteristics: Weight loss, arthritis, skin lesions, and a classic rash over the nose and malar region (butterfly rash) are common in DLE. Figure 12.28 is an example of the classic rash in the malar region. These features are present in approximately 25 to 40% of patients. Additionally, alopecia and vesiculobullous lesions are commonly found. Figure 12.29 depicts the scalp area of a patient with systemic lupus. Note the ulcers and scabs on the scalp.

The disease is associated with endothelial damage to the heart, resulting in an increased incidence of infective endocarditis. Other features of lupus erythematosus in-

APPLICATION

The dental profession is seeing a surge in the number of patients who present with varying oral symptoms related to hypersensitivity. Most professionals attempt to solve the mystery through trial and error by discontinuing dental products, foods, and other materials (e.g., soaps, detergents, cosmetics, drinks, environmental allergens) that their patients contact daily. Many clinicians, however, do not consider the possibility that intolerance or hypersensitivity could be the patient's problem with regard to oral symptoms. Stomatology Centers are specialty clinics that treat many such patients who come to the centers because their particular oral condition could not be diagnosed. These patients may have seen several other medical and dental practitioners before being referred to a specialty clinic. A reason for the tissue response is usually found, and many times, a hypersensitivity response is the diagnosis. This response may be categorized further into other subclassifications such as contact allergy, cinnamon allergy, toothpaste allergy, or metal allergy.

We are bombarded with so many chemicals and products daily that it is believed that the increase we are clinically observing is related to allergy/hypersensitivity reactions. The possibility that a generalized lip irritation, tissue sloughing. or gingival irritation may be linked to a hypersensitivity reaction is a viable consideration that clinicians should prudently include in their differential diagnosis. Read Clinical Protocol 6 for a checklist of possible flavoring agents and protocols that may be considered.

clude Raynaud's phenomenon, photosensitivity, giant cell arteritis, celiac disease, primary billary cirrhosis, facial and parotid swelling, and potential malignant changes. Central nervous system involvement is sometimes present, and seizures may occur that would warrant clinical consideration. The patient with external lesions may also be sensitive to sunlight.

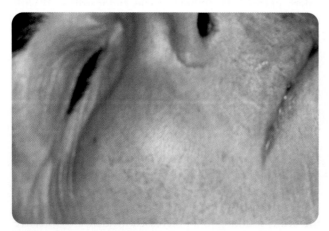

Figure 12.28.   Lupus Malar rash.

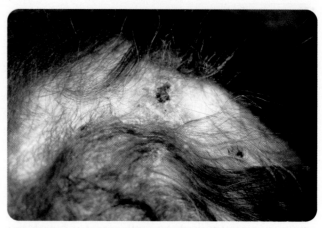

Figure 12.29.   Lupus erythematosus scalp lesion.

Perioral and Intraoral Considerations: Oral lesions are present in all forms of the disease in 25–40% of patients, but this is less evident in the milder form. The lesions are characterized by erythematous erosions or ulceration surrounded by a white rim with radiating keratotic striae. The most frequent sites of involvement are the hard and soft palate, buccal mucosa, and the vermillion border of the lips. The gingiva may take on a desquamative appearance, and there is often confusion with other mucosal diseases such as lichen planus, pemphigus, and pemphigoid. Figure 12.30 shows a discoid skin lesion above the eye associated with lupus), Figure 12.31 is an example of the ulcerative mucosa in systemic lupus. A biopsy and immunofluorescence are needed for a definitive diagnosis.

Significant Microscopic Features: Lymphocytic infiltrate, thickened basement membrane zones, and connective tissue are characteristic. The lymphocytic infiltrates are dispersed about appendages and vessels. Oral lesions may be found in all forms of the disease. Other key features of lupus include keratinocyte vacuolization, subepithelial periodic acid–Schiff-positive deposits, lamina propria edema, thickening of the basal cell layer membranes, and a severe perivascular lymphocytic infiltrate.

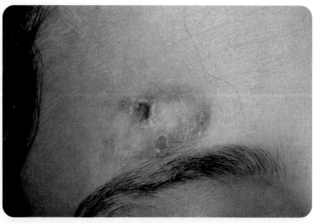

Figure 12.30.   Lupus skin lesion.

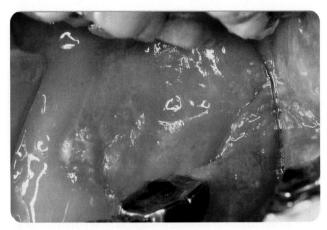

Figure 12.31. Discoid lupus oral lesion

Immunofluorescence is most helpful in differentiating lupus from other skin disorders such as lichen planus, pemphigus, and pemphigoid. Another diagnostic aid is a serologic test for circulating antibodies.

Dental Implications: The gingiva may be described as desquamative, and the general description of soreness is a common complaint of patients. In addition, other surfaces may be involved such as the oropharyngeal mucosa, the larynx, and the epiglottis. Patients may complain of severe dryness and other symptoms that are also found in Sjögren syndrome (Chapter 17, Part 1; see Clinical Protocol 4). When corticosteroids are used for extended periods, *Candida* infections may occur simultaneously. Treatment of the fungal infection would be needed (see Clinical Protocol 5).

Differential Diagnosis: Lupus must be distinguished from other skin disorders such as
• Erosive oral lichen planus—Chapter 13
• Pemphigus vulgaris—Chapter 11
• Benign mucous membrane pemphigoid—Chapter 11
• Erythematous candidiasis—Chapter 14
• Hypersensitivity reactions
  Some pharmaceutical agents have been implicated in the pathogenesis of drug-induced lupus erythematosus, and patients sometimes experience remission when these products are discontinued. The use of certain medications may present as similar to erythema multiforme, discussed above. Medications such as lovastatin, penicillamine, L-tryptophan, and procainamide have been implicated.

Treatment and Prognosis: Oral and skin lesions usually respond to topical and intralesionsal corticosteroids, depending on the severity. Hydroxychloroquine (Plaquenil sulfate) is often used as well as antiinflammatory agents for milder forms. Antibiotic prophylaxis may be used to prevent bacterial endocarditis if the patient has involvement of the endocardium or heart valves.

Additionally, the oral lesions are treated by topical corticosteroids and systemic steroids for SLE. Intralesional corticosteroids are sometimes used, with variable results. Antimalarial drugs (Plaquenil sulfate), gold salts, nonsteroidal antiinflammatory drugs (NSAIDs), and cyclosporine have been used in the treatment of lupus as well. Depending on the severity of the disease and the degree of systemic involvement, lupus is a chronic, progressive disease, and the treatment of symptoms related to lupus will vary. Renal failure is the most common cause of death. The 20-year survival rate is close to 70%. Topical corticosteroids and systemic steroids depending upon the severity treat the oral lesions.

NAME: Crohn's disease

Crohn's disease is mentioned here because of the associated oral aphthous ulcers seen as a chronic condition in patients. The disease was first described in 1932. It is a chronic disease that involves the gastointestinal tract from the mouth to the anus. The lesions are noncaseating epithelioid-type granulomas. The involved tissue may be fissured, and epithelial hyperplasia is usually present. Evidence suggests that there is a hereditary component. Crohn's disease is most common in young individuals.

Men exceed women in developing neoplasms by 2 to 1. Intestinal signs and symptoms include abdominal discomfort, anorexia, weight loss, and fever. Oral lesions are reported in up to 20% of the patient population. The lesions may manifest as lobular enlargement of the tongue, soft palate, and labial or buccal mucosa, which may appear to have a "cobble stoning" effect. The lips may be involved, enlarged gingival lesions may be present, and there is an increased incidence of aphthous ulcers. The lesions are usually slow healing and found in the oral vestibule at the base of the tissue folds. Figure 12.32 shows an ulceration in the maxillary retromolar area of a patient with Crohn's disease.

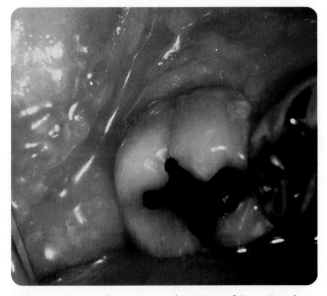

Figure 12.32. Crohn's Disease. (Courtesy of Terry Rees.)

The microscopic features include nonspecific focal aggregations of lymphocytes and regular perivascular infiltrates of inflammatory cells. Noncaseating epithelioid granulomas may be found, and multinucleated foreign body giant cells may or may not be present. The overlying epithelium may be normal, hyperplastic, or ulcerated.

The diagnosis for Crohn's is made on clinical signs, symptoms, and biopsy results, and the clinical appraisal alone is not sufficient to diagnose Crohn's disease. As presented throughout this chapter, many disease states have an ulcerative clinical appearance.

Management of the gut lesions is crucial in the success of treatment. Using systemic corticosteroids, sulfalazine, cyclosporine, or other antiinflammatory medications is the usual procedure. For oral lesions, the use of topical corticosteroids or intralesionsal corticosteroids is the treatment of choice. Crohn's disease is a chronic disease, and the patient may have remission periods with recurrent episodes.

NEOPLASMS

Neoplasia is a general term given to tissue that exhibits abnormal and uncontrolled growth. This section deals with neoplasms in relation to squamous cell carcinoma, since malignancies seen orally are, for the most part, squamous cell carcinoma. Chapter 5 has a comprehensive discussion of the types of cancers, staging, and the behavior and characteristics of various types of cancer. However, in Chapter 5, a neoplasm that does not spread to other tissues (i.e., does not metastasize) is described as benign. A neoplasm that spreads and invades other tissue or organs is termed *malignant* or may be referred to as *cancerous*. In understanding the names assigned to neoplasms, in most cases, the types of tissue that are involved can be determined simply by the name of the neoplasm. For example, tumors that arise from the epithelial tissue are termed *carcinomas*. If the epithelial tissue is of glandular origin, it is called an adenocarcinoma. The Latin root *adeno* means gland. A neoplasm of connective tissue, bone, nerve, or muscle is **a sarcoma**. The most common oral cancer is called the squamous cell carcinoma. The hygienist is sometimes the first person to see an early cancer, so the importance of detection and documentation cannot be overemphasized. When lesions are found and treated early, the patient's likelihood of recovery is increased immensely. The devastation of head and neck surgery can be minimized when early lesions are detected, and the patient's long-term health and long-term quality of life is increased (see Chapter 10).

NAME: Squamous cell carcinoma

Etiology: This section discusses ulcerative changes, since some SCC may have an ulcerlike appearance as they progress. The etiology of SCC is multifaceted. Lifestyle choices, environmental influences, genetic factors, infections (particularly by viruses), and various combinations of these and other items, may be responsible in the development of any type of cancer. Although no one cause is accepted in the development of oral cancer, there are factors that have been associated with the development of the disease. Sunlight, tobacco, alcohol, diet, stress, and the use of products such as betel quid in certain populations have a strong association. Infections that have been implicated include syphilis, candidosis, and viruses such as the human papilloma virus. Some chemical industrial hazards have been implicated, as evidenced by an increased cancer incidence in workers at woolen textile plants/chemical plants. A higher rate of cancer may be found in association with some mucosal disorders such as oral submucous fibrosis, lichen planus, and other chronic-type ulcerative lesions. In the past few years, inflammation in general has received much attention, and extensive research has focused on the impact of chronic inflammation at the cellular level affecting all areas of the body.

Method of Transmission: Oral cancer is not a contagious disease and has not been documented as such in the medical/dental literature. However, many recent studies have linked the human papilloma virus with certain types of cancers such as cervical cancer. In addition, HPV types 16, 18, 33, and 35 have been implicated in many head and neck cancers (Massano et al., 2006). Oral–genital sex has been implicated as a possible mode of transmission related to the HPV–cancer association (Gillison et al., 2000).

Epidemiology: The American Cancer Society cites estimates of 30,990 new cases of oral cancer, with 7,430 deaths per year due to the disease. SCCs encompass at least 90% of all oral malignancies. Oral and pharyngeal cancers account for approximately 3% of all cancers in the United States. Men exceed women in developing this neoplasm by 1.8 to 1. There has been an increase in SCC in women over the past decades. This is probably due to the increase in women who smoke and the use of tobacco products coupled with an increase in alcohol consumption. Approximately 90% of all oral cancers are carcinomas that arise from the surface stratified squamous epithelium. Data from the American Cancer Society (2006) indicate that the 5-year survival rate for localized stages (the cancer has not spread to other sites in the body) is 82%, with a 5-year survival rate for all stages combined at 59%. SCC typically affects an older population group. Half of all oral cancers are diagnosed in persons older than 68 years of age. However, statistics show an alarming increase in the number of cases involving those under the age of 40. Some 90% of patients with oral cancers use tobacco, and smokers are six times more likely to develop cancer than nonsmokers. Coupled with alcohol use, the risks are further increased; 75 to 80% of oral cancer patients drink alcohol frequently, placing them at 6 times the rate of nondrinkers. Interestingly, 25% of people who develop oral cancer have no risk factors. Blacks have a higher risk of oral and pharyngeal cancers, with oral cancer being the fourth most frequent site of cancer in this group. The incidence of oral cancer in Europe in people aged 20 to 39 years old has increased 6-fold. Studies report increased mortality rates for the past 2 decades in Eastern Europe (La Vecchia et al., 2004). This is also increasingly evident in statistics of SCC of the tongue in adults under the age of 40 in the United States (Schantz, 2002). Researchers have reported that cancer in younger patients tends to be more aggressive, with a poorer prognosis in these patients. It is speculated (Llewellyn et al., 2004) that because oral cancer is expected to occur in the older population, perhaps there is more of a delay in diagnosis and treatment in younger groups. Additionally, oral cancer is more often being discovered at advanced stages and requires more aggressive treatment. The prime areas for the development of oral cancer in the wet oral tissues are the following, in order of frequency: (1) tongue, (2) floor of the mouth, (3) salivary glands, and (4) gingiva. The lip is excluded in this data since it is not considered a "wet" oral tissue. The lip, however, is a high-risk area as well, and patients should be checked for cancer in this area and encouraged to wear lip balm with sunscreen (see Clinical Protocol 10 and Chapter 23).

Extraoral Characteristics:
The external features of squamous cell carcinoma and basal cell carcinoma are discussed fully in Chapters 5 and 23. In any oral examination, be sure to check the extraoral sites as well. Have the patient remove eyeglasses so that the area under the frames may be evaluated. This area is a prime location for basal cell carcinoma, and the patient may not view the area themselves in a mirror, without their glasses. The area under the frame is often totally missed. Hats and often wigs shield the areas on the head, and skin under these areas should be evaluated as well.

Perioral and Intraoral Characteristics:
SCC may show a wide variety of clinical appearances. Many SCC cases exhibit **erythroplakia**, which is a general clinical term for a red patch. Most all lesions having an erythroplakia component are found to be either dysplastic or malignant. Any lesion that has a mixture of red and white color and an ulcerated appearance is highly suspicious. (Erythroplakia and erythroleukoplakia are discussed fully in Chapter 14 and mentioned in Chapter 13.) Erythroplakia in addition to being red often is described as velvety in appearance. The lesions may be homogenous red or have a mixture of red and white components, in which case, it is termed **speckled erythroleukoplakia**. Any lesion in the oral cavity has the potential to be malignant or to change in form under certain circumstances. Therefore, every lesion deserves concern. The most frequent sites for oral cancer are found in what may be termed the "drainage" area, comprising the ventral and lateral border of the tongue, the floor of the mouth, the

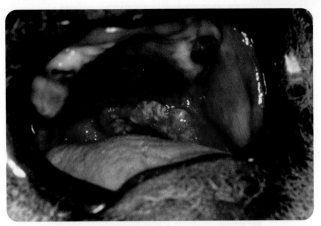

Figure 12.33.   Tonsillar squamous cell carcinoma. (Courtesy of Dr. Mike Brennan.)

adjacent lingual mucosa, lingual sulcus, and the retromolar region. The dorsum of the tongue is a low-risk area. The oral pharynx and tonsillar regions are often included in general head and neck cancer statistics. Figure 12.33 is an example of SCC of the tonsil, Figure 12.34 depicts SSC of the gingiva. Figure 12.35 shows SCC of the palate, and Figure 12.36 depicts SCC of the tongue, with trauma as well.

This area is one in which particular attention is warranted and it is overlooked in many cases. Evaluation should include the tonsil and pharyngeal region in a thorough intraoral examination and cancer screening. Although a malignant neoplasm may have many appearances, and any abnormal, unexplained, lesion should raise a red flag, SCC may initially appear as only a subtle change. Documentation and digital photography can greatly enhance the probability that small changes will be noticed. The lesion may be compared with previous photos and a subsequent referral should be made.

Distinguishing Characteristics:
Squamous cell carcinoma is a great imitator of other disease states. Early cancer can resemble many diseases or can appear essentially very benign initially. It is only after the tissue begins

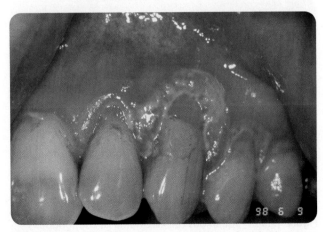

Figure 12.34.   Squamous cell carcinoma in the gingiva. (Courtesy of Dr. Terry Rees.)

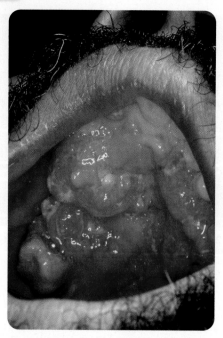

Figure 12.35.   Squamous cell carcinoma of the palate. (Courtesy of Dr. Michael Brennan.)

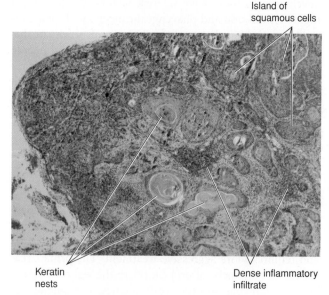

Island of squamous cells

Keratin nests

Dense inflammatory infiltrate

Figure 12.37.   Squamous cell carcinoma histology. (Courtesy of Dr. Harvey Kessler.)

to rapidly grow and change appearance that cancer may be suspected. Unlike other external areas of the body, the patient is usually not aware of these changes, since they are not visible areas. Unexplained lesions, continued enlargement, and a lesion that does not recede on its own should be evaluated by biopsy. Clinical Protocol 12 discusses various techniques that may be used in early cancer detection when there is a suspected change in tissue.

Microscopic Features: Depending upon the stage of the cancer, cells will present with hyperchromatism, pleomorphism, increased nuclear cytoplasmic ratio, premature keratinization, and formation of spheroidal masses of keratin deep within the epithelium. These nests are called

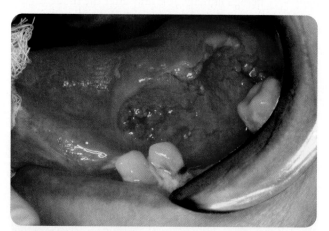

Figure 12.36.   Squamous cell carcinoma of the tongue. (Courtesy of Dr. Terry Rees.)

keratin pearls. Mitoses are typically increased in number and often abnormal in appearance. Figure 12.37 shows a histology slide that demonstrates the nests of cancerous cells, keratin production, and obvious invasive SCC.

Dental Implications: The dental implications related to SCC are extensive. The principles of detection and diagnosis of SCC are discussed throughout this book, and patients with previous SCCs who are on maintenance therapy must be considered. SCC may recur, and these patients should be carefully monitored for any tissue changes. The practitioner should be alerted to the increased risk of cancer development in patients who have a history of bone marrow transplantation, solid organ transplants, or any other reason for extensive immunosuppression (Sciubba, 2001). The current theory in cancer research is that head and neck cancers develop within a contiguous field of preneoplastic cells. Cells of a field show genetic alterations associated with the process of carcinogenesis even though the tissue appears clinically normal. In other words, even after the carcinoma has been removed, cells at the periphery but within the field may have a tendency to become invasive cancer. These cells all share genetic alterations. This differs from a cancer that may recur due to residual cancer cells left after surgery. Development of a secondary primary tumor in the same general area is also a possibility. The theory of **field carcinogenesis**, in practical terms, suggests that medical and dental practitioners should be alerted to any tissue changes in the surrounding areas when a patient has had any type of malignancy (Braakhuis et al., 2005).

Differential Diagnosis: Cancer in the early stages is often painless, white or red or variegated in color, and

Summary

- Ulcers may have many causes and may be factitial, traumatic, or iatrogenic.
- Necrotizing sialometaplasia is caused by trauma and salivary gland ischemia in a localized area.
- Tuberculosis is caused by *Mycobacterium tuberculosis* and is easily transmitted from one individual to another through coughing and sneezing.
- Syphilis consists of three stages with three types of oral lesions: primary stage, with a chancre type oral lesion; secondary stage, with mucous patch-type oral lesions; and tertiary stage, with a gumma-type lesion.
- Hutchinson's triad involves three factors in the infection of syphilis: inflammation of the cornea, eighth nerve deafness, and dental abnormalities.
- Gonorrhea is caused by *Neisseria gonorrhoeae* (gonococcus).
- Actinomycosis results in external draining fistulas and is caused by *Actinomyces israelii,* a gram-positive bacterium.
- Necrotizing ulcerative gingivitis produces a fiery red gingiva with bleeding and has a characteristic fetid odor.
- Deep fungal infections are produced by organisms found in the natural environment that may enter the body through cuts and the mucous membranes.
- Ulcerlike lesions may have an etiology that is infectious, autoimmune or traumatic, or in some cases malignant, which can be devastating.
- Recurrent aphthous ulcers appear on nonkeratinized tissue.
- Recurrent aphthous ulcers may appear in three types: minor, major, and herpetiform.
- A thorough health history, oral inspection, and the questioning nature of the dental hygienist will ensure that serious disease states are not overlooked.
- Some of the diseases discussed in this chapter are infectious and may continue to progress if not treated.
- Aphthous-like ulcers occur in Behçet syndrome, Reiter syndrome, PFAPA, and Crohn's disease.
- Reiter syndrome is a triad of arthritis, urethritis, and conjunctivitis.
- Many lesions have subtle appearances in the early stages, and it is important to evaluate any oral lesion thoroughly and to fully scrutinize those that lack an established cause.
- Erythema multiforme has characteristic "target lesions" or "iris lesions" on the skin.
- Hypersensitivity reactions may be related to medications and products that the patient is using, either systemically or topically.
- The dental hygienist is in a unique position to detect early premalignant and malignant lesions that are in the head and neck area.
- Squamous cell carcinoma may have varied appearances and must be detected early.
- Patients who have oral cancers detected in an early stage will have less surgery, less adjunctive therapy, and a higher rate of recovery long term.
- Patients who wear eyeglasses often view the facial area with their glasses on, and sometimes the rims of the glasses mask lesions lying under the frames.
- Having patients remove eyewear, hats, and anything obstructing the head and neck area allows the clinician a clear view of crucial areas.

may present as nodules, indurated masses, patches, or fissured or ulcerlike lesions. Essentially, cancer may have many faces. Early SCC may resemble other benign mucosal lesions. Unrecognized and untreated lesions progress to form the classic indurated fixed ulcer with raised and rolled edges and possible color variation. This emphasizes the importance of the role of the dental hygienist in early detection of cancerous lesions. Adoption of a healthy attitude toward thorough clinical examination and a questioning speculation toward any unaccountable lesion occurring in the oral cavity is critical. If an unexplained lesion does not subside within 2 weeks or if there is obvious concern initially, further examination and possible biopsy is warranted. We suggest that patients be considered for one or several options: (1) biopsied, (2) evaluated further (see Clinical Protocol 12) and referred,

or (3) rescheduled for a return visit to evaluate a suspicious area (such as an area that may be frictional).

Treatment and Prognosis: Treatment is primarily based on the stage of the lesions at initial diagnosis. Treatment may consist of surgical excision, radiation therapy, and/or chemotherapy, alone or in combination. The prognosis will depend upon the stage of the cancer but also the location. For example, the prognosis for floor-of-the-mouth cancers is less promising than the prognosis for cancers in the lip area. Additionally, health-related consultation should be part of the dental examination, such as reduction of frictional activities that promote tissue change, diet habits that are detrimental, smoking cessation, alcohol reduction (including alcohol-containing mouth rinses), and adoption of good health habits.

Critical Thinking Activity

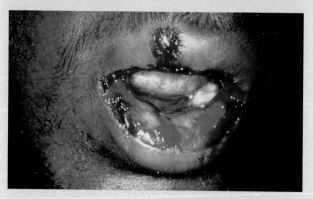

The figure depicts a heavy cocaine user. How is it possible that this person will be diagnosed as having erythema multiforme as well as having a factitial injury? Which diagnosis would you consider most appropriate?

(Courtesy of Dr. Terry Rees.)

INTERNET RESOURCES

National Library of Medicine Medline Plus
8600 Rockville Pike Bethesda, MD 20894
1-888-FIND-NLM (1-888-346-3656) or 301-594-5983
http://medlineplus.gov

Lupus Foundation
www.lupus.org

National Organization of Rare Diseases
http://www.rarediseases.org/

Centers for Disease Control and Prevention
Division of Sexually Transmitted Diseases Prevention
1-800-CDC-INFO (1-800-232-4636)
http://www.cdc.gov/std

American Social Health Association
P.O. Box 13827
Research Triangle Park, NC 27709-3827
919-361-8400
www.ashastd.org

PORTFOLIO ACTIVITIES

- Develop an information sheet for patients who suffer with chronic aphthous ulcers. Please use protocol A8 for Recurrent Aphthous Ulcers and individualize your information for various patients.
- Include "trigger" mechanisms and environmental factors associated with the condition. Clinical photos may be part of your educational information.
- Develop a procedure list for new patients and recall patients that would outline a thorough oral exam, a medical history update and help in screening visible external surfaces for skin cancer. Involve your entire office staff in this procedure.
- Develop a diet diary for the patient with aphthous ulcers using the clinical protocol A8 information.

Personalize the diet diary to your own clinic or office with name, contact information, etc.
- Determine the clinical protocol for your office on oral cancer. A set of guidelines that state your referral guidelines and procedures that will be developed and followed when evaluating any new lesion.
- Develop a patient education sheet for patients who are undergoing or have been through cancer surgery, radiation treatment and are having problems related to these factors. The clinical protocol on xerostomia would be most helpful to include as well as the protocol on radiation mucositis. You should include something on diet related suggestions as well.

Case Study

A 23-year-old male comes to your office for an appointment. His health is good, and he has no major complaints or problems. He has an appointment as a new patient, and his only oral complaint is about some swelling on the LL mandible region. He has noticed that he has some skin problems also on the same side. He complains about some exudates from the facial outbreaks. As you scan his face, the LL facial area does appear swollen, and the same area appears to have some surface lesions.

Critical thinking skills:

- What questions would you ask the patient?
- What possibilities of disease states would you consider for the facial lesions?

- Why would you not consider a dermatology condition such as acne?
- What features would you search for related to the skin lesions?

Additional Information:

- He had a third molar extraction a few months prior to the present appointment and has had no problems. Intraorally, the extraction site appears to be healing. There is some swelling in the 2nd and 3rd molar region, but he does not report any pain.
- What connections should be considered between his intraoral condition and the extraoral condition?
- What systemic problems or disease states would you consider that might be relevant in this case?

Additional information: You notice a small opening on the lower external jaw area.

What would you consider at this point?

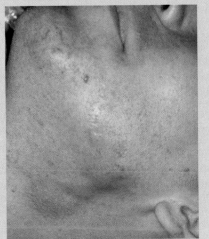
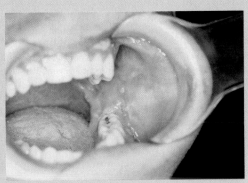

(Slides courtesy of Dr. John Jacoway)

REFERENCES

American Cancer Society, Inc. Oral Cancer publication 300208, 2006.

Avon SL. Oral mucosal lesions associated with use of quid. J Can Dent Assoc 2004;70(4):244–248.

Bulent A, et al. PFAPA syndrome mimicking familial Mediterranean fever: Report of a Turkish child. J Emer Med 2003;25(4):383–385.

Braakhuis BJ, Brakenhoff RH, Leemans CR. Second field tumors: a new opportunity for cancer prevention? Oncologist 2005;10:493–500.

Cawson RA, Odell EW. Essentials of oral pathology and oral medicine. 6th ed. London: Churchill Livingstone-Harcourt Brace and Company, 1998.

Cawson RA, Binnie WH, Eveson JW. Color atlas of oral disease—clinical and pathologic correlations. 2nd ed. London: Wolfe Publishing, 1994.

CDC, National Center for Infectious Diseases/Division of Bacterial and Mycotic Disease, Oct.12, 2005. *http://www.cdc.gov/ncidod/dbmd/diseaseinfo/histoplasmossi_t.htm*

Chambers MS, et al. Oral complications associated with aspergillosis in patients with a hematologic malignancy: presentation and treatment. Oral Surg Oral Med Oral Pathol 1995;79:599.

Chaudhary S, Kalra N, Gomber S. Tuberculous osteomyelitis of the mandible: a case report in a 4-year old child. Oral Surg Oral Med Oral Pathol Oral Radiol Endod 2004;97:603–606.

Danchenko N. Satia JA, Anthony SA. Epidemiology of systemic lupus erythematosus: a comparison of worldwide disease burden. Lupus 2006;15(5):308–318.

Eisen D, Lynch DP. The mouth-diagnosis and treatment. St. Louis: Mosby, 1998.

El-Hakim M, Chauvin P. Orofacial granulomatosis presenting as persistent lip swelling: review of 6 new cases. J Oral Maxillofac Surg 2004;62:114–117.

Eversole LR. Immunopathogenesis or oral lichen planus and recurrent aphthous stomatitis. Semin Cutan Med Surg 1997;14(4):284–294.

Health matters: syphilis fact sheet prepared by Office of Communications and Public Liaison National Institute of Allergy and Infectious Diseases National Institutes of Health. Bethesda, MD, December 2005.

Health matters: gonorrhea fact sheet prepared by Office of Communications and Public Liaison National Institute of Allergy and Infectious Diseases National Institutes of Health. Bethesda, MD, October 2004.

Herman WW, Konzelman JL, Thompson AL, Bonta CY. Update on recurrent aphthous stomatitis. Pract Hyg 2002;11(6):35–38.

Herrero R., et al. Human papillomavirus and oral cancer: The International Agency for Research on Cancer Multicenter Study. JNCI 2003;95(23):1772–1783.

Hochberg MC. Systemic lupus erythematosus. Rheum Dis Clin North Am 1990;16(3):617–639.

Jones AC, Bentsen TY, Freedman PD. Mucormycosis of the oral cavity. Oral Surg Oral Med Oral Pathol 1993;75:455.

La Vecchia C, Lucchini F, Negri E, Levi F. Trends in oral cancer mortality in Europe. Oral Oncol 2004;40:433–439.

Langlais R., Miller C. Color atlas of common oral diseases. Baltimore: Lippincott Williams & Wilkins, 2003.

Little J. Gonorrhea: update. Oral Surg Oral Med Oral Pathol Oral Radiol Endod 2006;101:139–145.

Lozada-Nur F, Gorsky M, Silverman S Jr. Oral erythema multiforme: clinical observations and treatment of 95 patients. Oral Surg Oral Med Oral Pathol 1989;67:36.

Llewellyn CD, Johnson NW, Warnakulasuriya S. Factors associated with delay in presentation among younger patients with oral cancer. Oral Surg Oral Med Oral Pathol 2004: 97:6, 707–713.

Marshall GS, Edwards KM, Lawton AR. PFAPA syndrome. Pediatr Infect Dis J 1989;8:658–659.

Massano J, Regateiro FS, Januario G, Ferreira A. Oral squamous cell carcinoma: review of prognostic and predictive factors. Oral Surg Oral Med Oral Pathol Oral Radiol Endod 2006;102:67–76.

Mignogna MD, Fedele S, Russo LL. The world cancer report and the burden of oral cancer. Eur J Cancer Prev 2004;13(2):139–142.

Millar JW, Johnston A, Lamb D. Allergic aspergillosis of the maxillary sinuses. Thorax 1981;36,710.

Molinari JA, Cottone JA, Chandrasekar PH. Tuberculosis in the 1990's: current implications for dentistry. Compend Contin Educ Dent 1993;14:276–292.

Murayama Y, Kurihara H, Nagai A, et al. Acute necrotizing ulcerative gingivitis: risk factors involving host defense mechanisms. Periodontology 2000 1994;6:116–124.

Nair U, Bartsch H, Nair J. Alert for an epidemic of oral cancer due to use of the betel quid substitutes gutkka and pan masala: a review of agents and causative mechanisms. Mutagenesis 2004;4:251–262.

Neville BW, Damm DD, Allen CM, Bouquot JE. Oral & Maxillofacial Pathology. Philadelphia: WB Saunders, 1995.

Ng KH, Siar CH. Review of oral histoplasmosis in Malaysians. Oral Surg Oral Med Oral Pathol 1996;81:303.

Ozcelik O, Haytac MC. Oral challenge test for the diagnosis of gingival hypersensitivity to apple: a case report. Oral Surg Oral Med Oral Pathol Oral Radiol Endod 2006;101:317–321.

Pinto A, Lindemeyer RG, Sollecito TP. The PFAPA syndrome in oral medicine: differential diagnosis and treatment. Oral Surg, Oral Med Oral Pathol Oral Radiol Endod 2006;102(1):35–39.

Plemons JM, Gonzales TS, Burkhart NW. Vesiculobullous diseases of the oral cavity. Periodontology 2000. 1999;21:158–175.

Popovsky JL, Camisa C. New and emerging therapies for diseases of the oral cavity. Dermatol Clin 2000;18(1):113–125.

Porth CM. Essentials of pathophysiology. Baltimore: Lippincott Williams & Wilkins, 2004.

Porter SR, Scully C. Pedersen A. Recurrent aphthous stomatitis. Crit Rev Oral Biol Med 1998;9:306–321.

Rees TD. Orofacial granulomatosis and related conditions. Periodontology 2000 1999;21:145–147.

Rees TD, Binnie WH. Recurrent aphthous stomatitis. Dermatol Clin 1996;14(2):243–256.

Regezi J, Sciubba J, Jordan R. Oral pathology—clinical pathologic correlations. 4th ed. St. Louis: WB Saunders, 2003.

Rivera-Hidalgo F, Stanford TW. Oral mucosal lesions caused by infective microorganisms 1. Viruses and bacteria. Periodontology 2000. 1999;21:106–124.

Rivera-Hidalgo, Shulman JD. The association of tobacco and other factors with recurrent aphthous stomatitis in an US adult population. Oral Dis 2004;10:335–345.

Rubin E, Gorstein F, Rubin R, et al. Rubin's pathology: clinicopathologic foundations of medicine. 4th ed. Baltimore: Lippincott Williams & Wilkins, 2005:1229–1231.

Samaranayake LP, Cheung LK, Samaranayake YH. Candidiasis and other fungal diseases of the mouth. Dermatol Ther 2002;15:251–269.

Schantz SP, Yu GP. Head and neck cancer incidence trends in young Americans, 1973-1997, with a special analysis for tongue cancer. Arch Otolaryngol Head Neck Surg. 2002;128(3):268–274.

Sciubba J. Oral cancer and its detection. JADA 2001; 132:12S–18S.

Scully C. Handbook of oral disease-diagnosis and management. London: Martin Duntz Ltd. Livery House Publishers, 1999.

Scully C, deAlmeida OP. Orofacial manifestations of the systemic mycoses. J Oral Med Oral Pathol Med 1992;21:289.

Shulman JD. An exploration of point, annual, and lifetime prevalence in characterizing recurrent aphthous stomatitis in USA children and youths. J Oral Pathol Med 2004;33:558–566.

Ship JA, Chavez EM, Doerr PA, et al. Recurrent aphthous stomatitis. Quintessence Intl 2000;31:95–112.

Silverman S. Demographics and occurrence of oral and pharyngeal cancers: the outcomes, the trends, the challenges. JADA 2001: 132.

Sook-Bin Woo, Sonis S. Recurrent aphthous ulcers: a review of diagnosis and treatment. JADA 1996;127:1202–1213.

Vicente M, et al. Immunoglobulin G subclass measurements in recurrent aphthous stomatitis. J Oral Pathol Med: 1996;25:538–540.

Watkins KV, Richmond AS, Langstein IM. Nonhealing extraction site due to Actinomyces naeslundii in patient with AIDS. Oral Surg Oral Med Oral Radiol Endod 1995;80:63–66.

Willard CC, Eusterman VD, Massengil PL. Allergic fungal sinusitis: report of 3 cases and review of the literature. Oral Surg Oral Med Oral Radiol Endo 2003;96(5):550–560.

Wilkins EM, Clinical practice of the dental hygienist. 9th ed. Baltimore: Lippincott Williams & Wilkins, 2005.

Yepes JF, Sullivan J, Pinto A. Tuberculosis: medical management update. Oral Surg Oral Med Oral Radiol Endo 2004;98:267–273.

Key Terms

- Angioedema
- Candidosis (candidiasis)
- Civatte bodies
- CREST syndrome
- Diascopy
- Dysphagia
- Ecchymoses
- Erythroplakia (erythroplasia)
- Fibrinous
- Giant cell epulis
- Hamartoma
- Hemangioma
- Hematoma
- Hereditary hemorrhagic telangiectasia
- Hypersensitivity
- Involution
- Kaposi's sarcoma
- Lichen planus
- Lingual varix
- Lichenoid reaction
- Lymphangioma
- Osler-Rendu-Weber disease
- Peripheral giant cell granuloma
- Perlèche
- Petechiae
- Phlebolith
- Plasma cell gingivitis
- Purpura
- Pyogenic granuloma
- Scleroderma
- Speckled leukoplakia (erythroplasia)
- Spongiosis
- Thrill
- Thrombosis
- Varices
- Varicosity
- Venous varix
- Violaceous

Chapter Objectives

1. Define the key terms used in this chapter.
2. List a variety of lesions that appear red to purple in color.
3. Describe the clinical features of each of the lesions discussed in the chapter.
4. Discuss the similarity and differences in the ecchymoses, petechiae, and purpura.
5. Describe the difference between a hypersensitivity reaction and an anaphylactic reaction.
6. Describe the clinical similarities and differences of the pyogenic granuloma and the peripheral giant cell granuloma.
7. Describe the etiology of the petechiae, ecchymoses, and purpura.
8. List and describe the two major acute forms of candidiasis that appear red in color and describe each.
9. Discuss and differentiate between a varicosity, a hematoma, and a lymphangioma. How would you determine the difference?
10. List the various forms of oral lichen planus (six forms). Describe each type.
11. Describe the difference between oral lichen planus and an oral lichenoid reaction.
12. List the treatment options for oral lichen planus.
13. Discuss the importance of lesions called erythroplakia and describe the characteristics of these types of lesions.
14. Describe the etiology and common locations of acquired vascular lesions.
15. List the significance of hereditary hemorrhagic telangiectasia with regard to the patient's general health and oral health.

Chapter Outline

TRAUMATIC OR INFLAMMATORY LESIONS

The oral cavity is an area of the body in which the tissues are subjected to constant forces, trauma, and tissue laceration. Most of the time, the trauma is mild. For example, occasional cheek bites, palatal injury caused by a sharp food product, or trauma from a new toothbrush are common occurrences. Most often, these injuries are small and heal within a day or so. However, chronic trauma and tissue irritation over an extended period produce a different type of tissue response. This includes an exuberance of tissue formed in response to the injury and often some damage caused to the surrounding tissue. This section discusses the types of injuries to the tissue that cause the tissue to produce more connective tissue, initiate an inflammatory response, and promote increased growth of the tissue.

NAME: Pyogenic granuloma

Etiology: Pyogenic granulomas are benign, inflammatory lesions that are exuberant tissue responses to trauma or local irritation. Other well-known names for these lesions include pregnancy granuloma, pregnancy tumor, or epulis gravidarum. The lesions often appear in pregnancy because of physiologic changes that take place during pregnancy due to the increase in hormones. The pyogenic granuloma is associated with trauma and reaction to a foreign substance in addition to hormonal changes.

Method of Transmission: Pyogenic granuloma is neither a contagious entity nor an infectious lesion. An irritant producing an inflammatory response usually initiates the inflammatory response.

Epidemiology: Puberty and pregnancy may make a person's tissue more susceptible to the development of a pyogenic granuloma. The oral pyogenic granuloma occurs more often in females than in males because of hormonal factors and usually in the second decade of life. Over 75% of oral granulomas appear on the gingiva.

Pathogenesis: A pyogenic granuloma results from chronic trauma or an irritation process. There are no specific pyogenic (pus-producing) organisms associated with the lesion, even though the term *pyogenic* would indicate a pus-producing lesion.

Extraoral Characteristics: Pyogenic granulomas may occur on other mucosal surfaces such as the eye, colon, or external body surfaces.

Perioral and Intraoral Characteristics: The lesion appears bright red in most instances, but the color can vary into shades of pink, depending upon the age of the lesion, with younger lesions appearing more red. At times, the inflammatory tissue will be ulcerated and then be replaced with a more fibrinous tissue, making it appear yellow. Initially, young pyogenic granulomas appear brighter red, with older lesions becoming various shades of pink with a somewhat more fibrotic appearance. The lesion can take various forms and appear more pedunculated (stalklike) or more sessile (flat-based) depending upon the location and cause. The surface of the lesion may be lobular, smooth, or even appear more papillary. Generally, the lesion occurs on the maxillary anterior gingiva, lower lip, tongue, and buccal mucosa. Lesions range in size from a few millimeters to several centimeters. Pyogenic granulomas are painless and without exudate. Figure 13.1 shows a pyogenic granuloma on the maxillary anterior arch. Figure 13.2 depicts a pyogenic granuloma on the lateral border of the tongue. Figure 13.3 shows the histology of a pyogenic granuloma. Note the multiple capillary channels within the specimen.

Distinguishing Characteristics: The combination of hyperplastic granulation tissue and the large number of capillaries cause the pyogenic granuloma to have its characteristic red color. The lesions occur in soft-tissue areas such as the gingiva.

Significant Microscopic Features: The pyogenic granuloma is not a true granulomatous inflammatory le-

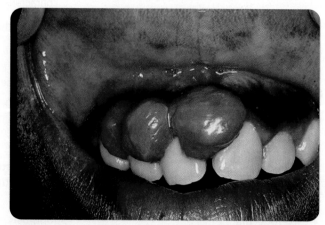

Figure 13.1. Pyogenic granuloma. (Courtesy of Dr. E.J. Burkes.)

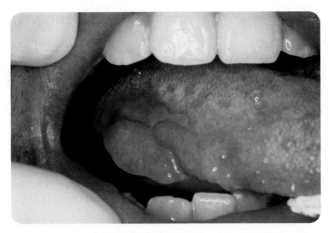

Figure 13.2. Pyogenic granuloma. (Courtesy of Dr. Terry Rees.)

sion, but rather an exuberant mass of hyperplastic granulation tissue. This condition involves a chronic inflammatory process and occasionally, there is some evidence of tissue repair. As the tissue repair occurs, the lesion becomes more **fibrinous** and may take on the characteristics of a fibrinous connective tissue appearance with a slightly yellow hue.

Dental Implications:
Pyogenic granulomas should be excised completely so that the lesion does not reoccur. Pyogenic granulomas that occur during pregnancy may exhibit shrinkage or completely diminish after the pregnancy.

Differential Diagnosis:
Other lesions that may be a part of a differential diagnosis:
1. The peripheral giant cell granuloma—Chapter 13
2. Fibroma—Chapter 17
3. Neoplasm—Any lesion should be considered a neoplasm until an etiology and diagnosis is determined

Treatment and Prognosis:
When the pyogenic granuloma occurs during pregnancy, the lesion often subsides after delivery when hormones are at a consistent and reduced level. If the lesion does not subside, it is surgically removed but may recur if all affected tissue has not been removed. Large defects may occur, depending upon the

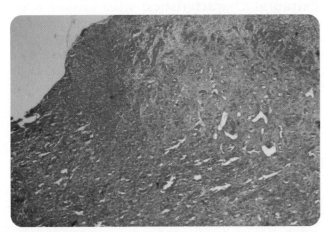

Figure 13.3. Pyogenic granuloma histology. (Courtesy of Dr. Denis Lynch.)

size of the lesion and the extent of tissue removal, and corrective surgery may be needed to restore the surrounding tissue to a normal appearance. The prognosis is excellent.

NAME: Peripheral giant cell granuloma.
The lesion also has been called a **giant cell epulis.**

Etiology:
Peripheral giant cell granulomas are reactive hyperplasic responses to tissue injury, producing an exuberance of tissue in the area of injury.

Method of Transmission:
The lesion is localized and not contagious.

Epidemiology:
The lesions may occur at any age, but most are reported to occur in the fifth to six decades of life. The lesion is less prominent in males, with about 60% occurring in females.

Pathogenesis:
Peripheral giant cell granuloma is a response to injury or trauma causing the connective tissue to respond with a more hyperplastic tissue. The lesions arise from the periodontal ligament or periosteum. Sometimes there is alveolar bone involvement with destruction if not treated. Precipitating factors include tooth extraction, plaque and calculus, faulty dental restorations, or dentures.

Extraoral Characteristics:
The peripheral giant cell granuloma is found on oral tissue and does not exhibit any extraoral characteristics unless the lesion becomes very large, with protruding tissue becoming visible in the anterior region.

Perioral and Intraoral Characteristics:
The lesion is found on the gingiva or edentulous ridge, and it is usually forward of the molar region. The lesions can be in the range of 1 cm and usually less than 2 cm. They are usually deep red or bluish purple and are reported to be more bluish than the pyogenic granuloma, which is often a deep red. They can be soft to somewhat firm and smooth in texture. Depending upon the degree of ulceration, they may bleed and are clinically very similar to the pyogenic granuloma, but can be distinguished by microscopic evaluation. Figure 13.4 depicts a peripheral giant cell granuloma between teeth 10 and 11.

Distinguishing Characteristics:
The lesion is distinguished by the multinucleated giant cells that make up the tissue when seen microscopically. Peripheral giant cell granuloma is microscopically similar to the central giant cell granuloma discussed in Chapter 18. The peripheral giant cell granuloma is found on the gingiva as opposed to the pyogenic granuloma, which can be found in any soft tissue location.

Significant Microscopic Features:
The peripheral giant cell granuloma is composed of fibroblasts, multinucleated giant cells with inflammatory cells within the lesion. The pyogenic granuloma and the peripheral giant cell gran-

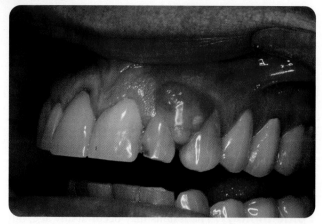

Figure 13.4. Peripheral giant cell granuloma. (Courtesy of Dr. Michael Brennan.)

uloma are distinguishable microscopically. The pyogenic granuloma is vascular, while the peripheral giant cell granuloma exhibits numerous multinucleated giant cells. Figure 13.5 depicts the histology of a peripheral giant cell granuloma. Note the abundant giant cells within the specimen.

Dental Implications: The peripheral giant cell granuloma can cause bone resorption. This is in contrast to the pyogenic granuloma. Depending upon the location, the peripheral giant cell granuloma may be observed radiographically when on the edentulous ridge.

Differential Diagnosis: Clinically, the appearance is very similar to that of the pyogenic granuloma. Considerations would be
1. Pyogenic granuloma—Chapter 13
2. Neoplasm—Chapter 17
3. Central giant cell granuloma—Chapter 18

Treatment and Prognosis: When the entire lesion has been completely removed, the prognosis is excellent. The periosteum and the periodontal ligament must be removed with the lesion to avoid recurrence. Along with the lesion removal, the local irritant must also be identified and removed.

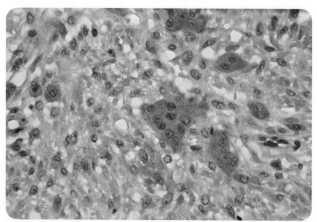

Figure 13.5. Histology of a peripheral giant cell granuloma. (Courtesy of Dr. Denis Lynch.)

NAME: Petechiae, ecchymoses, and purpura

Etiology: Petechiae, ecchymoses, and purpura are hemorrhages in the soft tissue due to either trauma or blood dyscrasias. When the cause is a blood dyscrasia, the problem is usually because of fewer platelets and/or clotting factor problems.

Transmission: The lesions that are identified as petechiae, ecchymoses, or purpura are not contagious and not transmitted to other individuals.

Epidemiology: Those of any age may be affected, and there is an equal predilection for males and females.

Pathogenesis: Both petechiae and ecchymoses arise from several sources. Traumatic injury is the major source, such as biting the oral tissues, trauma due to an object such as a finger (often used by patients who use disordered eating practices, see Clinical Protocol #9), fellatio, and factitial injuries (Chapter 12). Commonly this involves the cheek, tongue, palate, oropharyngeal areas, and lips. Additionally, the injury may be iatrogenic (Chapter 12), such as a dental procedure that causes ecchymoses from a hand piece or saliva ejector or just operator error such as anesthesia or impression tray misplacement. Dentures or poorly fitting appliances are another source of this type of injury. The second source of injury to consider is systemic disease such as blood dyscrasias. One such example would be the petechiae and ecchymoses associated with certain blood disorders such as monocytic leukemia and other forms of leukemia. Other blood dyscrasias also have oral manifestations producing petechiae, ecchymoses, and purpura (Chapter 9). The dental hygienist can be instrumental in referring the patient to a physician for treatment when a traumatic injury factor has been ruled out. Frequent nosebleeds, bruising, and evidence of frequent petechiae, ecchymoses, or purpura all warrant consideration of systemic disease. Figure 13.6 depicts petechiae at the midline, ecchymoses (area on the left side of the palate, left of the midline), and purpura (large area on the right side of the palate, right of the midline). Figure 13.7 shows petechiae on the palate due to trauma related to food.

Extraoral Characteristics: When pressure is applied, these lesions do not blanch. If blanching occurs, the practitioner would be curious about whether the lesion might be vascular. Since the hemorrhage is pooled blood in the area, the clinician should not be able to apply light pressure and stop the flow of blood to the area as would be possible with a venous-type lesion.

Perioral and Intraoral Characteristics: Bleeding that results from platelet deficiency occurs in small blood vessels and is characterized clinically by **petechiae**. Petechiae are defined as any tiny, perfectly round, purplish red spot that appears on the skin as a result of minute intradermal or submucosal hemorrhage. They are small, ranging from 1 to 2 mm and may be associated with certain disease states such as blood dyscrasia or trauma. The ecchymoses are much larger and broader. **Purpura** refers

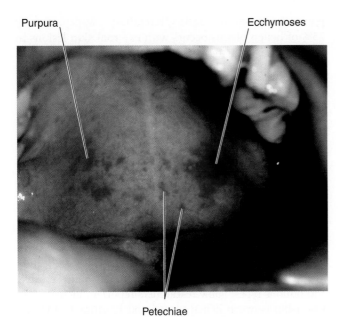

Figure 13.6. Petechiae, ecchymoses, and purpura. (Courtesy of Dr. Harvey Kessler.)

to focal, circumscribed hemorrhagic lesions that are larger than a petechia and less than 1 cm in the mucous membrane surfaces. Purpura may be associated with platelet abnormalities, bleeding disorders, trauma, or Rocky Mountain spotted fever. Purpura is a symptom rather than a disease entity. Depending upon the cause of the purpura, petechiae, or ecchymoses, the patient may also have associated nosebleeds, frequent bruises, and gingival bleeding. **Ecchymoses** may be described as hemorrhagic spots in the skin or mucous membrane caused by the extravasation of blood into the subcutaneous tissues. The skin areas are larger than purpura and measure over 1 cm. These lesions differ from the varicosities discussed below in this chapter, which involve a vein or vascular component. Ecchymoses, petechiae, and purpura are not in blood vessels but rather are located directly under the skin surface. Ecchymoses may be associated with bleeding disorders and hemophilia-related disorders. In hemorrhagic disease, the lesions can appear as blood blisters in the oral cavity.

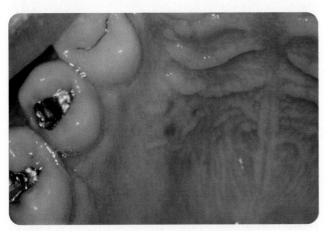

Figure 13.7. Petechiae. (Courtesy of Dr. Michael Brennan.)

Distinguishing Characteristics: Petechiae, ecchymoses, and purpura do not blanch and may be distinguished from the venous type lesions easily using **diascopy** (using a glass slide with applied pressure). Petechiae, ecchymoses, and purpura are pooled blood directly under the skin surface as opposed to varicosities discussed below in this chapter that involve venous blood flow, which may be stopped and observed under the slide.

Significant Microscopic Features: Not applicable

Dental Implications: Identification of blood disease and dyscrasias is important in seeking medical treatment for the patient. Additionally, those patients under care for blood diseases may need special care when dental treatment is necessary.

Differential Diagnosis: Some considerations may be

1. Blood platelet abnormalities—Chapter 9
2. Hemorrhagic diseases—Chapter 9
3. Trauma—Chapter 12
4. Bone marrow disorders such as myeloma—Chapter 5
5. Disordered Eating Practices—Clinical Protocol 9
6. Trauma induced by fellatio

Treatment and Prognosis: Treating the underlying cause or removing sources of trauma is needed to stop the development of petechiae, ecchymoses, and purpura. The prognosis depends upon the cause of the lesion, such as a traumatic lesion as opposed to one that is associated with disease states. These types of lesions associated with trauma usually subside within a week or more when the offending source is removed.

IMMUNE SYSTEM DISORDERS

The immune system (discussed in Chapter 4) is the body's major source of defense against disease. The immune system must recognize and differentiate the pathogens from the normal cells in our bodies. The conditions listed in this section are affected by the immune system, have oral manifestations, and appear in shades of red, blue, or purple.

NAME: Lichen planus

Etiology: Wilson (1869) originally documented cases of patients with oral lichen planus, depicting these individuals as highly-strung and overconscientious, with a tendency to worry excessively. Studies reported since Wilson's original documentation suggests anxiety and stress as factors contributing to the disease and subsequent recurrence of lichen planus. The disorder is a chronic, inflammatory mucocutaneous disease of unknown etiology. Lichen planus behaves more as a cell-mediated immune response, but in the past few years, lichen planus has been classified by some as an immune-related disease. Controversy exists among researchers, educators, and practitioners about the malignancy potential of lichen planus. Some researchers believe that any chronic lesions have the potential to trans-

APPLICATION

Areas of discoloration in the mouth and lip area are commonly observed in patients within a dental practice. The clinician must sort out the causes of these lesions and suggest a course of action. Sometimes the possibilities are numerous and using a systematic technique to question the patient is very helpful in determining the cause of the lesion.

1. If the patient is new, a complete health history is essential.
2. If the patient is a maintenance patient, an updated history is needed.
3. Be specific in identifying the lesion by showing the patient where the lesion is located.
4. Open a dialogue regarding the possibilities in etiology.
5. Determine whether the lesion is vascular or nonvascular.
6. Determine whether the patient has noticed the lesion:
   a. Ask when the person first noticed the area in question.
   b. Ask how long he or she believes the lesion has been present.
   c. Ask about relevant events that may have occurred at that time, such as a fall.

By involving the patient, the lesion can often be identified quickly, and the issue can be resolved with suggestions on how to avoid future injury. Injury that cannot be identified may require further tests. Intraoral photographs are priceless in documenting lesions and crucial for any follow-up evaluations.

form into malignancy given the time element and degree of the erosive nature (Eisen et al., 2005). Some researchers suggest that there is a high degree of misdiagnosis initially with regard to oral lichen planus (Lodi et al., 2005). The disease may be labeled lichen planus but may be premalignant or malignant from the beginning. This is usually due to relying on a clinical diagnosis rather than a tissue biopsy diagnosis. Additionally, the disease may begin as lichen planus and be followed with that diagnosis, but at some point, lesions become dysplastic or cancerous. The disease can appear similar to other mucosal diseases, and a careful diagnosis is crucial. A biopsy and immunofluorescence are needed for a definitive diagnosis.

Method of Transmission: Lichen planus is not a contagious disease. It cannot be transmitted to other individuals.

Epidemiology: Lichen planus affects approximately 0.5 to 2.5% of the population. Lichen planus usually occurs in midlife, at an average age of 57. However, reported cases have been documented in children and in the elderly. There is a female predilection, with reported figures ranging from 57 to 75%. A total of 48% of females are

postmenopausal or posthysterectomy. Approximately 25% of lichen planus occurs with external skin lesions in conjunction with the oral lesions. Figure 13.8 depicts a cutaneous lesion of lichen planus with purple papules and keratotic areas.

Pathogenesis: Lichen planus is often overlooked by practitioners and confused with other lesions, since its appearance can have many forms, and lichen planus is known to occur, then go into a remission state for periods of time, only to recur later. There are six forms of oral lichen planus; some of the lesions can be white, some red, and there is sometimes a mixture of colors. For this section since we are studying red lesions, we concentrate on forms that have a red appearance. The white lesions associated with lichen planus are discussed in Chapter 14. Andreasen (1968) divided lichen planus into six clinical forms. The classification includes reticular, papular, plaquelike, atrophic, erosive, and bullous types. Some researchers report an increased relationship between lichen planus and hepatitis C. Most of the increases in hepatitis have been reported in European countries (Carrozzo, 2002). Lichen planus occurs on the buccal mucosa, followed by the tongue, gingiva, lips, floor of the mouth, and palate. Lichen planus occurs on the buccal mucosa (about 90% of the cases), followed by the tongue (30%), gingival and alveolar ridge (13%). The lips, palate, and vermillion border are rarely seen (Scully et al., 2000).

Extraoral Characteristics: Cutaneous lesions of lichen planus present as keratotic, **violaceous**, pruritic plaques occurring most frequently on the flexor surfaces in from 30-50% of patients. Lesions of the genitalia are present in approximately 2% of patients with lichen planus, resulting in painful erosions of the vulva and vaginal areas of women. However, often no connection is made with the oral and genital symptoms by either dental or medical practitioners. The patient should let her gynecologist know that she has oral lichen planus so that she may be evaluated for genital lesions as well. Pineal and rectal lesions sometimes occur in patients with lichen planus, and the nail beds are sometimes involved, resulting in scarring of the fingernails and toenails.

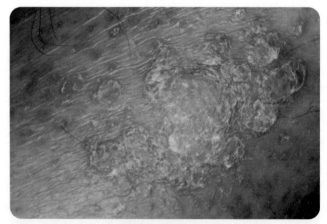

Figure 13.8. Cutaneous lichen planus on the arm of a patient. (Courtesy of Dr. Sumner Sapiro.)

Perioral and Intraoral Characteristics: Patients will exhibit either one or a combination of several forms of lichen planus, which are classified as reticular, plaque form, papular, erythematous or atrophic form, erosive-ulcerative form, and the bullous form.

- The reticular form of lichen planus is the classic form, and the lesions exhibit white striae called Wickham's striae. This form is discussed in Chapter 14.
- The papular form is discussed in Chapter 14.
- The plaque form resembles leukoplakia and is discussed in Chapter 14 as well.
- The atrophic form—The atrophic form appears as red patches with very fine white striae. This form often appears on the gingiva, with varying patterns of redness and striae.
- The bullous form of lichen planus ranges from a few millimeters to centimeters in diameter and is not usually seen clinically. However, this form may present with several of the specified types of oral lichen planus. Figure 13.9 depicts a bullous lichen planus lesion with erythematic tissue surrounding the bulla.
- Erosive forms can be very painful. The erosive form has been associated with increased malignancy, and chronic forms of this type should be carefully monitored with biopsies when changes occur. The lesions may be raw, red, and ulcerative, with pseudomembranous coverings. This form is often referred to as desquamative gingivitis, which is a general term for several mucosal disease states. Figure 13.10 shows erosive lichen planus with a pseudomembranous covering. Figure 13.11 also shows an erosive form of lichen planus.

Often a combination of forms is seen clinically. Another lesion associated with oral lichen planus and, unfortunately, very difficult to differentiate is what is termed a **lichenoid reaction.** If the lesion is a lichenoid reaction to a product, removal of the product usually causes the lesion to dissipate. Figure 13.12 depicts a reddened area opposite the molar area that is a lichenoid reaction to amalgam. Lichenoid reactions to dental materials occur in the

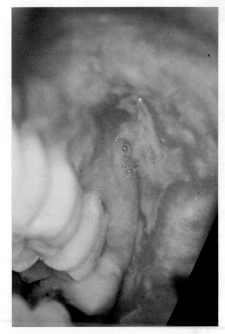

Figure 13.10. Erosive oral lichen planus. (Courtesy of Dr. Terry Rees.)

area of contact with the tissue. In this case, the reddened area is opposite an amalgam buccal restoration.

Esophageal lichen planus is reported with **dysphagia** (difficulty in swallowing) resulting from esophagitis and stricture formation. Esophageal lichen planus sometimes occurs after oral lichen planus has been diagnosed, and sometimes, patients complain about throat sensitivity without a definitive diagnosis being made.

Distinguishing Characteristics: One of the characteristics of lichen planus is Wickham's stria, which appears as a lacy, white pattern that resembles the lichen-type moss that is often seen on rocks (see Chapter 14). Additionally, lesions associated with lichen planus are usually purple, pruritic, polygonal papules when on the skin surface. Although the color varies, lichen planus is usually described with these terms (see Fig. 13.8).

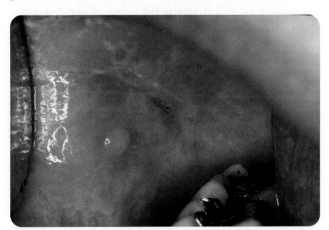

Figure 13.9. Bullous oral lichen planus. (Courtesy of Dr. Terry Rees.)

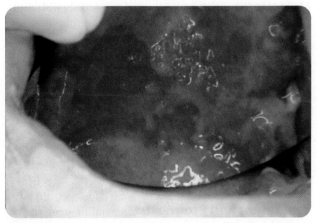

Figure 13.11. Erosive oral lichen planus. (Courtesy of Dr. Sumner Sapiro.)

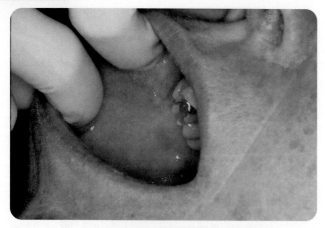

Figure 13.12. Lichenoid reaction.

Microscopic Features: The tissue exhibits liquefaction and degeneration of the basal cell layers and an increase in lymphocyte infiltrates. The basal cell layer typically has a bulbous or "saw-tooth" appearance. Degenerating epithelial cells, or **Civatte bodies,** are observed. Civatte bodies, observed microscopically, are eosinophilic ovoid bodies that are apoptotic (dying cells) or necrotic keratinocytes (epithelial cells that ultimately keratinize) at the basement membrane.

Dental Implications: Establishing a home regimen that works for the individual patient is important. Professional scaling and a prophy are essential in limiting the frequency of lesions. Homecare products that cause minimal abrasion and have low amounts of flavoring agents are best for lichen planus lesions, and a soft-bristle brush is recommended. The patient may react to a dental product such as amalgam or the materials of a gold crown. The reaction may be what is termed a "lichenoid reaction." The tissue in contact with the product will resemble lichen planus. Offending products include certain medications, and the patient may have a generalized erythematous appearance similar to lichen planus. Often, removal of the material or changing to another class of medication alleviates the problem. It is even difficult to differentiate the lichenoid reaction from true lichen planus histologically. Maintenance appointments at regular intervals with as little disruption to the tissues as possible are important for patients with mucosal disease. Air polishers are not recommended, and scaling with hand instruments is necessary in those with highly erosive lesions.

Differential Diagnosis: Differentiation from
- Lupus—Chapter 12
- Benign mucous membrane—Chapter 11
- Pemphigoid—Chapter 11
- Pemphigus vulgaris—Chapter 11
- Squamous cell carcinoma—Chapters 5 and 12
- Lichenoid reactions—Chapter 13

Treatment and Prognosis: Depending upon the patient, the disorder can be lifelong, but some patients can have one episode of oral lichen planus and not have any oral lesions again. Essentially, the disease is described as unpredictable. Because the condition has periods of remission and recurrence, many dental practitioners become frustrated with a lack of finality and progress. Since there is an increased risk of malignancy, the patient should be carefully monitored long term, and any changes in the tissue must be noted. Intraoral photographs are helpful in evaluating subtle tissue changes. There may be a need for increased biopsy, depending upon the changes. For mild, reticular forms, usually no treatment is needed. However, if the lesions become ulcerated or changes in form are noticed, a corticosteroid is usually prescribed.

The usual medications that are prescribed include fluocinonide, betamethasone dipropionate, and clobetasol propionate, and these medications have been found effective in the treatment of lichen planus. Sometimes with the erosive forms, intralesional corticosteroid injections may be beneficial. *Candida* is often a problem when corticosteroids are prescribed for extended periods, and the patient may need periodic treatment for *Candida* with antifungal medications. (See Clinical Protocol 6 for the recall guidelines for mucosal diseases.)

CRITICAL THINKING

What factors would you review with a patient if you suspected that person might have a lichenoid reaction? What factors might indicate that the person might have a reaction to a medication as opposed to a dental restoration reaction? What characteristics would you search for in your evaluation?

Points to Consider:

1. A person who is having a lichenoid reaction to a medication that is being taken systemically, such as one for hypertension, usually has lichen planus unilaterally.
2. A lichenoid reaction is usually in contact with the offending product, such as an amalgam restoration or crown. If the restoration is removed, the lesion will recede as well if this is the cause of the lesions. A lichenoid reaction is most often unilateral when caused by a specific dental material such as a cement, amalgam, or gold.
3. Remember, some patients have multiple disease states at any given time.

Be sure to consider all possible factors including diet and any other products that are used such as dental toothpaste and mouth rinses. Investigative questioning of the patient usually leads the clinician along the correct path.

NAME: Hypersensitivity reactions

Etiology: Hypersensitivity reactions appear to be delayed cell-mediated immune responses. Cell-mediated immune response is not the classic type 1 response that is associated with **angioedema** (edema of subcutaneous tissue such as wheals). Several varieties of contact allergies are known that affect the oral tissues and are considered orofacial disorders. **Plasma cell gingivitis** and allergic gingivostomatitis are terms that are associated with allergic responses to substances. Contact allergies and sensitivity to food products, flavoring agents, dental hygiene products, and even dental restorative products are all reported in the literature as causes. With more and more flavoring agents and combinations of products used by patients, increased numbers of cases are being reported and recognized as contact allergies. Additionally, orofacial granulomatosis that features noncaseating epithelioid granulomas in the lamina propria is reported in association with sodium benzoate and tartrazine additives in red wine, additives found in food products such as monosodium glutamate, and cinnamon aldehyde (Endo and Rees, 2006). The lips and face may be swollen. The gingiva is the prime area of involvement. Additionally, the buccal mucosa and tongue may appear enlarged, with folding leukoplakia (white-appearing tissue). A fiery red gingiva is characteristic of a hypersensitivity reaction and involves granular surface changes. Contact allergies are usually associated with dental products, such as toothpaste and mouth rinses, and specific foods, such as cinnamon, wheat, dairy products, chocolate, eggs, and peanuts. Many of the colas contain cinnamon aldehyde as do chewing gums,-especially the red ones. Some patients react to the ingredients found in toothpaste and the antitartar ingredients in tartar-control toothpaste with redness and sloughing. Ingredients, such as cinnamic aldehyde and cinnamon oil, and the preservatives such as benzoic acid, sodium benzoate, and methyl paraben, usually cause the sensitivity to toothpaste (see Clinical Protocol 6).

Method of Transmission:
The red lesions and erythematic tissue are localized and not contagious.

Epidemiology:
The responses to specific allergens can occur at any age and affect both sexes equally.

Pathogenesis:
A type lV hypersensitivity reaction is produced (see Chapter 4).

Extraoral Characteristics:
Hypersensitivity reactions may be external skin reactions as well as intraoral tissue reactions. Chapter 23 discusses some of the external skin reactions. With oral contact hypersensitivity reactions, the lips and the inner wet tissues may also be involved.

Perioral and Intraoral Characteristics:
The gingiva appears fiery red and somewhat bulbous. Figures 13.13A and B show the gingival tissue of a patient with cinnamon aldehyde allergies before and after discontinuing the cinnamon products, respectively.

The patient in Figure 13.13A was using multiple products with cinnamon, including soda, a toothpaste containing cinnamon, chewing gum, mints, and mouth rinses containing cinnamon. In this photo, a classic feature of

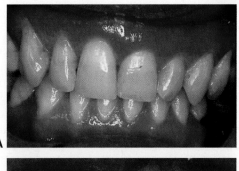

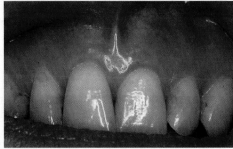

Figure 13.13. A. Cinnamon aldehyde allergy. **B.** Tissue after discontinuing cinnamon products. (Courtesy of Dr. Terry Rees.)

the contact allergy is clearing above the deeply red gingiva. This clearing indicates that the tissue is contacting the product up to this point, suggesting that a toothpaste or product consumed is responsible. Because the lip is folded over the vestibule, this clear area is protected from the offending product while other adjacent tissue is bathed in the product.

Distinguishing Characteristics:
Allergic-type tissue responses in the mouth related to dental products have a velvety, red appearance with distinctive clearing in areas where products do not contact the tissue. One such area is the oral vestibule, which is protected by the overlying tissue found in this area (Scully, 2006).

Significant Microscopic Features:
The key feature of the allergic response is plasma cells. The morphology is normal. The epithelium exhibits **spongiosis** (inflammatory intercellular edema of the epidermis) and inflammatory cells.

Dental Implications:
With any red, blue, or purple lesion, the underlying cause must be found. The dental implications consist of determining the offending source and discontinuing contact with the offending products.

Differential Diagnosis:
Consideration of the mucosal diseases such as
- Lichen planus—Chapter 13
- Lupus—Chapter 12
- Benign mucous membrane pemphigoid—Chapter 11
- Pemphigus vulgaris—Chapter 11
- Squamous cell carcinoma—Chapter 12
- Vitamin deficiency or anemia. When the tongue is involved in an allergic response, the fissuring and cobblestone effect may resemble that of a vitamin deficiency or anemia—Chapter 9

- Crohn's disease—Chapters 10 and 12
- Sarcoidosis
- Foreign body reaction—Chapter 3
- Deep mycotic infections—Chapter 12

Treatment and Prognosis: The correct diagnosis of the offending product or allergen is often through trial and error. The patient may discontinue use or contact with the agent, and the tissue is then evaluated again after a period of time. In the case of toothpaste and food allergy, a tissue response is usually evident within 2 weeks. Prognosis is excellent when the hypersensitivity agent is identified and its use is discontinued.

INFECTIONS

Infections that occur in the mouth have many different appearances such as redness, white colors, raised, eroded, and ulcerated. Infections may mimic other types of disease states as well, so providing a correct diagnosis is crucial. In previous chapters, fungal, bacterial, and viral lesions cause the tissue appearance to vary, depending upon the location and the type of agent present. This discussion involves those types of infections that may appear red or purple. *Candida* is discussed next because it is a fungal infection that exists and is commonly observed in patients. The appearance of oral candida is varied, with erosive lesions of both red and white patches occurring orally. Specifically, the red lesions are discussed in this chapter; the white lesions related to *Candida* are discussed in Chapter 14.

NAME: Candidosis (often referred to as Candidiasis)

Etiology: Candidiasis is a fungal infection caused by species of the genus *Candida*. *C. albicans* is the principal species associated with the oral infection. The fungus inhabits the gastrointestinal tract, the mouth, and the vagina. When the body systems are in harmony and the host is at an optimal level, the organism is not a problem. However, certain individuals may be more prone to the overgrowth of *Candida* than others, such as those in immunocompromised states of health and individuals taking certain medications that may alter the immune system, such as antibiotics for various conditions. Any time there is a disturbance in the normal bodily flora, an individual may be susceptible to developing a candidal infection. Endocrine disturbances and xerostomia predispose a person to the likelihood of developing *Candida* infection. The greater and more severe the candidiasis in this group of patients, the more difficult it is to manage the recurrence of the organism.

Transmission: *Candida* is not transmitted to another individual unless that person is susceptible as well. HIV and AIDS patients are especially vulnerable to the organism. Patients undergoing chemotherapy and radiation treatment are also more susceptible to *Candida* because of reduced immune system function.

Epidemiology: Pseudomembranous forms are found more in the elderly and young infants, while the erythematic forms are found more often in adults wearing dentures and appliances. There is an equal predilection of males and females.

Pathogenesis: *Candida* infections are usually superficial, but they can become deep fungal infections that affect the brain, heart, eyes, and kidneys when the individual is immunocompromised. Individuals who are taking antibiotics for extended periods of time destroy all of the "good" bacteria (organisms that compete with *Candida*), thereby allowing the unwanted *Candida* to become more numerous. Normally, *Candida* is kept in check within the body, but at times such as in the use of antibiotic therapy, the organisms may become more numerous. Individuals who are on antibiotics and those who may be in a debilitated state are more susceptible to oral *Candida*. *C. albicans* thrives in warm, moist areas, and certain conditions may make the host more prone to increased levels of the organisms. This is especially true for patients who are using corticosteroids for oral conditions such as lichen planus and other mucosal disorders in which inflammation is a key factor. Certain medical conditions predispose the patient to development of *Candida*, such as immunocompromised states, diabetes, hypoparathyroidism, and certain blood disorders. These conditions may make a person more vulnerable to *Candida*, and in some cases may have a genetic component to the development of *Candida* related to certain diseases. Generally, any health condition that causes a debilitated state would make persons more susceptible to *Candida*. (Refer to Box 13.1 for a listing of the more common predisposing factors associated with candidosis.)

Extraoral Characteristics: *Candida* is often found in elderly patients and is sometimes due to the loss of teeth and sagging tissue at the commissures. The loss of dimension at the commissures is a common problem in aging and they may sag and allow saliva to accumulate in the area. The damp tissue is a prime area for *Candida*. The general health of the elderly, decreased immune function, and poor dietary practices predispose patients to *Candida* infections. Other areas in the body are also prone to *Candida* such as the esophageal and vaginal tissues.

Perioral and Intraoral Characteristics: As mentioned above, *Candida* can have several different appearances. *Candida* may have a white appearance (pseudomembranous type) as well as a red color (erythematous type), depending upon the location and predisposing factors. *Candida* that appears white is discussed in more detail in Chapter 14 under white lesions. The white acute type of *Candida* infection (sometimes called thrush) may appear plaquelike or cottage cheese-like and usually is found in the pharynx, the tongue, and buccal mucosa as well as the mucosal folds. These lesions may be wiped off, and the surface that remains may appear red, raw, and ul-

Box 13.1	PREDISPOSING CONDITIONS ASSOCIATED WITH ORAL CANDIDIASIS

- Immunocompromised patients
  Elderly or very young age
  Cancer therapy
- Long-term corticosteroid therapy
  Cushing syndrome
  Treatment for mucosal diseases such as lichen planus, pemphigoid, pemphigus, lupus
- Endocrine candidiasis syndrome
  Diabetes
  Hypothyroidism
  Hypoparathyroidism
  Hypoadrenocorticism (Addison's disease)
  Hyperadrenalism
- Vitamin deficiencies
  Malnutrition
- Medications
  Antibiotics
  Corticosteroids
  Oral contraceptives
- Blood disorders
  Anemia
  Leukemia
- Genetic
  Congenital
- Appliances
  Dentures
  Decreased vertical dimension
  Poor hygiene practices
  Partials
  Retainers
- Oral environment
  Poor oral hygiene
  Xerostomia
  Stress
- Hormonal fluctuations
  Pregnancy
  Menopause

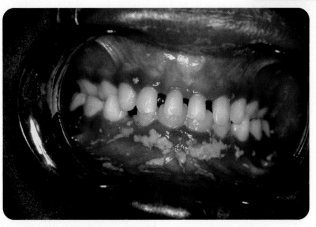

Figure 13.14. Erythematous *Candida*. (Courtesy of Dr. Michael Brennan.)

- Erythematous candidiasis—may arise due to chronic pseudomembranous candidiasis and is also strongly associated with HIV infection; this form appears as a red erythematous tissue
- Acute atrophic candidiasis—associated with broad-spectrum antibiotics; the patient may complain of a burning sensation and the tongue will have a red appearance
- Chronic atrophic (denture stomatitis)—diffuse erythematic lesions found under and around a denture, partial denture, or prostheses; Figure 13.15 shows *Candida*-infected, red tissue observed under a denture
- Angular cheilitis (also referred to as **perlèche**)—lesions are found at the commissures and appear red, dry, and rough; angular cheilitis lesions may occur in conjunction with oral *Candida*. Figure 13.16 shows angular cheilitis at the commissure, and the patient has an extremely dry mouth
- Median rhomboid glossitis—once thought to be a developmental defect of the tongue, but recent studies suggest a relationship between *C. albicans* and median rhomboid glossitis. Papillary atrophy is characteristic in the rhombus-shaped, well-demarcated, central denuded area of the tongue with a red appearance.

cerative. The raw appearance may occur, but in many cases the white area will be wiped off, with just visible denuded mucosa (this type is discussed in Chapter 14). The erythematous type has a bright red appearance. This chronic erythematous type is commonly found in denture wearers, with the usual sites being under the denture and on ridges. *Candida* may cause symptoms such as burning, and if xerostomia is involved, the patient may complain of dryness with changes in taste sensations. Figure 13.14 depicts erythematous tissue with pseudomembranous areas covering the gingiva.

- Pseudomembranous candidiasis—discussed in Chapter 14
- Chronic hyperplastic candidiasis—discussed in Chapter 14

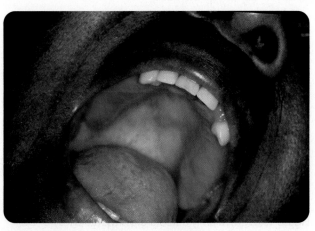

Figure 13.15. Partial denture stomatitis.

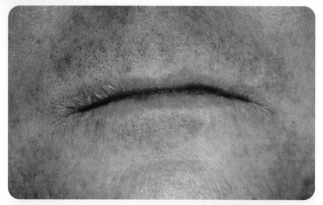

Figure 13.16. Perlèche. (Courtesy of Dr. Terry Rees.)

Median rhomboid glossitis is also described as hyperplastic candidiasis. Figure 13.17 depicts median rhomboid glossitis in the center part of the tongue forming rhomboid shaped lesions.

Distinguishing Characteristics: The white cheesy pseudomembranes associated with the pseudomembranous type can be wiped away to expose an erythematic, raw, denuded area.

Significant Microscopic Features: Many fungal hyphae are the prime diagnostic feature. Figure 13.18 depicts the histology of *Candida* with hyphae demonstrated.

Dental Implications: Common dental manifestations related to candidiasis include xerostomia (see Clinical Protocol 4) and poor oral hygiene. Optimal treatment emphasizes home care and compliance with procedures focused on treating existing *Candida* to ensure that the patient is not reinfected.

Differential Diagnosis: Diagnosis is usually based on microscopic examination of the tissues and membrane scrapings are placed in KOH solution (see Clinical Protocol 5). *Candida* hyphae are seen microscopically, and cultures may provide counts of the organisms. Since *Candida* can appear both white and red, the clinician must consider other possible lesions as well. Some considerations for red lesions include

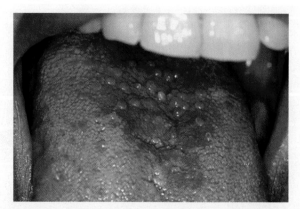

Figure 13.17. Median rhomboid glossitis. (Courtesy of Dr. Doron Aframian.)

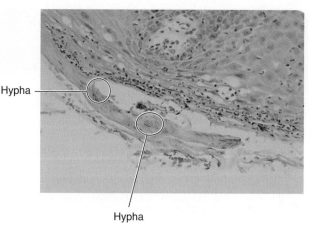

Figure 13.18. Histology of a lesion with *Candida* and hyphae

1. Lichen planus (Chapters 13 and 14)
2. Lupus (Chapter 12)
3. Pemphigus (Chapter 11)
4. Pemphigoid (Chapter 11)
5. Lichenoid reactions (Chapters 13 and 14)
6. Squamous cell carcinoma (Chapters 5 and 12)

Treatment and Prognosis: The treatment of choice is nystatin and clotrimazole oral or vaginal troches. Reinfection can occur if appliances, toothbrushes, and dentures are not treated along with the infected person. The organisms on the devices can cause *Candida* to infect the patient additional times. Cases have been reported in which partners are both prone to *Candida* and will continue to reinfect each other. See Clinical Protocol 5 for information on how to manage *Candida* infections. The prognosis depends on the health state of the patient.

Neoplasms

The terms neoplasm and tumor are used interchangeably and are classified as either malignant or benign. Benign neoplasms may vary in size and usually do not cause problems unless they begin to interfere with other tissues or organs. Malignant neoplasms do cause problems and also have the potential to spread to other parts of the body. They need to be surgically removed and may require adjunctive treatment with radiation or chemotherapy. Oncology is the study of tumors and their treatment.

Kaposi's Sarcoma

Kaposi's sarcoma is a malignant neoplasm occurring in the skin, oral tissues, and lymph nodes. The neoplasm is more common in patients who are in debilitated states such as those with AIDS and the elderly. Human herpesvirus 8 is associated with this sarcoma, and depending upon the stage, it may appear as a minor lesion. This tumor is discussed fully in Chapter 22. The lesions are mentioned here because of its blue to purple hue. (Figure

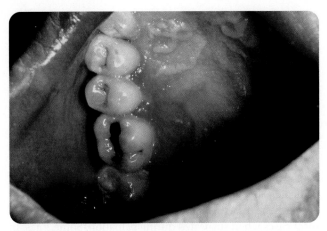

Figure 13.19. Kaposi's sarcoma. (Courtesy of Dr. Michael Brennan.)

13.19 shows the blue and bruised appearance of Kaposi's sarcoma opposite 3, 4, and 5 in the palatal region.)

NAME: Erythroplakia (Erythroplasia)

Etiology: The term **erythroplakia** refers to a red patch on oral mucous membranes. Erythroplakia encompasses several variations of both velvety red lesions and, sometimes, those containing a mixture of red and white lesions, which is referred to as **speckled leukoplakia** (discussed in more detail in Chapter 14). An increased incidence of erythroplakia is associated with tobacco and alcohol use. Dietary deficiencies and lifestyle factors may also be responsible in some cases. Additionally, chronic friction and exposure to irritants producing chronic inflammation are known to be sources.

Transmission: The lesion is not contagious.

Epidemiology: Erythroplakia lesions have a high rate of progressing to oral cancer, with most having dysplastic changes in the cells. At least 85% are usually severely dysplastic or frank malignancy (Scully, 2005). Incidence of malignant and premalignant lesions appears to increase after age 50, and as with all oral malignancy, there is a male gender predilection. The usual sites for erythroplakia are the floor of the mouth, the soft palate, and the buccal mucosa.

Pathogenesis: Erythroplakia is a generalized term that encompasses red, red and white, and variations of red and white lesions. The term *erythroplakia* is used to describe a lesion that is usually premalignant and occurs throughout the mouth. Leukoplakia (white lesions), which is more common that erythroplakia, is discussed in Chapter 14. When the epithelial cells no longer produce keratin (white lesions), they may undergo cellular changes and are more susceptible to malignancy, progressing to a more erythroplakic form. Although, white lesions can be malignant, the percentage of malignancy is greater with erythroplakia, or red lesions.

Extraoral Characteristics: Not applicable

Perioral and Intraoral Characteristics: Erythroplakia lesions may have a velvety red color or be dark pink. The surface areas are varied, sometimes appearing corrugated/pebbly and in some instances very smooth. The lesion may be broad and coalescing or it may be circumscribed and localized. Essentially, erythroplakia, along with squamous cell carcinoma, has many appearances. Figure 13.20 depicts the lateral border of the tongue with a velvety, reddened area that was found to be dysplasia. This lesion may be classified as erythroplakia. The lesions are often interspersed with lighter areas, representing keratosis. The lesions may be indurated (hardened) or they may be soft when palpated.

Distinguishing Characteristics: Deep, velvety red tissue is a distinguishing characteristic of this type of lesion.

Significant Microscopic Features: The lesions are considered premalignant and the earliest form of cancer. Approximately half of erythroplakias are cancerous. Most show severe dysplastic changes, and increased vascularity accounts for the red color of tissue.

Dental Implications: Erythroplakia-type lesions should be assessed for cancer cells via biopsy when warranted. The concern in most cases is when to biopsy the lesions. When a clear diagnosis is not present, the dilemma for the clinician is often confusing, and the question of the necessity for a biopsy arises. The clinician may have some concerns but not enough to biopsy. Any lesion should be guarded, watched carefully, or biopsied. In the initial evaluation, if an area of concern is detected, the clinician may want to use one of the abnormal cell detection devices. These devices detect questionable cells or abnormal tissue responses. One technique is the brush biopsy; another such device uses a rinse/light apparatus to detect cellular abnormality. See Clinical Protocol 12 for types of assessments and tests that may be used. When a cause cannot be determined and a lesion does not subside after

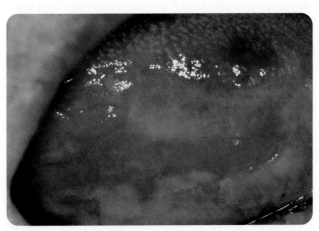

Figure 13.20. Erythroplakia. (Courtesy of Dr. Terry Rees.)

2 weeks, a biopsy should be performed. Additionally, if some abnormality is detected when using the brush biopsy or other abnormal cell detection devices, a biopsy should be performed.

Differential Diagnosis: Considerations are

- Squamous cell carcinoma—Chapter 12
- Kaposi's sarcoma—Chapter 22
- Systemic lupus erythematosus—Chapter 12
- Lichen planus—Chapter 13
- Pemphigoid—Chapter 11
- Pemphigus—Chapter 11
- Vascular-appearing lesions—Chapter 13
- Allergic reactions—Chapter 13
- Erythematous candidiasis—Chapter 13

Treatment and Prognosis: Treatment depends upon the histologic diagnosis. Any dysplastic areas are excised, depending upon the site, type, and results of the erythematous lesion biopsy. In some cases, radiation and chemotherapy are used. It is suggested that follow-up for any potentially malignant lesion be performed at 1 month, 3 months, and at 6- and 12-month intervals.

VASCULAR MALFORMATIONS

Vascular malformations comprise malformation of capillaries, veins, arteries, lymphatics, or combinations of these vascular structures. The malformations may be of two types:

1. Acquired
2. Congenital

There is often confusion in the differentiation of the congenital hemangioma and the congenital vascular malformations. Varicosities are discussed in the next section, and they are acquired lesions that are easily diagnosed and usually occur in specific locations. The congenital hemangioma is described in the section below and is a separate entity. Another lesion that may be confused with the hemangioma because of its similar vascular-like appearance is the lymphangioma that is discussed with the hemangioma. Congenital vascular malformations are described as a separate entity as well and are lesions that have some abnormality in the structure of the vessel.

NAME: Varicosities

Etiology: The varicosity, or varix, is an abnormally dilated and tortuous vein that is an acquired vascular malformation. They are found under the tongue (referred to as lingual varicosities), and sometimes are highly visible in older adults. The varicosity is thought to be a developmental abnormality and not associated with any systemic disease states. However, some association exists between varicosities found orally and those found in the legs of adults.

Method of Transmission: This is a localized lesion with no transmission factor.

Epidemiology: Varicosities are found in older adults, those over 60 years of age, and are rare in children. There is an equal predilection for males and females.

Pathogenesis: Varicosities indicate a weakness in the vessel wall. Since they are normally found in adults and not in children, they are associated with the aging process.

Perioral and Extraoral Characteristics: Some reports indicate a connection between enlarged veins in the legs and lingual varicosities. **Thrombosis blood clots** can occur in these lesions, and if this does occur, the lesion will be firmer on palpation. The formation of thrombosis is rare. Assessment of a thrombosis of the varicosity is needed in most cases when suspected during palpation. Sometimes, in older adults, the enlargement is found on the lower lip and is referred to as a **venous varix** (singular or solitary). The vessel wall becomes weak from chronic sun exposure. Figure 13.21 depicts a venous varix on the lower lip.

Intraoral Characteristics: The veins appear a dark blue to purple color and may be found on the lingual surface of the tongue, lips, or buccal mucosa. The practitioner may determine whether the lesion is vascular by compressing and releasing the area in question (diascopy) to determine blood flow and to differentiate between a vascular and nonvascular lesion. The varicosity that occurs under the tongue is termed **lingual varix**. Additionally, the term **varices** (plural) is given to varicosities that occur on the ventral surface of the tongue, termed *lingual varicosities*. Figure 13.22 is representative of lingual varicosities under the tongue.

Distinguishing Characteristics: The blood supply is disrupted by compression and resumes with release. A thrombus may be apparent in some cases and will seem firm when palpated.

Significant Microscopic Features: Not applicable

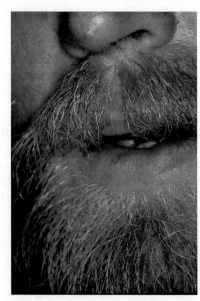

Figure 13.21. Varix.

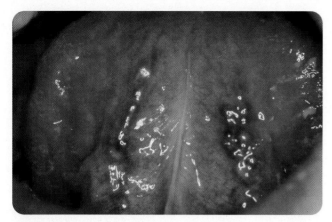

Figure 13.22. Lingual varicosity.

Dental Implications: There is no specific dental implication other than the appearance of the varicosity. Some patients object to the appearance of varicosities when they appear on the more visible areas such as the lip.

Differential Diagnosis: Other lesions, such as

1. Hematoma—(Chapter 13) The hematoma is not a vascular lesion. When pressure is applied, hematomas do not blanch, since they are an accumulation of blood in a specific area of the tissue, usually due to trauma. Figure 13.23 depicts a hematoma on the ventral surface of the tongue. The use of **diascopy** is helpful in determining whether the lesion will blanch upon pressure.
2. Hemangioma—(Chapter 13) Hemangioma is discussed further in the next session.
3. Lymphangioma—(Chapter 13) Discussed in the next section

Treatment and Prognosis: The varicosity requires no treatment unless it occurs in areas such as the lip or buccal mucosa and is of concern cosmetically to the pa-

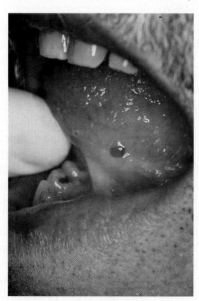

Figure 13.23. Hematoma.

tient. Formation of a thrombus would warrant surgical removal. The prognosis is excellent.

NAME: Congenital hemangioma (strawberry nevus)

Etiology: Hemangioma is one of the most common lesions in the mouth and is a benign proliferation of blood vessels, found in infancy and childhood. It consists of benign neoplasms composed of capillaries and venules. The hemangioma is a congenital entity usually present at birth or may be acquired through trauma in adulthood. The hemangioma is not a true neoplasm but may be a **hamartoma** or malformation. A hamartoma is a focal malformation consisting of an abnormal mixture of tissue elements or an abnormal amount or proportion of a single element normally present within a specific site.

Transmission: The lesion is localized and is not contagious.

Epidemiology: Although hemangiomas are found throughout the body, they tend to have a higher rate of occurrence in the head and neck region. They are found in approximately 2% of infants and are found more frequently in females. By age 2, 10% of the population exhibits a hemangioma with **involution** (return of an enlarged organ to normal size) occurring. The areas in which hemangiomas seem to occur more frequently are the tongue, lips, and buccal mucosa. Hemangiomas may be found in any soft tissue areas or bony intraoral locations.

Pathogenesis: Unlike neoplasms or tumors, the hemangioma does not exhibit unlimited growth. Many will dissipate, while others remain throughout life. When the lesions occur in adults, they are most likely the result of localized trauma and may be considered reactive lesions in these cases. The prime areas of trauma are the most susceptible sites such as the lip and tongue.

   Several classifications of hemangiomas are noted, but the two most widely encountered are

1. Capillary hemangiomas involving smaller capillaries, the most widely occurring type
2. Cavernous hemangiomas that contain larger blood vessels, termed the cavernous type.

Extraoral Characteristics: Depending upon the location and depth of the hemangioma, the color will vary from a dark pink in the deeper tissue areas to dark purple in superficial areas. The lesions may be single or multiple. Figure 13.24 shows a capillary hemangioma of the face.

Perioral and Intraoral Characteristics: The intraoral hemangioma usually appears as a deep blue to red enlargement, with a raised appearance. Figure 13.25 depicts a lingual vascular area on the posterior lateral border of the tongue that is a hemangioma.

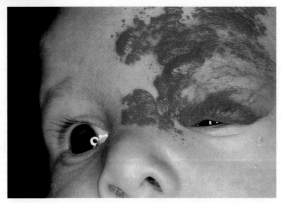

Figure 13.24. Hemangioma (Tasman W, Jaeger E. The Wills Eye Hospital Atlas of Clinical Ophthalomology, 2nd Edition. Philadelphia: Lippincott Williams & Wilkins,2001.)

Distinguishing Characteristics: Hemangiomas will blanch with pressure, allowing the practitioner to differentiate the vascular lesions from hematomas through diascopy.

Significant Microscopic Features: Hemangiomas appear as large blood-filled vascular channels in the underlying connective tissue. Cavernous hemangiomas exhibit large dilated blood vessels, while the capillary hemangioma demonstrates multiple capillary blood vessels. Figure 13.26 shows the histologic component of a cavernous hemangioma with multiple large dilated blood vessels filled with red blood cells.

Dental Implications: The hemangiomas are evaluated, clinically diagnosed, and watched closely. The only

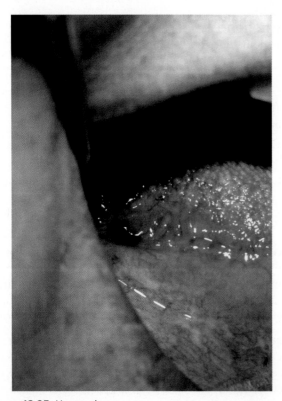

Figure 13.25. Hemangioma.

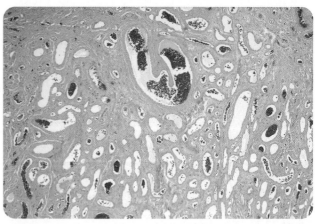

Figure 13.26. Histology of a cavernous hemangioma. (Courtesy of Dr. Harvey Kessler.)

foreseeable problem is the formation of a thrombus. When the thrombi exhibit calcification (the term **phlebolith** is given to a calcified thrombus) the lesion may need to be surgically removed.

Differential Diagnosis:

1. Malignant tumors such as Kaposi's sarcoma—Chapter 22
2. Varicosity—Chapter 13
3. Venous varix—Chapter 13
4. Hematoma—Chapter 13

Treatment and Prognosis: Some hemangiomas will involute; this is especially true for those found in children, and regression usually occurs within the first decade. Most require no treatment. Occasionally, lasers are recommended for troublesome areas as well as sclerosing solution. The prognosis is excellent. Monitoring of the area is needed, since some hemangiomas may enlarge, and development of thrombosis is possible.

LYMPHANGIOMA

Vascular malformations such as the **lymphangioma** occur during embryogenesis and are present at birth, consisting of lymphatic vessels. The lesions vary in size and location. Differentiation of vascular malformation and hemangiomas is often difficult clinically when they are subtle. Lymphangiomas are found on the tongue, buccal mucosa, and floor of the mouth, with the tongue being the most common site. Lymphangiomas present as multilocular lesions, often with some transparency observed. The lesions contain red blood cells within the channels and lymph tissue. It is thought that these lesions may actually be a combination of both hemangioma and lymphangioma. These lesions do not involute. Additionally, a **thrill** (pulsating of the lesion) may be observed in those that have arteriovenous malformations because of the high vascular flow of blood. Lymphangiomas are surgically removed, but with recurrences common. Figure 13.27 demonstrates a lymphangioma with multinodular surface and a variegated color pattern.

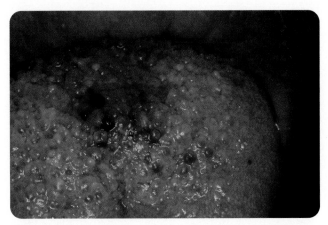

Figure 13.27. Lymphangioma. (Courtesy of Dr. Peter Jacobsen.)

NAME: Hereditary hemorrhagic telangiectasia (Osler-Rendu-Weber disease)

Etiology: Hereditary hemorrhagic telangiectasia is an autosomal dominant condition. In the usual sense, telangiectasias are dilated blood vessels that appear as what are commonly known as "spider veins." The blood vessels are small collections of dilated capillaries. These are more of a cosmetic problem for most people, but depending upon the severity of the condition, individuals may be affected to differing degrees.

Epidemiology: There is an equal predilection of males and females. The disease has, as a feature, abnormal dilations of vessels.

Transmission: This condition is not contagious.

Pathogenesis: The oral cavity and external surfaces are affected, and the bright red lesions may bleed profusely. Evidence is usually present at birth and tends to increase throughout life, with special prevalence in adolescence. Thus, diagnosis of the disease may occur at any time. Gastrointestinal bleeding may also be a problem. Another disease that exhibits telangiectasia is known as **scleroderma** (Chapter 23). The person with scleroderma exhibits certain characteristics that are part of the **CREST syndrome.** One of the similarities to hereditary hemorrhagic telangiectasia is the hemorrhagic lesions that occur in both diseases. The two need to be differentiated. CREST syndrome is a systemic sclerosis disease that not only exhibits telangiectasias, but also Raynaud's phenomenon, esophageal dysfunction, sclerodactyly (the skin becomes stiff and smooth), and formation of cutaneous nodules. Scleroderma and the CREST syndrome are discussed fully in Chapter 23.

Extraoral Characteristics: The skin lesions can appear on the palms, fingers, nail beds, face, and neck. Nasal areas are affected, and the patient may have severe nosebleeds. The skin lesions have a "spider vein" appearance, with fine red to pink lines (Chapter 23).

Perioral and Intraoral Characteristics: The lesions, usually bright red, occurring on the lips and ante-

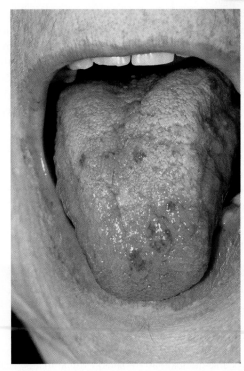

Figure 13.28. Telangiectasia. (Courtesy of Dr. Peter Jacobsen.)

rior tongue, can rupture, hemorrhage, and appear as an ulcer when traumatized. The papules are about 1 to 2 mm in size and will usually blanch. Figure 13.28 shows oral hereditary hemorrhagic telangiectasia on the dorsum of the tongue and lips. The lips, tongue, and gingival areas are most often affected. The lesions can appear obvious or more subtle in some instances, such as those found on the lips of the patient in Figure 13.29.

Distinguishing Characteristics: Patients who have hereditary hemorrhagic telangiectasia are suspected of the disease because of frequent epistaxis (nose bleeds). The spider veins are another distinguishing characteristic. Bright red hemorrhagic spots are seen in more extreme cases.

Microscopic Features: Microscopic features are dilated, thin-walled vascular spaces that contain erythrocytes.

Dental Implications: The lesions tend to bleed profusely when traumatized, causing a problem with dental

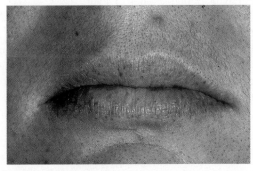

Figure 13.29. Telangiectasia (Langlais RP, Miller CS. Color Atlas of Common Oral Diseases. Philadelphia: Lee & Febiger, 1992, with permission.)

treatment for these patients. Depending upon the severity of the disease and the extent of the vascular malformations, a much more serious disease problem may exist, with malformations involving not only the capillaries, but also the venous, arterial, and lymphatic channels. There is a concern for brain abscesses and generalized infections. The patient may be premedicated for certain dental procedures depending upon the severity and extent of the procedure.

Differential Diagnosis:

1. Congenital hemangiomas—Chapter 13
2. Congenital vascular malformations—Chapter 13
3. Crest syndrome (scleroderma)

Prognosis and Treatment: The prognosis is guarded, depending upon the severity. The patient must be monitored throughout life in the severe forms. Anemia may result from blood loss, and there may be complications of the liver and spleen. Preventing hemorrhage is a key factor. This may be problematic in routine dental treatment such as scaling procedures, and precautions are needed, since any disruption of the tissues will cause bleeding. The extent of the bleeding depends upon the severity of the disease.

SUMMARY

- Pyogenic granulomas are benign, inflammatory lesions that are exuberant tissue responses to trauma or local irritation. Other well-known names for these lesions include pregnancy granuloma, pregnancy tumor, or epulis gravidarum.
- The peripheral giant cell granuloma is a reparative and reactive type of tissue response. The lesion also has been called a giant cell epulis. Peripheral giant cell granulomas are reactive hyperplasia responses to tissue injury, producing a tissue exuberance in the area of injury.
- Petechiae, ecchymoses, and purpura are hemorrhages in the soft tissue due to either trauma or blood dyscrasias.
- Lichen planus is classified as a cell-mediated immune response producing lesions in various forms that differ in appearance with both red and white lesions. Lichen planus may be a chronic disease with periods of remission.
- All of the disorders in Chapter 12 can have varying appearances; but for the most part, they all fall into the red, blue, or purple range of color.
- Depending upon the depth of a vascular lesion, the color variation is from pink to dark purple in hue.
- Hypersensitivity reactions may be caused by any source in the environment; examples are food products, dental products, environmental factors, insects, and medications.
- Hypersensitivity reactions appear to be delayed cell-mediated immune responses. The cell-mediated immune response is not the classic type I response that is associated with angioedema. Several varieties of contact allergies are known to occur that affect the oral tissues and are considered orofacial disorders.
- Candidiasis is a fungal infection caused by a species of the genus *Candida*. *Candida albicans* is the principal species associated with the oral infection.
- The terms *neoplasm* and *tumor* are used interchangeably and are classified as either malignant or benign.
- Erythroplakia refers to a red patch on oral mucous membranes. Erythroplakia encompasses several variations of both velvety red lesions and sometimes those containing a mixture of both red and white lesions, referred to as speckled leukoplakia.
- The varicosity or varix is an abnormally dilated and tortuous vein that is an acquired vascular malformation.
- The congenital hemangioma is a developmental anomaly of blood vessels found in infancy and childhood. It consists of benign neoplasms composed of capillaries and venules. The two types of hemangiomas are capillary and cavernous.
- Hereditary hemorrhagic telangiectasia is also known as Osler-Rendu-Weber disease and is an autosomal dominant condition. Multiple hemorrhagic lesions are usually observed.

PORTFOLIO ACTIVITIES

- Construct a list of medications that are known to cause a lichenoid reaction to use as a reference in your practice.
- Develop a "help" sheet with dental products that do not contain additives or promote allergic responses for patients. The material can be used for patient educational purposes when needed. Refer to Clinical Protocol 6.

- Construct a patient education sheet for your patients who have a problem with certain food products that contain preservatives and coloring additives. This will help the patient avoid future use of these products.

Case Study

A 34-year-old pregnant female is your next patient. This patient is almost 5 months pregnant, reports no complications during the pregnancy, takes no medications, and has scheduled an appointment for a routine cleaning of her remaining teeth on the advice of her obstetrician. She has no complaints but tells you that she does not floss. (See case study image 1).

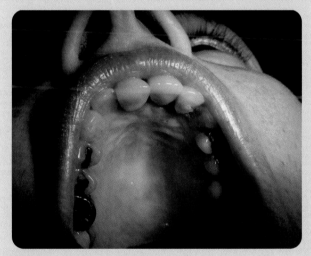

Figure 13.30. Courtesy of Dr. Doron Aframain

After examining her intraorally, your findings are the following:

1. The patient has fair oral hygiene, with minimum pocket depth in a 3–4 mm range.
2. The patient has 32 teeth.
3. She has multiple crowns and amalgam restorations.
4. The tissue appears normal except for the left hard palate near the rugae. You do notice some small areas of discoloration in multiple areas of the soft palate that are not very noticeable on first glance.

Given these findings, please answer the following questions:

A. The patient obviously has an area of concern in the left palate region. How would you describe the lesion?
B. How would you describe the color and texture of the lesion?

Is the lesion red? Would you classify the lesion as pedunculated or sessile? What do you think has caused this lesion? Is this serious, and would you be concerned? What questions would you ask the patient?

(continued)

CASE STUDY (continued)

Case study image 2: When you start asking the patient about the lesion on the palate, she states that she has another concern and shows you the stomach lesion (Figure 13.31).

When you ask how long the lesion has been there, she tells you that she always remembers having the lesion on her stomach. She comments that the dentist who placed her crowns commented on the palate lesion.

What do you observe in this slide? How would you describe the lesion on the stomach?

What questions do you have for this patient now?

What events could have caused the two lesions? Do you think that they are connected in source? Or, are they two separate issues?

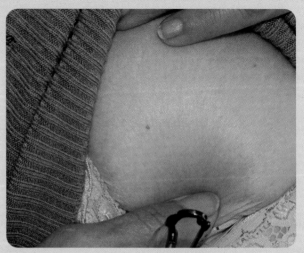

Figure 13.31. Courtesy of Dr. Doron Aframain

REFERENCES

Axell T, Samaranayake LP, Reichart PA, Olsen I. A proposal for reclassification of oral candidosis. Guest editorial. Oral Surg Oral Med Oral Pathol Oral Radiol Endod 1997;84:111–112.

Allen CM, Blozis GG. Oral mucosal reactions to cinnamon-flavored chewing gum. JADA 1988;116:664–667.

Abraham SC, Ravich WJ, Anhalt GJ, Yardley JH. Esophageal lichen planus. Am J Surg Pathol 2000;24(12):1678–1682.

Barbeau J, Seguin J, Goulet JP, et al. Reassessing the presence of Candida albicans in denture-related stomatitis. Oral Surg Oral Med Oral Pathol Oral Radiol Endod 2003;95:51–59.

Bosco AF, Bonfante S, Luize DS, et al. Periodontal plastic surgery associated with treatment for the removal of gingival overgrowth. J Periodontol 2006;77(5):922–928.

Budtz-Jorgensen E., Mojon P, Banon-Clement JM, Baehni P. Oral candidosis in long-term hospital care: comparison of endentulous and dentate subjects. Oral Dis 1996;2:285–290.

Burkhart NW, Burker EJ, Burkes EJ. Assessing the characteristics of patients with oral lichen planus. JADA 1996;127:648–662.

Burkhart NW, Burkes EJ, Burker EJ. Meeting the educational needs of patients with oral lichen planus. Gen Dent 1997;April:126–132.

Carrozzo M, Quadri R, Latorre P, et al. Molecular evidence that the hepatitis C virus replicates in the oral mucosa. J Hepatol 2002;37(3):364–369.

Cawson RA, Odell EW. Essentials of oral pathology and oral medicine. 6th ed. London: Churchill Livingstone–Harcourt Brace, 1998.

Cawson RA, Binnie WH, Eveson JW. Color atlas of oral disease—clinical and pathologic correlations. 2nd ed. London: Wolfe Publishing, 1994.

Chaparro-Avendano AV, Berini-Aytes L, Gay-Escoda C. Peripheral giant cell granuloma. A report of five cases and review of the literature. Med Oral Pathol Oral Cir Bucal 2005;10(1):53–57.

Eisen D. The clinical features, malignant potential and systemic associations of oral lichen planus: a study of 723 patients. J Am Acad Dermatol 2002:Feb:207–214.

Eisen D. Lynch DP. The mouth—diagnosis and treatment. St. Louis: Mosby, 1998.

Endo J, Rees TD. Clinical features of cinnamon-induced contact stomatitis. Compend Contin Educ Dent 2006; 27; 403–409; quiz 410, 412.

Fisher AA. Contact stomatitis. Dermatol Clin 1987;5:709–717.

Fowler CB. Benign and malignant neoplasms of the periodontium. Periodontology 2000.1999;21:33–83.

Gandolfo S, Richiardi L, Carrozzo M, et al. Risk of oral squamous cell carcinoma in 402 patients with oral lichen planus: a follow up study in an Italian population. Oral Oncol 2003;40(1):77–83.

Hood AF, Kwan TH, Mihm MC, Horn TD. Dermatopathology. 2nd ed. Boston: Little, Brown & Co., 1993.

Jafarzadeh H, Sanatkhani M, Montasham N. Oral pyogenic granuloma: a review. J Oral Sci 2006; 48:167–175.

Kaban LB, Mulliken JB. Vascular anomalies of the maxillofacial region. J Oral Maxillofac Surg 1986;44:203–213.

Kolokotronis A, Kioses V, Antoniades D, et al. Median rhomboid glossitis. An oral manifestation in patients infected with HIV. Oral Surg Oral Med Oral Pathol Oral Radiol Endod 1994;78:36–40.

Langlais R., Miller C. Color atlas of common oral diseases. Baltimore: Lippincott Williams & Wilkins, 2003.

Lodi G, Scully C, Carrozzo M, et al. Current controversies in oral lichen planus: report of an international consensus meeting. Part 1 Viral Infections and etiopathogenesis. Oral Surg Oral Med Oral Pathol Oral Radiol Endod 2005;100(2):164–178.

Nelville BW, Damm DD, Allen CM, Bouquot JE. Oral & maxillofacial pathology. Philadelphia: WB Saunders, 1995.

Plemons JM, Gonzales TS, Burkhart NW. Vesiculobullous diseases of the oral cavity. Periodontology 2000 1999;21:158–175.

Patton DW, Ferguson MM, Forsyth A, James J. Oro-facial granulomatosis: a possible allergic basis. Br J Oral Maxillofac Surg 1985;23:235–242.

Porth CM. Essentials of pathophysiology. Baltimore: Lippincott Williams & Wilkins, 2004.

Rees TD. Drugs and oral disorders. Periodontology 2000 1998;18:21–36.

Rees TD. Orofacial granulomatosis and related conditions. Periodontology 2000 1999;21:145–157.

Regezi J, Sciubba J, Jordan R. Oral pathology—clinical pathologic correlations. 4th ed. St. Louis: WB Saunders, 2003.

Sainio EL, Kanerva L. Contact allergens in toothpastes and a review of their hypersensitivity. Contact Derm 1995;33:100–105.

Samaranayake LP, Cheung LK, Samaranayake YH. Candidiasis and other fungal diseases of the mouth. Derm Ther 2002;15:251–269.

Sasmaz S, Karaoguz A, Uzel M, Coban YK. Pyogenic granuloma on the hand subsequent to friction blister in a hand surgeon. Dermatol Online J 2006;30:12(3):22.

Scully C. Reaction to cinnamon. Br Dent J 2006; 201:489.

Scully C, Felix DH. Oral medicine—update for the dental practitioner. Red and pigmented lesions. Br Dent J 2005;199:10.

Scully C, El-Kabir M, Samaranayake LP. Candida and oral candidosis: a review. Crit Rev Oral Biol Med 1994;5:125–157.

Scully, C. Handbook of oral disease—diagnosis and management. London: Martin Duntz Ltd. The Livery House Publishers, 1999.

Shulman JD, Beach MM, Rivera-Hidalgo FR. The prevalence of oral mucosal lesions in U.S. adults. Data from the Third National Health and Nutrition Examination Survey 1988–1994. JADA 2004;Sep:135.

Silverman RA. Hemangiomas and vascular malformations. Pediatr Clin North Am 1991;38:811–834.

Singh CN, Thakker M, Sires BS. Pyogenic granuloma associated with chronic actinomyces canaliculitis. Ophthal Plast Resonstr Surg 2006;22(3):224–225.

Sugerman PB, Savage NW. Oral lichen planus: causes, diagnosis and management. Aust Dent J 2002;47(4):290–297.

Wilkins EM, Clinical practice of the dental hygienist. 9th ed. Baltimore: Lippincott Williams & Wilkins, 2004.

White Lesions

Key Terms

- Ablated (ablation)
- Acanthosis
- Atopic/atopy
- Callus
- Coagulation necrosis
- Depapillated
- Dysplasia (epithelial)
- Erythroleukoplakia
- Leukoplakia
- Genokeratosis
- Hyphae
- Hyperkeratosis
- Koebner phenomenon
- Leukoplakia
- Nuclear hyperchromatism
- Pseudomembrane
- Premalignant lesion
- Proliferative verrucous leukoplakia
- Pruritic
- Retromolar trigone
- Reverse smoking
- Speckled leukoplakia
- Vacuolated
- Verrucous leukoplakia
- Vesiculobullous
- Wickham stria

Chapter Objectives

1. Define and use the key terms listed in this chapter.

2. Identify the etiology, method of transmission, and pathogenesis of the white lesions found in the oral cavity.

3. Describe the clinical features of the white lesions discussed in this chapter.

4. Discuss the cellular changes associated with chemical and physical reactions that result in white lesions.

5. List the clinical types of oral lichen planus.

6. Name the most common genokeratosis affecting oral mucosa.

7. Discuss the concept of oral premalignancy at both the cellular and clinical level.

8. Define epithelial dysplasia and note its characteristic cellular features.

9. List the two clinical features that increase the likelihood of a leukoplakia being dysplastic or an invasive carcinoma on biopsy.

10. List clinical changes in an otherwise homogeneous leukoplakia that would redefine it as nonhomogenous.

11. Provide a rationale for performing a biopsy on a leukoplakia.

12. Describe the dental implications of the white lesions discussed in this chapter.

CHAPTER OUTLINE

Diseases of the oral mucosa commonly manifest as white lesions, which is a change that is easily detected clinically. White lesions can be the result of **hyperkeratosis** (a thickening of the horny layer of the epidermis or mucosa by increased keratin production), necrosis of epithelial cells (usually caused by an injury), or ischemia (a defective blood supply to the tissues), which undermines the epithelium and results in whiteness. Any condition capable of stimulating keratin production can create a white lesion, since keratin (produced on the surface of the mucosa) turns white when hydrated by saliva.

Some white lesions are entirely innocuous and pose no health risk to patients, while others may be life threatening. The term **leukoplakia** (white patch) is often used to describe an undiagnosed white lesion. This term implies a premalignancy, meaning that untreated leukoplakia has the potential to progress to oral cancer. One should only use this term after formulating a differential diagnosis and ruling out other diseases that can manifest as white plaques. The conditions that mimic leukoplakia are discussed first, while leukoplakia is discussed fully later in the chapter.

VARIATIONS OF NORMAL

Some of the white lesions that are encountered within the oral cavity are variations of normal structures or tissues. These need to be recognized by the clinician to differentiate them from pathologic findings.

NAME: Fordyce granules

Etiology: Fordyce granules are normal sebaceous glands that are found in the oral mucosa. Sebaceous glands are also found in hair follicles of the skin, where they secrete an oily substance. Fordyce granules are a feature of normal development.

Method of Transmission: Not applicable

Epidemiology: Fordyce granules affect most of the adult population, as many as 80% in some studies. They are rarely found in children because sebaceous glands develop fully only under the influence of androgenic hormones produced at puberty. Males and females are affected equally (Regezi et al., 2003).

Pathogenesis: Not applicable

Extraoral characteristics: Not applicable

Perioral and Intraoral Characteristics: Fordyce granules appear as superficial yellowish to yellowish white, slightly elevated papules. (Fig. 14.1)

Fordyce granules are found most commonly on the buccal mucosa and are often bilaterally symmetrical. Patients may have a few to hundreds of Fordyce granules. Patients with these normal structures are asymptomatic.

Distinguishing Characteristics: Fordyce granules are very distinctive in their clinical presentation. Once the clinician has observed them in several patients, he or she is not likely to mistake them for anything else.

Significant Microscopic Features: Fordyce granules are normal sebaceous glands composed of lobules of rounded cells with abundant cleared, but coarsely granular, cytoplasm (Fig. 14.2).

Dental Implications: None

Differential Diagnosis: None

Treatment and Prognosis: Fordyce granules are normal anatomic findings that require no treatment.

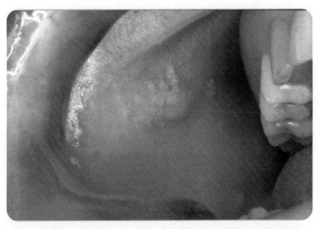

Figure 14.1. Fordyce granules. This characteristic presentation of Fordyce granules shows yellowish papules on the buccal mucosa.

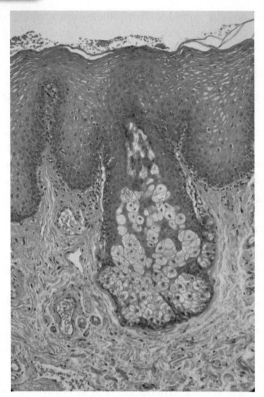

Figure 14.2. Fordyce granules. Histology image showing a normal sebaceous gland.

NAME: Leukoedema

Etiology: Leukoedema is sufficiently common that most authorities consider it a variation of normal rather than a pathologic condition.

Method of Transmission: Not applicable

Epidemiology: Leukoedema shows a remarkable racial predilection for African Americans and other darker-skinned individuals, but it also occurs in whites (Regezi et al., 2003). It affects males and females equally.

Pathogenesis: Leukoedema is a common mucosal anomaly characterized by intracellular edema and tissue whiteness.

Extraoral Characteristics: Not applicable

Perioral and Intraoral Characteristics: Leukoedema produces a whitish opaqueness, sometimes with fine wrinkles, of the mucosa (Fig. 14.3). Leukoedema is invariably found on the buccal mucosa and is often bilaterally symmetrical, a feature suggesting a developmental origin. It does not rub off and characteristically disappears when the mucosa is stretched. Normally, the condition can be diagnosed by its characteristic clinical features.

Distinguishing Characteristics: Leukoedema manifests as thin whitish plaques on the buccal mucosa that will dissipate when the tissue is stretched.

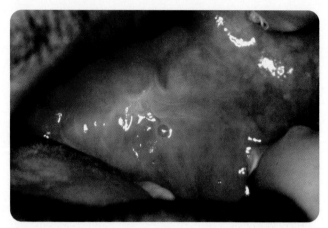

Figure 14.3. Leukoedema. Opaque whiteness of the buccal mucosa that disappears when the tissue is stretched is characteristic of leukoedema.

Significant Microscopic Features: The epithelium is thickened, and cells are **vacuolated** (having clear spaces within the cell) because of intracellular edema.

Dental Implications: None

Differential Diagnosis: The clinical features and racial predilection are distinctive. and there is usually no need for a differential diagnosis.

Treatment and Prognosis: No treatment is indicated.

TRAUMATIC AND INFLAMMATORY LESIONS

Oral white lesions are commonly associated with a traumatic or inflammatory process. Some have an unknown etiology, such as benign migratory glossitis, while others have a known cause, such as mechanical or chemical injury.

Name: Geographic tongue (GT) (benign migratory glossitis, erythema migrans)

Etiology: Unknown

Method of Transmission: Not applicable

Epidemiology: Geographic tongue is a relatively common mucosal disorder affecting as many as 2–3% of the population according to some studies. Rarely seen in children, geographic tongue is typically diagnosed in early to midadulthood. Females are affected about twice as often as males (Kelsch, July 2005). Many patients are **atopic** (highly allergic), but to date, there is no evidence that geographic tongue represents a hypersensitivity reaction.

Pathogenesis: Geographic tongue is an inflammatory condition, which is why it is included in this section; however, the cause of the inflammation is unknown.

Extraoral Characteristics: Not applicable

Perioral and Intraoral Characteristics: The clinical lesions of GT are characteristic and appear as **depapillated** areas (areas of atrophy with loss of filiform papillae). They are usually located on the dorsal surface of the tongue and are either erythematous or pink, surrounded by yellowish white lines that form the margins of the lesions (Fig. 14.4). Typically, lesions will heal, only to reappear at other tongue sites, which gives the illusion that the lesions are "migrating." Occasionally, the lesions remain stable. In addition, lesions may affect the ventral surface of the tongue. In rare instances, mucosal sites other than the tongue are affected (erythema migrans). Patients can be asymptomatic or complain of burning or sensitivity. GT is more common in patients who have psoriasis, but it is probably not an element of that condition. It may also be a component of a rare condition called Reiter syndrome, which consists of GT, urethritis, arthritis, and conjunctivitis.

Distinguishing Characteristics: Atrophic and often reddened patches with characteristic yellow-white borders on the dorsal and lateral tongue surfaces are characteristic of this condition.

Significant Microscopic Features: The clinical features of GT are usually sufficiently characteristic that a biopsy is not needed to establish the diagnosis. However, a biopsy does show inflammation of the connective tissue with neutrophils migrating through the epithelium forming small microabscesses.

Dental Implications: GT can be confused with other pathologic conditions. Patients may be alarmed by the appearance of GT when they first notice the condition.

Differential Diagnosis: Considerations include

1. Candidiasis, Chapters 13 and 14
2. Lichen planus, Chapters 13 and 14
3. Reiter syndrome, Chapter 12
4. Anemia, Chapter 9

Treatment and Prognosis: GT is not a premalignant condition. Asymptomatic patients do not require treatment; symptomatic patients are generally treated with topical corticosteroids to alleviate symptoms.

NAME: Frictional keratosis

Etiology: Physical irritation of the oral mucosa may produce whitish plaques known as frictional keratosis. Historically, white plaques that resulted from physical injury were considered leukoplakia and thought to be premalignant lesions (see the discussion on leukoplakia below in this chapter). However, there has never been convincing evidence that physical injury predisposes to oral malignancy, and accordingly, it is no longer appropriate to designate these lesions as leukoplakia. A white plaque that appears to be the result of physical irritation should currently be called frictional keratosis.

Method of Transmission: Not applicable

Epidemiology: Frictional keratosis is very common; however, there are no data on its prevalence.

Pathogenesis: The oral mucosa has a limited ability to respond to pathologic stimuli. One of its basic adaptive responses is to produce keratin as a protective mechanism against physical injury. This is analogous to a **callus** (over-production of keratin in the skin as a result of friction) of the skin.

Extraoral Characteristics: Not applicable

Perioral and Intraoral Characteristics: Frictional keratosis presents as a variably sized, whitish plaque that does not rub off (Fig. 14.5). Keratinization is a feature of chronicity, and an irritant can often be discerned on close clinical inspection.

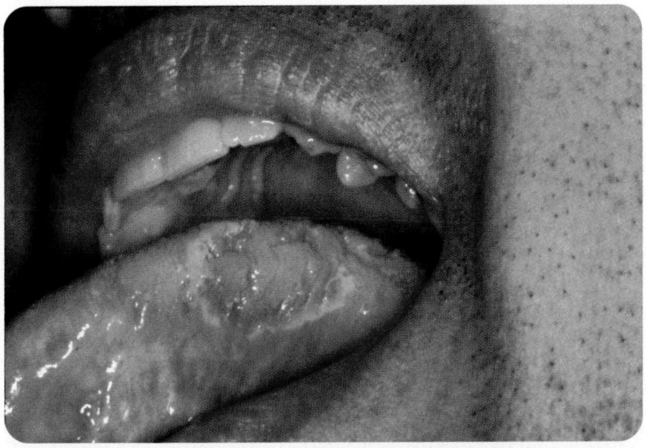

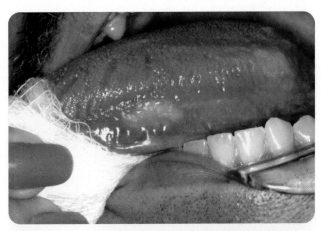

Figure 14.4. Geographic tongue (benign migratory glossitis). White borders surround a central depapillated area in this classic presentation of geographic tongue.

Figure 14.5. Frictional keratosis. This keratotic lesion is secondary to a fractured lingual cusp of a mandibular molar.

Distinguishing Characteristics: Frictional keratosis is a white plaque that does not rub off and usually has a cause-and-effect relationship with an irritant.

Significant Microscopic Features: None

Dental Implications: The cause of these lesions should be identified and eliminated. Factitious (self-inflicted) injuries are sometimes associated with psychiatric disorders. Lesions that do not resolve may be confused with other pathologic conditions, especially leukoplakia.

Differential Diagnosis: Considerations include

1. Leukoplakia, Chapter 14
2. Lichen planus, Chapters 13 and 14
3. Hyperplastic candidiasis, Chapter 14

Treatment and Prognosis: Because frictional keratosis is an adaptive response, the hyperkeratosis will resolve once the irritant is identified and removed. Clinical resolution confirms the presumptive clinical diagnosis.

NAME: Linea alba

Etiology: Linea alba is a localized form of frictional keratosis due to irritation of the cheek during function. This may indicate bruxism or clenching.

Method of Transmission: Not applicable

Epidemiology: Not applicable

Pathogenesis: Similar to frictional keratosis; linea alba is a reaction to irritation.

Extraoral Characteristics: Not applicable

Perioral and Intraoral Characteristics: Linea alba is a linear white line along the occlusal plane of the buccal mucosa (Fig. 14.6). Lesions are often bilateral, variably raised, and occasionally scalloped, corresponding to the embrasures between the teeth. Rarely, similar linear keratoses are seen on the lateral surfaces of the tongue.

Distinguishing Characteristics: The appearance of a linear white ridge on the buccal mucosa is characteristic of this condition.

Significant Microscopic Features: None

Dental Implications: None.

Differential Diagnosis: None

Treatment and Prognosis: No treatment is indicated. Linea alba is not considered premalignant.

NAME: Cheek chewing (morsicatio buccarum, morsicatio labiorum)

Etiology: Physical irritation (frictional keratosis) causes the lesions associated with cheek or lip chewing.

Method of Transmission: Not applicable

Epidemiology: Not applicable

Pathogenesis: Lesions are associated with overproduction of keratin and damage to the epithelium as a reaction to physical injury.

Extraoral Characteristics: Not applicable

Perioral and Intraoral Characteristics: Chronic cheek chewing induces hyperkeratosis and continued chewing abrades the tissue, leaving a whitish, irregular surface (Fig. 14.7). Lesions are often bilateral, and acute injury can produce areas of redness. Importantly, lesions are confined to the occlusal plane and are not located in the mucobuccal folds where it would be impossible to incur damage due to chewing. Similar lesions can be seen on the labial mucosa or lateral borders of the tongue.

Distinguishing Characteristics: The location of the lesion and the characteristic irregular, white plaques distinguish this condition from other similar lesions.

Significant Microscopic Features: None

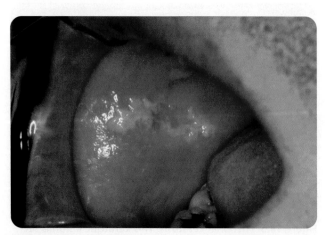

Figure 14.6. Linea alba. Note the linear elevated keratinized ridge of buccal mucosa.

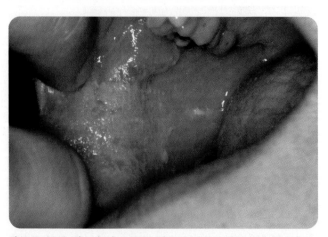

Figure 14.7. Cheek chewing. The macerated, white roughened surface of the buccal mucosa seen in this picture is the result of chronic cheek chewing.

APPLICATION

Many patients are not aware that they chew their cheeks or may not know of the severity. Very often, the patient will present with heavier areas of trauma during times of stress. Very limited research has been conducted with regard to the effects of chronic morsicatio buccarum. However, it is known that pathogens enter the body through any break in the tissue including the mucosa. It is easy to suggest that patients be advised to stop a cheek biting habit, but how does one go about doing it? In many instances, simply showing the patient the areas with a hand mirror or using intraoral photography will provide the awareness needed to assist the patient in decreasing or stopping the chewing.

The following approaches may be helpful in assisting the patient to stop the chewing:

1. Show the patient the area under the dental light. The light provides a clear view of the inside of the mouth for the patient.
2. Depending upon the appearance of the tissue, schedule an oral cancer screening (see Clinical Protocol 12).
3. Discuss whether the patient is under extreme stress at present. Suggest stress reduction techniques or help the patient find someone who may provide the needed guidance.
4. Take intraoral photographs of the area for comparison on future follow-up visits.
5. Determine the use of alcohol and tobacco, which may further place the patient at risk for oral cancer. This is of special concern because of the abraded areas.
6. Develop your own techniques for helping patients break these habits. Once patients are aware that they are chewing on the tissue, they become conscious of their own activity. A rubber band around the wrist or something worn that will remind them throughout the day is usually helpful. Stickers placed on key items that are seen throughout the day work well also. Small circles with "No" and the line through the word work well for some patients.
7. Monitor the abraded areas and be sure to evaluate the areas at a later date.

Dental Implications: Disruptive oral habits, such as cheek biting, should be discouraged.

Differential Diagnosis: These lesions are clinically distinct; however, one might consider white sponge nevus (discussed below in this chapter) in a differential diagnosis.

Treatment and Prognosis: The diagnosis can be made from the clinical features and confirmed by a patient history of cheek chewing. The clinical tissue changes are not considered premalignant; therefore, no treatment is indicated. The patient should be educated about the lesion and encouraged to cease the habit.

NAME: Nicotine stomatitis

Etiology: Heavy smokers often develop keratotic changes of their palatal mucosa. This occurs most frequently in pipe smokers. Heat may play a greater role than irritation from the combustion products of burnt tobacco, as is the case with **reverse smoking** (placing the lit end of the cigarette in the mouth and inhaling).

Method of Transmission: Not applicable

Epidemiology: Not applicable

Pathogenesis: The keratotic changes are a reaction of the palatal mucosa to irritation and heat from smoked tobacco.

Extraoral Characteristics: Not applicable

Perioral and Intraoral Characteristics: The irritation from smoking produces keratosis of the palatal mucosa and irritation of the minor salivary gland ducts as they exit onto the palate. This in turn produces inflammation and results in small elevations with central erythema (Fig. 14.8). Teeth are often significantly stained.

Distinguishing Characteristics: The whitish palate with small red dots (as shown in Fig. 14.8) combined with a history of smoking is characteristic of this condition.

Significant Microscopic Findings: None

Dental Implications: Although the lesion itself is not considered premalignant (except in the case of a lesion associated with reverse smoking), its presence can alert the clinician to the increased risk of development of oral carcinoma in the patient. The clinician can use the presence of the lesion as an educational opportunity to show the patient visible consequences of his or her tobacco habit. The patient should be offered tobacco cessation assistance.

Differential Diagnosis: This clinically distinct lesion does not require consideration of a differential diagnosis.

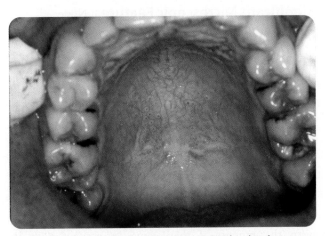

Figure 14.8. Nicotine stomatitis. Keratinized palatal mucosa with punctuate inflamed erythematic salivary gland ducts is characteristic of nicotine stomatitis.

Treatment and Prognosis: Nicotine stomatitis is diagnosed by its clinical features with confirmation of the patient's smoking habit. Palatal changes will resolve with smoking cessation. The lesion is not considered premalignant, except in the case of reverse smoking. Patients should be encouraged to stop smoking because the habit increases their overall risk of oral and other cancers.

NAME: Hairy tongue

Etiology: The etiology is unknown but there are several risk factors associated with its development, including

- Antibiotics
- Therapeutic radiation therapy
- Smoking
- Oxygenating mouth rinses/peroxide
- Overgrowth of oral flora

Method of Transmission: Not applicable

Epidemiology: Not applicable

Pathogenesis: Hairy tongue represents elongation of the filiform papillae of the dorsal tongue to the extent that the elongated projections look like hair. The reason for the elongation is unknown.

Extraoral Characteristics: Not applicable

Perioral and Intraoral Characteristics: The hair-like projections can be whitish or more commonly brown or black, representing pigments produced by oral flora or exogenous staining due to tobacco smoking (Fig. 14.9). Patients are asymptomatic but often complain of the unsightly appearance. The elongated papillae provide an environment that encourages continued growth of the oral flora which may result in halitosis. Infection with *Candida albicans* is also an occasional occurrence.

Distinguishing Characteristics: The elongated dorsal tongue papillae and white to brownish black coloration are characteristic of this condition.

Significant Microscopic Features: None

Differential Diagnosis: None

Treatment and Prognosis: Predisposing factors for this condition should be corrected if possible. Gentle physical debridement with a toothbrush or tongue scraper is helpful. Often, antimicrobial mouth rinses, such as chlorhexidine gluconate, are prescribed. Essential oil mouth rinses may also be recommended. If a candidal infection is present, antifungal therapy should be given.

NAME: Chemical and thermal burns

Etiology: Many chemicals or drugs are caustic and can burn the mucosa if they come in contact with it. Generally, this is caused by a group of chemicals that were not intended for topical placement on oral mucosa. The

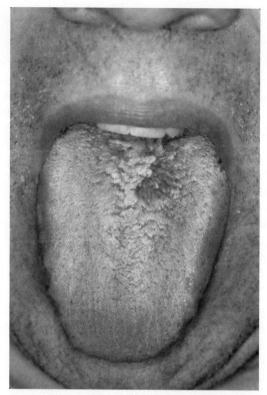

Figure 14.9. Hairy tongue. Note the elongated filiform papillae and discolored surface that are characteristic of this condition.

best example is aspirin burn, which occurs when patients place an aspirin tablet on the mucosa opposite a tooth that hurts. Many burns are produced by patients treating oral pain with numerous OTC medications or home remedies. Many different types of acids and alkalis can produce tissue necrosis, as can phenols, silver nitrate, and hydrogen peroxide. A variety of dental medicaments have also been implicated in mucosal chemical burns. Thermal burns can be caused by hot foods or implements placed in the mouth or by electric currents.

Method of Transmission: Not applicable

Epidemiology: Not applicable

Pathogenesis: Chemical and thermal burns often produce necrosis of the epithelium, which turns it white.

Extraoral Characteristics: Burns can occur on the extraoral skin, but these patients are not likely to present to a dental office for evaluation.

Perioral and Intraoral Characteristics: Most chemical and thermal burns manifest as white plaques of variable size (Fig. 14.10). Early or mild lesions do not rub off, whereas more severe lesions can often be removed with pressure from a tongue blade, leaving a raw and occasionally bleeding base. The ability to scrape a burn off depends upon the extent of the injury and is not a prerequisite clinical finding for the diagnosis.

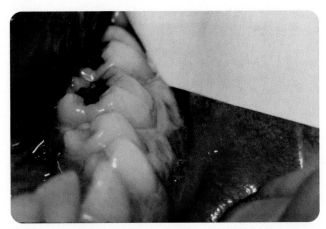

Figure 14.10. Chemical burn. This burn occurred when the patient placed an over-the-counter medication containing eugenol on the gingiva to relieve the pain of a toothache.

Distinguishing Characteristics: Chemical and thermal burns appear as localized white plaques that may or may not be rubbed off. A careful review of the patient's history with follow-up questions may uncover the actual event associated with the burn and thereby provide a definitive diagnosis.

Significant Microscopic Features: Burns produce **coagulation necrosis**, in which the cells become necrotic but maintain their original cellular outline (Fig. 14.11).

Dental Implications: These lesions may occasionally be confused with other pathologic conditions. In addition, the patient should be educated about the proper use of medications such as aspirin.

Differential Diagnosis: The diagnosis of a chemical or thermal burn can be established from the clinical features and identification of the offending chemical or hot substance. Other white lesions should be included in a differential diagnosis, including

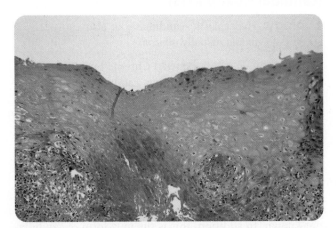

Figure 14.11. Coagulation necrosis. This histology slide depicts coagulation necrosis of the surface epithelium from a chemical burn. Note the cells within the epithelium that no longer have nuclei but still maintain their shape.

- Frictional keratosis, Chapter 14
- Hyperplastic candidiasis, Chapter 14
- Lichen planus, Chapters 13 and 14

Treatment and Prognosis: The lesion will heal once the offending chemical is withdrawn and/or the tissue is not traumatized by more hot substances.

INFECTIONS

Some white lesions arise from a known source of infection such as candidiasis, a fungal infection. Another example is the parulis that arises because of an acute infection due to a nonvital tooth or a periodontal pocket. In this section we discuss infections that manifest as white lesions, two specific forms of candidiasis (acute pseudomembranous candidiasis and chronic hyperplastic candidiasis) hairy leukoplakia and the parulis.

NAME: Acute pseudomembranous candidiasis (candidosis, moniliasis, thrush)

Etiology: Candidiasis is caused by species of *Candida*, usually *albicans*, which is a yeastlike fungus. Most patients harbor yeasts (*Candida* species) as part of their normal oral flora. Candidiasis usually represents an overgrowth of *Candida* that is already present in the mouth. The organism has extremely low virulence and tends not to produce infection in healthy patients. When it does cause disease, a variety of predisposing factors are present that appear to alter the oral environment or systemic status of the host and allow an opportunity for the organism to grow. The following are some of the more common factors that predispose an individual to infection with *C. albicans*:
- Systemic broad-spectrum antibiotic therapy
- Systemic, topical, or aerosolized corticosteroid use
- Smoking
- Xerostomia
- Immune system disorders
- Diabetes

Method of Transmission: While candidiasis is an infection, it is not highly transmissible. Candidiasis is considered an opportunistic infection.

Epidemiology: Candidiasis has a worldwide distribution and is commonly found in immunocompromised patients and the elderly who have other predisposing factors.

Pathogenesis: Acute pseudomembranous candidiasis, also known as thrush, is the most clinically characteristic form of yeast infection. This is the form of candidiasis commonly encountered in newborns who contract the infection from the birth canal. The infectious organisms either produce necrosis of the surface epithelium, which turns white and rubs off, or they produce erythema resulting from the body's reaction to the organism. The erythematic forms of this infection are discussed in Chapter 13.

Extraoral Characteristics: Candidiasis can occur in any epithelial surface of the body but is especially common in areas that are consistently warm and moist, such as the feet and areas where skin overlaps, for example in overweight persons where the rolls of skin and fat tissue overlap each other.

Perioral and Intraoral Characteristics: Acute pseudomembranous candidiasis manifests as multiple, raised, whitish, curdlike plaques with variable surrounding erythema (Fig. 14.12). The plaques are always multiple, and it is not unusual for large areas of the oral mucosa to be affected. Because it represents an infection, patients are almost always symptomatic and complain of pain, discomfort, or burning. The plaques can be scrapped off with a tongue blade or stiff instrument, hence the designation **pseudomembranous.** Many experts state that once a plaque is removed, it will reveal an erythematous or bleeding base. Most often, you will see erythema because without the dead plaque covering it, the inflammation in the underlying tissues, representing the body's reaction to the infection, can be seen.

Distinguishing Characteristics: The ability to scrape the pseudomembranes off is a diagnostic feature of this form of candidiasis. However, the dental hygienist almost never sees a "bleeding" base, since it would require scraping the tissues hard enough to remove the entire thickness of epithelium down into the underlying connective tissue.

Significant Microscopic Features: Candidal organisms typically grow on the surface of the mucosa and produce necrosis of superficial keratinocytes. As the cells die, they lie on the surface of the tissue as white plaques matted together by the **hyphae** (elongated form) of the organisms (Fig. 14.13).

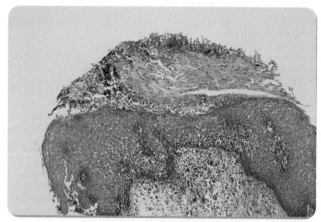

Figure 14.13. Pseudomembranous candidiasis. Histology slide of the necrotic surface cells in a pseudomembrane showing *Candida* organisms and a thickened epithelial surface.

Dental Implications: Candidiasis is an infection that needs to be diagnosed and treated. The tendency for this infection to occur in immunocompromised patients should prompt the dental professional to carefully review the patient's medical history for any sign of undiagnosed systemic problems.

Differential Diagnosis: Most white lesions that rub off are candidal infections, burns, or **vesiculobullous** (characterized by fluid filled blisters) diseases in which the epithelium sloughs.

Treatment and Prognosis: Once the diagnosis is established, a variety of effective antifungal medications are used for treatment. Many clinicians treat the infection with topical medications such as nystatin oral suspension or clotrimazole troches. Effective systemic medication is also available, such as fluconazole.

NAME: Chronic hyperplastic candidiasis (candidal leukoplakia)

Etiology: Hyperplastic candidiasis is also caused by a species of *Candida*, usually *albicans*.

Method of Transmission: Chronic hyperplastic candidiasis, like pseudomembranous candidiasis, is not considered to be highly transmissible.

Epidemiology: Chronic hyperplastic candidiasis is the rarest form of yeast infection.

Pathogenesis: There is experimental evidence that *C. albicans* may stimulate a hyperplastic reaction in the mucosal tissues of some individuals. The reason this type of response occurs in some individuals and not in others is not known. In addition, this is the only form of candidiasis that is considered to have a very low malignant transformation potential. Up to 15% of cases may progress into dysplastic lesions, which in turn may progress to cancer

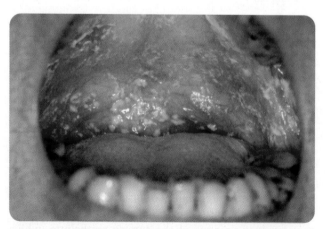

Figure 14.12. Pseudomembranous candidiasis. Multiple whitish plaques that scrape off leaving an erythematous base are characteristic of this form of candidiasis.

(Sitheeque and Samaranayake, 2003). (Refer to the discussion on epithelial dysplasia in the following section on leukoplakia.)

Extraoral Characteristics: Not applicable

Perioral and Intraoral Characteristics: Chronic hyperplastic candidiasis manifests as a thickened, often raised, whitish plaque that does not rub off. Lesions commonly affect the tongue or commissure (Fig. 14.14). The lesions have no distinctive clinical features and are indistinguishable from leukoplakia. In fact, another term for the condition is candidal leukoplakia.

Distinguishing Characteristics: Hyperplastic candidiasis cannot be clinically distinguished from other white lesions that do not wipe off.

Significant Microscopic Features: The diagnosis can only be established by a biopsy that demonstrates hyperkeratosis, epithelial hyperplasia, and the causative hyphae of the organism in the superficial keratin.

Dental Implications: This lesion is rare, but it is considered premalignant. Chronic forms of candidiasis are also an indication that the person's immune system may be deficient.

Differential Diagnosis: Chronic hyperplastic candidiasis is indistinguishable from leukoplakia.

Treatment and Prognosis: Treatments include systemic antifungals, topical application of vitamin A/retinoids and β-carotenes, laser surgery, and conventional surgical excision. The treatment of these lesions is somewhat controversial, because treatment does not universally result in resolution of the lesion. Furthermore, treatment does not necessarily prevent the development of epithelial dysplasia and progression to cancer (Sitheeque and Samaranayake, 2003). However, it is only this form of candidiasis that shows any malignant potential. The more common forms of erythematous or pseudomembranous candidiasis show no relation to oral cancer.

NAME: Hairy leukoplakia

Etiology: Hairy leukoplakia (HL) is caused by an infection with Epstein-Barr virus (EBV) secondary to immunosuppression. HL is linked to the immunosuppression that results from infection with the human immunodeficiency virus. However, HL is well documented in other immunosuppressed patients, as well; for example, those who are taking chemotherapy for malignancy or immunosuppression therapy for organ transplantation.

Method of Transmission: Not applicable

Epidemiology: HL occurs predominantly in HIV-infected patients. The incidence of HL has decreased significantly now that HIV-positive patients are treated with aggressive antiretroviral chemotherapy.

Pathogenesis: Unknown

Extraoral Characteristics: Not applicable

Perioral and Intraoral Characteristics: HL produces whitish plaques that do not rub off. They usually affect the lateral borders of the tongue, often bilaterally, where they appear as vertical, raised ridges or sometimes as irregular flattened lesions (Fig. 14.15). Rarely, HL will affect mucosal surfaces other than the tongue. Patients are typically asymptomatic.

Distinguishing Characteristics: HL characteristically presents as white plaques, often with vertical raised ridges, bilaterally on the tongue in immunosuppressed patients.

Significant Microscopic Features: The diagnosis of hairy leukoplakia is made by biopsy with demonstration of EBV in the surface epithelium. The name hairy leukoplakia comes from the histologic appearance, in which there is hyperkeratosis with exophytic extensions of keratin that appear somewhat like hair. Many of the su-

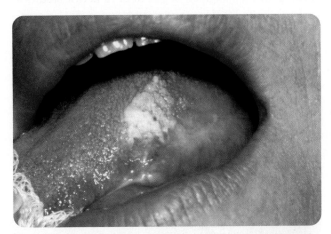

Figure 14.14. Chronic hyperplastic candidiasis. A characteristic white plaque that does not rub off is shown on the lateral border of the tongue.

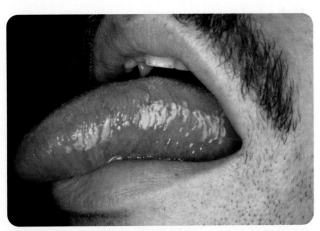

Figure 14.15. Hairy leukoplakia. The characteristic presentation of HL is bilateral white plaques along the lateral border of the tongue. This HL lesion is on the lateral border of the tongue in an HIV-positive male.

perficial keratinocytes show cytoplasmic clearing with intranuclear viral inclusions.

Dental Implications: HL is a significant diagnosis because it is a relatively accurate predictor of rapid progression from HIV latent infection to AIDS. (See also HIV/AIDS, Chapter 22.)

Differential Diagnosis: Several of the more keratotic white lesions discussed in this chapter are included in a differential diagnosis, including frictional keratosis, lichen planus, candidiasis, and thermal and chemical burns.

Treatment and Prognosis: Antiviral therapy often produces improvement or resolution of the lesion; however, recurrence is not uncommon. There is no evidence that hairy leukoplakia has the potential for malignant transformation.

Parulis

Parulis is a swelling of the gingiva caused by a draining sinus tract from an odontogenic infection of either periodontal or pulpal origin. The swelling is due to purulent exudate (pus), which is more yellowish than white. When pus is encountered clinically, the source of odontogenic infection should be determined and treated.

IMMUNE SYSTEM DISORDERS

A variety of skin conditions can also affect mucous membranes. Many of these are autoimmune disorders or immune-mediated inflammatory conditions.

NAME: Lichen planus (LP)

Etiology: LP is a chronic immune-mediated mucocutaneous disorder. T lymphocytes are recruited to the skin or oral mucosa where they produce damage to the surface epithelium.

Method of Transmission: Not applicable

Epidemiology: Lichen planus is the most common dermatologic condition that manifests with cutaneous as well as oral lesions. (Refer to Chapter 13 for detailed information on the epidemiology of lichen planus.)

Pathogenesis: While the reaction suggests that the body is reacting to an antigen within the surface epithelium, to date the specific antigen(s) has not been identified. Some authorities consider LP to be an autoimmune disorder; however, until an antigen is identified; it is premature to consider LP an autoimmune disease.

Extraoral Characteristics: The characteristic skin lesions are purplish, raised papules with a keratotic white surface pattern of very fine interlacing lines called **Wickham striae.** Lesions are also **pruritic** (itchy) and typically affect the legs and forearms.

Perioral and Intraoral Characteristics: LP is another condition that appears in a variety of clinical patterns, including white lesions, red lesions, and ulcers. This section focuses primarily on the white lesions, which are the most distinctive clinically. Other forms of this condition are discussed in Chapter 13 and are also mentioned in Chapter 23 regarding skin lesions. Two forms of lichen planus appear as white lesions, the reticular and plaque-like forms.

The *reticular or striate form* of LP is the most common and characteristic of the various presentations. It produces a lacy pattern of Wickham striae that do not rub off (Fig. 14.16). The lesions affect the buccal mucosa, usually bilaterally, but may also affect the gingiva. The reticular form of LP tends to be asymptomatic, but some patients will complain of a textural change. One of the most common sites to see LP is in the postbuccal mucosa in the lower mucobuccal fold, which is often traumatized from routine functioning. LP tends to affect sites prone to trauma, an occurrence known as the **Koebner phenomenon** (ability of a disease to affect chronically irritated tissue).

The *plaque* form of lichen planus is less common than the reticular form and manifests as a whitish plaque. This plaque has no clinically distinguishing features and appears similar to leukoplakia.

Distinguishing Characteristics: Wickham striae observed bilaterally on the buccal mucosa and possibly on the gingiva are characteristic of this disorder.

Significant Microscopic Features: The epithelium is hyperkeratotic, with irregular rete ridges that are often angular and described as "saw tooth." There is significant basal epithelial cell damage with liquefaction degeneration and an immune bandlike infiltrate of small lymphocytes in the underlying connective tissue.

Dental Implications: Lichen planus is often confused with other pathologic processes. Symptomatic patients require diagnosis and treatment. There is controversy regarding the premalignant nature of LP, and case studies as

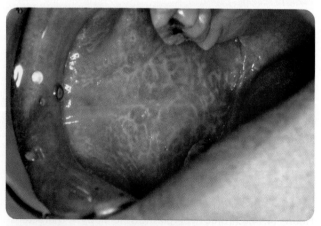

Figure 14.16. Lichen planus. Note the typical reticular or striate pattern of Wickham striae.

well as editorials are published on both sides of this issue. All agree that the lesions should be carefully monitored.

Differential Diagnosis: Other white lesions may have similar appearances such as:

1. Candidiasis, Chapter 14
2. Leukoplakia, Chapter 14

Treatment and Prognosis: The reticular and plaque forms of LP are generally asymptomatic, and patients usually do not require treatment unless the disease becomes erosive and symptomatic. Biopsy is usually not indicated unless a change occurs after a confirmed diagnosis is made. Erosive lesions are considered more suspicious, since they have been reported to become squamous cell carcinoma in some cases. However, the malignant potential of LP is controversial, and lesions not responding to traditional treatment, or lesions showing growth or a mass effect, should have a biopsy performed.

GENETIC OR CONGENITAL DISORDERS

Genokeratoses represent a variety of inherited oral mucosal disorders that produce keratinized (white) lesions of the oral mucosa. Because these lesions are inherited, they tend to appear at an early age or at birth and are often multifocal, affecting large areas of the oral mucosa. The most common condition of this type is white sponge nevus.

NAME: White sponge nevus (WSN)

Etiology: White sponge nevus is an inherited condition caused by the mutation of certain keratin genes. WSN is usually apparent in childhood but is sometimes not noticed until adolescence.

Method of Transmission: WSN follows an autosomal dominant inheritance pattern. Occasionally, cases appear in individuals with no family history of the disorder.

Epidemiology: This is a rare condition.

Pathogenesis: The disorder involves an autosomal dominant trait, and a diagnosis is made rapidly when a family history already exists.

Extraoral Characteristics: Rarely, WSN affects the upper aerodigestive tract mucosa and anogenital areas.

Perioral and Intraoral Characteristics: WSN tends to produce widespread keratinization of the buccal mucosa and often the labial mucosa (Fig. 14.17). The lesions do not rub off.

Distinguishing Characteristics: Widespread white plaques on the buccal and labial mucosa that do not rub off are characteristic of this disorder.

Significant Microscopic Features: Hyperkeratosis, **acanthosis** (thickening of the prickle cell layer of the ep-

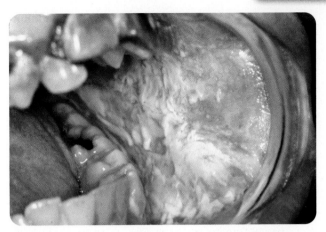

Figure 14.17. White sponge nevus. Observe the extensive keratotic plaques that extend into mucobuccal folds.

ithelium), and cytoplasmic clearing of the epithelial cells are microscopic findings related to this disorder.

Dental Implications: Occasionally, these lesions present as a cosmetic problem.

Differential Diagnosis: Because of the cheek involvement, the lesions show some similarity to cheek chewing. The lesions of WSN, however, invariably affect mucobuccal folds, sites that are virtually impossible to chew. Other possibilities include leukoedema, leukoplakia, and lichen planus, all discussed in this chapter.

Treatment and Prognosis: Once a diagnosis of WSN is confirmed, no other treatment is needed, and the prognosis is excellent.

PREMALIGNANT/MALIGNANT DISORDERS

A **premalignant** lesion can be defined as a clinically detectable morphologic tissue change that has a higher risk of developing into oral cancer than normal tissue. Oral leukoplakia is the most common form of premalignant lesion found in the oral cavity. A premalignant condition is defined as a generalized state associated with a significantly increased risk of cancer that can develop anywhere within the oral cavity, not just within a preexisting lesion (Reibel, 2003). Oral submucous fibrosis and oral lichen planus are examples of premalignant conditions. Oral lichen planus is discussed above; leukoplakia and oral submucous fibrosis are discussed below.

NAME: Leukoplakia

Leukoplakia is defined by the World Health Organization as "a white patch or plaque that does not rub off and that cannot be diagnosed clinically or pathologically as any specific disease." Accordingly, leukoplakia is a descriptive clinical term for a white patch with no clinically distinguishing features. It is also a diagnosis by exclusion. The term should only be used after a thorough differential diagnosis has been considered, and all specific conditions producing mucosal whiteness have been ruled out.

Etiology: Historically, chronic irritation was thought to be an etiologic factor in many leukoplakias. However, there has never been sound scientific documentation that physical irritation of tissues leads to malignancy. Therefore, white lesions that are clearly the result of physical irritation should not be diagnosed as leukoplakia but should be called frictional keratoses. The most important etiologic factor associated with leukoplakia is tobacco, both smoked and topical. Approximately 50% of leukoplakias in smokers will resolve with smoking cessation, and over 95% of spit tobacco lesions resolve with cessation (Wright, 2003). Leukoplakias do however occur in nonsmokers.

Method of Transmission: Not applicable

Epidemiology: Leukoplakia has a worldwide distribution and is found most commonly where tobacco use is prevalent and acceptable. It is typically found in less than 1% of nonsmokers but from 6% to as high as 60% of smokers in some studies. Men are more frequently affected, but with the social acceptance of smoking in women, more women are affected today.

Pathogenesis: Leukoplakia arises from genetic mutations to the epithelial cells following exposure to carcinogens (Chapter 5). Leukoplakia is considered a premalignant lesion (a lesion from which a malignant neoplasm may develop in a significant number of cases). Oral cancer does not arise from normal oral epithelial cells. Rather, as normal cells evolve into cancer, they develop microscopic changes that are known as epithelial dysplasia. Fortunately, dysplastic epithelium tends to produce clinically detectable alteration of the oral mucosa. These lesions tend to be white (leukoplakia) and/or red (erythroplakia). It is well documented that some untreated leukoplakias will progress into squamous cell carcinoma. However, many lesions take years to evolve into cancer, and some may never evolve. The significance of this slow progression is that many patients will have clinically detectable premalignant lesions that may persist for years (see Clinical Protocol 12 on early cancer detection devices). Detection and therapeutic intervention at the premalignant stage can potentially prevent the development of oral cancer. There are two clinical features of leukoplakia that can help to identify the dysplastic lesions: (1) the anatomic site involved and (2) whether or not the lesion is homogeneous. The overall likelihood that a leukoplakia will show microscopic evidence of dysplasia or invasive disease is 20%. Leukoplakias involving certain anatomic sites have a greater than 20% likelihood of showing dysplasia or invasion (Cawson et al., 2001). These are known as high-risk sites, and they correspond to sites prone to develop malignancy such as the lower lip, the floor of the mouth, the lateral and ventral tongue, the

retromolar trigone (the soft tissue area posterior to the mandibular molars toward the pharynx), and the lateral soft palate. The highest risk site is the floor of mouth and ventral tongue, where just over 40% of leukoplakias will show dysplasia/carcinoma. Presence on the lower lip increases the risk to 35% and on the lateral tongue to approximately 25% (Cawson et al., 2001). In addition, nonhomogeneous lesions (lesions containing redness, ulceration, or a verrucous surface architecture) will show evidence of dysplasia/carcinoma at a considerably higher rate (Cawson et al., 2001). Longitudinal studies have shown conclusively that some leukoplakias will progress to carcinoma if untreated, and traditionally this has occurred in approximately 5% of lesions. However, earlier studies did not distinguish between dysplastic and nondysplastic lesions. Newer studies have shown that approximately 1% of nondysplastic leukoplakias and 15% of dysplastic lesions will progress to carcinoma over time if untreated (Cowan et al., 2001).

Extraoral Characteristics: Not applicable

Perioral and Intraoral Characteristics: The clinical features of leukoplakia are highly variable, manifesting in a variety of shapes and sizes and affecting virtually any mucosal surface (Fig. 14.18). Lesions range from minute (millimeters) to several centimeters in size. Most lesions are single, but occasionally, multiple lesions are encountered. Most lesions are soft on palpation, but depending on the thickness of the surface keratin, some lesions feel leathery. Palpating a firm mass (induration) under the surface of the leukoplakia is a strong indicator that the lesion may represent invasive squamous cell carcinoma. Patients with leukoplakia are asymptomatic, and a thorough oral examination is the most important means of detection.

Leukoplakias in smokers can affect any site. The most commonly used spit tobacco that produces keratosis is snuff, and these lesions are often referred to as snuff dippers keratosis or snuff dippers pouch (Fig. 14.19). The

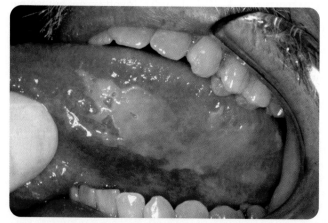

Figure 14.18. Leukoplakia. Shown is a characteristic leukoplakia of left lateral border of the tongue.

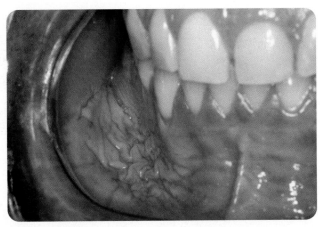

Figure 14.19. Snuff dippers keratosis. Classic presentation of snuff dippers keratosis at site of snuff placement.

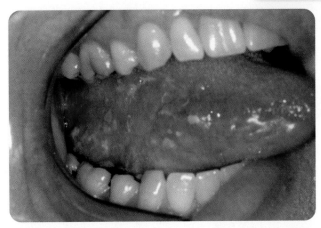

Figure 14.21. Speckled leukoplakia. This tongue lesion exhibits discrete red and white areas.

mucosa is often corrugated, and the adjacent teeth are usually stained and exhibit gingival recession.

Leukoplakias of the lower lip are invariably related to chronic sun damage and are termed actinic or solar keratosis (see Chapter 23 on skin lesions and Clinical Protocol 10). Sun damage to the lower lip produces atrophy of the vermilion border with loss of the sharp demarcation between the vermilion border and skin. The vermilion is variably white, with or without areas of erosion and/or crusting (Fig. 14.20).

Some authorities subclassify leukoplakia as homogeneous or nonhomogeneous. In some cases leukoplakias will also have areas of redness, ulceration, or a pebbly or verrucous surface. These later clinical changes make the lesion nonhomogeneous. These lesions have also been described as

(1) **Speckled leukoplakia (erythroleukoplakia).** These lesions exhibit both red and white components (Figs. 14.21 and 14.22). (See Chapter 13 for more on red lesions.)

(2) **Verrucous leukoplakia.** These lesions show an irregular or verrucous surface texture (Fig. 14.23).

(3) **Proliferative verrucous leukoplakia.** Proliferative verrucous leukoplakia is a particularly aggressive form of leukoplakia that tends to be multifocal and progressive and normally shows a high incidence of progression to carcinoma (Fig. 14.23). This form of leukoplakia exhibits a tendency to form on the gingival tissues, where it is associated with the greatest potential for malignant transformation (Shopper et al., 2004).

Distinguishing Characteristics: Leukoplakia is not clinically distinguishable from other white lesions that do not rub off.

Significant Microscopic Features: If large numbers of biopsies are performed on leukoplakias, approximately 80% will show hyperkeratosis (thickening of the stratum corneum layer), with or without acanthosis. The remaining 20% will show some grade of dysplasia, carcinoma in situ, or invasive squamous cell carcinoma (Waldron and Shafer, 1975). The most accurate predictor

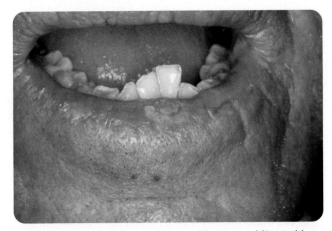

Figure 14.20. Actinic keratosis. Note the crusted lip and loss of a distinct vermilion border on this patient.

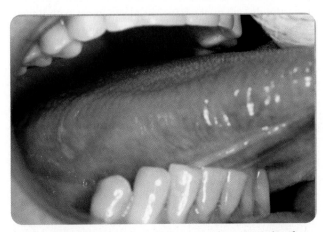

Figure 14.22. Speckled leukoplakia. Another example of a speckled leukoplakia or erythroleukoplakia with posterior white (leukoplakia) and anterior red (erythroplakia) portions.

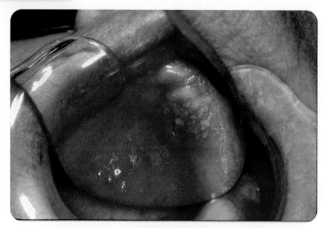

Figure 14.23. Proliferative verrucous leukoplakia. This white lesion on the alveolar ridge had a verrucous surface texture and was determined to be a proliferative verrucous leukoplakia. (Courtesy of Dr. John Wright.)

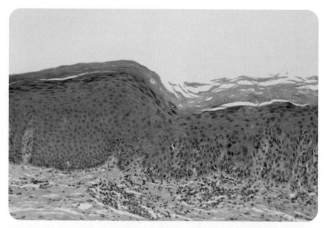

Figure 14.24. Mild epithelial dysplasia. Mild epithelial dysplasia on the right displaying minimal cytologic change and alteration of maturation compared with normal epithelium on the left.

of malignant progression is the presence of epithelial dysplasia. Dysplasia represents the morphologic changes the cells go through as they evolve from normal to malignant, and as such, it represents premalignant change. The presence of dysplasia can only be ascertained microscopically following a biopsy. The cellular features that characterize dysplasia are well recognized and include the following:

- Increase in cellular nuclear/cytoplasmic ratio
- Rounded or irregular rete ridges
- Altered maturation
- Increased mitoses, atypical mitoses, mitoses in upper layers of epithelium
- Pleomorphism (variation in size and shape)
- **Nuclear hyperchromatism** (chromosomal material that stains darkly when exposed to specific staining solutions)
- Enlarged nucleoli
- Loss of cellular cohesion
- Abnormal keratinization patterns

Not all features of dysplasia are present in all lesions; however, those present tend to occur in varying degrees. Accordingly, when assessing dysplasia, most pathologists subjectively grade the dysplasia according to its severity. Dysplasias are graded as mild, moderate, or severe. Figure 14.24 represents mild dysplasia, Figure 14.25 represents moderate dysplasia, and Figure 14.26 depicts severe dysplasia. Carcinoma in situ represents a lesion in which the cells look malignant but are still confined to the epithelium (in situ). Figure 14.27 shows carcinoma in situ, and Figure 14.28 depicts invasive cancer.

Ultimately, these abnormal cells will leave the epithelium and invade deeper structures, and this traditionally is when the process becomes malignant. The cellular features of premalignant and malignant lesions are similar; the main difference is the presence or absence of invasion.

Differential Diagnosis: In no other condition is differential diagnosis more important that in leukoplakia, because leukoplakia is a diagnosis by exclusion. Only after

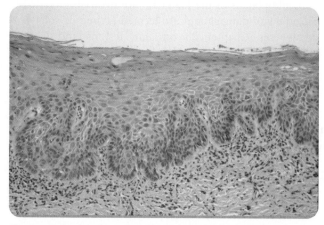

Figure 14.25. Moderate epithelial dysplasia. Moderate epithelial dysplasia displaying increasing cytologic atypia and alteration of maturation in the lower half of the epithelium.

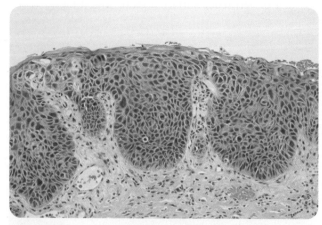

Figure 14.26. Severe epithelial dysplasia. Severe epithelial dysplasia displaying significant nuclear hyperchromatism, pleomorphism, and altered maturation affecting most of the epithelium.

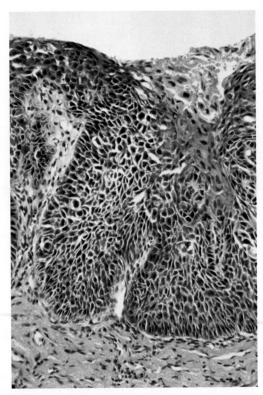

Figure 14.27. Carcinoma in situ.

all other white lesions are considered and ruled out is leukoplakia the appropriate clinical diagnosis. The speckled form of leukoplakia shows clinical features similar to those of pseudomembranous candidiasis, but unlike candidiasis, the speckled whitish elevations do not rub off.

Treatment and Prognosis: Biopsies should be performed on leukoplakias, since microscopic examination is the only way to accurately assess the presence of epithelial dysplasia. A small number of leukoplakias actually represent early invasive cancer, but one that was discovered before the cells could replicate sufficiently to produce a mass or swelling typically associated with cancer. The odds are

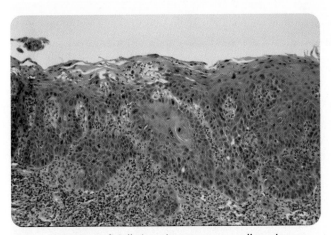

Figure 14.28. Superficially invasive squamous cell carcinoma. Note the penetration of the basement membrane by the cancer cells in this histology slide. (Courtesy of Dr. John Wright.)

in the patient's favor, as most leukoplakias are nondysplastic, but biopsy is mandatory to detect the ones that are dysplastic. Treatment decisions are best made following a biopsy and a determination of microscopic findings. Nondysplastic lesions are best managed by altering or eliminating risk factors such as tobacco use. With tobacco cessation, approximately 50% of leukoplakias associated with smoked tobacco and over 95% of those with spit tobacco regress (Cowan et al., 2001). Dysplastic lesions are ideally managed by risk factor modification and surgical removal. Lesions are either excised or **ablated** (removed completely) with laser therapy. While the likelihood of malignant progression can be substantially decreased by therapeutic intervention, as many as 50% of patients will experience "recurrence." This is due to either incomplete removal of the lesion or a process known as field cancerization (see also Chapter 12 under neoplasms). The basis of this process is that carcinogens in the mouth are unlikely to affect only a localized area. Rather they are likely to produce cellular changes all over the mouth (field), even though lesions may not be clinically apparent. The altered cells can continue to progress and ultimately produce additional lesions that may appear as a recurrence of the original lesion (Feller et al., 2006). Any patient who has been treated for a premalignant lesion has a significantly increased chance of developing additional lesions over time; therefore, continued clinical follow-up is mandatory.

NAME: Oral submucous fibrosis (OSF)

Etiology: As in many conditions that are considered premalignant, OSF is believed to have a multifactorial etiology. The following factors appear to be associated with an increased risk of developing this condition: (1) areca nut or betel nut chewing, (2) genetic predisposition and genetic mutation, and (3) nutritional deficiencies may play a role.

Method of Transmission: None

Epidemiology: It is estimated that 2.5 million individuals are affected by OSF around the world. Most of the cases are found in India, Southeast Asian countries, and Pacific island nations (Lountzis et al., 2006). OSF has also become a public health issue among immigrant populations located in the United Kingdom and South Africa (Lountzis et al., 2006). OSF is rare in the United States; however, because of the significant increase in Asian immigration, OSF is currently seen more frequently in the United States than it ever has been before.

Pathogenesis: Most cases develop in patients who chew some form of areca nut, usually betel quid, which is a form of topical tobacco mixed with slaked lime and areca nuts. Arecoline, a substance found in betel nuts, stimulates the production of collagen by fibroblasts. Other substances encourage the newly formed fibers to crosslink, enhancing their strength and inhibiting the body's attempts to break them down. Finally, studies suggest that genetic mutations occur in fibroblasts that are exposed to the chemicals in betel nut further stimulating the production of collagen fibers. This persists even after cessation of the habit. Three stages of clinical development have been identified and are discussed below along with perioral and intraoral characteristics.

Extraoral Characteristics: None

Perioral and Intraoral Characteristics: The first stage of development involves a generalized stomatitis that manifests as erythematous mucosal tissues that develop numerous vesicles and ulcers. An increase in melanin pigmentation and oral petechia may also be noted. The second stage or fibrosis stage is characterized by the progressive accumulation of collagen fibers in the mucosal tissues. Fibrous bands of tissue that form in the buccal and labial mucosa result in a white marblelike appearance and cause progressive limitation in opening the mouth (trismus) (Fig. 14.29).There is decreased flexibility of the tongue, soft palate, and uvula. Problems with speech, eating, and swallowing are common. The floor of the mouth becomes leathery, and the gingiva becomes fibrotic and pale. The third stage is characterized by the formation of premalignant leukoplakia lesions in about 25% of those affected by OSF (Lountzis et al., January 2006).

Distinguishing Characteristics: Patients who habitually chew betel nut have extensive dark (red or mahogany) staining of their teeth. The presence of this type of staining should prompt the dental professional to thoroughly investigate its cause.

Significant Microscopic Features: Early stages show edema, large fibroblasts, and inflammatory infiltrates. More advanced stages show dense bundles of collagen, decreased vascularity, and no edema.

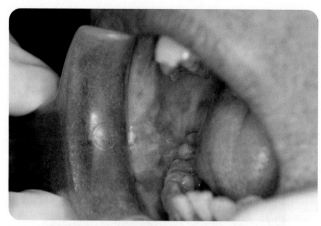

Figure 14.29. Oral submucous fibrosis. Note the white marbled appearance of the buccal mucosa. (Courtesy of Dr. John Wright.)

Dental Implications: Patients who habitually chew betel nut should be encouraged to stop the habit, have regular oral examinations, and receive appropriate education related to the complications of OSF.

Differential Diagnosis: OSF may present with manifestations that are similar to those seen in scleroderma (Chapter 23) and lichen planus (Chapters 13 and 14).

Treatment and Prognosis: There is no effective treatment for this condition, and the process is irreversible. The patient should be advised to stop chewing betel nut. Steroid injections may slow the progression of the disease. Surgery may be necessary to treat severe trismus by releasing the fibrous bands. The prognosis depends on the severity of the symptoms and whether the patient will cease chewing betel nut. The risk of developing squamous cell carcinoma within OSF is 7.6% (Lountzis et al., January 2006).

SUMMARY

- Fordyce's granules and leukoedema are examples of white oral lesions that are considered variations of normal tissues or structures.
- Geographic tongue is an inflammatory lesion of unknown etiology that is normally asymptomatic.
- Frictional keratosis is an adaptive response to chronic physical irritation that stimulates the production of keratin within the mucosa and results in a mucosal "callus."
- Linea alba is a specific form of frictional keratosis often associated with bruxing and/or clenching.

- Cheek chewing is another example of frictional keratosis that manifests in individuals who habitually chew on their cheeks.
- Nicotine stomatitis manifests as a whitening of the palatal mucosa with inflammation of the minor salivary gland ducts resulting in erythema.
- Elongation of the filiform papillae results in hairy tongue. The etiology of hairy tongue is unknown; however, some of the risk factors associated with its development include systemic antibiotic therapy and oxygenating mouth rinses.

(continued)

SUMMARY (continued)

- White lesions caused by chemical or thermal burns are common. Aspirin is the most common cause of chemical burns, while hot food is the most common cause of thermal burns.
- Acute pseudomembranous candidiasis presents as curdlike plaques on the mucosa that can be wiped off. Immune suppression is frequently associated with this infection.
- Chronic hyperplastic candidiasis is the least common form of candidal infection. These lesions have a slight potential to become dysplastic and to undergo malignant transformation.
- Hairy leukoplakia is caused by an infection with the Epstein-Barr virus and is associated with immunosuppression due to HIV infection, medications, or other immunosuppressive conditions.

- Reticular and plaque forms of lichen planus are associated with white oral lesions. These lesions are usually asymptomatic and tend to affect the buccal mucosa.
- White sponge nevus is a rare autosomal dominant genetic disorder that manifests as white plaques, usually found on the buccal and labial mucosa.
- Leukoplakia is a white lesion that cannot be diagnosed as any other condition. These are considered premalignant lesions and are commonly associated with tobacco use.
- Oral submucosa fibrosis is a premalignant condition that is associated with betel nut chewing. This condition may result in severe impairment of oral functions because of fibrosis and loss of tissue elasticity.

Critical Thinking Activity

A 45-year-old male patient is seen in your office today for routine prophylaxis. The patient is on a 3-month maintenance appointment schedule. As you review the notes, you read that the patient has diabetes type 2. He has allergies and uses a corticosteroid spray for seasonal allergic rhinitis. Last visit, he was treated by your office hygienist who practices on alternate days. Her notes indicate that the patient continues to be treated for oral fungal infections at least several times a year.

As you perform your oral examination, you notice a moderate amount of calculus, but minimal plaque. The patient is missing 22–28, which is sustained by a partial denture. His 3rd molars are missing, and all remaining molar teeth have MOD restorations. The oral tissue appears normal in most areas, but you do notice some white patchy areas in several locations. As you read the previous notes, the same scenario existed 3 months ago. The patient was given a nystatin rinse and asked to return within a few days. Although he did not return for another evaluation, he tells you that his wife checked his mouth and reported that the areas were completely gone within a few days.

A differential diagnosis of this lesion would include many conditions; however, in this scenario, the lesion is determined to be a *Candida* infection.

PORTFOLIO ACTIVITIES

1. Yeast infections are commonly seen in clinical practice, especially affecting the elderly. Volunteer to visit a nursing home in your community and present a discussion of yeast infections. Design a table clinic appropriate for your audience on intraoral yeast infections. Include how patients get these infections, predisposing factors, clinical features, and management.

2. Volunteer to give a presentation on the harmful effects of spit tobacco at your local high school. Organize a presentation including facts about oral cancer, the role of tobacco and spit tobacco, clinical features of cancer and their warning signs for patients, and management.

REFERENCES

Amagasa T, Yokoo E, Sato K, et al. A study of the clinical characteristics and treatment of oral carcinoma in situ. Oral Surg Oral Med Oral Pathol Oral Radiol Endod 1985;60:50–55.

Banoczy J, Csiba A: Occurrence of epithelial dysplasia in oral leukoplakia. Oral Surg Oral Med Oral Pathol Oral Radiol Endod 1976;42: 766–774.

Banoczy J, Sugar L. Progressive and regressive changes in Hungarian oral leukoplakias in the course of longitudinal studies. Community Dent Oral Epidemiol 1975;3:194–197.

Baric JM, Alman JE, Feldman RS, et al. Influence of cigarette, pipe smoking, removable partial dentures and age on oral leukoplakia. Oral Surg Oral Med Oral Pathol Oral Radiol Endod 1982;54:424–429.

Cawson RA, Binnie WH, Barrett AW, Wright JM. Oral disease: clinical and pathological correlations. 3rd ed. Edinburgh: Mosby International, 2001.

Cowan CG, Gregg TA, Napier SS, et al. Potentially malignant oral lesions in Northern Ireland: a 20-year population-based perspective of malignant transformation. Oral Dis 2001;7:18–24.

Feller L, Wood NH, Raubenheimer EJ. Proliferative verrucous leukoplakia and field cauterization: report of a case. J Int Acad Periodontol 2006;8(2):67–70.

Gupta PC, Mehta FS, Daftary DK, et al. Incidence rates of oral cancer and natural history of oral precancerous lesions in a 10-year follow-up study of Indian villagers. Commun Dent Oral Epidemiol 1980;8: 287–333.

Kelsch R. Geographic tongue. Last updated July 13, 2005. e medicine: Instant access to the minds of medicine. Available at: http://www. emedicine.com/derm/topic664.htm . Accessed December 24, 2006.

Kramer IRH, El-Labban N, Lee KW. The clinical features and risk of malignant transformation in sublingual keratosis. Br Dent J 1978;144: 171–180.

Mehta FS, Pindborg JJ, Gupta PC, et al. Epidemiologic and histologic study of oral cancer and leukoplakia among 50,915 villagers in India. Cancer 1969;24:832–849.

Mincer HH, Coleman SA, Hopkins KP. Observations on the clinical characteristics of oral lesions showing histologic epithelial dysplasia. Oral Surg Oral Med Oral Pathol Oral Radiol Endod 1972;33:389–399.

Neville BW, Damm DD, Allen CM, Bouquot JE. Oral and maxillofacial pathology. 2nd ed. Philadelphia: WB Saunders, 2002.

Regezi J, Sciubba J, Jordan R. Oral pathology—clinical pathologic correlations. 4th ed. St. Louis: WB Saunders, 2003.

Reibel J. Prognosis of oral pre-malignant lesions: significance of clinical, histopathological, and molecular biological characteristics. Crit Rev Oral Biol Med 2003;14(1):47–62.

Scully C. Candidiasis, mucosal. Last updated September 7, 2006. e medicine: Instant access to the minds of medicine. Available at: http://www.emedicine.com/derm/topic68.htm. Accessed December 24, 2006.

Shear M, Pindborg JJ: Verrucous hyperplasia of the oral mucosa. Cancer 1980;46:1855–1862.

Shopper TP, Brannon RB, Stalker WH. Proliferative verrucous leukoplakia: an aggressive form of oral leukoplakia. J Dent Hyg 2004;78(3):7.

Sitheeque MAM, Samaranayake LP. Chronic hyperplastic candidosis/candidiasis (candidal leukoplakia). Crit Rev Oral Biol Med 2003;14(4): 253–267.

Waldron CA, Shafer WG: Leukoplakia revisited. Cancer 1975;36: 1386–1392.

WHO Collaborating Center for Oral Precancerous Lesions. Definition of leukoplakia and related lesions: an aid to studies on oral precancer. Oral Surg Oral Med Oral Pathol Oral Radiol Endod 1978;46:518–539.

Wright BA, Wright JM, Binnie WH. Oral cancer: clinical and pathological correlations. Boca Raton: CRC Press, 1988.

Wright JM. Case of the month. Snuff dippers keratosis. Texas Dent J 2003;120:1181, 1186–1187.

Chapter
15

Pigmented Lesions

Key Terms

- **Amalgam tattoo**
- **Amelanotic melanoma**
- **Argyria**
- **Basal keratinocytes**
- **Biologic therapy**
- **Blue nevus**
- **Compound nevus**
- **Ephelis (pl, ephelides)**
- **Focal argyrosis**
- **Focal melanosis (oral melanotic macule)**
- **Intradermal nevus**
- **Intramucosal nevus**
- **Junctional nevus**
- **Labial melanotic macule**
- **Laugier-Hunziker syndrome**
- **Lentigo maligna**
- **Melanin**
- **Melanocytes**
- **Melanoma**
- **Melanosis**
- **Minocycline tissue staining (black bone stain)**
- **Nevus**
- **Oral submucosa fibrosis (OSF)**
- **Physiologic pigmentation**
- **Plumbism**
- **Quid**
- **Smoker's melanosis or smoking-associated melanosis**
- **Solar lentigines**

Chapter Objectives

1. Define and use the key terms in this chapter.
2. List three pigmented lesions that are physiologic and three pigmented lesions that are pathologic.
3. List three factors that contribute to the pigmentation of oral tissues.
4. Name six important factors that assist in a differential diagnosis of pigmented lesions.
5. Discuss the three origins of traumatic or inflammatory lesions.
6. Name two systemic diseases that may have pigmentation of the tissues as a sign of the actual disease.
7. Name four diseases involving an inflammatory process, which sometimes produces pigmentation.
8. Name four drugs that cause oral pigmentation.
9. List two diseases that may produce pigmentation of the lips.
10. Name three heavy metals that exhibit pigmentation of the tissues.
11. Discuss the types of antibiotics that may cause pigmentation of the oral tissues.

CHAPTER OUTLINE

Pigmented lesions may be physiologic or pathologic. Some are considered to be benign and some are extremely malignant. In early stages of both physiologic and pathologic lesions, it is often difficult to determine the seriousness of the lesion simply by a clinical examination. When a direct cause of a lesion cannot be determined, further investigation is always warranted, including a biopsy with microscopic examination of the tissue. In these cases, a thorough clinical examination and a full medical history of the patient are very important. Knowing the medical history of the patient, the medications that are being taken, and the lifestyle of the individual, is crucial in determining the pathogenesis of any lesion. The duration, location, clinical appearance, radiographic appearances, pathology reports, and self-reported changes are all important in the differential diagnosis. These steps are needed to distinguish a benign lesion from a malignant one. Another important factor related to a change in a lesion is the reality that, very often, what begins as a benign lesion takes a radical course into malignancy. Therefore, any changes in lesions should be taken seriously.

In this chapter, we explore the color variations of normal tissue versus tissue that has undergone pathologic changes. Some areas of pigmentation are localized, such as a benign amalgam tattoo. However, the early stages of the most malignant lesion, a melanoma, can also be localized and have a clinical appearance similar to that of an amalgam tattoo. Pigmented areas may be generalized, such as genetic and racial pigmentation, or they may be related to endocrine disorders, pregnancy, inflammatory conditions, trauma, or medications. All of the above may cause color variations. Pigmentation may also be due to the numbers of **melanocytes.** Melanocytes are found in or at the basal (deepest) layer of the epidermis and have long dendritic extensions that extend to the keratinocytes in the more superficial layers of the epidermis. The main function of melanocytes is to protect the skin from harmful ultraviolet rays by producing **melanin,** the black or brown substance that imparts color to the skin. Each melanocyte is able to produce granules of pigment called *melanosomes* that are then transferred along the dendritic processes to the keratinocytes, thereby coloring these cells. Hormones and genetics influence the amount of melanin and pigmentation produced. Additionally, the introduction of exogenous materials into the surrounding tissues may cause a pigmented lesion. An example of pigmentation due to an exogenous material is the pigmentation that occurs when amalgam fragments become embedded within the tissues. Another example is an embedded lead pencil point that may be incurred when a child puts the pencil in his or her mouth and falls, leaving the lead point or particles within the tissue.

Essentially, oral pigmentation is due to the following:

1. The number of melanocytes
2. The amount of melanin produced
3. The incorporation of a foreign substance introduced into the oral and perioral tissues

VARIATIONS OF NORMAL

Color changes in the mucosa depend upon the normal pigmentation of the skin, which may appear in varied hues depending upon racial and genetic factors. Racial pigmentation occurs to some degree in all ethnic groups and is due to an increase in melanin production, not to an increase in the number of melanocytes. Therefore, dark- and light-skinned individuals have a comparable number of melanocytes, with darker-skinned individuals producing more melanin than their lighter counterparts.

NAME: Physiologic pigmentation

Etiology: **Physiologic pigmentation** is usually found in the gingiva, but can occur throughout the mouth. Increased pigmentation may occur because of pregnancy and the increased levels of various hormones produced during pregnancy. Some pigmentation may occur in postmenopausal women taking hormone replacement therapy (HRT).

Method of Transmission: Not applicable

Epidemiology: There is no sex predilection or age preference related to physiologic pigmentation, and it may occur in any age group. Physiologic pigmentation is found most often in darker-skinned individuals. Approximately 5% of Caucasians are reported to have physiologic pigmentation.

Pathogenesis: Physiologic pigmentation occurs in certain individuals because of the tendency to produce melanin in varying amounts. The more production that occurs, the deeper the color, and depending upon the ethnicity of the individual, the color of the tissues will vary.

Just as the sun causes injury to the tissue, forcing us to produce more melanin and over time giving us tanned skin, the melanin production can occur in isolated areas, producing a focal pigmented area of tissue.

Extraoral Characteristics: Some pigmentation can occur extraorally and may be associated with disease states and with a genetic predisposition. These are discussed below in this chapter. Physiologic pigmentation may extend into the lip area as is seen in Figure 15.1A, which depicts the racial pigmentation of a black male. Note the inner lip pigmentation as well as the pigmentation around the gingival margin of tooth 27.

Perioral and Intraoral Characteristics: Oral melanin pigmentation may range from brown or black to dark blue. The deeper pigmentation is usually black. Figure 15.1B represents the physiologic pigmentation of the tongue. Figure 15.1C depicts the color variations in gingival tissue due to physiologic pigmentation.

Distinguishing Characteristics: Physiologic pigmented lesions do not blanch because they are due to melanin production and not to blood pooling within the tissues. In addition, the pigmentation is not caused by excess blood within a focal area such as the hematoma, ecchymosis, or petechiae that were discussed in Chapter 13.

Significant Microscopic Features: There is an increase of melanin pigmentation in **basal keratinocytes.** Melanin is also found in the connective tissue because of the dendritic processes of the melanocyte and the transfer of the melanin. The histologic section would show increased melanin in the epidermis, with unaltered numbers of melanocytes.

Dental Implications: Some patients complain about the cosmetic factors related to physiologic pigmentation when pigmentation is noticeable such as on the gingiva or perioral tissues. The tongue and gingiva may be visible when speaking and the appearance may be troublesome to the patient.

Differential Diagnosis: Pigmentation due to a serious disease should always be considered, such as the following:

1. Peutz-Jeghers syndrome, Chapters 10 and 15
2. Addison's disease, Chapter 7
3. Melanoma, Chapters 5 and 15

Treatment and Prognosis: The prognosis is excellent, and no treatment is required once a definitive diagnosis is confirmed. If the diagnosis is not clear and a clinical diagnosis cannot be made because the pigmentation

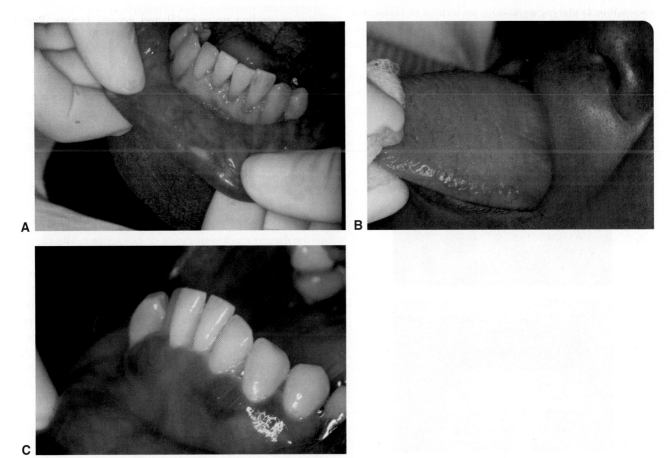

Figure 15.1. A. Physiologic pigmentation. **B.** Physiologic pigmentation of the tongue. **C.** Physiologic pigmentation of the gingiva.

does not exhibit the usual characteristics, further evaluation is needed. Follow-up should be performed when any changes occur that would require further examination.

Traumatic or Inflammatory Lesions

Traumatic lesions occur because of injury to the tissues, such as the amalgam that becomes embedded in the tissues during the restoration of a tooth, which produces a dark hue. Inflammatory pigmentation occurs because of chronic injury and assault to the tissue through the use of certain medications, chronic inflammation, or thermal changes. Certain chronic inflammatory diseases cause the body to react to constant injury or assault on the tissue by producing pigmentation. An example is the pigmentation sometimes produced because of chronic inflammation caused by oral lichen planus. Another example is the pigmentation caused by constant trauma to the tissue due to the heat and chemicals associated with smoking that result in smoker's melanosis.

Along with the common ways mentioned above, pigmentation may also occur from intentional incorporation of metallic particles used in some cultures as esthetic enhancement of the individual. Mani (1985) reported three cases of Ethiopian women who had tattooing of the upper gingivae performed as a traditional practice. Figure 15.2A shows intentional pigmentation, performed in childhood, of a 30-year-old female from Ethiopia. Figure 15.2B shows a 60-year-old woman from Arabia who has a tattoo on the lip, used to guard against bad luck.

In certain cultures this practice occurs, and clinicians who are in geographic areas where the practice is not known may mistake the tattooing for a type of pathology.

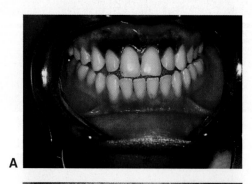

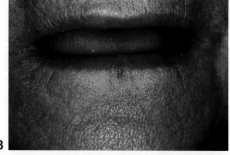

Figure 15.2.   A and **B.** Ethnic tattoo. (Courtesy of Dr. Doron Aframian.)

Tattooing of males is also practiced, but in this geographic location of Ethiopia, it is confined to the canines for males and more extensive gingival tattooing for the females. Intentional tattooing of this nature is performed in early childhood by using soot and abrasion of the tissue until the soot is embedded within the skin. This is accomplished after multiple attempts at abrasion and layering of the pigments.

The hygienist may observe a small oral tattoo on the lip, palate, or buccal mucosa caused by India ink or a graphite pencil. These unintentional tattoos are usually the result of childhood trauma and are most often caused by the child falling with a pen or pencil held in the mouth. Additionally, metal dust, broken dental burs, and any type of metal embedded into the tissue (such as titanium) may cause pigmentation through the release of ions. Several types of pigmented lesions are discussed in more depth in this section.

NAME: Amalgam tattoo (focal argyrosis)

Etiology: Amalgam tattoos occur because of amalgam particles becoming imbedded within the tissue.

Method of Transmission: Not applicable

Epidemiology: Amalgam tattoos may occur in all age groups, and there is no sex predilection.

Pathogenesis: Fragments of amalgam can become embedded within the tissues in several ways: Preparation of the tooth sometimes forces the particles down into the tissue; particles left in the surrounding areas could be driven down into the tissues by floss, routine tooth brushing, or scaling and polishing procedures. Additionally, endodontic procedures performed using amalgam can force the material into the tissues, and amalgam can fall into fresh extraction sites.

Extraoral Characteristics: Not applicable

Perioral and Intraoral Characteristics: The metal fragments are usually embedded in the surrounding tissue during tooth restoration or extractions. The clinical appearance of the amalgam tattoo remains within the areas that have been previously treated or in open wound areas. Therefore, you would expect to see the amalgam tattoos adjacent to a placed amalgam, previous restorative sites, or in a previous extraction site. Occasionally, the patient may have embedded amalgam fragments in uncommon areas, such as the buccal mucosa or floor of the mouth. The tissue becomes ulcerated or possibly has suffered an iatrogenic laceration during a dental procedure, allowing the fragments to become embedded in these unusual areas through breaks in the tissue.

The amalgam tattoo is diagnosed through both clinical appearance and radiographic appearance. Amalgam tattoos are usually localized, involving the gingiva and rarely the floor of the mouth. Since the tattoo is adjacent to previous amalgam restorations, the area that is involved is closer to the restoration and not in areas such as the floor of the mouth. The amalgam tattoo is localized and gray to blue/black and is found primarily on the gingivae and in areas next to restorative material. Confirmation can often be made with radiographs, and amalgam fragments may be seen on a radiograph.

Figure 15.3A shows an amalgam tattoo on the lower left gingiva. Figure 15.3B depicts amalgam fragments seen radiographically. Figure 15.3C depicts an amalgam tattoo in the retromolar area where amalgam entered the surgical site in the 2nd and 3rd molar region. Figure 15.3D shows amalgam fragments seen radiographically, and Figure 15.3E depicts an amalgam tattoo in the gingival tissue between the central and lateral teeth.

Distinguishing Characteristics: Opaque fragments of metal are apparent in radiographs where an amalgam tattoo is suspected and often confirm the diagnosis.

Significant Microscopic Features: Amalgam fragments embedded within the tissue specimen may be viewed through the microscope. Depending upon the age of the tattoo and the size of the discolored area, the fragments may be either focally located or dispersed throughout the specimen. Figure 15.3F depicts the histology of an amalgam tattoo. Particles of amalgam are evident, presenting as dark, opaque fragments.

Dental Implications: The cause of any pigmented area should be determined to rule out serious pathology such as melanoma.

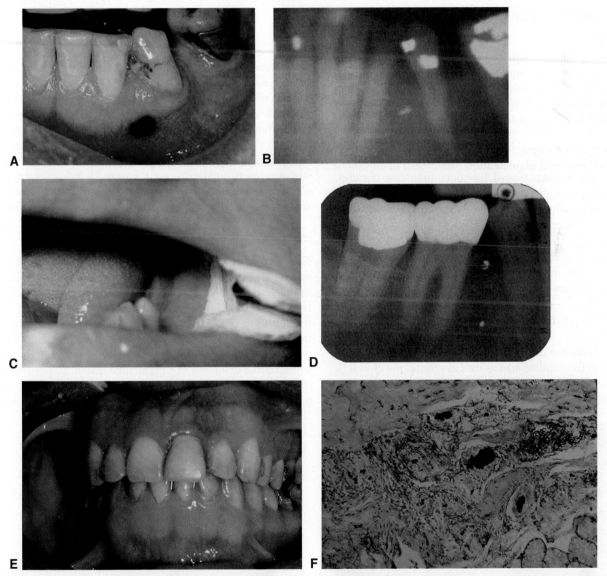

Figure 15.3. A. Amalgam tattoo. (Courtesy of Dr. William Carpenter) **B.** Amalgam tattoo seen on radiograph. (Courtesy of Dr. William Carpenter.) **C.** Amalgam tattoo. (Courtesy of Dr. Peter Jacobsen) **D.** Radiographic appearance of amalgam tattoo. **E.** Amalgam tattoo. (Courtesy of Dr. Peter Jacobsen) **F.** Histologic appearance of amalgam. (Courtesy of Dr. John Jacoway).

Differential Diagnosis: Early melanomas can sometimes be mistaken for amalgam tattoos, and this mistake has grave consequences for the patient. Further investigation is always warranted to rule out malignancy when there is any doubt regarding the cause.

Other considerations include:

1. Nevus, Chapter 15
2. Melanoma, Chapter 15
3. Cultural tattoos, Chapter 15

Treatment and Prognosis: No treatment is indicated for an amalgam tattoo, and the prognosis is excellent. The dental professional should document the location and clinical description of the tattoo and confirm the cause.

Other Metal Pigmentations

Metals can accumulate within the oral soft tissues as a result of either intentional or nonintentional systemic exposure or localized implantation. Some of these accumulations, such as the heavy metal pigmentations, are not seen very often anymore; others, such as titanium pigmentations, will become more common.

TITANIUM IMPLANTS

Implants have been placed for more than two decades, and the use of implants has become commonplace. Pigmentation of the oral tissue has been reported with regard to titanium plates used in maxillofacial surgery and with orthopedic implants. Breen and Stoker (1993) and Torgersen et al. (1995) have reported black staining from metallic wear and metal particles. Figure 15.4 depicts a patient who has multiple implants that have been in the mouth for 10 years or more. Note the gray-blue tissue around the gingiva and in the papillae from the canine to the first molar.

The tissue has a blue cast with some pigmentation occurring in the papillae area as well as around the crown. A blue-gray discoloration of tissue adjacent to titanium dental implants has occasionally been observed, apparently resulting from the accumulation of titanium ions in the tissue. The same phenomenon may account for some pigmentation found adjacent to dental amalgams, even though larger amalgam fragments may not be seen radiographically. Additionally, titanium dust may have been released during the original preparation of the crown for the implant. The titanium dust or particles may become dispersed through the tissue in differing degrees and exhibit the blue pigmentation that is present in Figure 15.4. Recent studies have reported cases of squamous cell carcinoma (SCC) around some dental implants in patients who have at least one known risk factor for SCC. Failing implants should be evaluated to rule out the presence of malignancy disguised as peri-implant disease (Czerninski et al., 2006). Additionally, abnormal appearances may indicate an existing problem, and the implant area should be watched carefully. Any ulceration or severe pigmentation may be a waring sign of further problems.

INTENTIONAL TATTOOING

Occasionally, the practitioner will find a patient who has had an oral tattoo. The patterns used may be objects or designs. Often a prime area for these tattoos is the oral vestibule tissue, since this area provides a flat, wider surface. Intentional tattooing is accomplished by using tattoo pens on the external surfaces of the body. Oral tattooing is less common than tattooing skin surfaces and often tissue piercing is involved as well. Figure 15.5 depicts a person who tattooed himself while viewing the area in a mirror, as evidenced by the inverted "N" seen in the lettering.

HEAVY METAL PIGMENTATION

Heavy metal pigmentation occurs with exposure to various types of heavy metals such as arsenic, bismuth, platinum, lead, silver, copper, and mercury; it can be problematic in the body and may cause pigmented lesions in the soft tissues. These are rarely seen because safety practices and regulations limit the use of heavy metals in the workplace and at home, but they should be considered in a differential diagnosis of a pigmented lesion. Exposure to these metals through excessive ingestion, inhalation, or prolonged cutaneous exposure may result in pigments ac-

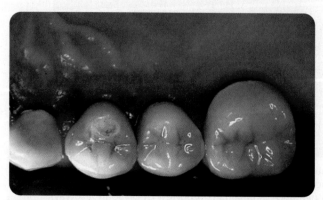

Figure 15.4. Titanium tattoo. (Courtesy of Dr. Terry Rees, Baylor College of Dentistry.)

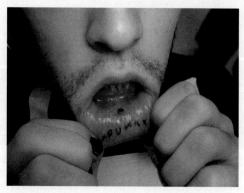

Figure 15.5. Intentional tattoo. (Courtesy of Dr. Kurt Summersgill.)

cumulating in the oral mucosa or in any cutaneous surface. Blood tests are always needed to determine the extent of the heavy metal accumulation in the body, and other procedures are needed to determine the amount of physical damage that the metals may have caused. Differential diagnoses include

1. **Argyria.** Argyria is the slate-gray or bluish discoloration of the skin caused by the accumulation of silver salts in the tissues. Silver was often used in the treatment of the nose and sinuses. Several metals are seen clinically as pigmentations and line stains. Discontinuing exposure to the metal is paramount. The prognosis is good when exposure is discontinued and the body levels of the substance are not high.

2. **Lead.** Lead poisoning in children, or **plumbism**, has been a significant problem in past decades and is usually due to environmental causes such as chipping paint, putty, plaster, pesticides, and lead-lined pipes. Lead line stain, sometimes referred to as Burtonian line, is often seen at the gingival margins when the lead proportion reaches certain levels. The common color of the line, often found in the premolar and molar gingiva, is blue, gray, or black. Figure 15.6 shows lead line stain along the gingival margins.

3. **Bismuth.** Bismuth was used to treat syphilis and produces a thin blue-black line. Diascopy may be used to differentiate heavy metals from common gingivitis around the margins. The lead line will become more accentuated when a glass slide is placed over the tissue, and the gingivitis line (due to inflammatory causes) will disappear (Lockhart, 1981). Further testing to confirm lead accumulation or differentiation from other heavy metals is needed, with blood levels documented.

PIGMENTATION ASSOCIATED WITH DRUGS

Oral pigmentation is associated with certain medications such as minocycline, tetracycline derivatives, azidothymidine (AZT), some oral contraceptives, hormone replacement medications, bleomycin, busulfan, clofazimine, and antimalarial medications. A wide range of such medications exists, with varying amounts of pigmentation produced. See Box 15.1 for a more extensive list of these medications and other substances.

NAME: Minocycline tissue staining (black bone staining)

Etiology: Minocycline tissue staining, or black bone staining, is caused by ingestion of minocycline, a semi-synthetic tetracycline that was introduced in the 1960s. The medication is used in the treatment of acne and other inflammatory and immune-mediated diseases. Since minocycline is a broad-spectrum antibiotic, it can be used in a wide variety of diseases. The medication is used in the treatment of acne and may be prescribed for long periods to treat the skin disorder. Dark staining of hard and soft tissues is associated with the medication when used long-

---

Box 15.1 — DRUGS AND OTHER SUBSTANCES CAUSING ORAL PIGMENTATION

Tobacco-related pigmentation
  Nicotine products
  Betel quid with tobacco
Addiction and "socially-used drugs"
  Heroin
  Bark and seed chewing
Heavy metals
  Lead
  Gold (chrysiasis)
  Silver (argyria)
  Arsenic
  Titanium
Hormone-related medications
  Oral contraceptives
  Hormone replacement therapy—Premarin
Antibiotics[a]
  Tetracycline
  Minocycline
Antimalarials
  Quinidine
  Chloroquine
Antitumor agents
  Busulfan (leukemia)
  Bleomycin
  Cyclophosphamide
  Nitrogen mustard
Medications used for specific diseases
  Zidovudine, AZT (antiviral treatment for AIDS)
  Ketoconazole (*Candida* infections, histoplasmosis)
  Clofazimine (leprosy)
  Amiodarone HCL (antidysrhythmic)

[a] Cephalosporins and penicillins may cause brown-black hairy tongue pigmentation due to *Candida* growth.

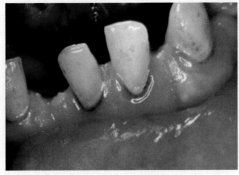

Figure 15.6. Lead-line stain. (Courtesy of Dr. Peter Lockhart, Carolinas Medical Center, Department of Oral Medicine.)

term. Studies suggest staining may occur not only with minocycline, but with other tetracycline-based medications as well. The oral manifestations of tetracycline staining have been well-documented.

Method of Transmission: Not applicable

Epidemiology: All age groups are affected; however, related staining is found more often in younger adults, since the medications are prescribed frequently in this age group and are widely used for the treatment of acne. There is no sex predilection.

Pathogenesis: Depending upon the medication, different sites may be affected orally and periorally. The alveolar area and bone areas of the gingiva (hard palate and attached gingiva) are affected most often with long-term use of minocycline. The staining occurs because of the accumulation of elements of the medication in the bone or the roots of the teeth that darken their color and thereby impart a darker color to the overlying tissues. These same elements can accumulate in soft tissues, also causing diffuse staining or deeper coloration.

Extraoral Characteristics: The sclera may become hyperpigmented, and the nail beds can exhibit staining as well. Pigmentation has been reported in other tissues such as the thyroid and the skin.

Perioral and Intraoral Characteristics: Minocycline pigmentation appears as generalized darker pigmented areas in the alveolar, palatal, and vestibule areas. Depending upon the severity of the staining, the lips may appear slightly darker or pigmented. Figure 15.7 depicts the accumulation of minocycline in the mucosa and bone, with a darkened area reaching the vestibule. The teeth exhibit a blue-gray color that is typical with this type of medication.

Distinguishing Characteristics: Minocycline staining manifests clinically as black to brown staining

that may be focal or generalized throughout the tissue toward the roots of the teeth.

Significant Microscopic Features: The typical microscopic features are fine brown spherical pigmented granules within the specimen.

Dental Implications: Minocycline that is prescribed for skin conditions over months or years may also affect the teeth and the oral mucosa. Patients may request bleaching and cosmetic dental procedures, depending upon the severity of the discoloration.

Differential Diagnosis: Physiologic pigmentation and disease states such as Addison's disease, melanoma, and Peutz Jeghers syndrome may have appearances similar to those of drug induced pigmentation such as minocycline staining.

Treatment and Prognosis: No treatment is needed, but discontinuing the medication when possible would diminish further staining. The prognosis is good when the medication is discontinued and further staining is not permitted.

AZT (ZIDOVUDINE, OR RETROVIR)

The buccal mucosa, tongue, palate, and nail beds may be affected with the use of zidovudine (AZT) for the treatment of AIDS. AZT may cause nail pigmentation in addition to mucosal pigmented areas such as those shown in Figure 15.8, which depicts heavy pigmentation of the tongue of a patient taking AZT for the treatment of AIDS.

NAME: Tobacco associated melanosis

Etiology: Tobacco-associated melanosis (smoker's melanosis) is caused by the use of tobacco products that stimulate the production of melanocytes within the tissue. Melanin functions as a defense mechanism against toxic agents penetrating the oral mucosa. Tobacco may be used in many different forms and is most often smoked or

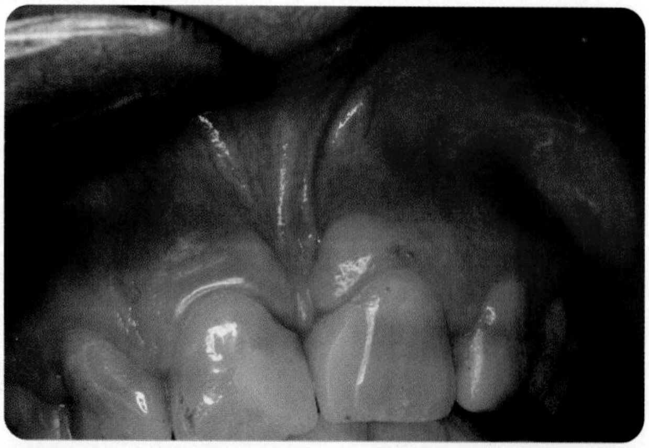

Figure 15.7. Minocycline—black bone staining. (Courtesy of Dr. Michael Brennan.)

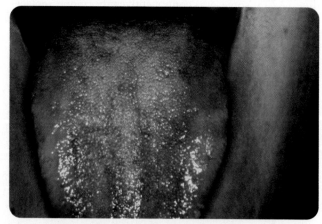

Figure 15.8. Pigmentation on the tongue from the use of AZT in the treatment of AIDS. (Courtesy of Dr. Terry Rees.)

chewed. Tobacco contains known carcinogens, and its relationship to oral cancer is well documented.

Method of Transmission: Smoker-associated melanosis is not contagious, since it is tobacco related.

Epidemiology: A higher percentage of women, especially those using contraceptives, is associated with smoker's melanosis. This is due to the increased hormone level associated with the development of melanosis in women. Any age group may be affected.

Pathogenesis: Smoking-associated melanosis is related to a component in tobacco that stimulates melanocytes to produce melanin. Since melanin is produced as a protective mechanism, toxic substances cause melanin to be produced to protect the tissue from heat and toxins. Most areas of the mucosa, gingiva, and palate can be affected. Women in childbearing years are more affected, supporting the role of a hormonal influence in the degree of pigmentation.

Extraoral Characteristics: Depending upon the degree of pigmentation, the lips may be affected, and the perioral tissue at the wet line of the lips may be involved. Existing physiologic pigmentation may be deepened as well.

Perioral and Intraoral Characteristics: Usually, light pigmentation occurs with the labial gingiva since this is a target region. The degree of pigmentation is associated with the amount of tobacco used and the physiologic component of the individual. Figure 15.9 shows smoking-associated melanosis, with the soft palate exhibiting the characteristic light brown pigmentation that is diffuse through the area. The tongue is also pigmented a soft brown with elongation of the filiform papillae.

Distinguishing Characteristics: The pigmentation that is produced has a diffuse, light brown color. Other disease states might have a similar appearance; therefore careful consideration of other possibilities and health states is very important in a final diagnosis.

Significant Microscopic Features: Increases in melanin production are evident in basal keratinocytes. The microscopic appearance is similar to that seen in physiologic pigmentation.

Dental Implications: Any tobacco product use increases the risk of oral cancer. Careful follow-up with the patient is crucial, and the patient should be educated about oral cancer and taught to do an oral cancer self-screening examination (see Clinical Protocol 11). Smoking cessation should be recommended by the hygienist and the dentist. If the office does not have a smoking cessation program, the patient should be referred to a special smoking cessation clinic. Many such clinics are associated with dental schools, hospitals, and private individuals. See Box 15.2 for a list of existing clinics and programs that enable the clinician to become certified as a tobacco treatment specialist.

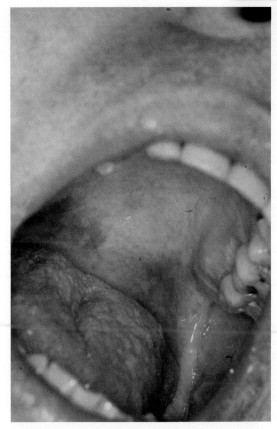

Figure 15.9. Smoking-associated melanosis of the soft palate with tongue pigments.

Differential Diagnosis: The following disease states have similar pigmentation appearances and should be considered:

1. Peutz-Jeghers syndrome, Chapter 10
2. Physiologic pigmentation, Chapter 15
3. Addison's disease, Chapter 10
4. Laugier-Hunziker syndrome, Chapter 15
5. Medication induced, Chapter 15

Treatment and Prognosis: Smoking cessation is the most appropriate treatment. Discontinued use of tobacco products results in less pigmentation and, finally, resolution in most cases. The prognosis is excellent when the patient stops using tobacco products. Long-term tobacco use in any form dramatically increases the patient's chance of oral cancer.

BETEL QUID USE

Tobacco is used in other forms, many of which have cultural origins. Tobacco is often combined with betel leaf in what is called a "**quid**." The term *quid* refers to a mixture of substances placed in the mouth and remaining in contact with the mucosa, usually containing one or both of the two basic ingredients, tobacco or areca nut, in raw or any manufactured or processed form (Zain et al., 1996). The betel quid is considered a specific variety of quid that

Box 15.2   SMOKING CESSATION CLINICS AND NATIONAL CONTACT INFORMATION

ORGANIZATIONS:

American Cancer Society
800 ACS-2345
www.cancer.org

American Heart Association
(800) 242-8721
www.americanheart.org

American Lung Association
(800) 586-4872
www.lungusa.com

Centers for Disease Control
www.cdc.gov/tobacco

The Oral Cancer Foundation
http://www.oralcancerfoundation.org

The World Health Organization
http://www.who.int/tobacco/en/

INTERNET RESOURCES

www.quitnet.org
www.webmd.com
www.outrageavenue.com
www.trytostop.org
National Registry and Master List of Certified Tobacco
   Treatment Specialists
http://www.umassmed.edu/behavmed/tobacco/specialists.cfm
American Dental Hygienists' Association in partnership
   with the Smoking Cessation Leadership Center
http://www.askadviserefer.org

MEDICAL AND DENTAL SCHOOLS PROVIDING SMOKING CESSATION CLINICS AND *TRAINING FOR PROFESSIONALS AS CERTIFIED TOBACCO TREATMENT SPECIALISTS

Baylor College of Dentistry, Dallas, Texas
214-828-8379
www.tambcd.edu/education
214-828-8379 (Smoking Cessation Clinic)

*The University of Medicine and Dentistry of New Jersey
   Tobacco Dependence Clinic
http://www.tobaccoclinic.org/
http://tobaccoprogram.org/trainreg5day.htm

*The University of Massachusetts Medical School
http://umassmed.edu/behavmed/tobacco/quit.cfm

*The University of Mississippi Medical Center
http://actcenter.umc.edu/

*Mayo Clinic-Rochester, Minnesota
http://mayoclinic.org/stop-smoking/rsttreatment.html
*http://mayoresearch.mayo.edu/mayo/research/ndc_
   education/tts_certification.cfm*
Tobacco Treatment Specialist Program 1-800-344-5984
The Mayo Clinic Nicotine Dependence Center Education
   Program, Rochester, Minn.
1-800-344-5984

Mayo Clinic-Jacksonville, Florida
http://mayoclinic.org/stop-smoking/

Mayo Clinic-Scottsdale, Arizona
http://mayoclinic.org/stop-smoking/scttreatment.html

Carolinas Healthcare System
http://www.carolinashealthcare.org/services/cancer/smoking.cfm
704-355-7808

*Facilities offering training for tobacco treatment specialists.

uses the betel leaf. Usually, there is a mixture of areca nut, slaked lime, catechu, several condiments such as flavoring agents, and often tobacco, wrapped in a betel leaf. Figure 15.10A depicts the ingredients used in a betel quid. The ingredients are placed on the leaf and then rolled into a quid. Figure 15.10B shows a finished quid.

Additionally, combinations of these products with or without tobacco may be used; some may be in the form of quid and others may be chewed, smoked, or rubbed into the oral tissues. Residents in Asia, Taiwan, Papua New Guinea, India, and neighboring countries commonly practice the use of these products. The quid is placed in the

mouth and held for extended periods. Quid is addictive, and the practice is culturally driven as well. When coupled with alcohol use, a person's chance of oral cancer is increased (Nair et al., 2004). A quid-induced lesion is associated with pigmentation, usually observed after long-term use and sometimes after only brief encounters with the products (Sarswathi et al., 2003). Tobacco with lime, betel quid with tobacco, betel quid without tobacco, and areca nut have been classified as carcinogenic to humans.

Oral submucosa fibrosis (OSF) is a premalignant condition seen predominantly in Southeast Asia with the use of betel nut, areca nut, and tobacco products discussed

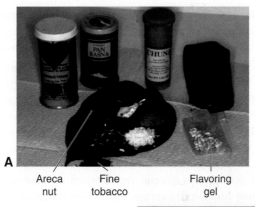
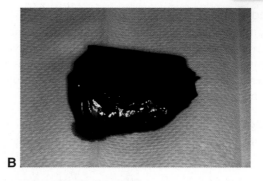

Areca nut   Fine tobacco   Flavoring gel

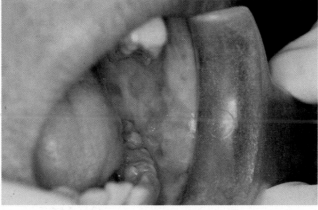

Figure 15.10. A. Betel quid use. **B.** Quid. **C.** Submucosa fibrosa with pigmentation. (Courtesy of Dr. John Jacoway.)

above. The mucosa loses its elasticity, and dense fibrous bands can often be palpated. It is typically progressive, and some patients develop carcinoma. Submucosa fibrosis may even be observed in the young, who may have only used quid products for a short period (Nair et al., 2004). Figure 15.10C depicts a 54-year-old woman from India who has used betel quid from late adolescence and was diagnosed with OSF. The pigmentation and white striation in the buccal mucosa region is due to the extensive use of betel quid. Often noted as well is the wrinkled appearance, thickening of the mucosa, and occasionally ulceration.

Betel quid use is becoming more common in the United States, increasing the likelihood that clinicians will observe this type of lesion in their practices. Also being introduced in the United States is the use of the sweet, flavored cigarettes called Bidis. Other tobacco products once found only in other countries are now more common in the United States. Careful counseling regarding the potential danger of the use of the products is clearly indicated.

CONGENITAL OR GENETIC DISORDERS

Congenital or genetic disorders are discussed thoroughly in Chapter 6. Chapter 23 presents the cutaneous pigmented-type lesions and the benign and malignant forms that may be part of the extraoral examination. However, some nevi may be perioral, affecting the lip area, and some are found intraorally. The patient may also, on occasion, have lip involvement that may affect the wet line of oral tissues.

NAME: Nevus

Etiology: Nevus (pl., nevi) is commonly referred to as a mole and infrequently seen orally. It is also known as pigmented nevus, melanocytic nevus, and nevomelanocytic nevus. The nevus is classified as benign but may appear similar to the early stage of melanoma. There are several different forms of a nevus including, in order of their frequency, the **intramucosal nevus,** the **blue nevus,** the **compound nevus,** and the **junctional nevus.** The pigmented intraoral lesion is also sometimes referred to as mucosal nevomelanocytic nevus, or melanocytic nevi. There is a genetic predisposition to the nevus, and most adults have from 20 to 40 distinguishable nevi present on the observable external skin surfaces.

Method of Transmission: Not applicable

Epidemiology: All age groups are affected with common moles, and many appear during childhood. However, individuals in predominately the third and fourth decades are most often reported and probably seek treatment for skin lesions at this time. There is no sex predilection. Approximately 20% are nonpigmented. Most nevi are located above the waist, with the head and neck affected most often. Most nevi are less than 6 mm in diameter. Caucasians are affected most often, followed by Asians and blacks. The intramucosal nevus is rare but may occur, causing concern because of the similar appearance of a malignant melanoma.

Pathogenesis: The nevus occurs from nevus cells in the epithelium, the basement membrane, the connective tissue, or a combination of these. Nevi are believed to originate because of melanocyte migration from the neural crest to the epithelium and dermis; or additionally, from the proliferation of melanocytes.

Extraoral Characteristics: The nevus may occur on any cutaneous surface. The extraoral nevus is discussed further in Chapter 23.

Perioral and Intraoral Characteristics: The intramucosal nevus is rare. Nevi are usually found in the palatal region and, to a lesser degree, in the buccal mucosa. Nevi may be seen clinically in shades of gray, brown, and blue. They are usually well circumscribed and slightly raised. The blue nevus is the second most frequent melanocytic nevus seen orally, accounting for 19–36% of all oral nevi. Blue nevi usually occur on the palate, followed by the buccal mucosa, and have been reported to become malignant in some instances. Because of the slight possibility of malignant transformation, all intraoral nevi are removed surgically. This is not only because of the transformation possibility but because it would be impossible to clinically differentiate a pigmented nevus from a melanoma.

Distinguishing Characteristics: A distinguishing characteristic of the nevus is the pigmented color of the lesion. Additionally, any nevus lesion may be elevated and should be recorded in three-dimensional documentation, such as 2 × 2 × 3 mm.

Significant Microscopic Features: Nevi are classified according to the location of the nevus cells in relation to the basal cell membrane. For instance, a junctional nevus is found between the epithelium and the connective tissue. A compound nevus has nevus cells that have proliferated with groups of cells that drop off into the underlying dermis. Since cells are now not only in the basement membrane, but also in the underlying dermis, they are referred to as a compound nevus. The third classification is the **intradermal nevus** or **intramucosal nevus**, and the nests are found in the connective tissue. When the nevus is found in the oral tissue, it is referred to as an intramucosal nevus. Figure 15.11A shows a nevus in the palatal region. Figure 15.11B shows the histology of the intramucosal nevus. Note the increased pigmentation of the nevus cells within the tissue. Figure 15.11C depicts the blue nevus.

Dental Implications: Although the cutaneous nevus is monitored and usually not removed unless suspicious, the intraoral nevus must be differentiated from a

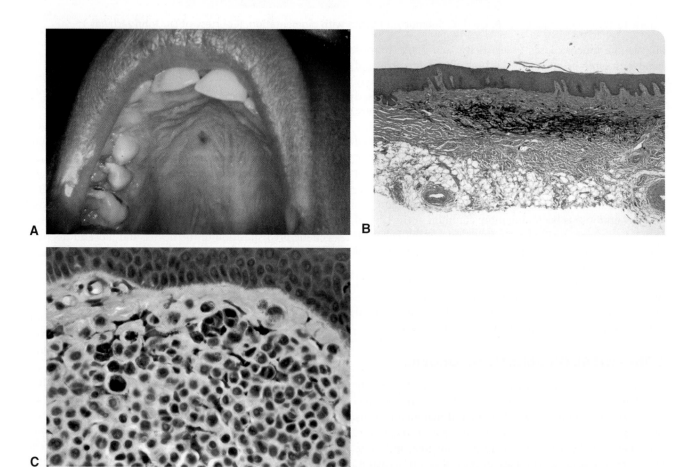

Figure 15.11. A. Palatal nevus. (Courtesy of Dr. Jeff Burkes) **B.** Histology of an intramucosal nevus. (Courtesy of Dr. John Wright) **C.** Histology of a blue nevus. (Courtesy of Dr. John Wright.)

melanoma through removal and biopsy. Melanoma is highly malignant and must be treated rapidly and totally removed.

Differential Diagnosis: Considerations include

1. Amalgam tattoos, Chapter 15
2. Melanoma, Chapter 15
3. Kaposi's sarcoma, Chapter 22
4. Hemangioma, Chapter 13

Treatment and Prognosis: Biopsy performed on the intraoral nevus, which is usually totally removed during the surgery.

NAME: Oral melanotic macule (focal melanosis)

Etiology: A focal pigmented lesion that occurs on the lip or the intraoral tissues is referred to as an oral melanotic macule or labial melanotic macule.

Method of Transmission: Not applicable

Epidemiology: Labial melanotic macules (occurring on the lips) most often are seen in childhood and the 20 to 30 age group. The intraoral lesions usually occur in patients older than 40. However, they may occur at any age and affect approximately 3% of the population, with the lip being the most common location. Focal melanosis is more commonly found in women.

Pathogenesis: The melanosis occurs on the vermillion border of the lip or the gingiva, because of postinflammatory or posttraumatic causes. Melanotic macules usually arise from three sources: an intraoral freckle, postinflammatory pigmentation, or disorders such as Addison's disease, Peutz-Jeghers syndrome, or Laugier-Hunziker syndrome.

Extraoral Characteristics: The macules appear as single lesions that are pigmented, flat, and well delineated.

Perioral and Intraoral Characteristics: Melanotic macules that occur on the buccal mucosa are usually multiple. The macules are most often seen on the lip, followed by the palate and gingival and buccal mucosa. When occurring on the lip, the appearance is that of a freckle, known as an **ephelis**. Ephelides (pl.) tend to be less than 0.5 cm and are associated with sun exposure, in contrast to the focal melanotic macule, which is not associated with solar damage. Figure 15.12A depicts a melanotic macule on the lip of a female. Figure 15.12B shows a melanotic macule on the lip of a male.

Ephelides are usually found in fair-skinned individuals, are due to sunlight exposure, occur in childhood, and have a tendency to diminish with age. The ephelides may be indistinguishable from melanotic macules without viewing them under the microscope. Histologically, ephelides have fewer melanocytes but have more melanosomes, which are larger in size. Using a sunscreen of 15 SPF will help to fade the ephelis. In contrast, **solar lentigos** are usually seen in older individuals, are much larger than ephelides, and tend to persist indefinitely even with sun protection (see Chapter 23). The macules are larger and appear more pigmented than ephelides. A good example is the backs of the hands of a fair individual who has been exposed to the sun over a period of time.

Distinguishing Characteristics: The melanotic macules are usually brown, deep blue/black, or black, and they are well-circumscribed with sharp, delineated borders.

Significant Microscopic Features: Melanin in the basal cell layer, lamina propria, or both are microscopic characteristics of a macule.

Dental Implications: When changes occur with these lesions, such as increased growth or shape, there could be a suspicion of a lesion that is characterized by early atypical melanocytes called **lentigo maligna**. These lesions exhibit atypical melanocytes in the epidermis with potential to invade the dermis layer. Changes in size, color, or border irregularity must be viewed with suspicion. These lesions are often seen on the faces of older individuals. The possibility of melanoma is always of concern with any lesion change, whether the macule is a freckle, melanotic

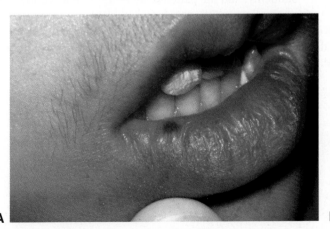

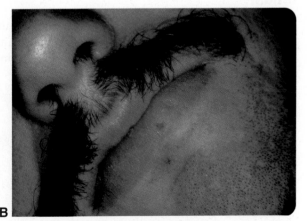

Figure 15.12. A. Macule. (Courtesy of Dr. Peter Jacobsen) **B.** Melanotic macule (Courtesy of Dr. E.J. Burkes.)

macule, or a lentigo maligna. Synonyms for the melanotic macules are Hutchinson freckle and melanotic freckle.

Differential Diagnosis: The differentiation of focal melanosis and ephelis is a prime consideration, and the following disease states are part of the differential diagnosis:

1. Addison's disease, Chapter 7
2. Peutz-Jeghers syndrome, Chapter 10
3. Laugier-Hunziker syndrome, Chapter 15
4. Melanoma, Chapter 15

Disease Associated Melanosis

Certain diseases are known to have hyperpigmentation as a characteristic. The different types of disease-associated melanosis listed below are highly correlated with oral pigmentation and are of prime concern in a differential diagnosis:

1. Addison's disease, Chapter 7
2. Peutz-Jeghers syndrome, Chapter 7
3. Lung diseases
4. Chronic lichen planus, Chapters 13 and 14
5. Polyostotic fibrous dysplasia, Chapter 10
6. Laugier-Hunziker syndrome, Chapter 15
7. Neurofibromatosis, Chapter 17
8. Albright's syndrome, Chapter 10
9. Kaposi's sarcoma, Chapter 23

Although all of the above-mentioned diseases are not discussed in detail here, they are mentioned in the general pathology section in relation to endocrine function and genetic disorders. Chapters 7 and 10 cover both endocrine and other diseases of concern in dentistry. The prognosis for the oral melanotic macule is excellent, and they are followed and monitored through documentation and photographs. No treatment is needed unless a biopsy is indicated because of changes or there is a question regarding the etiology of the macule.

NAME: Laugier-Hunziker syndrome (LHS, idiopathic lenticular mucocutaneous pigmentation)

Etiology: Some diseases and disorders have an unknown etiology with no history of a genetic or congenital etiology. One such disease, **Laugier-Hunziker syndrome**, has a distinct characteristic of pigmentation that mimics several of the pigmented lesions mentioned above. LHS is an acquired, benign, macular hyperpigmentation of the lips and oral mucosa, as well as nail pigmentation (Siponen and Salo, 2003). Although it is a benign condition, LHS may be confused with other pigmented diseases, and an incorrect diagnosis may occur. The patient may be treated for far more serious disease states.

Method of Transmission: Not applicable

Epidemiology: LHS was first described in 1970 with cases reported mostly in Caucasian populations. Women are affected more frequently than men, and the average age is reported to be 52.

Pathogenesis: LHS is thought to be linked to a functional alteration of the melanocytes that induce increased synthesis of melanosomes and their subsequent transport to the basal layer cells. The cause is unknown (Siponen and Salo, 2003).

Extraoral Characteristics: Nail involvement occurs in approximately 50% of patients. Figure 15.13A depicts a woman diagnosed with LHS with nail pigmentation.

Perioral and Intraoral Characteristics: Dark brown pigmentation is most often seen on the buccal mucosa and lips. The hard and the soft palate may also be involved and less frequently, the gingiva and the floor of the mouth. Figure 15.13B shows the same woman with pigmentation throughout the lip area. Figure 15.13C depicts the woman with pigmentation in the buccal mucosa.

Distinguishing Charactistics: The nail pigmentation is characteristic, containing bands or streaks of pigmentation. Racial pigmentation occurring orally or in the nails is not usually seen in Caucasians.

Significant Microscopic Features: Microscopically, basilar melanosis with increased numbers of melanophages in the lamina propria is normally present.

Dental Implications: The pigmentation may occur suddenly, and the patient may be apprehensive about the cause. Because the syndrome is often not recognized as LHS, the patient may face extensive testing, and the symptoms may be confused with many other disease states.

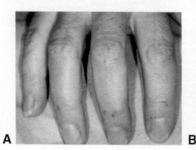 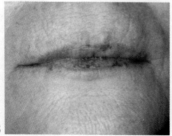 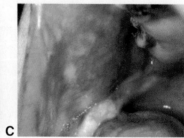

Figure 15.13. A–C. Laugier-Hunziker syndrome. (Courtesy of Dr. Maria Siponen).

Differential Diagnosis: Diseases that have pigmentation as a characteristic should be considered, such as

1. Addison's disease, Chapter 7
2. Peutz-Jeghers syndrome, Chapter 10
3. Smoking-associated melanosis, Chapter 15
4. Medications that produce pigmentation, Chapter 15
5. Physiologic pigmentation, Chapter 15
6. Heavy metal pigmentation, Chapter 15
7. Postinflammatory disorders, Chapter 15

Peutz-Jeghers disease involves gastrointestinal polyps, pigmentation of the hands and feet, gastrointestinal carcinoma, and genital and mammary tumors, thus differentiation is crucial to seeking treatment for patients with Peutz-Jeghers disease. Because of the pigmentation in both disorders, diagnostic differentiation is often a problem. Chapter 10, "Respiratory, Gastrointestinal, Neurologic, and Skeletal Disorders," includes a full description of this type of pigmentation.

Treatment and Prognosis: The syndrome is benign, but its importance is relevant to being included in the differential diagnoses of pigmentary disorders of the oral mucosa, since it may be confused with more serious diseases such as Addison's disease (Chapter 7) and Peutz-Jeghers disease. The correct diagnosis will avoid unnecessary tests, anxiety for the patient, and treatments that would not be needed.

NEOPLASMS

Neoplasms associated with pigmented lesions are rare and very aggressive, with an unpredictable pattern. The most common pigmented neoplasm in the oral cavity is the melanoma. Skin or external lesions are more common, but any pigmented lesion must be assessed to rule out the possibility of a malignancy. Oral melanoma is discussed next in this chapter and is also discussed as a cutaneous melanoma lesion fully in Chapter 5 and in Chapter 23 on skin diseases.

NAME: Oral melanoma

Etiology: Malignant oral melanomas of the head and neck region are rare and account for 0.2–0.5% of all melanomas (Sciubba, 2003; Meleti et al., 2006). The cutaneous melanoma rate is more pronounced in certain areas of the world where the sun is more intense. Oral melanoma occurs in the oral tissues that are not exposed to the sun, and the etiology is very different for oral melanomas and not as clearly understood. Although the etiology of the oral melanoma is unknown, tobacco use (Meleti, 2006), chronic irritation, formaldehyde exposure, familial history, and cytogenetic defects may play some role in its development. Most oral melanomas are preceded by a pigmented area, usually in the palate or the maxillary gingiva.

Method of Transmission: Not applicable

Epidemiology: Oral melanoma accounts for approximately 0.02–8% of all melanomas in Europe and the United States and 5% of all oral malignancies (Gao Man Gu et al., 2003). Melanomas usually occur in the fourth decade or later, with an average age of 56 (Barker et al., 1997), and the occurrence is extremely rare in children and young adults. Oral melanomas occur slightly more often in males. The rate of cutaneous melanomas among the young has dramatically increased in the past few years, and this continuing increase is discussed further in Chapter 23 on skin diseases. Ethnicity is a factor associated with the development of melanomas in general. For example, more melanomas are found in Japan (Takagi, 1974) and Uganda, with Native Americans and Latinos exhibiting higher rates in the United Sates. Tomicic and Wanebo (2003) suggest that the rarity of the melanoma makes progression in treatment difficult and advances slow. Researchers suggest that of those who were born in the year 2000, one in 75 persons will develop cutaneous melanoma in their lifetime, compared with only 4 in 10 million persons who will be diagnosed with oral melanoma. Oral melanomas are preceded by an area of melanosis 30–50% of the time (Kahn, 2005).

Pathogenesis: Sunlight, the environment and even genetic factors appear to influence the development and progression of melanomas. Several subtypes of melanomas exist: The in situ melanoma and the invasive-type melanoma. The in situ type may exist in a localized growth phase for months or years before becoming a more invasive form of melanoma with vertical growth patterns. The absence of pain in many cases is a factor in the failure of the patient to seek treatment, which results in not diagnosing a lesion until the later stages, which are associated with a poorer prognosis.

Extraoral Characteristics: The cutaneous lesions related to melanoma are discussed in Chapter 23 and in Chapter 5.

Perioral and Intraoral Characteristics: The most commonly affected sites are the hard palate and maxillary gingiva. The melanoma is usually a brown, red, black, and even black-bluish color and may be slightly raised, with irregular borders. The lesions may have a rapid growth pattern, with a deep invasive nature. Melanoma may appear exophytic or ulcerative, and the colors may be mixed, depending upon the stage of the neoplasm. Asymmetry and irregular borders are key signs related to melanomas. Enlarging masses whether pigmented or, as stated above, amelanotic (those that are more flesh color) lesions should have a biopsy performed to determine the diagnosis. Figure 15.14A depicts a malignant melanoma of the gingiva. Figure 15.14B depicts a malignant melanoma in the posterior retromolar area and buccal mucosa area. Figure 15.14C depicts the histologic specimen demonstrating malignant melanocytes.

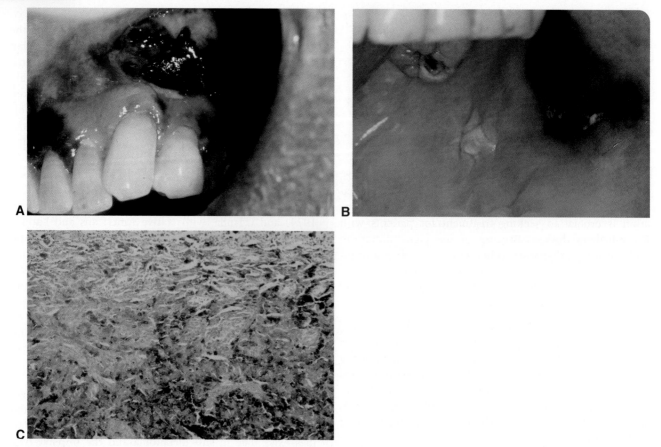

Figure 15.14. A and **B.** Melanoma. (Courtesy of Dr. John Jacoway) **C.** Histology of a melanoma. (Courtesy of Dr. John Jacoway.)

Although this discussion concerns pigmented lesions, in some cases melanomas may be light-colored as well, blending into the surrounding tissue, and may be referred to as an **amelanotic melanoma**. Some pigmentation may also be interspersed in the lesions and may precede the actual clinical manifestation of the amelanotic melanoma. Figure 15.15A depicts an amelanotic melanoma. Note the pigmented areas as well as the bulbous, papillary gingival tissue.

Distinguishing Characteristics: The intraoral melanoma may appear as a dark blue to black pigmented area with irregular borders increasing as the lesion continues to expand.

Significant Microscopic Features: The pathology shows malignant proliferation of melanocytes. Figure 15.15B shows the histology of the lesions, displaying a radical growth phase. The tumor is spreading laterally

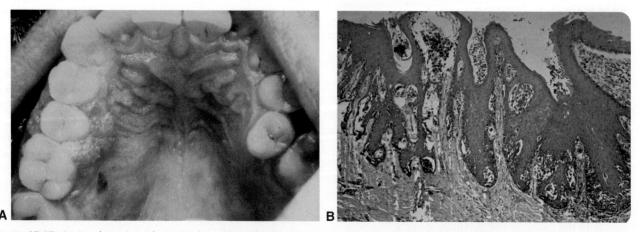

Figure 15.15. A. Amelanotic melanoma. (Courtesy of the U. S. Department of Veteran's Affairs.) **B.** Histology of an amelanotic melanoma. (Courtesy of the U. S. Department of Veteran's Affairs.)

APPLICATION

When a pigmented area is noticed anywhere in the mouth, several steps should be followed to determine the etiology of the area in question:

1. Is the pigmented lesion location one that follows the pattern of a specific known lesion? An example is a blue-black area that is adjacent to an amalgam. The likely diagnosis would be an amalgam tattoo. A blue-black lesion in the palate would not follow the normal pattern or location of an amalgam tattoo.
2. Is the lesion vascular or nonvascular? Does the lesion blanch? If the lesion does not blanch (using diascopy), the clinician categorizes the lesion as nonvascular.
3. Is the lesion erosive or does it have the appearance of an inflammatory lesion? Again, the lesion would be categorized as inflammatory or noninflammatory.
4. Does the health history indicate a disease state that might produce pigmented oral lesions such as Addison's disease or Peutz-Jeghers disease?
5. Does the patient know that the lesion is present? If so, further questioning may lead to a more definitive diagnosis. A childhood pencil injury in the palate is a prime example that may be discovered when fully questioning the patient.
6. If a radiograph has been taken, is there evidence in the radiograph, such as radiolucent spots suggesting metal fragments?
7. Do you have a photograph that was taken previously to offer a comparison?
8. Is there documented evidence of the previous size or shape of the lesion?
9. Upon questioning the patient, is there anything in the health history that would warrant the investigation of any disease states?
10. Are you able to confirm the cause of this lesion?
11. Is referral for a biopsy needed? Is follow-up recommended?

through the epithelium. The rounded collections of cells are the malignant melanocytes.

Dental Implications: The intraoral melanoma is a deadly lesion that should be recognized and removed in its earliest stage. Early melanomas may be confused with other pigmented lesions, and the poor prognosis has been attributed to the fact that there is often a delay in recognizing the lesion as a melanoma. Additionally, there is confusion with other lesions that are benign, causing a delay in treatment. Since pain is not a feature of the lesion, the patient may present at much later stages.

Differential Diagnosis: Several pigmented lesions should be evaluated when a diagnosis is being considered, including

1. Intramucosal nevus, Chapter 15
2. Amalgam tattoo, Chapter 15
3. Kaposi's sarcoma, Chapter 22
4. Physiologic pigmentation, Chapter 15
5. Melanotic macule, Chapter 15

Treatment and Prognosis: The rich vascular network found in the oral tissues makes the oral melanoma very aggressive with a much poorer prognosis; therefore, any pigmented lesion in the oral cavity should be viewed with suspicion. The growth rate and the tendency of oral melanomas to metastasize remain high. Therefore, early detection and treatment is of extreme importance. Excision of the oral melanoma is the course of action, with wide surgical margins because recurrence is common. Clear margins are critical in this type of neoplasm. Chemotherapy and radiation for head and neck cancers may be used as well, depending upon the size, location, and progressive nature of the lesion. Promising techniques are being used in some forms of cancer with **biologic therapy** that stimulates or restores the ability of the immune system to fight cancer, infections, and other disease states.

Oral melanomas are associated with a poor prognosis because of the tendency to metastasize to other organs and tissues. Five-year survival rates vary, with reports from 4.5 to 29%. Meleti et al. (2006) suggest that there is a 5-year survival rate of approximately 15%.

SUMMARY

- Physiologic pigmentation is a variant of normal. Physiologic pigmentation is found in varying degrees in all ethnic groups.
- Oral pigmentation is essentially due to: (1) the number of melanocytes, (2) the amount of melanin produced, or (3) the incorporation of a foreign substance introduced into the oral and perioral tissues.
- Amalgam tattoos result in amalgam particles within the oral tissues that produce a gray, blue, or black hue. Amalgam fragments may be seen on radiographs, which aids in the definitive diagnosis of an amalgam tattoo.
- A blue-gray pigmented area may be found from intentional tattooing performed in some cultures by using soot and metal dust, usually performed during childhood.
- Pigmentation appearance may occur in conjunction with some titanium implants.
- Minocycline staining, also referred to as black bone staining, results from injection of minocycline, which is a semisynthetic derivative of tetracycline. This medication is often used in the treatment of acne in adolescents and young adults.
- Tobacco-associated melanosis results from the long-term use of tobacco products. A soft brown pigmentation is produced, usually in the palate and buccal mucosa.
- Submucosus fibrosis is caused by betel quid and tobacco that is used in some cultures, and it is considered a premalignant condition.

- Heavy metal pigmentation is caused by the ingestion of heavy metals such as lead, bismuth, arsenic, and mercury. The exposure is usually occupational and occurs commonly through vapors. The disposition of lead in the tissue is referred to as "lead-line staining" and appears as a line at the gingival margin of the teeth.
- A nevus is commonly referred to as a mole. There are several classifications of the nevus: junctional, compound, intramucosal, and the blue nevus.
- The nevus found in oral tissues is called the intramucosal nevus.
- Oral melanotic macules or focal melanosis (freckles) are described as benign pigmented lesions and are usually found on the lips and the palate regions. The pigmentation may be associated with inflammation or sometimes disease states such as Peutz-Jeghers syndrome or Addison's disease.
- Certain disease states are associated with pigmented lesions and pigmented perioral tissue: Addison's disease, McCune-Albright disease, Peutz-Jeghers disease, and Laugier-Hunziker syndrome.
- The melanoma appears as a painless, usually fast-growing, blue-black lesion with a predilection for the gingiva. The amelanotic melanoma appears as more flesh colored, although some prior pigmented area is usually reported.
- Any pigmented lesion should be investigated and have a cause established.

Critical Thinking Activity

Figure 15.16 depicts a heavily pigmented area of the palate. The patient is a 40-year-old female who is a new patient. Pigmented areas are also found on the fingers of the patient, the lips, and the buccal mucosa.

1. What questions would you want to ask the patient during your examination of the oral tissues?
2. What facts would you expect to see on the health history that would help you make a determination or perhaps rule out a possible cause?
3. What external lesions would concern you or make you curious?

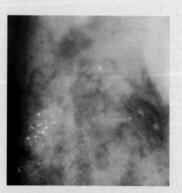

Figure 15.16. Critical thinking activity. (Courtesy of Dr. Maria Siponen)

PORTFOLIO 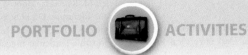 ACTIVITIES

- Develop a set of standards for your office on intraoral photographs to monitor lesions. If you do not have an intraoral photography system in place, discuss the benefits of having such a system with your peers and other staff members. Perhaps a short document on the benefits to both the patients and the staff for long-term health and for legal purposes could be a marketing tool for your office. Since many offices do not have a photography protocol for the office, this could be a major asset for your office.

- Research and make a list of the types of medications, diseases, and chemicals that may produce pigmented lesions. Use this chapter and other resources.
- Determine local dermatologists in your neighboring area who would like to have referrals from your office when a patient is found to need further evaluation. Your office may provide literature on common skin lesions and ways that they can protect themselves and family members from sun damage. See Clinical Protocol 10.

Case Study

The patient in the first slide is a new patient in your practice.

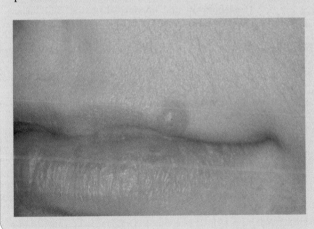

As you begin your extraoral exam, you notice the area on her lower lip. Using the slides presented, determine whether the raised area on her lip is of concern. Consider the following:

- What questions would you want to ask her?
- What characteristics of the lesion might make you concerned, or what characteristics might make you feel more comfortable with the fact that this is probably benign in nature?
- What does the histology of the lesion denote?
- What are some disease states that should be considered?
- Are there any tests or procedures that your office would recommend?

REFERENCES

Barker BF, Carpenter WM, Daniels TE, et al. Oral mucosal melanomas: The WESTOP Banff Workshop proceedings. Oral Surg Oral Med Oral Pathol Oral Radiol Endod 1997; 83:672–679.

Breen DJ, Stoker DJ. Titanium lines: a manifestation of metallosis and tissue response to titanium alloy mega prostheses at the knee. Clin Radiol 1993;47(4):274–277.

Cawson RA, Binnie WH, Eveson JW. Color atlas of oral disease—clinical and pathologic correlations. 2nd ed. London: Wolfe Publishing, 1994.

Cawson RA, Odell EW. Essentials of oral pathology and oral medicine. 6th ed. London: Churchill Livingstone–Harcourt Brace and Company, 1998.

Cheek CC, Heymann HO. Dental and oral decolorations associated with minocycline and other tetracycline analogs. J Esthet Dent 1999;11(1):43–48.

Coleman GC, Flaitz CM, Vincent SD. Differential diagnosis of oral soft tissue lesions. Tex Dent J 2002;119(6):484–488, 490–492, 494–503.

Eisen D. Lynch DP. The mouth—diagnosis and treatment. St. Louis: Mosby, 1998.

Gaeta GM, Satriano RA, Baroni A. Oral pigmented lesions. Clin Dermatol 2002;20(3):286–288.

Gorsky M, Epstein JB. Melanoma arising from the mucosal surfaces of the head and neck. Oral Surg Oral Med Oral Pathol Oral Radio Endod 1998;86(6):715–719.

Gu G, Epstein JB, Morton TH. Intraoral melanoma: long-term follow-up and implication for dental clinicians. A case report and literature review. Oral Surg Oral Med Oral Pathol Oral Radiol Endod 2003;96:404–413.

Hedin, CA, Axell T. Oral melanin pigmentation in 467 Thai and Malaysian people with special emphasis on smoker's melanosis. J Oral Pathol Med 1991;20(1):8–12.

Hood AF, Kwan TH, Mihm MC, Horn TD. Dermatopathology. 2nd ed. Boston: Little, Brown & Co., 1993.

Kahn MA, Weathers DR, Hoffman JG. Transformation of a benign pigmentation to primary oral melanoma. Oral Surg Oral Med Oral Pathol Oral Radiol Endod 2005;100:454–459

Kroumpouzos G, Frank EW, Albertini JG, et al. Lentigo maligna with spread onto oral mucosa. Arch Dermatol 2002;138(9):1216–1220.

Langford RJ, Frame JW. Tissue changes adjacent to titanium plates in patients. J Craniomaxillofac Surg 2002;30(2):103–107.

Langlais R., Miller C. Color atlas of common oral diseases. Baltimore: Lippincott Williams & Wilkins, 2003.

Lenane P, Powell FC. Oral pigmentation. J Eur Acad Dermatol Venereol 2000;14(6):448–465.

Lochary ME, Lockhart PB, Williams WT. Doxycycline and staining of permanent teeth. Pediatr Infect Dis J 1998;17(5):429–431.

Lockhart PB. Gingival pigmentation as the sole presenting sign of chronic lead poisoning in a mentally retarded adult. Oral Surg Oral Med Oral Pathol 1981;52:143–149.

Mani NJ. Gingival tattoo: a hitherto undescribed mucosal pigmentation. Quintessence Int 1985;2:157–159.

Martin JMM, Sharp I. Oral pigmentation secondary to treatment with mepacrine, with sparing of the denture bearing area. Br J Oral Maxillofac Surg 2004;42(4):351–353.

Mayall F, Wild DJ. A silver tattoo of the nasal mucosa after silver nitrate cautery. Laryngol Otol 1996;110(6):609–610.

Meleti M, Rene LC, Mooi WJ, et al. Oral malignant melanoma review of the literature. Oral Oncol 2006; Aug 22 [Epub ahead of print].

Mignogna MD, Lo Muzio L, Ruoppo E, et al. Oral manifestations of idiopathic lenticular mucocutaneous pigmentation (Laugier-Hunziker syndrome): a clinical, histopathologic and ultrastructural review of 12 cases. Oral Dis 1999;5(1):80–86.

Moore RT, Chae KA, Rhodes AR. Laugier and Hunziker pigmentation: a lentiginous proliferation of melanocytes. J Am Acad Dermatol 2004; 50(5 suppl):S70–S74.

Neville BW, Damm DD, Allen CM, Bouquot JE. Oral & maxillofacial pathology. Philadelphia: WB Saunders, 1995.

Owens BM, Johnson WW, Schuman NJ. Oral amalgam pigmentations (tattoos): a retrospective study. Quintessence Int 1992;23(12):805–810.

Penel N, Mallet Y, Mirabel X, et al. Primary mucosal melanoma of head and neck: prognostic value of clear margins. Laryngoscope 2006;116(6):993–995.

Perusse R, Morency R. Oral pigmentation induced by Premarin. Cutis 1991;48(1):61–64.

Pinto A, Raghavendra S, Lee R, et al. Epithelioid blue nevus of the oral mucosa: a rare histologic variant. Oral Surg Oral Med Oral Pathol Oral Radiol Endod 2003;96:429–436.

Porth CM. Essentials of pathophysiology. Baltimore: Lippincott Williams & Wilkins, 2004.

Regezi J, Sciubba J, Jordan R. Oral pathology—clinical pathologic correlations. 4th ed. St. Louis: WB Saunders, 2003.

Sarswathi TR, Kumar SN, Kavitha KM. Oral melanin pigmentation in smoked and smokeless tobacco users in India. Clinico-pathological study. Indian J Dent Res 2003;14(2):101–106.

Scully C. Handbook of oral disease—diagnosis and management. London: Martin Duntz Ltd. The Livery House Publishers, 1999.

Stedman's medical dictionary. 27th ed. Baltimore: Lippincott Williams & Wilkins, 2000.

Suresh L, Radfar L. Pregnancy and lactation. Oral Surg Oral Med Oral Pathol Oral Radiol Endod 2004;97:672–682.

Symvoulakis EK, Kyrmizakis DE, Drivas EI, et al. Oral mucosal melanoma: a malignant trap. Head Face Med 2006;28(2):7.

Takagi M, Ishikama G, Mori W. Primary malignant melanoma of the oral cavity in Japan. Cancer 1974;34:358–370.

Tomicic J, Wanebo HJ. Mucosal melanomas. Surg Clin North Am 2003;83(2):237–252.

Torgersen S, Gjerdet NR, Erichsen ES, Bang G. Metal particles and tissue changes adjacent to miniplates. A retrieval study. Acata Odontol Scand 1995;53(2):65–71.

Treister NS, Magalnick D, Sook-Bin W. Oral mucosal pigmentation secondary to minocycline therapy: report of two cases and review of the literature. Oral Surg Oral Med Oral Pathol Oral Radiol Endod 2004;97:718–725.

Ulusal BG, Karatas O, Yildiz AC, Oztan Y. Primary malignant melanoma of the maxillary gingiva. Dermatol Surg 2003;29:304–307.

Wilkins EM. Clinical practice of the dental hygienist. 9th ed. Baltimore: Lippincott Williams & Wilkins, 2005.

Zain RB, Ikeda N, Gupta PC, et al. Oral mucosal lesions associated with betel quid, areca nut and tobacco chewing habits: consensus from a workshop held in Kuala Lumpur, Malaysia, November 25–27, 1996.

16

Raised Lesions with a Rough or Papillary Surface

Key Terms

- Autoinoculation
- HPV, low risk
- HPV, high risk
- Keratinization
- Keratinocyte
- Mitosoid figures
- Parakeratotic
- Reservoir

Learning Outcomes

1. Define and use the key terms listed in this chapter.

2. Discuss the characteristics of the human papillomaviruses (HPV) and differentiate between the high-risk and low-risk types.

3. Describe the etiology, method of transmission, and pathogenesis of the lesions associated with HPV.

4. List the characteristics of the lesions caused by HPV and discuss their dental implications.

5. Describe the etiology, clinical characteristics, and dental implications associated with papillary hyperplasia.

6. Describe how papillary hyperplasia is usually treated.

7. Distinguish between papillary hyperplasia and papillary lesions caused by HPV.

8. Compare and contrast squamous cell carcinoma and keratoacanthoma.

9. Discuss the relationship between squamous cell carcinoma and verrucous carcinoma.

10. Identify the role of the dental hygienist in preventing cervical cancer.

CHAPTER OUTLINE

Raised lesions with a rough or papillary surface comprise a distinct group of oral mucosal masses that represent an epithelial abnormality. Among these are diverse malignancies, contagious infections (including viral proliferations associated with a large number of human papillomaviruses), sexually transmitted diseases (STDs), and reactive or inflammatory lesions. Since the most significant epithelial abnormality in the oral cavity is squamous cell carcinoma, all rough or papillary raised lesions should be managed as though they potentially could be squamous cell carcinomas. The goal of this chapter is to provide sufficient information to help the dental hygienist identify the clinical characteristics of these lesions and collaborate with other dental professionals to make appropriate recommendations for diagnostic and follow-up procedures.

INFECTIONS

The primary etiologic agent associated with lesions exhibiting a rough or papillary surface is the human papillomavirus (HPV). There are more than 100 different types and subtypes of HPV. Some of these are listed in Table 16.1 along with the disorders with which they are associated. Human papillomaviruses are members of the Papovaviridae family of viruses that produce epithelial tumors of the skin and/or mucous membranes. They are double-stranded DNA viruses that do not have an envelope surrounding them. They only affect humans, and humans are their only **reservoir** (substance or living host

within which an organism can multiply and develop). Some HPVs have been associated with benign lesions and are identified as **low-risk types**. These viruses normally inject their DNA into the nucleus of the host's cells, where it exists within the nucleus as a separate entity. Others, designated **high-risk types,** have been associated with carcinomas and infect the host's cells in a different manner. The viral DNA of high-risk types is integrated into the host's DNA, which results in malignant transformation of the host cell. Clinically, lesions associated with the human papillomavirus are exophytic, with a surface appearance that is cauliflower-like. As is the case with all infectious viruses, human papillomaviruses are transmissible, but their degree of infectivity varies from type to type. Benign lesions associated with HPV are discussed in this section.

NAME: Oral squamous papilloma (oral wart)

Etiology: Human papillomaviruses 2, 6, 11, and 57 (all low-risk types) have been associated with benign oral squamous papillomas (Regezi et al., 2003).

Method of Transmission: HPV is transmitted by direct contact between the virus and nonintact skin. They have very low infectivity. The virus can also be spread by **autoinoculation** (transfer from one site to another on the same person).

Epidemiology: There are no prevalence data for the oral lesions alone; however 7 to 10% of the population has some form of cutaneous or mucosal squamous papilloma (Gearhart et al., July 2006). Any age can be affected. There is equal distribution between the genders for oral and cutaneous lesions. Individuals who are immunosuppressed have a much higher risk of developing these lesions than those who do not have a compromised immune system. However, a higher number of females are infected with anogenital HPV than males (Gearhart et al., July 2006). See the application following this section for information about HPV and cervical cancer.

Pathogenesis: Lesions associated with this virus are believed to arise from the proliferation of infected basal **keratinocytes** (living precursors to the dead keratin-filled

Table 16.1	EPITHELIAL DISEASE AND ASSOCIATED HUMAN PAPILLOMAVIRUS TYPES

Disease	Human Papillomavirus Types[a]
Verruca vulgaris (common wart)	1, 2, 4, 26, 27, 40, 41
Focal epithelial hyperplasia	13, 32
Condyloma acuminatum	6, 11, 16, 18
Squamous papilloma	2, 6, 11, 57
Verrucous carcinoma	2, 6, 11, 16, 18
Keratoacanthoma	Possible 9, 11, 13, 16, 18, 24, 25, 33, 37, 57

[a]HPV types listed are the most common ones associated with the lesions; others are possible.

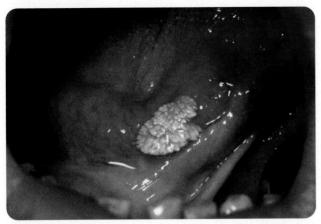

Figure 16.1. Oral squamous papilloma. The white finger-like projections covering the surface of this growth on the ventral surface of the tongue are characteristic of the squamous papilloma.

cells of the stratum corneum on the outermost layer of the skin) (Gearhart et al., July 2006).

Extraoral Characteristics: Not applicable

Perioral and Intraoral Characteristics: Oral squamous papillomas manifest as painless, exophytic, well-circumscribed, pedunculated, or sessile masses. These masses may have a cauliflower-like surface texture or they may consist of many finger- or hairlike projections. They range in color from white to pink and can be found on the lips or any mucosal surface, however, they are seen more often on the hard and soft palates and the tongue (Fig. 16.1).

Distinguishing Characteristics: The cauliflower-like appearance of oral squamous papilloma suggests an infection with HPV.

Significant Microscopic Features: The surface exhibits a proliferation of parakeratinized squamous epithelium with fingerlike projections (Fig. 16.2).

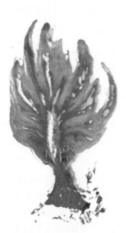

Figure 16.2. Oral squamous papilloma. Photomicrograph showing fingerlike projections on a pedunculated lesion.

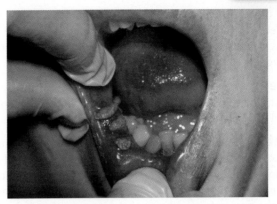

Figure 16.3. Verruca vulgaris. Multiple oral lesions in a 9-year-old who had similar lesions on his hands.

Dental Implications: These lesions should be removed because of the association of some forms of HPV with oral malignancies.

Differential Diagnosis: Any of the other forms of HPV infection need to be considered in a differential diagnosis, including

1. Verruca vulgaris, Chapter 23
2. Condyloma acuminatum, Chapter 16
3. Verrucous carcinoma, Chapter 16
4. Focal epithelial hyperplasia, Chapter 16

Treatment and Prognosis: Conservative surgical excision usually suffices to treat this lesion. The risk of recurrence is low except in those individuals who are immunosuppressed and therefore have a considerably higher risk.

VERRUCA VULGARIS

The verruca vulgaris lesion is also known as the common wart. It can be caused by several of the human papillomaviruses, specifically 2, 4, 6, and 40 (all low-risk types). The virus enters through a break in the skin, and a wart forms. Oral lesions are usually caused by autoinoculation from the fingers to the mouth. Any time the clinician observes a verrucal-papillary lesion in the mouth, he or she should perform a quick examination of the patient's fingers for a similar lesion.

The virus enters the mucosa through a break in the surface epithelium usually caused by trauma. Figure 16.3 depicts multiple verrucae in a 9-year-old boy who had a habit of biting his cuticles. Surgical excision is the treatment of choice for these lesions. Approximately two thirds of the lesions have been reported to disappear spontaneously, presumably because of the effectiveness of the patient's immune system in combating the virus.

NAME: Condyloma acuminatum (genital or venereal warts)

Etiology: Approximately 30 different types of HPV can infect the anogenital tract; however, HPV subtypes 6 and

11 (low-risk types) are the most common causes of this infection. HPV subtypes 16 and 18 (high-risk types) are less commonly associated with condyloma acuminatum (Higgins et al., July 2006).

Method of Transmission: HPV is transmitted by direct (oral-oral or oral-genital) contact between the virus and compromised skin or mucous membranes.

Pathogenesis: An estimated two-thirds of individuals who have sexual contact with an infected partner will develop genital warts, making this a highly infectious condition. The epithelial cells of the oral mucosal membranes or the mucosal membranes of the anogenital tract harbor the virus. Proliferation of the virus depends on the process of **keratinization** (production of keratin within the cells) (Regezi et al., 2003).

Extraoral Characteristics: These lesions can occur on any mucosal surface in the anogenital area. The clinical appearance is of multiple flat, pinkish, exophytic growths with sessile bases and rough cauliflower-like surfaces.

Perioral and Intraoral Characteristics: Intraoral lesions can be quite extensive and occur in those sites that are frequently traumatized during fellatio or cunnilingus, such as the labial and lingual frenula and the soft palate and oropharynx. However, almost any oral site can be affected. The lesions begin as papular growths that enlarge and coalesce, becoming nodular, pink, exophytic growths with a rough papillary surface (Fig. 16.4).

Distinguishing Characteristics: The cauliflower-like appearance of the lesion suggests an HPV infection.

Significant Microscopic Features: The surface of the lesion is covered by stratified squamous epithelium that is either **parakeratotic** (cells that have retained their nuclei after they should have been lost) or nonkeratinized. There is marked thickening of the basal layer and the stratum spinosum of the epithelium (Fig. 16.5).

Dental Implications: Diagnosis and treatment of this condition will help to prevent transmission of the virus.

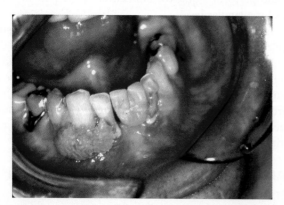

Figure 16.4. Condyloma acuminatum. Recurrent lesions exhibit the characteristic nodular growth with a rough papillary surface.

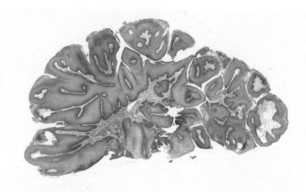

Figure 16.5. Condyloma acuminatum. Photomicrograph showing the histology of condyloma acuminatum. Note the more rounded projections of epithelium compared with the more pointed projections of the squamous papilloma.

This infection is more common in immunosuppressed patients, and the clinician should carefully evaluate the patient's assessment data for other indications that would suggest a medical referral.

Differential Diagnosis: Any of the verrucal-papillary lesions should be considered in a differential diagnosis. However, the flatter, less papillary appearance of this infection is more consistent with focal epithelial hyperplasia.

Treatment and Prognosis: Oral lesions are usually removed surgically using scalpel, laser, cryosurgery, or electrosurgery. Recurrences are common. Patients who are exposed to HPV 16 or 18 have an increased risk of developing anogenital carcinomas. In addition, recent research has suggested a link between HPV 16 and oral and oropharyngeal carcinomas (Ritchie et al., 2003; De Petrini et al., 2006). Interestingly, these studies also suggest that the presence of HPV 16 in these cancers correlate with a better overall survival rate (Ritchie et al., 2003; De Petrini et al., 2006). The significance of this information is not clear, and more research is needed.

NAME: Focal epithelial hyperplasia (Heck's disease)

Etiology: HPV 13 and 32 (low-risk types) have been implicated in the development of this condition.

Method of Transmission: HPV 13 or 32 is transmitted in a manner similar to that of other human papilloma viruses, by surface contact with the virus through a break in the mucosal barrier. This is frequently due to localized trauma.

Epidemiology: Focal epithelial hyperplasia was first identified in 1965 in Native North Americans. It has since been identified in many population groups around the world. All ages can be affected, but the condition is somewhat more common in younger age groups. It affects both genders equally.

APPLICATION

HPV AND CERVICAL CANCER

The American Cancer Society estimates that there will be 9710 new cases of invasive cervical cancer and four times that many cases of cervical carcinoma in situ (noninvasive) in the United States in 2006. In addition, they estimate that 3700 American women will die from cervical cancer in 2006 (ACS, 2006). Cervical cancer was one of the major causes of cancer deaths in women in the United States before the Pap test became available in 1955. From 1955 to 1992 there was a 74% drop in the rate of cervical cancer deaths because of early detection (ACS, 2006). Recently, researchers have made dramatic advances in understanding the cause of, and in finding potential preventive strategies for, cervical cancer.

The most important risk factor for cervical cancer has been found to be infection with an HPV virus. The high-risk human papilloma viruses that are associated with most cervical cancers are HPV 16, 18, 31, 33, and 45. Approximately 66% are caused by HPV 16 and 18. HPV is sexually transmitted by skin-to-skin contact during vaginal and anal intercourse and by genital-oral contact. Using condoms and otherwise practicing "safe sex" has not been shown to be an effective preventive measure for HPV transmission because it is transmitted by skin-to-skin contact in addition to mucosal contact. Most women who are infected by the virus are never aware of their infection, and their immune system is able to eliminate it. In some women the virus stays in the cells. A small percentage of the women who retain the virus will develop cervical cancer. It is not known why some women with the virus develop cervical cancer while others do not, but researchers have identified several additional risk factors that coupled with HPV infection may increase the risk of developing cervical cancer. These include

- Smoking
- HIV infection
- Coinfection with *Chlamydia*
- Diet (being overweight, diet low in fruits and vegetables)
- Long-term oral contraceptive use (5+ years)
- Multiple full-term pregnancies
- Family history of cervical cancer

The CDC estimates that 20 million people are currently infected with HPV, including about 75% of the reproductive age population. The CDC also expects up to 5.5 million new infections each year (CDC, 2006). The numbers are staggering, but a new vaccine has been developed that has been shown to be 100% effective in preventing the initial infection with HPV 16 and 18 (high-risk types that cause 70% of cervical cancers) and 99% effective in preventing infection with HPV 6 and 11 (low-risk types that cause 90% of genital warts) (ACS, 2006). The vaccine, called Gardasil, has been approved for use in young women to prevent infection with these viruses. It is recommended that girls ages 11 and 12 be vaccinated before they become sexually active. In addition, women between the ages of 13 and 26 should also be vaccinated as a sort of "catch-up" to try to cover as many as possible against the virus (SGO, 2006). It is important to understand that once a woman has become infected with the virus, the vaccine is no longer of any use: it can neither treat an established infection nor prevent cancer in someone who has the infection. The vaccine can only be used to prevent the initial infection. The vaccine is given in three doses over a 1-year period, the second injection is given 2 months after the first, and the third is given 4 months later (ACS, 2006).

Why is it important for the dental professional to be aware of this vaccine? Dental offices see many young children two or more times per year. Therefore, dental hygienists are in an excellent position to educate the parents of young girls about this excellent opportunity to prevent a terrible disease. Many parents are not likely to think that they have to worry about their 11- and 12-year-old girls being sexually active. However, this is not the point in question. The point is to vaccinate before there is any chance of exposure. Dental hygienists are also in a good position to talk to the 13- to 26-year-old women who may also want to take advantage of this vaccine.

Pathogenesis: Introduction of the virus into the mucous membranes causes proliferation of the keratinized cells in the stratum spinosum.

Extraoral Characteristics: Not applicable

Perioral and Intraoral Characteristics: The lesions of focal epithelial hyperplasia display a pink to whitish, somewhat translucent, surface that is only slightly cauliflower-like. They are soft on palpation, as they generally have less keratin than the other HPV-related lesions. The lesions most commonly affect the lips, tongue, and buccal mucosa, where they appear as numerous discrete papular or nodular growths (Fig. 16.6).

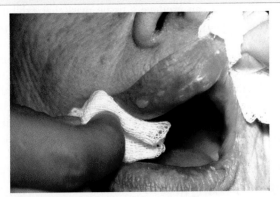

Figure 16.6. Focal epithelial hyperplasia. Lesions on the upper lip appear whitish, translucent, and much less papillary than other HPV-related lesions.

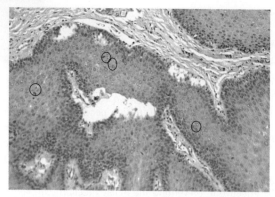

Figure 16.7. Focal epithelial hyperplasia. Photomicrograph showing mitosoid figures *(circled)* in the midspinous zone.

Distinguishing Characteristics: These lesions may be more generalized within the oral cavity than the other forms of HPV.

Significant Microscopic Features: The hallmark of focal epithelial hyperplasia is the presence of **mitosoid figures** (cells in which the nuclear DNA has fragmented, resulting in a cell that looks like it is undergoing mitosis) in the middle of the spinous layer of the epithelium (Fig. 16.7).

Dental Implications: None

Differential Diagnosis: All of the verrucal or papillary type lesions previously discussed would be considered in a differential diagnosis. In addition, the oral lesions associated with Cowden syndrome (Chapter 17) and Crohn's disease (Chapter 10) may have a similar intraoral appearance, and they should also be considered.

Treatment and Prognosis: Treatment is not always necessary. Conservative excision may be done to establish a diagnosis. Often these lesions will resolve spontaneously without any treatment. Malignant transformation is unlikely.

INFLAMMATORY OR REACTIVE LESIONS WITH A PAPILLARY CONFIGURATION

Hyperplasia is a form of cellular adaptation to chronic injury. Often this can produce a tissue mass that exhibits a rough or papillary surface. Most examples of reactive hyperplasias exhibit a smooth surface; however, it is not unusual to see some of these growths present with a somewhat rough or papillary surface. Most of these lesions are discussed under the clinical characteristics that they most often exhibit and are found within other chapters. One form of reactive hyperplasia, papillary hyperplasia, almost always exhibits a papillary surface and, therefore, is discussed in this section.

NAME: Papillary hyperplasia (inflammatory papillary hyperplasia)

Etiology: Papillary hyperplasia is a reactive tissue proliferation due to mild, persistent trauma caused almost exclusively by the rubbing of an ill-fitting denture on the mucosa during function.

Method of Transmission: Not applicable

Epidemiology: Papillary hyperplasia can occur in any age group but most often occurs in the elderly, because these are the patients who are more likely to wear dentures, especially ill-fitting dentures. The longer a patient keeps a denture without having it evaluated for proper fit by a dentist, the more likely this lesion is to occur. The lesion occurs equally in both males and females.

Pathogenesis: Papillary hyperplasia develops over time as a patient's denture becomes increasingly more loose-fitting as a result of the normal process of bone remodeling after loss of the teeth. As more and more bone is lost over time, the denture becomes increasingly likely to slip and rub during mastication. The chronic rubbing of the denture on the soft tissues of the mucosa overlying the bone results in a broad field of small papules in the areas directly beneath the denture. The condition is more common on the maxillary mucosa than on the mandibular mucosa, possibly because patients are more likely to keep their maxillary dentures in their mouths longer and because the maxillary denture covers a greater area of soft tissue.

Extraoral Characteristics: Not applicable

Perioral and Intraoral Characteristics: The lesion most commonly appears on the palatal mucosa as a field of pink to bright red, clustered papules that are firm to palpation (Fig. 16.8).

Distinguishing Characteristics: This condition is always related to the presence of dentures or oral appliances.

Significant Microscopic Features: A thickened or thinned epithelium covers cores of proliferative fibrovascular connective tissue. Numerous capillaries are present

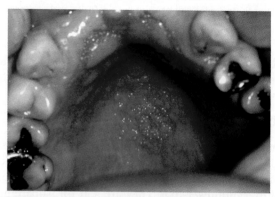

Figure 16.8. Papillary hyperplasia. This patient has been wearing a temporary partial to replace the maxillary incisors for several years. The poor fit associated with this type of prosthesis is often related to the development of papillary hyperplasia. Note the clusters of pink papules covering the surface of the hard palate.

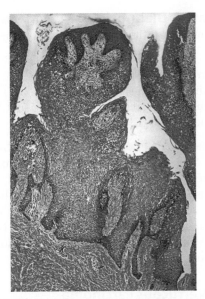

Figure 16.9. Papillary hyperplasia. Photomicrograph showing increased connective tissue rather than proliferating exophytic epithelium causing the papillary appearance. (Courtesy of Dr. Valerie A. Murrah.)

in the connective tissue. This, combined with thinned epithelium, results in a reddish appearance to the tissue (Fig. 16.9).

Dental Implications: Patients who exhibit this condition should be treated with a soft denture reline material prior to surgical removal of the lesion and fabrication of a new denture. They should also be educated on the proper use and care of their dentures, including the fact that dentures must be removed from the mouth for a period of time every day.

Differential Diagnosis: Although the clinical appearance of this lesion and its association with a denture strongly suggests papillary hyperplasia, other more serious conditions such as early verrucous carcinoma (Chapter 16) must be considered and ruled out.

Treatment and Prognosis: The lesions should not be surgically excised without the fabrication of a new denture, since mechanical trauma related to functioning of an ill-fitting denture will simply result in recurrence. New dentures should never be fabricated over papillary hyperplasia, as the impressions for the new denture will incorporate the papillary configurations and will increase the likelihood that the new denture will not fit as well. Papillary hyperplasia is frequently associated with candidiasis, indicating that both the soft tissue and the denture surface needs to be treated with an antifungal agent. (Refer to Clinical Protocol 5.)

The prognosis is excellent, as long as new dentures are fabricated following removal of the lesion and the patient is educated about the necessity of periodic evaluations to check the fit of the denture and the health of the underlying mucosa.

NEOPLASMS ASSOCIATED WITH A ROUGH OR PAPILLARY SURFACE

The genetic material of the high-risk HPV types 16 and 18 is typically added or combined with the host's DNA in malignant lesions. Integration of the viral DNA into the host cell's DNA is considered a hallmark of malignant transformation (Gearhart et al., 2006). Proteins made by the viral DNA of high-risk types have been shown to inactivate the host's tumor suppressor proteins, resulting in unregulated host cell proliferation and malignant transformation. Two conditions are discussed in this section. Keratoacanthoma is considered a benign lesion even though it exhibits some characteristics associated with a malignant lesion, and verrucous carcinoma is a low-grade epithelial malignancy.

NAME: Keratoacanthoma

Etiology: The exact cause of keratoacanthoma is not clear. Keratoacanthomas are somewhat controversial lesions in that some experts regard them as benign and others regard them as a low-grade variant of invasive squamous cell carcinoma (Chuang and Brashear, 2006).

Exposure of the affected area to sunlight is strongly associated with the development of this lesion. Other possible factors include the presence of chromosomal abnormalities in the skin, occupational exposure to tar and/or pitch, a compromised immune status, and exposure to several forms of HPV, including types 9, 11, 13, 16, 18, 24, 25, 33, 37 and 57.

Epidemiology: The peak incidence of this lesion occurs in those over the age of 60 years. It is rarely found in anyone under the age of 20. It is uncommon in darker-skinned individuals and is seen more often in males than females (Chuang and Brashear, 2006).

Pathogenesis: These lesions originate from the pilosebaceous glands (sebaceous glands associated with hair follicles). The lesions are usually solitary and begin as firm, skin-colored, or reddish papules that rapidly progress to dome-shaped nodules, about 1 to 2 cm in size, over a period of several weeks. This tumor frequently undergoes spontaneous regression.

Extraoral Characteristics: Most keratoacanthomas arise on the sun-exposed skin of the face, neck, and upper extremities. The dome-shaped nodules display a smooth shiny surface with a central crater containing a core or plug of keratin.

Perioral and Intraoral Characteristics: Keratoacanthomas are most frequently detected by the dental team on the edge of the vermilion border of the lower lip (Fig. 16.10). These lesions are not found on mucous membranes within the oral cavity.

Distinguishing Characteristics: The clinical appearance and location of the keratoacanthoma may help to differentiate it from other lesions. However, the uncer-

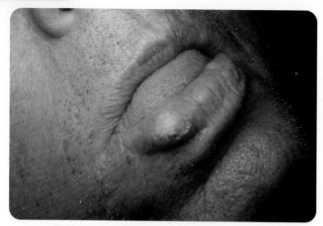

Figure 16.10. Keratoacanthoma. Note the keratin within the central area of the lesion. (Courtesy of Dr. Amy Brooks.)

tain relationship between this and squamous cell carcinoma indicates the need for prompt identification and treatment.

Significant Microscopic Features: The keratoacanthoma is a symmetrical lesion of well-differentiated squamous epithelium. There is cupping of the edges of the normal epidermis that extends over a central crater filled with keratin. A prominent inflammatory cell infiltrate is present in the dermis, adjacent to the invading epithelium of the lesion (Fig. 16.11). Of utmost importance is the histologic similiarity between the keratoacanthoma and well-differentiated, low-grade squamous cell carcinoma, which makes distinguishing between the two difficult at the very least.

Dental Implications: Observation of a lesion with this general appearance during an extraoral examination should prompt a medical referral by the dental healthcare provider. In addition, patients who develop keratoacanthomas are at higher risk for developing subsequent nonmelanoma skin cancer; therefore, patients should be educated about prevention and self-examination. (Refer to Clinical Protocol 10 for information related to preventing skin cancer.)

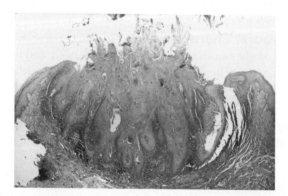

Figure 16.11. Keratoacanthoma. Note the cup-shaped appearance, central keratin, and the extensive infiltrate of inflammatory cells below the epithelium. (Courtesy of Dr. Valerie A. Murrah.)

Differential Diagnosis: Differential diagnoses of keratoacanthoma in its typical location on the lower lip include

1. Recurrent herpes labialis, Chapter 11
2. Syphilis chancre, Chapter 12
3. Squamous cell carcinoma, Chapters 5 and 12
4. Actinic cheilitis, Chapter 14

Treatment and Prognosis: Surgical excision is the treatment of choice. Since the biologic behavior of an individual keratoacanthoma cannot be predicted, many dermatologists consider treatment of keratoacanthoma to be equivalent to treatment for squamous cell carcinoma (Chuang and Brashear, 2006). The prognosis is excellent with complete surgical removal. Untreated lesions usually regress spontaneously leaving a scar.

NAME: Verrucous carcinoma

Etiology: Most verrucous carcinomas appear to be related to the use of spit tobacco, either snuff or chewing tobacco. Spit tobacco contains various carcinogens including: polonium-210, tobacco-specific N-nitrosamines, volatile aldehydes, and polycyclic aromatic hydrocarbons. Mucous membrane exposure to alcohol also appears to be a factor in the etiology of verrucous carcinoma. In addition, several forms of human papillomavirus have been found within lesions of verrucous carcinoma.

Method of Transmission: Verrucous carcinomas are not thought to be contagious, although a variety of human papillomavirus types have been localized within them.

Epidemiology: Verrucous carcinoma occurs primarily in males over the age of 55. Data on the frequency of verrucous carcinoma are not available; however, it is estimated that 7 to 13 million people use spit tobacco in the United States every year, making the potential for the development of this lesion significant (Dolev and Kimball, 2006).

Pathogenesis: Verrucous carcinoma most often develops at the site of placement of the tobacco quid. This association is so strong that this type of carcinoma has often been termed "snuff dippers' cancer" when it appears in the oral cavity. Verrucous carcinomas are slow-growing lesions. Although they invade adjacent structures, they do not tend to metastasize.

Extraoral Characteristics: Not applicable

Perioral and Intraoral Characteristics: Early lesions appear as white patches, whereas more fully developed lesions display a cauliflower-like papillary appearance that spreads over a large area of the mucosa. There may be fissuring and ulceration of the lesions. In addition, squamous cell carcinomas have been reported to develop within verrucous carcinoma lesions. Verrucous carcinoma

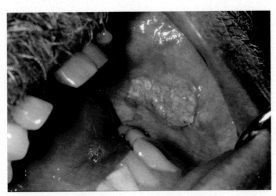

Figure 16.12. Verrucous carcinoma. Verrucous carcinoma of the left buccal mucosa in a male patient who was a long time tobacco chewer and smoker. Note the areas of leukoplakia surrounding the lesion.

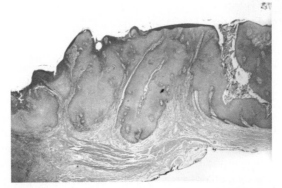

Figure 16.13. Verrucous carcinoma. Photomicrograph showing the invagination of epithelium, the invasive downgrowth of the epithelium, and the chronic inflammatory cells just below the invading epithelium.

is usually found on the vestibular mucosa, alveolar ridge, and gingiva, as well as the buccal mucosa (Fig. 16.12).

Distinguishing Characteristics: The general appearance of verrucous carcinoma coupled with a history of spit tobacco use suggests this lesion; however, a biopsy must be performed for a definitive diagnosis.

Significant Microscopic Features: The lesion displays a highly keratinized surface that is undulating and markedly papillary, with deep invaginations of the mucosa (Fig. 16.13). In most cases, one observes a chronic inflammatory cell infiltrate immediately adjacent to the margins of the invading neoplasm.

Dental Implications: Verrucous carcinoma often forms within longstanding leukoplakia associated with spit tobacco. The dental hygienist is in an excellent posi-

tion to educate patients about the effects of spit tobacco use and counsel them about tobacco cessation.

Differential Diagnosis: Any of the papillary lesions are included in a differential diagnosis of verrucous carcinoma, including

1. Condyloma acuminatum, Chapter 16
2. Oral squamous papilloma, Chapter 16
3. Verruca vulgaris, Chapter 16
4. Leukoplakia, Chapter 14

Treatment and Prognosis: Surgical removal is the treatment of choice. Cryotherapy (freezing) also has a high cure rate for well-circumscribed lesions. Most patients have a good prognosis, as metastasis is rare. However, if squamous cell carcinoma is identified within the verrucous carcinoma, the prognosis becomes much less favorable.

SUMMARY

- HPV is the primary etiologic agent associated with verrucous or papillary lesions. There are over 100 different types of HPV.
- Low-risk HPV types are associated with benign epithelial lesions, while high-risk types are associated with malignant lesions, such as verrucous carcinoma and squamous cell carcinoma.
- Oral squamous papillomas are associated with low-risk HPV and can be spread by autoinoculation. They appear as exophytic, pedunculated, or sessile masses covered with fingerlike projections.
- Verruca vulgaris (common wart) can present in the oral cavity and is usually associated with autoinoculation from a lesion on the hands.
- Condyloma acuminatum is a sexually transmitted disease that is caused by 30 or more types of HPV. The le-

sions can affect the genitals and/or the mouth, depending on where the virus contacts the skin. Infection with high-risk types of HPV, and retention of the virus within the cells, increases the individual's risk of developing squamous cell carcinoma in the future.

- Over 90% of cases of cervical cancer are thought to be caused by high-risk HPV. A vaccine to prevent infection with specific HPV types (6, 11, 16, and 18) is available. The vaccine can prevent 100% of infections with HPV 16 and 18 and 99% of infections with HPV 6 and 11.
- Focal epithelial hyperplasia presents in the oral cavity as numerous discrete papular or nodular growths that are much less papillary than other lesions caused by HPV. Numerous mitosoid figures in the epidermis are characteristic microscopic features of this disorder.

(continued)

SUMMARY *(continued)*

- Papillary hyperplasia is an inflammatory lesion caused by wearing an ill-fitting denture. It may be accompanied by an infection with *Candida albicans*. The lesion must be removed before a new denture can be made.
- The keratoacanthoma is a benign lesion that originates in a pilosebaceous gland. Its development is associated with exposure to sunlight and some forms of HPV, among other factors. This lesion is histologically very similar to squamous cell carcinoma, and experts are undecided as to whether this is actually a low-grade form of squamous cell carcinoma or a benign lesion. The lesion appears as a papule that rapidly grows to form a dome-shaped nodule with a central plug of keratin.

The lesion usually regresses without treatment; however, patients who have had keratoacanthoma have a higher risk of developing skin cancer in the same area.

- Verrucous carcinoma is a slow-growing epithelial cancer that invades local structures but does not tend to metastasize. These cancers often develop in a preexisting leukoplakia that is associated with spit tobacco use. In addition, HPV has been found within the lesions, possibly linking this form of cancer to an infection with HPV. Squamous cell carcinoma development has been observed within these lesions.

PORTFOLIO POSSIBILITIES

1. Construct separate patient education sheets for patients with verruca vulgaris, condyloma acuminatum, and inflammatory papillary hyperplasia. Describe the causes of these conditions in terms that are easily understandable. Delineate the reason(s) that surgical treatment(s) is(are) required. Finally, discuss appropriate lifestyle changes that will prevent the patient from acquiring recurrences of the lesions.
2. Construct a pamphlet for education of high school students concerning oral lesions caused by human papillomavirus. Include information about HPV transmissibility and the use of smokeless tobacco in the etiology of verrucous carcinoma.
3. Write a patient information pamphlet on appropriate denture care. In it, discuss the interrelationship between loose dentures and papillary hyperplasia, the ill effects of leaving one's dentures in at night, and the sequelae of failing to get periodic oral examinations by a dentist despite the fact that the patient no longer has teeth.

Critical Thinking Activity

A 70-year-old male and 50-year spit tobacco user displays a rough white verrucous lesion of the mandibular vestibule measuring 2.0 × 2.5 cm. The lesion is very firm to palpation. The patient doesn't want to quit his habit.

a. Should the practitioner ask the patient to move his quid of spit tobacco around to different places in the vestibule and then have the patient return in 2 weeks to look for regression?

b. In what situation, if any, would this type of recommendation be appropriate?

c. Could some method other than a biopsy be used to determine the identity of a thick verrucous white lesion found on the oral mucosa?

Case Study

A 45-year-old male, Mr. G, arrives at your office for a routine checkup and prophylaxis. He complains of a white bump that has never been there before. He admits to picking off portions of the bump, but it always comes back to its regular size, in fact, it seems to the patient that the lesion has recently been increasing in size. The patient is not quite sure how long the lesion has been present, but says that he thinks it is approximately 6 months, because he was sure it was not present at the last dental appointment. You confirm this by reviewing the chart notes of the previous appointment, as your office prides itself on meticulous notes regarding maintenance examinations. The patient indicates that the lesion is nonpainful but is bothersome to him, and he feels it may "show" when he speaks. You listen intently and tell Mr. G that his complaint will be addressed as soon as you have completed your assessment. The extraoral examination is unremarkable except for the lesions pictured in Figure 16.14. During the intraoral examination you note a white papillary lesion on the mucosal portion of the right lower lip (Fig. 16.15).

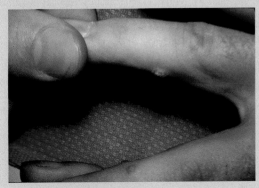

Figure 16.14. Extraoral findings.

1. What are the critical parts of the health history that you would want to review at this point?
2. Develop a differential diagnosis for this lesion.
3. What part do your extraoral findings play in determining a differential diagnosis?
4. What do you think the most likely diagnosis for the oral lesion will be when it is biopsied?

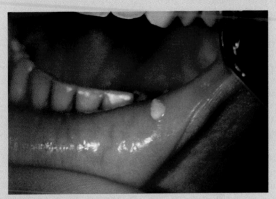

Figure 16.15. Intraoral findings.

INTERNET RESOURCES

The following are web sites that have good information about women's topics.

- American Cancer Society
  Web site: *www.cancer.org*
- American Social Health Association
  Web site: *www.ashastd.org*
- CancerCare
  Web site: *www.cancercare.org*
- Centers for Disease Control and Prevention
  Web site: *www.cdc.gov/cancer/nbccedp/index.htm*
- Eyes on the Prize
  Web site: *www.eyesontheprize.org*
- Gynecologic Cancer Foundation
  Web site: *www.thegcf.org*
- National Cancer Institute
  Web site: *www.cancer.gov/cancerinfo/types/cervical/*

- National Cervical Cancer Coalition
  Web site: *www.nccc-online.org*
- OncoLink
  Web site: *www.oncolink.com*
- Society of Gynecologic Oncologists
  Web site: *www.sgo.org*
- The Agency for Healthcare Research and Quality
  Web site: *www.ahrq.gov*
- The American Society for Colposcopy and Cervical Pathology
  Web site: *www.asccp.org*
- The Witness Project of Harlem
  Web site: *www.witnessprojectharlem.org*
- U.S. Food and Drug Administration's Office of Women's Health
  Web site: *www.fda.gov/womens/*
- Women's Cancer Network
  Web site: *www.wcn.org*

REFERENCES

Ackerman LV. Verrucous carcinoma of the oral cavity. Surgery 1948; 23:670–678.

American Cancer Society (ACS). Cervical cancer. 2006. available at: http://www.cancer.org. Accessed November 29, 2006.

Antonelli JR, Pann FV, Witko A. Inflammatory papillary hyperplasia: supraperiosteal excision by the blade–loop technique. Gen Dent 1998;46(4):390–397.

Archard HO, Heck JW, Stanley HR. Focal epithelial hyperplasia: an unusual oral mucosal lesion found in Indian children. Oral Surg Oral Med Oral Pathol 1965;20:201–212.

Barrellier P, Louis MY, Babin E. The use of cryotherapy in oral pathology. Our experience in 36 cases. 1992;93(5):345–348. French.

Baumgarth N, Szubin R, Dolganov GM, et al. Highly tissue substructure—specific effects of human papilloma virus in mucosa of HIV-infected patients revealed by laser-dissection microscopy. Am J Pathol 2004;165(3):707–718.

Bhasker SN, Beasley JD, Cutright DE. Inflammatory papillary hyperplasia of the oral mucosa: report of 341 cases. J Am Dent Assoc 1970;81(4): 949–952.

CDC. Cancer—cervical cancer statistics. Centers for Disease Control and Prevention. Available at: http://www.cdc.gov/cancer/cervical/statistics/. Accessed November 29, 2006.

Chuang TY, Brashear R. Keratoacanthoma. Last updated September 18, 2006. e medicine: Instant Access to the Minds of Medicine. Available at: http://www.emedicine.com/derm/topic206.htm. Accessed November 28, 2006.

Clausen OP, Beigi M, Bolund L. Keratoacanthomas frequently show chromosomal aberrations as assessed by comparative genomic hybridization. J Invest Dermatol 2002;119:1367–1372.

Dolev J, Kimball AB. Smokeless tobacco lesions. Last updated May 24, 2006. e medicine: Instant Access to the Minds of Medicine. Available at: http://www.emedicine.com/derm/topic652.htm. Accessed November 26, 2006.

Eisenberg E, Rosenberg B, Krutchkoff DJ. Verrucous carcinoma: a possible viral pathogenesis. Oral Surg Oral Med Oral Pathol 1985;59:52–57.

Eversole LR, Laipis PJ. Oral squamous papillomas detection of HPV DNA by in situ hybridization. Oral Surg Oral Med Oral Pathol 1988;44(3): 216–221.

Gearhart PA, Randall TC, Buckley RM. Human papillomavirus. Last updated July 6, 2006. e medicine: Instant Access to the Minds of Medicine. Available at: http://www.emedicine.com/med/topic1037.htm. Accessed November 25, 2006.

Henley JD, Summerlin DJ, Tomich CE. Condyloma acuminatum and condyloma-like lesions of the oral cavity: a study of 11 cases with an intraductal component. Histopathology 2004;44(3):216–221.

Higgins RV, Naumann W, Hall J. Condyloma acuminatum. Last updated July 6, 2006. e medicine: Instant Access to the Minds of Medicine. Available at: http://www.emedicine.com/med/topic3293.htm.

Kellokoski J, Syrjanen S, Syrjanen K, Yliskoski M. Oral mucosal changes in women with genital HPV infection. J Oral Pathol Med 1990;19(3): 142–148.

Kellokoski JK, Syrjanen SM, Chang F, et al. Southern blot hybridization and PCR in detection of oral human papillomavirus (HPV) infections in women with genital HPV infections. Oral Pathol Med 1992;21(10): 459–464.

Kui LL, Xiu HZ, Ning LY. Condyloma acuminatum and human papillomavirus infection in the oral mucosa of children. Pediatr Dent 2003; 25(2):149–153.

Lutzner M, Kuffer R, Blanchet-Bardon C, Croissant O. Different papillomaviruses as the causes of oral warts. Arch Dermatol 1982;118(6): 393–399.

MCCoy JM, Waldron CA. Verrucous carcinoma of the oral cavity: a review of forty-nine cases. Oral Surg Oral Med Oral Pathol 1981;52: 623–629.

Medina JE, Dichtel W, Luna MA. Verrucous-squamous carcinomas of the oral cavity: a clinicopathologic study of 104 cases. Arch Otolaryngol 1984;110:437–440.

Neville BW, Damm DD, Allen CM, Bouquot JE. Oral & maxillofacial pathology. 2nd ed. Philadelphia: WB Saunders, 2002.

Panici PB, Scambia G, Perrone L, et al. Oral condyloma lesions in patients with extensive genital human papillomavirus infection. Am J Obstet Gynecol 1992;167(2):451–458.

Regezi J, Sciubba J, Jordan R. Oral pathology—clinical pathologic correlations. 4th ed. St. Louis: WB Saunders, 2003.

Shroyer KR, Greer RO, Frankhouser CA, et al. Detection of human papillomavirus DNA in oral verrucous carcinomas by polymerase chain reaction. Mod Pathol 1993;6:669–672.

The Society of Gynecologic Oncologists (SGO). Statement on a cervical cancer vaccine. Available at: http://www.cervicalcancercampaign.org/CervicalCancerVaccinePosition.doc . Accessed November 29, 2006.

Syrjanen S, Puranen G. Human papillomavirus infections in children: the potential role of maternal transmission. Crit Rev Oral Biol Med 2000;11(2):259–274. Review.

Wysocki GP, Hardie J, Ultrastructural studies of intraoral verruca vulgaris. Oral Surg Oral Med Oral Pathol 1979;47(1):58–62.

Key Terms

- Adjuvant therapy
- Café-au-lait macule
- Choristoma
- Crepitus
- Cyst
- Cystic hygroma
- Dysphonia
- Fluctuant
- Foliate papilla
- Gingivectomy
- Hamartoma
- Keratoconjunctivitis sicca
- Mutation
- Mycobacteria
- Myoepithelial cells
- Neoplasm
- Oophoritis
- Orchitis
- Parotitis
- Perineural invasion
- Photophobia
- Prognosis
- Proliferation
- Syndrome
- Teratoid cyst
- Trismus
- Tumor
- Xerophthalmia
- Xylitol

Learning Outcomes

1. Define and use the key terms listed in this chapter.

2. Identify the different types of processes associated with the development of soft tissue enlargements.

3. Identify the extraoral manifestations associated with Cowden syndrome, sarcoidosis, Sjögren syndrome, neurofibromatosis, MEN type IIIB, and lymphangiomas.

4. Identify distinguishing characteristics for traumatic neuroma, denture-induced fibrous hyperplasia, peripheral ossifying fibroma, generalized gingival hyperplasia, bacterial sialadenitis, Sjögren syndrome, minor salivary gland tumors, neurofibromatosis, and lymphangioma.

5. Name three medications that are associated with the development of gingival hyperplasia.

6. Identify the circumstances under which traumatic or inflammatory lesions have the highest potential for recurrence after surgical removal.

7. Describe the role of dental biofilm in exacerbating the hyperplastic process that takes place in generalized gingival hyperplasia.

8. List the structures in the oral cavity that are most likely to contain hyperplastic lymphoid tissues.

9. Identify the complications associated with mumps.

10. Discuss treatment options for Sjögren syndrome and other forms of xerostomia.

11. List the soft tissue tumors that occur most frequently on the tongue.

12. Identify the most common soft tissue sarcoma found in children.

13. Discuss complications of parotid gland surgery or removal, including Frey syndrome.

14. Differentiate salivary gland tumors according to whether they arise more frequently in the major or minor salivary glands.

15. State the diagnostic criteria for neurofibromatosis.

16. Describe the malignant conditions associated with neurofibromatosis, MEN III syndrome, and Cowden syndrome.

17. Identify the soft tissue neoplasms for which adjuvant radiation or chemotherapy is often recommended.

CHAPTER OUTLINE

This chapter introduces the clinical, microscopic, and diagnostic aspects of both benign and malignant soft tissue enlargements. Soft tissue enlargements originate from several sources, some of which include epithelial tissue, connective tissue, and neural tissue. Some of the lesions are traumatic or reactive, which means they are associated with an inflammatory process. Others are associated with a neoplastic process, which can be caused by inherited mutations. They may also be associated with genetic damage from an environmental source or from a change in the individual's ability to repair damaged DNA or suppress tumor formation. Still others are developmental, caused by an error in morphogenesis, the abnormal development of a tissue or organ. Often these mimic a neoplastic process, but they are not true neoplasms because they do not exhibit uncontrolled growth. Instead, they grow as the individual grows, in a pattern that is consistent with the specific tissue. The descriptive name, **hamartoma**, is given to a lesion comprising an excessive abnormally arranged mass of normal tissue at any given site. For example, vascular tissues are normally found all over the body, but a

vascular malformation (Chapter 13) is a disarrayed mass of vascular tissues and is therefore a hamartoma. The term **choristoma** is given to this type of lesion when it occurs as a well-formed entity in an area where it would <u>not</u> be expected to be found. For example, Fordyce granules are well-formed sebaceous glands that develop within the buccal mucosa, which is not where they are customarily found. Developmental anomalies are often present at birth (congenital) or they may develop as the individual ages. Soft tissue enlargements exhibit a wide variety of clinical manifestations. Large lesions may be clinically visible, while smaller lesions may only be detectable when palpated. The art of palpation must be developed over time so that the clinician is able to reliably distinguish normal from abnormal (see the application below). Occasionally, specific lesions are associated with very distinct characteristics that help to differentiate them from other lesions. More often, soft tissue enlargements exhibit a generic clinical appearance that offers little direction toward discovering a diagnosis. Because of this, most soft tissue enlargements require a biopsy to determine a definitive diagnosis.

TRAUMATIC OR INFLAMMATORY LESIONS

Hyperplastic traumatic or inflammatory lesions are usually associated with a specific cause or event that initiates an adaptive response in the tissues that initiates enlargement (see Chapter 2). The cause can be as simple as a cheek bite or an ill-fitting denture that causes chronic irritation or it can be complex, such as extensive facial trauma related to a motor vehicle accident. In any case, hyperplastic tissue forms as an overexuberant response to the injury. The disorders in this section are all associated with acute or chronic trauma or inflammation.

NAME: Traumatic neuroma

Etiology: Traumatic neuromas result from chronic or acute trauma that severs nerve tissue. One of the most common causes of traumatic neuroma in the oral cavity is the injection of local anesthetics prior to dental procedures. Surgical procedures such as tooth extraction may also be associated with development of a traumatic neuroma.

Method of Transmission: Not applicable

Epidemiology: Neuromas can occur in any age group, but most often occur in adults.

Pathogenesis: Trauma to the nerve is followed by ineffective unregulated nerve regeneration, which results in enlargement.

Extraoral Characteristics: Not applicable

Perioral and Intraoral Characteristics: Traumatic neuromas appear as small firm nodules covered by nor-

---

APPLICATION

Palpation is defined as using the sense of touch to examine anatomic structures or areas for size, shape, consistency, texture, and other characteristics. This is a learned skill that must be practiced many times before a clinician can feel somewhat confident about his or her findings. It is important to develop a systematic method for palpating the structures of the head, neck, and oral cavity. Some suggestions for this are outlined in Chapter 1. Clinicians should be looking for the following while performing palpations:

- Differences (size, shape, consistency, and texture, among others) between structures that occur on opposite sides. For example: submandibular lymph nodes on the right side may be enlarged, while those on the left are nonpalpable, or the left parotid gland may be hard or doughy to palpation, while the right gland is not. These differences could be significant and should be noted.
- Tenderness. Before beginning palpation, the clinician should ask the patient to report any feelings of tenderness or pain. In addition, it may be helpful for the patient to report any sort of difference between sensations

felt in one area and those felt in other areas. Problems associated with nerve damage, such as paresthesia, may be discovered in this fashion.

- Variations in temperature. Be aware of the temperature of structures as they are palpated. A rise in the temperature can indicate increased blood supply to the area and may be associated with abnormalities, such as vascular malformations or infections.
- Alterations in color. Color changes during palpation of an area should also be noted. Color changes can indicate a vascular lesion or perhaps an inflammatory reaction if the tissue blanches upon palpation.
- Sounds. The clinician should be aware of any sounds that are produced when tissues are palpated. Fluid movement from one part of a lesion to another may cause a crackling sound, or crepitus.

Identification of abnormalities during palpation is just the first step. Formulating a differential diagnosis is the next step. The process then of determining a definitive diagnosis from a differential diagnosis was discussed in Chapter 1.

---

mal mucosa. The nodules are usually painful when palpated but otherwise may produce no symptoms. These lesions are found most often on surfaces that are traumatized frequently, such as the tongue (Fig. 17.1), lower lip and alveolar ridge, or in the area of the mental foramen.

Distinguishing Characteristics: Although not always present, pain on palpation is characteristic of this lesion and may help to differentiate it from similar lesions.

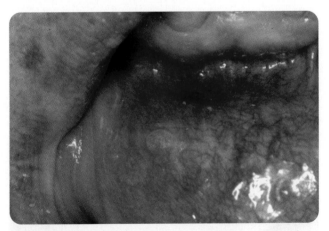

Figure 17.1. Traumatic neuroma. Careful examination of the lower vestibule detected the small nodular growth depicted in this photograph. Microscopic examination determined this to be a neuroma. (Courtesy of Dr. James Sciubba.)

Significant Microscopic Features: Irregular nerve bundles can be seen within dense fibrous connective tissue. Inflammatory cells are rarely seen within the lesion.

Dental Implications: Careful avoidance of the area during dental or dental hygiene therapy is indicated to reduce the chance of eliciting or exacerbating pain.

Differential Diagnosis: The appearance of this lesion is similar to that of many of the other soft tissue enlargements; thus biopsy is necessary for a definitive diagnosis. The presence of pain on palpation should make the clinician suspect a traumatic neuroma, especially if there is a history of trauma. The following lesions should be considered in a differential diagnosis:

1. Neurofibroma, Chapter 17
2. Neurilemmoma, Chapter 17
3. Fibroma, Chapter 17

Treatment and Prognosis: Surgical removal of the neuroma is the usual treatment. There is a low rate of recurrence; therefore, the prognosis is excellent. In some cases, pain persists even after surgical removal of the neuroma.

NAME: Fibroma (focal fibrous hyperplasia, irritation fibroma, traumatic fibroma)

Etiology: Fibromas are not considered true neoplasms, but rather reactive responses to chronic trauma or irritation. One specific form of this condition is called "denture-induced fibrous hyperplasia" (sometimes called "epulis fissuratum") and results from wearing an ill-fitting denture.

Method of Transmission: None

Epidemiology: Fibromas are the most common tumors found in the oral cavity. The peak incidence of this lesion occurs in the fourth to sixth decades, and it is seen more frequently in females than in males. Denture-induced fibrous hyperplasia is seen more often in the older population, since this condition only occurs in denture patients. Older patients in nursing homes are particularly vulnerable, since dental care is not always provided in these facilities.

Pathogenesis: Chronic or recurrent trauma causes a reactive hyperplasia, resulting in a fibrous connective tissue enlargement that appears similar to the surrounding tissues. The affected areas are frequently re-traumatized, adding to the proliferation of the tissues.

Extraoral Characteristics: Not applicable

Perioral and Intraoral Characteristics: The growths are usually nodular and exophytic. They may be pedunculated. They have a smooth surface texture and firm consistency and are about the same color or slightly lighter in color than the surrounding tissues. The surface of the lesion may be ulcerated if it is continually traumatized. Although the lesions can be found on any mucosal surface, they are usually found in areas of the oral cavity that are frequently traumatized, such as the tongue, buccal mucosa, and lips (Fig. 17.2). Figure 17.3 shows a fibroma in the palatal region. Denture-induced fibrous hyperplasia is characterized by exuberant growth of tissue under and around a denture, often involving the tissues in the vestibule. The tissue normally takes on a folded appearance, with the flange of the denture fitting between the folds (Fig. 17.4).

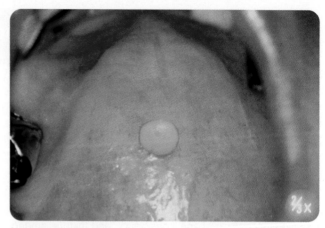

Figure 17.3. This fibroma has developed on the hard palate.

Distinguishing Characteristics: Fibromas can look like any other soft tissue tumor. However, denture-induced fibrous hyperplasia is always be associated with a denture, which can help in developing a differential diagnosis.

Significant Microscopic Features: The histologic appearance is that of a nodular excess of collagen fibers with sparse amounts of inflammatory cells.

Dental Implications: The most important dental implication is determining the cause of the irritation or trauma and removing it. Removing the source will not result in complete resolution of the lesion, but may result in reduction in size because of a reduction in the amount of inflammation present in the tissue.

Patients who have dentures should be advised to seek routine dental care in the form of soft tissue examinations and oral cancer screenings. In addition, dentures do not "fit" an individual for the rest of his or her life, the alveolar bone remodels over time, and the denture teeth wear down from use, so they need to be evaluated routinely for fit and function. Eventually, all dentures must be relined

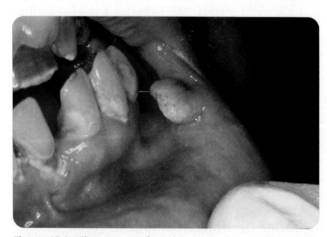

Figure 17.2. Fibromas are found in areas that are frequently traumatized, such as the lip in this picture. (Courtesy of Dr. Michael Brennan.)

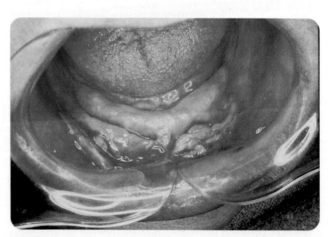

Figure 17.4. Denture-induced fibrous hyperplasia. Note the folds of fibrous tissue within which the flange of the mandibular denture rests.

or replaced. Wearing the denture too often also plays a part in the development of denture-induced fibrous hyperplasia. Dentures should always be left out of the mouth for a period of time every day. One of the problems associated with denture-induced fibrous hyperplasia is the tendency for these areas to develop fungal infections (candidosis) that require treating the denture along with the soft tissue. Patients should be shown how to care for their dentures and for the soft tissues that support them. Refer to Clinical Protocol 11 for information about how to care for a denture.

Differential Diagnosis:
The traumatic fibroma is clinically similar to many of the other soft tissue enlargements. A definitive diagnosis depends on histologic findings after a biopsy. Some of the most likely lesions included in the differential diagnosis include

1. Neurofibroma, Chapter 17
2. Neurilemmoma, Chapter 17
3. Lipoma, Chapter 17
4. Peripheral occifying fibroma, Chapter 17

The surface of denture-induced fibrous hyperplasia may be rough or papillary, in which case it can resemble verrucous carcinoma (Chapter 16) or verruca vulgaris (Chapter 16).

Treatment and Prognosis:
Surgical removal of the fibroma is the treatment of choice. However, recurrence is likely if the source of the trauma is not removed. Surgical removal is also indicated for denture-induced fibrous hyperplasia. In addition, a new, better-fitting denture should be constructed, and the patient should be advised concerning correct methods of denture care. The prognosis for both forms of this lesion is excellent if the source of the irritation is removed. If the source is not eliminated, there is a good risk of recurrence.

COWDEN SYNDROME (MULTIPLE HAMARTOMA SYNDROME)

Cowden syndrome is an autosomal dominant syndrome characterized by a variety of systemic, cutaneous, and oral manifestations. This is a rare disorder; however, since it has severe health implications, a discussion of the basic manifestations is appropriate. Almost all of the individuals affected by this genetic disorder develop facial papules, small 1 to 5 mm, flat-topped, flesh-colored growths. Many also have similar lesions on the hands and feet. Some 80% of patients also exhibit oral papules that are 1 to 3 mm in size, smooth-surfaced, and about the same color, or a little lighter than, the surrounding tissues. The oral lesions are histologically the same as fibromas. The most notable systemic manifestations include thyroid cancer and breast cancer. Approximately 7% of patients will have a thyroid malignancy and 20 to 36% of women will be diagnosed with breast cancer (Miller, 2005). Men with this disorder also have a higher risk of breast cancer. These cancers do not develop until the individual is an adult, and the dental professional may be the first healthcare provider to discover the cutaneous and oral manifestations, which are rather nonspecific. Therefore, the clinician should suspect this disorder if multiple fibroma-like lesions are present and should make an appropriate medical referral. In addition, these patients should be monitored closely for the development of thyroid, breast, and other cancers.

NAME: Peripheral ossifying fibroma

Etiology:
Peripheral fibroma is a reactive hyperplastic lesion that appears exclusively on the gingiva and is thought to originate from submucosal connective tissue or the periodontal ligament.

Method of Transmission: None

Epidemiology:
This is a common oral lesion that occurs in any gender and at any age.

Pathogenesis:
In most cases a local factor such as calculus or some other type of foreign body initiates the hyperplastic process.

Extraoral Characteristics: None

Perioral and Intraoral Characteristics:
Peripheral ossifying fibroma presents as a well-defined, firm, pedunculated or sessile, exophytic mass on the attached gingiva. It is usually smooth-surfaced and covered with normal mucosa, but it may have a rougher or papillary surface texture instead. These lesions are usually less than 1 cm in size. Lesions have a tendency to become traumatized the larger they get, so at times, the surface may be ulcerated. Most peripheral ossifying fibromas are located in interdental papilla areas (Figs. 17.5 and 17.6).

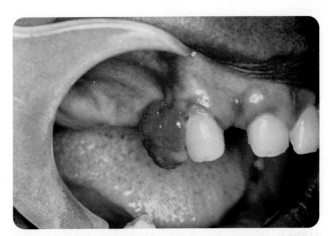

Figure 17.5. Peripheral fibroma. Note the papillary surface texture of this peripheral fibroma. The color of this lesion is darker than normal, making this peripheral fibroma look very similar to a pyogenic granuloma.

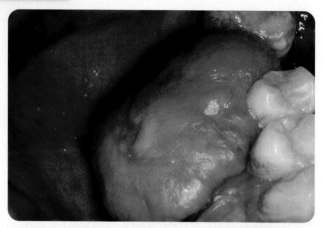

Figure 17.6. Peripheral ossifying fibroma. This exophytic growth arises from the attached gingiva. Note the ulcerated surface.

Distinguishing Characteristics: The peripheral ossifying fibroma is found exclusively on the attached gingiva.

Significant Microscopic Features:

- The peripheral ossifying fibroma contains bone and deposits of cementum within an excessive collagenized connective tissue containing spindle-shaped fibrohistiocyte cells and variable amounts of inflammatory cells. The surface is frequently ulcerated.
- The giant cell fibroma contains many multinucleated fibroblasts.
- The peripheral odontogenic fibroma is distinguished by the presence of odontogenic epithelium within the connective tissue.

The three subtypes cannot be differentiated on a clinical basis, and a biopsy is necessary for a definitive diagnosis.

Dental Implications: The peripheral ossifying fibroma is a reactive lesion; thus it is important to try to identify the source of irritation or trauma and eliminate it.

Differential Diagnosis: Other soft tissue enlargements that form on the attached gingiva are included in the differential diagnosis. These include the following:

1. Pyogenic granuloma, Chapter 13
2. Peripheral giant cell granuloma, Chapter 13
3. Fibroma, Chapter 17
4. Traumatic neuroma, Chapter 17

Treatment and Prognosis: This lesion is treated by local excision with no recurrence usually expected. The prognosis is good if the underlying local factors are removed.

NAME: Generalized gingival hyperplasia

Etiology: Generalized gingival hyperplasia is a generic term used to describe an overgrowth of gingival tissues caused by a number of diverse factors. The most common cause of hyperplastic gingiva is an exuberant response to chronic inflammation associated with dental biofilm or other local factors such as calculus. Some cases of gingival hyperplasia are associated with specific drugs, notably the anticonvulsant *phenytoin* (used in the treatment of epilepsy), *calcium channel blockers* (used for treating cardiovascular conditions), and *cyclosporine* (used as an immunosuppressant in patients who have had organ or tissue transplants). Hormone changes in puberty and pregnancy have also been associated with an overgrowth of gingival tissues due to an exaggerated response to local factors, specifically, dental biofilm. Two other etiologic factors associated with this condition are discussed in previous chapters (leukemia, Chapter 9, and inherited traits, Chapter 6); both may cause generalized gingival enlargement. Information on these two etiologic factors is not repeated in this chapter. Refer to Chapters 6 and 9 for a review of this information, if necessary.

Method of Transmission: Not applicable

Epidemiology: Gingival hyperplasia associated with phenytoin is estimated to occur in 50% of those taking the medication, 27% of those taking cyclosporine, and 10–20% of those taking calcium channel blockers. There are no epidemiologic data available regarding hyperplasia related to hormone fluctuations or dental biofilm infections. There is equal distribution among ages, between genders, and across racial groups.

Pathogenesis: The mechanism that causes drug-induced and hormone-related gingival hyperplasia is not known. Some individuals may be more susceptible to the condition than others, and it is thought that this may be related to the presence of excessive amounts of keratinocyte growth factor, a type of fibroblast growth factor. Whatever the mechanism, poor oral hygiene plays a significant role in the development of gingival hyperplasia. Individuals who have inadequate oral hygiene and are taking drugs associated with this condition, or who are going through hormonal changes, have a higher risk of developing this condition than individuals who have good oral hygiene.

Extraoral Characteristics: Not applicable

Perioral and Intraoral Characteristics: The hyperplasia can be generalized or it can be limited to a localized area. It can range in severity from mild enlargement of the interdental papilla to being so severe it covers most of the coronal surfaces of the teeth. Hyperplasia that is associated with hormonal changes is usually more inflammatory and presents with edema and erythema. Drug-induced hyperplasia is often more fibrotic and presents as firm enlargement of the gingival tissues (Fig. 17.7). If oral hygiene is inadequate, the tissues appear inflamed and edematous in either case.

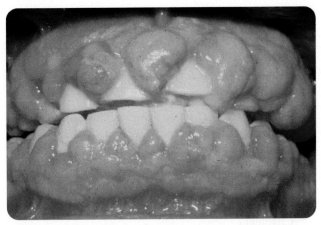

Figure 17.7. Generalized drug-induced gingival hyperplasia. In this case, the hyperplastic process is associated with the drug cyclosporine. (Courtesy of Dr. Terry Rees.)

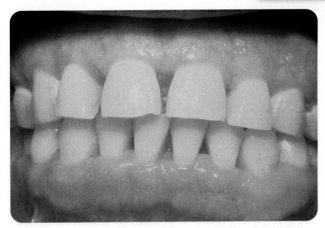

Figure 17.8. Generalized gingival hyperplasia. Same patient as in Figure 17.7 after discontinuing medication, showing resolution of the hyperplasia. (Courtesy of Dr. Terry Rees.)

Distinguishing Characteristics: The clinical appearance of generalized gingival hyperplasia, coupled with a history of taking the specific drugs or hormonal changes, distinguishes this condition from others.

Significant Microscopic Features: Excess amounts of fibrous connective tissue are seen, with or without inflammation.

Dental Implications: The clinician should obtain a thorough medical history and identify risk factors associated with this condition. Dental biofilm is associated with exacerbation of this condition, so patient instruction in oral hygiene is crucial, because it is much easier to prevent this condition than to treat it once it is established.

Differential Diagnosis: No differential diagnosis is necessary because this is a descriptive term; however, the cause of the hyperplasia must be determined. Some etiologic agents that should be considered in addition to hormones and drugs include

1. Leukemia, Chapter 9
2. Dental biofilm infections (periodontitis or gingivitis)
3. Hereditary gingival fibromatosis, Chapter 6

Treatment and Prognosis: Discontinuance of the offending drug, especially cyclosporine, often results in reduction or resolution of the hyperplasia (Fig. 17.8). Increased efforts toward oral hygiene that result in the reduction of biofilm will reduce the inflammatory component of the hyperplasia. Surgical removal of the excess tissue, **gingivectomy,** may be required when there is little or no resolution of the condition after oral hygiene has improved. The prognosis depends on the cause of the hyperplasia. Hormone-induced hyperplasia may resolve when hormones come back into balance. Drug-induced hyperplasia may resolve after discontinuing the drug. However, discontinuing the drug might not be an option, in which

case there is a high probability that the hyperplasia will recur, even after surgical removal.

NAME: Lymphoid hyperplasia

Etiology: Lymphoid hyperplasia (proliferation of lymph cells within lymph tissues) is a reactive response of the immune system caused by infectious agents or foreign substances that invade the body.

Method of Transmission: The infectious agents are transmitted according to their individual characteristics. The hyperplastic response is not transmissible, but is specific for the individual host and depends on the status of the host's immune system and other individual traits.

Epidemiology: This lesion is found in patients of all ages and both sexes.

Pathogenesis: Lymphoid tissue is involved in both the identification and processing of viruses, bacteria, and other invaders of the host. Lymphoid hyperplasia increases the chance that the host will be able to defeat invading agents by providing more cells to destroy them. Acute infections, such as HIV, may cause lymphoid tissues to respond very aggressively as seen in Figure 17.9, which depicts the tonsil area of an individual with HIV.

Extraoral Characteristics: Lymphadenopathy is the abnormal enlargement of lymph nodes anywhere in the body.

Perioral and Intraoral Characteristics: Lymphoid tissue is abundant within the mouth (soft palate, hard palate, ventral surface of the tongue, and floor of the mouth) and is especially dense in Waldeyer's ring (Chapter 4). Lymphoid hyperplasia presents clinically with varying enlargements of the lymphoid tissue, which may appear bulbous, have a papillary or smooth surface, and in most cases be the same color

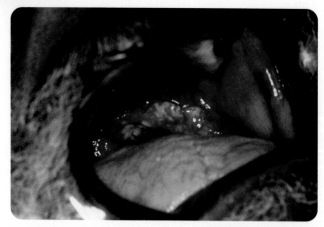

Figure 17.9. Lymphoid hyperplasia. HIV-related lymphoid enlargement of the tonsil.

or slightly lighter than the surrounding tissue. Hyperplasia may involve the lymphoid tissue in the tonsillar region, which may result in bulbous, enlarged tonsils (Fig. 17.10), or, it may occur in the posterior portion of the lateral border of the tongue mixed with the **foliate papilla** (folds of tissue containing taste buds, that are located on the posterior lateral border of the tongue). When hyperplasia occurs in this area, it can become traumatized and appear very suspicious for oral cancer, which is common at this site as well.

Distinguishing Characteristics: The location of the hyperplastic tissue in areas associated with lymphoid tissue suggests lymphoid hyperplasia, but other entities should be ruled out.

Significant Microscopic Features: Proliferation of lymphocytes is evident as well as the presence of numerous macrophages.

Dental Implications: Identification of the hyperplastic tissue is important to rule out more serious conditions such as cancer. The tonsillar region should always be included in the oral cancer examination. This region is of-

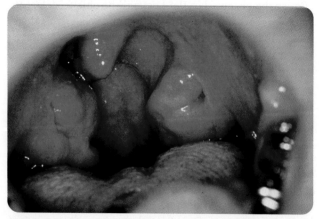

Figure 17.10. Lymphoid hyperplasia. Note the asymmetrical enlargement of the tonsils associated with lymphoid hyperplasia. (Courtesy of Dr. Michael Brennan.)

ten neglected and believed to be beyond the dental practitioner's area of expertise. Any abnormality that is observed should be followed with further evaluations on a periodic basis. In addition, patients may need to be referred to a physician for evaluation for systemic conditions such as infections.

Differential Diagnosis: Any of the disorders that could present as enlargement of lymphoid, tissue or look similar to this, need to be ruled out. Some of these include

1. Carcinoma, Chapter 5
2. Lymphoma, Chapter 9
3. Fibroma and denture-induced fibrous hyperplasia, Chapter17

Treatment and Prognosis: Treatment is not necessary unless the tissue becomes large enough to impede oral functions such as eating or is chronically traumatized. The prognosis is good. Biopsy may be needed to distinguish what appears to be a hyperplasia malignancy.

NAME: Sarcoidosis

Etiology: Sarcoidosis is a multisystem inflammatory disease of unknown etiology that results in the formation of granulomas within affected organs and tissues. Current research supports evidence that this is neither a neoplastic nor an autoimmune disorder. In addition, pathogenic organisms have not been consistently associated with sarcoidosis, although **mycobacteria** (gram-positive, aerobic, nonmotile rods) and Epstein-Barr virus have been suggested. There is some evidence that both genetic and environmental factors play a role in the development of sarcoidosis.

Method of Transmission: It is unknown whether or not this disease is transmissible; however, most believe that it is not passed from person to person.

Epidemiology: Five to 40 of every 100,000 individuals are estimated to be affected by this disease. The prevalence is higher in African Americans than in Caucasians, and females are affected more often than males. The incidence of sarcoidosis peaks between the ages of 25 to 35 years. Females experience a second peak between 45 to 65 years of age.

Pathogenesis: Sarcoidosis is characterized by an exaggerated immune response to an unknown antigen or antigens within the organs that are affected. Lymphocytes, macrophages, mast cells, and natural killer cells perpetuate the immune response and cause a chronic inflammatory process that results in the formation of granulomas. (See Chapter 3 for a review of the chronic inflammatory process.)

Extraoral Characteristics: Sarcoidosis can affect any organ, but the respiratory system is the main target. Respiratory manifestations include shortness of breath

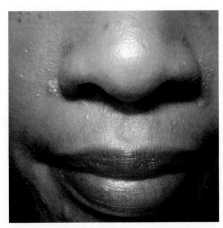

Figure 17.11. Sarcoidosis. Maculopapular rash on the face of an individual who has sarcoidosis. (From Goodheart HP. Goodheart's photoguide of common skin disorders. 2nd ed. Philadelphia: Lippincott Williams & Wilkins, 2003.)

and a persistent cough. Progressive disease can result in respiratory failure. Ocular involvement can cause cataracts, glaucoma, or blindness. Dermatologic manifestations include a maculopapular rash (rash consisting of raised papules surrounded by flat areas of erythema) that can occur on the limbs, face, and buttocks (Fig. 17.11). In addition, painful inflammation of subcutaneous adipose tissues (*erythema nodosum*) may be seen on the arms and the legs, especially on the shins. Granulomas are often found in the liver but usually are not associated with abnormal liver function.

Perioral and Intraoral Characteristics: Salivary gland enlargement, especially of the parotid gland, and xerostomia are possible in sarcoidosis. Other oral lesions present as either firm or spongy papular or nodular growths found on the gingiva, lips, palate, buccal mucosa, or tongue (Fig. 17.12).

Distinguishing Features: Not applicable

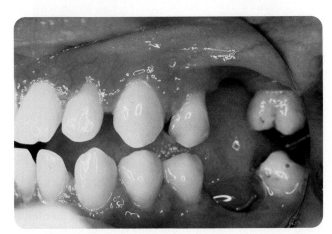

Figure 17.12. Sarcoidosis. Note the small papular growths on the free and attached gingiva in this individual. (Courtesy of Dr. Terry Rees.)

Significant Microscopic Features: Granulomas surrounded by an intense infiltrate of lymphocytes and multinucleated foreign body giant cells are characteristic of sarcoidosis.

Dental Implications: The patient should be encouraged to adhere to a good oral hygiene regimen because of the potential for involvement of the gingival tissues. If xerostomia is present, the patient should be counseled on how to manage the associated symptoms (see Clinical Protocol 4).

Differential Diagnosis: Any other condition associated with parotid gland enlargement needs to be considered, including the following:

1. Papillary cystadenoma lymphomatosum, Chapter 17
2. Chronic alcoholism can cause a diffuse parotid gland enlargement similar to that seen in sarcoidosis. A careful personal/medical and dental history might give the clinician clues as to whether this is a consideration.
3. Diabetes, Chapter 7
4. Eating disorders. Patients with eating disorders may exhibit parotid gland enlargement. The presence of other signs and symptoms of eating disorders such as enamel erosion would help to suggest this diagnosis.
5. Salivary neoplasms, Chapter 17
6. Sjögren syndrome, Chapter 17

In addition, oral mucosal lesions associated with sarcoidosis may resemble those seen in Crohn's disease (Chapter 10) and some deep fungal infections (Chapter 12).

Treatment and Prognosis: Patients often experience spontaneous resolution of the disease. Many other patients live a long productive life with few if any symptoms or manifestations. Still others experience intermittent exacerbations of the disease and require treatment with corticosteroids. These patients must be evaluated for disease manifestations by a physician on a regular basis. Topical steroids may help manage oral lesions. The prognosis is good for those affected by sarcoidosis. Death due to sarcoidosis occurs in less than 5% of untreated patients and is usually associated with respiratory failure or right heart failure.

Ranula

Ranula is a descriptive term used to describe a swelling in the floor of the mouth that resembles a frog's belly (Fig. 17.13). The term usually refers to a swelling that is caused by obstruction of the submandibular or sublingual salivary glands, which results in the development of an inflammatory response. In this case, the ranula is the clinical manifestation of a mucocele (see Chapter 11). Obstruction of the duct can be associated with trauma or with a sialolith (salivary duct stone). If the lesion herni-

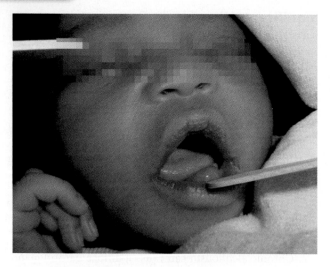

Figure 17.13. Ranula.

ates through the mylohyoid muscle, it is called a "plunging ranula" and appears in the area of the neck.

INFECTIONS

Oral infections can cause soft tissue enlargements. Edema from the inflammatory process can affect any of the oral tissues. This section focuses on infections that cause enlargement of the salivary glands. The parotid gland is affected more often than the other major glands. Parotid enlargement may be clinically visible when the clinician stands in front of the patient and assesses facial symmetry and fullness. The patient may also report feelings of pressure and a sense of fullness.

NAME: Mumps (viral sialadenitis)

Etiology: Mumps is caused by a paramyxovirus.

Method of Transmission: Mumps is transmitted by direct contact with the saliva or saliva droplets of an infected person.

Epidemiology: In 1964 more than 200,000 cases of mumps were reported. This number dropped dramatically with the introduction of a vaccination against the virus that causes mumps. In 2005, only 291 cases were reported across the United States (Curtis and Sinert, 2006).

Pathogenesis: Mumps has an incubation period of 14–25 days; then nonspecific symptoms of low-grade fever, malaise, headache, and chills occur and last anywhere from 3 to 5 days. After this, the patient may experience swelling of the salivary glands. The most common presentation is a **parotitis** (inflammation of the parotid gland), which occurs in 30–40% of patients. Other reported sites of infection are the testes, pancreas, eyes,

ovaries, central nervous system, joints, and kidneys. A patient is considered infectious from about 3 days before the onset up to 4 days into active parotitis. Infections can be asymptomatic in up to 20% of persons.

Extraoral Characteristics: In addition to the general systemic manifestations of the infection, specific complications can occur. This virus can potentially affect any glandular tissue within the body. Some of the tissues that may be affected include the liver, pancreas, kidney, and nervous system. Encephalitis is a rare complication, but it accounts for the 1.4% mortality rate associated with the disease. The sex organs, testes and ovaries, can also be affected if the infection occurs postpuberty. **Orchitis** is the term used to describe inflammation of the testes, and **oophoritis** describes inflammation of the ovaries. Rarely, male sterility can result from this type of inflammation.

Perioral and Intraoral Characteristics: Swelling can occur in any of the major salivary glands, but the parotid gland is affected more often than the others (Fig. 17.14). The classic presentation in the parotid gland includes swelling that lifts the ear lobe upward and outward. There may be erythema surrounding the salivary ducts (Wharton's and/or Stensen's). The patient may complain of pain when chewing or when eating foods that stimulate the salivary glands. Pain may also occur in and around the ear because of pressure from the swelling.

Distinguishing Characteristics: The presence of swelling of the salivary glands, in addition to the systemic manifestations associated with viral infections, strongly suggests this condition.

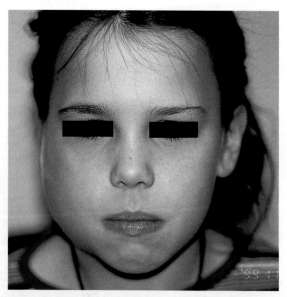

Figure 17.14. Mumps. A unilateral swelling of the parotid gland is clinically evident in this child who has mumps. (From Fleisher GR, Ludwig W, Baskin MN. Atlas of pediatric emergency medicine. Philadelphia: Lippincott Williams & Wilkins, 2004.)

Significant Microscopic Features: The mumps virus can be isolated from urine, blood and nasopharyngeal and buccal swabs for up to 7 days before and 9 days following the appearance of salivary gland swelling.

Dental Implications: It is important to recognize the manifestations of this infection so that the patient can be referred for medical evaluation.

Differential Diagnosis: No differential diagnosis is necessary, as mumps is easily diagnosed from the symptoms and a history of exposure to the virus.

Treatment and Prognosis: Treatment is focused on relieving the general symptoms associated with a viral infection and includes bed rest, plenty of fluids, and analgesics for pain and fever. The prognosis is excellent, and most individuals recover completely. Rarely, the infection results in the complications noted above.

NAME: Bacterial sialadenitis

Etiology: Pathogens that have been associated with bacterial sialadenitis include *Staphylococcus aureus, Streptococcus viridans, Streptococcus pneumoniae,* and *Haemophilus influenzae,* among others.

Epidemiology: This infection tends to appear in older, debilitated patients because this population group has more of the risk factors than any other age group.

Method of Transmission: This infection is not transmitted from person to person.

Pathogenesis: Bacterial sialadenitis develops from an overgrowth of bacteria in a gland that is not producing adequate amounts of saliva (xerostomia) to keep the bacterial population under control. The overgrowth of bacteria causes acinar and ductal inflammation and can lead to the destruction of these cells over time. The xerostomia that predisposes an individual to this infection is often related to medications, connective tissue disorders that include Sjögren syndrome as a component, postradiation therapy side effects, side effects related to salivary gland surgery, and inadequate hydration.

Extraoral Characteristics: Systemic manifestations of fever, malaise, and headache are often present.

Perioral and Intraoral Characteristics: Painful swelling of the affected gland is the classic clinical feature of this infection. **Trismus** (persistent contraction of the masseter muscle) is common, as is painful chewing. Purulent exudate may be present at the duct orifice, and exudate may be expressed from the gland with gentle pressure.

Distinguishing Characteristics: Inflammation of the salivary ducts and the presence of purulent exudate are characteristic of this infection.

Significant Microscopic Features: Not applicable

Dental Implications: Xerostomia is one of the major risk factors for developing this infection. Patients who have xerostomia should be monitored closely. In addition, they should be educated about various strategies that can be used to alleviate xerostomia. (See Clinical Protocol 4 for additional information.)

Differential Diagnosis: The characteristic features of this infection make a differential diagnosis unnecessary.

Treatment and Prognosis: This infection may be difficult to treat. The exudate coming from the gland should be cultured to determine the specific bacteria responsible, so that the appropriate antibiotic can be prescribed. Analgesics are used to help decrease pain, and moist compresses, rehydration, and stimulation of salivary flow are helpful in alleviating discomfort. The prognosis is good in most cases. Occasionally, the infection may extend into the tissues surrounding the gland and cause spread of the infection into the neck or within the ear.

IMMUNE SYSTEM DISORDERS

Parotid enlargement can result from an immune system disorder. Many connective tissue disorders associated with immune system dysfunction include salivary gland dysfunction, with or without enlargement, as one of their elements.

NAME: Sjögren syndrome

Etiology: Sjögren syndrome is an autoimmune disorder.

Method of Transmission: Not applicable

Epidemiology: Sjögren syndrome is the second most common connective tissue disorder after lupus erythematosus. It affects about 3% of the population. About 90% of patients with Sjögren syndrome are women between the ages of 30 and 65 years.

Pathogenesis: The destruction of the exocrine glands, especially the salivary and lacrimal glands, is caused by activated T cells that infiltrate the glands (for reasons that are not clear) and attack the acinar cells and the gland ducts. The presence of the large numbers of T cells causes glandular enlargement, and destruction of the acini causes loss of function. There are two forms of the disease, primary and secondary. *Primary Sjögren syndrome* occurs as isolated destruction of the lacrimal and salivary glands, while *secondary Sjögren syndrome* occurs in conjunction with another autoimmune disorder. The most common associated disorder is rheumatoid arthritis (Chapter 10); others include systemic lupus erythematosus (Chapter 12) and scleroderma (Chapter 23).

Extraoral Characteristics: Changes in the lacrimal gland cause **keratoconjunctivitis sicca** (**xerophthalmia**, or "dry eyes"), which is associated with blurring of vision, burning, and itching. Most patients complain of severe **photophobia** (sensitivity to light) and a feeling that there is something in their eyes. If this condition is not managed correctly, the cornea can become eroded and ulcerated, and permanent damage can result. While the salivary and lacrimal glands are affected most often, any mucosal surface is at risk. This has implications within the intestinal, respiratory, and genitourinary tracts. Pulmonary disease and frequent infections often manifest when the mucus-producing cells of the bronchi are involved. The mucus becomes very thick and sticky and is more prone to colonization by pathogenic bacteria. Gastrointestinal (GI) problems might include dysphagia (difficult or painful swallowing) and inflammation of the mucosal surfaces of the GI tract due to inadequate and abnormal secretions. Liver disease, kidney disease, and inflammation of the thyroid have all been reported with Sjögren syndrome. Secondary Sjögren syndrome presents identically but with the additional manifestations of the concurrent connective tissue disorder.

Perioral and Intraoral Characteristics: The most significant oral manifestation of Sjögren syndrome is xerostomia, which varies in severity from individual to individual. Patients complain of difficulty swallowing, altered taste, and difficulty wearing prosthetic devices such as dentures. Xerostomia may cause the oral tissues to atrophy and the tongue to become more fissured. The parotid glands and/or the submandibular glands become enlarged in about 50% of patients with this disorder. The enlargement is usually bilateral and symmetrical and may recur and regress many times over the course of the disease (Fig. 17.15).

Distinguishing Characteristics: The most common clinical presentation of secondary Sjögren syndrome is a triad manifestation of rheumatoid arthritis, xerostomia, and keratoconjunctivitis.

Significant Microscopic Features: Heavy lymphocyte infiltration that replaces major salivary gland tissue is characteristic of Sjögren syndrome.

Dental Implications: Xerostomia increases the patient's risk for dental caries, periodontal disease, and infections such as candidiasis (Chapters 13 and 14). Refer to Clinical Protocol 4 for more information on the management of xerostomia. These patients should also be periodically monitored for neoplastic changes in the parotid gland (see below).

Differential Diagnosis: The differential diagnosis of a diffuse parotid enlargement includes the following conditions:

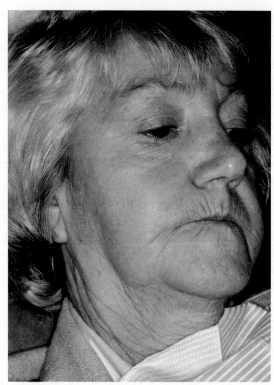

Figure 17.15. Sjögren syndrome. This patient had bilateral swelling of the parotid glands associated with Sjögren syndrome. Note the redness surrounding the eyes, which indicates keratoconjunctivitis sicca.

1. Papillary cystadenoma lymphomatosum, Chapter 17
2. Alcoholism. Chronic alcoholism can cause a diffuse parotid gland enlargement similar to that seen in Sjögren syndrome. A careful personal/medical and dental history might give the clinician clues about whether this is a consideration.
3. Diabetes, Chapter 7
4. Eating disorders. Patients with eating disorders may exhibit parotid gland enlargement. The presence of other signs and symptoms of eating disorders such as enamel erosion would suggest this diagnosis.
5. Salivary neoplasms, Chapter 17

An assessment of salivary function, including, but not limited to, salivary flow rate of individual glands and of the oral cavity as a whole (stimulated and unstimulated) is the mode of assessment used most often. Biopsy of labial minor salivary glands, or sometimes the parotid gland is often done to demonstrate lymphocyte infiltration. There are also blood tests that measure specific levels of autoantibodies particular to several of the autoimmune diseases, including Sjögren syndrome, which can help to create a more definitive diagnosis.

Treatment and Prognosis: Sjögren syndrome is usually treated by managing the symptoms of the disease. This includes the use of artificial saliva and tears, the extensive use of fluoride for caries prevention, and home care and diet modifications. Using fluoride varnish at every 3-month maintenance appointment is an excellent therapy for the Sjögren's patient. Another simple modification is the introduction of **xylitol** (an artificial sweetener)—sweetened chewing gum. Chewing gum physically stimulates saliva production, and the xylitol itself stimulates saliva production. Bacteria ingest xylitol over sucrose, but they are unable to metabolize it, so the number of bacteria and the level of acid in the mouth drop. Research on drugs that stimulate saliva production shows mixed results. When drugs are used, they should be used with caution, and their effectiveness should be monitored. Sjögren syndrome is a chronic condition that requires long-term management and lifestyle adaptations. The prognosis is normally good with strict adherence to modifications. The prognosis is complicated by the fact that about 6 to 10% of cases are associated with a malignant transformation of the altered glandular tissue to lymphoma.

SOFT TISSUE NEOPLASMS

Neoplastic soft tissue enlargements are often associated with specific gene mutations that may be inherited or created by environmental factors. Soft tissue neoplasms can be either benign or malignant. Benign neoplastic growths are usually well circumscribed and often *encapsulated* (surrounded by a fibrous tissue capsule). These may invade local tissues, but they are not able to metastasize. Malignant soft tissue growths invade local tissues and can metastasize to any part of the body. Malignant cells replace normal functioning cells of an organ or tissue and can result in the death of the individual. Benign and malignant soft tissue neoplasms are derived from one or more of the tissues found in the body. Chapter 5 discusses the general characteristics of neoplastic growths. Table 5.2 lists the nomenclature for both benign and malignant neoplasms and may be referred to for review of this information.

NAME: Fibromatosis (desmoid tumor)

Etiology: There is no specific etiology associated with most of these neoplasms. They may be associated with mutation of the cell's DNA or disruption of another defense against uncontrolled growth of cells. At one time they were thought to be reactive lesions, because they occasionally appeared at a site where a previous surgical procedure was performed.

Method of Transmission: Several forms of fibromatosis (myofibromatosis, familial adenomatous polyposis, and multicentric fibromatosis) are considered inherited conditions.

Epidemiology: These neoplasms are more frequent in those under the age of 40, with children and young adults

affected most often. Females are more likely to have aggressive fibromatosis than males.

Pathogenesis: Fibromatosis represents a group of lesions that exhibit a somewhat aggressive behavior. They are more destructive than benign neoplasms but have no ability to metastasize.

Extraoral Characteristics: These growths can occur in any area of the body. In the head and neck area, these lesions appear as enlarging masses that are firm to palpation when found in soft tissues. They may also be found centrally located within bone, where expansion of the cortical bone may be observed.

Perioral and Intraoral Characteristics: Fibromatosis manifests as a slowly enlarging soft tissue mass when observed in the oral cavity (Fig. 17.16).Facial asymmetry can be expected as the lesions enlarge. The soft tissues surrounding the mandible are commonly affected. If the bone of the mandible is affected, the lesions appear as ill-defined radiolucencies. Expansion of the cortical bone may occur.

Distinguishing Characteristics: Not applicable

Significant Microscopic Features: Spindle-shaped cells growing in bundles are characteristic of fibromatosis.

Dental Implications: Early diagnosis of any enlarging mass is crucial to obtaining a favorable treatment outcome. The dental hygienist is in an excellent position to provide thorough examinations, which can identify abnormal growths when they are small.

Differential Diagnosis: Any of the soft tissue tumors would have to be ruled out by biopsy. Specifically, fibromatosis must be differentiated from fibrosarcoma. The differentiation between the two depends largely on tumor behavior and somewhat less on the histology of the lesion.

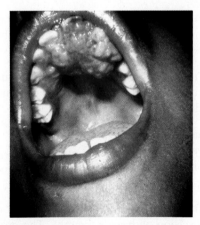

Figure 17.16. Fibromatosis. This palatal lesion is an example of an aggressive fibromatosis. (Courtesy of Dr. John Jacoway.)

Treatment and Prognosis: The treatment of choice is aggressive surgical excision. Chemotherapeutic agents (anticancer drugs) are sometimes used in addition to the surgery because there is a high rate of recurrence with these tumors. The tumors have been known to regress spontaneously, but, in general, they have a recurrence rate of approximately 25% in the head and neck area. Deaths have been reported due to recurrence and locally aggressive invasion of vital tissues.

NAME: Fibrosarcoma

Etiology: The development of fibrosarcoma may be linked to previous radiation therapy or burn injury.

Method of Transmission: Not applicable

Epidemiology: This rare neoplasm occurs more often in young adults and children and slightly more often in males.

Pathogenesis: Fibrosarcoma is a malignant tumor of fibroblasts that can occur in soft tissues or within bone. Fibrosarcoma is characterized by a proliferation of fibroblasts. It usually arises about 10 years after radiation therapy or about 30 years after a burn injury.

Extraoral Characteristics: The most common extraoral presentation of fibrosarcoma is in the thigh bone around the knee joint.

Perioral and Intraoral Characteristics: Most of these lesions present as gradually enlarging, painless masses. Ulceration of the surface, secondary to trauma, may occur as the lesion enlarges.

Distinguishing Characteristics: Not applicable

Significant Microscopic Features: Proliferating spindle cells are arranged in a herringbone pattern, and mitotic figures are commonly observed.

Dental Implications: Early identification of enlarging soft tissue masses is of utmost importance in obtaining a favorable treatment outcome.

Differential Diagnosis: Any of the soft tissue tumors need to be ruled out by biopsy. The neoplasms most likely to be considered include

1. Fibromatosis, Chapter 17
2. Leiomyosarcoma, Chapter 17
3. Melanoma, Chapters 5 and 15
4. Spindle cell carcinoma

Treatment and Prognosis: The treatment of choice is surgical excision with wide margins. The prognosis is guarded. There is local recurrence in 50 to 75% of cases, and this is the most common cause of death. Distant metastasis occurs in 20 to 40% of cases, with spread occurring more commonly to the lungs. The 5-year survival rate is 50 to 70%.

NAME: Neurilemoma (Schwannoma)

Etiology: The neurilemoma arises from proliferation of the Schwann cells of the nerve sheath.

Method of Transmission: Not applicable

Epidemiology: Neurilemomas are found most often in individuals between the ages of 20 and 50 years. They present in the oral cavity in both genders in equal numbers.

Pathogenesis: This is a slow-growing tumor that can occur in soft tissues or within bone. As the Schwann cells proliferate they become surrounded by a fibrous capsule. The nerve does not become entangled with the tumor but is pushed aside as the tumor grows.

Extraoral Characteristics: Neurilemomas usually appear as small, smooth-surfaced, firm, nodular growths in the head and neck area and on the flexor surfaces of the arms and legs. The lesions are normally painless unless they are very large or they impinge on vital tissues (Kao, 2006). One form, the acoustic neurilemoma, affects the eighth cranial nerve at about the position of the internal auditory meatus. These can cause tinnitus (ringing in the ears) and deafness.

Perioral and Intraoral Characteristics: Intraoral neurilemomas manifest as smooth-surfaced submucosal masses (Fig. 17.17). The lesions can occur anywhere in the mouth but occur most frequently on the tongue. They can also occur within the bone of the maxilla or mandible, where they appear as well-defined radiolucencies. Bone lesions are often associated with pain and paresthesia (numbness).

Distinguishing Characteristics: Not applicable

Significant Microscopic Features: The neurilemoma is a mass of spindle-shaped cells surrounded by a

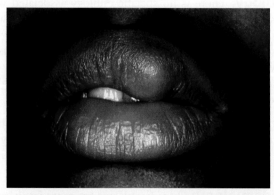

Figure 17.17. Neurilemoma of the lip. The lip is not a common location in which to find this lesion. (Courtesy of Dr. Jacob Jacoway.)

fibrous capsule composed of residual nerve fibers and the connective tissue that forms the support structure for the peripheral nerves.

Dental Implications: Accurate interpretation of radiographic findings in areas where a patient reports pain and/or paresthesia may be essential to detect this neoplasm, when it arises in bone.

Differential Diagnosis: Any of the soft tissue tumors must be ruled out by biopsy. The most likely soft tissue growths that should be considered include

1. Neurofibroma, Chapter 17
2. Leiomyoma, Chapter 17
3. Traumatic fibroma, Chapter 17
4. Lipoma, Chapter 17

Treatment and Prognosis: The treatment of choice is surgical excision. There is little chance of recurrence, and the prognosis is excellent.

NAME: Neurofibroma

Etiology: The solitary neurofibroma is a benign neoplasm that originates from the Schwann cells and/or connective tissue cells that support the peripheral nerves. Neurofibromatosis (*von Recklinghausen's disease of the skin*) is an inherited syndrome characterized by multiple neurofibromas and other abnormalities. The solitary form of neurofibroma and the form associated with the inherited syndrome display similar clinical and microscopic appearances. Neurofibromatosis is discussed below in this chapter with other genetic disorders.

Method of Transmission: Not applicable

Epidemiology: The average age for developing a solitary oral neurofibroma is 45 years. There is no predilection for any race or gender.

Pathogenesis: The solitary neurofibroma may be found on any nerve, where it presents as a slow-growing, painless mass.

Extraoral Characteristics: Solitary neurofibromas may affect skin, major nerve plexuses, and the gastrointestinal tract, among others. The cutaneous presentation is a soft, nodular, sessile, or pedunculated growth. They are usually small, ranging in size from a few millimeters to several centimeters.

Perioral and Intraoral Characteristics: Intraorally, the tumor manifests as a slow-growing, smooth-surfaced, asymptomatic mass. It is most commonly located on the tongue or buccal mucosa; however, it can be located at any intraoral site (Fig. 17.18). Occasionally, the tumor may be found within the bone of the maxilla or mandible, where it can cause extensive expansion and destruction of the bone.

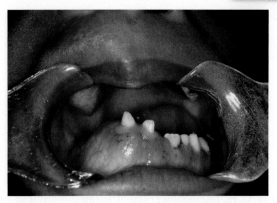

Figure 17.18. Neurofibroma. This neurofibroma of the gingiva has caused significant deformity. If this had been detected earlier, it might have been easily removed. The solitary lesions have little chance of recurring. (Courtesy of Dr. John Jacoway.)

Distinguishing Characteristics: Not applicable

Significant Microscopic Features: Neurofibromas are composed of spindle cells in a delicate connective tissue matrix. Neurofibromas may be diffuse, with no apparent margins, or they may be well circumscribed. Mast cells are usually found within the lesion.

Dental Implications: The presence of multiple neurofibromas may indicate a relatively common genetic disorder called neurofibromatosis. The dental hygienist may be in a unique position to detect these lesions and request referral of the patient for medical evaluation.

Differential Diagnosis: Any of the soft tissue enlargements must be ruled out, including:

1. Neurilemoma, Chapter 17
2. Leiomyoma, Chapter 17
3. Traumatic fibroma, Chapter 17
4. Lipoma, Chapter 17

In addition, in the case of diffuse lesions of the tongue, other causes of macroglossia such as amyloidosis (Chapter 9) or lymphangioma (Chapter 17) need to be ruled out.

Treatment and Prognosis: Surgical excision is the preferred treatment. Solitary neurofibromas have little chance of recurrence and thus have an excellent prognosis.

Neoplasms of Smooth Muscle

The leiomyoma is a benign neoplasm of smooth muscle that is commonly found in the muscular layer of the gut and in the uterus. Rarely, leiomyomas are found in the oral cavity, where they present as a slow-growing, painless, smooth-surfaced mass that is usually less than 2 cm in diameter. They can be found in any intraoral site; however, the tongue, hard palate, and buccal mucosa are fre-

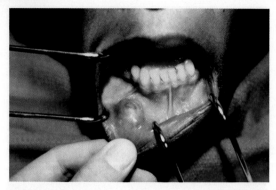

Figure 17.19. Leiomyomas present as smooth-surfaced submucosal masses, such as this leiomyoma in the lip.

quently involved. Figure 17.19 shows a leiomyoma of the labial mucosa. Surgical removal is the treatment of choice, and the chance of recurrence is negligible.

The leiomyosarcoma is a malignant neoplasm of smooth muscle that occurs most often in the deep tissues of the extremities and within the muscular layers of the esophagus. It occurs infrequently within the oral cavity, where the tissue of origin is the smooth muscle associated with the walls of blood vessels. The lesions usually manifest as painful masses in the jaws or gingival tissues. The treatment of choice is surgical excision with wide margins. Local recurrence of the tumor is seen in 30% of cases, and metastasis to the cervical lymph nodes or to the lungs is reported in more than 50% of cases. The long-term prognosis is poor.

Neoplasms of Striated Muscle Cells

The rhabdomyoma is a benign neoplastic growth of striated muscle cells. These tumors are very rare but tend to form in the soft tissues of the head and neck more frequently than in other areas. They appear as painless submucosal swellings of the floor of the mouth, tongue, and soft palate (Fig. 17.20). Surgical removal is the treatment

of choice, and there is little chance of recurrence. The malignant counterpart of the rhabdomyoma is the rhabdomyosarcoma.

NAME: Rhabdomyosarcoma

Etiology: The rhabdomyosarcoma is a malignant tumor of striated muscle that has an unknown etiology. Several genetic syndromes, including neurofibromatosis and nevoid basal cell carcinoma syndrome, and several environmental agents, including parental use of marijuana or cocaine and intrauterine exposure to x-radiation, have been associated with an increased risk of developing this tumor.

Method of Transmission: Not applicable

Epidemiology: Rhabdomyosarcoma is the most common soft tissue sarcoma seen in children. Approximately 87% of cases are seen in children under the age of 15 years. Some 250 cases, about 6 individuals out of 1 million, are diagnosed every year in the United States. The tumor occurs equally in all ethnic groups and is slightly more common in males.

Pathogenesis: Rhabdomyosarcoma presents as a rapidly growing mass. The lungs, bone, and bone marrow are the most common sites for metastasis.

Extraoral Characteristics: These tumors are found most often in the head and neck area, extremities, and the genitourinary tract. Symptoms are usually related to the location of the tumor. The growths may be palpable if superficially located. One of the most common sites of involvement in the head and neck is the orbital area (33% of cases) (Fig. 17.21). Deeper growths may not be discovered until they are very large and become symptomatic.

Perioral and Intraoral Characteristics: When this lesion develops intraorally, it is found on the hard and soft palates and the tongue more frequently than in other areas. Symptoms of pain and paresthesia may be present,

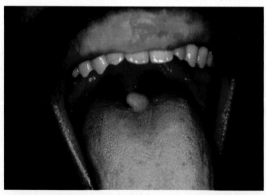

Figure 17.20. Rhabdomyoma. This is an example of a rhabdomyoma on the dorsal surface of the tongue. (Courtesy of Dr. Valerie A. Murrah.)

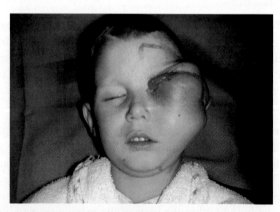

Figure 17.21. Periorbital rhabdomyosarcoma is a rapidly growing tumor seen most often in young children. (Courtesy of Dr. John Jacoway.)

especially if the jaw is involved. Lesions located within the jaws appear radiographically as ill-defined radiolucencies.

Distinguishing Characteristics: Rapidly growing soft tissue masses in the orbital region should alert the clinician to the possibility of rhabdomyosarcoma.

Significant Microscopic Features: There are three main histologic forms of this neoplasm, ranging from neoplasms with well-differentiated cells that exhibit the striations normally seen in striated muscle to oddly shaped cells that exhibit few if any striations.

Dental Implications: Any soft tissue enlargement that has not been identified and does not resolve over a 2-week period should be biopsied. Patients should have dental evaluations prior to starting chemotherapy and/or radiation therapy. (Refer to Chapter 5 for a review of the procedures that need to be done prior to chemotherapy or radiation therapy.)

Differential Diagnosis: Other tumors that manifest as rapidly growing enlargements need to be considered in a differential diagnosis. These include

1. Myofibroma, Chapter 17
2. Ewing sarcoma, Chapter 18
3. Lymphoma, Chapter 9
4. Osteosarcoma, Chapter 18

Treatment and Prognosis: The standard treatment for rhabdomyosarcoma is complete surgical removal combined with chemotherapy and radiation therapy. The prognosis varies widely, according to the location of the tumor, its histologic characteristics, and whether there has been metastasis. The 5-year survival rate for localized disease is more than 80%, while that for metastatic disease is less than 30% (Cripe, 2006).

Neoplasms of Fat Tissue

The lipoma is a benign neoplasm of adipose cells. This neoplasm is considered the most common soft tissue tumor in the body, and it can occur in any tissue or organ; however, it is rare in the oral cavity. Intraorally, lipoma appears as a superficial, smooth-surfaced, soft, palpable mass that often imparts a yellowish color to the overlying mucosa (Fig. 17.22). This tumor is found more often in adults around the age of 50 years. Surgical removal is the treatment of choice, and recurrence is not a factor.

The malignant counterpart of the lipoma is the liposarcoma. Like the lipoma, the liposarcoma is rarely found in the oral cavity. Surgical excision is the treatment of choice, and the prognosis is normally good; however, the tumor has a tendency to recur, and the prognosis becomes less favorable with each recurrence. These patients should

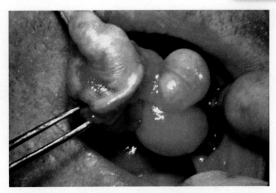

Figure 17.22. This lipoma is being excised from the buccal mucosa. The lipoma is the small, smooth-surfaced, yellowish mass to the right of center in the photograph.

be followed closely by a dental professional to facilitate the early discovery of any recurrent lesions.

Salivary Gland Neoplasms

Salivary gland tumors constitute a relatively uncommon, but important, set of soft tissue lesions. In addition to the major salivary glands (parotid, submandibular, and sublingual), hundreds of minor salivary glands exist throughout the oral mucosa. Salivary gland neoplasms, both benign and malignant, usually present as smooth-surfaced masses of the soft tissue; therefore, the role of palpation in the detection of these tumors and in their clinical characterization is paramount. If tumors arise in the major salivary glands, it is often necessary to remove the entire gland to remove the tumor. In the case of the parotid gland, the facial nerve may have to be sacrificed. Complications of facial nerve damage are identical or similar to those seen in Bell's palsy (Chapter 10). The dental hygienist may have to educate the patient about methods of managing the complications associated with facial nerve damage if present.

NAME: Pleomorphic adenoma (mixed tumor)

Etiology: The pleomorphic adenoma is a benign neoplasm that arises from the proliferation of two different types of salivary gland cells, ductal and **myoepithelial** (contractile cells of epithelial origin). Alterations in chromosome 8 may be associated with the development of this neoplasm.

Method of Transmission: Not applicable

Epidemiology: This is the most common benign salivary gland neoplasm, accounting for about 80% of these tumors. They have been reported in all age groups but predominate in middle-aged individuals, from 30 to 50 years. Most studies report a slight female predilection.

Pathogenesis: Pleomorphic adenomas typically arise as slow-growing, firm masses that are slightly compressi-

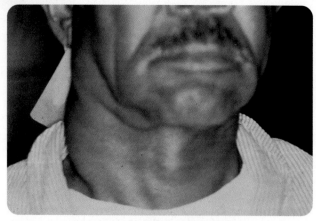

Figure 17.23. Pleomorphic adenoma presents as an enlargement of a salivary gland. The parotid gland is the gland most commonly involved. (Courtesy of Dr. Carolyn Bentley.)

ble. Pleomorphic adenomas have a tendency to recur; in addition, there is a slight chance that they will undergo malignant transformation (carcinoma ex pleomorphic adnoma).

Extraoral Characteristics: Not applicable

Perioral and Intraoral Characteristics: This neoplastic growth affects the parotid gland more often than any of the other major salivary glands, but it is not uncommon to find it in any of the major glands. It manifests as a painless, slow-growing, firm mass, usually found in the lower superficial lobe of the parotid near the angle of the mandible (Fig. 17.23). Within the oral cavity, the pleomorphic adenoma appears as a firm, nodular growth covered by intact mucosa, most often found on the palate (Fig. 17.24), followed by the upper lip and buccal mucosa. The tumors are mobile when found in the soft tissues but are not mobile when found on the palate.

Distinguishing Characteristics: Not applicable

Significant Microscopic Features: These tumors have a wide range of histologic presentations, with varying amounts of ductal versus myoepithelial cells and various patterns of growth. The pleomorphic adenoma is frequently surrounded by a capsule that may have nests of neoplastic cells extending through it. This is thought to be the reason for its high recurrence rate.

Dental Implications: Pleomorphic adenomas are difficult to remove completely; therefore, it is essential to monitor these patients periodically for recurrences.

Differential Diagnosis: Other salivary gland tumors must be ruled out; in addition, the following conditions should receive consideration:

1. Lymphoma, Chapter 9
2. Sarcoidosis, Chapter 17
3. Lymphadenopathy, mentioned in many chapters in association with many disorders
4. Peripheral nerve sheath tumors

Intraoral involvement of the minor salivary glands can mimic other soft tissue enlargements, and lesions such as the lipoma (Chapter 17) and necrotizing sialometaplasia (Chapter 12) should also be included in a differential diagnosis.

Treatment and Prognosis: Complete surgical removal is recommended, with enough adjacent tissue removed with the tumor to ensure that there are no remaining nests of cells. Excision of parotid tumors normally requires techniques that allow the facial nerve to be preserved. Tumors located on the palate may require the removal of some bone. The prognosis is excellent for pleomorphic adenomas that have been removed completely. Failure to adequately treat pleomorphic adenomas can result in significant morbidity due to extensive growth (Fig. 17.25), or in malignant transformation of the tumor. The likelihood of malignant transformation increases with the

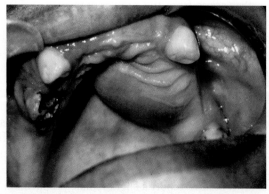

Figure 17.24. Pleomorphic adenoma. When this lesion is found intraorally, it is seen on the palate (as shown here) more than in any other area.

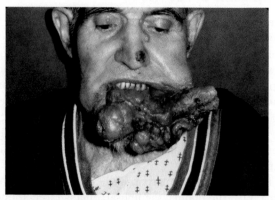

Figure 17.25. Pleomorphic adenoma. When treated early, the prognosis for pleomorphic adenoma is excellent. However, failure to treat these neoplastic growths can result in extensive deformity as seen in this picture. (Courtesy of Dr. Robert J. Gorlin.)

duration of the tumor, the number of recurrences, and the age of the patient.

CARCINOMA EX-MIXED TUMOR

This rare malignant lesion develops within an already existing mixed tumor (pleomorphic adenoma). Most of these are found in the parotid gland (68%), while about 18% are found in the minor salivary glands. Surgical removal is the treatment of choice, but there is a 50% chance of recurrence. The 15-year survival rate is approximately 20%. Prompt identification and removal of pleomorphic adenomas drastically reduces the occurrence of these tumors.

FREY SYNDROME

The parotid gland may have to be totally removed (parotidectomy) to obtain complete surgical excision of any neoplastic growth in the gland. Frey syndrome is a common complication of this surgical procedure and represents a unique example of how nerve regeneration can go awry. In this case, the parasympathetic nerves that innervate the parotid gland are severed during the surgery, after which they may undergo abnormal regeneration and join with the sympathetic nerves that innervate the facial sweat glands. This abnormal regeneration causes about 50% of patients to report symptoms of facial sweating when their salivary glands are stimulated. In rare cases, the facial sweating can be copious; however, there are no serious problems associated with this condition. Medical therapies are available to manage Frey syndrome, for example, the use of local botulinum toxin (botox) injections.

NAME: Papillary cystadenoma lymphomatosum (Warthin's tumor)

Etiology: The etiology of these tumors is unknown, although multiple studies have shown a strong relationship of up to eight times the normal risk between smoking and the development of this tumor.

Method of Transmission: Not applicable

Epidemiology: Warthin's tumor is the second most common benign parotid gland tumor. It usually appears in individuals between 40 and 70 years of age. The tumor is seen most often in Caucasian male smokers.

Pathogenesis: The pathogenesis of Warthin's tumor is largely unknown. These tumors may originate from the entrapment of salivary gland cells within lymph nodes as the nodes are developing. Another possibility is that they develop from a proliferation of salivary gland tissue associated with lymphoid hyperplasia due to chronic inflammation. There is speculation that damage to mitochondrial DNA in the cells of the parotid gland may initiate the neoplastic process. The damage is thought to be associated with chemicals formed in the oral environment as a result of exposure to tobacco smoke when the tumor occurs in smokers.

Extraoral Characteristics: Not applicable

Perioral and Intraoral Characteristics: Warthin's tumors present as slow-growing, rubbery or firm, painless masses, usually found in the tail of the parotid gland near the angle of the mandible (Fig. 17.26). There is a tendency for this tumor to appear bilaterally.

Distinguishing Characteristics: Not applicable

Significant Microscopic Features: The tumor is named for its microscopic appearance. Cystic spaces contain papillary projections that are lined by columnar cells, which are in turn supported by an underlying layer of lymphoid tissue.

Dental Implications: Patients who have a history of smoking have a much higher risk of developing this neoplasm. The dental professional should take this into consideration when performing extraoral and perioral palpations. In addition, since these tend to appear bilaterally, if one parotid gland is found to have a palpable mass the opposite gland should be thoroughly palpated. The decrease in risk for this tumor can be mentioned as a benefit associated with smoking cessation.

Differential Diagnosis: Any of the salivary gland tumors that present as slow-growing masses or neoplasms that manifest as enlarged lymph nodes must be ruled out, including the following:

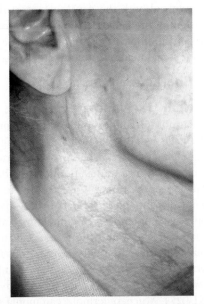

Figure 17.26. Papillary cystadenoma lymphomatosum. Note the subtle swelling at the angle of the mandible where the tail of the parotid gland is located. This is the classic presentation of this tumor.

1. Pleomorphic adenoma, Chapter 17
2. Lymphoma, Chapter 9
3. Mucoepidermal carcinoma, Chapter 17

In addition, one should consider infectious diseases that manifest in the parotid gland, such as mumps, and metabolic conditions such as malnutrition (including malnutrition caused by eating disorders and chronic alcoholism), and diabetes mellitus in the differential diagnosis.

Treatment and Prognosis: Surgical removal of the tumor is the treatment of choice. The prognosis is excellent. There is a chance of recurrence, but many feel that these recurrent tumors may actually be new primary lesions, especially if the patient has continued to smoke. There have been rare reports of malignant transformation within the tumors.

NAME: Mucoepidermoid carcinoma

Etiology: The etiology of mucoepidermoid carcinoma is not known.

Method of Transmission: Not applicable

Epidemiology: Mucoepidermoid carcinoma is the most common malignant salivary gland tumor in the United States. The highest numbers of cases occur in individuals during their second to seventh decade of life. This tumor is also considered the most common salivary gland malignancy in children. Slightly more females than males are affected.

Pathogenesis: The tumors are thought to arise from proliferation of undifferentiated excretory stem cells (stem cells involved with the development of the excretory duct system of the glands). The proliferation may be caused by inactivation of tumor suppressor genes or deletion of chromosomal material, among other possibilities.

Extraoral Characteristics: Not applicable

Perioral and Intraoral Characteristics: This malignant neoplasm is found most often in the parotid gland, where it manifests as an asymptomatic swelling. The lesion may exist for several years before it is reported by the patient or before it comes to the attention of a healthcare provider. The longer the tumor is present, the more likely that symptoms of pain and facial nerve paralysis or palsy will develop. Mucoepidermoid carcinoma may also affect the submandibular gland and the minor salivary glands found throughout the oral cavity. Minor salivary gland mucoepidermoid carcinomas appear as asymptomatic swellings, which may be fluctuant and slightly blue in color (Fig. 17.27). Mucoepidermoid carcinoma may also appear within the bone of the maxilla or more commonly the mandible, where it will present as a unilocular or multilocular radiolucency.

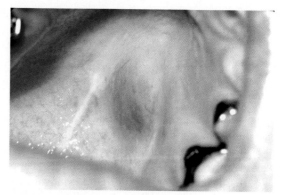

Figure 17.27. Note the bluish color of this palatal mucoepidermoid carcinoma. Significant amounts of underlying bone may have to be removed with this lesion if it is found to be a high-grade carcinoma.

Distinguishing Characteristics: Not applicable

Significant Microscopic Features: Mucoepidermoid carcinoma is composed of a combination of mucus-secreting cells and epidermoid cells. These tumors exhibit varying degrees of aggressiveness from low-grade to high-grade, depending on their cellular composition. The more aggressive tumors have fewer mucus-secreting cells, while the less aggressive tumors have many mucus-secreting cells.

Dental Implications: These tumors can be present for several years before they are noticed by the patient, therefore, oral cancer screening examinations should include palpation of all of the major salivary glands to identify abnormalities at an early stage.

Differential Diagnosis: The major entities in the differential diagnosis are other benign and malignant salivary gland tumors such as pleomorphic adenoma and polymorphus low-grade adenocarcinoma. In addition, an intraoral differential diagnosis includes the following:

1. Mucocele, Chapter 11
2. Neurofibroma, Chapter 17
3. Neurilemoma
4. Lymphoma, Chapter 9

Treatment and Prognosis: This tumor is treated by surgical removal. The extent of the surgery depends on the size and grade of the tumor. Low-grade parotid tumors may require partial removal of the gland with the tumor, while saving the facial nerve. High-grade parotid tumors may require total removal of the gland and sacrifice of the facial nerve. Surgical removal of lesions affecting the minor salivary glands also depends on the tumor grade and can be conservative in low-grade lesions or can require the removal of large amounts of normal tissue, including underlying bone, in high-grade lesions. If there is evidence of metastasis, lymph nodes in the neck may have to be removed. Postsurgical radiation is often indicated as **adjuvant therapy** (additional treatment to enhance the primary therapy) for high-grade tumors.

The prognosis depends primarily on the grade of the tumor. Patients with low-grade tumors have a very good prognosis, with more than 95% of patients surviving 5 years. In contrast, only 40% of patients with high-grade tumors survive 5 years.

NAME: Acinic cell carcinoma

Etiology: The etiology of acinic cell carcinoma is unknown.

Epidemiology: The mean age for development of this tumor is 45 years, but it can be found any time between the ages of 20 to 70 years. Acinic cell carcinoma appears equally in women and in men.

Pathogenesis: Acinic cell carcinomas arise from serous cells within the major salivary glands. Mutations in chromosomal DNA are thought to initiate the neoplastic process. The parotid gland is affected most often, followed by the submandibular gland and then minor salivary glands.

Extraoral Characteristics: Not applicable

Perioral and Intraoral Characteristics: When found in the parotid or submandibular glands, these tumors present as slow-growing hard masses. In parotid tumors, facial nerve paralysis occurs infrequently but indicates a less than favorable prognosis. Minor salivary gland tumors appear as slow-growing masses on the palate, buccal mucosa, or lips more often than any other intraoral area (Fig. 17.28). Pain can be a symptom no matter where this tumor is located and is not related to the degree of tumor involvement; it does not indicate a less favorable prognosis.

Distinguishing Characteristics: Not applicable

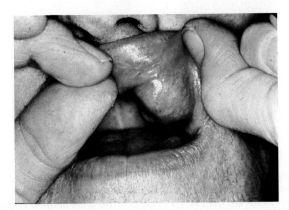

Figure 17.28. Acinic cell carcinoma. This malignancy usually arises in the major salivary glands; however, here it is pictured in the upper lip.

Significant Microscopic Features: Acinic cell carcinoma is characterized by a highly variable microscopic appearance.

Dental Implications: As noted above, these tumors are slow growing, and the dental hygienist may be the first person to detect this neoplasm during a periodic oral examination.

Differential Diagnosis: Clinically, acinic cell carcinoma may present as a painless mass similar to other salivary gland and soft tissue tumors. Biopsy is necessary to differentiate between these entities.

Treatment and Prognosis: Acinic cell carcinoma is a low-grade carcinoma with a relatively good chance of local recurrence, but only a slight chance of distant metastasis. Involvement of the parotid gland results in partial or total removal of the gland (often sacrificing the facial nerve in a total parotidectomy), depending on the location of the tumor. The entire submandibular gland is removed when tumors are found in this location. Minor salivary gland tumors are treated with surgical excision of the tumor including an adequate margin of normal surrounding tissue.

Prognosis is similar to that of mucoepidermoid carcinoma, which is generally good. About one third of patients have a local recurrence, and distant metastasis develops in about 15%. The 5-year survival rate is about 90%. At 20 years, the survival rate is about 55%.

Minor Salivary Gland Malignancies

Polymorphous low-grade adenocarcinoma (PLGA) and adenoid cystic carcinoma are malignant tumors that primarily affect the minor salivary glands. Low-grade mucoepidermoid carcinoma, discussed above, is also frequently seen within the minor salivary glands.

NAME: Polymorphous low-grade adenocarcinoma (PLGA)

Etiology: The etiology of PLGA and other salivary neoplasms may be associated with various genetic mutations and the overproduction of specific gene products including the protein, p63.

Method of Transmission: Not applicable

Epidemiology: This lesion appears most frequently at about 60 years of age (range between 40 and 80 years of age).

Pathogenesis: Proliferation of salivary duct cells results in a slow-growing, submucosal mass.

Extraoral Characteristics: Not applicable

Perioral and Intraoral Characteristics: The palate is the most frequent site for PLGA. It presents as a

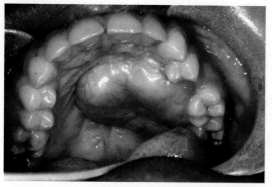

Figure 17.29. Polymorphous low-grade adenocarcinoma is found most often as a slow-growing mass in the hard palate as seen in this example. (Courtesy of Dr. George Blakey.)

slow-growing, smooth-surfaced, painless mass that may exist for years before discovery leads to diagnosis and treatment (Fig. 17.29). Large tumors may become ulcerated because of secondary trauma.

Distinguishing Characteristics: Not applicable

Significant Microscopic Features: The ductal cells of this malignant neoplasm display different growth patterns, hence the name polymorphous.

Dental Implications: One of the first signs of a palatal growth might be a denture that starts to feel uncomfortable or loose. All denture patients should be encouraged to have periodic oral examinations to detect abnormalities in the early stages.

Differential Diagnosis: Biopsy is necessary to determine a definitive diagnosis for this soft tissue neoplasm. However, the following conditions should be included in a differential diagnosis:

1. Lymphoma, Chapter 9
2. Fibroma, Chapter 17
3. Neurofibroma, Chapter 17
4. Neurilemoma, Chapter 17
5. Adenoid cystic carcinoma, Chapter 17
6. Mucoepidermic carcinoma, Chapter 17

Treatment and Prognosis: Surgical excision with wide margins is the treatment of choice for PLGA. Local recurrence has been reported but is usually managed by reexcision. Metastasis is considered an uncommon occurrence.

NAME: Adenoid cystic carcinoma

Etiology: The etiology of adenoid cystic carcinoma is unknown; however, some evidence supports an association with mutations on chromosomes 6 and 12 and deletion of genetic material from chromosome 19.

Method of Transmission: Not applicable

Epidemiology: This neoplasm is seen most frequently in the 40- to 60-year age group. Most studies have shown that gender distribution is equal.

Pathogenesis: Adenoid cystic carcinoma is a high-grade malignant tumor. This tumor arises most frequently within the minor salivary glands, followed by the parotid gland and the submandibular gland. The tumors are usually nonencapsulated and infiltrate the surrounding normal tissue.

Extraoral Characteristics: Not applicable

Perioral and Intraoral Characteristics: Parotid gland tumors present as firm, well-defined masses within the gland. They are slow-growing and may be tender on palpation. Facial nerve involvement may indicate that the tumor is in an advanced stage. Intraoral tumors occur on the palate more frequently than any other surface, although these tumors can occur anywhere in the oral cavity (Fig. 17.30).Often the mucosal surface of lesions of adenoid cystic carcinoma are ulcerated, especially the lesions located on the palate. Pain may be reported prior to any clinical evidence of the growth. In addition, palatal lesions may cause destruction of the underlying bone.

Distinguishing Characteristics: Intraoral lesions often manifest with pain as an early symptom.

Significant Microscopic Features: Adenoid cystic carcinoma is composed of cystic spaces and clusters of cells that form ductlike structures. The lesions have a tendency to invade the tissues surrounding nerve fibers (**perineural invasion**), which may account for the difficulty in managing adenoid cystic carcinoma.

Dental Implications: Radiation therapy is almost always recommended. Therefore, all dental procedures

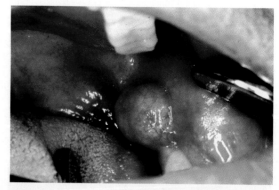

Figure 17.30. Adenoid cystic carcinoma. Minor salivary glands are affected by this malignancy more often then the major salivary glands. The palate is the most common location for the development of adenoid cystic carcinoma, but it can occur on any intraoral surface as evidenced by this tumor found on the buccal mucosa.

need to be accomplished prior to the radiation therapy. In addition, the patient needs to be instructed about the long-term management of xerostomia and other oral side effects of radiation.

Differential Diagnosis: Any soft tissue enlargement, especially those associated with surface ulceration, should be considered in a differential diagnosis of adenoid cystic carcinoma. The following are included:

1. Lymphoma, Chapter 9
2. Necrotizing sialometaplasia, Chapter 12
3. Traumatic fibroma, Chapter 17

Treatment and Prognosis: Surgical excision is the treatment of choice for adenoid cystic carcinoma. Removal of tumors within the parotid gland may require sacrifice of the facial nerve. Intraoral tumors should be removed with wide surgical margins. Removal of underlying bone may be necessary with palatal lesions. Adjuvant radiation therapy is recommended for most tumors. Studies show that immunotherapy, in addition to surgery and radiation therapy, may prove useful in the future.

This tumor has a good 5-year prognosis and a poor 20-year prognosis.

GENETIC AND CONGENITAL DISORDERS

Soft tissue enlargements in the oral cavity are often associated with genetic abnormalities or congenital malformations. Some of these are neoplastic, with the proliferative process being initiated by genetic abnormalities that cause the production of defective proteins or inhibit the action of tumor suppressor or caretaker genes. Other enlargements are caused by abnormal development of tissues, such as lymphatic vessels, or the development of epithelium-lined cavities (cysts) that are derived from remnants of early epithelial tissues.

NAME: Neurofibromatosis, type 1 (von Recklinghausen's disease of the skin)

Etiology: This is an inherited disorder that is associated with a mutation of the *NF1* gene (neurofibromatosis-1 gene) on chromosome 17. New genetic mutations that occur spontaneously, without any hereditary influence, may account for up to 50% of cases.

Method of Transmission: Neurofibromatosis is transmitted through an autosomal dominant inheritance pattern, or it occurs as a new mutation.

Epidemiology: It is estimated that 1 of every 3000 individuals throughout the world is affected by this disorder. However, many feel that this estimate is low because of misdiagnosis or nonidentification of cases in which the manifestations are very mild. All races and ethnic groups are equally affected as are both genders.

Pathogenesis: Genetic abnormalities in the *NF1* gene cause decreased production of neurofibromin, a substance that functions as a tumor suppressor. The manifestations of this deficiency range from mild to severe and appear in organs and tissues throughout the body.

Extraoral Characteristics: The typical manifestations associated with neurofibromatosis include the following:

- Multiple neurofibromas, including small superficial cutaneous and subcutaneous lesions (Fig. 17.31), large cutaneous and subcutaneous lesions, and plexiform neurofibromas. Plexiform neurofibromas are large, diffuse growths that invade deeper tissues and can cause pain and destruction of bone.
- **Café-au-lait macules** (flat areas of hyperpigmented skin) are usually the first manifestation of this disorder, appearing in early childhood and increasing in number and size throughout life (Fig. 17.32). In addition, patients almost always present with axillary (under the arms) or inguinal (groin area) freckles that develop sometime during childhood.
- Lisch nodules (freckling within the iris of the eye) are also seen frequently in this condition (Fig. 17.33).
- Individuals usually have a short stature and other bone abnormalities, which include: thinning of the cortical bone leading to bowing of the legs, sphenoid dysplasia, which can lead to herniation of the brain through the defective sphenoid bone, scoliosis (curvature of the spine), and destruction of the knee joints.
- Seizures due to intracranial neurofibromas are present in 4 to 7% of cases.
- Many individuals have learning disabilities and may have poor eye–hand coordination.

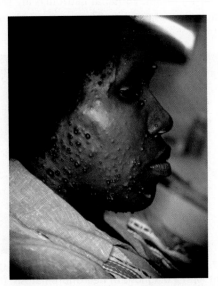

Figure 17.31. Neurofibromatosis. This female patient presented with multiple neurofibromas on the face and other cutaneous surfaces.

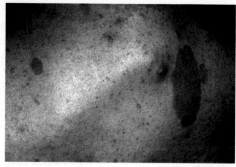

Figure 17.32. Multiple café-au-lait macules are seen on the upper back of an individual diagnosed with neurofibromatosis. (From Goodheart HP. Goodheart's photoguide of common skin disorders. 2nd ed. Philadelphia: Lippincott Williams & Wilkins, 2003.)

• Hypertension is often associated with growths in the adrenal gland or a specific form of kidney disease that is common in these individuals.

Diagnosis of this condition usually depends on identifying the clinical manifestations and knowing the genetic background of the individual. Included in the diagnostic criteria are the following: (1) a first-degree relative with the condition, (2) six or more café-au-lait macules or freckling in the axillary or inguinal regions, (3) Lisch nodules, (4) optic glioma, (5) the presence of two or more neurofibromas or one plexiform neurofibroma, and (6) characteristic bone changes. An individual who meets any two or more of these criteria is highly suspected to have the condition. Individuals who have neurofibromatosis have a 10% lifetime risk for developing malignant peripheral nerve sheath tumors or a neurosarcoma within a preexisting neurofibroma.

Perioral and Intraoral Characteristics:
Neurofibromas and café-au-lait macules can appear on the face and lips. Multiple intraoral neuromas are seen in approximately 25% of patients. These appear on any intrao-

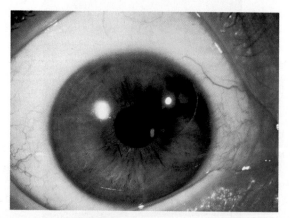

Figure 17.33. Lisch nodules. Freckling seen within the iris is consistent with a diagnosis of neurofibromatosis. (From Tasman W, Jaeger E. The Wills Eye Hospital atlas of clinical ophthalmology. 2nd ed. Baltimore: Lippincott Williams & Wilkins, 2001.)

ral surface as well-defined, painless, submucosal nodules. Lesions of the tongue can appear as macroglossia.

Distinguishing Characteristics: The cutaneous manifestations, including: multiple café-au-lait macules, Lisch nodules, and axillary or inguinal freckling, are characteristic of this disease.

Significant Microscopic Features: See the microscopic features of the solitary neurofibroma.

Dental Implications: The appearance of neurofibromas in the oral and perioral area is common. Problems associated with the development of these lesions include impairment of mastication, swallowing, and speaking. Lesions can become chronically traumatized if they are near the plane of occlusion. The growths may complicate the patient's attempts to maintain good oral hygiene. The hygienist may be asked to suggest home care modifications to alleviate this problem. Dental healthcare providers should evaluate the oral soft tissues and bone for any clinical or radiographic changes indicating malignant transformation of these tumors.

Differential Diagnosis: This disease is not easily confused with any other disorder.

Treatment and Prognosis: Neurofibromatosis is a genetic disorder and therefore cannot be treated in the strict sense of the word. Management of neurofibromatosis includes frequent examination of the skin for new lesions and assessment of already present lesions for the development of malignant changes. Surgical resection of lesions that are causing problems because of their location or for cosmetic reasons is beneficial. However, in many cases there are so many lesions that it is impossible to remove them all. The tendency for the lesions to recur makes surgical management even more difficult. Children should have an annual evaluation of the spine to identify and treat scoliosis in the early stages. All patients should have periodic assessment of their blood pressure to identify kidney problems. Patients with this genetic disorder should receive genetic counseling to help with future life choices (Pletcher, 2006).

Generally speaking, neurofibromatosis decreases life expectancy by about 15 years. This is due to the complications of hypertension and the increased chance of a malignancy occurring (Pletcher, 2006).

NAME: Multiple endocrine neoplasia syndrome, type III (MEN-III)

Etiology: MEN-2B is a genetic disorder caused by mutation of a protooncogene (called *RET*) that is located on chromosome 10.

Method of Transmission: The genetic mutation can be inherited as an autosomal dominant trait or it can occur spontaneously as a new mutation.

Epidemiology: MEN-III is estimated to occur in 1 of every 5,000 to 10,000 individuals. The disorder is distributed equally among racial and ethnic groups, but is seen twice as often in males than in females.

Pathogenesis: Mutation and subsequent activation of the *RET* protooncogene causes hyperplasia of the target cells that are located in the thyroid and adrenal glands and in mucosal tissues, which leads to tumor formation in these tissues.

Extraoral Characteristics: Most of these individuals have a tall, slender body with long arms often referred to as a *marfanoid* body type because of the similarity to the body type seen in Marfan syndrome (Chapter 6). Aggressive thyroid cancer (medullary thyroid carcinoma) can appear as early as 1 year of age, with 5% of cases occurring prior to the age of 5 years. Adrenal gland tumors also occur early in these patients, and constant medical follow-up is required to watch for neoplastic changes. Adrenal gland tumors cause flushing, heart palpitations, diffuse sweating, and diarrhea. Mucosal neuromas may occur on any mucosal surface and are often seen on the eyelids or the cornea.

Perioral and Intraoral Characteristics: Mucosal neuromas can be found on the lips, tongue, and any other oral mucosal surface. The lips may appear puffy and protuberant because of multiple neuromas. The palate may be high-arched and narrow, a finding that is not related to the presence of neuromas but to the general marfanoid body type that is manifest. The tongue is a common location for formation of multiple neuromas and macroglossia due to these tumors is often seen (Fig. 17.34).

Distinguishing Characteristics: Mucosal neuromas, pheochromocytomas, and medullary carcinoma of the thyroid are the distinctive elements of this syndrome.

Significant Microscopic Features: The mucosal neuromas display marked hyperplasia of nerve bundles in a loose connective tissue background.

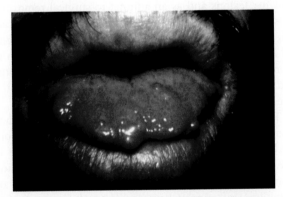

Figure 17.34. Multiple endocrine neoplasia syndrome, type 2B. Multiple mucosal neuromas indicate this disorder. Pictured here are several mucosal neuromas on the tongue of an individual with MEN-III.

Dental Implications: The dental hygienist may be the first healthcare provider to detect mucosal neuromas in a young child during a routine oral examination. It is important to recognize the possibility of this diagnosis to make an appropriate medical referral. Prompt diagnosis of this condition is crucial in preventing thyroid cancer and ensuring that the individual has every chance of a long life.

Differential Diagnosis: The mucosal neuromas associated with MEN-2B resemble the neurofibroma, fibroma, and lipoma (all in Chapter 17). If macroglossia is present, congenital malformations such as lymphangioma and hemangioma and metabolic conditions such as amyloidosis should be considered in the differential diagnosis.

Treatment and Prognosis: Treatment of the syndrome includes prophylactic removal of the thyroid, often prior to the age of 5 years (Ferry et al., 2006), followed by continual monitoring of blood calcitonin levels. Increased levels of calcitonin indicate a recurrence of the thyroid tumor. Adrenal gland tumors are benign, but have the ability to cause significant hypertension and other cardiovascular problems. Surgical removal of these tumors is also recommended. Mucosal neuromas are usually surgically excised and are not expected to recur.

The prognosis is good if the disease is identified early and the thyroid prophylactically removed. If medullary carcinoma of the thyroid does occur, the prognosis is poor, with a 5-year survival rate of only 50%.

NAME: Lymphangioma

Etiology: The etiology of lymphangiomas is unknown. Some may be associated with an inherited trait that has yet to be identified.

Method of Transmission: Lymphangioma may have a genetic tendency relative to its congenital presentation, but otherwise, it is not transmissible.

Epidemiology: Lymphangiomas are relatively rare in the United States, accounting for about 4% of all vascular tumors (Fernandez and Schwartz, 2005). Lymphangioma affects Caucasians more often than other races but affects males and females equally. It is usually evident at birth or in early childhood.

Pathogenesis: Lymphangioma is a congenital malformation of lymphatic vessels thought to be associated with islands of misplaced embryologic lymph tissue that develop independently of the lymph system and grow as the child grows. These growths are considered hamartomas. The lesions do not regress as the child ages. Lymphangiomas may be superficial or located deep within tissues.

Extraoral Characteristics: The most common location of lymphangioma is the head and neck area. One specific form of lymphangioma, **cystic hygroma**, affects the

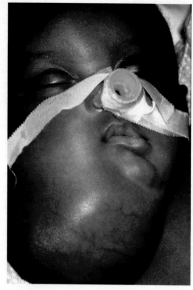

Figure 17.35. A large cystic hygroma in the neck of an infant. (Courtesy of Dr. John Jacoway.)

neck and submandibular spaces (Fig. 17.35). Cystic hygromas may cause respiratory obstruction and become life-threatening. Rapid enlargement of a cystic hygroma can occur when there is trauma to the area or when there is a respiratory or oral infection that results in an inflammatory response.

Perioral and Intraoral Characteristics: Superficial lymphangiomas present as painless nodules that may be translucent or bluish and have a pebbly or bubbly surface that looks somewhat like cooked tapioca. Blood vessels that may develop within the lesion can impart a darker red to blue color (Fig. 17.36). Deeper lesions present as submucosal swellings that are poorly-defined and distort the local anatomy. When these lesions are palpated, movement of the lymph fluid within them may produce a crackling

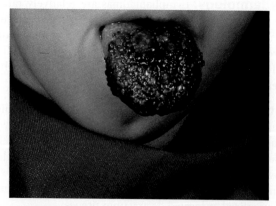

Figure 17.36. Lymphangioma. Note the bluish color caused by the growth of blood vessels within the lesion and the pebbly surface of this superficial lymphangioma of the tongue. (Courtesy of Dr. Robert J. Gorlin.)

sound (**crepitus**). The tongue and buccal mucosa are the most common sites for lymphangiomas in the oral cavity. Large tongue lesions can cause macroglossia.

Distinguishing Characteristics: The pebbly surface texture of superficial lesions and evidence of crepitus on palpation are significant features that can help to identify this lesion.

Significant Microscopic Features: The lesion is composed of endothelial-lined, thin-walled channels that are found just beneath the epithelial surface.

Dental Implications: Patients who have had surgical removal of a lymphangioma may have damage to the facial, lingual, or hypoglossal nerves. The dental hygienist is in an excellent position to help the patient learn how to manage the complications associated with some of this damage.

Differential Diagnosis: Most of the other soft tissue enlargements that present in the oral cavity may need to be differentiated from this lesion. Some of those include

1. Hemangioma, Chapter 13
2. Mucocele and ranula, Chapter 11
3. Dermoid cyst, Chapter 17
4. Branchial cleft cyst, Chapter 17
5. Cellulitis, Chapter 3
6. Thyroglossal duct cyst, Chapter 17

Treatment and Prognosis: Treatment depends on the size, location, and composition of the malformation. Small lesions may not need to be treated at all unless they create a cosmetic problem. Surgical removal of lymphangiomas is the treatment of choice for other lesions, even though there is a 20 to 40% postsurgery recurrence rate. Large lesions in the tongue can be difficult to manage because it is not desirable to remove large portions of the tongue. In cases like this, other therapies can be used in conjunction with surgery to produce a better result. Other therapies that are gaining acceptance are *laser therapy* and *sclerotherapy*. Laser therapy is used to control the size of growing lesions and as an adjunct to surgical removal in most cases. Some small superficial lesions may be eradicated with laser therapy alone. Sclerotherapy uses chemical agents injected directly into the lesion to cause an inflammatory reaction that results in scar tissue formation and subsequent destruction of the lesion or reduction in size.

The prognosis for small, isolated lesions is excellent. The prognoses for larger lesions and the cystic hygroma are based on the location and size of the lesion and its involvement with adjacent vital structures. Complications from surgery occur frequently and include airway obstruction, infections, hematomas, and nerve damage. Mortality rates from the lesions or from complications of surgery range from 2 to 12%.

SOFT TISSUE DEVELOPMENTAL CYSTS

The formation of these developmental **cysts** (epithelial-lined, fluid-filled cavities) is associated with remnants of epithelial tissues left after embryologic development of the structures is completed. These lesions all present as smooth-surfaced masses that are somewhat rubbery to palpation. They are only visualized easily when they have grown to a fairly large size. However, they can be detected much earlier in the course of their development by thorough head and neck examinations performed by the dental hygienist or dentist. Failure to include palpation as an examination method will often lead to missing these lesions.

NAME: Cervical lymphoepithelial cyst (branchial cleft cyst)

Etiology: Historically, this lesion was thought to develop from remnants of the second branchial arch. A more recent theory suggests that it arises from parotid gland epithelium that becomes entrapped within cervical lymph nodes.

Method of Transmission: None

Epidemiology: These lesions are usually detected in young adults between the ages of 10 and 40 years, and there is no gender predilection.

Pathogenesis: Parotid gland epithelium that is trapped within a cervical lymph node begins to proliferate and eventually forms a cyst. The cyst enlarges as the epithelial cells continue to proliferate.

Extraoral Characteristics: The cervical lymphoepithelial cyst is normally located along the anterior border of the sternocleidomastoid muscle. It is soft and **fluctuant** (manifests a wavelike feeling) when palpated. It is seen more often on the left side but can be found anywhere in the general vicinity of the sternocleidomastoid muscle (Fig. 17.37). Occasionally, lesions will become infected, and formation of an abscess within the cyst is possible. In most cases the cysts are asymptomatic, but drainage to the exterior surface of the skin may develop.

Perioral and Intraoral Characteristics: The intraoral counterpart is called a lymphoepithelial cyst and is commonly found in the floor of the mouth and the posterior lateral border of the tongue.

Distinguishing Characteristics: The intraoral lesions often have a pale yellowish hue.

Significant Microscopic Features: The epithelium lining the cyst is composed of stratified squamous and/or pseudostratified columnar epithelium supported by connective tissue containing lymphoid cells.

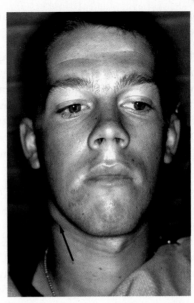

Figure 17.37. Cervical lymphoepithelial cyst. This lesion presents as a right neck mass in the area of the anterior border of the sternocleidomastoid muscle.

Dental Implications: It is essential for the dental healthcare provider to consistently provide examinations that include palpation of the neck and soft tissues of the face to detect abnormalities at an early stage.

Differential Diagnosis: Any soft tissue enlargement that could occur in this area should be considered in a differential diagnosis. Some of the more likely lesions include the following:

1. Lymphadenopathy, which occurs as a symptom or sign of many disorders and diseases and is found in conditions discussed throughout this text
2. Vascular neoplasm or malformation, Chapter 13
3. Lipoma, Chapter 17
4. Cystic hygroma, Chapter 17

Treatment and Prognosis: Complete surgical excision is recommended. The prognosis is good; however, untreated lesions are prone to recurrent infections and abscess formation.

NAME: Thyroglossal tract cyst

Etiology: This cyst results from a proliferation of remnants of epithelial cells that lined the thyroglossal tract during embryonic development.

Method of Transmission: None

Epidemiology: The cyst is considered the most common of the developmental cysts of the neck, making up 2 to 4% of all neck masses. Thyroglossal tract cysts are seen more often in children. The lesion is seen equally among males and females and among ethnic groups.

Pathogenesis: This cyst originates in the embryologic development of the thyroid gland, which occurs within the posterior portion of the tongue at the foramen caecum. The immature thyroid tissue migrates down an epithelial duct or tract to its permanent location at the level of the thyroid cartilage at about the 7th week of embryonic development. Although the thyroglossal duct epithelium normally undergoes atrophy, occasionally remnants remain and proliferate, forming the thyroglossal tract cyst.

Extraoral Characteristics: Most of these cysts are found in the midline of the neck where they appear as well-circumscribed, nontender, mobile masses, usually between 2 and 4 cm in diameter (Fig. 17.38). Often dysphagia and **dysphonia** (a change in voice quality) accompany larger lesions. In addition, airway restriction is noted occasionally. The lesions have a tendency to become infected, and draining fistula tracts may develop because of the infection.

Perioral and Intraoral Characteristics: About 2% of these lesions develop within the tongue itself (lingual thyroid). Rarely, these will appear in the suprahyoid position as a swelling of the floor of the mouth.

Distinguishing Characteristics: Not applicable

Significant Microscopic Features: The lesion displays a central cavity lined with stratified squamous, columnar, and/or cuboidal cells. Some thyroglossal tract cysts contain actual thyroid tissues peripheral to the epithelial lining.

Dental Implications: Lesions located on the posterior dorsal surface of the tongue should not be removed until it is known what they are, because there is a chance

that a mass in this location may contain the patient's only thyroid tissue.

Differential Diagnosis: As noted above, biopsy is the only way to definitively diagnose any of these lesions. A few lesions that would be included in a differential diagnosis of this condition include

1. Dermoid cyst, Chapter 17
2. Thyroid neoplasms, which are clinically similar to the thyroglossal tract cyst; biopsy is the only way to determine a definitive diagnosis of this type of lesion.
3. Branchial cyst, Chapter 17
4. Epidermoid cyst, which has clinical features identical to the dermoid cyst, but does not have dermal appendages within the cyst wall.
5. Goiter, Chapter 7

Treatment and Prognosis: Complete surgical excision using the sistrunk procedure is the treatment of choice after testing to determine the presence of other functioning thyroid tissues in the normal location. If complete excision is not accomplished, there is a 3 to 5% chance of recurrence. Recurrence is also associated with a history of repeated infections. Prognosis is normally excellent if the cyst is completely excised. There is a very slight risk of malignant transformation of this lesion, especially if it has recurred after excision and has a history of repeated infection.

NAME: Dermoid cyst

Etiology: Dermoid cysts result from the entrapment of epithelial cells along the lines of embryonic closure or fusion. They are, therefore, located in the midline in the head and neck region.

Method of Transmission: None

Epidemiology: This is an uncommon oral cyst that usually appears between the ages of 10 and 30 years. It is seen equally in males and females and across all ethnic groups.

Pathogenesis: These cysts develop from bits of epithelium that are trapped in embryonic lines of fusion. Proliferation of this epithelium leads to the development of an epithelial-lined cavity containing sebaceous glands, sweat glands, hair follicles, and sometimes toothlike structures.

Extraoral Characteristics: The related teratoid cysts are uncommon tumors that can develop in any area of the body.

Perioral and Intraoral Characteristics: The dermoid cyst develops as a painless, slow-growing soft, doughy, midline mass, primarily in the floor of the mouth (Fig. 17.39). It can be located superior to the mylohyoid muscle and cause the tongue to be displaced superiorly and posteriorly, or it can be located inferior to the muscle and appear as a swelling in the midline of the neck.

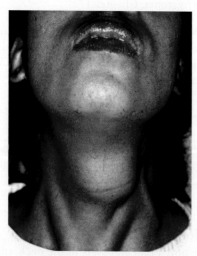

Figure 17.38. The fluctuant mass seen in midline of the neck is a thyroglossal tract cyst.

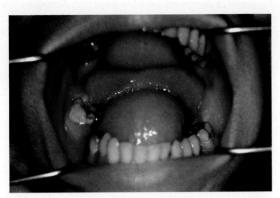

Figure 17.39. Dermoid cyst. When this cyst occurs intraorally, it is seen in the floor of the mouth.

Distinguishing Characteristics: None

Significant Microscopic Features: The dermoid cyst displays a central cavity lined by orthokeratotic stratified squamous epithelium supported by a connective tissue wall containing sebaceous glands, sweat glands, and hair follicles. Large amounts of keratin and sebum from the glands in the connective tissue wall fill the cavity. If this cyst contains elements from all three embryonic germ layers it is called a **teratoid cyst**.

Dental Implications: If this lesion is located in the floor of the mouth it can impair chewing, swallowing, and speaking. Patients may present with this as a reason for seeking dental care.

Differential Diagnosis: Some of the disorders that are included in a differential diagnosis of this type of lesion include

1. Thyroglossal tract cyst, Chapter 17
2. Salivary gland enlargements (including ranula), Chapter 17
3. Salivary gland neoplasms, Chapter 17
4. Cystic hygroma, Chapter 17

Treatment and Prognosis: Treatment is surgical excision. The prognosis is excellent. There is a slight chance of malignant transformation in dermoid cysts that have been present for a long time.

SUMMARY

- Soft tissue enlargements are associated with reactive (traumatic), genetic, neoplastic, or developmental processes. The lesions arise from epithelial, endothelial, or connective tissues, and they can be benign or malignant.
- Lesions that are associated with trauma or inflammation can be linked to a specific cause that initiates the adaptive hyperplastic cellular response.
- Traumatic neuromas occur in areas where a nerve has been traumatized. Pain on palpation is often associated with this lesion.
- Fibromas are the most common soft tissue tumor found in the oral cavity. They occur most often in areas that are traumatized frequently. Denture-induced fibrous hyperplasia is a variant of the same process.
- Cowden syndrome is characterized by multiple facial and oral fibrous papules. Individuals with this disorder have a higher than normal risk of developing thyroid and breast cancers.
- The peripheral ossifying fibroma (three histologic forms) is a reactive lesion found exclusively on the attached gingiva.
- Drug-induced generalized gingival hyperplasia is associated with phenytoin, calcium channel blockers, and some immunosuppressants (cyclosporine). Hormone-related gingival hyperplasia usually occurs when hormone imbalances or spikes occur in different stages of life, such as pregnancy and puberty. The presence of dental biofilm enhances the hyperplastic process.
- Lymphoid hyperplasia is a reactive response that is part of the normal immune system function. Waldeyer's ring and the posterior lateral and dorsal portions of the tongue are common places to find lymphoid hyperplasia.
- Sarcoidosis is a multisystem inflammatory disease that may manifest with salivary gland enlargement, nodular growths on the oral mucosal surfaces, and xerostomia.
- Mumps is a viral infection of the glandular tissues, most often affecting the parotid gland.
- Individuals with xerostomia have the highest risk of developing bacterial sialadenitis, which is characterized by painful swelling of the gland and a purulent exudate from the gland orifice.
- Sjögren syndrome occurs in a primary form as isolated destruction of exocrine glands (salivary and lacrimal specifically) or as a secondary form combined with another autoimmune disorder such as rheumatoid arthritis.
- Fibromatosis is an aggressive benign tumor that has no potential for metastasis.
- Most oral soft tissue neoplasms present as slow growing, painless masses that cannot be differentiated from each other on the basis of clinical appearance or behavior alone. A biopsy is necessary to obtain a definitive diagnosis.
- The neurilemoma, neurofibroma, neuroma, fibroma, and lymphangioma frequently appear as submucosal swellings on the tongue.
- The leiomyoma (benign) and leiomyosarcoma (malignant) are neoplasms of smooth muscle tissue. The rhabdomyoma (benign) and rhabdomyosarcoma (malignant) are neoplasms of striated muscle. The rhabdomyosarcoma is the most common soft tissue sarcoma seen in children.
- The pleomorphic adenoma is the most common form of benign salivary gland neoplasm. It affects the major salivary glands more often, but may also be found in the minor glands.
- Frey syndrome is often seen in individuals who have had parotid gland surgery. It is characterized by facial sweating on the affected side when nervous stimulation of the salivary glands occurs.
- Papillary cystadenoma lymphomatosum is a relatively common salivary gland tumor associated with smoking tobacco, which develops most often in the tail of the parotid.
- Mucoepidermoid carcinoma is the most common salivary gland malignancy in the United States, affecting the major and minor salivary glands.
- Neurofibromatosis is a common genetic disorder that manifests with very distinctive cutaneous and oral conditions. Café-au-lait macules (six or more), Lisch nodules, and multiple neurofibromas are elements of the diagnostic criteria.
- Multiple endocrine neoplasia syndromes, specifically MEN-III, present with multiple mucosal neuromas and other general physical findings. Early identification of individuals with this disorder is crucial to prevent the development of a very aggressive thyroid cancer.
- Lymphangiomas are hamartomatous tumors that may present intraorally with a pebbled surface and crepitus on palpation. Cystic hygromas are a form of lymphangioma that affects the large spaces of the neck and can produce respiratory distress.
- The cervical lymphoepithelial cyst, dermoid cyst, and thyroglossal tract cyst are all developmental cysts associated with the proliferation of entrapped embryonic epithelial tissues. They are most commonly observed in the neck region or the floor of the mouth.

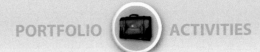

PORTFOLIO ACTIVITIES

1. Prepare an office manual segment that illustrates correct palpation techniques for detecting masses of the neck and intraoral masses that could be cysts or neoplasms.
2. Prepare an office manual segment listing the contact numbers for those practitioners who may need to be contacted for management of your patient who presents with a mass that could be a benign or malignant mesenchymal tumor. These contact numbers would include, but not be limited to, numbers for a(n)
   - Oral and maxillofacial surgeon
   - Oral and maxillofacial pathologist
   - Oncologist
   - Otolaryngologist
   - Hospital or imaging facility that could provide MRI (magnetic resonance imaging) or CT (computerized tomography)

Critical Thinking Activity

1. What characteristics would you need to observe in a lesion or what information would you have to have about a lesion before you would recommend that it be biopsied? Why?

Case Study

Carlos, a 25-year-old man, comes to your school's dental hygiene clinic for an initial appointment. His health history is unremarkable except for the fact that he quit smoking 4 years ago. He is taking no medication at this time but does report an allergy to aspirin. His vital signs are within normal limits. There are no positive findings from the extraoral examination. However, during the intraoral examination you discover the tongue lesion depicted in Figure 17.40.

1. Write a clinical description of this lesion from what you can observe.
2. Develop a preliminary differential diagnosis for this lesion from what you observe in the figure.
3. What would you like to ask this patient about this lesion?
4. As you continue your examination you palpate the tongue and feel a wavelike movement or vibration with very slight crackling (crepitus) as you palpate the lesion. The lesion does not blanch when palpated. The patient reports no pain and tells you that the lesion has been there as long as he can remember. He also states that it was much smaller when he was young, but that it got larger when he was a teenager. It hasn't gotten any larger for quite a few years now though.

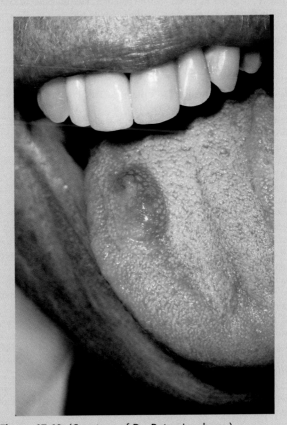

Figure 17.40. (Courtesy of Dr. Peter Jacobsen.)

(continued)

CASE STUDY (continued)

5. What important information has he just relayed to you and what could it mean?

6. Determine the most likely diagnosis from your differential diagnosis.

7. Is there any way that you can obtain a definitive diagnosis for this lesion without performing a biopsy?

REFERENCES

Atkinson JC, Fox PC. Sjogren's syndrome: oral and dental considerations. JADA 1993;124:74–86.

American Academy of Periodontology—Academy report. Drug-associated gingival enlargement—informational paper. J Periodontol 2004; 75:1424–1431.

Bagan JV, Penarrocha M, Vera-Sempere F. Cowden syndrome: Clinical and pathological considerations in two new cases. J Oral Maxillofac Surg 1989;47:291–294.

Batal H, Chou L, Cottrell D. Sarcoidosis: medical and dental implications. Oral Surg Oral Med Oral Pathol Oral Radiol Endod 1999; 88: 386–390.

Bhattacharyya I, Cohen D. Oral neurofibroma. Last updated April 14, 2006. e medicine: Instant Access to the Minds of Medicine. Available at: *http://www.emedicine.com/derm/topic674.htm*. Accessed November 10, 2006.

Bouquot JE, Wrobleski GJ. Papillary (pebbled) masses of the oral mucosa: more than simple papillomas. Pract Periodont Aesthetic Dent 1996;8(6):533–543.

Buchner A., Begleiter A, Hanse LS. The predominance of epulis fissuratum in females. Quintessence Int 1984;15:699–702.

Cawson RA, Odell EW. Essentials of oral pathology and oral medicine. 6th ed. London: Churchill Livingstone–Harcourt Brace, 1998.

Cawson RA, Binnie WH, Eveson JW. Color atlas of oral disease—clinical and pathologic correlations. 2nd ed. London: Wolfe Publishing, 1994.

Christopoulos P, Sklavounou A, Patrikiou A. True fibroma of the oral mucosa: a case report. Int J Oral Maxillofac Surg 1994;23:98–99.

Cripe TP. Rhabdomyosarcoma. Last updated October 4, 2006. e medicine: Instant Access to the Minds of Medicine. Available at: *http://www.emedicine.com/ped/topic2005.htm*. Accessed November 10, 2006.

Curtis KA, Sinert R. Mumps. Last updated July 12, 2006. e medicine: Instant Access to the Minds of Medicine. Available at: http://www.emedicine.com/emerg/topic324.htm. Accessed November 21, 2006.

de Ru JA, Plantinga RF, Majoor MHJM, et al. Warthin's tumour and smoking. B-ENT 2005;1(2):63–66.

Dunleavy KM, Waes CV, Kass E, et al. Lymphomas of the head and neck. Last updated October 3, 2005. e medicine: Instant Access to the Minds of Medicine. Available at: http://www.emedicine.com/ent/topic742.htm . Accessed November 23, 2006.

Edwards S, Helman JI. Oral lymphangiomas. E medicine: Instant Access to the Minds of Medicine. Available at: http://www.emedicine.com/derm/topic650.htm . Accessed November 23, 2006.

Eisen D. Lynch DP. The mouth—diagnosis and treatment. St. Louis: Mosby, 1998.

El-Naggar AK, Batsakis JG, Luna MA, et al. DNA flow cytometry of acinic cell carcinomas of major salivary glands. J Laryngol Otol 1990; 104(5):410–416.

El-Naggar AK, Abdul-Krim, Hurr K, et al. Genetic alterations in acinic cell carcinoma of the parotid gland determined by microsatellite analysis. Cancer Genet Cytogenet 1998;102(1):19–24.

Epivatanos A, Lordanides S, Zaraboukas T, Antoniades D. Adenoid cystic carcinoma and polymorphous lowgrade adenocarcinoma of minor salivary glands: a comparative immunohistochemical study using the epithelial membrane and carcinoembryonic antibodies. Oral Dis 2005;11(3):175–180.

Fernandez G, Schwartz RA. Lymphangioma. Last updated November 8, 2005. e medicine: Instant Access to the Minds of Medicine. Available at: http://www.emedicine.com/derm/topic866.htm. Accessed November 10, 2006.

Ferry RJ, Radebold K, Koch CA, Chronsos GP. Multiple endocrine neoplasia . Last updated July 27, 2006. e medicine: Instant Access to the Minds of Medicine. Available at: *http://www.emedicine.com/ped/topic1496.htm*. Accessed November 12, 2006.

Foundation for Sarcoidosis Research. (2006) Available at: http://www.stopsarcoidosis.org/sarcoidosis/diseasefacts.htm. Accessed November 24, 2006.

Fowler CB. Benign and malignant neoplasms of the periodontium. Periodontology 2000 1999;21:33–83.

Furlong MA, Fanburg-Smith JC, Childers ELB. Lipoma of the oral and maxillofacial region: site and subclassification of 125 cases. Oral Surg Oral Med Oral Pathol Oral Radiol Endod 2004;98(r4),441–450.

Hallmon W. Rossman J. The role of drugs in the pathogenesis of gingival overgrowth. A collective review of current concepts. Periodontology 2000 1999;21:176–196.

Hood AF, Kwan TH, Mihm MC, Horn TD. Dermatopathology. 2nd ed. Boston: Little, Brown & Co., 1993.

Inampudi P, Jacobson JA, Fessell DP, et al. Soft-tissue lipomas: accuracy of sonography in diagnosis with pathologic correlation. Radiology 2004;233(3):763–767.

Kamangar N, Shorr AF. Sarcoidosis. Last updated May 31, 2006. e medicine: Instant Access to the Minds of Medicine. Available at: http://www.emedicine.com/med/topic2063.htm. Accessed November 27, 2006.

Kao GF. Neurilemoma Last updated April 12, 2006. e medicine: Instant Access to the Minds of Medicine. Available at: *http://www.emedicine.com/derm/topic285.htm* . Accessed November 12, 2006.

Karia VR, Arora ML, Worrell RV, D'Silva KJ. Rhabdomyomas. Last updated November 22, 2006. e medicine: Instant Access to the Minds of Medicine. Available at: *http://www.emedicine.com/med/topic2021.htm*. Accessed November 22, 2006.

Keogh PV, McDonnell D, Toner M. Intraosseous mandibular lipoma (IML): a case report and review of the literature. J Ir Dent Assoc 2004;50(3):132–134.

Klussmann JP, Wittekindt C, Preuss SF, et al. High risk for bilateral Warthin tumor in heavy smokers—review of 185 cases. ACTA Oto-Laryngol 2006;126(11):1213–1217.

Kotwall CA. Smoking as an etiologic factor in the development of Warthin's tumor of the parotid gland. Am J Surg 1992;164(6): 202–224.

Langlais R., Miller C. Color atlas of common oral diseases. 3rd ed. Baltimore: Lippincott Williams & Wilkins, 2003.

Laszlo S, Bürger H, Vormoor J, et al. Aggressive fibromatosis involving the mandible—case report and review of the literature. Oral Surg Oral Pathol Oral Radiol Endod 2005;99(1):30–38.

Lewis PD, Fradley SR, Griffiths AP, et al. Mitochdrial DNA mutations in the parotid gland of cigarette smokers and non-smokers. Mutat Res 2002;518(1):47–54.

Lozada-Nur F, Vacharotayangul P. Drug-induced gingival hyperplasia, Last updated August 23, 2005. e medicine: Instant Access to the Minds of Medicine. Available at: *http://www.emedicine.com/derm/topic645.htm* . Accessed November 15, 2006.

Martins C, Fonseca I, Roque L, et al. Cytogenetic similarities between two types of salivary gland carcinomas: adenoid cystic carcinoma and polymorphous lowgrade adenocarcinoma. Cancer Genet Cytogenet 2001;128(2):130–136.

Miller C. Cowden disease (multiple hamartoma syndrome). Last updated June 2, 2005. e medicine: Instant Access to the Minds of Medicine. Available at: http://www.emedicine.com/derm/topic86.htm. Accessed November 10, 2006.

Mino M, Pilchbz, Faquin WC. Expression of KIT (CD 117) neoplasms of the head and neck: An ancillary marker for adenoid cystic carcinoma. Mod Pathol 2003;16(12):1224–1231.

Najera MP, Al-Hashimi I, Plemons JM, et al. Prevalence of periodontal disease in patients with Sjogren's syndrome. Oral Surg Oral Med Oral Pathol Oral Radiol Endod 1997;83:53–57.

Neville BW, Damm DD, Allen CM, Bouquot JE. Oral & Maxillofacial Pathology. Philadelphia: WB Saunders, 1995.

Pickett F, Gurenlian.J. The medical history: clinical implications and emergency prevention in dental settings. Baltimore: Lippincott Williams & Wilkins, 2005.

Pinkston JA, Cole P. Cigarette smoking and Warthin's tumor. Am J Epidemiol 1996;144(2):183–187.

Pletcher BA. Neurofibromatosis. Last updated May 2, 2006. e medicine: Instant Access to the Minds of Medicine. Available at: *http://www.emedicine.com/ped/topic2418.htm* . Accessed November 12, 2006.

Poetsch M, Zimmermann A, Wolf E, Kleist B. Loss of heterozygosity occurs predominantly, but not exclusively, in the epithelial compartment of pleomorphic adenoma. Neoplasia 2005;7(7):688–695.

Porth CM. Essentials of pathophysiology. Baltimore: Lippincott Williams & Wilkins, 2004.

Przewozny T, Stankiewicz C, Narozny W, Kuczkowski J. Warthin's tumor of the parotid gland. epidemiological and clinical analysis of 127 cases. Otolaryngol Pol 2004;58(3):583–592.

Qualman SJ, Coffin CM, Newton WA, et al. Current practice in pediatric pathology: Intergroup Rhabdomyosarcoma Study: update for pathologists. Pediatr Dev Pathol 1998;1(6)550–561.

Rees T. Orofacial granulomatosis and related conditions. Periodontology 2000, 1999;21:145–157.

Regezi J, Sciubba J, Jordan R. Oral pathology—clinical pathologic correlations. 4th ed. St. Louis: WB Saunders, 2003.

Rubin E, Gorstein F, Rubin R, et al. Rubin's pathology: clinicopathologic foundations of medicine. 4th ed. Baltimore: Lippincott Williams & Wilkins, 2005.

Rutherford S, Hampton GM, Frierson HF, Moskluk CA. Mapping of candidate tumor suppressor genes on chromosome 12 in adenoid cystic carcinoma. LAB Invest 2005;85(9):1076–1085.

Schwartz RA, Trovato MJ. Desmoid tumor. Last updated June 12, 2006. e medicine: Instant Access to the Minds of Medicine. Available at: http://www.emedicine.com/derm/topic778.htm. Accessed November 27, 2006.

Scully C. Handbook of oral disease—diagnosis and management. London: Martin Duntz Ltd. The Livery House Publishers, 1999.

Stedman's medical dictionary. 27th ed. Baltimore: Lippincott Williams & Wilkins, 2000.

Tewfik TL, Yoskowitch A. Congenital malformations, neck. Last updated June 12, 2006. e medicine: Instant Access to the Minds of Medicine. Available at: http://www.emedicine.com/ent/topic323.htm . Accessed November 27, 2006.

Teymoortash A, Krasnewicz Y, Werner JA. Clinical features of cystadenolymphoma (Warthin's tumor) of the parotid gland: a retrospective comparative study of 96 cases. Oral Oncol 2006;42(6):569–573.

Toida M, Shimokawa K, Makita H, et al. Intraoral minor salivary gland tumors: a clinical pathological study of 82 cases. Int J Oral Maxillofac Surg 2005;34(5):528–532.

Vivino FB, Al-Hashimi I, Khan Z, et al. Pilocarpine tablets for the treatment of dry mouth and dry eye symptoms in patients with Sjogren syndrome. Arch Intern Med 1999;159:174–181.

Wagner AL, Hagg J. Parotid, pleomorphic adenoma. Last updated April 8, 2005. e medicine: Instant Access to the Minds of Medicine. Available at: *http://www.emedicine.com/radio/topic531.htm* . *Accessed November 12, 2006.*

Waldron CA. Mixed tumors (pleomorphic adenoma) and myoepithelioma. In: Ellis GL, Auclair PL, Gnepp DR, ed. Surgical pathology of the salivary glands. Philadelphia: WB Saunders, 1991:135–164.

Wilkins EM, Clinical practice of the dental hygienist. 9th ed. Baltimore: Lippincott Williams & Wilkins, 2004.

Yi-Fang Z, YuLin J, Xin-Ming C, Wen-Fen Z. Clinical review of 580 ranulas. Oral Surg Oral Med Oral Pathol Oral Radiol Endod 2004;98: 281–287.

Yih W-Y, Kratochvil FJ, Stewart JCB. Intraoral minor salivary gland neoplasms: review of 213 cases. JOMS 2005; 63(6): 805–810.

Zhong L, Zhao S, Chen G, Ping F. Ultrasonic appearance of lipoma in the oral and maxillofacial region. Oral Surg Oral Med Oral Pathol Oral Radiol Endod 2004;98(6):738–740.

18

Hard Tissue Enlargements

Key Terms

- Ameloblastoma
- Calcifying epithelial odontogenic tumor
- Cementoossifying fibroma
- Central giant cell granuloma
- Chondroma
- Chondrosarcoma
- Chronic osteomyelitis with proliferative periostitis
- Dysesthesia
- Ewing's sarcoma
- Exostosis/exostoses
- Liesegang rings
- Mandibular tori
- Neoperiostosis
- Odontogenic tumor
- Osteosarcoma
- Ossifying fibroma
- Parosteal osteosarcoma
- Pindborg tumor
- Subpontic osseous proliferation
- Tonus palatinus

Chapter Objectives

1. Use and define the key terms listed in this chapter.

2. Name three areas in which bony growths may occur in the mouth and state the correct term for each growth of bone.

3. List the types of osteomyelitis that may occur in the oral tissues.

4. State the etiology of the ameloblastoma.

5. Compare and differentiate between the CEOT and the ameloblastoma.

6. Describe the clinical and radiographic characteristics of the osteosarcoma.

7. List the radiographic characteristics of the central giant cell granuloma and the clinical signs that would suggest such a lesion.

8. Describe the radiographic appearance of the osteosarcoma, chondrosarcoma, and Ewing's sarcoma.

9. Describe three of the clinical signs that may be associated with each of the following: osteosarcoma, chondrosarcoma, and Ewing's sarcoma.

Chapter Outline

Hard tissue enlargements are found periodically in the mouth and must be evaluated to determine whether there is pathology. Some are benign, and others are malignant. The suffix "oma" refers to a tumor or neoplasm, as discussed in Chapter 5. The prefix "osteo" (bone forming), added to the root word "sarcoma" (neoplasm of connective tissue) is one example of the various word forms that are joined together to name a disease. Osteosarcoma, discussed below in this chapter, is a malignant neoplasm of connective tissue that is considered very aggressive. Very common types of hard tissue enlargements such as the torus palatinus, mandibular torus, and exostosis are benign lesions. Other enlargements such as the sarcoma-type lesions and those that cause expansion with tissue destruction such as the ameloblastoma will be discussed in this chapter. Other than the torus palatinus, mandibular torus, and exostoses that are almost always diagnosed clinically, the diagnoses of many other lesions must be confirmed by directly viewing their cells under the microscope. In other instances, radiographs or special tests may be needed to determine the etiology of the lesion. This chapter discusses the types of hard tissue lesions the practitioner may consider in clinical evaluations.

VARIATIONS OF NORMAL

These lesions find their origin from the bone and have a firm to hard texture. Three benign findings, the mandibular tori, the torus palatinus, and general exostosis are detailed in this section. Occasionally, these lesions exhibit an unusual clinical presentation, in which case, biopsy or other tests may be needed to ensure a correct diagnosis. However, for the most part, these growths are very evident clinically and can be easily diagnosed.

Name: Torus palatinus and/or mandibular torus

Etiology: Both of these conditions appear to be associated with a genetic and ethnic predisposition for their development. In addition, masticatory stresses from bruxing and clenching have been suggested as contributing factors in their etiology. Environmental factors related to injuries, such as burns and blunt force trauma affecting the bone, have also been implicated.

Method of Transmission: Not applicable

Epidemiology: The growths are usually found in adults and occur after puberty. There is a female predilection of 2:1 for the torus palatinus, but mandibular tori are reported to occur more frequently in males. The palatal growth is found in higher numbers of Asians, Eskimos, and Native Americans. Recent studies (Al Quaran, 2006) examined 338 patients in Jordan. The researchers reported that 13.9% of the study participants had tori. The highest prevalence was for mandibular tori, with 20 of 47 study participants having bony growths in the mandible. Torus palatinus was slightly less common, 14 of the 47 participants. A larger Turkish study of schoolchildren (Yildiz, 2005) reported a study group of 1943 children from age 5 to 15 years. The prevalence rate was 30.9%, and torus palatinus was significantly more frequent in females than in males. Depending upon the region of the world, and the ethnicity of the population, the prevalence varies considerably. Reports in the United States place the prevalence rates for torus palatinus at a much higher rate of up to 25% and the mandibular tori at a slightly lower rate of about 10 to 12%.

Pathogenesis: The torus palatinus and mandibular tori are comprised of normal compact bone and usually appear after puberty and continue to enlarge throughout adulthood. Some lesions can become very large and may interfere with normal function.

Extraoral Characteristics: Not applicable

Perioral and Intraoral Characteristics: The torus palatinus is found in the midline of the hard palate where the growths may be large, lobulated, or in some cases, very subtle. In many cases, the elevation may not be apparent until the clinician palpates the area and notices a slight rise of elevation and firmness. The growths appear radiopaque on diagnostic radiographs because of the dense bone. Mandibular tori develop along the lingual aspect of the mandible and are usually bilateral, although occasionally they are unilateral. Figure 18.1A depicts torus palatinus. Figure 18.1B shows mandibular tori (note the varying size of the mass of bone within the picture). Figure 18.1C depicts a mandibular torus that is more isolated to the right and middle of the mandible.

Distinguishing Characteristics: The location and clinical characteristics of these lesions are distinctive. In comparison to a tumor that would produce sudden and rapid growth, mandibular tori and the torus palatinus do not appear suddenly and do grow rapidly.

Significant Microscopic Features: Mature, dense, lamellar cortical bone is characteristic of the his-

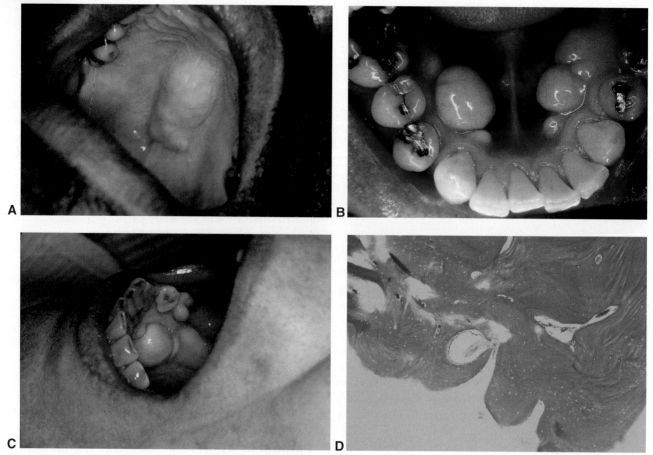

Figure 18.1. A. Torus palatinus. **B.** Mandibular tori. (Courtesy of Dr. Sumner Sapiro.) **C.** Mandibular tori. **D.** Histology of the torus.

tology seen in torus palatinus and mandibular tori. Figure 18.1D shows the histology of a torus palatinus demonstrating the dense, mature cortical bone of the specimen.

Dental Implications: Bony growths may interfere with speech, eating, and toothbrushing. On occasion, the growths may need to be removed for comfort and for the placement of dental appliances.

Differential Diagnosis: The torus palatinus and mandibular torus are usually diagnosed clinically because of their characteristic features and their location, unless they exhibit an uncommon appearance that may warrant further evaluation.

Treatment and Prognosis: The growths may become traumatized due to normal oral function. Standard treatment for this type of irritation is the same as for any other mucosal surface trauma. The growths normally pose no problem, and treatment is not usually needed.

Name: Exostosis

Etiology: Exostosis (pl., exostoses) represents an asymptomatic, exuberant growth of compact bone, occurring along the facial surfaces of the maxilla and the mandible. The growth can be single or may consist of

multiple nodules composed of dense compact bone. The growth originates because of irritation and occlusal forces. Solitary exostosis is a single protuberance, usually due to frictional causes such as an ill-fitting dental prosthesis or bruxism.

Method of Transmission: Not applicable

Epidemiology: Exostosis occurs equally in males and females and is found more frequently in adults.

Pathogenesis: Exostosis has been reported in correlation with skin grafts, dental work such as bridges, and stressors, such as bruxism. Occasionally, a solitary bony growth may occur, usually in response to a local irritation factor. The growths have been known to occur under the pontics of fixed bridges (**subpontic osseous proliferation**). The pontic replaces the missing tooth and has an open area under it, allowing the individual to clean the area more easily. In subpontic osseous proliferation, excess bone grows up into this opening, making oral hygiene procedures difficult.

Extraoral Characteristics: Not applicable

Perioral and Intraoral Characteristics: The bony growths tend to occur along the facial aspect of the maxilla and the mandible and manifest as lobulated, un-

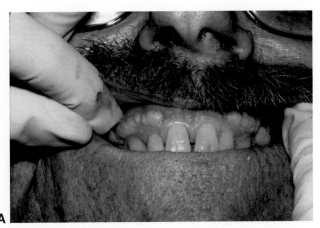
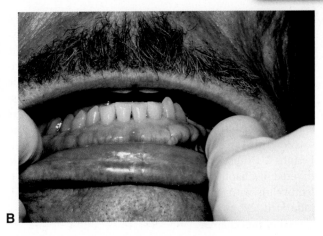

A **B**

Figure 18.2. **A.** Maxillary exostosis. **B.** Mandibular exostosis.

even solid bony growths. The posterior region is affected most often. The tissue appears a normal color unless the area has been traumatized. Figure 18.2A shows the multiple lobulated body growths in maxillary exostoses, and Figure 18.2B shows the multiple lobulated bony growths in mandibular exostoses.

Distinguishing Characteristics: The location and appearance of these lesions are characteristic.

Significant Microscopic Features: Mature hyperplastic cortical and trabecular bone are characteristic of the exostosis.

Dental Implications: It is important to determine if there are any direct causes associated with the development of the excess bone, such as bruxism. In this case, limiting excessive occlusal forces through the use of appliances or behavior modification would be optimal. Growths may need to be removed if dentures or other dental appliances are required.

Differential Diagnosis: The growths are usually diagnosed by their clinical appearance. Radiographs are sometimes helpful, especially in the case of a solitary exostosis, to rule out conditions that do not present as radiopaque lesions. Exostosis is a very hard, bony growth as are some malignancies. Some possible considerations of a solitary exostosis in a differential diagnosis are

1. Osteosarcoma, Chapter 18
2. Chondrosarcoma, Chapter 18
3. Ewing's sarcoma, Chapter 18

Treatment and Prognosis: There is no treatment recommended for exostosis unless the growth interferes with dentures or there is continuous injury to the site producing chronic inflammation. If bruxism is a factor, night guards may be fabricated for the patient, to lower occlusal forces. Exostosis usually presents no problems and is left alone unless the area becomes highly irritated or other disease states are suspected.

APPLICATION

Exostosis may be very subtle, or patients may exhibit large areas of bony growths in both the maxillary and mandibular arches. Evaluating the patient for occlusion problems, bruxism, and stress-related clenching is part of a thorough oral examination. An evaluation of the patient's eating and sleeping patterns may give the clinician a good indication of whether the patient may be bruxing while sleeping and waking with tight or sore muscles. Determining bruxism early and providing a night guard can dramatically decrease the amount of damage that is occurring to the oral structures. Stress reduction and behavior modification techniques can be learned and greatly affect overall health in general. Unless a healthcare practitioner calls these conditions to the patient's attention, they often go unnoticed or undiagnosed and cause increasing problems.

INFECTIONS

Infections may occur throughout the body affecting many tissues and organs. The next section discusses the hard tissue enlargements that are caused by infection and produce changes in the bone and the surrounding tissues. One such broad category is osteomyelitis. Osteomyelitis is an inflammatory process of the bone and bone marrow caused by an infection. The initial infection is normally from a bacterial source: staphylococci, streptococci, actinomyces, and other organisms. Abscesses, periodontal infections, jaw fractures, and cysts are often involved in the initiation of osteomyelitis. The condition can be acute osteomyelitis or it may become chronic osteomyelitis, due to the absence of treatment or the use of improper treatment. The difference between acute and chronic osteomyelitis is often related to the virulence of the bacteria involved. Acute osteomyelitis is always highly destructive. Several categories of chronic osteomyelitis exist, affecting different areas in the mouth. Chronic focal sclerosing osteomyelitis (condensing osteitis) is usually found as an area of radiodensity at the apex of a tooth, while diffuse sclerosing osteomyelitis exhibits more radiodensity throughout the jaw area. The bony sclerosis is a reaction to either an inflamed or a devitalized pulp, and the tooth will invariably be nonvital. Due to the radiographic appearances of the various forms of osteomyelitis, some lesions appear radiolucent while others appear radiopaque. Both chronic osteomyelitis and acute osteomyelitis are discussed in Chapter 20, "Radiolucent Lesions." Diffuse and focal sclerosing osteomyelitis are covered in Chapter 19, "Radiopaque Lesions." Chronic osteomyelitis with proliferative periostitis produces a hard, indurated, exophytic mass, and for this reason, it is discussed in this chapter.

Name: Chronic osteomyelitis with proliferative periostitis (Garré osteomyelitis)

Etiology: Chronic osteomyelitis with proliferative periostitis is described as a proliferative inflammatory response of the periosteum to infection or other irritants. The lesion can originate from odontogenic factors, such as a periapical abscess or periodontal infection, or from nonodontogenic factors, such as bacteremia, oral surgery, or jaw fractures.

Method of Transmission: Not applicable

Epidemiology: Chronic osteomyelitis with proliferative periostitis is seen more often in children and young adults, with a mean age of 13 years; there is no sex predilection.

Pathogenesis: Chronic osteomyelitis with proliferative periostitis occurs when an infection, usually of odontogenic origin, passes through the cortex of the bone and involves the periosteum. The infection stimulates the periosteum to become hyperplastic and causes the body to lay down bone on the surface of the cortical bone to wall off the infection, which results in enlargement of the bone. This type of bone growth produces a characteristic layering of bone (onionskin pattern) that is observed on the surface of the cortical bone on a radiograph. This onionskin effect is also referred to as **neoperiostosis** (described by Eversole et al., 1979).

Extraoral Characteristics: Not applicable

Perioral and Intraoral Characteristics: The lesion appears as an asymptomatic, unilateral, bony, hard protuberance with normal tissue covering the growth. It usually involves the posterior regions of the mandible. Radiographs of the lesion show evidence of neoperiostosis. Figure 18.3 depicts proliferative periostitis in an 8-year-old boy. The image on the left was taken at the initial examination and shows the classic appearance of neoperiostosis or onionskin pattern. The image on the right was taken 12 months later, after endodontic therapy, and shows resolution of the lesion. The initial diagnosis was

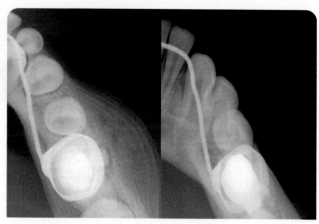

Start of treatment   12 month recall

Figure 18.3. Proliferative periostitis. (Courtesy of Dr. J. Craig Baumgartner.)

pulpal necrosis with a provisional diagnosis of chronic osteomyelitis with proliferative periostitis. The bony enlargement of 3 to 4 cm in diameter and 1.5 cm in depth is evident on the radiograph.

Distinguishing Characteristics: The onionskin pattern of the bone growth, presence of a dental infection, and young age of the patient are characteristic features of this condition.

Significant Microscopic Features: The microscopic appearance is that of newly formed bone consisting of osteoid and primitive bone in a fibrous connective tissue stroma that is scantly infiltrated by lymphocytes and plasma cells. The vital bone is oriented perpendicular to the surface epithelium.

Dental Implications: Tooth mobility may be a problem, depending upon the degree of advancement and stage of treatment related to chronic osteomyelitis with proliferative periostitis. The source of the irritation must be removed. Endodontic treatment has been successful in some cases, but extraction of the tooth may be necessary in other situations.

Differential Diagnosis: Neoperiostosis also occurs in the following conditions, which should be considered in the differential diagnosis:

1. Ewing's sarcoma, Chapter 18
2. Osteogenic sarcoma, Chapter 18
3. Congenital syphilis, Chapter 12
4. Fluorosis, Chapter 21

Treatment and Prognosis: The treatment protocol for chronic osteomyelitis with proliferative periostitis is the identification of the bacteria involved and subsequent removal of the tooth or teeth or endodontic treatment in the area affected. The use of antibiotics is often required as part of the course of treatment. The prognosis is good, and the bone will resolve over time. Osteomyelitis is further discussed in Chapter 19.

NEOPLASMS

Neoplasms are new growths of tissue that may be either benign or malignant. Neoplasms provide no benefit to the host. The lesion or tumor will continue to expand and grow even after any known stimulus is removed (see Chapter 5). The following section discusses neoplasms that appear as firm or hard nodules in the mouth.

Name: Ameloblastoma

Etiology: The **ameloblastoma** is classified as an **odontogenic tumor.** Odontogenic tumors arise from epithelial or mesenchymal remnants of tooth-forming tissues, such as the remnants of the rests of the enamel organ, the rests of Malassez, rest of Serres, or the reduced-enamel epithelium. They may also be formed from the epithelial lining of an odontogenic cyst, such as the dentigerous cyst (Chapter 20).

Method of Transmission: Not applicable

Epidemiology: Ameloblastomas are the most commonly occurring odontogenic tumors. Most occur in adults from 20 to 50 years of age, predominately in the fourth and fifth decades. There is no sex predilection. Approximately 80% occur in the mandibular molar region around impacted 3rd molars, reaching the angle of the mandible. The tumor can occur in the maxilla as well.

Pathogenesis: The ameloblastoma presents as a multilocular or unilocular lesion comprised of epithelial cells. There are several types of ameloblastoma, including follicular, plexiform, desmoplastic, acanthomatous, basal cell, granular cell, and peripheral. Ameloblastomas may also be extraosseous, but these are very rare. Malignancy is also rare, occurring in less than 1% of all ameloblastomas. Normally, ameloblastomas are considered benign growths, even though they are locally aggressive, invasive, and expansive.

Extraoral Characteristics: The expanding ameloblastoma may cause facial asymmetry, which might be the first indication that a tumor exists. Until discovered on radiographs, the lesions are usually asymptomatic.

Perioral and Intraoral Characteristics: The ameloblastoma appears as a painless swelling, usually in the posterior mandibular region. Buccal and lingual expansion in the area is frequently present upon clinical examination. The ameloblastoma may cause root resorption, and teeth may become mobile as the neoplasm expands. When viewed on a radiograph, ameloblastomas appear as multilocular and sometimes unilocular, radiolucencies with well-defined, scalloped margins. The multilocular lesions exhibit a characteristic "soap-bubble" appearance. Figure 18.4A shows a radiograph of an ameloblastoma in the left mandibular region. Note the multilocular appear-

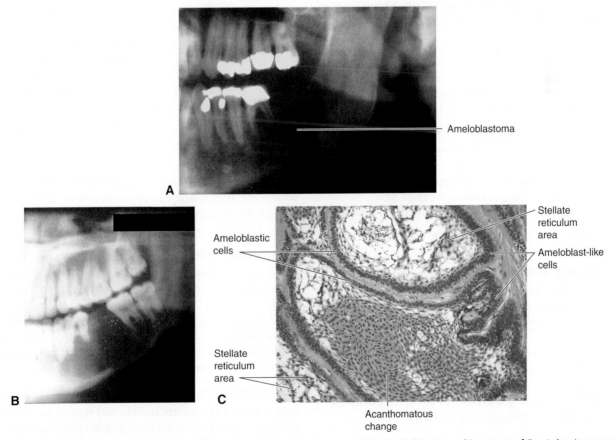

Figure 18.4. A. Ameloblastoma intraoral. (Courtesy of Dr. John Jacoway.) **B.** Ameloblastoma (Courtesy of Dr. John Jacoway.) **C.** Ameloblastoma histology (Courtesy of Dr. Harvey Kessler.)

ance of the lesion. Figure 18.4B depicts an ameloblastoma in the mandibular molar region. Figure 18.4C depicts the histology of an ameloblastoma.

Distinguishing Characteristics: The "soap-bubble" radiographic appearance and well-defined scalloped margins are characteristic features of this lesion.

Significant Microscopic Features: The ameloblastoma appears as palisading columnar cells around epithelial nests resembling the enamel organ. Elements of the stellate reticulum of the enamel organ are present. Depending upon the type of ameloblastoma, there may be nests of tumor cells or tumor islands. Peripheral cells resemble ameloblasts with reverse polarity of their nuclei. The islands resemble the stellate reticulum of the enamel organ. The lesion is unencapsulated. Figure 18.4C depicts the histology of an acanthomatous-type ameloblastoma. Note the labeled appearance of the ameloblast-like cells and the appearance of stellate reticulum-like areas noted on the slide. Peripheral cells resemble ameloblasts with reverse polarity of their nuclei. The islands resemble the stellate reticulum of the enamel organ.

Dental Implications: Although the ameloblastoma is a localized unencapsulated lesion, it can break through the cranial cavity by expansion, making it life threatening. When ameloblastomas are discovered in the maxilla, they can result in death due to direct extension into vital structures. The lesions also become more difficult to manage when they spread through the bone into the soft tissues.

Differential Diagnosis: Differentiation of this lesion from cysts and other radiolucent lesions is required and is determined through biopsy. Any of the tumors that exhibit a multilocular or unilateral appearance on radiographs should be considered, such as

1. Calcifying epithelial odontogenic tumor, Chapter 18
2. Odontogenic myxoma, Chapter 20
3. Dentigerous cyst, Chapter 20
4. Odontogenic keratocyst, Chapter 20
5. Central giant cell granuloma, Chapter 18
6. Ossifying fibroma, Chapter 18

The only way to obtain a definitive diagnosis of any of these lesions is through biopsy.

Treatment and Prognosis: Excision is the course of action. The tumor requires wide excision with clear margins to lessen the chance of recurrence. Careful radiographic follow-up is necessary to ensure early detection of any recurrence. The prognosis is good when timely treatment is rendered, but ameloblastomas may recur, and untreated ameloblastomas can result in death.

Name: Calcifying epithelial odontogenic tumor (CEOT) or (Pindborg tumor)

Etiology: The **calcifying epithelial odontogenic tumor (CEOT)** or **Pinborg tumor** (Pinborg, 1955) is an odontogenic tumor probably originating from remnants of the enamel organ. Although the precise origin is not known, it is associated with unerupted teeth.

Method of Transmission: Not applicable

Epidemiology: The CEOT can occur in any age group, but is usually found in 20- to 50-year-olds; it occurs equally in males and females. The CEOT accounts for about 1% of all odontogenic tumors and occurs less frequently than the ameloblastoma. The mandible is affected twice as often as the maxilla. Peripheral (extraosseous) odontogenic tumors are rare, with recent reports in the United States of 2.2% reported to be CEOTs.

Pathogenesis: The CEOT is a benign but locally invasive tumor, occurring in both intraosseous (94%) and extraosseous (6%) sites. This lesion is much less aggressive than the ameloblastoma, but like the ameloblastoma, the CEOT is locally invasive.

External Characteristics: A large CEOT may produce clinically observable facial asymmetry resulting from expansion of the jaw.

Perioral and Intraoral Characteristics: The CEOT manifests as a slow-growing, painless jaw expansion, usually in the molar and premolar region of the mandible. A maxillary CEOT tends to grow more rapidly than one in the mandible and does not remain as well confined. These lesions are often associated with impacted teeth. Radiographically, the CEOT appears as a multilocular radiolucent lesion with variable amounts of calcification. Figure 18.5A is a radiograph of a CEOT with diffuse opaque calcifications in the crown region of the unerupted lower right third molar.

Distinguishing Characteristics: A distinct entity, referred to as **Liesegang rings,** may be visible microscopically when calcification within the CEOT is dense enough. The rings represent calcified deposits forming within the tumor islands of the specimen. Figure 18.5B depicts the histology of a CEOT and shows a closer view of the Liesegang rings.

Significant Microscopic Features: The CEOT is made up of islands and sheets of polyhedral epithelial cells in a noninflamed connective tissue stroma. Deposits of hyaline (enamel protein) that resemble amyloidlike material are components of the CEOT. Figure 18.5C depicts the histology of a CEOT with areas of hyaline (amyloid), epithelial cells, clumps of polyhedral tumor cells with indistinct borders, and some calcifications.

Dental Implications: These tumors are usually discovered when the patient notices and reports facial asymmetry or during a routine radiographic examination. The potential of identifying lesions such as this emphasizes the need for periodic clinical and radiographic dental evalua-

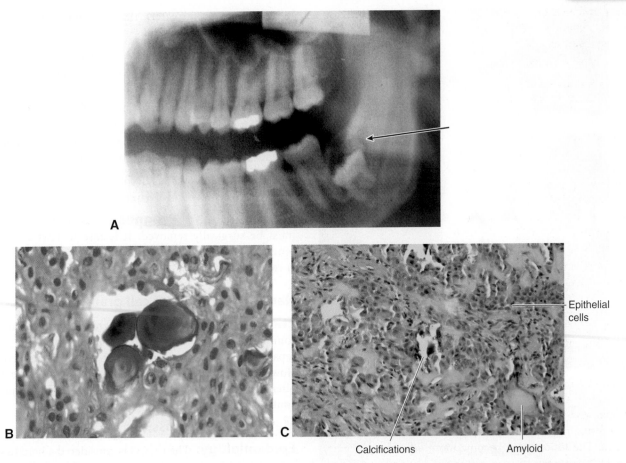

Figure 18.5. A. Calcifying epithelial odontogenic tumor. (Courtesy of Dr. Harvey Kessler.) **B.** Calcifying epithelial odontogenic tumor histology (Courtesy of Dr. Harvey Kessler.) **C.** Calcifying epithelial odontogenic tumor histology. (Courtesy of Dr. John Jacoway.)

tions. The patient should be followed closely for any sign of recurrence.

Differential Diagnosis: Since the CEOT may be radiolucent or may contain foci of calcification, the differential diagnosis is sometimes not readily apparent. In addition to cysts, fibromas, and tumors, the following are considerations:

1. Odontogenic keratocyst, Chapter 20
2. Dentigerous cysts, Chapter 20
3. Ameloblastoma, Chapter 18

Treatment and Prognosis: Surgical removal of the tumor with a wide margin of normal tissue is the required procedure. The prognosis is excellent.

Name: Ossifying fibroma (cementoossifying fibroma)

Etiology: The **ossifying fibroma**, or **cementoossifying fibroma** is a benign neoplasm, composed o-f cementum-like calcifications and bony components. The cause is not known.

Method of Transmission: Not applicable

Epidemiology: The ossifying fibroma occurs most commonly in the third and fourth decades of life. This lesion generally occurs in the premolar and molar regions of the mandible. There is a high female predilection of 5 to 1.

Pathogenesis: Ossifying fibromas are most often slow growing, painless, and expansile.

Extraoral Characteristics: Larger ossifying fibromas may cause swelling and facial asymmetry.

Perioral and Intraoral Characteristics: The larger versions of this lesion may appear as a nonpainful swelling. Otherwise, the lesion may be clinically undetectable but may appear on a radiograph during a routine examination. The radiographic appearance is of a well-circumscribed radiolucency with variable density. Sclerotic borders may be evident in the radiograph, depending on the amount of calcification present. Root resorption or root divergence may be noted. The ossifying fibroma on the radiograph shown in Figure 18.6A clearly presents a radiopaque lesion at the apical area of the maxillary left molar region, with evident root divergence (diverging roots).

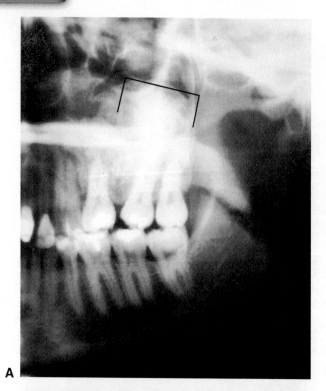

A

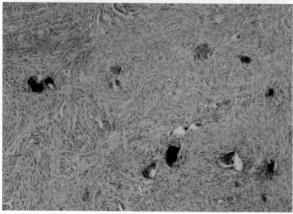

B

Figure 18.6. A. Cementoossifying fibroma radiograph. (Courtesy of Dr. John Jacoway.) **B.** Cementoossifying fibroma histology. (Courtesy of Dr. John Jacoway.)

Distinguishing Characteristics: Radiographic lesions appear as well-defined, unilocular, radiolucent lesions with radiopaque calcifications. Diverging roots may be evident, or the lesion may appear dense and calcified.

Significant Microscopic Features: The histologic features appear as vascular, cellular, fibrous connective tissue with bone fragments that are both mature and immature. The collagen fibers are arranged in what is termed a "storiform pattern." The bone is immature, and osteoblasts are often seen. The tumor may be encapsulated, with fibrous tissue surrounding the perimeter of the lesion. Figure 18.6B depicts the histology of an ossifying fibroma, demonstrating the areas of calcified bony material within the specimen. The tissue specimen ex-

hibits the storiform pattern that is characteristic of this type of lesion.

Dental Implications: The lesion is removed, and a complete diagnosis is made after the specimen is viewed microscopically.

Differential Diagnosis: The challenge with an ossifying fibroma is differentiating it from fibrous dysplasia (Chapter 10), which is the primary entity in a differential diagnosis. The following are also considerations:

1. Focal cementoosseous dysplasia, Chapter 20
2. Focal osteomyelitis, Chapter 20

Treatment and Prognosis: Ossifying fibromas must be surgically removed. It is rare to have a recurrence, and they do not become malignant. The prognosis is excellent.

Name: Central giant cell granuloma (CGCG)

Etiology: The **central giant cell granuloma** was, and in some areas still is, believed to be a reactive lesion or a reparative response to trauma or other local factors. However, many feel that because of its unpredictable and often aggressive nature it is a true neoplasm. This topic is controversial and is still being debated.

Method of Transmission: Not applicable

Epidemiology: The CGCG is considered a hard tissue enlargement accounting for fewer than 7% of all benign tumors of the jaws. There is a 65 to 75% prevalence for the mandible, where the CGCG is most often found anterior to the molar teeth and sometimes in the molar area. The ramus of the mandible is not a common site for the development of a CGCG. Although the lesion can appear at any age, it favors the under 20 age group, and there is a female predilection of 2:1. A recent study by Kruse-Losler et al. found 76.9 % of study participants to be under the age of 30, with a female to male ratio of 1.8:1. Additionally, 69.2% of the lesions occurred in the mandible, with 57.7% appearing as unilocular lesions.

Pathogenesis: The CGCG lesion is usually discovered on radiographs, appearing as a radiolucent lesion with expanding margins. The first indication of the CGCG may be mobility or expansion of teeth. The lesions demonstrate aggressive behavior and are classified as neoplasms.

Extraoral Characteristics: While most cases occur within the maxilla and the mandible, CGCG can also affect small long bones, such as those of the hands and feet, and facial bones.

Perioral and Intraoral Characteristics: The lesion usually manifests as a painless expansion of the jaw, usually anterior to the first molar. If the lesion penetrates and protrudes through the cortical bone, it then appears as a soft tissue, flat-based nodule with a blue-to-purple

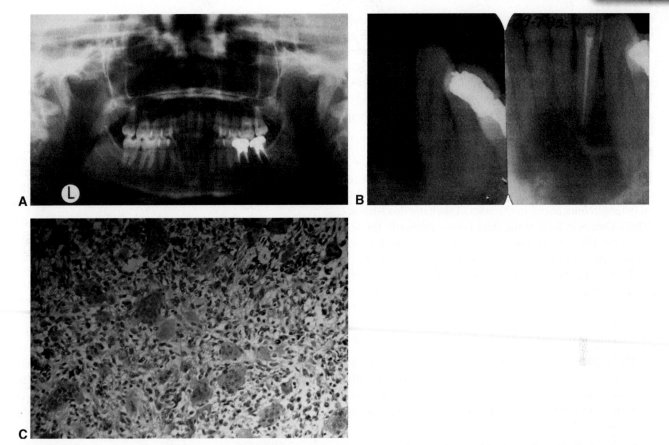

Figure 18.7. A. Radiographic view of a CGCG. (Courtesy of Dr. John Jacoway.) **B.** Radiographic view of CGCG. (Courtesy of Dr. John Jacoway.) **C.** Histology of a CGCG. (Courtesy of Dr. John Jacoway.)

color. There is usually no pain associated with the CGCG. The teeth may exhibit divergence. The radiographic appearance of the CGCG is of a radiolucent, multilocular or less often unilocular lesion with scalloped and expanding margins. Figure 18.7A depicts a radiographic slide of a central giant cell granuloma in the lower right mandibular region. Figure 18.7B shows a CGCG with a subsequent recurrence in the anterior region 22 years later.

Distinguishing Characteristics: The expansion of bone is a key feature of this lesion. The color variation of a blue-gray hue is sometimes a distinguishing characteristic for those patients who are seen clinically for perforation of the cortical bone plate.

Significant Microscopic Features: The lesion shows spindle-shaped mesenchymal cells with focal aggregates of small-multinucleated giant cells. The stroma is that of fibroblast and fibrosis. Figure 18.7C shows the histology of a CGCG with multinucleated giant cells.

Dental Implications: Aggressive lesions may recur, and complete removal is indicated. The possibility of other systemic disease needs to be eliminated, and all factors evaluated.

Differential Diagnosis: Tests may be needed to rule out other disorders that may be associated with the

CGCG, such as bone cyst, fibrous dysplasia, chondroblastoma, and osteoid osteoma. It is difficult to differentiate between the CGCG and other multilocular lesions, such as early ameloblastomas. Additionally, in the early development, it is difficult to differentiate other lesions, such as the small focal cyst lesions. Other lesions to be considered are

1. Hyperparathyroidism (Brown's tumors), Chapter 7
2. Cherubism, Chapter 10
3. Giant cell tumors involving Paget's disease, Chapter 10
4. Aneurysmal bone cysts, Chapter 19
5. Ameloblastoma, Chapter 18
6. Odontogenic keratocyst, Chapter 20

Treatment and Prognosis: Excision by curettage is the recommended treatment. A recurrence rate of 15–20% is noted. The more aggressive lesions tend to reoccur more often. Those occurring in children may have a higher rate of recurrence. The prognosis is good with complete removal.

Name: Osteosarcoma (osteogenic sarcoma)

Etiology: **Osteosarcoma** is the most common primary malignant tumor found in bone and accounts for 20% of all bone tumors (McMains, 2005). Gene tests find that mutations of the *Rb* gene and the *p53* gene are common in these neoplasms (Chapter 5). In older persons, osteosarcoma is most often associated with Paget's disease or past radiation exposure for treatment of other diseases. Increased osteosarcomas have been found in painters who at one time painted radium watch dials and wetted their brushes with saliva.

Method of Transmission: Not applicable

Epidemiology: This tumor accounts for about 25% of all sarcomas. Approximately 5 to 10% of all cases of skeletal osteosarcoma occur in the jaws (Takehana dos Santos, 2002). Osteosarcoma of the long bones, primarily the femur and tibia, most commonly occurs in the second decade age group and a decade later for osteosarcoma of the jaws, with the mean age being 35. Males are affected more often than females, with a predilection of 2:1. Worldwide, osteosarcomas affect about 1 per 100,000 persons per year. The mandible is affected more often than the maxilla, with most arising in the body of the mandible.

Pathogenesis: Although most osteosarcomas arise in the long bones, this sarcoma can be found in the maxilla and mandible. The mandible is more commonly affected with the prime areas being the body, symphysis, and an-

gle. A variant of osteosarcoma is **parosteal osteosarcoma**, a tumor that grows from the external surface of the bone. This type of osteosarcoma grows slowly and metastasizes late. The prognosis for this type is better than that for osteogenic sarcoma.

Extraoral Characteristics: Lung metastasis may occur with osteosarcoma.

Perioral and Intraoral Characteristics: The clinical symptoms may include pain, swelling, loose teeth, or numbness. **Dysesthesia** (a condition in which a disagreeable sensation is produced by ordinary stimuli) is also reported. Patients complaining of burning mouth syndrome often report unusual sensations that they have noticed, such as tingling and numbness in a specific area. In many cases of osteosarcoma, the radiographic appearance may be described as a "sunburst" pattern. When the neoplasm involves teeth, a widened periodontal ligament space and root resorption, called "spiking resorption" because the roots have a tapered appearance. Figure 18.8A, demonstrates the intraoral characteristics of an osteosarcoma in a 28-year-old white male. The tissue around teeth 19 and 20, as well as the distal retromolar, appears to be expansile. Figure 18.8B depicts the radiographic view of an osteosarcoma of the same patient, demonstrating the

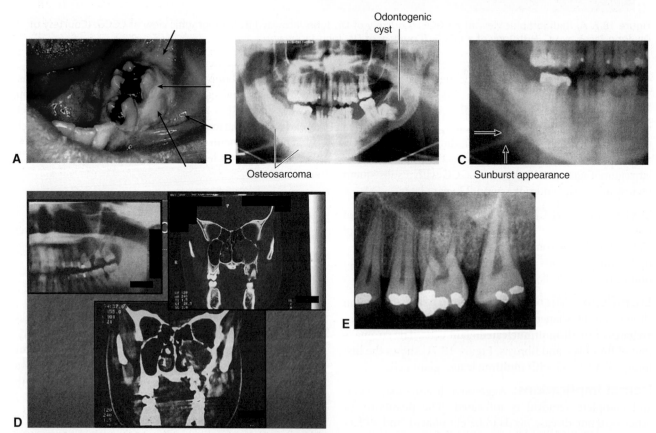

Figure 18.8. A. Clinical view of osteosarcoma. (Courtesy of Dr. John Svirsky.) **B.** Radiographic view of osteosarcoma. (Courtesy of Dr. John Svirsky.) **C.** Radiographic view of osteosarcoma. (Courtesy of Dr. John Svirsky.) **D.** Radiographic view, scans of osteosarcoma-(Courtesy of Dr. John Svirsky.) **E.** Radiographic view of osteosarcoma. (Courtesy of Dr. John W. Preece.)

osteosarcoma on the left mandibular region with heavy bone growth in the molar region. Note the "sunburst" appearance of bone radiating around the inferior mandibular region. An obvious cystic structure is also present on the opposite side in the distal molar region of tooth 31–32 area. Figure 18.8C shows the sunburst appearance in significant detail in the same patient. Figure 18.8D depicts an osteosarcoma found in a 32-year-old black male. View 1 represents the area on the upper left premolar region, with obvious destruction of the orbital floor. Views 2 and 3 show the scan with the tumor breaking though the left orbital area of the maxilla. Figure 18.8E represents the widening of the periodontal ligament in an osteosarcoma.

Distinguishing Characteristics: Symmetrical widening of the periodontal ligament of one or several teeth is often seen. Additionally, the typical "sunburst" or "spiking" seen radiographically are other distinguishing characteristics. Although other disease states may cause a widening of the periodontal ligament, osteosarcoma may be a strong consideration when pain and swelling have been reported.

Significant Microscopic Features: Pleomorphic malignant spindle cells, tumor giant cells, and mitoses are common features. The tumor produces bone matrix that is focally calcified. Also present are malignant cells producing osteoid. There is better differentiation of the osteosarcomas of the oral region than of the long bones such as the femur.

Dental Implications: The dental implications include tooth mobility, swelling, and pain. The patient may complain of nasal obstruction and paresthesia. The growth can affect the trigeminal nerve, causing paraesthesia. Fractures may be observed as well. Early radiographic evidence may be a widening of the periodontal ligament space as shown in Figure 18.8E.

Differential Diagnosis: CT scans and MRI techniques are needed to determine the extent of the lesion. Other neoplasms would be considered in the differential diagnosis depending upon the radiographic extent of the lesion and its radiolucent and radiopaque qualities. In addition, the following are also to be considered in the differential diagnosis:

1. Chronic osteomyelitis, Chapter 19
2. Metastatic carcinomas, Chapters 10, 17
3. CEOT, Chapter 18
4. Chondrosarcoma, Chapter 18
5. Ewing's sarcoma, Chapter 18

Treatment and Prognosis: Chemotherapy and surgical removal of the affected bone is the treatment of choice, with negative margins obtained around the periphery of the specimen. Poor rates of survival are correlated with the inability to obtain clear or negative margins during surgery. Survival varies, and reports are approximately 20% for 5 years, depending upon the extent of the lesion at the time of treatment.

Name: Chondrosarcoma

Etiology: **Chondrosarcoma** is a malignant tumor of cartilage. There is some evidence of a genetic predisposition. Rarely, these tumors can form within preexisting benign chondromas. Postradiation chondrosarcoma has been seen in individuals receiving more than 7000-rad dosages.

Epidemiology: Chondrosarcomas are much less common than osteosarcoma. Less than 1% of the chondrosarcomas found in the body are seen in the maxilla or the mandible. Chondrosarcomas arise in the third decade through the sixth decade of life, with most tumors reported to occur after the age of 40. A secondary form of chondrosarcoma occurs in younger patients between the ages of 20 and 40 years. Slightly more males are affected than females (ratio of 1.5 to 2:1). Chondrosarcoma is the second most frequently occurring primary sarcoma of bone, accounting for approximately 26% of all primary osseous sarcomas. Overall, 8 cases per 1 million population are reported (Hide, 2005).

Method of Transmission: Not applicable

Pathogenesis: Most chondrosarcomas arise in the pelvis, femur, ribs, and craniofacial bone. The presenting features are not consistent, and reports of pain and no pain, with swelling and no swelling, appear to be equal. If untreated or inadequately treated, these lesions can become large and extend into vital structures, causing death. Metastasis to the lungs or other bones is more common in high-grade chondrosarcomas than in the lower grades.

Extraoral Characteristics: Depending upon the location of the chondrosarcoma and the extent of the lesion, external swelling and asymmetry may be visible due to the growth of the tumor.

Intraoral and Perioral Characteristics: The most common oral site for development of these lesions is the maxilla, followed by the mandible. Maxillary involvement manifests as a painless swelling of the affected bone, with possible ulceration of the overlying mucosa. The patient may complain of headache, nasal problems, and separation and/or loosening of the teeth. Figure 18.9A shows a clinical view of a chondrosarcoma with evident bone expansion and mucosal ulceration. Figure 18.9B depicts a radiographic view of a chondrosarcoma showing a radiolucent/opaque destructive process causing widening of the periodontal ligament space (PDL) of an adjacent tooth as well as displacement of adjacent teeth; this is called root divergence. When found in the mandible, they usually involve the premolar and molar regions but may be found in the symphysis and the coronoid and condylar processes. Usually discovered radiographically, the chondrosarcoma may appear as a multilocular or a focal radi-

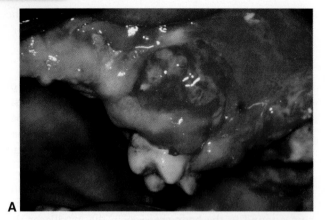

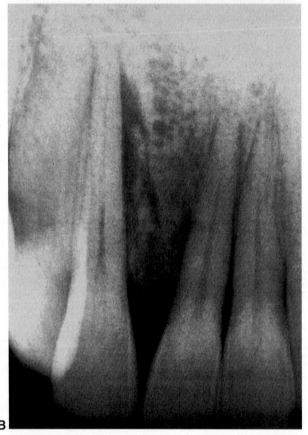

Figure 18.9. A. Clinical view of a chondrosarcoma. (Courtesy of Dr. Shabnum Meer.) **B.** Radiographic view of a chondrosarcoma. (Courtesy of Dr. Michael Kahn.)

olucent lesion, sometimes with opaque features. Widening of the periodontal ligament space of affected teeth is another feature commonly seen.

Microscopic Features: Chondrosarcomas are well differentiated with cellular atypia. Multiple cells in the lacunae and cellular pleomorphism are the common features. The chondrosarcomas are graded with the increasing incidence of metastasis.

Dental Implications: Chondrosarcomas may cause teeth to become mobile. Monitoring the patient periodically for signs of a recurrence is crucial.

Differential Diagnosis: Considerations include

1. Chondroma: The **chondroma** is a benign neoplasm of cartilage tissue that may exhibit features similar to those of the chondrosarcoma. Although rare in the oral cavity, the chondroma affects some of the same sites as the chondrosarcoma but appears even later in life. Histologically, chondromas are masses of hyaline cartilage containing mononuclear chondrocytes. The chondroma is mentioned in the differential diagnosis because differentiation of chondrosarcoma and chondroma can sometimes be difficult. The chondrosarcoma is similar to the chondroma but cellular atypia is present in the chondrosarcoma specimen.
2. Pleomorphic adenoma, Chapter 17
3. Osteosarcoma, Chapter 18

Treatment and Prognosis: Surgical excision, which can be extensive, depending upon the size of the lesion, is the treatment of choice. MRI scans are the most reliable tool in diagnosing the extent of the lesion. These tumors are radioresistant, meaning that radiation therapy is not a treatment option. A 5-year survival rate of 90% is reported for low-grade tumor but only 29% for high-grade. If the tumor recurs, it is usually found 5 to 10 years postsurgery.

Name: Ewing's sarcoma

Etiology: **Ewing's sarcoma** is a malignant bone tumor of unknown origin; however, a neural or neuroectodermal origin is suspected. A relationship between the development of this tumor and past irradiation or childhood diseases that required chemotherapy may exist. Radiation-induced Ewing's sarcoma is determined by several factors: (1) whether the past radiation occurred at least 5 years prior to the existing state, (2) if the malignancy is in the same area as the past irradiated field, and (3) if the tumor meets criteria of being histologically different from the originally treated disease.

Method of Transmission: Not applicable

Epidemiology: Ewing's sarcoma is a malignant bone tumor constituting approximately 4 to 6% of all primary bone tumors and is the second most common malignant bone tumor in children. Approximately 4% of these tumors occur in the head and neck area. This tumor usually affects the under 20 age group, with the sarcoma occurring most often in children. White males are affected more often than females, but in head and neck cases, there is a nearly equal distribution.

Pathogenesis: This tumor is thought to arise from primitive elements of the bone marrow or mesenchymal cells. Most are also associated with a translocation of genetic material between chromosomes 11 and 22. Both osseous and extraosseous subtypes of Ewing's sarcoma exist.

Extraoral Characteristics: During childhood, the lesions of Ewing's sarcoma usually involve the long bones such as the femur, tibia, and humerus. When the tumor arises later in life, it affects the pelvic area and the femur more often. A soft tissue in the area of the tumor may be clinically evident.

Perioral and Intraoral Characteristics: When Ewing's sarcoma is found in the mouth, the lesions usually involve pain, swelling, numbness, and often tooth mobility. One may also encounter a soft tissue mass in the affected area. The ramus of the mandible is the most common intraoral location for this tumor. Often there is destruction of the alveolar bone and ulceration of the overlying gingiva. The growing tumor may cause facial asymmetry. The lesion appears radiographically as a "moth-eaten radiolucency" or as an infection in the bone, with destruction or erosion of the cortical bone. Additionally, it may exhibit an "onionskin" appearance.

Distinguishing Characteristics: The most distinguishing feature of Ewing's sarcoma is the enlarging mass or swelling that is usually present.

Significant Microscopic Features: A sheetlike proliferation of small round cells resembling very large mature lymphocytes is common. The cells are dark staining, with a rim of cytoplasm and appear vacuolated.

Dental Implications: Any hard tissue growth should be evaluated and diagnosed through biopsy and additional warranted tests.

Differential Diagnosis: Considerations in a differential diagnosis include

1. Chondrosarcoma, Chapter 18
2. Metastatic cancer. All chapters cover this aspect since this is a risk with most malignancies.
3. Leukemia, Chapter 9
4. Lymphoma, Chapter 9

Treatment and Prognosis: Surgery, radiation, and chemotherapy are the standard treatment. A survival rate of 60 to 80% has been reported in cases of Ewing's sarcoma; however, the survival rate has continued to improve. Approximately 20% of those affected will experience metastasis, commonly involving the lungs.

SUMMARY

- The hard tissue enlargements covered in this chapter can be benign or very serious tissue enlargements that are life threatening.
- As with any disease state, early diagnosis is the key to successful treatment and recovery.
- Sometimes subtle changes that the patient may notice such as pressure, loose teeth, or pain may be the first sign of a bone tumor.
- Some lesions are clinically evident; others may be seen initially on radiographs.
- Careful review of the medical history and radiographs along with a thorough clinical examination are all keys in the evaluation of a patient's health.
- Torus palatinus and mandibular tori are composed of normal compact bone and pose no problems in most situations.
- Exostoses are asymptomatic, exuberant, compact bone growths that occur along the maxilla and the mandible. The growths can be single or multiple nodules composed of dense, compact bone.
- Chronic osteomyelitis with proliferative periostitis is described as a proliferative inflammatory response of periosteum to infection, caused by other irritants.

- Odontogenic tumors arise from epithelial tissue or from mesenchymal remnants of tooth-forming tissues.
- The ameloblastoma is classified as an odontogenic tumor.
- The calcifying epithelial odontogenic tumor has an odontogenic origin. The CEOT is found more often in the mandible, and there is no gender predilection.
- CEOT has distinct concentric calcified deposits known as Liesegang rings.
- The ossifying fibroma, or cementoossifying fibroma, is a benign neoplasm, composed of cementum-like calcifications and bony components.
- The central giant cell granuloma can grow outside of bone and penetrate through into the soft tissue.
- The osteosarcoma is the most common primary malignant tumor found in bone and accounts for 20% of all bone tumors. In some cases of osteosarcoma, the radiographic appearance may be described as a "sunburst" pattern or a "spiking resorption."
- Chondrosarcoma is a malignant tumor of cartilage.
- Ewing's sarcoma is a malignant bone tumor of unknown origin.

Critical Thinking Activity

1. Early osteosarcoma can present with radiographic evidence of widening of the periodontal ligament space.

   A. How do you know if the widened periodontal ligament space that you see on one of your patient's radiographs is NOT an osteosarcoma?

   B. What additional information would help to rule out an osteosarcoma?
   C. Should you refer everyone with widened periodontal ligament spaces for a biopsy?
   D. What other conditions can present with a widened periodontal ligament space?

Case Study

New patient Kasa Lovelace, a Native American female, age 45, presents for her first ever full mouth radiographic survey. You have everything set up, including plastic positioning devices and bite-wing tabs. You ask Kasa to remove any removable appliances if she has them and you begin the survey. You find that you cannot position the first maxillary molar film because Kasa cannot bite down. Finally, frustrated, you look in her mouth and discover the growths in the slide shown below

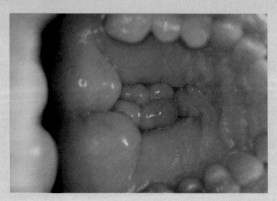

Answer the following questions:

1. What is your best guess as to the identity of this lesion?
2. What questions would you want to ask Kasa?
3. Would you expect the tissue to be completely firm in all areas?
4. What factors may have contributed to the development of this growth?
5. Would Kasa experience any complications related to this growth other than the problem with positioning radiographic films? Should she have this removed?
6. What are your options for completing your radiographic procedure at this point?

PORTFOLIO POSSIBILITIES

1. Gather some information for patient education on one of the sarcomas including its development, treatment, and prognosis.

2. Consider the fact that until a clinician discovers the torus, the patient may not even be aware of its existence. Once pointed out, the patient may wonder why it is there and if it is a type of pathology. The patient may even touch the area constantly with the tongue and actually irritate the torus. Research tori and collect color slides with various types of torus palatinus, mandibular tori, and exostosis.

Write an explanation of the process that could be presented to the patient when a torus or tori are diagnosed.

3. Many of the diseases discussed in this chapter are diagnosed through radiographs.

If your office does not have a written policy on the use of radiographs, the rationale for taking them, and stated intervals, this could be an excellent project to develop as a team. Perhaps the written guidelines could be given to new patients with your own stated philosophy regarding their importance in the dental office.

REFERENCES

Al-Bayaty HF, Murti PR, Thomson ERE, Deen M. Painful, rapidly growing mass of the mandible. Oral Surg Oral Med Oral Pathol Oral Radiol Endod 2003;95:7–11.

Al Quran FA, Al-Dwairi ZN. Torus palatinus and torus mandibularis in edentulous patients. J Contemp Dent Pract 2006;7(2):112–119.

Kruse-Lösler B, Diallo R, Gaertner C, et al. Central giant cell granuloma of the jaws: a clinical, radiologic, and histopathologic study of 26 cases. Oral Surg Oral Med Oral Pathol Oral Radiol Endod 2006;101:346–354.

Buchner A, Merrell PW, Carpenter WM. Relative frequency of peripheral odontogenic tumors: a study of 45 new cases and comparison with studies from the literature. J Oral Pathol Med 2006;35(7):385–391.

Cawson RA, Odell EW. Essentials of oral pathology and oral medicine. 6th ed. London: Churchill Livingstone–Harcourt Brace and Company Ltd, 1998.

Cawson RA, Binnie WH, Eveson JW. Color atlas of oral disease—clinical and pathologic correlations. 2nd ed. London: Wolfe Publishing, 1994.

Eisen D. Lynch DP. The mouth—diagnosis and treatment. St. Louis: 1998.

Eversole LR, Leider AS, Corwin JO, Karian BK. Proliferative periostitis of Garre: its differentiation from other neoperiostoses. J Oral Surg 1979;37:725–731.

Fowler CB. Benign and malignant neoplasms of the periodontium. Periodontology 2000 1999;21:33–83.

Hegtvedt AK, Terry BC, Burkes EJ, et al. Skin graft vestibuloplasty exostosis: a report of two cases. Oral Surg Oral Med Oral Pathol 1990;69:149–152.

Hide, G. Chondrosarcoma. Aug 11, 2005. Available at http://www.emedicine.com/radio/topic 168.htm. Accessed August 3, 2006.

Hood AF, Kwan TH, Mihm MC, Horn TD. Dermatopathology. 2nd ed. Boston: Little, Brown & Co, 1993.

Jacobson HLJ, Baumgartner JC, Marshall JG, Beeler WJ. Proliferative periostitis of Garre: report of a case. Oral Surg Oral Med Oral Pathol Oral Radiol Endod 2002;94:111–114.

Kalcioglu MT, Oncel S, Miman MC, et al. A case of Ewing's sarcoma in the mandible and the skull base. Kulak Burum Bogaz Ihtis Derg 2003;11(5):144–147.

Ladeindi AL, Ajayi OF, Ogunlewe MO, et al. Odontogenic tumors: a review of 319 cases in a Nigerian teaching hospital. Oral Surg Oral Med Oral Pathol Oral Radiol Endod 2005;99(2):191–195.

Langlais R, Miller C. Color atlas of common oral diseases. Baltimore: Lippincott Williams & Wilkins, 2003.

Mardinger O, Givol N, Talmi YP, Taicher S. Osteosarcoma of the jaw. The Chaim Sheba Medical Center Experience. Oral Surg Oral Med Oral Pathol Oral Radiol Endod 2001;91:445–451.

McMains KC, Gourin CG. Pathology: sarcomas of the head and neck. Nov. 14, 2005. Available at http://www.emedicine.com/ent//topic 675.htm. Accessed August 1, 2006.

Neville BW, Damm DD, Allen CM, Bouquot JE. Oral & maxillofacial pathology. Philadelphia: WB Saunders, 1995.

Pinborg JJ. Calcifying epithelial odontogenic tumor. Acta Pathol Microbiol Scan Suppl 1955;111:71

Pickett F, Gurenlian J. The medical history: clinical implications and emergency prevention in dental settings. Baltimore: Lippincott Williams & Wilkins, 2005.

Pinborg JJ. Calcifying epithelial odontogenic tumor. Acta Pathol Microbiol Scand Suppl 1955;111:71.

Porth CM. Essentials of pathophysiology. Baltimore: Lippincott Williams & Wilkins, 2004.

Regezi J, Sciubba J, Jordan R. Oral pathology—clinical pathologic correlations. 4th ed. St. Louis: WB Saunders, 2003.

Rinaggio J. Duffey D, McGuff HS. Differentiated chondrosarcoma of the larynx. Oral Surg Oral Med Oral Pathol Oral Radiol Endod 2004;97:369–375.

Rubin E. Essential pathology. 3rd ed. Baltimore: Lippincott Williams & Wilkins, 2001.

Scully C. Handbook of oral disease—diagnosis and management. London: Martin Duntz Ltd. The Livery House Publishers, 1999.

Seah YH. Torus palatinus and torus mandibularis: a review of the literature. Aust Dent J 1995;40(5):318–321.

Shulman JD, Beach MM, Rivera-Hidalgo F. The prevalence of oral mucosal lesions in U.S. adults. JADA 2004;135:1279–1286.

Stedman's medical dictionary. 27th ed. Baltimore: Lippincott Williams & Wilkins, 2000.

Suzuki K, Yoshida H, Onizawa K, Onobori M. Metastatic osteosarcoma to the mandibular gingiva: a case report. J Oral Maxillofac Surg 1999;57:864–868.

Terry BC, Jacoway JR. Management of central giant cell lesions. Oral Maxillofac Surg Clin North Am 1994;6:579–600.

Takehana dos Santos D, Cavalcanti MG. Osteosarcoma of the temporomandibular joint: report of 2 cases. Oral Surg Oral Med Oral Pathol Oral Radiol Endod 2002;94:641–647.

Wilkins EM. Clinical practice of the dental hygienist. 9th ed. Baltimore: Lippincott Williams & Wilkins, 2004.

Yazdizadeh M, Tapia JL, Baharvand M, Radfar L. A case of neurofibromatosis—Noonan syndrome with a central giant cell granuloma. Oral Surg Oral Med Oral Pathol Oral Radiol Endod 2004;98:316–320.

Yildiz E, Deniz M, Ceyhan O. Prevalence of torus palatinus in Turkish schoolchildren. Surg Radiol Anat 2005;27(5):368–371.

Zorzan G, Tulio A, Bertolini F, Sesenna E. Osteosarcoma of the mandibular condyle: case report. J Oral Maxillofac Surg 2001;59:574–577.

19

Radiopaque Lesions

Key Terms

- **Albers-Schönberg disease**
- **Ankylosis**
- **Cementoblastoma**
- **Endosteal**
- **Focal sclerosing osteomyelitis (condensing osteitis)**
- **Gardner syndrome**
- **Hamartomas**
- **Metastatic calcifications**
- **Odontoma**
- **Osteoma**
- **Osteopetrosis**
- **Periosteal**
- **Phleboliths**
- **Polyposis**
- **Tonsilloliths**

Chapter Objectives

1. Define and use the key terms discussed in this chapter.
2. State the most common location for finding focal sclerosing osteomyelitis.
3. List the various interventions that are indicated in the treatment of focal sclerosing osteomyelitis.
4. Discuss the etiology of diffuse sclerosing osteomyelitis and state the primary cause of the bone lesions.
5. List the significance of discovering an osteoma in a clinical patient.
6. Differentiate between the compound and the complex odontoma.
7. Describe the clinical significance of the cementoblastoma and its effect on the tooth structure.
8. Name and define two types of osteomas.
9. State the origin of osteopetrosis, along with two dental conditions that are associated with the disease.
10. Describe Gardner syndrome and state the importance of its early detection to the patient and the relatives of the patient.
11. List the possible calcifications that may be seen on a Panorex within the submandibular and neck region and discuss the importance of these findings.

Chapter Outline

As discussed in Chapter 18, some lesions not only appear clinically, but may also be seen on a radiograph. Other lesions may only be obvious on a radiograph, without exhibiting a clinical appearance. The conditions discussed in this chapter may be seen on a radiograph in various stages of development and are classified as radiopaque lesions. Some of these lesions may be completely opaque, while others may have radiopaque qualities, with varying amounts of radiolucent qualities as well depending on the stage of development.

TRAUMATIC OR INFLAMMATORY LESIONS

This section contains a discussion of focal sclerosing osteomyelitis that occurs because of a reaction to a low-grade inflammatory stimulus. The stimulus may be due to pulpitis, or an inflammatory process that causes a reaction in the bone. Also discussed in this section is osteomyelitis with diffuse lesions that may be caused by a microorganism of low virulence. The microorganism gains entry through the caries process, periodontal disease, or through some other port of entry into the tissues.

Name: Focal sclerosing osteomyelitis (condensing osteitis)

Etiology: Focal sclerosing osteomyelitis is an inflammatory reaction that usually involves pulpal inflammation and necrosis. However, it can be associated with a normal tooth as well.

Method of Transmission: Not applicable

Epidemiology: The mandibular molar teeth are usually the prime regions involved, and the first molar is most affected. Younger age groups are most often reported with focal sclerosing osteomyelitis, and the individuals tend to be under 20 years of age. There is no gender difference with focal sclerosing osteomyelitis as the condition is due to necrosis.

Pathogenesis: Focal sclerosing osteomyelitis is sometimes referred to as sclerotic bone and bony scar. Local inflammation from pulpitis or pulpal necrosis is often termed "condensing osteitis." The lesion is usually a reaction to some type of trauma or an inflammatory reaction to some stimulus, such as longstanding pulpal involvement. The term "focal," used in the name of this lesion indicates that it is usually isolated to one area, normally involving the apex of the tooth. Figure 19.1 depicts focal sclerosing osteomyelitis (condensing osteomyelitis) in the apical area of the molar.

Extraoral Characteristics: Not applicable

Perioral and Intraoral Characteristics: The lesions are usually noticed during examination of the radiographs, and the patient may be asymptomatic. The radiograph sometimes exhibits a varying radiopaque area at the apex of the tooth and the surrounding area.

Distinguishing Characteristics: Sclerotic bone without inflammation is usually characteristic; however, depending upon the extent of the lesions, inflammatory lesions may appear with different degrees of lucency. These lesions produce a combination of dense bone and radiolucent patches that may be diffuse and do not exhibit a completely focal opaque appearance.

Significant Microscopic Features: The histologic features of focal sclerosing osteomyelitis include sclerotic trabeculae and fibrous marrow with few lymphocytes.

Dental Implications: The tooth must be treated, and the caries removed. Endodontic treatment may be rendered, depending upon the damage to the tooth.

Differential Diagnosis: Other disease states that may be considered are

1. Periapical cementoosseous dysplasia, Chapter 20
2. Cementoblastoma, Chapter 19
3. Osteoma, Chapter 19
4. Complex odontoma, Chapter 19

Treatment and Prognosis: The tooth involved is treated by endodontics, extraction, or restoration. In some cases, there may be no treatment rendered, and this is approached and determined on an individual basis. The prognosis of the tooth depends upon the involvement of necrosis or infection, but the osteomyelitis may resolve once the stimulus is removed. Osteomyelitis may be a continuing problem manifesting for varying lengths of

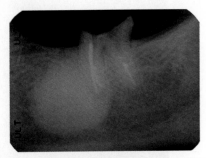

Figure 19.1. Focal sclerosing osteomyelitis (condensing osteitis). (Courtesy of Dr. Harvey Kessler.)

time or the sclerotic bone alone may be present indefinitely.

OSTEOMYELITIS WITH DIFFUSE LESIONS

Infections that appear radiopaque may have varying amounts of density and can extend throughout each quadrant of the mouth. Any osteomyelitis can be focal or diffuse, depending upon the extent of the bony involvement. If large areas of bone are involved, it is technically diffuse. Any osteomyelitis may be sclerosing (producing opaque areas), but many are not sclerosing and appear mostly as radiolucent. True osteomyelitis, whether focal, diffuse, sclerosing, or nonsclerosing, is normally caused by infection. Osteomyelitis that appears diffuse occurs mostly in the mandible, particularly the angle of the mandible, and can extend throughout the affected quadrant. The infection is caused by microorganisms and a resulting inflammatory reaction process. This can arise from periodontal disease, which allows bacteria to enter into the bone region. We have discussed focal sclerosing osteomyelitis in which there is pulpal involvement in an isolated area due to a known stimulus that produces a physiologic bone reaction. Chronic osteomyelitis may include a wider area; the bacteria may be more infectious, and it sometimes involves a long-term, low-grade inflammatory reaction. Figure 19.2 shows osteomyelitis with diffuse lesions exhibiting both opaque and radiolucent areas in the right and left mandibular regions. Diffuse osteomyelitis may occur in a large isolated site or there can be extensive coverage in an entire quadrant as depicted in Figure 19.2.

NEOPLASMS

Neoplasms related to radiopaque lesions, including the cementoblastoma, the odontoma, and the osteomas, are discussed in this section. The radiopaque nature of these lesions makes diagnosis clinically challenging. As previously discussed, diffuse sclerosing osteomyelitis can exhibit both a radiopaque and a radiolucent appearance, depending upon the extent of the lesions and the stage of development. Likewise, some neoplasms may have a varied appearance depending upon their stage of development.

Name: Cementoblastoma

Etiology: Cementoblastoma, also called true cementoma, or true tumor of cementum, is a benign odontogenic tumor. The tumor is characterized by proliferating cementum-like tissue.

Method of Transmission: Not applicable

Epidemiology: Cementoblastomas are usually found in young adults under 25 years of age. There is no gender predilection. The tumors account for 0.08 to 2.6% of all odontogenic tumors (Ohki, 2004). The posterior mandible is the most common site of occurrence, but the maxilla is more common when multiple teeth are involved.

Pathogenesis: Cementoblastoma is a true neoplasm of cementoblasts. The lesions may produce pain, and the tooth remains vital. The cementoblastoma is attached to the tooth root and appears radiographically as an opaque calcified mass. Figure 19.3A depicts a mass of calcification at the apices of a molar.

Extraoral Characteristics: Not applicable

Perioral and Intraoral Characteristics: There may be normal pulp tissue that is vital, but because of the disruption of normal neural impulse transmission, the tooth will not test vital with an electric pulp tester. Figure 19.3B shows a cementoblastoma in the mandibular right region and depicts the radiolucent area around the calcification.

Distinguishing Characteristics: When viewed radiographically, the calcified mass has a radiolucent halo around the outer perimeter, which is the periodontal ligament space. Since the calcified mass engulfs the root of the tooth (referred to as **ankylosis**), it is visible on the ra-

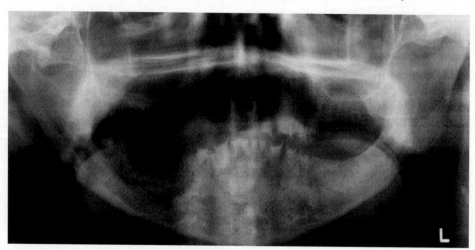

Figure 19.2. Diffuse osteomyelitis. (Courtesy of Dr. Enrique Plantin.)

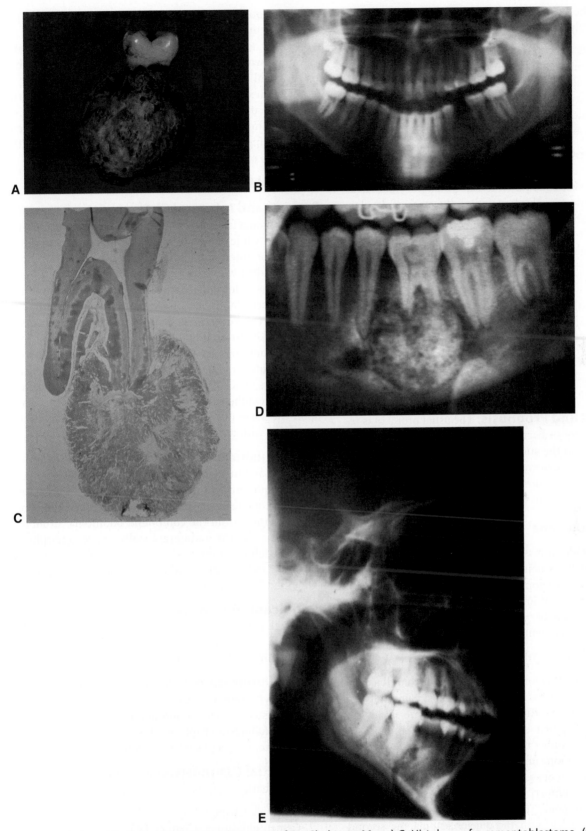

Figure 19.3. A and **B.** Cementoblastoma. (Courtesy of Dr. Shabnum Meer.) **C.** Histology of a cementoblastoma. (Courtesy of Dr. John Jacoway.) **D** and **E.** Cementoblastoma. (Courtesy of Dr. Shabnum Meer.)

diograph. The patient may be with or without pain, and there is usually swelling.

Significant Microscopic Features: The cementoblastoma exhibits dense mineralized cementum with many reversal lines, irregular lacunae, and cellular fibrovascular stromata. Figure 19.3C depicts the histology of the cementoblastoma with the attachment of the tumor at the apical area of the tooth.

Dental Implications: The patient may present to the dental practitioner with only symptoms of pain. Therefore, the clinician will be required to categorize the characteristics of the lesion involved, including the stage of development, the vitality of the tooth, and the factors that would indicate that the lesion is a cementoblastoma. Figure 19.3D depicts a large cementoblastoma of the mandibular molar region. Figure 19.3E represents a large cementoblastoma of the mandible, extending from the molar region forward.

Differential Diagnosis: Considerations may include some of the other radiopaque lesions such as

1. Focal sclerosing osteomyelitis, Chapter 19
2. Hypercementosis, Chapter 21
3. Osteoblastoma, Chapter 19
4. Odontoma, Chapter 19

Treatment and Prognosis: The usual protocol is removal of the tooth because of the unlimited growth potential related to the attached calcified mass. This growth potential makes removal necessary even though the tooth tests vital. The prognosis is excellent, without usual recurrence as long as the mass is totally removed.

Name: Odontoma

Etiology: **Odontomas** are mixed odontogenic tumors comprised of both epithelial and mesenchymal tissues. Odontomas are developmental anomalies and are **hamartomas** (composed of an abnormal mixture of tissue elements). In the case of odontomas, the tissue involved is a mixture of enamel, dentin, cementum, and pulp.

Method of Transmission: Not applicable

Epidemiology: Odontomas are the most common type of odontogenic tumors. The age group most commonly affected is individuals under age 20, and there is no sex predilection (Buchner et al., 2006). Recent results from studies to determine the relative frequency of central odontogenic tumors in relation to all biopsy specimens submitted to a biopsy service, reviewed 91,178 dental cases. Of that number, 1,088 biopsy results were central odontogenic tumors. The odontoma was the most common type (75.9%), with the ameloblastoma the second most commonly found (Buchner et al., 2006).

Pathogenesis: The odontoma is a mixture of both epithelial and mesenchymal dental hard tissues. Two forms of the odontoma exist:

1. Compound odontoma: resembles small teeth and appears in a collection of calcified material. Figure 19.4A depicts a clinical view of the complex odontoma with toothlike structures at the surface of the gingival tissue of an adult.
2. Complex odontoma: consists of a collection of hard tissue and includes deposits of enamel, dentin, cementum, and pulp all together in a masslike calcified form. Figure 19.4B shows a complex odontoma with a mass of calcified structures of the odontoma.

Extraoral Characteristics: Not applicable

Perioral and Intraoral Characteristics: The complex odontoma is usually found in the posterior mandibular region, while the compound odontoma is most often seen in the anterior maxilla. The compound odontoma may be evident when normal eruption patterns do not occur and may block the permanent tooth from erupting. This is especially noticeable when the failure to erupt is unilateral. Figure 19.4C depicts an unerupted permanent tooth blocked by an odontoma.

The odontomas are usually asymptomatic and discovered on routine radiographs. The complex odontoma usually appears on a radiograph as a calcified mass and sometimes may exhibit some radiolucent properties, depending upon the stage of development. Figure 19.4D shows an odontoma with a calcified mass in the mandible.

Distinguishing Characteristics: The complex odontoma and the compound odontoma may be found on a radiograph during a dental examination. However, further histology tests are needed to differentiate the complex odontoma from the compound odontoma. Complex odontomas appear radiographically more amorphous (without definite form or shape) and as solitary forms of indistinct radiopacities, rather than toothlike structures (Oner and Pocan, 2006).

Significant Microscopic Features: The elements of enamel, dentin, cementum, and pulp are present in the odontoma. The separate structures may be observed in a tissue sample and viewed under the microscope.

Dental Implications: The odontoma may be seen in Gardner syndrome (discussed in the next section) along with the osteoma. The odontoma may impinge on teeth, causing a failure to erupt (see Fig. 19.4C) and may also grow in size, causing facial asymmetry.

Differential Diagnosis: Other entities that should be considered are

1. Osteoma, Chapter 19
2. Cementoblastoma, Chapter 19
3. Periapical cementoosseous dysplasia, Chapter 20

Treatment and Prognosis: Excision is the treatment of choice; the prognosis is excellent without incidence of recurrence.

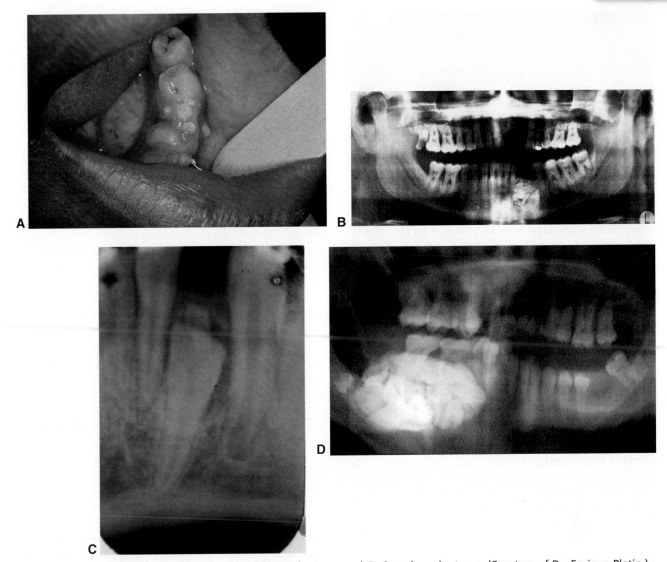

Figure 19.4. A. Complex odontoma. (Courtesy of Dr. John Jacoway.) **B.** Complex odontoma. (Courtesy of Dr. Enrique Platin.) **C.** Compound odontoma preventing eruption. (Courtesy of Dr. John Jacoway.) **D.** Odontoma. (Courtesy of Dr. A. Yusuf Oner.)

Name: Osteoma

Etiology: The origin of the osteoma is unknown, but trauma, infections, and developmental defects have been suggested as possible causes.

Method of Transmission: Not applicable

Epidemiology: Osteomas occur in the second to fifth decade of life, and males are affected more often than females. The growths may occur in the maxilla and mandible, the skull, and the sinuses (Bilkay et al., 2004).

Pathogenesis: The **osteoma** is a benign tumor consisting of mature compact or cancellous bone. Osteomas may be classified as either **periosteal**, occurring on the surfaces of bone, or **endosteal**, occurring in the bone. Although rare, the osteoma may also occur in other facial bones, such as the sinus areas. The osteoma is slow growing, but may eventually reach larger sizes, causing expan-

sion and deformity. The patient sometimes notes facial asymmetry. Osteomas are considered hamartomas along with the odontoma, and both may occur in relation to Gardner syndrome. Multiple osteomas are the hallmark of Gardner syndrome (discussed in the next section).

Extraoral Characteristics: Depending upon the size of the osteoma, some swelling may be noticed extraorally, which may be subtle since the lesion is slow growing. The patient may report noticing this for years before the actual diagnosis.

Perioral and Intraoral Characteristics: Osteomas appear radiographically as a dense opaque growth on the bone. The bony growths may be in the condyle, mandible and maxilla, or even in the sinus region. Depending upon the size, the patient may be asymptomatic or may experience headaches, sinusitis, or vague related symptoms. Osteomas may be confused radi-

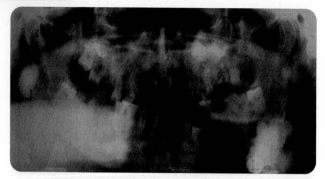

Figure 19.5. Gardner syndrome osteomas. (Courtesy of Dr. Enrique Platin.)

ographically with odontomas and often must be differentiated histologically by biopsy. Figure 19.5 depicts an osteoma in multiple areas of the maxilla and mandible.

Distinguishing Characteristics: Osteomas usually exhibit certain characteristics, such as a sharply defined radiopaque structure with clumped calcifications that resemble toothlike structures. A radiolucent rim is sometimes seen on the periphery of the lesion.

Significant Microscopic Features: Osteoclast and osteoblast activity and normal bone pattern are evident. Depending upon the type of osteoma, the bone pattern varies. Compact and cancellous bone osteomas are both possible.

Dental Implications: The dental implications make differentiation of an osteoma especially important in the early diagnosis of Gardner syndrome. The presence of osteomas and odontomas may indicate Gardner syndrome and thus the need for further tests (see Gardner syndrome).

Differential Diagnosis: Osteomas may have characteristics that appear similar to those of the complex odontoma. Supernumerary teeth, osteomas, and odontomas are also common occurrences in Gardner syndrome. Radiographically, an osteoma is sometimes similar to the complex odontoma; however, viewing the tissue under the microscope will differentiate the two.

The following would be considered as possible diagnoses:

1. Exostoses, Chapter 18
2. Cementoblastoma, Chapter 19
3. Odontoma, Chapter 19
4. Focal sclerosing osteomyelitis, Chapter 19

Treatment and Prognosis: Observation is the protocol for very small osteomas, with careful monitoring in some cases and surgery for the larger, more extensive, lesions. The prognosis is excellent when the osteoma is removed, and recurrence is usually not a problem. A biopsy and histologic diagnosis is necessary to differentiate the lesions from other pathology, thus the lesions are usually removed anyway for complete diagnosis. Osteomas re-

main benign, but they may be associated with other disease states, such as Gardner syndrome. Referral to a medical doctor is necessary when there is an indication of Gardner syndrome. Intestinal resection is often performed when there are intestinal polyps indicating Gardner syndrome.

GARDNER SYNDROME

Gardner syndrome is inherited as an autosomal dominant disorder characterized by polyposis coli (**polyposis**) associated with multiple hard and soft tissue tumors. The syndrome manifests osteomas of the bones and sometimes odontomas, epidermoid cysts, supernumerary teeth, other benign tumors of the skin and soft tissues, gastrointestinal polyps and multiple polyps. Figure 19.5 depicts osteomas in a Panorex, exhibiting the sharply defined, clumped radiopaque structures of Gardner syndrome.

If left untreated or unrecognized, the polyps associated with Gardner syndrome usually develop into malignant invasive adenocarcinoma in the gastrointestinal tract and the stomach by the fourth decade or before. Polyposis coli occurs in approximately 1 in 8000 individuals and is the most common form of the hereditary polyposis syndromes (Oner and Pocan, 2006). Gardner syndrome may produce both osteomas and odontomas in both the mandible and maxilla, although the mandible is the favored location. Facial bones may also be involved and develop osteomas leading to facial asymmetry. When recognizing an osteoma, and especially multiple osteomas, the clinician should be aware that the osteoma is the hallmark of Gardner syndrome. Early treatment of the patient with Gardner syndrome is crucial, since there is a fatal outcome of malignancy in relation to the polyps that accompany the syndrome. The polyps have a 100% risk of undergoing malignant transformation (Bilkay et al. 2004). Family members should be advised to have screenings for Gardner syndrome as well, since it is a variant of familial adenomatous polyposis. As a dental professional, the clinician can play a crucial role in the recognition of the disorder in association with the osteomas and odontomas that may be found during a routine dental visit.

Osteomas may produce few or no symptoms, and they may only be discovered during a dental visit, becoming apparent on a routine radiograph. Larger, more significant osteomas may cause problems as they impinge upon surrounding tissues and produce some extraoral facial swelling. Providing treatment at the earliest stage in Gardner syndrome is very important in the prognosis of the disease for both the patient and family members.

CONGENITAL OR GENETIC DISORDERS

Congenital or genetic disorders related to radiopaque lesions are sometimes not diagnosed until the clinician takes a radiograph or the patient exhibits some symptom indicating that there may be a problem. Sometimes, in mild cases involving bone disorders, the person may not experience problems until later in life. The disease discussed below, osteopetrosis, is such a disease that may go undetected until the patient has a radiograph or there are problems encountered during an extraction.

Name: Osteopetrosis

Etiology: Osteopetrosis, also known as **Albers-Schönberg disease** and marble bone disease, is a congenital sclerosing disease of bone, characterized by osteoclastic dysfunction.

Method of Transmission: Osteopetrosis has a hereditary component that is expressed as an autosomal recessive and autosomal dominant disorder, depending upon the type of osteopetrosis.

Epidemiology: The age of the individual affected will vary with the type of osteopetrosis diagnosed. Several types of osteopetrosis may occur. One type may be evident in the infant and a second form, the intermediate type, may become obvious in the first decade of life. The benign form may become apparent as increasing bone disturbances occur in midlife. Osteopetrosis occurs equally in males and females. The development of osteopetrosis occurs almost exclusively in the mandible (Barry and Ryan, 2003).

Pathogenesis: Osteopetrosis is a genetic disease with varying degrees of bone involvement. The disorder is characterized by a noted increase in the density of the bone, due to reduced osteoclastic activity, along with defective bone resorption. As discussed above, the condition is hereditary and is categorized into several groups. The first type, found in infants, has a fatal outcome within several years. A second, intermediate type involves an autosomal recessive form of osteopetrosis as well and is very aggressive. The third type is an autosomal dominant type, which manifests noted bone involvement. Obviously, the second and third types may be found clinically as the disorder progresses. The recessive type is found in approximately one per 200,000 (Filho et al., 2004). The benign type has been reported in approximately 50 cases.

Extraoral Characteristics: Prognathic profiles are often a clinical sign of osteopetrosis. These are shown in Figure 19.6, which shows the advanced stage of osteopetrosis with dense, generalized sclerosis of the mandible.

Perioral and Intraoral Characteristics: Radiographically, there is skeletal density due to diffuse sclerosing of all the bones. Clinically, there is delayed tooth eruption, enamel hypoplasia, defects in the periodontal membrane, and thickened lamina dura. Bone fractures and osteomyelitis are also problems for the patient. The infantile form of the disorder often exhibits frontal bossing, snub nose, and facial deformity.

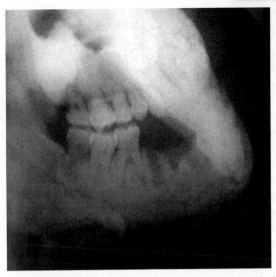

Figure 19.6. Osteopetrosis. (Courtesy of Dr. John Wright.)

In the adult form, the bone becomes more involved as the patient ages, and multiple bone fractures, anemia, and malformation of dental crown and root canals are evident, with pseudoodontomas often present. Osteomyelitis is another complication, and bone fractures are common as well. Often, osteopetrosis is diagnosed when these types of events occur, and at a time when radiographs are routinely made (Filho et al., 2004).

Distinguishing Characteristics: Radiographs show increased bone density with an amorphous aspect, marrow space encroachment, and malformed teeth that may appear clinically as the odontoma discussed above.

Significant Microscopic Features: Histologically, there is evidence of decreased in osteoclastic function. Additionally, there is a deficiency of bone resorption and bone remodeling, and increased bone density. Diagnosis is made on the history of previous fractures and the radiographic findings of osteosclerosis, along with the histologic results.

Dental Implications: The relevance to the clinician of osteopetrosis is great, because approximately 10% of patients report osteomyelitis in conjunction with the osteopetrosis. An existing dental problem may cause the patient to seek treatment, and the osteopetrosis may be diagnosed during routine treatment. Osteomyelitis may be a complication in tooth extraction or trauma, and bone fractures may occur during extractions. Often delayed tooth eruption is a clinical manifestation in children.

Differential Diagnosis:

1. Paget's disease, Chapter 10
2. Hyperparathyroidism, Chapter 7
3. Acromegaly, Chapter 7
4. Malignant bone disease, Chapter 18

The main concern related to this disease is a failure to recognize the disorder when treating the patient for extractions. The patient may suffer multiple bone fractures when pressure is applied.

Prognosis: It is suggested (Filho et al 2004) that the patient who is diagnosed with osteopetrosis in any form be seen in a dental school for treatment related to the teeth or oral structures, since a multidisciplinary approach is needed for adequate care. Antibiotics are prescribed when needed, as in the case of osteomyelitis with incision and drainage. Hyperbaric oxygen is often recommended as an adjunct treatment in the case of osteomyelitis. Prophylaxis with fluoride is recommended to aid against caries, and restorative dental procedures are part of the protocol. The infantile form has a poor prognosis, with most dying from anemia or infection. The adult form has a better prognosis and may be diagnosed during routine dental examinations as the disease progresses.

OTHER RADIOPAQUE ENTITIES

Another entity that should be discussed under radiopaque lesions is the calcification that is sometimes witnessed on a Panorex in the carotid and lymph node locations. These lesions may not have any symptoms and may not even be palpable, but may be clearly visible on the Panorex. The carotid calcification can cause significant vascular occlusion leading to a stroke; therefore, early detection and identification may save the person's life.

Calcified lymph nodes are typically evidence of past infection rather than metastatic disease, such as carcinoma. In the presence of an elevated serum calcium level, such calcifications may be referred to as **metastatic calcifications.** This term means calcification that is occurring in nonosseous tissue (i.e., nonbone, such as the lymph tissue) and tissue that is not degenerated or necrotic. The cells of these organs secrete acidic materials, and under certain conditions, in instances of hypercalcemia, the alteration in pH causes precipitation of calcium salts in these sites. In the past, the most common cause for calcified nodes was tuberculous lymphadenitis (scrofula). At present, it is more likely due to some other infectious process, with multiple recurrences eventually producing fibrosis within the node that subsequently calcifies. Additional radiographic surveys may be needed to determine that the calcifications are in the lymph nodes and not the carotid artery, which could be a serious medical problem.

Figure 19.7A shows a carotid calcification detected on a routine Panorex. A closer view of this calcification is shown in Figure 19.7B.

Carotid calcifications are rarely reported, but many may be overlooked in the dental office because of their subtle appearance in most cases. Other calcifications appear in a Panorex and may be noted as well, such as calcified lymph nodes, **phleboliths** (a calcified deposit in a venous wall or thrombus), submandibular salivary gland sialoliths and **tonsilloliths** (concretion in a tonsil crypt) (Pornprasertsuk-Damrongsri and Thanakum, 2006). Normal anatomy and artifact must be differentiated as well and sometimes must be differentiated from normal tiss ue, when the appearance is questionable. Pornprasertsuk-Damrongsri and Thanakum (2006) also found higher rates of hypertension, diabetes mellitus, and hyperlipidemia in patients who were confirmed to have carotid artery calcifications.

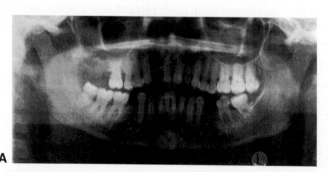
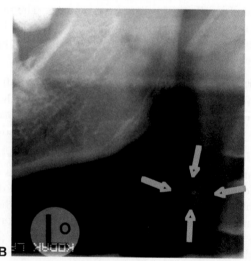

Figure 19.7. A and **B.** Carotid artery calcification. (Courtesy of Dr. Enrique Platin.)

APPLICATION

As discussed above, osteopetrosis is a good example of a disorder that is beyond the routine treatment for a dental practice, since treatment involves a multidisciplinary approach. Many individuals are involved in both the diagnosis and the treatment of these patients. Some crucial specialty areas are radiology, pathology, oral surgery, periodontology, prosthodontics, and specialists in treating bone diseases. Additionally, the hygienist, nutritionist, and others who would be involved in both medicine and dentistry for the care of the patient with osteopetrosis, would need to provide adjunctive care.

The best place to find all the specialists together is a medical and dental school or a teaching hospital that accommodates all the various specialists in one area. The patient would be assured of the best possible care with many specialists planning his or her care. The general practitioner and possibly the dental hygienist may be the first professionals to recognize that there is a problem such as osteopetrosis and should refer the patient to the correct facility for initial treatment.

SUMMARY

- In many cases, radiopaque lesions are complicated to diagnose because there is often not much clinical evidence manifested during an oral examination. Therefore, a radiograph is necessary to provide the needed diagnostic information related to these disease states.
- The clinician can play a powerful role in detecting obvious changes in dental conditions and, most importantly, those subtle changes that can affect the life of the patient.
- Disorders that have radiopaque lesions as part of other syndromes, such as Gardner syndrome, have profound effects on many areas of the body, making early diagnosis and treatment crucial.
- Gardner syndrome is an inherited autosomal dominant disorder that involves the osteoma and sometimes odontomas, epidermoid cysts, supernumerary teeth, and other benign tumors of the skin and soft tissues, and multiple polyps as part of the disease state.
- The polyposis coli (polyposis) in Gardner syndrome have a 100% risk of undergoing malignant transformation.
- The complex odontomas are usually found in the posterior mandibular region, while the compound odontomas are most often seen in the anterior maxilla.
- The compound odontoma may be evident when normal eruption patterns do not occur and may block the permanent tooth from erupting. Odontomas are mixed odontogenic tumors composed of both epithelial and mesenchymal tissues. Odontomas are developmental anomalies and are hamartomas (composed of abnormal mixtures of tissue elements).
- Osteomas appear radiographically as dense opaque growths on the bone.
- Focal sclerosing osteomyelitis usually involves pulpal inflammation and necrosis of the pulp. Any osteomyelitis may be sclerosing (producing opaque areas), but many are not sclerosing and appear radiolucent or a mixture of opaque and radiolucent.
- Cementoblastoma, also called true cementoma, or true tumor of cementum, is a benign odontogenic tumor.
- Osteopetrosis is a genetic disease occurring with varying degrees of bone involvement. Osteopetrosis requires a multidisciplinary approach, and the treatment involves many specialists in both medical and dental fields.

PORTFOLIO POSSIBILITIES

Research the vast array of resources in your area that provide both dental treatment and medical treatment in one facility. The facilities should be able to treat patients who are diagnosed with diseases such as osteopetrosis and Gardner syndrome.

- Make a list of the facilities with each specialty area noted.
- Acquaint yourself with key individuals who would be willing to treat special needs patients upon the referral of your office.

- Design a letter stating that your practice is referring a patient with suspected disease. A specific form letter is appropriate and could be modified for each patient's needs.
- If there are no facilities close to your practice, find ones that are within a reasonable travel distance for a patient.

Critical Thinking Activity

You have just finished a maintenance appointment with a patient who was recently referred to an oral surgeon for the extraction of #17 and #32. Upon evaluation of the patient's radiograph, the oral surgeon became suspicious of some areas in the radiograph and the patient was referred for some additional tests. The patient was ultimately diagnosed with osteopetrosis, also known as Albers-Schönberg disease. Fractures are common, and care with extractions is needed because of the fragility of the bones. The disease causes an increase in bone density and reduction of marrow spaces.

- Do you think the patient has a defective function of the osteoclasts or the osteoblasts?
- What is the cause of osteopetrosis?
- Can you explain the function of both osteoclasts and osteoblasts?
- Can you explain how the patient would develop the characteristic prognathic profile?

Case Study

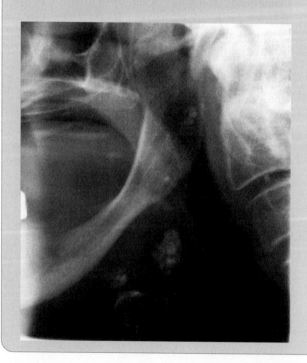

The slide presented is of a 57-year-old male who was seeking routine dental treatment at a clinic. He had no obvious health problems and was taking no medications. He needed a routine prophylaxis and dental examination. During routine radiographs, the clinician noticed that small opaque areas were evident on the Panorex in the posterior mandible and neck area.

What would you have considered in viewing this radiograph?

What are some possibilities?

REFERENCES

Barry CP, Ryan CD. Osteomyelitis of the maxilla secondary to osteopetrosis: report of a case. Oral Surg Oral Med Oral Pathol Oral Radiol Endod 2003;95:12–15.

Bilkay U, Erdem O, Ozek C, et al. Benign osteoma with Gardner syndrome: review of the literature and report of a case. J Craniofac Surg 2004;15 (3):506–509.

Buchner A, Merrell PW, Carpenter WM. Relative frequency of central odontogenic tumors: a study of 1,088 cases from Northern California and comparison to studies from other parts of the world. J Oral Maxillofac Surg 2006;64(9):1343–1352.

Cawson RA, Binnie WH, Eveson JW. Color atlas of oral disease—clinical and pathologic correlations. 2nd ed. London: Wolfe Publishing, 1994.

Cawson RA, Odell EW. Essentials of oral pathology and oral medicine. 6th ed. London: Churchill Livingstone–Harcourt Brace and Company Ltd., 1998.

Eisen D. Lynch DP. The mouth—diagnosis and treatment. St. Louis: Mosby, 1998.

Hood AF, Kwan TH, Mihm MC, Horn TD. Dermatopathology. 2nd ed. Boston: Little, Brown & Co., 1993.

Filho P, Chaves MD, Vieira EH, et al. Osteopetrosis of the jaws. Gen Dent 2004;52(3):240–242.

Kaugars GE, Miller ME, Abbey LM: Odontomas, Oral Surg Oral Med Oral Pathol 1989;76:172.

Langlais R., Miller C. Color atlas of common oral diseases. Baltimore: Lippincott Williams & Wilkins, 2003.

Mohn A, Capanna R, Delli Pizzi C, et al. Autosomal malignant osteopetrosis: from diagnosis to therapy. Minerva Pediatr 2004;56(1): 115–118.

Neville BW, Damm DD, Allen CM, Bouquot JE. Oral & maxillofacial pathology. 2nd ed. Philadelphia: WB Saunders, 2001.

Ohki K, Kumamoto H, Nitta Y, et al. Benign cementoblastoma involving multiple maxillary teeth: report of a case with a review of the literature. Oral Surg Oral Med Oral Pathol Oral Radiol Endod 2004;97:53–58.

Oner AY, Pocan S. Gardner's syndrome: a case report. Br Dent J 2006;24;200(12):666–667.

Pacifici L, Tallarico M, Bartoli A, et al. Benign cementoblastoma: a clinical case of conservative surgical treatment of the involved tooth. Minerva Stomatol 2004;53(11–12):685–691.

Pickett F, Gurenlian J. The medical history: clinical implications and emergency prevention in dental settings. Baltimore: Lippincott Williams & Wilkins, 2005.

Pornprasertsuk-Damrongsri S, Thanakun S. Carotid artery calcification detected on panoramic radiographs in a group of Thai population. Oral Surg Oral Med Oral Pathol Oral Radiol Endod 2005;101(1):110–115.

Porth CM. Essentials of pathophysiology. Baltimore: Lippincott Williams & Wilkins, 2004.

Regezi J, Sciubba J, Jordan R. Oral pathology—clinical pathologic correlations. 4th ed. St. Louis: WB Saunders, 2003.

Rubin E. Essential pathology. 3rd ed. Baltimore: Lippincott Williams & Wilkins, 2001.

Scully C. Handbook of oral disease—diagnosis and management. London: Martin Duntz Ltd. The Livery House Publishers, 1999.

Sayan NB, Ucok C, Karasu HA, Gunhan O. Peripheral osteoma of the oral and maxillofacial region: a study of 35 new cases. J Oral Maxillofac Surg 2002;60(11):1299–1301.

Stedman's medical dictionary. 27th ed. Baltimore: Lippincott Williams & Wilkins, 2000.

Ulmansky M. Hjorting-Hansen E, et al. Benign cementoblastoma: a review and five new cases. Oral Surg Oral Med Oral Pathol 1994;77:48–55.

Wilkins EM. Clinical practice of the dental hygienist. 9th ed. Baltimore: Lippincott Williams & Wilkins, 2004.

Wright JM. Reactive, dysplastic and neoplastic conditions of periodontal ligament origin. Periodontology 2000 1999;21:7–15.

Younai F, Eisenbud L, Sciubba JJ. Osteopetrosis: a case report including gross and microscopic findings in the mandible at autopsy. Oral Surg Oral Med Oral Pathol 1988;65:214–221.

20 Radiolucent Lesions

Key Terms

- Aneurysmal bone cyst
- Bohn's nodules
- Botryoid odontogenic cyst
- Caseous necrosis
- Cementoma
- Cyst
- Epithelial rests
- Florid cementooseous dysplasia
- Focal cementooseous dysplasia
- Lumen
- Nevoid basal cell carcinoma syndrome
- Nonvital tooth
- Odontogenic cysts
- Paradental cyst
- Periapical cementooseous dysplasia
- Periapical granuloma
- Precystic epithelial proliferation
- Primordial cyst
- Pseudocyst
- Radicular cyst
- Residual cysts
- Rests of Malassez
- Rests of Serres
- Sequestrum

Chapter Objectives

1. Define and use the key terms listed in this chapter.
2. Describe how a cyst develops.
3. Describe the origin and identifying characteristics of the radicular cyst.
4. List and describe the three types of cementooseous dysplasia.
5. State the characteristics of the aneurysmal bone cyst.
6. Compare and contrast the traumatic bone cyst and the aneurysmal bone cyst.
7. Describe the radiographic characteristics of the dentigerous cyst and the odontogenic keratocyst.
8. Discuss the radiographic appearance of the lateral periodontal cyst.
9. List the factors involved in the nevoid basal cell carcinoma syndrome.
10. Note the two forms of the odontogenic keratocyst.
11. State the histologic finding that is a key diagnostic feature of the calcifying odontogenic cyst.
12. Identify the location of the globulomaxillary cyst.
13. Discuss the origin of the static bone cyst.
14. List and describe the three classifications of Langerhans cell disease.

Chapter Outline

As discussed in Chapter 19, lesions that are radiopaque appear to have a dense, white presentation on the radiograph. Oftentimes, lesions may have a combined radiopaque and radiolucent appearance, depending upon the stage of calcification involved. An example is the cementoblastoma, which manifests a halo effect with the radiolucent lesion appearing as a darker area on the radiograph and forming a definite contrast between the lesion, the bone, and the existing tissue. This chapter discusses the development of these types of cysts and the common cysts that the dental hygienist may view on a radiograph. Radiolucent lesions that are seen clinically, such as bone cysts, cementoosseous dysplasia, and certain neoplasms are also discussed.

Odontogenic cysts are cysts with an epithelial lining composed of the remnants of the tooth-forming organ, such as the rests of Malassez (rests of the root sheath of Hertwig), glands of Serres (rests of the dental lamina), and reduced enamel epithelium (remnants of the enamel organ). Odontogenic cysts, including the radicular cysts, are presented in the next section.

TRAUMATIC OR INFLAMMATORY LESIONS

Traumatic and inflammatory lesions develop in an attempt by the body to isolate offending tissue or pathogens to maintain homeostasis. This occurs in the entities that are discussed in the next section. The body is miraculous in its attempt to isolate any foreign substance that may

threaten homeostasis. The cells perform this feat in several ways. One way is accomplished by the antigen and antibody responses discussed in Chapter 4. In another method, the body's attempt to protect the area of tissue may result in trying to isolate a foreign body from the surrounding tissue through the formation of a **cyst**. The cyst eventually seals the invader off from other tissue.

When inflammation is present, such as occurs in caries, which is followed by infection of the pulp, the epithelium begins to proliferate (grow and reproduce similar cells), form a distinct circle, and eventually close itself off from the surrounding tissue. The **lumen**, or center of the cyst, becomes fluid filled due to the buildup of osmotic pressure in the core of the cyst. The membrane of the cyst allows fluid to enter the cyst core in an attempt to equalize the osmotic pressure with that of the surrounding tissue, and eventually the cyst expands in size. As bone is resorbed by osteoclasts and bone resorbing factors, the cyst can expand and continue to fill with fluid and increase in size. **Pseudocysts** have an accumulation of fluid in a cystlike structure, but they do not have an epithelial lining, which is a characteristic of a true cyst.

Figure 20.1 is an excellent example of the development of an inflammatory odontogenic cyst in its early formation. One of the theories for this development states that inflammation in the bone can stimulate rests of odontogenic epithelium to proliferate and become cystic (Shear, 1992). These rests (small clusters of cells) are termed **epithelial rests**. For this reason, certain cysts such as the **radicular cyst** are known as inflammatory cysts. In these cysts, the inflammation comes first and induces epithelial proliferation of the epithelial rests, which have been dormant since tooth development, to begin cyst formation. These remnants become disorganized after tooth development until stimulated by some force, such as caries or pulpal infection. Figure 20.1 depicts a normal rest without much associated inflammation and then a proliferating

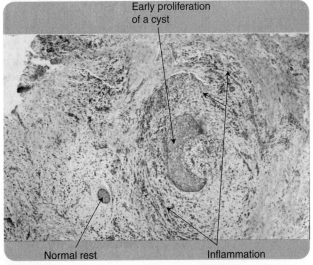

Figure 20.1. The formation of a cyst. (Courtesy of Dr. John Jacoway.)

Box 20.1   ODONTOGENIC CYSTS

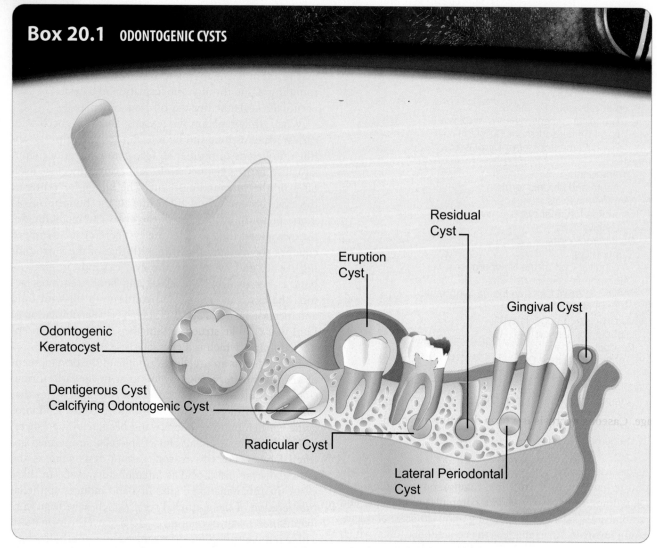

rest surrounded by inflammation. This is sometimes called "**precystic**" **epithelial proliferation.** In other words, the structure of the proliferating rest is associated with inflammation and is growing and beginning to circle in this earliest developmental stage. The **periapical granuloma** is the first stage of an inflammatory process, and ultimately as it progresses, it will lead to the radicular cyst. This cyst originates from the rests of Malassez, which are the remnants of the root sheath of Hertwig, responsible for the formation of the roots of the teeth. The rests have lain dormant until stimulated. Box 20.1 depicts the location of most odontogenic cysts (those cysts formed from the remnants of the tooth-forming organ).

Name: Periapical Granuloma

Etiology: The periapical granuloma or dental granuloma (also called apical periodontitis) is the result of necrotic pulp tissue and byproducts resulting from an inflammatory process, which has damaged the tissue at the apex of the tooth. The cause may be trauma, injury to the pulp through dental procedures, caries, periodontal dis-

ease that has affected the root area severely, or fractures to the tooth. All of these may contribute to the inflammatory process. The process of bone destruction in periapical lesions is not well established, but periapical inflammatory processes result in resorption of bone surrounding the roots of the affected teeth (Menezes et al., 2006).

APPLICATION

You have just discovered a radiolucent lesion in the apical area of 30 on Mrs. J. The dentist had viewed the radiograph, and he has confirmed that the patient has a probable lateral periodontal cyst, although this would need to be confirmed through biopsy. She is leaving for an extensive trip soon and is worried about this development. Her question to you is what caused the cyst to develop.

Use the material presented in this chapter, including Box 20.1, to discuss how you would explain to a patient how and why a cyst has developed.

Method of transmission: Not applicable

Epidemiology: Any age group may be affected by a periapical granuloma, and there is equal gender distribution. Since it is caused by damage to the tooth, anyone may be affected.

Pathogenesis: The diseased tissue from the tooth causes chronically inflamed granulation tissue to accumulate in the apical area of the tooth. The mobilizations of host defense mechanisms kill the invading microorganisms and also destroy normal tissue components, inducing bone resorption. As the pulp develops necrosis (cell death or irreversible damage), the tooth may slowly die and eventually become a **nonvital tooth** (a tooth that has essentially died or is dying because of a pulp that is no longer viable). If chronic inflammation occurs and chemical mediators are present, there may be stimulation of epithelial rests as discussed above. In this case, the granuloma will develop into the radicular cyst as the epithelium begins to separate and wall itself off from surrounding tissue. The bacteria produce toxic products, making the inflammatory process progress in granuloma formation. The granuloma is not the same as the entity that involves granulomatous inflammation, such as those involved in tuberculosis that develop caseous necrosis as the granulomas age. **Caseous necrosis** is a term denoting a necrotic tissue resembling cheese, made of a mixture of protein and fat.

Extraoral Characteristics: Not applicable

Perioral and Intraoral Characteristics: The periapical granuloma is the accumulation of granulation tissue that is focused at the apical area of a nonvital tooth. The lesion cannot be distinguished from the radicular cyst discussed in the next section, since by all appearances, they are the same radiographically. The tooth may be asymptomatic, but in most cases, complaints such as sensitivity or pain do exist. The tooth will test nonvital in most cases, depending upon the degree of damage to the pulp. Figure 20.2 depicts a periapical granuloma at the apex of the anterior teeth with radiolucent, well-demarcated lesions at the apex.

Distinguishing Characteristics: The dental granuloma is seen radiographically as a round or ovoid translucent lesion. The size of the lesion may vary from several millimeters to larger, more advanced lesions encompassing larger areas.

Significant Microscopic Features: The microscopic features of the granuloma are those of inflamed granulation tissue. The inflammatory response consists of a defense mechanism in response to bacterial components. Therefore, there is a lymphocytic infiltrate of plasma cells, neutrophils, histiocytes, and eosinophils.

Dental Implications: Vitality testing is crucial, since the tooth will test nonvital when obvious radiographic ev-

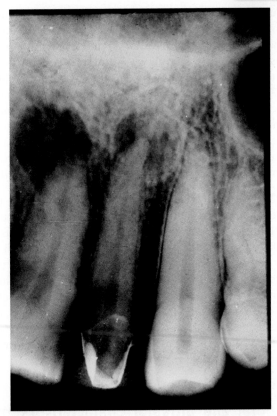

Figure 20.2. Periapical granuloma. (Courtesy of Dr. John Jacoway.)

idence is apparent. If the tooth is nonvital, endodontic treatment is needed.

Differential Diagnosis: In a nonvital tooth, radicular cyst (next section) would be considered.

Treatment and Pronosis: Endodontic treatment is the usual procedure for granulomas. The prognosis is good if all the granuloma is removed.

Name: Radicular Cyst (apical periodontal cyst or periapical cyst)

Etiology: The radicular cyst is always associated with a nonvital tooth, and the common causes are caries, trauma, or periodontal disease. The inflammatory process and necrosis of the pulp cause the epithelial proliferation that a cyst needs to develop. Epithelial rests remain quiescent throughout life but may be stimulated or triggered to proliferate when an inflammatory process develops, such as caries or inflammation of the pulpal tissue.

Epidemiology: The radicular cyst is the most commonly occurring cyst of the jaws, with most reported in the maxillary region. Radicular cysts occur more frequently in the maxillae and most often are discovered during routine dental examination of radiographs. Results from studies by Jones et al. (2006) indicate that the radicular cyst was the most commonly occurring of all odontogenic cysts in a specimen population of 55,446, of which 7,121 were diagnosed as odontogenic cysts. The patient usually reports no pain. Although radicular cysts are the most commonly occurring cysts, the reported incidence varies from less than 50% (Jones et al., 2006) to as much as 75% of reported cysts. The differentiation of the periapical granuloma and the radicular cyst cannot be made clinically but must be made through biopsy and microscopic interpretation. Jones reported that there was a sharp increase up until the third decade, with a decrease thereafter. Equal gender distribution was also reported.

Pathogenesis: Radicular cysts are derived from the **rests of Malassez**, found in the developing tooth structure of the periodontal ligament. These cells from the rests of Malassez serve as the source of the epithelium that lines the cavities of lesions that become radicular cysts. As discussed above, initially, a granuloma is produced, which then stimulates the cells of the odontogenic epithelial residues or rests within the periodontal ligament (i.e., the rests of Malassez). These rests lie dormant until some trigger mechanism such as inflammation causes epithelial proliferation and ultimately, the formation of a cyst.

Extraoral Characteristics: Not applicable

Perioral and Intraoral Characteristics: The radicular cyst may be found in any region of the mandible and maxilla, but it generally favors the maxillary anterior region at the apex of a nonvital tooth. The patient may experience no pain and is usually not aware of the cyst until it is diagnosed radiographically. The radiograph may show obvious evidence of root resorption (discussed in Chapter 21), depending upon the size and stage of devel-

opment of the cyst. This type of root resorption appears as a blunting of the root surface, usually at the apices of the tooth. Figure 20.3A depicts the radiographic appearance of a radicular cyst. The radicular cyst appears as a well-circumscribed radiolucent lesion attached to a tooth root. In some cases, the cyst may appear lateral to the apex when a lateral pulp canal is involved.

Distinguishing Characteristics: The radicular cyst cannot be differentiated from the periapical granuloma by a radiograph. A pulp-testing device is used as a diagnostic tool; however, a biopsy is needed to confirm a radicular cyst. Identification can only be made through microscopic examination, since other disease states have very similar radiographic appearances (see differential diagnoses below).

Significant Microscopic Features: The epithelial lining of the radicular cyst is composed of nonkeratinized-stratified squamous epithelium varying in thickness. The lumen may contain necrotic debris and inflammatory infiltrate. Figure 20.3B represents the histology of the radicular cyst, depicting the inflammatory cell infiltrate and the nonkeratinized epithelial lining.

Dental Implications: Failure to remove the radicular cyst completely results in recurrence.

Differential Diagnosis: The radicular cyst is usually discovered on a radiograph, but the radiolucent characteristics are not diagnostic, since other entities may appear similar. Periapical central giant cell granulomas are sometimes misdiagnosed as radicular cysts (Lombardi et al., 2006). The radicular cyst is always associated with a nonvital tooth.

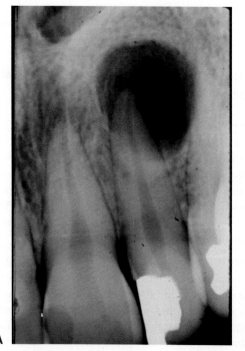
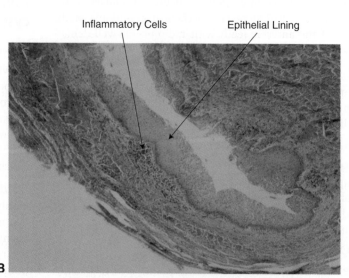

Figure 20.3. A. Radicular cyst. **B.** Radicular cyst histology. (Both courtesy of Dr. John Jacoway.)

1. Periapical granuloma, Chapter 20
2. Central giant cell granuloma, Chapter 18
3. Newly developing periapical cementoosseous dysplasia, Chapter 20
4. Traumatic bone cysts (when in the posterior region), Chapter 20

Treatment and Prognosis: Treatment usually involves several options: removal by extraction, surgery with curettage, and most commonly root canal therapy, the treatment of choice. Treatment may also include surgery, apicoectomy, or extraction. The prognosis is good with complete removal. Failure to remove the entire cyst results in what is called a **residual cyst.** This cyst develops after the stimulating inflammatory products have been removed. The cyst can produce extensive weakening and invasion of the bone. If fragments remain, the residual cyst may be a concern.

Name: Aneurysmal Bone Cyst

Etiology: The **aneurysmal bone cyst** is considered a pseudocyst, in that it appears as a cyst, but unlike the epithelium-lined true cyst, the aneurysmal bone cyst does not have the epithelium-lined lumen. This lesion is a benign lesion that is blood filled. It is suggested that this type of bone cyst arises from prior trauma, and recent research suggests some genetic components (Leithner et al., 2004). Cytogenetic research suggests chromosomal alterations. Some literature suggests that it may well be a tumor rather than a reactive lesion. However, this is still under consideration and research.

Method of Transmission: Not applicable

Epidemiology: Aneurysmal bone cysts are found in individuals under 30 years of age, with a peak incidence in the second decade of life (Rattan and Goyal, 2006). The bone cysts are rare and account for about 1–2% of primary biopsies on bone tumors (Perrotti et al., 2004). A slight female predilection is common. The mandible is more involved than the maxilla, and they are more common in the posterior regions of the mouth.

Pathogenesis: The pathogenesis is unclear about whether there is a preexisting lesion or whether the bone cyst develops because of dilated vessels.

Extraoral Characteristics: Extraoral swelling is reported in extensive lesions producing swelling.

Perioral and Intraoral Characteristics: The patient usually notices swelling with or without pain. The radiographic features of an aneurysmal bone cyst include a multilocular lesion, described as having a "soap bubble" appearance. Figure 20.4 demonstrates the honeycomb or soap bubble appearance of the aneurysmal bone cyst.

Distinguishing Characteristics: Aneurysmal bone cysts exhibit some key radiographic appearances as de-

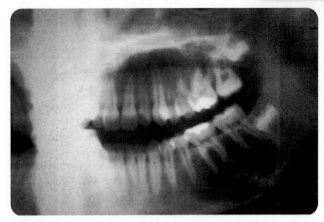

Figure 20.4. Aneurysmal bone cyst. (Courtesy of Dr. Shabnum Meer.)

scribed above. The lesion presents as expansile, with thin peripheral bone that is blood filled, without the presence of what is called bruit (a purring sound at the suspected area of aneurysmal cyst), thrill (a vibration), or pulse pressure (Rattan and Goyal, 2006). A vascular type of lesion has a pulse sensation.

Significant Microscopic Features: The nonepithelial lining is composed of immature connective tissue and scattered multinucleated giant cells. A thin layer of a bony shell often covers the blood-filled cavity.

Dental Implications: Aneurysmal bone cysts may cause the teeth to become displaced or loose because of bone expansion.

Differential Diagnosis: The prime considerations are

1. Odontogenic keratocyst, Chapter 20
2. Central giant cell granuloma, Chapter 18
3. Ameloblastic fibroma, Chapter, 20
4. Ameloblastoma, Chapter 18

Treatment and Prognosis: Excision and curettage is the treatment of choice. When the lesion is removed completely, the prognosis is good. There may be recurrence if any lesion remains, and the rate of this recurrence is usually very high.

Name: Traumatic Bone Cyst

Etiology: Traumatic bone cyst (also called simple bone cyst) is as the name implies; that is, it is thought to be caused by trauma. As mentioned above, this cyst is not considered a true cyst because it is not epithelium lined.

Method of Transmission: Not applicable

Epidemiology: The traumatic bone cyst is usually found in the 10- to 20-year-old age group, although they have also been reported in a wide range of ages. There is no gender preference. The most common site for a traumatic bone cyst is in the mandible (Dvori et al., 2006).

Pathogenesis: The traumatic bone cyst was originally thought to be a hematoma (Chapter 13), probably induced by trauma, which does not heal and subsequently liquefies and becomes a cyst. Since it is not epithelium lined, it fits more in the category of a pseudocyst. Another cause that has been suggested is calcium deficiency.

Extraoral Characteristics: The traumatic bone cysts may cause extraoral swelling if the lesion is large enough or has existed long enough.

Perioral and Intraoral Characteristics: Increased swelling in the mouth may be observed, but pain is not usually a factor. The lesions are discovered on radiographs, with the patient reporting no pain or other symptoms. The radiographic appearance is that of a scalloping cyst with well-delineated radiolucent characteristics. Margins may be very sharp in some areas and ill-defined in others. The cyst is also often seen scalloping between the teeth. Figure 20.5 depicts a traumatic bone cyst in a large area of the mandible, manifesting a scalloped appearance that reaches between the teeth in a honeycomb radiographic appearance.

Distinguishing Characteristics: When questioning the patient about a radiolucent lesion, the patient will often report previous trauma to the area in question. When the lesion is opened, the escape of blood from the lesion indicates that it was blood filled, which suggests a traumatic bone cyst.

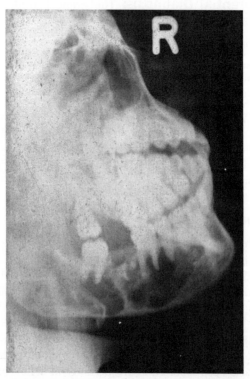

Figure 20.5. Traumatic bone cyst. (Courtesy of Dr. Shabnum Meer.)

Significant Microscopic Features: When viewing the traumatic bone cyst, an epithelial component is not present, since there is no epithelial lining. Bone and blood products are generally seen.

Dental Implications: The traumatic bone cyst may continue to expand and increase in size when not detected in the early stages. The lesion must be drained to begin healing.

Differential Diagnosis: Cases have been reported of florid cementoosseous dysplasia (discussed in Chapter 20) as a differential diagnosis in connection with these types of lesions.

Treatment and Prognosis: The usual treatment involves opening the cyst. Once the blood cavity is emptied, the bone will repair itself over time. There is a good prognosis with no recurrence.

Name: Cementoosseous Dysplasia

The term "cementoosseous dysplasia" represents three types of lesions that are believed to fall under this heading and are variants of the same category. These variants include

1. Periapical cementoosseous dysplasia
2. Focal cementoosseous dysplasia
3. Florid cementoosseous dysplasia

The more recent term, "periapical cementoosseous dysplasia," has generally replaced the term cementoma, in descriptions of these lesions.

Etiology: The etiology of these lesions is unknown, but it is considered a reactive process.

Method of Transmission: Not applicable

Epidemiology: Periapical cementoosseous dysplasia is a reactive process that is not contagious and is considered benign. Occurrence is usually in the over 30 age group and around middle age. Women are affected most often, particularly middle-aged black women (Regezi et al., 2003).

Pathogenesis: Some researchers suggest that cementoosseous dysplastic conditions are developmental and related to a defect in the bone and/or cementum remodeling in adulthood, and others consider them only reactionary type entities.

Extraoral Characteristics: Not applicable

Perioral and Intraoral Characteristics: The patient is usually asymptomatic, and the lesions are discovered on routine radiographs. Figure 20.6A shows the progression of periapical cementoosseous dysplasia over a 20-year period.

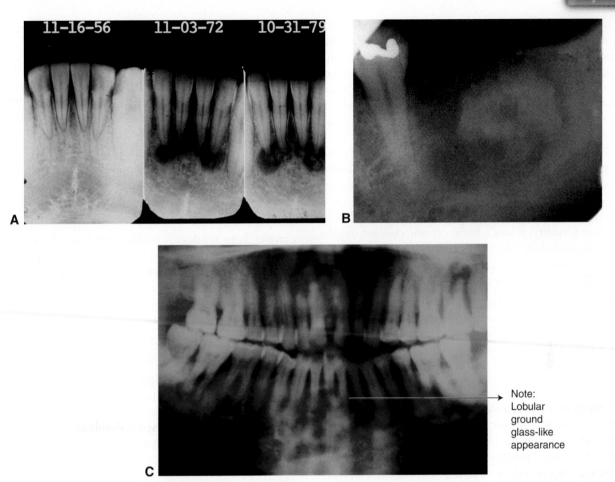

Figure 20.6. A. Progression of peripheral cementoosseous dysplasia (cementoma). (Courtesy of Dr. John Jacoway.) **B.** Focal osseous dysplasia. (Courtesy of Dr. Enrique Platin.) **C.** Florid cementoosseous dysplasia. (Courtesy of Dr. Michael Brennan.)

Distinguishing Characteristics: Periapical cementoosseous dysplasia occurs at the apex of vital teeth, with a propensity for the anterior mandibular teeth. The cementoma is asymptomatic and not usually noticed until seen on a radiograph.

Significant Microscopic Features: The histology of the periapical cementoosseous dysplasia is that of fibrous connective tissue that can be seen with bone and cementum in varying quantities. The three types of cementoosseous dysplasia are indistinguishable histologically.

Dental Implications: The vitality of the tooth is important, since the tooth tests vital with periapical cementoosseous dysplasia.

Differential Diagnosis: The diagnosis of periapical cementoosseous dysplasia depends upon the stage of development of the lesions. The initial diagnosis is important, since in the early stages, there may be a radiolucent appearance that would appear more cystlike. As the lesion calcifies and becomes more opaque, the lesion may appear more as a tumor. Additional considerations are

1. Odontoma, Chapter 19
2. Cementoossifying fibroma, Chapter 17

Treatment and Prognosis: Periapical cementoosseous dysplasia requires no treatment, and extraction or surgery is not required since the teeth remain vital.

FOCAL CEMENTOOSSEOUS DYSPLASIA

Focal cementoosseous dysplasia is believed to be closely related to periapical cementoosseous dysplasia, with most experts claiming that they are indeed variants of the same entity. Most cases occur in females around the fourth to fifth decade of life. In contrast to the periapical cementoosseous dysplasia, the focal cementoosseous dysplasia occurs most often in whites rather than blacks (Neville et al., 1999). The term "focal" is used when the lesion occurs in areas other than at the apex of the tooth as shown in Figure 20.6B. The lesions can also be radiolucent progressing to a more radiopaque lesion. Again, just as generally occurs with the periapical cementoosseous dysplasia lesion, the focal version is usually discovered on a radiograph.

FLORID CEMENTOOSSEOUS DYSPLASIA

Florid cementoosseous dysplasia is the third type of cementoosseous dysplasia to be discussed. Adult black women and Asian women are most affected with this type of cementoosseous dysplasia, and a familial tendency is reported (Singer et al., 2005). The disorder can affect any quadrant of the mouth and is sometimes seen in all quadrants at the same time. Clinically, there may be evidence of a yellow bonelike material, and during surgical removal, it is difficult to separate the material from the bone. The radiograph may have a more "ground glass" type of appearance as seen in Figure 20.6C.

The radiographic appearance of florid cementoosseous dysplasia is one of progressing lucent and opaque quality, which is described as lobular. The differentiation between florid cementoosseous dysplasia and simple bone cyst is not simple, and in some cases, a bone cyst is reported when in actuality, it was a florid cementoosseous dysplasia with secondary infections. The treatment is observation, and osteomyelitis can be a complication in severe cases. Differential diagnosis may include

1. Paget's disease, Chapter 10
2. Osteomas of Gardner syndrome, Chapter 19
3. Simple bone cyst, Chapter 20
4. Chronic diffuse osteomyelitis, Chapter 19

INFECTIONS

Infections of the mouth can be extensive enough to penetrate into the bone. Many are caused by periodontal problems, fractures, breaks in the mucosa, and bacteria that enter the bone. Two types of infections discussed in this section are acute osteomyelitis and chronic osteomyelitis.

Acute osteomyelitis exhibits an acute inflammatory response with the general signs of an inflammatory process. The patient may complain of pain and swelling with lymphadenopathy. Chronic osteomyelitis results when acute osteomyelitis is not resolved.

Name: Osteomyelitis—acute and chronic forms

Etiology: A periapical abscess is most often the cause of the acute form of osteomyelitis. There may be specific bacteria involved in the occurrence, such as staphylococci, actinomyces, and streptococci. Fractures, trauma, and surgery including extractions (see Chapter 3 covering alveolar osteitis) can also allow bacteria to enter the bone. If the acute form is not addressed completely, the chronic form usually follows. The chronic form may additionally be caused by a long-term inflammatory reaction from some stimulus, such as a systemic disease affecting the bone. Most cases of osteomyelitis are infectious, and any organism may be involved. Bone radiated for head and neck cancer is especially susceptible to osteonecrosis (see Chapter 5). The decreased blood supply and radiation exposure to the bone places the patient at a high risk for infections.

Method of Transmission: The acute form of osteomyelitis may have several infectious organisms involved in the disease process (see pathogenesis, below).

Epidemiology: Osteomyelitis can occur in any age group. Both sexes are equally affected.

Pathogenesis: Staphylococci and streptococci are the bacteria most commonly involved in the origin of osteomyelitis. The difference between acute and chronic osteomyelitis is often the virulence of the bacteria involved. Acute osteomyelitis is always destructive and painful.

Extraoral Characteristics: Lymphadenopathy, fever, and pain are often symptoms of osteomyelitis and are especially noted in the acute form.

Perioral and Intraoral Characteristics: An acute infection may not produce the destruction that the chronic form produces, because it has not been present long enough. In the chronic form, more evident patches of necrotic bone and diffuse radiolucent lesions are seen, and the lesions appear more mottled, with a sclerotic appearance on the radiograph. Figure 20.7 shows osteomyelitis in the posterior molar region.

Distinguishing Characteristics: The radiographic appearance is a distinguishing characteristic.

Significant Microscopic Features: The specimen shows loss of osteocytes from their lacunae and bacterial colonization with the presence of predominately necrotic bone. Abscess formation occurs containing **sequestrum** (necrotic bone that has broken away from the vital bone; pl., sequestra).

Dental Implications: The patient may have pain and lymphadenopathy. Addressing the cause of the osteomyelitis is paramount. The correct antibiotic is needed to treat the infection; therefore, identification through laboratory tests is crucial.

Differential Diagnosis: The pain, lymphadenopathy, and radiographic appearance usually indicate osteomyelitis. The clinical appearance along with the existence of an open area allowing bacteria to enter the site, such as occurs with caries or in extraction sites, allow a more definitive diagnosis.

Treatment and Prognosis: Drainage and antibiotics are needed to treat the acute form of osteomyelitis. The chronic form is more difficult to manage because of necrosis. Surgery is indicated, with antibiotic coverage. In acute osteomyelitis, antibiotics are very effective, but chronic osteomyelitis usually requires surgery, antibiotics, and drainage.

DEVELOPMENTAL CYSTS

As mentioned in the beginning of the chapter, a cyst is defined as an epithelium-lined cavity that contains a serous or semisolid material. The odontogenic cyst arises primarily in the soft tissue and bone (see Box 20.1). Traumatic and inflammatory lesions and infections have been discussed up to this point; developmental cysts are the topic of this section.

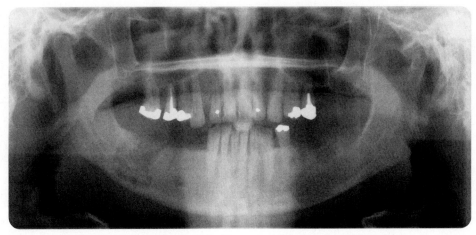

Figure 20.7. Panoramic radiograph showing osteomyelitis. (Courtesy of Dr. Michael Bornstein.)

Name: Lateral periodontal cyst (botryoid odontogenic cyst)

Etiology: Lateral periodontal cysts are odontogenic, nonkeratinized developmental cysts, believed to be developed from the dental lamina remnants (rests of Malassez) from within bone.

APPLICATION

Recently there have been reports linking osteomyelitis to bisphosphonate use (see Chapter 10). Bisphosphonates are used in the management of metastatic disease and in the treatment of osteoporosis (Nase and Suzuki, 2006). Reports indicate a rise in osteonecrosis of the jaws associated with these medications; thus as this usage continues to increase, the clinician may see more cases related to osteomyelitis in the dental office (Ruggiero et al., 2004). The goal of this research is to help identify osteonecrosis in patients early and prevent advancement of damage to the bone (Otomo-Corgel, 2006).

In addition to the new focus on bisphosphonates, cases of methicillin-resistant *Staphylococcus aureus* (MRSA) infection are also being reported, and this organism has been known to affect any bone (Arnold et al., 2006). As the name implies, concern exists regarding the currently available antimicrobial agents and the fact that they may become ineffective in treating systemic infections, including osteomyelitis. This could be a concern when osteomyelitis affects the maxillae and mandible (Appelbaum, 2006). With third molar extractions, implants, and other penetrations within the bone, this could be a very real possibility, especially if the patient reports previous episodes with MRSA.

Method of Transmission: Not applicable

Epidemiology: The lateral periodontal cyst is usually found in individuals in the third decade of life and beyond, and there is a male predilection. The mandibular premolar and cuspid area is favored, followed by the maxillary premolar and cuspid region. In a recent study (Jones et al., 2006), data from 55,446 specimens were reviewed, and 7,121 specimens were odontogenic cysts. Lateral periodontal cysts represented 0.4% of the diagnosed cysts, with an average age range of 48.2 years.

Pathogenesis: The lateral cyst is found mostly in the mandibular cuspid and premolar region on the lateral surface of the tooth.

Extraoral Characteristics: Not applicable

Perioral and Intraoral Characteristics: The lateral periodontal cyst is asymptomatic in most cases and is not usually noticed until seen on a radiograph. The cyst is usually unilocular, round or oval, and a well-delineated lesion. Figure 20.8A shows a lateral periodontal cyst.

Distinguishing Characteristics: The teeth associated with the lateral periodontal cyst are vital. When a multilocular cyst is present, it is called a variant of the lateral periodontal cyst and is known as the **botryoid odontogenic cyst.**

Significant Microscopic Features: The thin lining of the cyst consists of cuboidal epithelium. The cyst demonstrates clusters and whorls of cells, some of which have clear cytoplasm.

Dental Implications: The cyst should be identified as a lateral periodontal cyst, since it is necessary to rule out an inflammatory-type lesion or a more serious type of cyst or tumor, such as the odontogenic keratocyst discussed below in this chapter.

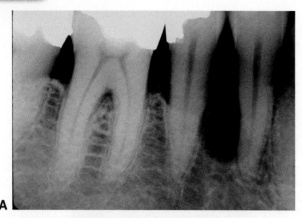
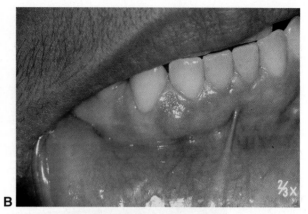

Figure 20.8. A. Lateral periodontal cyst. (Courtesy of Dr. Carolyn Bentley.) **B.** Gingival cyst in an adult. (Courtesy of Dr. John Jacoway.)

Differential Diagnosis: When occurring in the lateral location of premolars and cuspid area, the following are considerations:

1. The radicular cyst, Chapter 20
2. The odontogenic keratocyst, Chapter 20

Treatment and Prognosis: Surgical excision and pathologic review is the treatment of choice. The prognosis is excellent.

GINGIVAL CYST

The gingival cyst is the soft tissue counterpart to the lateral periodontal cyst. Both the gingival and the lateral periodontal cyst are developmental cysts. The gingival cyst may occur at a later age around the fifth to sixth decade, occurring predominately in the mandible 60% of the time, with a slight female predilection (Jones et al., 2006). The **rests of Serres** (originating from the dental lamina, occurring from the epithelial connection between the mucosa and the enamel organ) is believed to be the source for the gingival counterpart to the lateral periodontal cyst when trapped within the soft tissue (Regezi et al., 2003). Figure 20.8B shows the soft tissue counterpart known as the gingival cyst.

Name: Dentigerous cyst

Etiology: Dentigerous cysts are odontogenic in development and arise from a cystic change in the dental follicle following crown formation. The reduced enamel epithelium results from the remnants of the enamel organ. The dentigerous cyst is always associated with the crown of an impacted or unerupted tooth, supernumerary tooth, or odontoma.

Method of Transmission: Not applicable

Epidemiology: The dentigerous cyst is the second most commonly occurring odontogenic cyst, following the most common radicular cyst. However, dentigerous cysts are the most commonly occurring developmental cyst of the jaw. Dentigerous cysts are usually found in a young age group, especially in those with unerupted third molars. Recent reports by Jones (2006) found that 81.6% of the cysts in a patient population of 1,292 diagnosed dentigerous cysts occurred in the mandible. The remainder occurred in the anterior maxilla. A male gender preference was reported at 1.86 to 1.

Pathogenesis: Dentigerous cysts are also known as follicular cysts and are found around the crown of unerupted third molars, canines, and unerupted teeth. The cyst has an accumulation of fluid between the completely formed crown of a tooth and the reduced-enamel epithelium. The attachment is at the cementoenamel junction.

The **paradental cyst** is derived from the enamel epithelium and is thought to be a variant of the dentigerous cyst. An enamel projection is present in the bifurcation area of the third molars, which is thought to stimulate cyst production. The histology is similar to that of the dentigerous cyst with some inflammation. The appearance is often observed, and the prime areas are third molars for adults and unerupted first molars in children; however, other posterior teeth may be involved as well. Extraction of a third molar with curettage of the cyst is performed with close follow-up.

Extraoral Characteristics: Not applicable

Perioral and Intraoral Characteristics: The dentigerous cyst is usually only evident on radiographs, with no symptoms of pain or discomfort reported. On radiographs, it is well-circumscribed, unilocular, and sometimes multilocular. Figure 20.9A shows a dentigerous cyst around an impacted tooth. Figure 20.9B shows a dentigerous cyst in the distal area of a third molar.

Distinguishing Characteristics: On radiograph the dentigerous cyst is well-circumscribed, unilocular, and sometimes multilocular.

Significant Microscopic Features: The thin lining of the dentigerous cyst is composed of stratified squamous epithelium, varying in thickness, which is usually a few

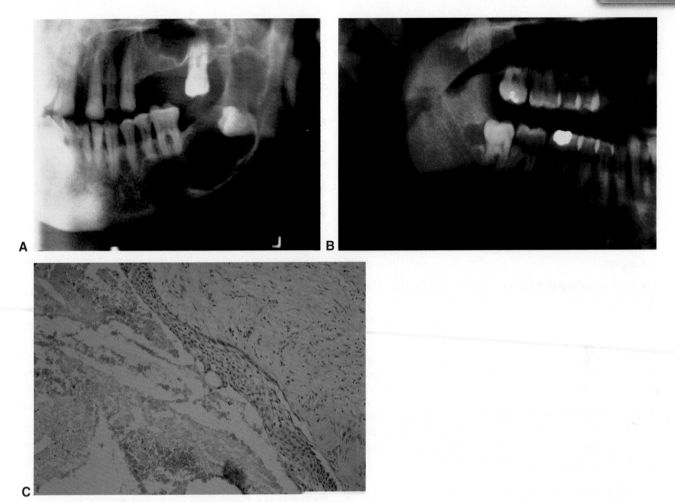

Figure 20.9. A. Dentigerous cyst (Courtesy of Dr. John Jacoway.) **B.** Dentigerous cyst (Courtesy of Dr. Michael Brennan.) **C.** Dentigerous cyst histology. (Courtesy of Dr. John Jacoway.)

cell layers thick. The epithelial lining is nonkeratinized. Some lining may contain mucous cells and/or ciliated columnar respiratory-type epithelium. The fibrous connective tissue wall varies in thickness and may exhibit inflammation. Odontogenic epithelium or dental lamina remnants may be seen as well. Figure 20.9C shows the histology of a dentigerous cyst with a cyst lining of epithelial tissue several layers thick.

Dental Implications: Delayed tooth eruption is a common theme. The dentigerous cyst can become quite large and has the potential to displace teeth and resorb roots. Dentigerous cysts continue to grow and expand; therefore, early diagnosis is imperative.

Differential Diagnosis: Other possible lesions to consider are

1. Odontogenic keratocyst, Chapter 20
2. Ameloblastoma, Chapter 18
3. Adenomatoid odontogenic tumor, Chapter 20

Treatment and Prognosis: Complete removal of the cyst is indicated, since the recurrence is high when this is not accomplished. The prognosis is excellent, but

the patient should be followed closely, since the slight possibility for subsequent tumors, such as the ameloblastoma or mucoepidermoid carcinoma, exists.

Name: Eruption cyst

Etiology: The eruption cyst is considered a variant of the dentigerous cyst and is caused by the accumulation of fluid or blood between the crown of an erupting tooth and the reduced enamel organ, due to trauma.

Method of Transmission: Not applicable

Epidemiology: The eruption cyst is not gender specific. Most occur in deciduous teeth and permanent molars of children (Sciubba et al., 2001).

Pathogenesis: The eruption cyst is considered a variant of the dentigerous cyst. It is painless and is found around the crown of an unerupted tooth. The cysts are probably unreported in most cases, since the cyst will rupture following eruption of the relevant tooth.

Extraoral Characteristics: Not applicable

Perioral and Intraoral Characteristics: The tissue of the eruption cyst may have a darker appearance and appear elevated. The eruption cyst is seen as a smooth bluish swelling (domelike) on the crest of the alveolar ridge. The radiographic finding of an eruption cyst is an enlarged follicular space.

Distinguishing Characteristics: The cysts may have a bluish cast due to the inflammatory inner core and blood accumulation. Figure 20.10 shows an eruption cyst. Note the blue hue of the lesion.

Significant Microscopic Features: The microscopic feature is a blood- and fluid-filled cavity. Normal oral mucosa on the surface is found with cyst epithelium containing heavy inflammatory infiltrate covering the inner aspect.

Dental Implications: The only dental implication is the failure of the tooth to erupt; therefore, the cyst may be opened to hasten the event. Most eruption cysts are left to dissipate on their own.

Differential Diagnosis: The radiograph of the area confirms the pending tooth eruption, and the eruption cyst around the tooth.

Treatment and Prognosis: No treatment is necessary; however on occasion, removal of the overlying tissue could facilitate a quicker eruption. The tooth eventually erupts through the tissue, and the cyst disappears.

GINGIVAL CYST OF THE NEWBORN (BOHN'S NODULES OR DENTAL LAMINA CYSTS OF THE NEWBORN)

Another consideration with regard to the clinical appearance of eruption cysts are the gingival cysts that occur on the ridges of the oral tissues in the newborn (**Bohn's nodules**). The nodules are multiple small cysts found at the junction of the hard and soft palates and along buccal and lingual dental ridges. The nodules usually disappear and rupture over time and are of no concern. The usual clinical scenario is the worried mother who believes that her

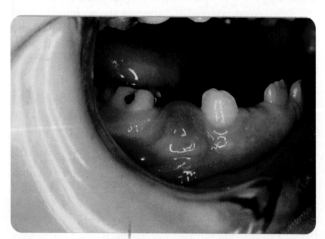

Figure 20.10. Eruption cyst. (Courtesy of Dr. John Jacoway.)

baby's teeth are erupting too early and seeks evaluation. Epstein's pearls or palatine cysts of the newborn are similar developmental cysts occurring in the line of fusion in the midline of the palate. They are inclusion cysts and require no treatment.

Name: Odontogenic keratocysts

Etiology: The odontogenic keratocyst develops from the dental lamina or its remnants.

Method of Transmission: Not applicable

Epidemiology: The odontogenic keratocyst is three times more likely to be found in the mandible, and in a study by Jones (2006), 96% of the cases with known site of presentation, the mandible was the most frequently occurring site. There is a male predilection. In an evaluation of 55,446 specimens submitted over a 30-year period (Jones et al., 2006), it was calculated that 828 were odontogenic cysts, with 464 in males and 364 in females, a ratio of 1.27 to 1. The age group affected ranged from 5 years to 92 years, with an average age of occurrence at 41 years. The odontogenic keratocyst is the third most commonly occurring odontogenic cyst, preceded by the radicular cyst (seen most frequently) and the dentigerous cyst (the second most common).

Pathogenesis: The source of the odontogenic keratocyst is the dental lamina and differentiated parts of the dental enamel organ.

Extraoral Characteristics: Not applicable

Perioral and Intraoral Characteristics: Odontogenic keratocysts occur most often in the posterior mandibular region and can occupy most of the ramus in some cases. In late stages of development of the odontogenic keratocysts, the cyst may become large enough to displace teeth and extend through the cancellous bone into the oral cavity. As the jaw becomes weakened, a fracture is more likely to occur.

Radiographically, the lesions can be multilocular or unilocular, well-circumscribed on the radiograph, and radiolucent, with a scalloped appearance. The appearance closely resembles that of an ameloblastoma in certain cases. Figure 20.11A shows an odontogenic keratocyst in ramus. Figure 20.11B shows an odontogenic keratocyst, and Figure 20.11C depicts the histology of the keratocyst.

Distinguishing Characteristics: Not applicable

Significant Microscopic Features: The basal cell layer may be cuboidal or columnar. The basal cell layer has hyperchromatic nuclei and the corrugated surface is parakeratinized and in some cases orthokeratinized. The parakeratinized cysts may occur more often because of the thin, friable fibrous capsule. In most cases, there is epithelial budding and the existence of daughter cysts. The odontogenic keratocysts that are associated with nevoid

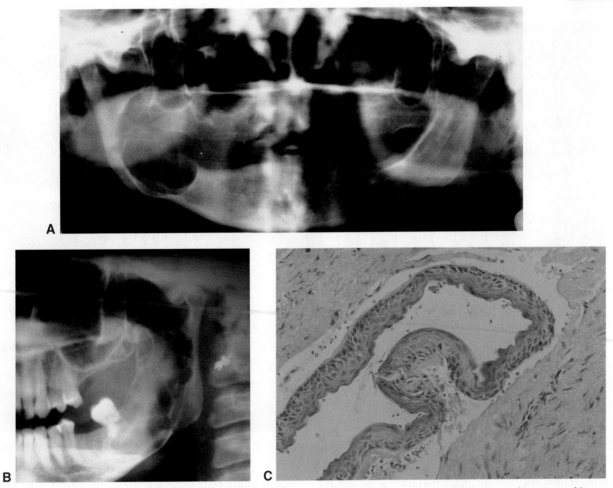

Figure 20.11. A. Radiograph of odontogenic keratocyst (Courtesy of Dr. John Jacoway.) **B.** Odontogenic keratocyst (Courtesy of Dr. John Jacoway.) **C.** Histology of odontogenic keratocyst. (Courtesy of Dr. John Jacoway.)

basal cell carcinoma syndrome, discussed next in this chapter, tend to have more daughter cysts or satellite cysts; the recurrence rate is higher because of this fragmented cellular proliferation.

Dental Implications: Although the odontogenic keratocysts can radiographically resemble other cysts, the microscopic interpretation is unique once a specimen is submitted. The association with nevoid basal cell carcinoma syndrome is especially important in a diagnosis, and the cysts have very aggressive behavior. Therefore, prompt treatment is required.

Differential Diagnosis: When associated with teeth, the following are considerations:

1. The radicular cyst, Chapter 20
2. Dentigerous cyst, Chapter 20
3. Ameloblastoma, Chapter 18
4. Adenomatoid odontogenic tumor, Chapter 20
5. Central giant cell granuloma, Chapter 18

Treatment and Prognosis: Since recurrence is high (as much as 60%), careful removal of the entire structure is crucial.

NEVOID BASAL CELL CARCINOMA SYNDROME

Also known as Gorlin-Goltz syndrome, **nevoid basal cell carcinoma syndrome** is a prime concern for patients diagnosed with odontogenic keratocyst due to a close association of the cysts with this syndrome. This syndrome is an inherited autosomal dominant disorder with a male predilection of 3 to 1 (Melo, 2004). The syndrome has five main components: nevoid basal cell carcinoma, jaw cysts, congenital skeletal anomalies, ectopic calcifications, and palmar and plantar pits. The patient will have nevi or small basal cell carcinomas on cutaneous areas, as shown in Figure 20.12A.

Additionally, there are other reported characteristics associated with this disease including a wide nasal bridge and frontal bossing, milia (Chapter 23), potential for mental retardation, ovarian fibromas, and increased incidence of cleft lip and palate. Figure 20.12B illustrates the presence of odontogenic keratocyst. Figure 20.12C illustrates the pitted areas of the palms.

THE PRIMORDIAL CYST

The term "primordial" is a synonym for odontogenic keratocyst (Neville et al., 1995). The preferred term is "odon-

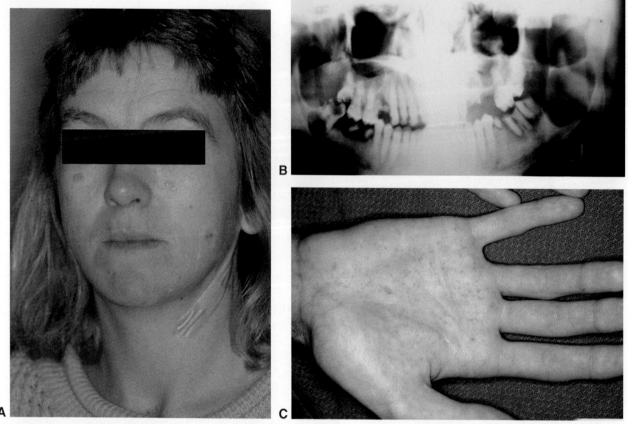

Figure 20.12. A Facial basal cell carcinoma. **B.** Odontogenic keratocyst. **C.** Plantar palmar pits in nevoid basal cell syndrome. (All courtesy of Dr. John Jacoway.)

togenic keratocyst," but the older literature separates the two entities into odontogenic keratocysts and primordial cysts.

The primordial cyst technically develops in place of the existing tooth or before any calcification of the tooth. The prime location for the primordial cyst is development in the third molar region. Histologically, the primordial cyst is almost always diagnosed as an odontogenic keratocyst. This type of cyst is usually painless and found on routine radiographic examination. The cysts are usually diagnosed in young adults and children.

Name: Calcifying odontogenic cyst

Etiology: The calcifying odontogenic cyst is believed to be derived from the reduced-enamel epithelium or dental lamina remnants.

Method of Transmission: Not applicable

Epidemiology: The calcifying odontogenic cyst may occur at any age, but it is most often found in the second decade and usually in individuals under the age of 40. Jones et al. (2006) reported results from a patient population of 7,121 odontogenic cysts. The patient age groups for finding calcifying odontogenic cysts were 5–79 years, with an average age of 41.5. Jones et al. report the cysts occuring more often in males. Others (Regazi et al., 2003) report them occuring more often in females. Calcifying

odontogenic cysts occur equally in the mandible and maxilla, with a propensity toward the anterior regions.

Pathogenesis: The calcifying odontogenic cyst (sometimes called the Gorlin cyst, as reported in 1962) is seen radiographically with varying amounts of radiodensity.

Extraoral Characteristics: Not applicable

Perioral and Intraoral Characteristics: The calcifying odontogenic cysts may be found as masses within the oral tissues, but this is rarely observed. When they do occur, they may resemble a gingival cyst or a peripheral giant cell fibroma. These cysts can occur in any location and present as an expansile intraosseous lesion or tender gingival swelling. Radiographically, the calcifying odontogenic cysts are unilocular or multilocular radiolucencies that exhibit clearly defined margins. Mixtures of calcifications and radiolucent properties are usually seen on the radiograph. Figure 20.13 depicts a radiograph of a calcifying odontogenic cyst.

Distinguishing Characteristics: The presence of "ghost cells" when the specimen is viewed microscopically is a diagnostic feature of the calcifying odontogenic cyst. Root divergence is often observed.

Significant Microscopic Features: As mentioned above, a key feature of this type of cyst is the presence of

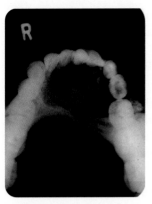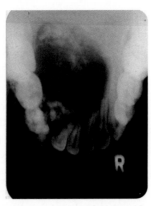

Figure 20.13. Calcifying odontogenic cyst. (Courtesy of Dr. Shabnum Meer.)

ghost cells with dystrophic calcification. The ghost cells are composed of keratin with lost nucleus. These types of cells may be found in other odontogenic tumors also. Calcifications may be seen as well and may exhibit larger areas of opacities. The microscopic appearance may resemble that of the ameloblastoma in some cases. There is a neoplastic lesion resembling the ameloblastoma called epithelial odontogenic ghost cell tumor that is a more solid variant with very aggressive behavior.

Dental Implications: Definitive diagnosis is important to rule out more aggressive lesions, and complete removal is necessary.

Differential Diagnosis: The diagnosis depends upon microscopic examination, but to begin a differential diagnosis, the radiographic appearance is initially evaluated. The degree of the radiolucent and radiopaque qualities determines the order of the following differential diagnoses:

1. Dentigerous cyst, Chapter 20
2. Odontogenic keratocyst, Chapter 20
3. Ameloblastoma, Chapter 18
4. Adenomatoid odontogenic tumor, Chapter 20
5. Odontoma, Chapter 19

Treatment and Prognosis: Surgical excision is recommended for the cystic type of calcifying odontogenic cyst. The neoplastic type must be treated as an ameloblastoma with aggressive protocol. The prognosis is good, although recurrence is sometimes seen.

Name: Globulomaxillary cyst

Etiology: The globulomaxillary cyst is believed to be odontogenic in origin and may represent multiple types of cysts such as a periapical or lateral periodontal cyst, radicular cysts, and odontogenic keratocyst, as well as others. Originally, the cyst was thought to be epithelium trapped during the fusion of the globular portion of the medial nasal process and the maxillary process and was called a fissural cyst and later termed odontogenic in origin. However, since there is no fusion between median nasal and the maxillary process, this etiology is no longer viable (Haring et al., 2006).

Method of Transmission: Not applicable

Epidemiology: Not applicable, since the cysts may be multiple variations and most are discussed within Chapter 20.

Pathogenesis: Globulomaxillary cyst is a vague term for a lesion in the globulomaxillary region between the maxillary lateral incisor and canine. The location of the cyst is linked to the name globulomaxillary. A biopsy is necessary to determine the origin and diagnosis of the determined lesion to classify the cyst.

Extraoral Characteristics: Extraoral characteristics do not occur unless the lesion is extremely large.

Perioral and Intraoral Characteristics: The cyst may be an inverted pear-shaped lesion because of the location, causing divergence of the tooth roots. It is circumscribed and radiolucent. Vitality of the pulp provides some evidence about the type of cyst.

A classic radiographic characteristic of the cyst is the divergence of the roots when the lesion is large enough to cause this factor. Figure 20.14 shows a globulomaxillary cyst in which root divergence is noted.

Distinguishing Characteristics: The location and the pear-shaped configuration of the globulomaxillary cyst give it a classic type of presentation. However, a biopsy is needed to determine the cyst type. Possible cysts

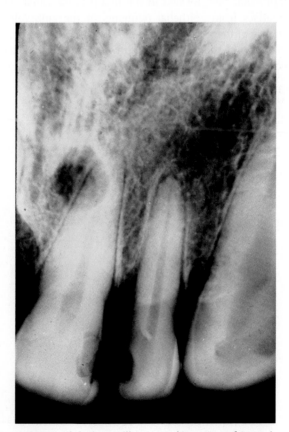

Figure 20.14. Globulomaxillary cyst. (Courtesy of Dr. John Jacoway.)

are radicular, giant cell granulomas, calcifying odontogenic cysts, odontogenic myxomas, etc.

Significant Microscopic Features: The tissue sample provides evidence as to which type of cyst has occurred in this location. Again, the term "globulomaxillary" applies to location, with varying cysts occurring in an anatomic sense.

Dental Implications: The vitality of the teeth involved, such as the lateral and cuspid, must be evaluated. Endodontic therapy should be administered when necessary.

Differential Diagnosis: Considerations include

1. Odontogenic keratocyst, Chapter 20
2. Lateral periodontal cyst, Chapter 20

Treatment and Prognosis: Surgical removal is the treatment of choice, and the prognosis is good, depending upon the type of cyst. Recurrence is rare. Any resemblance to the odontogenic keratocyst should be evaluated frequently because of the higher recurrence rate involved with these cysts.

Name: Nasopalatine canal cyst (incisive canal cyst, also nasopalatine duct cyst)

Etiology: The nasopalatine canal cyst is considered a developmental cyst, located in the nasopalatine canal. This cyst arises from epithelial remnants of the embryologic structure of the nasopalatine ducts, and the structure connects the oral and nasal cavities in the area of the incisive canal, probably because of infection or some stimulation.

Method of Transmission: Not applicable

Epidemiology: It is the most common cyst that is not of odontogenic origin and occurs in about 1% of the population. The nasopalatine cyst is most commonly seen in the fourth to sixth decades, and there is a male predilection (Righini et al., 2004).

Pathogenesis: The nasopalatine cyst is also known as the incisive canal cyst, and when located in the incisive papilla, it is called cyst of palatine papilla. The cysts are developmental and are located within the nasopalatine canal proximity or the incisive papillae.

Extraoral Characteristics: The size and extent of the cyst determine any extraoral characteristics such as swelling and elevation of the external surfaces around the nose and lip areas.

Perioral and Intraoral Characteristics: The patient may complain of pain, tenderness, and swelling, and drainage may be noted in the maxillary incisor region. When the lesion develops in the soft tissues of the incisive papillae, it is referred to as a cyst of the incisive canal. Usually, the lesion has a dark-red to bluish hue.

Radiographically, the nasopalatine cyst is seen between the maxillary central incisors. The lesion is a well-circumscribed radiolucent lesion, which may have a sclerotic border. Figure 20.15A shows a nasopalatine cyst above the maxillary central incisors.

Distinguishing Characteristics: When drainage occurs with the nasopalatine cyst, the patient may complain of a foul, salty taste. The patient may also experience pain, discomfort, and burning.

Significant Microscopic Features: The lining of the cyst is composed of stratified squamous epithelium

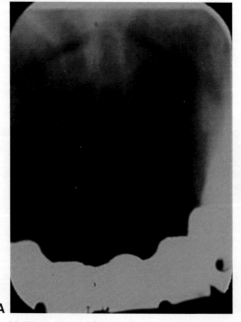
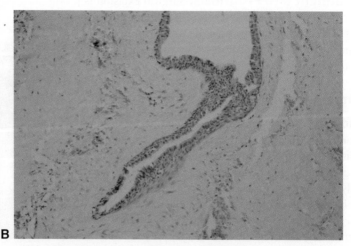

Figure 20.15. A. Nasopalatine duct cyst. (Courtesy of Frieda Pickett, RDH.) **B.** Histology of the nasopalatine duct cyst (Courtesy of Dr. John Jacoway.)

(most common), pseudostratified columnar epithelium, simple columnar epithelium, or simple cuboidal epithelium. Nerves and small vessels may be found in the connective tissue wall. Figure 20.15B depicts the histology of a nasopalatine cyst containing a flattened cuboidal epithelial lining.

Dental Implications: The cyst is not radiographically diagnostic and must be removed for microscopic evaluation.

Differential Diagnosis: Other cysts may be considered such as

1. Radicular, Chapter 20
2. Periapical granulomas, Chapter 20
3. Median palatine cyst, Chapter 20

Treatment and Prognosis: Complete surgical removal is needed. The prognosis is good, and the recurrence rate is low with complete removal.

MEDIAN PALATINE CYST

The median palatine cyst is located in the same vicinity as the nasopalatine cyst but is more apically centered toward the midline of the hard palate. The lesion is lined by stratified squamous epithelium and is surrounded by dense connective tissue. The median palatine cyst is a fissural cyst that develops from entrapped epithelium along the embryonic line of fusion. It may be difficult to differentiate the nasopalatine cyst with the median palatine cyst. The patient may complain of pain and expansion of the palate. Surgical removal is indicated as treatment. Figure 20.16 shows a median palatine cyst.

Name: Static bone cyst (also known as Stafne's bone defect, and static defect)

Etiology: This type of lesion is not a true cyst; although by all appearances on a radiograph, it does resemble a cyst. Technically, the static bone cyst is a defect in the mandible that surrounds salivary gland tissue. It is believed to be entrapment of the salivary gland tissue and is not lined by epithelium.

Method of Transmission: Not applicable

Epidemiology: The static bone cyst is seen in adults, and most static bone cysts are unilateral and believed to be present from birth. Studies have reported cases involving children as well, although few cases are reported in the literature (Campos et al., 2004).

Pathogenesis: It is believed that the static bone results from lingual mandibular cortical bone erosion from hyperplastic salivary gland tissue or entrapment of salivary gland tissue during the development of the mandible.

Extraoral Characteristics: Not applicable

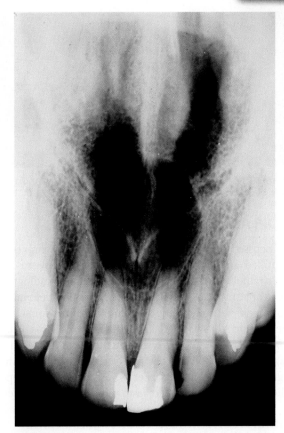

Figure 20.16. Median palatine cyst. (Courtesy of Dr. John Jacoway.)

Perioral and Intraoral Characteristics: The static bone cyst is asymptomatic and is usually discovered when a Panorex film is taken. On a radiograph, the bone cyst is seen as radiolucency in the posterior mandible below the mandibular canal. The static bone cyst is a sharply circumscribed, oval, radiolucent lesion with a sclerotic border.

Distinguishing Characteristics: The static bone cyst is usually found at the angle of the mandible.

Significant Microscopic Features: The static bone cyst is a defect, which if biopsied, may contain submandibular gland tissue, some blood vessel, muscle, and fat.

Dental Implications: The static bone cyst is usually diagnosed clinically by using radiographs; however, when the location is superior to the mandibular canal, a biopsy may be needed to rule out pathology.

Differential Diagnosis: The location and the appearance of the lesion is confirmation in most cases. Radiographs are followed long-term for any changes.

Treatment and Progress: The static bone cyst is noted and followed. Figure 20.17 illustrates a static bone cyst at the angle of the mandible.

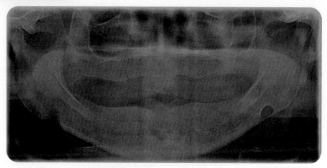

Figure 20.17. Static bone cyst. (Courtesy of Dr. Shabnum Meer.)

NEOPLASMS

As discussed in previous chapters, a neoplasm exhibits uncontrolled growth. This chapter discusses neoplasms that have a radiolucent appearance when viewed on a radiograph. The neoplasms discussed in this section are the adenomatoid odontogenic tumor, the odontogenic myxoma, the ameloblastic fibroma, and Langerhans cell disease. All of these neoplasms exhibit growth potential, and they each appear radiolucent on radiographs. Certain neoplasms may originate from metastatic cancer as well and will also appear radiolucent. This type of neoplasm is discussed in Chapter 5.

Name: Adenomatoid odontogenic tumor (AOT)

Etiology: Once thought to be a variant of the ameloblastoma, the AOT is now classified as an encapsulated benign epithelial odontogenic tumor.

Method of Transmission: Not applicable

Epidemiology: The AOT is usually seen between the ages of 5 and 30 years. Most patients are under 20 years of age. There is a female predilection of 2:1, and some experts report an even larger percentage of females with the tumor. The anterior maxilla is the favored location. AOTs are found associated with impacted teeth (Batra et al., 2005).

Pathogenesis: The AOT is a benign epithelial tumor with a dense fibrous connective tissue capsule, which does not recur once removed. It is a benign tumor and commonly appears in the anterior portion of the maxilla. This tumor is seen as a unilocular radiolucency, usually around the crown of a tooth. Seen less often is the form located between the roots of several erupted teeth.

Extraoral Characteristics: Swelling in the facial area is sometimes reported causing flaring of the nasolabial fold and extending beyond the facial contour.

Perioral and Intraoral Characteristics: As the tumor expands and increases in size, there may be root displacement and a bony hard expansion with an eggshell cracking appearance over the protrusion.

For the most part, this tumor appears radiolucent on radiograph but may exhibit small opaque foci within the

tumor. The number and size of the foci determine the radiographic appearance of the lesion. Figure 20.18A shows the radiographic view of an AOT. Figure 20.18B depicts the intraoral AOT.

Distinguishing Characteristics: The microscopic features of this tumor are distinguishing characteristics. The glandular or ductlike features forming a rosette pattern clearly differentiates the AOT from others.

Significant Microscopic Features: As mentioned above, the rosettes and ductlike features are somewhat characteristic of this tumor. These patterns are composed of ductlike structures of columnar epithelial cells. The nuclei of the cells are polarized away from the central spaces. Figure 20.18C depicts the histology of the oral AOT, demonstrating the rosette pattern.

Dental Implications: Facial asymmetry is one of the first signs to be noticed by the patient as the tumor increases in size. The tumor expands and should be excised.

Differential Diagnosis: Considerations include

1. The dentigerous cyst because of the occurrence around impacted teeth, Chapter 20
2. The calcifying epithelial odontogenic tumor when calcifications are present, Chapter 18
3. The ameloblastoma, Chapter 18

Treatment and Prognosis: Complete removal of the tumor is necessary, and the prognosis is excellent without any recurrence.

Name: Odontogenic myxoma

Etiology: The odontogenic myxoma is derived from odontogenic ectomesenchyme, and it originates in the periodontal ligament or dental pulp.

Method of Transmission: Not applicable

Epidemiology: Odontogenic myxoma usually occurs in the 10- to 30-year-old age group. It is rare in the over 50-year-old age group. There is no gender preference for this lesion (Ogutcen-Toller et al., 2006). Myxomas are seen equally in the maxilla and the mandible.

Pathogenesis: Myxomas are benign neoplasms that are capable of rapid growth and are very persistent. Root resorption and displacement may be seen in some cases. This is not an encapsulated tumor.

Extraoral Characteristics: Depending upon the size of the myxoma, swelling may occur in isolated areas.

Perioral and Intraoral Characteristics: Radiographically, the tumors can be unilocular or multilocular, and the radiolucencies may have a scalloped appearance. Myxomas have also been described as having a "step ladder" or "honeycombed" appearance. The margins

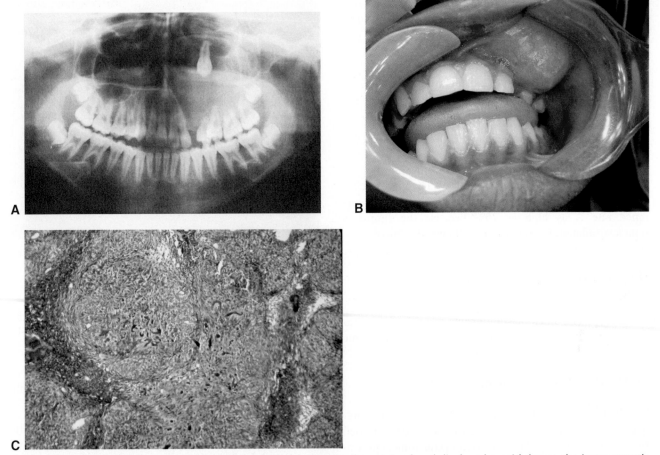

Figure 20.18. A and **B.** Adenomatoid odontogenic tumor **A.** Note the retained and displaced cuspid due to the large growth of the tumor (Courtesy of Dr. Shabnum Meer). **B.** The tumor fills the labial space above tooth #11 and tooth #12 (Courtesy of Dr. Shabnum Meer). **C.** The classic Rosett pattern is depicted (Courtesy of Dr. James Sciubba.)

may be well defined or they may be diffuse. Figure 20.19 illustrates a myxoma in the lower right molar region. Note the soap bubble appearance around the molar and bicuspid regions.

Distinguishing Characteristics: Not applicable

Significant Microscopic Features: The features are stellate-shaped cells and fine collagen fibrils. The specimen is gelatinous and pulplike.

Dental Implications: Enlarged dental follicles or the dental papilla of a developing tooth may be mistaken for

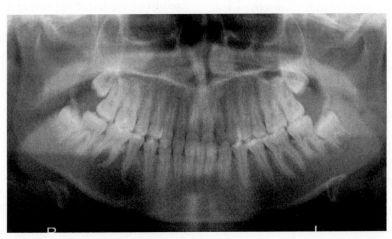

Figure 20.19. Odontogenic myxoma. (Courtesy of Dr. Enrique Platin.)

the myxomas upon microscopic examination. They also can be confused with other myxoid jaw neoplasms. The tumors can become quite large, causing tooth displacement.

Differential Diagnosis: Considerations include

1. Odontogenic fibroma, Chapter 17
2. Ameloblastoma, Chapter 18
3. Hemangiomas of bone, Chapter 20

Treatment and Prognosis: The myxoma is removed surgically with chemical cautery. The highly gelatinous material makes removal difficult, and the recurrence rate is as high as 25% because the tumor is nonencapsulated. Fragments are difficult to remove.

Name: Ameloblastic fibroma (Fibroodontoma)

Etiology: The ameloblastic fibroma is a mixed odontogenic tumor that is believed to originate from odontogenic ectomesenchyme and odontogenic epithelium.

Method of Transmission: Not applicable

Epidemiology: Ameloblastic fibromas are seen infrequently. A recent study by Buchner et al. (2006) reported the relative frequency of central odontogenic tumors in relation to all biopsy specimens submitted to a biopsy service. After excluding the odontomas, which accounted for 75.9% of all odontogenic tumors, the ameloblastic fibromas (accounting for 6.5%) were seen less frequently than ameloblastomas (48.5%), myxomas (9.2%), and adenomatoid odontogenic tumors (7.3%). The lesions are usually seen early in life before the age of 20, but some have been reported in the third and fourth decades. The posterior mandible is the most common site. There is no gender preference.

Pathogenesis: The lesions are composed of neoplastic epithelium and neoplastic myxomatous connective tissue and are usually associated with third molars (Regezi, 2003).

Extraoral Characteristics: Depending upon the expansion, some external swelling may be present.

Perioral and Intraoral Characteristics: The patient usually experiences no pain with any swelling that may occur. The ameloblastic fibroma has potential for extensive growth causing jaw expansion. Occasionally, there may be calcified material containing enamel and dentin. At this point, the lesion is identified as the ameloblastic fibroodontoma.

Radiographically, the lesion can be unilocular or multilocular. It is normally well defined and usually associ-

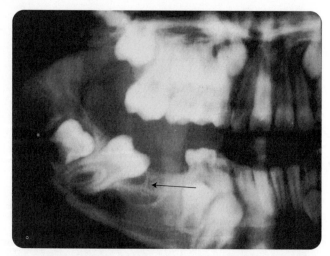

Figure 20.20. Radiograph of ameloblastic fibroma. (Courtesy of Dr. Harvey Kessler.)

ated with an unerupted tooth. Figure 20.20 illustrates the ameloblastic fibroma seen in the molar region as a well-circumscribed lesion with a sclerotic border.

Distinguishing Characteristics: The histology of the ameloblastic fibroma is unusual and highly diagnostic (see below for details).

Significant Microscopic Features: The ameloblastic fibroma is composed of long strands and islands of odontogenic epithelium set in an immature cellular matrix resembling the dental papilla or developing dental pulp. The strands are usually only two cells thick of cuboidal or columnar cells. The stroma sets it apart from the ameloblastoma. The ameloblastic fibroma presents as a pulplike stroma with islands of ameloblastic epithelium. The tall columnar cells resemble ameloblasts around stellate reticulum.

Dental Implications: Generally, the ameloblastic fibroma is asymptomatic.

Differential Diagnosis: Other entities are considered when the lesion appears to deviate from normal radiologic patterns, and the size of the lesion or age of the patient may be out of the usual range. The ameloblastic fibroma may appear as the early stages of the following:

1. Ameloblastoma, Chapter 18
2. Odontogenic myxoma, Chapter 20
3. Dentigerous cyst, Chapter 20
4. Odontoma, Chapter 19
5. Dentigerous cyst, Chapter 20
6. Myxoma, Chapter 20
7. Odontogenic keratocyst, Chapter 20
8. Central giant cell granuloma, Chapter 18

Treatment and Prognosis: Conservative excision is the treatment of choice. Recurrence is seen in approximately 20% of cases. Some recurrences of ameloblastic fibrosarcomas have been reported in previously benign cases of ameloblastic fibromas.

Name: Langerhans cell disease

Etiology: The basic cause of this disease, formally called histocytosis X, is unknown. It involves proliferation of the Langerhans cells, which normally reside in the epidermis and mucosa. The other cells involved are the histocytes and eosinophils. Specifically identified are Birbeck granules and a few macrophages. In some cases, a neoplastic transformation is believed responsible for this disease. An immune response has also been implicated. Additionally, a neoplastic process and a reactive process have been suggested as causal.

Method of Transmission: Not applicable

Epidemiology: Langerhans cell disease usually involves young adults and children. Over 50% are under the age of 10. However, the age range can extend to older adults. Males are affected more than females (Buchmann et al., 2006).

Pathogenesis: Three distinct disorders are involved in the disease: They include

1. Eosinophilic granuloma—This disorder occurs in young adults or adults. Bone lesions are present exhibiting well-defined radiolucent lesions. When found in the mouth, the posterior mandible is most often affected, which results in displaced teeth and fractures (described as floating teeth). Oral ulcerations are usually present. Figure 20.21A illustrates a radiograph that exhibits floating teeth and bone destruction. Figure 20.21B is a photomicrograph illustrating eosinophilic granuloma in Langerhans cell disease (eosinophilic granuloma).
2. Hand-Schüller-Christian disease—This variant is termed "multifocal eosinophilic granuloma." This disorder primarily affects children, usually under 5 years old, and results in diabetes insipidus, punched out lesions, and ophthalmus. Skin lesions may or may not be present. The patient may have persistent oral lesions including gingival ulcerations. Halitosis and difficulty healing are also characteristic. Skull lesions exhibit a "punched-out" appearance (Mortellaro et al., 2006). Figure 20.21C illustrates the skull lesions that have a "punched out" appearance.
3. Letterer-Siwe disease—Infants are especially affected by this disease. A rash may be the first sign of the disorder. Ear infections, lymphadenopathy, fever, ane-

mia, and other infections are all known to occur. Bone lesions may or may not be seen radiographically. The disease has been associated with a lymphoma. The course of the disease is extremely rapid, with a poor prognosis.

Extraoral Characteristics: Poor healing is common with Langerhans cell disease, dermatologic conditions may be evident, and all bones of the body may be affected. Lymphadenopathy may be present, cranial bones may be involved, and the cutaneous areas may involve rashes and erythematic lesions. Radiographically, the bone lesions resemble a "punched out" appearance with sharply demarcated lesions.

Perioral and Intraoral Characteristics: The disease may involve one or more multiple bones in the body, including the bones around the teeth, contributing to loosening (also, called "floating teeth"). Tenderness, pain, and swelling are common complaints. The patients may overlap in the above stated symptoms and may or may not exhibit the stated characteristic symptoms, depending upon the stage and type of the disorder.

Distinguishing Characteristics: A key characteristic of Langerhans cell disease is premature loosening and exfoliation of teeth in children.

Significant Microscopic Features: The microscopic features involve large histiocytoid cells mixed with eosinophils. Birbeck granules within the Langerhans cells are diagnostic factors. These cells have large abundant cytoplasm and are arranged in sheets.

Dental Implications: Lesions that occur periapically can be confused with periapical cyst or granulomas. Tooth vitality would still be present.

Differential Diagnosis: Some considerations are

1. Juvenile periodontitis
2. Leukemia, Chapter 9
3. Malignant neoplasms, discussed throughout the book
4. Multiple myeloma, considered when well-circumscribed radiolucencies are present

Treatment and Prognosis: The treatment depends upon the involvement of the disease and the age of the patient. Conservative surgical treatment is sometimes the only treatment. However, in more extensive disease involvement, chemotherapy may be needed as well. Additionally, bone marrow transplantation may be done; but essentially, the more widespread the lesions, the poorer the prognosis.

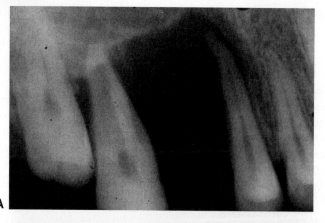

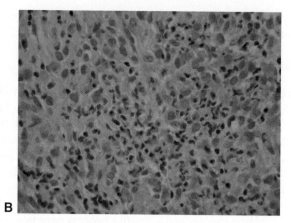

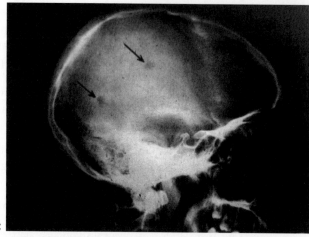

Figure 20.21. A. Radiograph of Langerhans cell disease demonstrates the loss of teeth. **B.** Photomicrograph illustrating eosinophilic and Langerhans cells. **C.** Slide demonstrates the "punched-out" skull lesions associated with Langerhans cell disease. (All courtesy of Dr. Shabnum Meer.)

SUMMARY

- Cysts are fluid filled cavities lined with epithelium.
- The cementoblastoma has a halo affect, with the radiolucent lesion appearing as a darker area on the radiograph, with definite contrast between the lesion, the bone, and the existing tissue.
- Odontogenic cysts are cysts with an epithelial lining that is formed from the remnants of the tooth-forming organ: the rests of Malassez (rests of the root sheath of Hertwig), glands of Serres (rests of the dental lamina), and reduced enamel epithelium (remnants of the enamel organ).
- The periapical granuloma or dental granuloma (also called apical periodontitis) is the result of necrotic pulp tissue and byproducts resulting from an inflammatory process that has damaged the tissue at the apex of the tooth.
- The radicular cyst is always associated with a nonvital tooth, and the common causes are caries, trauma, or periodontal disease.
- Periapical cementoosseous dysplasia is also called cementoma, but the term has been replaced with the more current term periapical cementoosseous dysplasia in recent years.
- Three variants of cementoosseous dysplasia are periapical cementoosseous dysplasia, focal cementoosseous dysplasia, and florid cementoosseous dysplasia.
- A periapical abscess most often is the cause of the acute form of osteomyelitis.
- The traumatic bone cyst (also called the simple bone cyst) is thought to be caused by trauma. This cyst is not considered a true cyst because it is not epithelium lined.
- Lateral periodontal cysts are odontogenic, nonkeratinized developmental cysts and are believed to be developed from the dental lamina remnants (rests of Malassez) from within bone.
- Dentigerous cysts are odontogenic in development and arise from a cystic change in the dental follicle after crown formation.

(continued)

SUMMARY *(continued)*

- The eruption cyst is considered a variant of the dentigerous cyst and is caused by the accumulation of fluid or blood between the crown of an erupting tooth and the reduced enamel organ, caused by trauma.
- The aneurysmal bone cyst is considered a pseudocyst in that it appears as a cyst, but unlike the true cyst, the aneurysmal bone cyst does not have the epithelium-lined lumen.
- Gingival cyst of the newborn occurs on the ridges of the oral tissues in the newborn. The nodules are multiple small cysts found at the junction of the hard and soft palates and along buccal and lingual dental ridges.
- The odontogenic keratocyst is developed from the dental lamina or its remnants.
- Nevoid basal cell carcinoma syndrome, also known as Gorlin-Goltz syndrome, is of prime concern, since the odontogenic keratocyst is associated with this syndrome, resulting in patients having multiple jaw cysts and basal cell carcinoma.
- Calcifying odontogenic cyst is believed to be derived from the reduced enamel epithelium or dental lamina remnants.
- The nasopalatine canal cyst is a developmental cyst located in the nasopalatine canal. This cyst arises from epithelial remnants of the embryologic structure of the nasopalatine ducts, probably caused by infection or stimulation.
- The globulomaxillary cyst is believed to be odontogenic in origin and may represent a periapical or lateral periodontal cyst.
- Technically, the static bone cyst is a defect in the mandible that surrounds salivary gland tissue. It is believed to be entrapment of the salivary gland tissue and is not lined by epithelium.
- The adenomatoid odontogenic tumor is now classified as an encapsulated benign epithelial odontogenic tumor.
- The odontogenic myxoma is derived from odontogenic ectomesenchyme and originates in the periodontal ligament or dental pulp.
- The ameloblastic fibroma is a mixed odontogenic tumor that is believed to originate from odontogenic ectomesenchyme and odontogenic epithelium.
- Langerhans cell disease has three distinct subgroups: eosinophilic granuloma, Hand-Schüller-Christian syndrome, and Letterer-Siwe disease.

Critical Thinking Activities

Please study the slide provided in Figure 20.11B.

Study the object in the middle right side of the slide.

Does the small white area have anything to do with the odontogenic keratocyst in the ramus?

Is it in the spinal column?

What purpose does it serve?

Why is it appearing as a white object?

Would it cause damage to the tissues?

Should the person have this removed?

PORTFOLIO POSSIBILITIES

1. Design a chart with the most commonly seen types of cysts, using radiographs and diagrams for patients to understand where these cysts occur and how they differ in a differential diagnosis from other more common cysts. This chart gives the patient some sense of how the clinician arrives at the diagnosis. The radiographs could be enlarged for easier viewing.
2. Develop patient instructions for each commonly seen cyst. The material could provide information that is specific to each cyst and contain your office logo or referral information.

Case Study

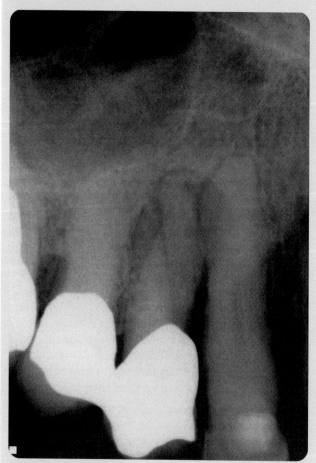

The photo presented in this exercise is of a 73-year-old male who was on holiday from Germany visiting his daughter in the United States. He is a healthy male with no apparent health problems and is taking no medications. After a 10-hour flight and arrival in the United States, he began to have severe pain in the tooth 5 area. Clinically, the apical area on the gingiva was raised, erythematic, fluctuant, and painful when pressure was applied. There is no mobility. His daughter became concerned and brought him in to see the doctor when the pain did not subside. The patient did not speak English, and his daughter served as an interpreter. On radiography, there is an obvious radiolucent lesion above the apices of tooth 5.

What would be your opinion of the lesion?

What do you think has caused the radiolucent lesion?

What do you believe would relieve the pain and pressure of the lesion?

Are there factors that may have contributed to the sudden appearance of this lesion?

Figure CT-1. Courtesy of Dr. Kathryn Savitsky.

REFERENCES

Althof PA, Ohmori K, Zhou M, et al. Cytogenetic and molecular cytogenetic findings in 43 aneurysmal bone cysts: aberrations of 17p mapped to 17p13.2 by fluorescence in situ hybridization. Mod Pathol 2004;17(5):518–525.

Appelbaum PC. MRSA—the tip of the iceberg. Clin Microbiol Infect 2006;12(Suppl 2):3–10.

Arnold SR, Elias D, Buckingham SC, et al. Changing patterns of acute hematogenous osteomyelitis and septic arthritis: emergence of community-associated methicillin-resistant staphylococcus aureus. J Pediatr Orthop 2006;26(6):703–708.

Batra P, Prasad S, Parkash H. Adenomatoid odontogenic tumour: review and case report. J Can Dent Assoc 2005;71(4):250–253.

Binnie WH. Periodontal cysts and epulides. Periodontology 2000 1999;21:16–32.

Buchner A. The central (intraosseous) calcifying odontogenic cyst: an analysis of 215 cases. J Oral Maxillofac Surg 1991;49:330–339.

Campos PS, Panella J, Crusoe-Rebello IM, Mandibular ramus-related Stafne's bone cavity. Dentomaxillofac Radiol 2004;33(1):63–66.

Cawson RA, Binnie WH, Eveson JW. Color atlas of oral disease—clinical and pathologic correlations. 2nd ed. London: Wolfe Publishing, 1994.

Cawson RA, Odell EW. Essentials of oral pathology and oral medicine. 6th ed. London: Churchill Livingstone–Harcourt Brace and Company Ltd. 1998.

Cebeci AR, Kamburoglu K, Oztas B. Diffuse sclerosing osteomyelitis in the maxilla: case report. Dent Update 2004;31(7):405–406, 409.

Chi AC, Owings JR Jr, Muller S. Peripheral odontogenic keratocyst: report of two cases and review of the literature. Oral Surg Oral Med Oral Pathol Oral Radiol Endod 2004;99(1):71-78.

Eisen D, Lynch DP. The mouth—diagnosis and treatment. St. Louis: Mosby, 1998.

Hood AF, Kwan TH, Mihm MC, Horn TD. Dermatopathology. 2nd ed. Boston: Little, Brown & Co., 1993.

Ellis MW, Hospenthal DR, Dooley DP, et al. Natural history of community-acquired methicillin-resistant staphylococcus aurens colonization and infection in soldiers. Clin Infect Dis 2004;39(7): 971–979.

Dvori S, Shohat Y, Taicher S. Simple bone cyst in the mandible—a rare occurrence in an elderly patient. Refuat Hapeh Vehashinayim 2006;(1):27–30, 69.

Fowler CB. Benign and malignant neoplasms of the periodontium. Periodontology 2000 1999;21:33–83.

Haring P, Filippi A, Bornstein MM, et al. The "globulomaxillary cyst": a specific entity or a myth? Schweiz Monatsschr Zahnmed 2006;116(4):380–397.

High AS, Hirschmann PN. Symptomatic residual radicular cysts. J Oral Pathol 1988;17:70–72.

Jones AV, Craig GT, Franklin CD. Range and demographics of odontogenic cysts diagnosed in a UK population over a 30-year period. J Oral Pathol Med 2006;3598:500–507.

Langlais R, Miller C. Color atlas of common oral diseases. Baltimore: Lippincott Williams & Wilkins, 2003.

Leithner A, Machacek F, Haas OA, et al. Aneurysmal bone cyst: a hereditary disease? J Pediatr Orthop B 2004;13(3):214–217.

Lombardi T, Bischof M, Nedir R, et al. Periapical central giant cell granuloma misdiagnosed as odontogenic cyst. Int Endod J 2006;39(6):510–515.

Melo ESA, Kawamura JY, Alves CAF, et al. Imaging modality correlations of an odontogenic keratocyst in the nevoid basal cell carcinoma syndrome: a family case report. Oral Surg Oral Med Oral Pathol Oral Radiol Endod 2004;98:232–236.

Menezes R, Bramante CM, da Silva Paiva KB, et al. Receptor activator NFkappaB-ligand and osteoprotegerin protein expression in human periapical cysts and granulomas. Oral Surg Oral Med Oral Pathol Oral Radiol Endod 2006;102(3):404–409.

Nair PNR, Pajarola G, Luder HU. Ciliated epithelium-lined radicular cysts. Oral Surg Oral Med Oral Pathol Oral Radiol Endod 2002;94:485–493.

Nair PNR, Pajarola G, Schroeder HE. Types and incidence of human periapical lesions obtained with extracted teeth. Oral Surg Oral Med Oral Pathol 1996;81:93–102.

Nakamura N, Mitsuyasu T, Mitsuyasu Y, et al. Marsupialization for odontogenic keratocysts: Long-term follow-up analysis of the effects and changes in growth characteristics. Oral Surg Oral Med Oral Pathol Oral Radio Endod 2002;94:543–553.

Nase JB, Suzuki JB. Osteonecrosis of the jaw and oral bisphosphonate treatment. JADA 2006;137:115–119.

Nelville BW, Damm DD, Allen CM, Bouquot JE. Oral & maxillofacial pathology. 2nd ed. Philadelphia: WB Saunders, 2002.

Otomo-Corgel J. Biophosphonate use and oral health. Dimensions of Dental Hygiene. 2006;4(6):32,34.

Ogutcen-Toller M, Sener I, Kasap V, Cakir-Ozkan N. Maxillary myxoma: surgical treatment and reconstruction with buccal fat pad flap: a case report. J Contemp Dent Pract 2006;15;7(1):107–116.

Perrotti V, Rubini C, Fioroni M, Piattelli A. Solid aneurysmal bone cyst of the mandible. Int J Pediatr Otorhinolaryngol 2004;68(10):1339–1344.

Pickett F, Gurenlian J. The medical history: clinical implications and emergency prevention in dental settings. Baltimore: Lippincott Williams & Wilkins, 2005.

Pippi R, Della RC, Sfasciotti GL. Periapical cemental (fibrous) dysplasia: clinical, radiographic and pathologic aspects in 7 reported cases. Minerva Stomatol 2004;53(4):135–141.

Porth CM. Essentials of pathophysiology. Baltimore: Lippincott Williams & Wilkins, 2004.

Regezi J, Sciubba J, Jordan R. Oral pathology—clinical pathologic correlations, 4th ed. St. Louis: WB Saunders, 2003.

Rubin E. Essential pathology. 3rd ed. Baltimore: Lippincott Williams & Wilkins, 2001.

Sciubba JJ, Fantasia JE, Kahn LE. Atlas of tumour pathology: tumours of the jaw. Third Series. Fasciole 29, Washington DC: AFIP, 2001:49.

Scully C. Handbook of oral disease—diagnosis and management. London: Martin Duntz Ltd. The Livery House Publishers, 1999.

Ruggiero SL, Mebrotra B, Rosenberg TJ, Engroff SL. Osteonecrosis of the jaws associated with the use of bisphosphonates: a review of 63 cases. J Oral Maxillofac Surg 2004;62:527–534.

Simon JHS. Incidence of periapical cysts in relation to root canal. J Endod 1980;6:845–848.

Shear M. Cysts of the oral regions. 3rd ed. Oxford, Wright, 1992.

Singer SR, Mapparapu M, Rinaggio J. Florid cementoosseous dysplasia and chronic diffuse osteomyelitis: report of a simultaneous presentation and review of the literature. J Am Dent Assoc 2005;136(7):927–931.

Stedman's medical dictionary. 27th ed. Baltimore: Lippincott Williams & Wilkins, 2000.

Su L, Weathers D, Waldron C. Distinguishing features of focal cementoosseous dysplasias and cemento-ossifying fibromas: 1. A pathological spectrum of 316 cases. Oral Surg Oral Med Oral Pathol Oral Radiol Endod 1997;84(3):301–309.

Trodahl JN. Ameloblastic fibroma: a survey of cases from the Armed Forces Institute of Pathology. Oral Surg Oral Med Oral Pathol Radiol Endod 1972;33:547–558.

Tsukamoto GT, Makino T, Kikuchi T, et al. A comparative study of odontogenic keratocysts associated with and not associated with an impacted mandibular third molar. Oral Surg Oral Med Oral Pathol Oral Radiol Endod 2002;94:272–275.

Wilkins EM. Clinical practice of the dental hygienist. 9th ed. Baltimore: Lippincott Williams & Wilkins, 2004.

Wright JM. Reactive, dysplastic and neoplastic conditions of periodontal ligament origin. Periodontology 2000 1999;21:7–15.

21

Abnormalities of the Teeth

Key Terms

- **Autosomal**
- **Coloboma**
- **Coronal**
- **Dominant**
- **Ectoderm**
- **Follicular**
- **Gastroesophageal reflux**
- **Heterozygous**
- **Hiatal hernia**
- **Homozygous**
- **Kindred**
- **Parafunctional**
- **Pathognomonic**
- **Penetrance/penetrant**
- **Percussion**
- **Prophylactic**
- **Radicular**
- **Recessive**
- **Stellate reticulum**
- **Tensile strength**
- **Venereal disease (sexually transmitted disease [STD])**
- **X-linked**

Objectives

1. Define and use the key terms listed in this chapter.

2. List the three main categories of traumatic influences that produce an alteration in the appearance of the teeth and note how they can be differentiated from one another.

3. Discuss the characteristic clinical features associated with a pulp polyp.

4. Describe the differences seen in the radiographs that help to distinguish internal resorption from external resorption.

5. Describe the clinical presentation of inflammatory induced enamel hypoplasia and how it differs from the developmental abnormalities that affect enamel formation.

6. Note the location of the most commonly missing tooth and discuss the genetically linked syndrome that is associated with multiple missing teeth.

7. Discuss hyperdontia and note the genetically linked syndrome associated with a markedly increased number of teeth (above the normal number of 32).

8. Note the tooth (other than the third molar) that is most commonly affected by microdontia.

9. Discuss the primary clinical concern when performing an occlusal adjustment on teeth affected with talon cusp or dens evaginatus.

10. List the pertinent radiographic features that allow distinction of gemination from fusion.

11. Define enamel pearl and note the common dental condition for which it may be mistaken.

12. Discuss the disease process involved with excessive hypercementosis on multiple teeth.

13. Describe the radiographic features associated with amelogenesis imperfecta and dentinogenesis imperfecta.

14. List four conditions that alter the structure of teeth and may lead to the development of periapical radiolucent lesions without an obvious cause being seen in the tooth crown.

15. Note the scientific names for the alteration in tooth structure described as "rootless teeth" and "ghost teeth."

16. State the level of fluoride concentration in the drinking water at which dental fluorosis typically occurs.

17. Discuss how tetracycline may be associated with discoloration of the teeth when administered during the period of tooth formation.

Chapter Outline

Pathologic changes affecting the teeth may be caused by (1) genetic influences, (2) environmental factors, (3) disease processes, (4) metabolic disturbances, or (5) nongenetically linked defects in the normal development and growth of the teeth. In most cases, the pathologic process will produce clearly visible evidence in the teeth that heralds the presence of an abnormality. In some cases, however, the teeth may appear entirely normal on casual observation, and additional clinical correlation or microscopic evaluation of the teeth may be necessary to identify the nature of the process.

Pathologic changes affecting the teeth can be grouped into two broad categories: (1) changes occurring during the initial growth and development of the tooth (developmental abnormalities), and (2) changes occurring after tooth development when the tooth has completely erupted into the oral cavity (postdevelopmental abnormalities). The abnormalities that occur during the initial growth and developmental process are by far the more numerous. The abnormalities that occur following tooth eruption are relatively few and are typically limited to the traumatic and inflammatory categories.

POSTDEVELOPMENTAL ABNORMALITIES OF THE TEETH

Traumatic Conditions

ATTRITION

Attrition is defined as the wearing away of tooth structure caused by tooth-to-tooth contact. Some attrition occurs in all individuals over the course of time as part of the normal functional aging process. It is produced by the ordinary forces of occlusion and the abrasive stresses of mastication. The areas most affected by attrition are the occlusal surfaces of the posterior teeth and the incisal edges of the anterior teeth. Attrition also occurs at the interproximal contact points of the teeth and over time can result in small reductions in arch length. Therefore, attrition should only be regarded as pathologic when the loss of tooth structure is severe and out of proportion to expectations considering the age of the patient.

Certainly the nature of the individual diet must also be considered, as it will affect the amount of attrition seen in a particular patient. Diets high in coarse, unrefined foods would be expected to produce greater attrition. Excessive grinding of the teeth (bruxism) and other **parafunctional** dental habits have also been implicated in severe attrition. Environmental factors may also play a role in the rate and extent of attrition. For example, people exposed to abrasive aerosols, such as those living in sandy desert climates, may show increased attrition relative to other populations. Attrition may be accelerated when developmental abnormalities affecting the surface hardness of the teeth are present. Abrasion and erosion (see below) are often seen in conjunction with attrition and can increase the severity of the loss of tooth structure.

Attrition can typically be recognized by a flattening of the normal rounded contour of the tooth in the affected area (Fig. 21.1). The surface of the flattened area usually appears burnished or polished relative to the adjacent unworn tooth surface. The area of faceting will show direct contact with an occluding tooth in the opposite dental arch. Even when excessive, attrition rarely causes symptoms for the patient, although occasionally a patient may complain of thermal sensitivity. The process proceeds at a slow enough rate to allow deposition of secondary dentin, insulating the dental pulp from noxious stimuli.

Abfraction

Abfraction is considered a subcategory of attrition by some authors, but the concept is not universally accepted as a cause of loss of tooth structure. Abfraction is defined as the loss of tooth structure in the cervical neck area of the teeth, which is produced by the transmission of forces generated during occlusion and mastication (chewing). Dentin is known to have a greater **tensile strength** than enamel. Because of this greater tensile strength, when stresses are applied to the tooth during occlusion and mastication, the dentin is better able than enamel to deform and rebound to its normal shape. This produces stress along the dentinoenamel junction. At the cervical

area of the tooth, the enamel thins considerably as it curves inward to abut the root surface. Thus, this combination of curvature, thinning of the enamel, and flexing of the dentinoenamel junction with the application of occlusal forces is theorized to produce cracking within the crystalline rodlike enamel structure. With repeated stresses, the enamel may eventually separate from the dentin completely and be lost. Abfraction typically appears as wedge-shaped areas of enamel loss. It is hypothesized to occur more often when the forces of occlusion are applied eccentrically, such as occurs in lateral jaw movements or in the grinding pattern associated with bruxism.

ABRASION

Abrasion is defined as the pathologic wearing away of tooth structure due to external factors that are mechanical and usually frictional. It typically occurs in the setting of a regularly repeated action performed over a long period of time. Inappropriate toothbrushing is probably the most common cause of abrasion. Increased attention to patient oral hygiene habits by dental professionals, accompanied by advocacy of the use of soft bristle toothbrushes and the development of less abrasive toothpastes has decreased the incidence of this type of abrasion; however, it still is seen with some frequency. Since cementum is softer and less resistant to abrasion than enamel, the exposed root surfaces in patients with gingival recession or periodontal disease are the most prone to develop this type of abrasion. It usually presents as a linear, V-shaped or U-shaped depression in the tooth structure just above the free gingival margin. The defect tends to be oriented parallel to the occlusal surface of the involved tooth.

Abrasion may be produced by other individual habits, which may be related to the patient's occupation. In this situation, the abrasion is associated with the use of the teeth as a "tool" or to assist the individual in repetitive tasks related to their job (Fig. 21.2). Thus, hairdressers

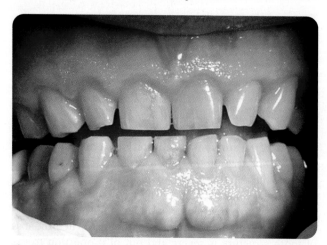

Figure 21.1. Attrition. Note the short height of the clinical crowns of the anterior teeth in both the maxilla and mandible. There is also flattening of the canine and premolar cusp tips.

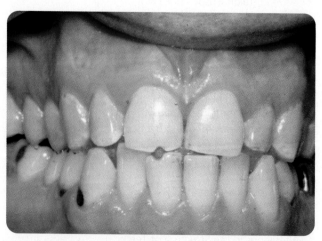

Figure 21.2. Abrasion. Distinctive notching of the maxillary and mandibular central incisors. The patient was an electrician and used his teeth to strip protective plastic covering from electrical wire.

(opening bobby pins), carpenters (holding nails), tailors and seamstresses (holding pins and needles, biting thread), and electricians (stripping electrical wire) among others have been reported to show an increased incidence of abrasion. When abrasion is occupation associated, it is often seen to primarily affect the anterior teeth and it may be limited to a single tooth in each arch. Nonoccupational habits often reported to be associated with abrasion include pipe smoking, tobacco chewing, and misusing other dental hygiene aids, such as dental floss and toothpicks.

As with attrition, developmental defects that alter the composition or hardness of tooth structure may predispose a patient to develop abrasion. In addition, the rate of loss of tooth structure may be more rapid. Even when abrasion occurs over a relatively short period of time, patients are seldom symptomatic.

EROSION

Erosion is defined as the loss of tooth structure produced by the contact of chemical agents with the tooth. Dental caries, although produced by the acidic byproducts of the activity of oral bacteria, is a separate category of disease and is not considered a form of erosion. Highly acidic foods and liquids are most often implicated in the production of erosion, but other chemicals have occasionally been shown to produce it. Chelating agents, such as EDTA, have specifically been implicated. Susceptibility to erosion, at least in part, is influenced by the quantity and quality of salivary flow. Normal saliva contains bicarbonate, which has a natural buffering effect, reducing the acidity of materials that pass through the oral cavity. Also, since prolonged and repeated contact of the acidic materials with tooth structure is customarily required for erosion to occur, adequate salivary flow should hinder erosion by diluting and washing the acidic materials away from contact with the tooth. In fact, saliva is known to facilitate remineralization of enamel surfaces that show early erosion or carious involvement. Thus, patients with decreased salivary flow would be expected to show an increased incidence of erosion, and loss of tooth structure.

Despite the generally protective effects of saliva, patients with normal salivary flow may still show evidence of erosion. This may be due to idiosyncrasies in the individual diet, personal habits, or medical conditions. In all instances though, the quantity of acidic material is so great that it overwhelms the ability of the saliva to compensate. Ingestion of large quantities of sugar-containing carbonated beverages has been implicated as a significant etiologic factor. Citrus fruit and juices are other potential sources of highly acidic material. In one instance, severe erosion of the maxillary and mandibular teeth was noted in a patient who would habitually suck on a lemon wedge held against the anterior teeth by the lips. Another unusual case highlights erosion seen in competitive swimmers who practiced daily for long periods in a swimming pool with inadequately controlled pH. Medical conditions that predispose a patient to

repeated episodes of vomiting are additional etiologic factors in the production of erosion. The best known and most often reported of these is anorexia nervosa/bulimia, but pregnancy and alcoholism are also established as potential factors. **Gastroesophageal reflux** and **hiatal hernia** likely account for a small number of cases as well. When erosion is produced by contact with gastric secretions, it is termed "perimolysis." As with attrition and abrasion, concurrent developmental defects affecting the hardness of tooth structure may accelerate the process of erosion.

Clinically, erosion may resemble attrition and abrasion to some extent, producing a smooth and polished-appearing depression in the tooth surface. Multiple teeth are normally affected. Unlike attrition, it does not tend to be seen in areas where there is occlusal contact of the teeth, although severe cases of erosion may involve occlusal surfaces. Erosion may be distinguished from abrasion, since it typically produces a broader and more rounded area of depression than the linear, V-shaped areas that typify abrasion (Fig. 21.3). However, since erosion may predispose to abrasion by softening the tooth surface, the two processes are often seen in concert. While erosion may be seen on any tooth surface, it typically is found in the gingival third area of the teeth where the normal periodontal architecture may provide a somewhat protected environment for prolonged contact of the chemical agent with the tooth surface. The root surface and cementoenamel junction areas of the teeth are most susceptible to the effects of erosion. In general, erosion associated with acidic dietary foods and liquids tends to affect the labial and buccal surfaces of the teeth more prominently, while erosion associated with repeated vomiting is seen to produce more damaging effects on the lingual and palatal surfaces. Thus, the areas of involvement with erosion may produce significant clues about the cause of erosion. Another prominent

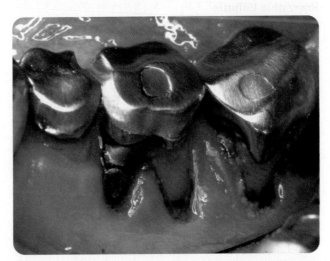

Figure 21.3. Erosion. Note the diffuse flattening of the exposed root surfaces on the facial surface of the premolar and molar teeth. The patient placed smokeless tobacco in this area regularly over a prolonged period. Some abrasion from the rough texture of the smokeless tobacco is also present.

diagnostic sign associated with erosion is protrusion of amalgam restorations above the level of the surrounding tooth structure. In this scenario, the metallic amalgam restoration is immune to the effects of the chemical agent, while the surrounding tooth structure is eroded, producing the characteristic "elevation" of the filling material. In severe cases of erosion, thermal sensitivity may be reported, but many patients are entirely asymptomatic.

Inflammatory Conditions

PULPITIS

By definition, pulpitis is inflammation involving the dental pulp. Pulpitis is exceedingly common, and nearly every individual will suffer symptoms of pulpitis at some time during his or her life. The inflammation within the dental pulp may be produced by a variety of stimuli. Dental caries is the most common. External trauma, trauma from occlusion and mastication, invasive and noninvasive dental procedures, and extreme temperature changes may produce pulpitis as well. Attrition, abrasion, and erosion are occasionally implicated. The involved tooth may show an obvious source for the pulpal inflammation (e.g., carious lesion, fracture) or it may appear entirely normal clinically. Unless pulpal necrosis has occurred with spread of the inflammatory process through the root apex and into the **radicular** bone, radiographs will appear normal. Occasionally, teeth affected by pulpitis will show a slight widening of the periodontal ligament space at the apical region of the tooth. Therefore, in many instances, pulpitis can only be recognized by the symptoms reported by the patient (i.e., a toothache).

Pulpitis can be divided into three subcategories: reversible pulpitis, irreversible pulpitis, and hyperplastic pulpitis. These three subcategories have clinical features that usually allow rapid and dependable diagnosis.

Reversible Pulpitis

In reversible pulpitis, as the name indicates, it is expected that the inflammation of the pulp will resolve and the tooth will eventually return to a normal condition. Pain is the presenting symptom, and it typically is instigated by cold only. Heat may elicit the pain on occasion but usually not without cold sensitivity being present as well. In very rare instances, sweets or tart food may initiate the pain, but **percussion** of the tooth (striking a tooth with short, sharp blows to elicit pain) normally does not. The pain is not usually described as severe but is sharp. A particularly distinctive characteristic of reversible pulpitis is that the pain is very sudden in onset with application of the stimulus and almost as sudden in disappearance once the stimulus is discontinued. The total duration of the pain is classically described as only a few seconds following stimulus removal. An inciting stimulus for the pain is a required criterion, as the pain associated with reversible pulpitis is never spontaneous.

Irreversible Pulpitis

If the inflammation of the dental pulp persists, the condition may progress from reversible to irreversible pulpitis. The hallmark feature of irreversible pulpitis is the presence of pain that lingers or is continuous following removal of an inciting stimulus. Pain may still be initiated by cold but is also more reliably produced by heat, among other stimuli. In contrast to reversible pulpitis, the pain may be initiated only by heat without corresponding cold sensitivity. The pain is more often described as severe, in addition to being sharp, and it may worsen when the patient lies down. Percussion of the tooth may elicit the pain response. In irreversible pulpitis, an initiating stimulus for the pain is not always necessary, and spontaneous onset of pain in particular heralds the presence of irreversible inflammatory changes. Once the inflammation in the dental pulp has progressed to irreversible pulpitis, endodontic therapy becomes necessary.

Hyperplastic Pulpitis

Hyperplastic pulpitis, often referred to as chronic hyperplastic pulpitis, is a form of pulpitis with a characteristic clinical presentation. It has also been termed pulp polyp. It is always seen in association with a tooth that has a large carious lesion. The deciduous and permanent molar teeth are the most commonly involved, and patients tend to be children, adolescents, or young adults. The carious lesion almost always involves a major portion of the occlusal surface and has progressed to the point of destroying the roof of the underlying pulp chamber, exposing the pulp tissue to the oral environment. The pulpal tissue is irritated and inflamed. However, because the roof of the pulp chamber has been destroyed by the carious process, the pulp tissue is able to expand in response to the inflammation, unlike the other forms of pulpitis in which the irritated and inflamed pulp tissue is nearly completely enclosed by dentin. Thus, the pulp tissue is able to become hyperplastic, with a mass of granulation tissue welling up out of the pulp chamber. Clinically this presents as a bright red, dome-shaped mass of tissue occupying the carious defect in the occlusal surface. Pain is usually not present, although occasionally patients complain of some sensitivity when they try to chew on the affected side. However, touching the surface of the dome-shaped red lesion with the tip of an explorer may elicit a sharp, stabbing pain and bleeding. Treatment requires endodontic therapy or extraction.

PULP STONES

Pulp stones are abnormalities of the teeth that, for the most part, are clinically insignificant. However, they are occasionally noticed in dental radiographs, usually as an incidental finding.. On the radiograph, they present as round to oval areas of opacity within the radiolucent area that defines the pulp chamber or root canal space (Fig. 21.4). Unless there is another reason for inflammation involving the dental pulp, the teeth that show pulp stones are predictably asymptomatic. The etiology of pulp stones is not known with certainty. Studies done in the first half of the 20th century suggest that the formation of pulp stones may be a physiologic process representing the nor-

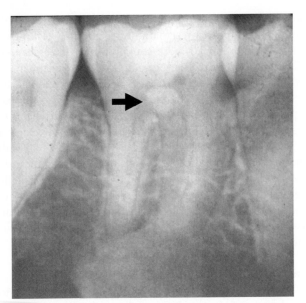

Figure 21.4. Pulp stone. A rounded area of radiopacity is seen within the pulp chamber of the molar tooth. Note the large restoration encroaching on the dental pulp as a likely source of pulpal inflammation.

mal aging process of the dental pulp. These studies showed that the incidence of pulp stones increased with advancing age of the patient, with more than 90% of teeth examined in the 50- to 70-year-old age group showing some evidence of pulp stone formation. The actual mechanism of pulp stone formation is also uncertain but is theorized to involve calcification around a nidus of altered cells within the pulp tissue. The most likely cause of the cellular alteration appears to be inflammation of the pulp tissue. Since pulp stones are clinically innocuous and are most often discovered as an incidental finding, no treatment is necessary. The only significant untoward effect of pulp stones occurs when a particularly large pulp stone interferes with conventional endodontic procedures.

Internal Resorption

Internal resorption is defined as the destruction of tooth structure that is initiated from within the pulp chamber or root canal. This is a rare occurrence compared to the far more frequently observed process of external resorption (discussed below). Usually, a single tooth is affected. While the exact cause of internal resorption is not known in all cases, a significant number of cases are believed to result from injury to the pulp tissues. This injury causes an influx of inflammatory cells, some of which transform into osteoclast-like cells that then destroy the dental hard tissue from within (Fig. 21.5A). Dental caries and traumatic episodes have been most often implicated in initiating the inflammation. The resorptive process may stabilize and remain at a fixed size or it may be progressive, eventually perforating the external tooth surface unless treatment intervenes.

Teeth affected by internal resorption are usually asymptomatic. Most are discovered as an incidental finding in a radiograph taken for some other reason. The resorption

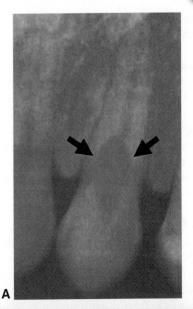

A

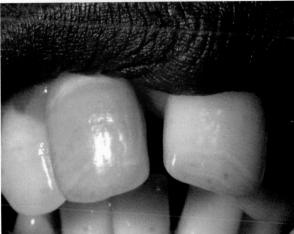

B

Figure 21.5. Internal resorption. **A.** Note the bulbous radiolucent enlargement of the pulp. **B.** Pink discoloration of the crown is due to enlargement of the pulp chamber associated with internal resorption.

presents as a bulbous radiolucent enlargement of the pulp that is commonly symmetric and clearly visualized against the surrounding opaque tooth structure. The margins of the lucent area are often sharply defined, but may be hazy. The resorption is seen most often in the cervical neck area of the tooth at the level of the cementoenamel junction; however, it can occur anywhere within the pulp system. If it involves primarily the **coronal** pulp chamber, thinning of the dentin may occur to the extent that the highly vascularized pulp tissue can be visualized through the translucent enamel. The crown of the tooth exhibits a pink to light red discoloration (Fig. 21.5B). This presentation is sometimes referred to as the "pink tooth of Mummery" and is considered diagnostic for internal resorption. Teeth affected by internal resorption can be successfully treated with endodontic therapy in many cases. Once perforation of the external surface has occurred, treatment options are more limited, and extraction is regularly the treatment of choice. Heroic attempts at restoration of the area of perforation have been attempted with varying results.

External Resorption

External resorption is defined as the destruction of tooth structure that is initiated from outside the tooth. In contrast to internal resorption, it is commonly observed. In some studies, critical evaluation of large numbers of radiographs revealed some external resorption to be present in all patients. Thus, external resorption should not be considered a pathologic process unless a significant portion of tooth structure has been destroyed. The main impetus for external resorption is also thought to be trauma. However, a larger proportion of cases of external resorption have no identifiable causal factor. These cases are classified as **idiopathic** external resorption. Destruction of tooth structure in external resorption is believed to be initiated by cells that originate in the periodontal ligament. These cells differentiate into osteoclast-like cells to destroy tooth structure. Numerous specific local factors in addition to trauma have been shown to be associated with external resorption, but they all can be divided, from an etiologic standpoint, into two categories: (1) conditions that generate inflammation on the external tooth surface and (2) conditions that produce pressure against the periodontal ligament. Conditions generating inflammation include periapical pathosis secondary to inflammatory pulpal disease, periodontal infections, periodontal treatment, endodontic treatment, surgical procedures (e.g., bone grafts, biopsy procedures, reimplantation of avulsed teeth), and some bleaching procedures. Specific infections have also been implicated, particularly herpes zoster. Conditions producing pressure against the periodontal ligament include pathologic processes (e.g., cysts, tumors, fibroosseous diseases, condensing osteitis), pressure from adjacent impacted or erupting teeth, orthodontic care, and perhaps even traumatic occlusion.

External resorption affects multiple teeth more commonly than does internal resorption, but involvement of only a single tooth also occurs. Any area of the tooth may be affected, although most cases involve the lower one half of the tooth. Resorption of the crown is unusual unless the tooth is impacted or the resorption encroaches on the crown structure from an area of cervical involvement. When the cervical area of the tooth is involved, resorption can be exceptionally destructive and rapid, threatening to produce amputation of the crown. Radiographically, external resorption is generally characterized by an asymmetric radiolucency that has a ragged or "moth-eaten" border where it abuts against tooth structure. Where tooth structure is actively being destroyed, the lucent area may show variation in the degree of lucency, producing a mottled or mixed radiolucent-radiopaque appearance as shown in Figure 21.6A. Alternatively, some cases of external resorption manifest simply as loss of tooth root length. In this situation, a clearly defined radiolucent defect is not appreciated, and the tooth roots just seem abnormally short. The root tip area often seems blunted. This radiographic presentation of external resorption tends to be produced more commonly by processes that place pressure on the periodontal ligament. Treatment of external resorption depends entirely on the location of the resorptive defect, the amount of resorption, and the patient's symptoms. Obviously any factors predisposing to resorption must be eliminated first. If the resorptive defect is in an accessible area, restorative procedures may halt the process. Large areas of resorption that significantly weaken the tooth or its surrounding support will usually necessitate extraction (Fig. 21.6B and C). External resorption that presents as shortening of the root without an associated radiolucent defect does not require any treatment as long as the tooth is not excessively mobile.

Enamel Hypoplasia

While most cases of enamel hypoplasia are linked directly to developmental abnormalities of the teeth, it is sometimes produced by inflammation. The inflammation involves the **follicular** tissues that surround the crown at the time of production and/or calcification of enamel matrix. This type of enamel hypoplasia is almost always seen involving premolar teeth, although it can affect any of the permanent teeth that have a deciduous tooth precursor. Permanent molar teeth are rarely affected. The deciduous tooth develops a periapical inflammatory lesion, which is most often a periapical abscess secondary to a carious lesion. Traumatic injury to the deciduous tooth, particularly of the type that tends to drive the tooth into the alveolar bone, has also been implicated as a causative factor. The crown of the permanent tooth, developing immediately beneath the roots of the deciduous tooth, becomes engulfed in the noxious environment produced by the periapical inflammation, injuring the enamel-forming cells of the tooth bud. The severity of involvement of the developing tooth crown can be quite variable and depends on the size, extent, and duration of the infection; the individual resistance of the patient; and the stage of growth of the involved developing tooth. This explains why the anterior teeth (incisors and canines) are so rarely involved. The anterior permanent teeth begin crown development shortly after birth, and enamel formation is complete by about age 5. Since the anterior deciduous teeth are less prone to develop carious lesions, the enamel on the underlying teeth is ordinarily fully formed before periapical inflammation can develop.

Inflammation-induced enamel hypoplasia most commonly affects only a single tooth, in contrast to developmental hypoplasia, in which multiple teeth are habitually involved. The involved tooth is often referred to as a Turner's tooth. The degree of enamel hypoplasia can be minimal and difficult to recognize, presenting only as a discoloration of the enamel surface. This is typically seen when the initiating infection is mild or is successfully treated without delay. The hypoplasia can also be severe, producing considerable alteration of the normal crown

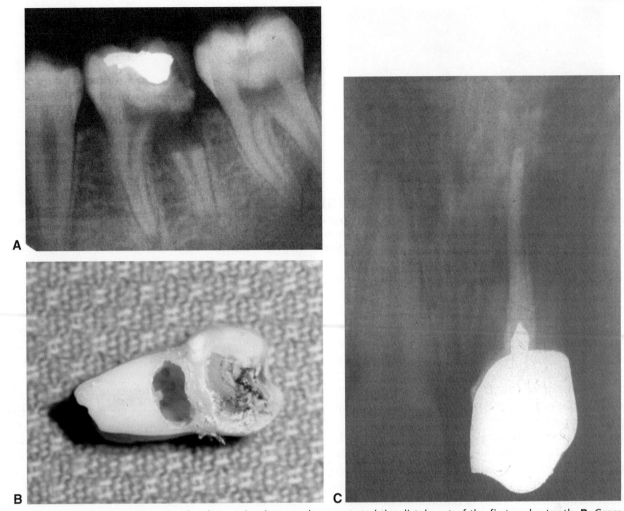

Figure 21.6. External resorption. **A.** The destruction has nearly amputated the distal root of the first molar tooth. **B.** Gross specimen of extracted tooth shows the extent of destruction of tooth structure. Soft tissue has been cleaned from the resorptive defect. **C.** Another case shows the extent of resorption possible. Nearly the entire hard tissue of the root has been resorbed, and the tooth was highly mobile, being retained in the alveolus only by the endodontic filling material. The patient gave a history of severe trauma to the tooth many years previously.

form. In this situation, radiographic evidence of loss of enamel is evident. Most commonly, the hypoplasia presents as areas of pitting, grooving, or shallow cavitation, disrupting the normally smooth and shiny enamel surface. Large areas of loss of enamel may be seen. In some instances, small, but multiple discrete areas of involvement on a single crown may be noted. If the enamel hypoplasia is severe, is unaesthetic, or the patient develops symptoms, restorative procedures remedy the situation in most cases.

DEVELOPMENTAL ABNORMALITIES OF THE TEETH

Alterations in Number of Teeth

DECREASED NUMBER OF TEETH/ANODONTIA

A decrease in the number of teeth is termed "anodontia." Anodontia may be complete or partial. Complete anodontia

requires a failure of formation of all teeth, which is very rare. Partial anodontia is common and is defined as a failure of formation of one or more teeth as depicted in Figure 21.7A and B. If six or more teeth are missing, the condition may be referred to as oligodontia. Hypodontia describes a situation in which one to five teeth do not develop.

Before classifying the absence of teeth as anodontia, the dental history of the patient must be considered, and a radiographic examination may be necessary. True anodontia is the failure of development of a tooth. The extraction of teeth may give the incorrect impression that teeth are developmentally missing. This condition is termed "false anodontia." An unerupted or impacted tooth may present as a clinically missing tooth with no dental history of prior extraction, also simulating true anodontia. Radiographs will prove that the tooth did develop appropriately. This is sometimes referred to as "pseudoanodontia."

Bilateral symmetry is commonly seen in anodontia, but on occasion, a single tooth on only one side of the jaws is

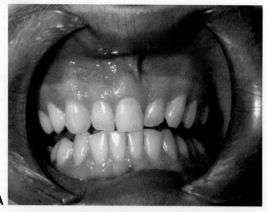
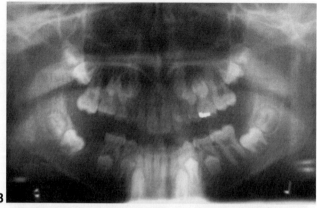

Figure 21.7. Partial anodontia. A. Only one maxillary central incisor tooth is present. The patient gives no history of tooth extraction in this area. (Photograph courtesy of Dr. Theodore Zislis.) **B.** The right mandibular first molar is missing. The other first molars are all present. There was no history of extraction or surgery in the right mandible.

absent. The teeth most commonly found to be developmentally missing are the maxillary and mandibular third molars. The maxillary lateral incisors are the second most commonly missing teeth. Mandibular second premolars are also often absent. The permanent first molar appears to be the least likely to be found developmentally missing. In the deciduous dentition, the maxillary lateral incisor is the tooth most commonly absent. In most cases when anodontia affects the deciduous dentition, the corresponding permanent successor also fails to form.

In most cases of anodontia, the lack of formation of the teeth is not associated with an identifiable systemic or genetic disease. However, some genetically inherited conditions are consistently connected with anodontia, and the failure of tooth formation may be the clinical characteristic that allows initial recognition of the associated syndrome.

DECREASED NUMBER OF TEETH ASSOCIATED WITH SYNDROMES

Hereditary Hypohidrotic Ectodermal Dysplasia

Ectodermal dysplasia is the most common of the genetic diseases that produce a decrease in the number of teeth. The oligodontia (discussed above) associated with ectodermal dysplasia is so striking that it is often the distinguishing feature that facilitates initial recognition of the genetic disease. A variety of genetic patterns of inheritance are known to exist. However, in most instances, it is an **X-linked** syndrome, meaning that the gene that produces the clinical manifestations is carried on the X (female) chromosome. In this form, it is also a **recessive** characteristic, since features of the disease are not seen in the patient if a normal gene is present on the matching X chromosome. However, males have only one X chromosome, thus if they inherit a defective gene from their mother, they will show manifestations of the syndrome. Females are only seen to be affected when they inherit a defective gene from both parents, which occasionally occurs. Affected female patients are said to be **homozygous** for the disorder (both X chromosomes carry the defective

gene), and the manifestations of the disease are particularly severe in this situation. Some **homozygous** females show almost complete anodontia. A female with one affected X chromosome and one normal X chromosome is a heterozygote. These patients typically do not show oligodontia, although sometimes they may be missing one or two teeth. Other manifestations of the disease are also typically absent in the **heterozygous** female. However, these women are carriers of the defective gene and can pass the disease on to their children. Most patients with hypohidrotic ectodermal dysplasia are, therefore, males.

As the name indicates, patients with hereditary hypohidrotic ectodermal dysplasia show defects of a variety of structures that are derived from the **ectoderm**. The skin is soft, smooth, thin, and seems dry. Teeth are ectodermally derived structures; therefore, in addition to exhibiting oligodontia, the teeth that do form in patients with ectodermal dysplasia are often misshapen. Cone-shaped anterior teeth are particularly common. Hair is another structure that is derived from the ectoderm, producing a distinguishing facial appearance. The scalp hair is very fine, blond, and sparse in distribution. Eyebrows and eyelashes are also sparse and may be nearly completely absent (Fig. 21.8A–C). Interestingly though, most male patients develop a nearly normal facial hair distribution as they progress through puberty. For unexplained reasons, patients also typically have large, protruding, blubbery lips out of proportion to other facial features. Sweat glands are also affected by the genetic deficiency, and patients with ectodermal dysplasia may show heat intolerance due to their inability to lose heat through the sweating mechanism. The failure of the salivary glands to form may be a component of the disease, and, when present, patients may complain of a dry mouth. This appears to be an uncommon manifestation; however if it is present, the patient may be at increased risk of developing dental caries and periodontal disease.

Incontinentia Pigmenti (Bloch-Sulzberger Disease)

Failure of formation of teeth is a characteristic associated with numerous other genetically linked diseases and syn-

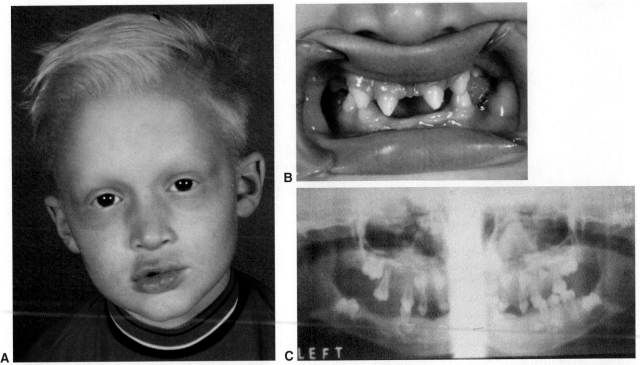

Figure 21.8. Ectodermal dysplasia. **A.** Young male patient shows characteristic facial appearance, with sparse fine blond hair, absence of eyebrows and eyelashes, and large lips. (Photograph courtesy of Dr. Robert Acterberg.) **B.** Intraoral clinical appearance of the same patient. Note multiple missing teeth. The anterior teeth have a cone-shaped crown morphology that is also commonly present in these patients. (Photograph courtesy of Dr. Robert Acterberg.) **C.** Panoramic radiograph of same patient reveals extensive number of congenitally missing teeth. (Photograph courtesy of Dr. Robert Acterberg.)

dromes. More than 30 syndromes are currently included on this list. In most of these diseases, the anodontia is a nominal component, with only a few teeth at most found missing, and the absence of the teeth does not usually contribute to the recognition of the disease process as it does in hereditary hypohidrotic ectodermal dysplasia. Incontinentia pigmenti seems to be the most likely of these diverse syndromes to produce a significant anodontia. Incontinentia pigmenti is also known as Bloch-Sulzberger disease. It is an **X-linked, dominant** genetic disease. As such, most patients are females. It is thought that the condition may be lethal in most males that inherit the defective gene, resulting in spontaneous abortion of the fetus or death during childbirth or in the early neonatal period. The disease manifests with skin abnormalities, neurologic disorders, and bone defects. The teeth are affected in 60–80% of patients. Partial anodontia is usual but not an overly prominent component. Peg shaped anterior teeth are a common accompanying feature, and tooth eruption may exhibit a generalized delay.

INCREASED NUMBER OF TEETH/HYPERDONTIA

An increase in the number of teeth is termed "hyperdontia." It is a relatively common occurrence. The category of hyperdontia may be subdivided into supernumerary teeth and accessory teeth. Supernumerary teeth are additional teeth that at least approach the normal expected size of the adjacent teeth in the area. The crown form of a supernumerary tooth is usually identifiable as a specific class (i.e., incisor, canine, premolar, or molar). Supernumerary teeth tend to occur in specific sites within the jaws. While they can be multiple in a single site, they usually present as a single extra tooth per quadrant but show a significant propensity to bilateral symmetry with another supernumerary tooth being found in the same general location on the opposite side of the jaw. Accessory teeth, on the other hand, are diminutive, appearing as miniature replicas of a tooth. They often show a conical crown form rather than mimicking the occlusal form of the adjacent teeth, as is found with supernumerary teeth (Fig. 21.9A–C).

Accessory teeth tend to occur with greatest frequency on the buccal or palatal aspect of the maxillary molar teeth. There may be multiple accessory teeth in one area, and while occasionally bilaterally symmetrical, they are more often limited to a single quadrant. Fusion of the accessory tooth to the adjacent normal tooth occurs occasionally. Accessory teeth in the maxillary molar region are often referred to as "paramolars."

Statistically, the most common supernumerary tooth is the mesiodens. There is some evidence of **autosomal dominant** genetic inheritance associated with the presence of a mesiodens. It is found in the anterior maxilla, in many cases in the midline between the central incisor teeth. It presents as a single tooth most frequently, but occasionally it occurs in pairs. It often presents with a peg-shaped

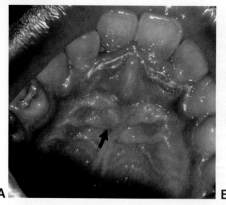
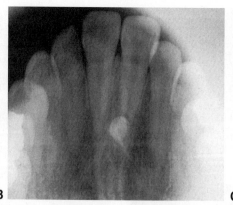
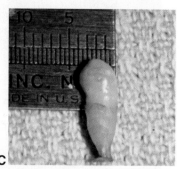

Figure 21.9. Accessory tooth. **A.** Clinical appearance of diminutive tooth in the rugae area of the hard palate. **B.** Occlusal radiograph of the accessory tooth seen in **A**. **C.** Extracted tooth as seen in **A** is only 4 mm in width.

or conical crown form rather than the typical appearance of a central incisor. Many mesiodens are impacted, and up to 50% of impacted ones appear upside down on periapical radiographs. In some instances, the mesiodens may erupt into the oral cavity, often on the palatal aspect. Early eruption of a mesiodens may block normal eruption of the permanent central incisor or cause significant crowding and malocclusion in the anterior area. The unaesthetic appearance normally prompts removal (Fig. 21.10A and B).

Distomolars are supernumerary molar teeth that occur distal to the third molars as shown in Figure 21.11. They are the second most common supernumerary teeth. They typically show the normal crown anatomy of a molar but are slightly smaller in overall dimensions. The mandibular premolar area is another common site of preference for the development of supernumerary teeth (Fig. 21.12). Supernumerary teeth are rare in the deciduous dentition, but when it does occur, the lateral incisor is the site most affected.

INCREASED NUMBER OF TEETH ASSOCIATED WITH SYNDROMES

In most cases of hyperdontia, the formation of extra teeth is not associated with a readily identifiable genetic disease. However, as in anodontia, some genetically inherited conditions are consistently connected with hyperdontia, and the presence of supernumerary teeth can be so dramatic that it becomes the clinical characteristic that allows initial recognition of the associated syndrome.

Cleidocranial Dysplasia (Dysostosis)

Previously called "cleidocranial dysostosis," cleidocranial dysplasia is now the preferred terminology for this genetic disease. In most cases, affected individuals have an affected parent, indicating that the disease is transmitted as an autosomal dominant trait. In up to 40% of cases though, neither parent of the affected individual shows evidence of the disease, suggesting that a good proportion of cases arise as new mutations in the individual patient's genetic makeup. The disease produces a wide array of clinical features that assist in its identification. While the

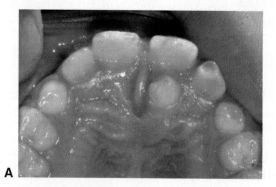

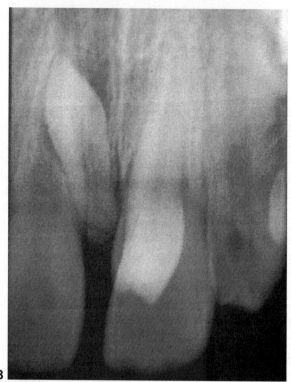

Figure 21.10. Hyperdontia. **A.** A mesiodens has erupted palatal to the left maxillary central incisor tooth. **B.** A radiograph of the area seen clinically in **A** reveals a second, impacted mesiodens present upside down in the maxilla behind the right maxillary central incisor.

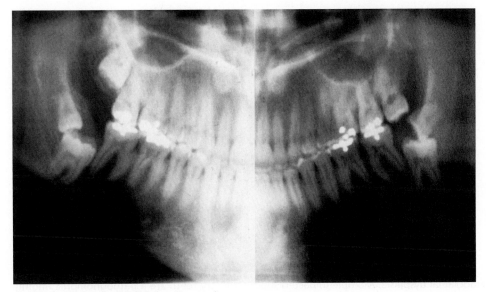

Figure 21.11. Hyperdontia. Bilateral mandibular distomolars are present.

name of the disease seems to indicate that only the clavicle (*cleido*) and the skull (*cranial*) are affected, membranous bones throughout the skeleton appear to be involved. Affected individuals are typically short in stature with the average height of males and females reportedly 5'2" and 4'10", respectively. The oral findings are truly remarkable and produce a **pathognomonic** (clearly recognizable) radiographic appearance that is diagnostic for this condition. The midface area is often deficient, resulting in the appearance of overdevelopment of the lower jaw. The palate is often cleft. The most striking radiographic feature, however, is the presence of multiple impacted supernumerary teeth (Fig. 21.13). Patients routinely have 10 or more supernumerary teeth. The sheer number of teeth present within the jaws produces overcrowding that prevents eruption of both the regular adult dentition and the supernumerary teeth. Moreover, the teeth of patients with cleidocranial dysplasia lack deposition of cellular cementum on the roots, further hindering eruption. Due to this lack of eruption of the permanent teeth, deciduous teeth are retained well past the normal expected age of exfoliation.

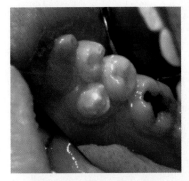

Figure 21.12. Hyperdontia. A supernumerary mandibular premolar has erupted lingual to the normally positioned premolars in the left mandible. (Photo is taken in intraoral mirror.)

Gardner Syndrome

Gardner syndrome is a disease process that may present with head and neck manifestations, including hyperdontia, which is vitally important for the dental healthcare practitioner to recognize. While the degree of hyperdontia is not as spectacular as is seen in cleidocranial dysplasia, the presence of supernumerary teeth in concert with other characteristic features seen on dental panoramic radiographs may be enough to alert the vigilant observer to the presence of the disease (Fig. 21.14).

Gardner syndrome is a genetic disease that is transmitted as an autosomal dominant trait. The disease is highly **penetrant**, meaning that patients who inherit the defective gene from a parent will normally show many, if not all, of the characteristic features. The dental findings include multiple supernumerary teeth that are often impacted. Multiple odontomas may be seen as well. Other features of the disease include multiple epidermoid cysts of the skin, which are particularly common in the neck, and desmoid tumors found principally in the abdominal area but occasionally found in other soft tissue sites as well. Multiple osteomas involving the skull, face, and jaws is a distinguishing feature. The angle and ramus areas of the mandible are often involved, producing irregularly dense radiopaque masses on dental panoramic films that are not seen in any other disease process. This feature in particular heralds the presence of Gardner syndrome. The primary characteristic feature of Gardner syndrome, and the feature that makes its recognition so important, is the presence of numerous polyps in the large intestine and rectum. In aggregate, these polyps have a virtual 100% incidence of eventual transformation to cancer. There is such a strong association of the development of cancer in these patients that individuals diagnosed with the syndrome often undergo **prophylactic** removal of the colon, sometimes in the very early adult years. Recognition of the characteristic head and neck manifestations is so important because development

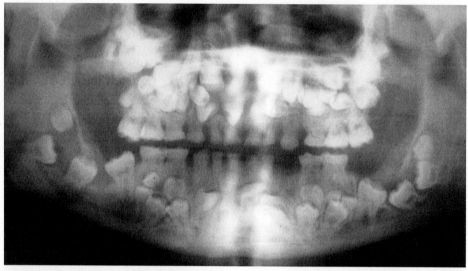

Figure 21.13. Cleidocranial dysplasia. Multiple impacted supernumerary teeth are a pathognomonic finding. As many as 50 teeth may be present. (Photograph courtesy of Dr. William Binnie.)

of the head and neck abnormalities typically precedes development of the colonic polyps. Early diagnosis of the syndrome, coupled with early bowel removal, may therefore be a life-saving procedure.

Other Syndromes Exhibiting Hyperdontia

The formation of supernumerary teeth is a characteristic associated with a number of other genetically linked syndromes. At least 16 additional syndromes other than cleidocranial dysplasia and Gardner syndrome are currently included on the list. In most of these syndromes, the hyperdontia is not a prominent component, with only an occasional supernumerary tooth being found. Therefore, the presence of supernumerary teeth will not usually allow ready recognition of the disease process as it does in cleidocranial dysplasia and Gardner syndrome. Paradoxically, many of the genetic diseases that are associated with supernumerary teeth also show up on the list of genetic syndromes that can produce a decreased number of teeth. These include Crouzon syndrome, Down syndrome, Ehlers-Danlos syndrome, Hallermann-Streiff syndrome,

Orofacialdigital (type I) syndrome, and Sturge-Weber syndrome.

Alterations in Size of Teeth

DECREASED SIZE OF TEETH/MICRODONTIA

Microdontia is a decrease in the size of the teeth relative to what is considered the normal range for each class of tooth. Microdontia may be generalized, affecting the entire dentition, or it may be localized, affecting only one or a few teeth.

A true generalized microdontia is relatively rare. Most cases of true generalized microdontia are associated with pituitary dwarfs. These individuals either lack growth hormone production by the pituitary gland or their tissues do not respond appropriately to the presence of growth hormone. Since growth hormone is responsible for growth of all the tissues of the body, these individuals are well proportioned but are smaller in every respect, including the teeth. Patients with Down syndrome have also

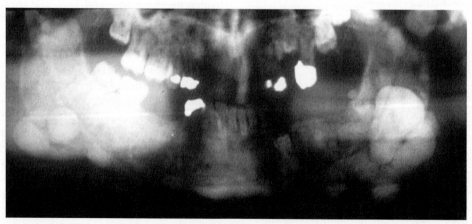

Figure 21.14. Gardner Syndrome. The panoramic radiograph shows large osteomas involving the angle and ramus areas of the mandible bilaterally, a diagnostic feature. Several supernumerary premolar teeth are also seen.

been reported to have a true generalized microdontia in some instances.

Perhaps more common than a true generalized microdontia is relative generalized microdontia. In this situation, the teeth are on the small end of the normal size range, but the bone of the jaw is larger than normal. The teeth therefore appear small when viewed in the context of the size of the jaw, but actual measurements show them to be within the normal range.

Localized microdontia is seen far more commonly. In general, the teeth usually affected by localized microdontia are the same as the teeth most commonly missing in cases of hypodontia. Thus, third molars are most often affected, with maxillary lateral incisors being the second most often involved. When the lateral incisor is affected, it often assumes a peg-shaped crown form. These teeth are sometimes referred to as peg laterals (Fig. 21.15 A and B). Bilateral symmetry is often noted in localized microdontia.

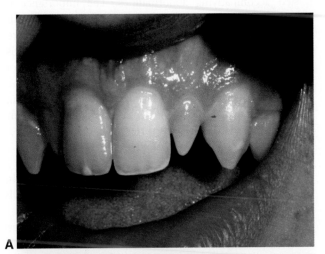

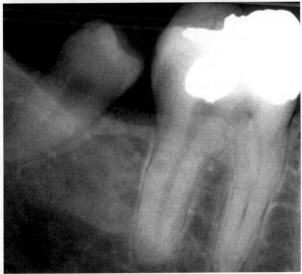

Figure 21.15. Microdontia. **A.** The lateral incisors are involved bilaterally. Note the conical crown form. These teeth are sometimes referred to as peg lateral incisors. **B.** A mandibular third molar is severely reduced in size. (Photograph courtesy of Dr. John Wright.)

INCREASED SIZE OF TEETH/MACRODONTIA

Macrodontia is an increase in the size of the teeth relative to what is considered the normal range for each class of tooth. As with microdontia, macrodontia may be generalized, affecting the entire dentition, or it may be localized, affecting only one or a few teeth.

True generalized macrodontia is unusual. Most cases are associated with pituitary giantism. These patients typically have a tumor of the pituitary gland that secretes excess quantities of growth hormone. The excess growth hormone stimulates overgrowth of all tissues in the body. These individuals are well proportioned but larger in every respect, including the teeth. Pituitary giants typically are extraordinarily tall, with many attaining a height of more than 8 feet.

Relative generalized macrodontia is also known to occur. As with relative generalized microdontia, this is due to a lack of coordination between tooth size and jaw size, with the jaw being smaller than average while the teeth are on the large end of the spectrum of normal size. The illusion, then, is that all the teeth are excessively large.

Localized macrodontia is relatively rare. Only isolated teeth tend to be affected, and usually only a single tooth is involved. However, bilateral symmetry may be seen with this condition (Fig. 21.16).

A developmental anomaly of unknown etiology that may produce localized macrodontia affecting many teeth is hemifacial hyperplasia. In this disease, one half of the face enlarges relative to the opposite side, and in many cases, the enlargement is present at birth. The growth on the enlarged side keeps pace with the growth on the unaffected side, resulting in continual facial asymmetry that is evident throughout the childhood years and into adult life. Typically the canine, premolar, and molar teeth on the affected side in both the maxilla and the mandible will show evidence of macrodontia. The affected teeth may also erupt ahead of the corresponding teeth on the unaffected side.

Macrodontia may be simulated by other dental anomalies. Close clinical observation, along with radiographic evaluation, will usually allow accurate diagnosis. Fusion of teeth, particularly when the fusion occurs between a normal tooth and a supernumerary tooth, is the most likely anomaly to be misinterpreted as macrodontia. Gemination may produce similar confusion if minimal separation of the crowns of the geminated tooth is present.

Alterations in Shape (Morphology) of Teeth

There are a variety of abnormalities affecting the teeth that produce recognizable clinical and/or radiographic changes without affecting the structural integrity or hardness of the tooth. These are referred to as changes in the morphology of the teeth. Abnormalities affecting the crown of the tooth are easily recognized because of the unusual clinical appearance of the crown as it is viewed in the oral

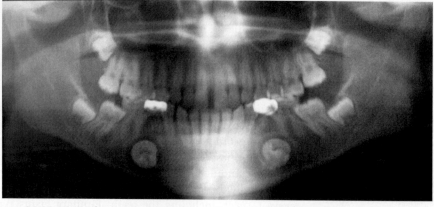
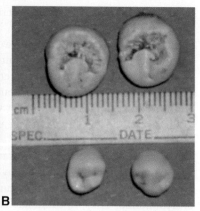

Figure 21.16. Macrodontia. **A.** Panoramic radiograph shows impacted macrodont premolars. Compare macrodont size with size of normal erupted premolars. **B.** Extracted specimens from "**A**" allow measurable comparison of size of macrodonts compared to normal mandibular premolar teeth.

cavity. Abnormalities affecting the roots of the teeth generally require radiographic analysis for recognition.

ABNORMALITIES AFFECTING THE CROWNS OF TEETH

Shovel-Shaped Incisors

Shovel-shaping of the incisor teeth is an aberration that is of no clinical significance and can go completely unrecognized without adverse consequences. The affected teeth show markedly thickened mesial and distal marginal ridges that extend apically from the incisal edge, eventually blending into the lingual surface. When the tooth is viewed from above the incisal edge, the lingual surface resembles the blade of a shovel, accounting for the descriptive name applied to this morphologic variation. Characteristic shovel-shaping is depicted in Figure 21.17. The radiographic appearance of the involved teeth is typically unremarkable. Patients with shovel-shaping of the incisor teeth may have

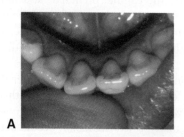
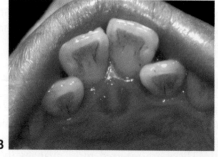

Figure 21.17. Shovel-shaped incisors. **A.** The mandibular incisors show prominent mesial and distal marginal ridges, producing the characteristic shovel shape on the lingual surface. **B.** The maxillary incisor teeth in the same patient.

other associated abnormalities of the teeth. Dens invaginatus and dens evaginatus (see below) are the most commonly reported accompanying abnormalities. The importance of shovel-shaped incisors lies only in its anthropologic implications. Shovel-shaped incisors are seen with increased frequency in East Asian populations, Siberian Eskimos, Alaskan Eskimos, and Native Americans. This distribution of populations affected with shovel-shaped incisors is sometimes cited as evidence of an ancient land bridge spanning the current Bering Sea that allowed Asian populations to migrate and populate the Western Hemisphere.

Accessory Cusps

Accessory cusps are supplementary cusps that alter the expected surface anatomy of a tooth. They are typically nonfunctional and can affect any tooth.

Cusp of Carabelli. The cusp of Carabelli is the best known and most common of the accessory cusps. In fact, it is so common that it is considered part of the normal anatomy of the maxillary first molar tooth in certain populations. It is found as an elevation on the palatal surface of the mesiolingual cusp. It may be very small and rudimentary or it may be prominent enough to produce a groove in the lingual surface of the mesiolingual cusp. When a groove is present, it may predispose the area to the development of a carious lesion. The cusp of Carabelli is also seen frequently on the deciduous second molar tooth, and its presence in the deciduous dentition is a good indication that it will also be seen in the permanent dentition. It is far less frequently found on permanent second and third molar teeth. The prevalence of the cusp of Carabelli is highest in Caucasians, and is rarely reported in Asian populations. Some studies report that it is more common in male patients. The cusp of Carabelli is not normally visualized on radiographic examination.

Talon Cusp. The talon cusp is an accessory cusp that arises from the cingulum area of an incisor or canine tooth. It is markedly elongated to the point that the tip of the elongated cusp may approach the level of the incisal edge of the tooth. The elongated cusp is normally fused to the lingual surface of the affected tooth, producing a three-pronged appearance (Fig. 21.18A). A groove may be present at the points where the accessory cusp fuses with the lingual surface and may dispose the area to development of a carious lesion. This accessory cusp is termed a talon cusp because, when viewed from the incisal aspect, the prominent three-pronged, T-shaped pattern evident on the lingual surface roughly resembles the talon shape seen in the claws of birds of prey. The talon cusp most often affects a single tooth, but bilateral involvement sometimes occurs. The elongated cusp usually contains a pulpal extension, and adjustment of the height of the accessory cusp may result in pulp exposure, necessitating endodontic therapy. Occasionally the length of a talon cusp may interfere with occlusion, blocking the normal overbite relationship of the anterior teeth. Reduction of the talon cusp is necessary in this circumstance. On rare occasions, a talon cusp has been seen to arise from the facial surface of a tooth rather than the lingual side. Because this cusp is quite prominent, it usually produces a characteristic radiographic appearance, with the additional cusp

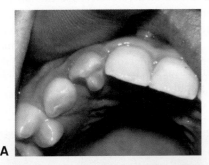

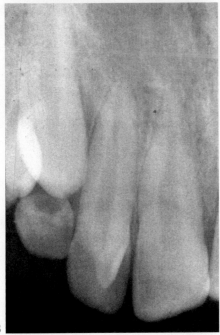

Figure 21.18. Talon cusp. **A.** The right maxillary lateral incisor shows a markedly elongated cingulum cusp, producing the talonlike architecture when viewed from the incisal. **B.** Radiographic features of the talon cusp seen in **A.**

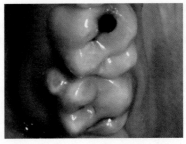

Figure 21.19. Doak's cusp. An accessory cusp is present on the mesiobuccal cusp of the maxillary second molar tooth.

being easily visualized on periapical radiographs as depicted in Figure 21.18B.

Doak's Cusp. Doak's cusp is an accessory cusp that is found on the facial surface of maxillary molar teeth (Fig. 21.19). As with most accessory cusps, an increased incidence of caries may be seen in the groove that often is present at the point where the accessory cusp fuses with the facial surface. A pulp horn normally extends into the cuspal elevation, limiting the ability to reduce the cusp height for restorative or aesthetic purposes. It is often not visualized on radiographic evaluation.

Dens Evaginatus. "Dens evaginatus" is a term used to describe an anomalous cusp that emanates from the central groove on the occlusal surface of posterior teeth as depicted in Figure 21.20. The premolar teeth are affected most often, with molar teeth being only occasionally involved. Mandibular teeth are affected with greater regularity than maxillary teeth. Bilateral involvement is generally the rule. Dens evaginatus is seen with increased frequency in Asians. The accessory cusp may interfere with normal occlusion if it is of sufficient size. It normally contains a pulpal extension, and adjustment of the occlusion requires caution to prevent pulp exposure. It is often difficult to identify this cusp on periapical or panoramic radiographs unless it is first noticed clinically. Shovel-shaping of the incisor teeth is a common accompanying feature.

Gemination

Gemination is defined as the attempt by a single tooth germ to produce two teeth. In the past it was also referred

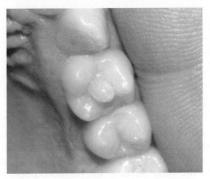

Figure 21.20. Dens evaginatus. An accessory cusp emanates from the central groove in the occlusal table of a maxillary premolar.

to as "twinning" by some researchers. On clinical observation, if the visible crowns are counted, a supernumerary tooth may seem to be present, fused to the adjacent normal tooth. However, radiographic evaluation reveals the diagnostic features. The root canal system, which appears essentially normal within the root area, splits as it ascends toward the crown. Thus, the two crowns appear to arise from a single root, having separate pulp chambers but sharing the same root canal (Fig. 21.21A and B). In many instances both the root and the root canal space may appear slightly enlarged relative to the adjacent unaffected

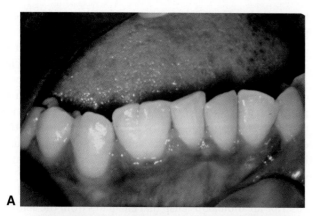

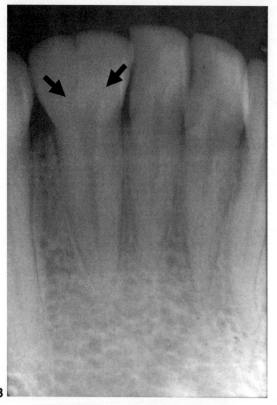

Figure 21.21. Gemination. **A.** The right mandibular lateral incisor appears much larger than the other mandibular incisors and has a prominent groove in the incisal edge that blends into the facial surface. **B.** The radiograph of the right mandibular lateral incisor shows a single root with an attempt to form two crowns. Note the splitting of the pulp in the coronal area.

teeth. The maxillary incisors are the most commonly affected teeth. The incidence of gemination decreases dramatically from anterior to posterior, with gemination involving the molars being basically nonexistent. In the deciduous dentition, the mandibular incisors are more commonly involved than the maxillary. There does appear to be a hereditary tendency in the incidence of gemination.

Fusion

Fusion occurs when tooth buds develop in such close proximity that contact occurs as the dentinal matrix is formed and calcified. The crowns of the two teeth are found to be inextricably joined by the shared dentin. On clinical observation, when counting the number of visible crowns, a tooth appears to be missing. Again, radiographic evaluation reveals the diagnostic features. Two complete root complexes, each containing a separate root canal system, are present. The two roots merge as they ascend occlusally, producing a single composite crown. Typically the root canal systems remain separate within the fused crown structure. Because this abnormality results from the linking of two adjacent normal teeth, the composite crown produced may appear larger than normal and, before radiographic examination, may initially be interpreted as a macrodont (Fig. 21.22). Like gemination, fusion is seen most commonly in the anterior regions of the jaws. In contrast to gemination, however, it is more

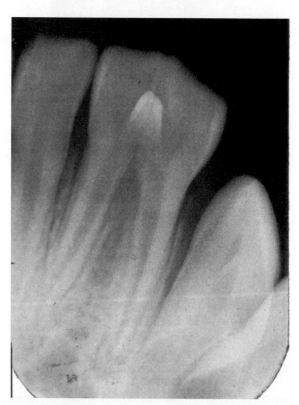

Figure 21.22. Fusion. The mandibular central and lateral incisors are fused. Note two separate root structures with fusion of the crowns of the teeth only.

commonly found in the deciduous dentition than in the permanent teeth.

Congenital Syphilis

Abnormalities in the morphology of the teeth produced by the **venereal** disease syphilis are decidedly rare in the modern era. In the past, particularly prior to the development of antibiotics, these abnormalities were seen with much greater frequency. The tooth abnormalities produced by syphilis are seen only when the infection is passed from the infected pregnant mother to the fetus. This is believed to occur following 4 months in utero. The causative organisms, *Treponema pallidum,* cross the placental barrier at that time. These spirochetes have an affinity for the developing tooth germs and produce distinctive alterations in the shape of the teeth that are developing in the neonatal period. Incisor and first permanent molar teeth are typically affected. In the incisor teeth, the organisms are believed to produce loss of the developing middle mammelon of the incisal edge. At eruption, the tooth is seen to have marked narrowing of the width of the incisal edge, producing a screwdriver shape. The middle portion of the incisal edge is often notched. These teeth are referred to as "Hutchinson's incisors" (Fig. 21.23A).

The first permanent molar also shows severe alteration of the occlusal anatomy of the tooth when it erupts, with the normal five cusp architecture being replaced by an excessive number of small supernumerary cusps on a constricted occlusal table. Because of this "knobby" occlusal pattern, these teeth are referred to as "mulberry molars" (Fig. 21.23B).

The infected child, born into the second stage of syphilitic infection, shows multiple other anomalies that facilitate recognition of the disease. In addition to the tooth abnormalities, deafness due to loss of function of the eighth cranial nerve and opacification of the cornea with loss of eyesight are common manifestations. This constellation of findings is referred to as "Hutchinson's triad."

Lobodontia

Lobodontia is a genetically transmitted disease that is named for the distinctive alteration of crown morphology that it produces. Studies of several afflicted **kindreds** (families) suggest that it is transmitted as an autosomal dominant trait. The teeth appear to be the only structures affected, with no associated abnormalities reported in other body areas or systems. Lobodontia was originally described by Keene and Dahlberg in 1973. They noted multiple anomalies of the dentition that they felt resembled the teeth of a wolf (*lobo,* wolf). Other authors have suggested that the affected teeth resemble those of dogs. The most prominent change seen in the crowns of affected teeth is the elongation of some of the cusp tips while other cusps are reduced in height. The buccal cusps are more commonly elongated, although the molars typically show

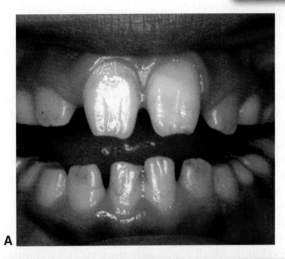

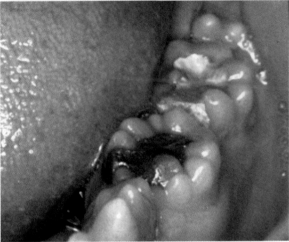

Figure 21.23. Syphilis. **A.** The incisor teeth show narrowing of the width of the incisal edge with a screwdriver-like shape. This feature is termed Hutchinson's incisors. **B.** The molar teeth, despite having been restored, show multiple irregularly distributed small cusps. This feature is termed "mulberry molars." (Both photographs courtesy of Dr. William Binnie.)

multiple affected cusps. The anterior teeth may also show elongation of the cingulum area, and a pit or invagination in the cingulum area often accompanies the elongated cingulum cusp. The elongated cusp tips are often very pointed and almost fanglike in appearance. Generally the teeth are smaller than average. All of the teeth may be affected, or limited involvement of only some teeth may be seen. On radiographic evaluation, additional characteristic features may be noted. The roots of all teeth tend to be narrowed. The molar teeth, rather than being multirooted, have a single, tapering root that also appears narrower than normal and contains a single root canal space. This creates the illusion of an overly large, bulbous crown on top of the tapering root that produces an "ice cream cone" appearance.

Treatment of patients with lobodontia may prove difficult, although the problems are not insurmountable. The elongated cusp tips may contain a correspondingly elongated pulp horn and reduction of the elongated cusps for aesthetic purposes, particularly in the anterior region, may result in pulp exposure and the need for endodontic therapy. Likewise, intracoronal preparations risk pulp exposure. Periapical radiolucent lesions may develop due to the invaginations that are commonly seen in the cingulum area of the anterior teeth. The conical root form of the molar teeth often makes these patients poor candidates for fixed bridge abutments should prosthodontic replacement of teeth become necessary. Otherwise, treatment is routine and is often directed at improvement of the aesthetics.

Globodontia

Globodontia may be confused with lobodontia because of the name similarity, but it is a separate condition. Unlike lobodontia, which affects only the teeth, globodontia is a component of the oculo-oto-dental syndrome, a genetic disease process that produces distinctive abnormalities of other body systems that are consistently present in the affected patients. Oculo-oto-dental syndrome is transmitted as an autosomal dominant disease, and it has been definitively mapped to a specific gene found on chromosome 20 (20q13.1). The findings other than abnormalities of the shape of the teeth that are associated with oculo-oto-dental syndrome include **colobomas** of the iris and retina (absence or defect of some portion of the eye tissues) and progressive sensorineural deafness for high-frequency sounds.

The tooth abnormality associated with oculo-oto-dental syndrome consists of bizarre, greatly enlarged teeth (macrodontia). Interestingly, the condition appears to affect all of the teeth except the incisors. The crowns are decidedly rounded, bulbous, or globelike, accounting for the descriptive name used for this tooth abnormality. The typical fissured anatomy of the occlusal table of the posterior teeth is nearly obliterated, with the occlusal surface having a convex dome-shaped appearance. On radiographic examination, the molar teeth show taurodontism (discussed below). In addition, the pulps of the involved teeth appear larger than usual. Congenitally missing teeth may also be associated with this syndrome.

ABNORMALITIES AFFECTING THE ROOTS OF THE TEETH

Abnormalities affecting the roots of the teeth can be grouped into two categories: (1) abnormalities produced by alterations in Hertwig's epithelial root sheath, the structure that directs the growth and form of the root, and (2) abnormalities produced by overproduction of cementum on the surface of the root. Abnormalities affecting the roots are generally not evident on clinical examination; however, they are detected in the subsequent dental radiographs.

Accessory Roots (Supernumerary Roots)

Accessory roots are a fairly commonly observed irregularity of root form that is sometimes referred to as "supernumerary roots." It is believed to be produced by overprolif-

eration of a segment of Hertwig's epithelial root sheath, resulting in extraneous root formation as shown in Figure 21.24. The molar teeth are the most commonly affected, but it can involve any tooth in either arch. The incidence varies among different races. Accessory roots are an inconsequential finding in most cases. It becomes significant only should endodontic therapy or extraction of the involved tooth become necessary. Since the accessory root is often smaller and thinner than the adjacent roots, locating and obturating the root canal space during endodontic therapy may be more difficult. The small, thin nature of the accessory root also makes it more prone to accidental fracture during extraction of the tooth, producing an increased incidence of complications during such procedures. Because of the reduction in size and overlap with the other roots of the tooth, accessory roots may not be easily visualized on radiographs.

Dilaceration

Dilaceration is defined as a markedly abnormal curvature in the shape of the root (Fig. 21.25). It can affect any tooth and can be seen at any level of the root. It is believed to be caused most often by trauma to the area of the developing tooth that slightly displaces the position of the already calcified portion of the tooth, without affecting Hertwig's root sheath. Pathologic conditions occurring adjacent to a developing tooth have also reportedly produced dilacerations. Teeth exhibiting dilacerations may show a delay or failure of eruption that requires dental intervention. Otherwise, dilaceration is clinically insignificant in most instances. As with accessory roots, however, significant problems can be encountered should endodontic therapy or extraction be necessary in a tooth with a dilacerated root. It has also been suggested that teeth with dilacerated roots may be less desirable for use as an abutment tooth for a fixed bridge or less amenable to orthodontic movement.

Enamel Pearl

Enamel pearls are abnormalities of root formation that are of particular importance for dental hygienists and periodontists. Enamel pearls are likely produced by an abnor-

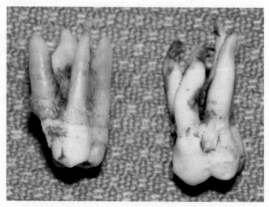

Figure 21.24. Accessory roots. Maxillary molar teeth showing four roots rather than the customary three.

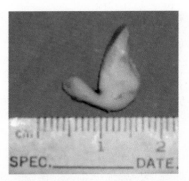

Figure 21.25. Dilaceration. A maxillary lateral incisor showing excessive curvature of the root. There was a history of trauma to the area as a very young child.

mality in Hertwig's epithelial root sheath in which an area of **stellate reticulum** (the middle layer of enamel organ) is retained between the two layers of epithelium that normally comprise the root sheath. The presence of the stellate reticulum allows differentiation of the root sheath cells into ameloblasts, leading to the formation of a small area of enamel on the external root surface. The enamel typically forms as a small, rounded, nodular elevation that produces an area of increased radiopacity on the radiograph. In many instances, a dentin core exists within the nodular elevation, and a pulp horn may also be present. The enamel pearl is most commonly found in the furcation area of molar teeth, but it can occur anywhere along the root surface down to the midroot level. It is rarely encountered in the lower one half of the root. Maxillary teeth are involved more often than mandibular teeth, and Asian populations appear to be affected more commonly than other races. When the enamel pearl occurs in the furcation area, it may disrupt the normal epithelial attachment apparatus in the area, producing a periodontal defect. Periodontal probing of the area reveals an excrescence on the root surface in the area (Fig. 21.26), and the radiograph shows an area of increased opacity, all of which often adds up to the mistaken impression that the periodontal defect is due to calculus deposition. Scaling may be performed in an attempt to remove the adherent material, which is solidly fused to the root surface and cannot be dislodged. Repeated attempts at removal with ever-increasing application of force to the scaler may eventually

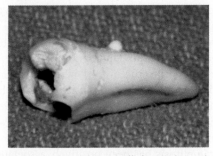

Figure 21.26. Enamel pearl. A small dome shaped nodule is present firmly attached to the root surface. Note the bright white surface of the nodule has the same color and translucency as the enamel on the crown.

result in breakage of the instrument. Once recognized as an enamel pearl, treatment may prove problematic when it is present in the furcation area. Surgical removal may be deemed necessary to correct the periodontal problem but may result in pulp exposure if a pulp horn is present within the core of the enamel pearl. In such situations, endodontic therapy may become necessary.

Taurodontism

Taurodonts are believed to occur because of a failure of proliferation of that portion of Hertwig's epithelial root sheath that is responsible for development of the morphologic form of the roots. Since this occurs only in multi-rooted teeth, taurodontism is seen almost exclusively in molar teeth. They are called taurodonts because they show some resemblance to the teeth seen in bulls. The body of the tooth is enlarged at the expense of the roots. The typical cervical constriction in the cementoenamel junction area is reduced or may be entirely absent. This gives the superior portion of the tooth a rectangular appearance on radiographic appraisal. The pulp chamber is enlarged and appears to penetrate more deeply into the root area. The roots are shortened, often markedly so. Three types of taurodont teeth are described. Hypotaurodonts show only slight shortening of the roots with a mild increase in size of the pulp chamber, and the changes may be subtle enough that the condition goes unrecognized. Mesotaurodonts show obvious shortening of the roots with a corresponding increase in size of the pulp chamber, and hypertaurodonts show severe root shortening. Taurodontism primarily affects the permanent teeth. While it may be unilateral in occurrence, it is often seen in a bilaterally symmetrical pattern (Fig. 21.27A–C). Taurodontism has been identified as a component of some genetically based syndromes. Down syndrome is the disease most often noted in association with taurodontism.

Concrescence

Concrescence is a rare abnormality that is similar to fusion. In contrast to fusion, however, the union of the affected teeth is not via the dentin but due to overproduction of cementum on the root surface of two or more teeth that are positioned in close proximity as depicted in Figure 21.28. The teeth therefore tend to be joined in the apical region and the abnormality is discovered on radiographs. In fusion, the crowns tend to be conjoined rather than the roots, allowing rapid recognition and delineation of the two processes. Concrescence occurs most frequently in the posterior regions of the jaws, and the maxilla is affected more often than the mandible. Concrescence normally has little clinical significance unless extraction of the involved teeth becomes necessary.

Hypercementosis

Hypercementosis is defined as excessive production of cementum on the root surface. It may involve only a single tooth, it may affect multiple teeth in the same area, or it

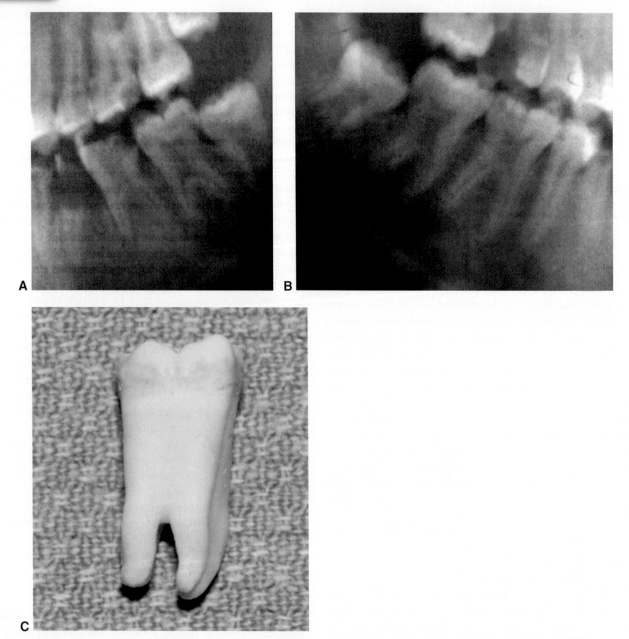

Figure 21.27. Taurodontism. **A.** The left mandibular molar teeth show elongation of the pulp chamber with marked shortening of the roots. **B.** The right mandibular molar teeth in the same patient show similar changes. **C.** An extracted molar showing the general rectangular shape of the elongated pulp chamber.

may be seen in multiple quadrants. When it is seen in multiple quadrants, a metabolic abnormality may be identifiable as the underlying cause. Hypercementosis, if particularly excessive, could eventuate in concrescence, particularly if multiple adjacent teeth are producing excessive amounts of cementum. Clustering of cases in some family groups suggests a hereditary influence in the development of hypercementosis. The apical one third of the root is affected, and the process does not appear to involve other areas of the root without involvement of the apical area. The incidence of hypercementosis increases with aging, and children are rarely affected. The premolar teeth are statistically the most commonly involved. Diagnosis is made via dental radiographs. The root end of the tooth appears enlarged and often is bulbous at the tip. Characteristically, a thin radiolucent rim separates the affected area from the surrounding alveolar bone. This lucent halo blends into the normal periodontal membrane space in those areas of the tooth unaffected by the hypercementosis, indicating that the periodontal membrane is maintained intact around the area of excessive cementum production (Fig. 21.29A and B).

Hypercementosis has been positively associated with a number of disease processes that show alterations in bone metabolism. Paget's disease of bone, acromegaly, and pituitary giantism are included in this group. Paget's disease

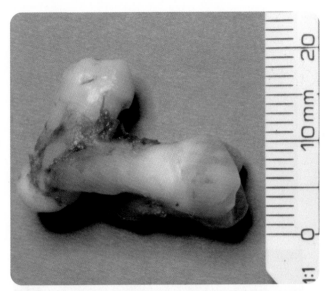

Figure 21.28. Concrescence. The teeth are fused by the cementum of the roots.

in particular has a very strong association, to the point that patients presenting with multiple teeth showing hypercementosis should be sent for serum alkaline phosphatase analysis to rule out Paget's disease. Inflammatory stimulation of the cementum-producing cells of the periodontal ligament may also result in hypercementosis. This is evidenced by the presence of hypercementosis, albeit mild, in a large number of cases of long-standing periapical granuloma. Teeth found to be in traumatic occlusion and, ironically, nonfunctional teeth (teeth without an op-

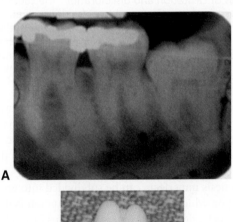

A

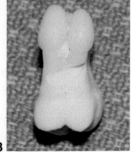

B

Figure 21.29. Hypercementosis. **A.** There is a marked thickening of the cementum around the distal root of the first molar tooth. **B.** Gross specimen of extracted tooth shows thickening of the cementum at the root tip area of a molar.

posing tooth in occlusion) may also show hypercementosis. Hypercementosis is of limited clinical significance and does not compromise normal function in most instances. If extraction becomes necessary, difficulty may ensue, and surgical extraction may be necessary if the degree of hypercementosis is substantial. The dental hygienist must have a good clinical understanding of the features of hypercementosis to distinguish it from cementoblastoma, a true neoplastic proliferation of cementum. In hypercementosis the root maintains its general form, but it is enlarged, and the root tip area can be visualized in the bone. In cementoblastoma, the proliferation of cementum obscures the form of the root which seems to "disappear" into the radiopaque lesion that surrounds the apex area. Thus, the root tip of the involved tooth is not clearly visualized in cementoblastoma.

Alterations in the Structure of Teeth

Defects in the function of the cells that are responsible for the development and calcification of the teeth can result in pathologic conditions. These abnormalities generally affect the structural integrity of the tooth, the hardness of the calcified components of tooth structure, or the normal anatomic arrangement and structural interrelationships of the different layers of the tooth. The affected teeth may appear entirely normal in the shape of the crown and root when viewed clinically in the oral cavity or on radiographic examination. In some instances, however, the alteration in the structure of the calcified components produces clinical and/or radiographic changes that can be visualized as well. Most of the disease processes included in this category have a genetic basis.

Enamel Hypoplasia

Systemic illness, nutritional deficiencies, and environmental factors may produce structural defects of the enamel that are not hereditary but are still considered developmental. These defects are seen only when the associated causative disorder occurs during the period of tooth bud development and calcification.

Any systemic illness that produces a high fever may be implicated. The fever is thought to obstruct the ability of the ameloblastic cells to lay down the organic matrix that serves as the scaffold for enamel calcification. Without the organic matrix, calcification cannot subsequently occur, and the defect is produced. However, only the ameloblasts active at the time of the fever are affected. The defect appears clinically as a line or groove in the enamel surface that runs in an arc shaped pattern roughly parallel to the incisal/occlusal line. Because the fever affects the body as a whole, all the teeth that are developing at that time are affected. Since the crowns of different teeth begin formation at separate ages, they will be at different stages of development when the fever occurs. The hypoplastic defect, therefore, is found at different levels on adjacent teeth. In general, the linear defect appears closer to the incisal/occlusal surface the further posteriorly the teeth are located, with one exception. The first permanent molars begin calcification at birth and hypoplastic defects in these teeth will be found at close to the same level of the crown as seen in the central incisor teeth. A good estimate of the age at which the illness occurred can be made by correlating the position of the defect in the enamel surface with knowledge of the timetable of tooth formation and calcification. In general, teeth with enamel hypoplasia associated with a high fever will not show significant alteration in the overall shape of the teeth.

Malnutrition may cause enamel hypoplasia as a result of the lack of the materials required by the cells to produce the enamel matrix. Alternatively, calcification of adequately formed enamel matrix may be hindered by inadequate calcium, phosphates, or other required elements in the diet. Metabolic disorders that alter the ability to absorb nutrients from the digestive system are also included in this group as causes of enamel hypoplasia. Malabsorption syndromes, liver disease, hypoparathyroid states, and renal disease are all included in this category. The enamel defects seen may vary from very mild to quite severe, depending on the degree of malnutrition present and its duration. If the degree or duration of the malnutrition is substantial, the teeth may show significant alteration of the crown shape in addition to a reduction of the enamel hardness.

Environmental factors that may produce enamel hypoplasia include an array of chemicals and medications. The teeth may be minimally or severely affected, depending on the age of the patient at initiation of therapy, the dose of the agent ingested, and its duration of usage. Changes may range from alterations of surface color or translucency to actual pitting, grooving, or cavitation (Fig. 21.30). Chemotherapeutic drugs used in the treatment of childhood malignancies are implicated in this category, since they inhibit the normal cellular mechanisms involved in matrix deposition and calcification. In some cases of enamel hypoplasia the tooth becomes discolored in addition to exhibiting the enamel deficiencies, and it is the change in color of the tooth that leads to identification of the cause. Fluoride and tetracycline medications are the best known causative agents and are discussed in the section on alteration of the color of teeth. Local trauma and x-radiation are also known factors in producing enamel hypoplasia.

Amelogenesis Imperfecta

In amelogenesis imperfecta, the enamel covering of the crowns of the teeth is found to be defective. The dentin and cementum are not affected. Systemic illness, malnutrition, and environmental factors play no role in its cause; instead, the condition is caused by the defective development of enamel, which has a genetic basis. Enamel development is a three-stage process that begins with enamel matrix depo-

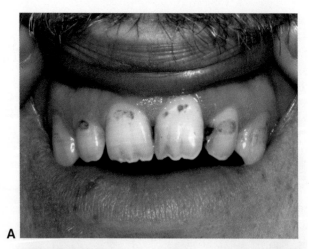

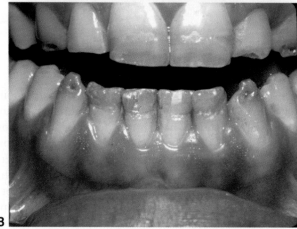

Figure 21.30. Enamel hypoplasia. **A.** The teeth show multiple areas of cavitation and discoloration. The cause of the hypoplasia in this patient could not be determined. **B.** Note the linear groovelike defects at differing levels in the enamel surfaces of multiple teeth. The maxillary central and lateral incisors have been previously restored for aesthetic reasons. The patient gave a history of life-threatening pneumonia with high fever at age 6 months.

sition, transitioning to mineralization of the matrix, and ending with final hardening (maturation) of the enamel layers. Each stage is controlled by separate genetic mechanisms, and a defect in the genetic control at any of the three stages will produce amelogenesis imperfecta. Therefore, amelogenesis imperfecta can be subdivided into groups depending on which stage of enamel production is disrupted by the genetic defect. Numerous variations of amelogenesis imperfecta are known, and the clinical manifestations are so diverse that an entire text could be devoted to describing all of the types that might be seen. For that reason, this discussion emphasizes the general patterns seen in the main subgroups.

The largest of the subgroups is composed of those genetic defects that affect deposition of enamel matrix. Seven separate disorders have been identified in this group. These disorders show a variety of genetic inheritance patterns, with autosomal dominant, autosomal recessive, and X-linked dominant disorders all having been verified. The enamel defects seen in this category are quite varied and may present with localized or generalized pitting of the enamel surfaces, or they may simply manifest as an alteration of the surface color combined with a loss of translucency. In the most severe form of hypoplastic amelogenesis imperfecta, enamel completely fails to form. Luckily this last type is a rare form of amelogenesis imperfecta transmitted as an autosomal recessive trait.

Hypocalcified forms of amelogenesis imperfecta affect the deposition of inorganic elements onto the organic enamel matrix. This is an uncommon form of amelogenesis imperfecta, and only two types have been identified. Both types tend to show diffuse involvement of the teeth. Autosomal dominant and autosomal recessive inheritance are seen in these two forms. Both tend to manifest clinically as a diffuse, mottled color change of the enamel.

The hypomaturation type of amelogenesis imperfecta comprises four separate genetically determined disease processes. Because the defects are limited to the final hardening of the enamel surfaces, the clinical presentation typically shows alterations in the surface color, with loss of translucency of the enamel. Pitting or cavitation is generally not present in the hypomaturation types. Diffuse involvement is generally seen, and two of the genetic patterns produce a distinctive "snow-capped" appearance in the enamel. Autosomal recessive and X-linked recessive inheritance patterns have been confirmed in two of the types. The specific genetic mode of inheritance in the remaining two types has not been definitively proven.

A final group of disorders appears to combine defects in both the deposition of enamel matrix and its maturation once the limited matrix is calcified. Two different types are known, both of which show an autosomal dominant mode of inheritance. Some evidence suggests that the two syndromes may represent two ends of the spectrum of a single disease. Color change in the enamel surface is normally seen, and pitting defects may also manifest. In addition to amelogenesis imperfecta, affected individuals show taurodontism.

Regardless of the stage at which enamel formation is disrupted, the clinical complaints of the affected patients are usually quite similar. Aesthetic concerns are often an early complaint. This is due to the presentation of multiple anterior teeth with significant color variations and/or surface defects. The specific pattern seen depends on the type of amelogenesis imperfecta that is present in the individual patient. Early loss of enamel structure often occurs, with patients noting that the enamel seems to "flake off" the tooth surface. This tends to occur easily, seemingly unprovoked by the patient. Simple chewing may result in loss of portions of the enamel. The use of ultrasonic scaling instruments may produce separation of the enamel in some of the types as well. The problem is manifested in both the deciduous and permanent dentition in most cases. Older patients also often complain that their teeth have come to appear more yellow as they age. This is the

result of continual loss of the whiter, translucent enamel, allowing the underlying duller, yellow color of the dentin to be seen (Fig. 21.31A and B).

The radiographic pattern seen in amelogenesis imperfecta will vary depending on the specific subtype encountered, but in general, the enamel seen on the radiographs appears thinner than normal, and its density more closely approximates that of the dentin in many of the forms. Therefore, no sharp demarcation between enamel and dentin may be evident. Older patients may exhibit complete loss of evidence of enamel.

Treatment of amelogenesis imperfecta normally centers on correction of the aesthetic concerns. Some patients have sensitivity due to loss of the enamel surface with exposure of the underlying dentin.

Dens Invaginatus (Dens in Dente)

Dens invaginatus is also commonly referred to as "dens-in-dente." This accurately describes the anomaly as a

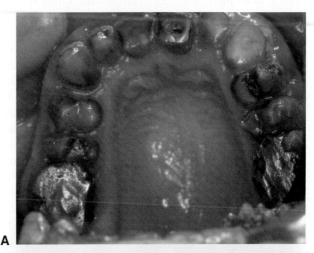

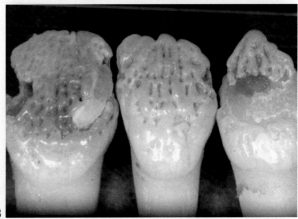

Figure 21.31. Amelogenesis imperfecta. **A.** The enamel has been lost from nearly all the teeth, resulting in a prominent yellowish color of the dentition and more rapid attrition and abrasion. **B.** Another type of amelogenesis imperfecta shows diffuse pitting defects of the enamel surface. Note areas where the enamel has flaked off of the underlying yellow-brown dentin surface. (Both photographs courtesy of Dr. William Binnie.)

tooth forming inside a tooth. It results from an abnormality in the enamel organ that produces an invagination of the enamel surface. While the actual calcified structures of the different layers of the tooth are unaffected, the customary anatomic layering of the enamel and dentin is disrupted. This causes enamel, which is normally found only on the external surface of the crown, to be found internally within the crown substructure in dens invaginatus. The invagination of the enamel surface may be minimal and difficult to recognize either clinically or radiographically. In this situation the affected tooth looks entirely normal morphologically (Fig. 21.32A).

In other instances, the invagination is sizeable, clearly altering the normal tooth shape both on clinical observation and in the dental radiographs. Two types of dens invaginatus are recognized: the more common coronal type and the rare radicular type (Fig. 21.32B and C).

Coronal dens invaginatus is a relatively common abnormality of tooth formation, reported in one study to be present in an incredible 10% of all patients. Other studies report much lower frequencies of occurrence, usually less than 1%. The maxillary lateral incisor is the most commonly affected tooth, and maxillary teeth in general tend to be affected more often than their mandibular counterparts. Molar teeth, regardless of arch, are only rarely involved. Unilateral or bilateral involvement is possible. In occasional instances, the defect is seen in more than one tooth on the same side rather than bilaterally. In teeth that are minimally affected, the area of invagination may not be overtly obvious on clinical examination. It will sometimes be visible as a pit in the enamel surface in an area that would otherwise be expected to be entirely smooth.

In maxillary incisor teeth, this is typically seen on the palatal surface in the cingulum area. The cingulum may even appear enlarged and is sometimes quite prominent. In the more severely affected forms, the cingulum area may be enlarged and elongated to the extent that a talon cusp architecture is manifest. The more severe the invagination of the enamel, the more the normal shape of the tooth is distorted. In its most severe form, the invagination will extend all the way into the root area, often perforating the lateral portion of the root and providing direct communication from the tooth surface into the alveolar bone. In minimally affected teeth the radiographic findings may be decidedly subtle, but in the most severe cases, a characteristic radiographic appearance is present. An area of increased opacity with the same density as the external enamel surface is visible in the central area of the crown and may extend down into the root structure.

Coronal dens invaginatus is clinically significant because in some instances the area of enamel invagination is deep enough to communicate directly with the dental pulp. This causes an opening to arise from the surface of the tooth into the vital portion of the tooth, allowing unimpeded access to the pulp by the microorganisms of the oral cavity. Pulpal necrosis with spread to involve the periapical region ensues, and patients may exhibit large periapical radiolucent lesions without an obvious cause. When the enamel invagination extends very deeply into the root area and perforates the root surface, the pulp chamber and root canal typically are separate from the defect, and the tooth may respond normally to vitality tests. In this situation, the normal pulpal architecture can be

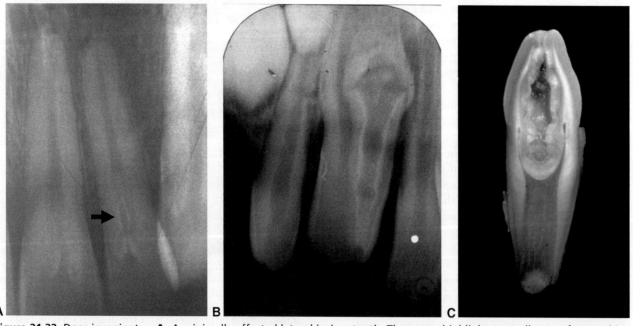

Figure 21.32. Dens invaginatus. A. A minimally affected lateral incisor tooth. The *arrow* highlights a small area of enamel invaginating from a pit in the cingulum area. **B.** A severely affected incisor results in marked deformation of the tooth shape. **C.** A cross section through the tooth shows the invaginating enamel within the crown of the tooth.

seen in a radiograph, with a layer of dentin separating it from the clearly visible, malformed area of the root.

Treatment of coronal dens invaginatus depends entirely on the depth of penetration of the enamel defect, whether or not it communicates with the dental pulp, and whether or not perforation of the root surface is present. If the invaginating defect is shallow and does not penetrate the pulp or perforate the root, simple restoration of the defect is advocated to prevent carious involvement. If the defect is deep enough to involve the dental pulp, endodontic therapy is warranted and may allow retention of the tooth. When root perforation is present, the situation is often very difficult to handle, and attempting conventional root canal therapy on the enamel tract may or may not alleviate the problem. Surgical endodontic therapy often ensues, and ultimately extraction of the tooth may be necessary.

Radicular dens invaginatus is quite rare. While the cause is not known with certainty, it likely represents an invagination arising from proliferation of Hertwig's epithelial root sheath. The defect typically originates on the lateral surface of the root. The enamel formed within the invaginating defect arises from ameloblastic differentiation of the root sheath that is analogous to formation of an enamel pearl. Radiographically, the defect may be difficult to visualize. Radicular dens invaginatus should be suspected though when there is an enlargement of the root without obvious cause. Treatment depends on the location of the defect along the root. If the defect is near the cementoenamel junction, it can become exposed to the oral environment, with resultant severe periodontal problems. In such instances, restoration is possible. When the defect occurs deeper on the root surface, no treatment is usually necessary.

Dentinogenesis Imperfecta (Hereditary Opalescent Dentin)

Dentinogenesis imperfecta is a hereditary disease that, as the name suggests, results in defective dentin formation. The dentin that is formed in patients with this disease has significantly fewer dentinal tubules than normal dentin. The tubules that are present are larger in diameter. In addition, the dentinoenamel junction is less convoluted, which reduces the mechanical retention of the enamel to the underlying dentin. For this reason, loss of enamel structure, which may mimic amelogenesis imperfecta, is a common additional finding in dentinogenesis imperfecta. Dentinogenesis imperfecta shows an autosomal dominant hereditary pattern. Caucasians are disproportionately affected. The deciduous dentition is usually most severely affected, but the permanent teeth are invariably involved as well. In the permanent dentition, the later in life the teeth begin development, the less severe are the effects. Second and third molar teeth thus may show little evidence of the disease in some patients.

The characteristics of the teeth in individuals with dentinogenesis imperfecta are distinguishing. They appear discolored, usually in shades of brown to gray, and they

have a distinctive, almost silvery sheen in the early stages of the disease (Fig. 21.33A).

As enamel is lost from the surface, the dentin becomes more clearly visualized and the teeth have a yellow color. A thin, white-to-gray "outline," representing areas of retained enamel, is often present around the exposed yellow dentin. Since dentin is softer and less resistant to wear than enamel, once it becomes exposed, the teeth may show pronounced attrition, with loss of vertical dimension of occlusion. The radiographic appearance is also quite distinctive. The crowns appear bulbous because of a constriction at the cementoenamel junction area (Fig. 21.33B). Enamel may or may not be visualized covering the crown on the radiographs, depending on the degree of loss of the enamel already experienced. Quite characteristically, the pulp chambers and root canals are absent or greatly reduced in size. This is believed to result from excessive production of secondary dentin that obliterates the pulp tissue.

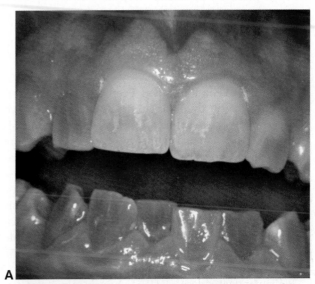

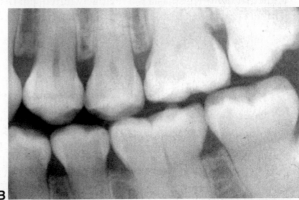

Figure 21.33. Dentinogenesis imperfecta. A. Clinical appearance of the teeth with markedly brown, opalescent appearance. The maxillary central incisors had previously been restored for aesthetic reasons. **B.** FA bitewing radiograph reveals the bulbous nature of the crowns, with constriction at the cervical neck of the tooth and obliteration of the pulp chambers and root canals.

The secondary dentin formation is stimulated by direct exposure of dentinal surfaces to the oral environment as a result of early enamel loss. The sclerotic changes in the pulp tissue may result in pulpal necrosis, eventuating in a periapical radiolucency without an obvious cause.

Treatment of patients with dentinogenesis imperfecta can be problematic. The loss of enamel may necessitate restoration of the teeth, but intracoronal restorations are often poorly retained. Crown coverage of involved teeth has also been advocated but predisposes the restored teeth to root fracture. If periapical inflammatory lesions occur, conventional root canal procedures may not be an option because of the obliteration of the pulp chambers and root canals, and surgical endodontic therapy may become necessary instead.

The dental changes associated with dentinogenesis imperfecta may be the only abnormality seen in a patient, but a large number of patients with these changes will prove to have an associated systemic disease of bone known as osteogenesis imperfecta. While the dental changes seen in these two disease processes are essentially identical, genetic analysis indicates that they are entirely separate diseases.

Dentinal Dysplasia ("Rootless Teeth")

The name "dentin dysplasia" actually is applied to two disorders of tooth development, both of which result in alterations in the structure of dentin. These two forms are sublabeled (1) radicular dentin dysplasia (dentin dysplasia, type I) and (2) coronal dentin dysplasia (dentin dysplasia, type II). Neither of these two types is normally associated with dentinogenesis imperfecta or osteogenesis imperfecta. Certain other systemic diseases have been associated with tooth abnormalities that can closely mimic dentinal dysplasia. These diseases all seem to have one thing in common—a disruption in calcium control.

Radicular dentin dysplasia is a relatively infrequent disorder that shows an autosomal dominant pattern of transmission. It affects only the formation of the root by inducing disorganization in the deposition of the root dentin. When present in its most severe form it produces an immediately recognizable radiographic picture consisting of a normally developed crown with minimal or no root formation. For this reason, the disorder is sometimes referred to as "rootless teeth." A range of affectation may be seen however, and the classic radiographic features are not present in all instances. In many cases the disorder may be recognized by roots that appear somewhat shorter and more tapered than normally expected combined with an abnormality in the shape of the pulp chamber and an absence of root canals. In its mildest form the root length is within normal range, and the only indication of the disease may be the existence of a large pulp stone in the pulp chamber. Variation in the time of onset of the disease most likely accounts for the range in severity of root affectation. If the onset of the disease occurs very early in the cycle of root development, the roots will be severely shortened. If it occurs very late, the root will approach normal size (Fig. 21.34A and B).

As with dentinogenesis imperfecta, the deciduous dentition is more severely affected than the permanent teeth. In the permanent dentition, considerable variability in the degree of involvement of the teeth may be seen within the same individual. One or only a few teeth may show evidence of the disease, with the remainder appearing normal radiographically. However, the entire dentition may be uniformly affected. Clinically, the teeth appear normal when visualized intraorally. Early and otherwise unexplainable mobility is a common presenting symptom, and the diagnosis is subsequently established when radiographs of the loose teeth are made. Premature loss of teeth, both deciduous and permanent, is also commonly cited as a presenting symptom in the most severe forms of radicular dentin dysplasia. The pulp chamber assumes a characteristic form in those teeth that have a shortened but sustainable root length, and it is described as a cres-

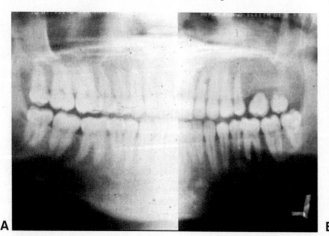 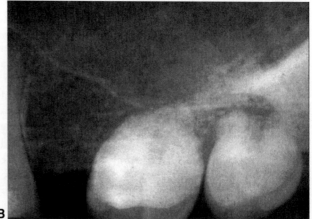

A   **B**

Figure 21.34. Dentin dysplasia. **A.** A local area of involvement in the left maxilla is present. The first molar had been lost several years previously due to excessive mobility. **B.** A periapical radiograph of same patient as in **A** shows the almost complete lack of root development associated with the involved molar teeth.

cent-shaped lucency in the area of the cementoenamel junction. The root apical to the crescent-shaped lucency appears uniformly calcified without evidence of a root canal space. Due to the disorganization of dentin deposition with obliteration of the root canals, pulpal necrosis may occur with development of a periapical radiolucent lesion with no apparent cause. In affected teeth that have a nearly normal root length, the disorder is difficult to recognize and may go undiagnosed. The pulp chamber may appear normal in size. Notably, a large pulp stone is present in the pulp chamber, usually at the point where it funnels into the root canal area. The root appears bulbous in this region, but the enlargement is isolated to the area that surrounds the stone.

Treatment of radicular dentin dysplasia may be problematic, as there is little satisfactory recourse when root length is severely compromised. Extraction may be necessary if spontaneous loss of the involved teeth does not occur. Because of the extreme disorganization of the dentin and the lack of a negotiable root canal system, conventional endodontic therapy is often not a viable option. Creation of a canal space using rotary instruments with subsequent conventional endodontic filling has been attempted with some success. If the root length is sufficient and it is expected that the tooth can be retained, surgical endodontic therapy may also be an option, particularly in the presence of periapical pathosis.

Coronal dentin dysplasia shows many features in concert with dentinogenesis imperfecta, except that it appears to affect only the deciduous teeth significantly. Minimal changes are noted in the permanent dentition. The disease follows an autosomal dominant pattern of inheritance. The deciduous teeth have a brown-to-gray discoloration of the crown, with an opalescent sheen similar to that seen in dentinogenesis imperfecta. There is a constriction of the tooth at the cementoenamel junction area that makes the crown appear bulbous on radiographs. The pulp chambers and root canals are obliterated prematurely, but root length is not altered as it is in radicular dentin dysplasia. However, the roots may appear thinner than expected. Therefore, an original misinterpretation of the abnormality as dentinogenesis imperfecta is not unexpected. With eruption of the permanent teeth, that diagnosis becomes suspect. The permanent teeth are normal in color, do not show cervical constriction, and the pulp chamber and root canal spaces can be visualized on the radiographs. In fact, in contrast to dentinogenesis imperfecta, the pulp chamber typically appears enlarged and mimics the pattern seen in taurodontism. The pulp chamber extends apically into the superior portion of the root, creating a radiolucent area that is larger than expected for the involved tooth. The lucent pulp chamber is often described as rectangular to flame-shaped. Pulp stones may be seen within the enlarged pulp chamber.

Treatment of coronal dentin dysplasia is generally less problematic than that involved with radicular dentin dys-

plasia. The same problems encountered for dentinogenesis imperfecta are seen in trying to maintain the deciduous dentition, but once the permanent teeth erupt, treatment becomes easier. There is still an increased incidence of periapical inflammatory lesions associated with coronal dentin dysplasia. Since the pulp chambers are not obliterated, conventional endodontic therapy can be performed as needed on the permanent teeth. Pulp stones, if present, may increase the difficulty of conventional endodontic procedures to some degree.

Regional Odontodysplasia ("Ghost Teeth")

Regional odontodysplasia is a developmental abnormality that affects all of the calcified structures of the involved teeth. It does not show a recognizable hereditary pattern of transmission, but instead is believed to be caused by a locally decreased blood supply to the developing tooth buds. This theory accounts for the typical clinical presentation in which several neighboring teeth in a limited region of the jaws are affected. In nearly all instances, the teeth involved are found to receive their blood supply from the same alveolar artery branch. Teeth that receive their blood supply from a different arterial branch but are immediately adjacent to the involved teeth appear entirely normal and unaffected. Without adequate blood supply, the inorganic elements necessary for calcification of the enamel and dentin matrices cannot reach the developing tooth, and the result is a poorly mineralized and incompletely formed tooth. Both clinically and radiographically, the teeth appear deformed. On clinical examination the teeth show an irregular surface with discoloration in shades of gray to brown and may be mistaken for several of the other developmental abnormalities that alter the structure of the teeth. However, the radiographic appearance in regional odontodysplasia is diagnostic and easily recognized. The outline of the crown is irregular, and the pulp chamber appears markedly enlarged. A thin, malformed layer of poorly mineralized dentin is usually present, but it may be difficult to discern on the radiograph. The enamel is equally thin and irregular in outline. The roots are short and poorly formed; the apex is wide open. Thus the overall appearance on radiographic examination is that of a mere phantom of a normal tooth, and the condition is often referred to as "ghost teeth" (Fig. 21.35A and B).

Statistically, the most common area involved with regional odontodysplasia is the anterior maxilla, with the central incisor, lateral incisor, and canine teeth unilaterally being affected. All of these teeth are supplied by the anterior superior alveolar artery, a branch of the internal maxillary artery. Teeth affected with regional odontodysplasia, because of poor root development, often do not erupt. If the deciduous dentition is seen to be affected, their permanent successors are often involved. Most cases are diagnosed in the preteenage years. Involvement occurs more commonly in maxillary teeth than in mandibular teeth. On rare occasions, an apparently normal tooth will

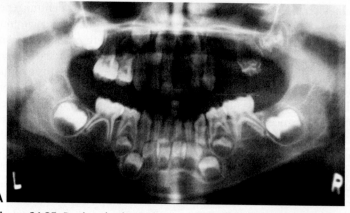
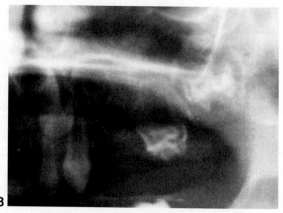

Figure 21.35. Regional odontodysplasia. **A.** The panoramic radiograph shows that the affected teeth are limited to the right posterior maxillary quadrant. **B.** A closeup view of the right maxilla reveals that the premolar and molar teeth are all affected. Note the irregular outlines of the crowns of the molar teeth.

be seen between adjacent teeth affected by regional odontodysplasia. Cases of involvement of both the maxillary and mandibular teeth on the same side have been reported as well as bilateral involvement in the same jaw.

Treatment of teeth affected with regional odontodysplasia is difficult, and ultimately extraction becomes necessary in a large number of cases. The extreme thinness of the enamel and dentin precludes intracoronal restorations or crown preparation in most instances. Endodontic therapy likewise can be difficult if root formation is minimal and the root apex is unformed. Early extraction of the involved teeth should be avoided, however, since the presence of teeth is necessary for normal growth and development of the bone of the alveolar process. Therefore, heroic attempts may be made to retain the teeth affected by regional odontodysplasia for as long as possible. Once the patient completes growth, extraction of the teeth with prosthodontic replacement can be accomplished in the later teenage or early adult years.

Vitamin D-Resistant Rickets (Hypophosphatemia)

Vitamin D-resistant rickets is also known as hypophosphatemia. It is a hereditary disease that inhibits the body's ability to control and retain phosphates in the blood, resulting in a metabolic disturbance that affects all the calcified structures in the body. The disease is transmitted as an X-linked dominant trait; thus there are an excess number of females affected because it is thought that most males that inherit the defective gene die in utero, at birth, or shortly thereafter. The clinical manifestations closely resemble those seen in classic rickets, a disease produced by inadequate dietary amounts of vitamin D. Unlike classic rickets, however, patients with vitamin D-resistant rickets do not show improvement with vitamin D therapy. Patients tend to be short in stature and commonly show bowing of the legs, due to an inability of the weakened bones to support the body's weight. Serum phosphate levels are also below normal.

As might be expected, vitamin D-resistant rickets also affects the structural relationships of the different parts of the tooth. On clinical observation the teeth may show only subtle evidence of the disease. They appear normal in size, shape, and color. The time of eruption is often delayed. Patients will sometimes present with a dental abscess or other periapical pathology without an apparent cause for death of the pulp tissue. This symptom is directly related to the disease process. The deficiency in calcification involving the dentin results in abnormally extended pulp horns that often reach up to the dentinoenamel junction. Enamel defects, attrition, or shallow carious lesions allow exposure of the pulp horn, with unimpeded ingress of the oral microflora directly into the pulp chamber. Pulpal necrosis with development of a periapical radiolucency ensues. Radiographs may reveal the overelongated pulp horns and allow an accurate diagnosis to be made. The mandibular incisor teeth tend to show the radiographic changes most clearly, and the radiographic picture has been described as a "crow's foot" pulp because of the three-pronged appearance of the pulp horns in these teeth (Fig. 21.36).

Treatment of teeth affected by vitamin D-resistant rickets includes regular follow-up to monitor for periapical lesions. The hardness of the teeth is not affected, and the teeth are not prone to develop carious lesions. Restoration of carious lesions must be performed with great care, as exposure of the elongated pulp horns with routine intracoronal cavity preparation can easily occur. Prevention of carious lesions is therefore of particular concern, and sealants might be considered particularly beneficial for these patients. Endodontic treatment is performed when the teeth become pulpally involved.

Hypophosphatasia

Hypophosphatasia is a hereditary disease that shows a variety of patterns of inheritance. Autosomal dominant and autosomal recessive forms have been identified, with numerous different mutations within the gene linked to production of symptoms of the disease. The autosomal recessive pattern of inheritance shows the most severe effects and manifests earliest in life. The genetic defect alters pro-

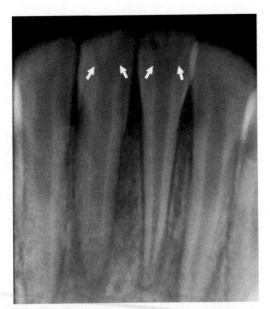

Figure 21.36. Vitamin D-resistant rickets. Pulp horns in the anterior mandibular teeth extend to the incisal edge. *Arrows* point out the "crow's foot" pattern seen in the superior portion of the pulp chamber.

duction of alkaline phosphatase, an enzyme that functions in bone metabolism as well as in numerous other tissues. The patients show defects in bone deposition and calcification. Regardless of the inheritance pattern, the younger the patient is at the onset of the initial symptoms, the more severe the disease tends to be in its overall manifestation. Afflicted individuals tend to be short of stature with bowing of the legs, producing a clinical picture similar to that seen in rickets. The skull fails to calcify completely. Other symptoms are linked to an excessive calcium level in the blood, with calcification in the kidneys being a common complaint.

The dental changes associated with hypophosphatasia are related to the inability of the cells of the periodontal ligament to produce cellular cementum. In the absence of cellular cementum, the periodontal attachment fibers cannot attach to the root surface, resulting in premature loss of teeth. The deciduous dentition in particular is affected. The inability to properly calcify the other layers of the tooth results in teeth with thin enamel and dentin and large pulp chambers. Radiographically, these teeth may appear as a shell of their normal form.

Dental treatment of patients with hypophosphatasia can be a challenge. The absence of cellular cementum makes retention of the teeth in the alveolus difficult, and the only option for treatment often is replacement of lost teeth with removable appliances. Because of the defect in bone formation, the alveolar ridges may show incomplete development, further hampering prosthodontic rehabilitation.

Alterations in the Color of Teeth

The color of the teeth may be altered by adherence of pigmented materials to the external surface. In this situation, scaling of the teeth will allow relatively simple removal of the pigment, and the underlying normal tooth color will be restored, allowing easy recognition that the condition is caused by an external concretion. The products of cigarette, cigar, or pipe smoking are the most common external pigments encountered. As discussed above, alterations in the structure of the enamel and dentin may also produce color changes in the teeth. Lastly, incorporation of pigments into the calcified portions of the tooth or spillage of blood into the dentinal tubules may result in a color change. In these situations cleaning, scaling, or polishing of the teeth will not remove the pigmentation, identifying it as a permanent intrinsic stain.

Fluorosis

Fluorosis was one of the earliest recognized conditions to produce an unsightly color change in the teeth. It was first perceived as a significant finding in communities in Colorado and was originally referred to as "Colorado brown stain" because of the typical color exhibited by the affected teeth. Detailed study of several populations affected revealed that the condition was caused by an excess quantity of fluoride in the drinking water. The extent of involvement was found to depend entirely on the total concentration of fluoride in the water, with severe effects routinely found when the fluoride levels exceeded 5 parts of fluoride per million parts of water. Lesser quantities of fluoride produced less discoloration, with levels of 1 part per million usually showing no deleterious effects on the color of the teeth. At lower fluoride concentrations, the color alteration is often found to be patchy. Enamel hypoplasia will accompany the brown discoloration at very high fluoride levels, with visible pitting of the enamel surface. A chalky surface with loss of translucence due to enamel hypoplasia is present at lower concentrations of fluoride (Fig. 21.37). Many other areas in the United States have also been found to have natural fluoride levels

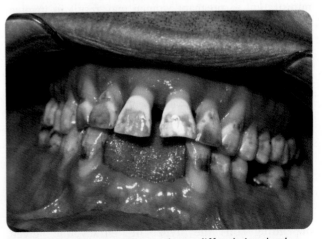

Figure 21.37. Fluorosis. The teeth are diffusely involved. Note areas of chalky white enamel that lack the typical luster of enamel alternating with areas of yellow-brown discoloration. The patient grew up in West Texas in an area of high natural fluoride concentration in the water.

exceeding 1 part per million; therefore, the problem is not limited to Colorado.

Interestingly, the teeth affected with fluorosis were found to have fewer caries than teeth without fluorosis. Even in the presence of enamel hypoplasia associated with very high levels of fluoride, an increase in carious lesions did not accompany the problem. Eventually, fluoride was proven to protect against the development of caries when present in sufficient concentration. Today, many toothpastes contain fluoride as an anticaries additive. In addition, most communities in the United States supplement their drinking water supply with fluoride, maintaining a level of approximately 1 part per million, as a public health initiative to prevent tooth decay.

Since teeth affected by fluorosis show lower carious activity, these patients tend to have fewer treatment needs overall. The discoloration is a major aesthetic problem for many patients, however. In the past, vital bleaching of the anterior teeth was often attempted to try to lighten the brown discoloration and improve the appearance, with quite variable results depending on the degree of involvement. For the most severely involved, crowning of the anterior teeth was often the only solution. Today, porcelain veneers offer a distinct improvement in the options available to patients with fluorosis.

Tetracycline Staining

Tetracycline is an antibiotic medication developed in the mid-20th century. Tetracycline was useful because it seemed to penetrate into bone better than penicillin, therefore, it was used as the drug of choice by many practitioners for infections involving bone. After its usage became more widespread and it was being increasingly prescribed for children, it became known that the tetracycline was also incorporated into any teeth that were undergoing calcification at the time that the medication was administered. Tetracycline can cross the placental barrier, and administration to pregnant women may result in involvement of the deciduous teeth of the developing infant. The affected teeth show a distinctive yellow-to-brown discoloration (Fig. 21.38A). The degree of involvement of the teeth was found to depend on the age at which the medication was administered, the dosage given, and the length of time the medication was taken. High doses of tetracycline also produced enamel hypoplasia because the incorporation of tetracycline disrupted the normal hydroxyapatite crystal structure of the enamel. Because of the deleterious effects on the teeth, the use of tetracyclines is now discouraged in pregnant women and in children under 8 years of age.

The color of the affected teeth was also found to vary, depending on the type of tetracycline given. Oxytetracycline tends to produce a yellow discoloration while chlortetracycline generates a gray-brown color. Minocycline, a newer synthetic preparation, produces a green to gray to black color (Fig. 21.38B,C) and has been reported to produce discoloration of the teeth even after they are fully formed.

When viewed under ultraviolet light, teeth that have tetracycline incorporated into their crystalline structure will fluoresce a yellow to yellow-green color. As stated above, with the recognition of the deleterious aesthetic effects of the use of tetracycline in children, its administration was significantly curtailed to the point that severe tetracycline staining of the teeth is not commonly seen today. Tetracycline is still used quite often in the teenage years to treat severe forms of acne. In many instances, the roots of the teenager's teeth are still forming when the tetracycline is administered. The fact that tetracycline was taken may be evident at the time of extraction of the wisdom teeth, when a bright yellow tetracycline ring is seen in the roots of the extracted third molars (Fig. 21.38D). However, if this acne treatment is instituted slightly too early and the roots in the area of the cementoenamel junction are still forming, the tetracycline discoloration may be seen as a dark area visible through the translucent free gingival margin at the neck of the tooth (Fig. 21.38C). This is particularly problematic with minocycline, which tends to produce a much darker discoloration of the tooth structure.

Hemolytic Anemia and Erythroblastosis Fetalis

Hemolytic anemia is defined as a systemic condition in which there is excessive and premature destruction (hemolysis) of red blood cells throughout the circulation. Hemolytic anemia can be produced by a variety of medical conditions, and a complete medical workup is often necessary to determine the specific cause. Conditions that are known to cause hemolytic anemia may be grouped into two categories: (1) systemic conditions that destroy red blood cells and (2) functional defects within the red blood cells themselves. Systemic conditions include overwhelming infections, toxins (cobra venom, brown recluse spider venom), enlargement of the spleen, chronic liver disease, hematologic malignancies such as leukemia and lymphoma, certain vitamin deficiencies (folic acid, vitamin B_{12}), some autoimmune diseases (specifically lupus erythematosus), and transfusion reactions. Functional defects of the red blood cells include hereditary diseases that affect the shape of the red blood cells (e.g., spherocytosis, ellipsocytosis), disorders of hemoglobin (e.g., sickle cell disease, thalassemia), and enzyme deficiencies (e.g., glucose-6-phosphatase deficiency).

Changes in the color of the teeth are produced by breakdown products of the destroyed red blood cells. Breakage of blood vessels within the dental pulp allows spillage of the hemolyzing red blood cells into the dentinal tubules. Degeneration of the spilled red blood cells results in eventual degradation to hemosiderin, a brown pigment that in sufficient quantity can appear black. Since the degenerating red cells are within the dentinal tubules and cannot be phagocytized and removed, the brown-to-black discoloration is permanent and may be seen through

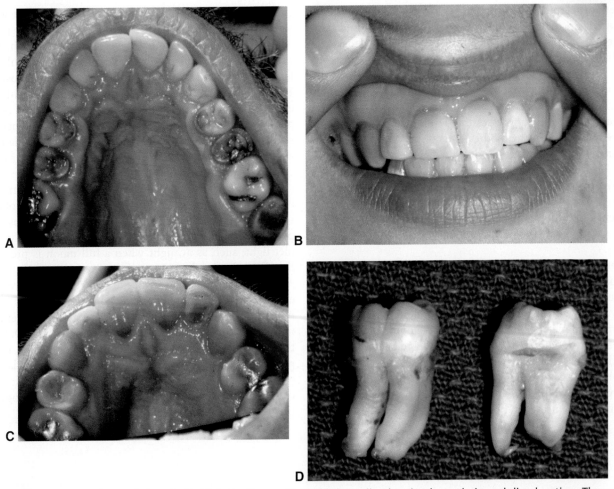

Figure 21.38. Tetracycline staining. **A.** Multiple teeth are affected bilaterally, showing hypoplasia and discoloration. The patient took tetracycline for a prolonged period about age 5. Note that the first molar teeth, which complete crown formation prior to that age, are not affected. **B.** There is discoloration at the cervical neck area of the central incisor teeth. The patient had a history of minocycline administration. **C.** Palatal view of same patient as in **B** reveals more clearly the dark brown staining associated with minocycline. **D.** A bright yellow tetracycline ring is seen in the midroot area of these extracted third molar teeth. The patient took tetracycline for treatment of acne as a teenager.

the overlying translucent calcified layers. In addition, hemolytic anemia results in accumulation of bilirubin in the blood. Bilirubin is another breakdown product of red blood cell hemolysis. At elevated levels in the blood, it can be deposited in the calcified structure of teeth that are developing at the same time, producing a permanent blue-to-black discoloration. Adults tend to be most commonly affected by hemolytic anemia. Because the pulp chambers are often reduced in size in adults due to gradual deposition of secondary dentin, the discoloration associated with hemolytic anemia in this population is most often noted at the cervical areas of the teeth, which show a brown-to-black hue that may resemble the pattern seen in minocycline staining.

In the past, perhaps the most common manifestation of the hemolytic anemias was a condition termed erythroblastosis fetalis. The cause of this condition was found to be an incompatibility of the blood type of a developing fetus with the blood type of the mother. The mother's blood type was found to be Rh negative. The affected child was typically the second child born to the mother. The blood type of the firstborn child proved to be Rh positive, and the mother developed antibodies against Rh-positive blood at the time of delivery of the first child when the blood of the Rh-positive baby was mixed with her own. On becoming pregnant a second time, the blood of the second child, also Rh positive, is attacked by the previously developed antibodies in the mother's blood, which cross the placental barrier and produce widespread hemolysis in the baby. The breakdown of red cells causes an excess of circulating bilirubin in the blood, with deposition into the calcified tooth structures of the developing teeth. This produces pigmentation of the teeth that is analogous to the process in the other hemolytic anemias. In erythroblastosis fetalis, however, only the deciduous dentition is involved, and the pigmentation is severe, with all the crowns of the teeth being diffusely discolored. The discoloration may vary from green to blue to brown to black. An additional finding in erythroblastosis fetalis is a hypoplastic line in the enamel surface in the area of the teeth developing at the time of hemolysis. This is typically present on the deciduous canine or molar teeth and has been called the "Rh hump." Presently, erythroblastosis fetalis is rarely seen. Prenatal testing of the fetal blood type in Rh-negative mothers reveals the incompatibility in blood types in the first pregnancy and antiantigen gamma globulin is administered to the mother at delivery. The gamma globulin suppresses the development of Rh-positive antibodies in the mother's blood, preventing a future hemolytic crisis in subsequent pregnancies.

Treatment of teeth affected by hemolytic anemia is usually unnecessary unless there is significant visible discoloration that causes aesthetic concerns. It that case treatment typically involves restorative procedures directed at masking the areas of discoloration.

Porphyria (Congenital Erythropoietic Porphyria)

Congenital erythropoietic porphyria is a rare genetically transmitted disease. It is inherited as an autosomal recessive trait, with the defective gene producing a disorder in porphyrin metabolism. Porphyrins are an integral component of hemoglobin and are found in large quantity in the red blood cells. The genetic defect causes increased synthesis and excretion of porphyrins. Uroporphyrins, a byproduct of porphyrin metabolism, accumulate in the skin, blood, urine, and other body tissues. Deposition oc-

curs in the bone and teeth as well. Patients present with significant photosensitivity because the sun's rays react with the uroporphyrins that have been deposited in the skin. This results in the development of vesiculobullous lesions of the skin, even with only minimal sun exposure. The large blisterlike lesions rupture and then heal with increased pigmentation, scarring, and mutilation. A compensatory response of the body is hirsutism and hypertrichosis—an increased proliferation and growth of hair in an attempt to protect the skin surfaces from further exposure to the damaging rays of the sun.

Oral findings in congenital erythropoietic porphyria include a reddish brown to gray to black discoloration of the teeth, depending on the quantity of uroporphyrins deposited in them. When these teeth are exposed to ultraviolet light, such as at night when a full moon is present, they fluoresce bright red.

As an autosomal recessive trait, congenital erythropoietic porphyria tends to occur in population groups with limited diversity, in which the recessive gene is present in more individuals than in the general population. During the 19th century, in several isolated areas of Europe, such population groups were known to exist. The constellation of findings associated with congenital erythropoietic porphyria may be responsible, therefore, for the mythology of the werewolf that originated from these locales.

SUMMARY

- This chapter details the various pathologic processes that affect the hard structures of the teeth.
- Pathology involving the teeth can be subdivided into those conditions that occur following normal growth and development of the teeth (postdevelopmental abnormalities) and those processes that occur during the period of tooth formation (developmental abnormalities). The developmental conditions are by far the most numerous.
- Postdevelopmental pathology typically produces obvious changes in the appearance of the tooth, either clinically

or on radiographic examination, and normally manifests as a loss of tooth structure.
- While pathologic changes in the teeth of developmental etiology also normally produce some change in the appearance of the tooth, in a number of the developmental abnormalities the teeth may appear entirely normal on clinical evaluation.
- Developmental defects in the teeth can affect the number of teeth, the size of teeth, the shape of the teeth, the structural makeup of the teeth, or the color of the teeth.

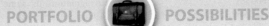

PORTFOLIO POSSIBILITIES

- Construct a patient education sheet for the parents of children who reside in an area where fluoride is not routinely added to the water supply, and the dentist may want to prescribe fluoride supplements for the children to decrease caries incidence. Include facts about the potential for tooth discoloration with excess fluoride and the need to strictly follow the dentist's or hygienist's instructions regarding dosage and frequency of administration.
- Develop an educational fact sheet that details the aesthetic restorative options available for patients with unaesthetic discoloration of the teeth. List the advantages and disadvantages for each restorative method suggested (whitening kits, in-office bleaching, veneers, crown placement).

- Construct a fact sheet for parents of adolescent children that emphasizes the typical dental changes seen in erosion caused by repeated vomiting associated with eating disorders. Include names and addresses of local resources and facilities that are available to assist in treatment of children with anorexia nervosa and bulimia.
- Create a visual aid (chart, drawing, or diagram) that can be given to parents of young children to illustrate the position of the developing permanent teeth in relation to the overlying deciduous teeth. Using the visual aid, devise a script that explains why early treatment of dental disease in deciduous teeth is important to prevent inflammatory induced enamel hypoplasia in the permanent dentition.

REFERENCES

Abbott PV. Labial and palatal "talon cusps" on the same tooth: a case report. Oral Surg Oral Med Oral Pathol Oral Radiol Endod 1998;85(6):726–730.

Acs G, Pokala P, Cozzi E. Shovel incisors, three-rooted molars, talon cusp, and supernumerary tooth in one patient. Pediatr Dent 1992;14(4):263–264.

Aldred MJ, Crawford PJ. Amelogenesis imperfecta—towards a new classification. Oral Dis 1995;1(1):2–5.

Aldred MJ, Savarirayan R, Crawford PJ. Amelogenesis imperfecta: a classification and catalogue for the 21st century. Oral Dis 2003;9(1):19–23.

Aldred MJ, Savarirayan R, Lamande SR, Crawford PJ. Clinical and radiographic features of a family with autosomal dominant amelogenesis imperfecta with taurodontism. Oral Dis 2002;8(1):62–68.

Alpaslan G, Alpaslan C, Gogen H, et al. Disturbances in oral and dental structures in patients with pediatric lymphoma after chemotherapy: a preliminary report. Oral Surg Oral Med Oral Pathol Oral Radiol Endod 1999;87(3):317–321.

Ansari G, Reid JS. Dentinal dysplasia type I: review of the literature and report of a family. ASDC J Dent Child 1997;64(6):429–434.

Archard HO, Witkop CJ. Hereditary hypophosphatemia (vitamin D-resistant rickets) presenting primary dental manifestations. Oral Surg Oral Med Oral Pathol 1966;22:184–193.

Atasu M, Genc A, Ercalik S. Enamel hypoplasia and essential staining of teeth from erythroblastosis fetalis. J Clin Pediatr Dent 1998;22(3):249–252.

Badger GR. Three-rooted mandibular first primary molar. Oral Surg Oral Med Oral Pathol 1982;53(5):547.

Bentley EM, Ellwood RP, Davies RM. Fluoride ingestion from toothpaste by young children. Br Dent J 1999;186(9):460–462.

Bodin I, Julin P, Thomsson M. Hyperdontia: frequency and distribution of supernumerary teeth among 21,609 patients. Dentomaxillofac Radiol 1978;7:15–17.

Bowles WH. Protection against minocycline pigment formation by ascorbic acid (vitamin C). J Esthet Dent 1998, 10(4):182–186.

Brook AH, Winder M. Lobodontia: a rare inherited dental anomaly. Br Dent J 1979;147(8):213–215.

Burt BA. The changing patterns of systemic fluoride intake. J Dent Res 1992;71(5):1228–1237.

Caliskan MK, Turkun M. Prognosis of permanent teeth with internal resorption: a clinical review. Endod Dent Traumatol 1997;13(2):75–81.

Cangialosi TJ. Management of a maxillary central incisor impacted by a supernumerary tooth. JADA 1982;105(5):812–814.

Cavanha AO. A new rare type of enamel pearl. Oral Surg Oral Med Oral Pathol 1967;23(2):213–214.

Cavanha AO. Enamel pearls. Oral Surg Oral Med Oral Pathol 1965;19:373–382.

Celik E, Aydinlik E. Effect of a dilacerated root on stress distribution to the tooth and supporting tissues. J Prosthet Dent 1991;65(6):771–777.

Cheek CC, Heymann HO. Dental and oral discolorations associated with minocycline and other tetracycline analogs. J Esthet Dent 1999;11(1):43–48.

Chiappinelli JA, Walton RE. Tooth discoloration resulting from long-term tetracycline therapy: a case report. Quintessence Int 1992;23(8):539–541.

Ciola B, Bahn SL, Goviea GL. Radiographic manifestations of an unusual combination types I and type II dentin dysplasia. Oral Surg Oral Med Oral Pathol 1978;45(2):317–322.

Crawford PJ, Aldred MJ. Amelogenesis imperfecta: autosomal dominant hypomaturation-hypoplasia type with taurodontism. Br Dent J 1988;164(3):71–73.

Croll TP. Esthetic correction for teeth with fluorosis and fluorosis-like enamel dysmineralization. J Esthet Dent 1998;10(1):21–29.

Dahllof G, Rozell B, Forsberg C-M, et al. Histologic changes in dental morphology induced by high dose chemotherapy and total body irradiation. Oral Surg Oral Med Oral Pathol 1994;77(1):56–60.

Dankner E, Harari D, Rotstein I. Conservative treatment of dens evaginatus of anterior teeth. Endod Dent Traumatol 1996;12(4):206–208.

Dankner E, Harari D, Rotstein I. Dens evaginatus of anterior teeth. Literature review and radiographic survey of 15,000 teeth. Oral Surg Oral Med Oral Pathol Oral Radiol Endod 1996;81(4):472–475.

Dayan D, Heifferman A, Gorski M, et al. Tooth discoloration—extrinsic and intrinsic factors. Quintessence Int 1983;14(2):195–199.

De Sousa SM, Bramante CM. Dens invaginatus: treatment choices. Endod Dent Traumatol 1998;14(4):152–158.

Duncan K, Crawford PJ. Transposition and fusion in the primary dentition: report of case. ASDC J Dent Child 1996;63(5):365–367.

Duncan WK, Helpin ML. Bilateral fusion and gemination: a literature analysis and case report. Oral Surg Oral Med Oral Pathol 1987;64(1):82–87.

Duncan WK, Perkins TM, O' Carroll MK, et al. Type I dentin dysplasia: report of two cases. Ann Dent 1991;50(2):18–21.

Durr DP, Campos CA, Ayers CS. Clinical significance of taurodontism. J Am Dent Assoc 1980;100(3):378–381.

Eccles JD. Tooth surface loss from abrasion, attrition and erosion. Dent Update 1982;9(7):373–374, 376–378, 380–381.

Elfenbaum A. Unusual brown teeth. Dent Dig 1969;75:20–22.

Eugster EA, Pescovitz OH. Gigantism. J Clin Endocrinol Metab 1999;84:4379–4384.

Fadavi S, Rowold E. Familial hypophosphatemic vitamin D-resistant rickets: review of the literature and report of case. ASDC J Dent Child 1990;57:212–215.

Fayle SA, Pollard MA. Congenital erythropoietic porphyria—oral manifestations and dental treatment in childhood: a case report. Quintessence Int 1994;25:551–554.

Gallant CM. Inverted mesiodens. Dent Radiogr Photogr 1980;53(2):31.

Gartner AH, Mack T, Somerlott RG, et al. Differential diagnosis of internal and external root resorption. J Endod 1976;2(11):329–334.

Geist JR. Dens evaginatus. Case report and review of the literature. Oral Surg Oral Med Oral Pathol 1989;67(5):628–631.

Goldman HM. Anomalies of teeth (part I). Compend Contin Educ Dent 1981;2(6):358–367.

Goldman HM. Anomalies of teeth (part II). Compend Contin Educ Dent 1982;3(1):25–33.

Goldstein AR. Enamel pearls as contributing factor in periodontal breakdown. J Am Dent Assoc 1979;99(2):210–211.

Gorlin RJ. Otodental syndrome, oculo-facio-cardio-dental (OFCD) syndrome, and lobodontia: dental disorders of interest to the pediatric radiologist. Pediatr Radiol 1998;28(10):802–804.

Gound TG, Maixner D. Nonsurgical management of a dilacerated maxillary lateral incisor with type III dens invaginatus: a case report. J Endod 2004;30(6):448–451.

Gound TG. Dens invaginatus—a pathway to pulpal pathology: a literature review. Pract Periodont Aesthet Dent 1997;9(5):585–594.

Grippo JO, Simring M. Dental 'erosion' revisited. J Am Dent Assoc 1995;126(5):619–620, 623–624; 627–630.

Grippo JO. Abfractions: a new classification of hard tissue lesions of teeth. J Esthet Dent 1991;3(1):14–19.

Grover PS, Lorton L. Gemination and twinning in the permanent dentition. Oral Surg Oral Med Oral Pathol 1985;59(3):313–318.

Hattab FN, Yassin OM, Al-Nimri KS. Talon cusp in permanent dentition associated with other dental anomalies: review of literature and reports of seven cases. ASDC J Dent Child 1996;63(5):368–376.

Heimler A, Sciubba J, Lieber E, et al. An unusual presentation of opalescent dentin and Brandywine isolate hereditary opalescent dentin in an Ashkenazic Jewish family. Oral Surg Oral Med Oral Pathol 1985;59(6):608–615.

Heller KE, Eklund SA, Burt BA. Dental caries and dental fluorosis at varying water fluoride concentrations. J Public Health Dent 1997;57(3):136–143.

Hillmann G, Geurtsen W. Pathohistology of undecalcified primary teeth in vitamin D-resistant rickets: review and report of two cases. Oral Surg Oral Med Oral Pathol Oral Radiol Endod 1996;82:218–224.

House RC, Grisius R, Bliziotes MM, et al. Perimolysis: unveiling the surreptitious vomiter. Oral Surg Oral Med Oral Pathol 1981;51(2):152–155.

Hulsmann M. Dens invaginatus: aetiology, classification, prevalence, diagnosis, and treatment considerations. Int Endod J 1997;30(2):79–90.

Hyman JL, Cohn ME. The predictive value of endodontic diagnostic tests. Oral Surg Oral Med Oral Pathol 1984;58:343–346.

Imfeld T. Dental erosion. Definition, classification and links. Eur J Oral Sci 1996;104(2-Pt 2):151–155.

Joshi N, Parkash H. Oral rehabilitation in dentinogenesis imperfecta with overdentures: case report. J Clin Pediatr Dent 1998;22(2):99–102.

Kalk WW, Batenburg RH, Vissink A. Dentin dysplasia type I: five cases within one family. Oral Surg Oral Med Oral Pathol Oral Radiol Endod 1998;86(2):175–178.

Kelleher M, Bishop K. Tooth surface loss: an overview. Br Dent J 1999;186(2):61–66.

Kessler HP, Kraut RA. Dentigerous cyst associated with an impacted mesiodens. Gen Dent 1989;37(1):47–49.

Kharat DU, Saini TS, Mokeem S. Shovel-shaped incisors and associated invagination in some Asian and African populations. J Dent 1990;18(4):216–220.

Killian CM, Croll TP. Dental twinning anomalies: the nomenclature enigma. Quintessence Int 1990;21(7):571–576.

Kindelan JD, Rysiecki G, Childs WP. Hypodontia: genotype or environment? A case report of monozygotic twins. Br J Orthodont 1998;25(3):175–178.

Kosowicz J, Rzymski K. Abnormalities of tooth development in pituitary dwarfism. Oral Surg Oral Med Oral Pathol 1977;44:853–863.

Lamberts SWJ, de Herder WW, van der Lely AJ. Pituitary insufficiency. Lancet 1998;352:127–134.

Lee WC, Eakle WS. Stress-induced cervical lesions: review of advances in the past 10 years. J Prosthet Dent 1996;75(5):487–494.

Leider AS, Garbarino VE. Generalized hypercementosis. Oral Surg Oral Med Oral Pathol 1987;63(3):375–380.

Levitas TC. Gemination, fusion, twinning and concrescence. ASDC J Dent Child 1965;32:93–100.

Llamas R, Jimenez-Planas A. Taurodontism in premolars. Oral Surg Oral Med Oral Pathol 1993;75(4):501–505.

Lykogeorgos T, Duncan K, Crawford PJ, Aldred MJ. Unusual manifestations in X-linked amelogenesis imperfecta. Int J Paediatr Dent 2003;13(5):356–361.

Maragakis GM. Crown dilaceration of permanent incisors following trauma to their primary predecessors. J Clin Pediatr Dent 1995; 20(1):49–52.

Mason C, Rule DC, Hopper C. Multiple supernumeraries: the importance of clinical and radiographic follow-up. Dentomaxillofac Radiol 1996;25(2):109–113.

McCulloch KJ, Mills CM, Greenfeld RS, et al. Dens evaginatus: review of the literature and report of several clinical cases. J Can Dent Assoc 1998;64(2):104–106, 110–113.

McWhorter AG, Seale NS. Prevalence of dental abscess in a population of children with vitamin D-resistant rickets. Pediatr Dent 1991;13:91–96.

Melnick M, Eastman JR, Goldblatt LI, et al. Dentin dysplasia, type II: a rare autosomal dominant disorder. Oral Surg Oral Med Oral Pathol 1977;44(4):592–599.

Morley KR, Tompson BD. The palatally impacted mesiodens. J Can Dent Assoc 1983;49(8):571–574.

Morse DR. Age-related changes of the dental pulp complex and their relationship to systemic aging. Oral Surg Oral Med Oral Pathol 1991;72:721–745.

Moskow BS, Canut PM. Studies on root enamel (2). Enamel pearls. A review of their morphology, localization, nomenclature, occurrence, classification, histogenesis and incidence. J Clin Periodontol 1990;17(5):275–281.

Moss-Salentijn L, Hendricks-Klyvert M. Calcified structures in human dental pulps. J Endod 1988;14:184–189.

Murayama T, Iwatsubo R, Akiyama S, et al. Familial hypophosphatemic vitamin D-resistant rickets: dental findings and histologic study of teeth. Oral Surg Oral Med Oral Pathol Oral Radiol Endod 2000;90:310–316.

Neville BW, Damm DD, Allen CM, Bouquot JE. Oral and Maxillofacial Pathology. 2nd ed. Philadelphia: WB Saunders, 2002.

Nguyen AM, Tiffee JC, Arnold R. Pyramidal molar roots and canine-like morphologic features in multiple family members: a case report. Oral Surg Oral Med Oral Pathol 1996;82:411–416.

O' Carroll MK, Duncan WK. Dentin dysplasia type I. Radiologic and genetic perspectives in a six-generation family. Oral Surg Oral Med Oral Pathol 1994;78(3):375–381.

O' Carroll MK, Duncan WK, Perkins TM. Dentin dysplasia: review of the literature and a proposed subclassification based on radiographic findings. Oral Surg Oral Med Oral Pathol 1991;72(1):119–125.

Oguz A, Cetiner S, Karadeniz C, et al. Long-term effects of chemotherapy on orodental structures in children with non-Hodgkin's lymphoma. Eur J Oral Sci 2004;112(1):8–11.

Olsson A, Matsson L, Blomquist HK, et al. Hypophosphatasia affecting the permanent dentition. J Oral Pathol Med 1996;25:343–347.

Ooshima T, Ishida R, Mishima K, et al. The prevalence of developmental anomalies of teeth and their association with tooth size in the primary and permanent dentitions of 1650 Japanese children. Int J Paediatr Dent 1996;6(2):87–94.

Owens BM, Gallien GS. Noncarious dental "abfraction" lesions in an aging population. Compend Contin Educ Dent 1995;16(6):552, 554, 557–558.

Pajari U, Lanning M. Developmental defects of teeth in survivors of childhood ALL are related to the therapy and age at diagnosis. Med Pediatr Oncol 1995;24(5):310–314.

Payne M, Craig GT. A radicular dens invaginatus. Br Dent J 1990;169(3–4):94–95.

Pindborg JJ. Aetiology of developmental enamel defects not related to fluorosis. Int Dent J 1982;32:123–134.

Plagmann H-H, Kocher T, Kuhrau N, Caliebe A. Periodontal manifestation of hypophosphatasia. A family case report. J Clin Periodontol 1994;21:710–716.

Ranta H, Lukinmaa PL, Waltimo J. Heritable dentin defects: nosology, pathology, and treatment. Am J Med Genet 1993;45(2):193–200.

Regezi JA, Sciubba JJ, Pogrel MA. Atlas of oral and maxillofacial pathology. Philadelphia: WB Saunders, 2000.

Ruprecht A, Batniji S, El-Neweihi E. Double teeth: the incidence of gemination and fusion. J Pedod 1985;9(4):332–337.

Ruprecht A, Batniji S, El-Neweihi E. The incidence of taurodontism in dental patients. Oral Surg Oral Med Oral Pathol 1987;63(6):743–747.

Rushton MA. Anomalies of human dentine. Br Dent J 1955;98(12): 431–444.

Saini TS, Kharat DU, Mokeem S. Prevalence of shovel-shaped incisors in Saudi Arabian dental patients. Oral Surg Oral Med Oral Pathol 1990;70(4):540–544.

Sapp JP, Eversole LR, Wysocki GP. Contemporary oral and maxillofacial pathology. St. Louis: Mosby, 1997.

Schalk-van der Weide Y, Steen WHA, Bosman F. Distribution of missing teeth and tooth morphology in patients with oligodontia. ASDC J Dent Child 1992;59(2):133–140.

Schalk-van der Weide Y, Steen WHA, Bosman F. Taurodontism and length of teeth in patients with oligodontia. J Oral Rehabil 1993;20(4):401–412.

Scheiner MA, Sampson WJ. Supernumerary teeth: a review of the literature and four case reports. Aust Dent J 1997;42(3):160–165.

Scully C, Bagan J-V. Adverse drug reactions in the orofacial region. Crit Rev Oral Biol Med 2004;15(4):221–239.

Sedano HO, Gorlin RJ. Familial occurrence of mesiodens. Oral Surg Oral Med Oral Pathol 1969;27(3):360–361.

Seow WK, Needleman HL, Holm IA. Effect of familial hypophosphatemic rickets on dental development: a controlled, longitudinal study. Pediatr Dent 1995;17:346–350.

Seow WK, Perham S, Young WG, et al. Dilaceration of a primary maxillary incisor associated with neonatal laryngoscopy. Pediatr Dent 1990;12(5):321–324.

Seow WK. Clinical diagnosis and management strategies of amelogenesis imperfecta variants. Pediatr Dent 1993;15(6):384–393.

Seow WK. Enamel hypoplasia in the primary dentition: a review. ASDC J Dent Child 1991;58(6):441–452.

Sim TPC. Management of dens evaginatus: evaluation of two prophylactic treatment methods. Endod Dent Traumatol 1996;12(3):137–140.

Steidler NE, Radden BG, Reade PC. Dentinal dysplasia: a clinicopathological study of eight cases and review of the literature. Br J Oral Maxillofac Surg 1984;22(4):274–286.

Stewart DJ, Kinirons MJ. Globodontia: a rarely reported dental anomaly. Br Dent J 1982;152(8):287–288.

Sutton PR. Double shovel-shaped teeth associated with a supernumerary incisor. Aust Dent J 1973;18(1):32.

Takinami S, Kaga M, Yahata H, et al. Radiation-induced hypoplasia of the teeth and mandible. A case report. Oral Surg Oral Med Oral Pathol 1994;78(3):382–384.

Tanaka T, Murakami T. Radiological features of hereditary opalescent dentin. Dentomaxillofac Radiol 1998;27(4):251–253.

Tatum RC, Fraga A, Saini R, et al. Mesiodens and supernumerary central incisors: early diagnosis and treatment to avoid extensive orthodontic treatment—two cases. Compend Contin Educ Dent 1983;4(3): 271–276, 278.

Thorburn DN, Ferguson MM. Familial ogee roots, tooth mobility, oligodontia, and microdontia. Oral Surg Oral Med Oral Pathol 1992;74(5):576–581.

Tidwell E, Cunningham CJ. Dentinal dysplasia: endodontic treatment, with case report. J Endod 1979;5(12):372–376.

Tonder KJH. Vascular reactions in the dental pulp during inflammation. Acta Odontol Scand 1983;41:247–256.

Tronstad L. Recent development in endodontic research. Scand J Dent Res 1992;100:52–59.

Uyeno DS, Lugo A. Dens evaginatus: a review. ASDC J Dent Child 1996;63(5):328–332.

Van Dis ML, Allen CM. Dentinal dysplasia type I: a report of four cases. Dentomaxillofac Radiol 1989;18(3):128–131.

Vieira H, Gregory-Evans K, Lim N, et al. First genomic localization of oculo-oto-dental syndrome with linkage to chromosome 20q13.1. Invest Ophthalmol Vis Sci 2002;43(8):2540–2545.

Witcop CJ. Hereditary defects of dentin. Dent Clin North Am 1975;19(1):25–45.

Witkop CJ Jr. Amelogenesis imperfecta, dentinogenesis imperfecta and dentin dysplasia revisited: problems in classification. J Oral Pathol 1988;17(9–10):547–553.

Witkop CJ Jr. Partial expression of sex-linked recessive amelogenesis imperfecta in females compatible with the Lyon hypothesis. Oral Surg Oral Med Oral Pathol 1967;23(2):174–182.

Younes SA, Al-Shammery AR, El-Angbawi MF. Three-rooted permanent mandibular first molars of Asian and black groups in the Middle East. Oral Surg Oral Med Oral Pathol 1990;69(1):102–105.

Yusof WZ. Non-syndrome multiple supernumerary teeth: literature review. J Can Dent Assoc 1990;56(2):147–149.

Zhu JF, Marcushamer M, King DL, et al. Supernumerary and congenitally absent teeth: a literature review. J Clin Pediatr Dent 1996;20(2):87–95.

Zvolanek JW, Spotts TM. Supernumerary mandibular premolars: report of cases. JADA 1985;110(5):721–723.

Chapter Objectives

1. List six oral lesions associated with HIV infection.

2. Describe the clinical features of pseudomembranous candidiasis.

3. List two other clinical conditions that should be included in a differential diagnosis of a patient with hairy leukoplakia.

4. Describe the clinical appearance of human papillomavirus lesions within the oral cavity.

5. List the two most common malignancies associated with HIV infection.

6. List the most common location for Kaposi's sarcoma lesions within the oral cavity of an immunocompromised patient.

7. Compare and contrast the clinical appearance and common characteristics of minor versus major aphthous ulcers.

8. List current treatment modalities for the management of patients with recurrent herpetic stomatitis.

9. Describe the clinical features of linear gingival erythema.

10. Discuss the clinical presentation of patients with necrotizing ulcerative periodontitis.

Chapter Outline

Oral lesions are often the first indicators of a potential systemic illness, and as a result, oral healthcare providers are in a unique position to provide initial intervention, diagnosis, and treatment of HIV-related illnesses. Although the overall incidence of oral manifestations related to HIV infection has decreased with the use of highly active antiretroviral therapy (Ives et al., 2001; Patton et al., 2000; Ceballos-Salobrena et al., 2000), oral lesions remain a significant cause of morbidity and mortality in HIV-seropositive patients. Factors that increase the probability of developing oral lesions include CD4 counts less than 200 cells/mm^3, viral load more than 3000 copies/mL, xerostomia, poor oral hygiene and smoking (Tappuni et al., 2001; Aquirre et al., 1999). The following discussion covers the most commonly encountered oral manifestations seen in association with HIV infection.

CANDIDIASIS

Candidiasis is a common intraoral condition that may be the first manifestation of potential HIV infection and is often a recurrent problem in HIV/AIDS patients (Silverman et al., 1996). Intraoral candidiasis is most frequently caused by *Candida albicans*; however, other species may be involved including *C. tropicalis, C. glabrata, C. krusei*, and *C. parapsilosis* (Redding et al., 2000). Oral lesions associated with candidiasis can be classified as pseudomembranous, hyperplastic, or atrophic (erythematous), and may manifest as chronic angular cheilitis.

The pseudomembranous form is characterized by creamy yellow or white, curdlike deposits that may be easily wiped away, exposing red or bleeding surfaces beneath (Fig. 22.1). Patients may complain of a burning sensation or an altered taste sensation, but many patients are asymptomatic. Occasionally, the infection may progress to involve the esophagus, resulting in discomfort, difficulty in swallowing, nausea, chest pain, and weight loss. The hyperplastic form of candidiasis is also white, but the lesions are not easily removed. It occurs as firm white lesions that may be mistaken for hairy leukoplakia when present on the tongue (Fig. 22.2). Erythematous or atrophic candidiasis produces a generalized or patchy erythema that is most frequently observed on the palate and the tongue. Its distribution often follows the pattern of a removable appliance if present (Fig. 22.3). Angular cheilitis affects the corners of the mouth, where patients may complain of cracking, redness, and swelling (Fig. 22.4).

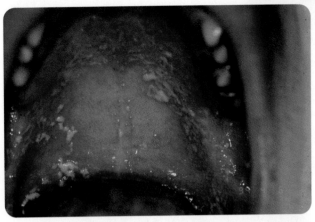

Figure 22.1. Pseudomembranous candidiasis. Yellow, curdlike lesions that rub off easily.

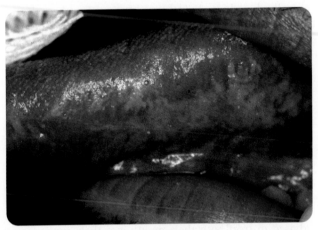

Figure 22.2. Hyperplastic candidiasis. Firm white lesion that is not easily removed.

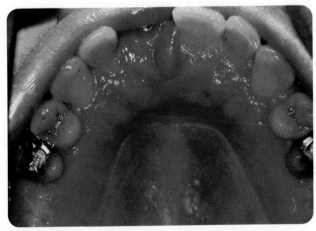

Figure 22.3. Atrophic candidiasis. Erythema following outline of temporary removable partial denture.

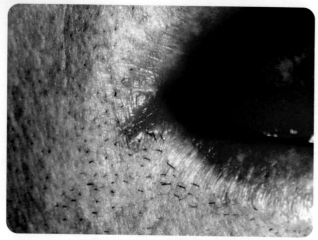

Figure 22.4. Angular cheilitis. Erythema, cracking, and fissuring of the corners of the mouth.

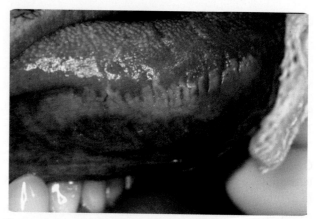

Figure 22.5. Hairy leukoplakia. White lesion on lateral border of the tongue with corrugated surface.

The presence of candidiasis can be confirmed through a culture or smear; however, most patients are treated empirically, based on clinical presentation. Esophageal candidiasis that is refractory to treatment may require endoscopy. Topical antifungals are useful in the treatment of patients with oral candidiasis including both rinses and lozenges or troches. Nystatin is the most common rinse used to manage patients with oral candidiasis, while both nystatin and clotrimazole are available as lozenges. Care must be taken when using topical medications over prolonged periods, because the sugar content in these formulations is often high enough to contribute to caries in xerostomic patients. Angular cheilitis is often managed with nystatin ointment or cream applied directly to the corners of the mouth. Patients with removable appliances such as dentures, nightguards, or orthodontic retainers should be advised to treat both their mouth and their appliance to reduce the chance of reinfection. Ketoconazole, fluconazole, and itraconazole are the most common systemic antifungals used to treat oral candidiasis; however, resistant cases may respond to amphotericin B administered orally or intravenously (Queiroz-Telles et al., 2001; Menon et al., 2001; Vazquez, 2000; Linpiyawan et al., 2000; Powderly et al., 1995; Redding et al., 1992).

HAIRY LEUKOPLAKIA

Oral hairy leukoplakia was originally described in 1984. It manifests as nonpainful, bilateral white plaques on the lateral borders of the tongue (Fig. 22.5). The lesions have a corrugated or shaggy appearance with accentuated vertical folds, resulting in a relatively distinct clinical appearance. Ectopic lesions have been observed on the labial and buccal mucosa. Hairy leukoplakia is usually diagnosed by clinical appearance; however, the differential diagnosis must include hyperplastic candidiasis and frictional hyperkeratosis (Scully et al., 1999). Hairy leukoplakia is associated with Epstein-Barr virus, a member of the herpesvirus family and, as a result, fails to respond to antifungal therapy. Lesions may be observed in any im-

munocompromised patient, including those with HIV/AIDS, solid organ transplant patients, and patients using medications designed to suppress the immune system (Nicolatou et al., 1999).

Hairy leukoplakia is often not treated specifically, and the lesions usually resolve with initiation of antiretroviral therapy for HIV infection. Although patients are most frequently asymptomatic, the presence of oral lesions may be an aesthetic concern and occasionally interfere with function. Current treatment modalities include topical application medications including podophyllin and retinoic acid, systemic antivirals, and surgical removal (Gowdey et al., 1995; Lozada-Nur and Costa, 1992; Glick and Pliskin, 1990). All of these treatment modalities may fail to predictably prevent recurrence, and as a result, patients often require additional treatment.

HUMAN PAPILLOMA VIRUS LESIONS

Of the more than 100 human papilloma virus (HPV) types currently identified, 24 are associated with oral lesions (Terai et al., 1999). Each of these organisms has the ability to infect stratified squamous epithelium and induce proliferative changes that can result in both benign and potentially malignant changes (Eversole, 2000). HPV is present in the normal mucosa in approximately one third of the general population and is shed in the saliva. The modes of transmission include reactivation of latent virus acquired earlier in life, autoinoculation from skin and facial lesions, or sexual transmission. Despite highly active antiretroviral therapy, the incidence of HPV-associated oral warts appears to be increasing (King et al., 2002; Greenspan et al., 2001).

Three human types of benign warts related to HPV infection occur in the oral cavity, including verruca vulgaris (HPV types 2 and 4), squamous papilloma, and condyloma acuminatum (HPV types 6 and 11) (Syrjanen, 2003; Piattelli et al., 2001). Focal epithelial hyperplasia (referred to as Heck's disease in children) is associated with types 13 and 32 and has been described in HIV-infected patients as resulting in multiple nodular lesions (Moerman et al.,

2001). Each of these lesions varies slightly in histologic appearance, but all produce epithelial proliferations demonstrating superficial keratinocytes with pyknotic nuclei surrounded by clear zones (koilocytes), a classic microscopic feature of HPV infection.

Oral lesions most commonly related to HPV infection manifest as singular or, more frequently, multiple papillomas or wartlike lesions that are nonpainful (Fig. 22.6). The lesions can be nodular with a smooth surface, may possess an irregular or cauliflower appearance, or may be shaggy lesions with fingerlike projections. The lesions are most commonly seen on the nonkeratinizing mucosa, including the labial mucosa, soft palate, floor of the mouth, and lateral borders of the tongue. Oral condyloma acuminatum is a sexually transmitted condition in which HPV appears to be a major etiologic agent (Newland, 2000). It generally appears 1 to 3 months following exposure and often accompanies anogenital involvement. A recent study showed that HIV-positive subjects were much more likely to have an oral HPV infection, to be infected with more than one type of HPV, and to be infected with a high-risk type of HPV than HIV-negative subjects (Kreimer et al., 2004). The prevalence of oral warts in HIV-positive patients is estimated to be between 1 and 4%.

Treatment of patients with oral HPV lesions may include surgical removal, cryotherapy, laser ablation, or electrocautery. In addition, keratolytic agents applied topically such as podophyllin resin and intralesional injections of interferon or cidofovir have shown therapeutic benefit (Lozada-Nur et al., 2001; Eversole, 2000; Ishida and Ramos-e-Silva, 1998). Recurrence following removal as well as the development of new lesions is likely, and patients may require repeated episodes of treatment.

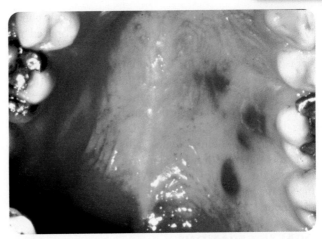

Figure 22.7. Kaposi's sarcoma. Flat, nonpainful purple lesion on the palate.

MALIGNANCIES OR NEOPLASTIC LESIONS

Kaposi's sarcoma (KS) is the most common AIDS-associated neoplasia and remains a significant cause of morbidity and mortality in HIV-infected patients. The lesions manifest as an angiomatous malignancy of the skin and mucosa that may spread to the lungs, liver, or gastrointestinal tract. It appears to be associated with a sexually transmitted virus (human herpesvirus 8). The oral cavity is the first site of involvement in 20–70% of cases, and the hard palate and gingiva are the most frequently affected sites (Gorsky and Epstein, 2000). Early lesions occur as nonpainful, purple-to-red macules that may be focal or diffuse and are easily overlooked (Fig. 22.7). As the lesions progress, they may become nodular and exophytic, interfering with function and/or aesthetics (Scully et al., 1991) (Fig. 22.8). Along with medical management of the patient including initiation of antiretroviral therapy and chemotherapy/radiation, dental treatment may include laser excision, cryotherapy, or intralesional injections with vinblastine (Flaitz et al., 1995; Epstein et al., 1989).

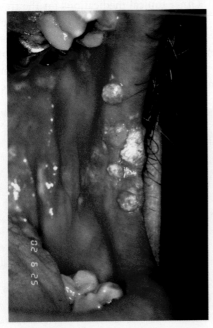

Figure 22.6. Human papillomavirus lesions. Multiple wartlike lesions within the oral cavity.

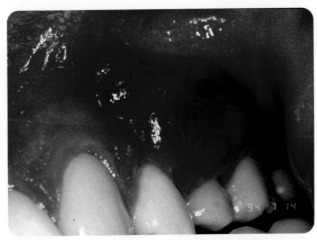

Figure 22.8. Kaposi's sarcoma. Exophytic mass that interferes with function.

Non-Hodgkin's lymphoma is another neoplastic condition seen more frequently in immunocompromised patients. Oral lesions occur in approximately 4% of HIV patients with non-Hodgkin's lymphoma, and the mouth may be the first site of involvement. Patients present with rapidly growing, painful masses that are often ulcerated and most frequently appear on the gingiva or palate (Lozada-Nur et al., 1996) (Fig. 22.9). Diagnosis is confirmed through biopsy and histologic evaluation, and patients are generally referred for medical management. Therapy often includes the use of radiation or chemotherapy, necessitating evaluation and stabilization of dental needs prior to treatment.

ORAL ULCERATIONS

Oral ulcerations are common in the immunocompromised patient and severity, response to therapy, as well as the propensity for recurrence may be different from that in the general population (MacPhail and Greenspan, 1997). The most common ulcerations manifest primarily as recurrent aphthae and herpes simplex virus type 1 lesions (MacPhail et al., 1992). Substantially less common are ulcerations related to cytomegalovirus (CMV) infection, fungal infections such as histoplasmosis and cryptococcosis, and bacterial infections such as tuberculosis and syphilis. Because the clinical appearance may be similar in many of these lesions, biopsy and/or culture of persistent, atypical-appearing ulcerations may be indicated to arrive at a definitive diagnosis and appropriate treatment.

Recurrent aphthae are common oral lesions affecting approximately 10–20% of the general population (Ship et al., 2000). Most patients report a history of recurrent lesions developing prior to the age of 30, and a possible familial predisposition exists. A potential systemic etiology should be considered in patients who spontaneously develop chronic, severe episodes that do not respond to therapy. Aphthae are classified according to size and duration into three groups: minor aphthae, major aphthae, and herpetiform aphthae. Minor aphthae are small lesions

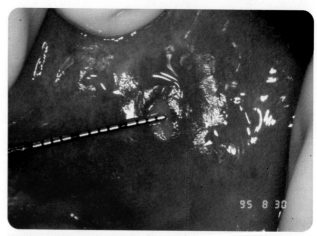

Figure 22.10. Minor aphthous ulcer. Small ulceration with fibrinous coating and red halo.

(<5 mm in diameter) that occur as single or multiple ulcerations. Minor aphthae generally affect the mobile mucosa (tongue, floor of mouth, soft palate, and buccal/labial mucosa) and manifest as superficial erosions with a fibrinous covering, often surrounded by a red halo (Fig. 22.10). The lesions persist for 7–14 days and can cause significant discomfort. Major aphthae are characterized by larger, painful ulcerations that persist for up to 6 weeks and initially heal with scarring (Fig. 22.11). Herpetiform aphthae occur as crops of small ulcers that coalesce and may be mistaken for herpes simplex virus lesions.

Aphthae respond well to topical steroid therapy, including the use of fluocinonide, clobetasol, and betamethasone; however, patients should be closely monitored for subsequent development of candidiasis (MacPhail et al., 1992; Eisen and Lynch, 2001; Muzio et al., 2001). Other topical medications for the treatment of aphthae include chlorhexidine and amlexanox (Khandwala et al., 1997). Intralesional injections with triamcinolone may be useful for isolated persistent lesions, and systemic steroid therapy including prednisone is useful for patients with severe outbreaks. Systemic thalido-

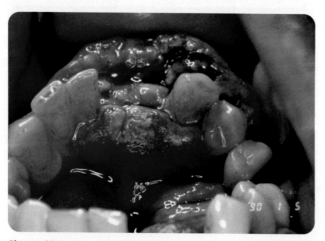

Figure 22.9. Non-Hodgkin's lymphoma. Large mass involving mandibular anterior gingiva.

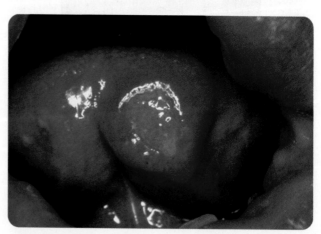

Figure 22.11. Major aphthous ulcer. Large ulceration with indurated borders.

mide has also shown therapeutic efficacy in patients with recalcitrant lesions (Calabrese et al., 2000; Jacobson et al., 1997).

Recurrent herpetic stomatitis is characterized by multiple, small vesicles, which quickly rupture to form ulcerations. These ulcerations often coalesce, creating a larger lesion that is associated with significant discomfort (Fig. 22.12). Traditionally affecting primarily the palate and attached gingiva or the vermillion border, patients who are significantly immunosuppressed may have lesions involving any mucosal surface. Recurrent herpetic stomatitis is caused by herpes simplex virus type 1, and most lesions respond to systemic antiviral therapy including acyclovir, valacyclovir, or famiciclovir (Itin and Lautenschlager, 1997; Flaitz et al., 1996). Topical therapy with penciclovir may be useful in some patients (Femiano et al., 2001). Intravenous administration of foscarnet may be indicated in patients whose lesions are recalcitrant to therapy with acyclovir.

In contrast to recurrent aphthous and recurrent herpetic stomatitis, oral ulcerations associated with cytomegalovirus (CMV) are more frequently seen in patients with AIDS nearing the advanced stages of the disease. Approximately 50% of the general population and 90% of patients with HIV are carriers of the virus that causes CMV-related disease. When HIV weakens a patient's immune defenses, CMV can attack several parts of the body, most frequently involving the retina, colon, and esophagus. Within the oral cavity, CMV lesions occur as painful oral ulcerations with irregular or punched out borders, persistent, and covered by a pseudomembrane (Syrjanens et al., 1999; Reichart, 1997; Firth et al., 1994; Jones et al., 1993; Schubert et al., 1993). Diagnosis frequently requires a viral culture or biopsy of the lesion. Treatment is best managed by physicians and may include the use of ganciclovir, foscarnet, and cidofovir (Salmon-Ceron, 2001; Naesen and DeClercq, 2001).

Histoplasmosis and cryptococcosis are both fungal infections that may manifest within the oral cavity as per-

sistent ulcerations. Histoplasmosis is a fungal infection caused by the organism *Histoplasma capsulatum* in which over 30% of patients demonstrate oral lesions (Gomes Ferreira et al., 2001; Piluso et al., 1996; Chinn et al., 1995). The lesions occur most frequently on the gingiva, tongue, buccal mucosa, and soft palate and manifest as granulomatous appearing ulcerations with indurated borders covered by a nonspecific gray membrane. Cryptococcosis is another deep fungal infection, caused by the organism *Cryptococcus neoformans,* which can manifest intraorally as a nonspecific ulceration (Schmidt-Westhausen et al., 1995). Both of these conditions require assessment for systemic disease and are best managed by physicians. Treatment frequently includes the use of systemic antifungals including ketoconazole, fluconazole, itraconazole, or amphotericin B.

Other, more infrequent causes of intraoral ulcerations result from bacterial infections including tuberculosis and syphilis (Anil et al., 2000). Once identified through culture or biopsy, patients require referral to a physician for a medical evaluation and treatment.

PERIODONTAL DISEASES

Chronic gingivitis and periodontitis remain as the most common forms of periodontal disease affecting the general population as well as HIV infected patients. Although less frequently encountered, three atypical forms of periodontal disease have been associated with HIV infection: including linear gingival erythema, necrotizing ulcerative gingivitis, and necrotizing ulcerative periodontitis (Narani and Epstein, 2001; Ryder, 2000; Grbic and Lamster, 1997).

Linear gingival erythema generally manifests as a persistent, generalized band of erythema involving the marginal and papillary gingiva. The lesions are nonpainful and can range in appearance from a distinct band of bright red gingiva to more subtle and diffuse erythema (Fig. 22.13). Occasionally, lesions extend into the attached gin-

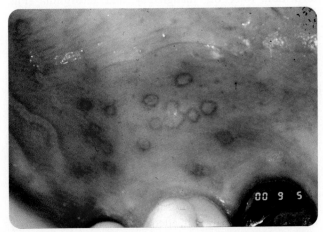

Figure 22.12. Recurrent herpetic stomatitis. Multiple small ulcerations on hard palate.

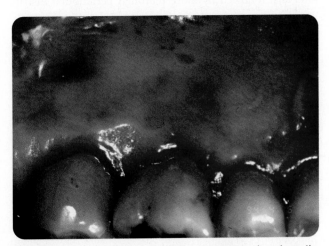

Figure 22.13. Linear gingival erythema. Marginal and papillary erythema that does not resolve despite periodontal debridement.

giva and manifest as petechia-like patches that are often accompanied by bleeding. A distinguishing feature of linear gingival erythema is that it is often refractory to treatment and persists despite both adequate personal oral home care and periodontal debridement. Treatment is directed toward improving oral hygiene, periodontal debridement, the use of topical chemotherapeutic agents such as chlorhexidine rinses, and supportive periodontal therapy at shorter intervals to monitor progression. Antifungals are occasionally useful in nonresponsive patients.

Necrotizing ulcerative gingivitis is characterized by rapid onset of periodontal destruction, including marked necrosis and ulceration of the marginal and papillary gingiva (Holmstrup and Westergaard, 1998). Patients generally experience severe pain, spontaneous bleeding, and a distinct oral malodor. Destruction of the interdental tissue results in open interproximal areas and soft tissue craters, making future oral self-care more difficult (Fig. 22.14). Lesions may occur throughout the dentition; however, the mandibular incisor and maxillary molar regions are most commonly affected.

Necrotizing ulcerative periodontitis (NUP) occurs as the disease progresses to involve the underlying bone and supporting tissues (Fig. 22.15). It has been reported in 0–5% of the HIV-seropositive population and is associated with advanced immune suppression and CD4 counts often below 100/mm^3. Patients often complain of deep bone pain as soft-tissue destruction occurs very rapidly, exposing underlying alveolar bone (Novak, 1999). The exposed bone quickly becomes necrotic and may eventually slough away as a sequestrum or require surgical debridement. Alveolar ridge defects are common following NUP, and tooth loss is common.

Pain control and management of infection through sequential episodes of periodontal debridement and antimicrobial therapy are cornerstones of treatment. Therapy often begins with gentle debridement performed at frequent intervals, followed by more thorough periodontal instru-

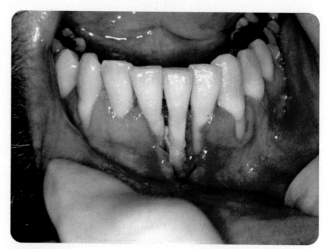

Figure 22.15. Acute necrotizing periodontitis. Infection resulting in exposure of bone.

mentation. Topical antimicrobials including chlorhexidine and povidone–iodine are useful as rinses or for subgingival irrigation. Systemic antibiotics are indicated, especially if signs of systemic involvement are present, including swelling and lymphadenopathy, or if bone exposure is apparent. Metronidazole has been shown particularly effective in the management of patients with NUP; however, care must be taken to monitor for potential secondary candidiasis (Robinson, 1997). In addition, patients must be advised to avoid the use of alcohol during metronidazole therapy. Healing is often dramatic, with a rapid reduction in erythema and ulceration. However, oral hygiene remains complicated by residual soft tissue craters and open interproximal spaces. The need for regular and frequent supportive periodontal care is of extreme importance in patients with a history of NUP (Hofer et al., 2002).

SALIVARY GLAND DISEASE AND XEROSTOMIA

Patients with HIV infection may present with enlargement of the salivary glands due to several factors, including cyst formation, infection, malignancy, and xerostomia (Fig. 22.16). Enmeshed within the intraparotid lymph nodes formed during embryonic development, salivary gland tissue may demonstrate epithelial proliferation leading to lymphoepithelial cyst formation (Patel and Mandel, 2001; Mandel and Hong, 1999). The swelling is usually bilateral and nonpainful and usually does not require treatment; however, care must be taken to rule out other conditions such as infection (cytomegalovirus) and neoplasias (lymphoma). As a result, radiographic imaging of the glands and fine needle biopsy may be indicated.

Xerostomia is a common complaint in patients with HIV/AIDS (Younai et al., 2001; Navazesh et al., 2000). As in the general population, salivary hypofunction is most frequently caused by side effects associated with a variety of medications. Patients may complain of an inability to eat comfortably, and the oral tissues may be easily trau-

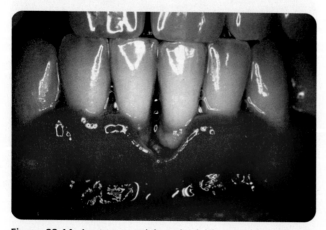

Figure 22.14. Acute necrotizing gingivitis. Loss of papillae in mandibular anterior region with associated attachment loss.

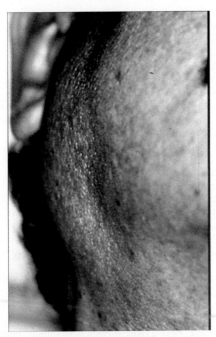

Figure 22.16. Salivary gland swelling due to lymphoepithelial cyst formation in parotid gland.

matized, resulting in nonspecific ulcerations. Candidiasis is more common in xerostomic patients, and caries can become a significant concern. Patients should be encouraged to increase their intake of water throughout the day and may find relief through the use of salivary substitutes or oral lubricants. Systemic medications such as pilocarpine and cevimeline increase secretions and may be useful in patients without significant gastrointestinal problems. Home fluoride therapy as well as regular professional dental care are essential in reducing the risk of caries and periodontal disease.

SUMMARY

Oral lesions occur frequently and are often early manifestations of patients with HIV infection or AIDS. Many of the intraoral conditions can be managed well in the dental office, providing patients with a continuum of care that is extremely important. As the population of patients living with HIV/AIDS increases and patients live longer and healthier lives, the need for routine comprehensive dental care is critical. Through knowledge, skills, and understanding, dental care providers can be prepared to meet the challenge.

REFERENCES

Anil S, Ellepola AN, Samaranayake LP, Beena VT. Tuberculosis ulcer of the tongue as presenting feature of pulmonary tuberculosis and HIV infection. Gen Dent 2000;48:458–461.

Aquirre JM, Echebarria MA, Ocina E, et al. Reduction of HIV-associated oral lesions after highly active antiretroviral therapy. Oral Surg Oral Med Oral Pathol Oral Radiol Endod 1999;88:114–115.

Calabrese L, Fleischer AB. Thalidomide: current and potential clinical applications. Am J Med 2000;108:487–495.

Ceballos-Salobrena A, Gaitan-Cepeda LA, Ceballos-Garcia L, Lezama-Del Valle D. Oral lesions in HIV/AIDS patients undergoing highly active antiretroviral treatment including protease inhibitors: a new face of oral AIDS? AIDS Patient Care STDS 2000;14:627–635.

Chinn H, Chernoff DN, Migliorati CA, et al. Oral histoplasmosis in HIV-infected patients. A report of 2 cases. Oral Surg Oral Med Oral Pathol 1995;79:710–714.

Eisen D, Lynch DP. Selecting topical and systemic agents for recurrent aphthous stomatitis. Cutis 2001;68:201–206.

Epstein JB, Lozada-Nur F, McLeod WA, Spinelli J. Oral Kaposi's sarcoma in acquired immunodeficiency syndrome. Review of management and report of the efficacy of intralesional vinblastine. Cancer 1989;64:2424–2430.

Eversole LR. Papillary lesions of the oral cavity: relationship to human papillomaviruses. J Calif Dent Assoc 2000;28:922–927.

Femiano F, Gombos F, Scully C. Recurrent herpes labialis: efficacy of topical therapy with penciclovir compared with acyclovir. Oral Dis 2001;7:31–33.

Firth NA, Rich AM, Reade PC. Oral mucosal ulceration due to cytomegalovirus associated with human immunodeficiency virus infection. Care report and brief review. Aust Dent J 1994;39:273–275.

Flaitz CM, Nichols CM, Hicks MJ. Herpesviridae-associated with persistent mucocutaneous ulcers in acquired immunodeficiency syndrome. A clinicopathologic study. Oral Surg Oral Med Oral Pathol Oral Radiol Endod 1996;81:433–441.

Flaitz CM, Nichols CM, Hicks MJ. Role of intralesional vinblastine administration in the treatment of intraoral Kaposi's sarcoma in AIDS. Eur J Cancer B Oral Oncol 1995;31B:280–285.

Glick M, Pliskin ME. Regression of oral hairy leukoplakia after oral administration of acyclovir. Gen Dent 1990;38:374–375.

Gomes Ferreira O, Vieira Fernandes A, Sebastiao Borges A, et al. Orofacial manifestations of histoplasmosis in HIV-positive patients: a case report. Med Oral 2001;6:101–105.

Gorsky M, Epstein JB. A case series of acquired immunodeficiency syndrome in patients with initial neoplastic diagnoses of intraoral Kaposi's sarcoma. Oral Surg Oral Med Oral Pathol Oral Radiol Endod 2000;90:612–617.

Gowdey G, Lee RK, Carpenter WM. Treatment of HIV-related hairy leukoplakia with podophyllum resin 25% solution. Oral Surg Oral Med Oral Pathol 1995;79:64–67.

Grbic JT, Lamster IB. Oral manifestations of HIV infection. AIDS Patient Care STDS 1997;11:18–24.

Greenspan D, Canchola AJ, MacPhail LA, et al. Effect of highly active antiretroviral therapy on frequency of oral warts. Lancet 2001;357:1411–1412.

Hofer D, Hammerle CH, Grassi M, Lang NP. Long-term results of supportive periodontal therapy (SPT) in HIV-seropositive and HIV-seronegative patients. J Clin Periodontol 2002;29:630–637.

Holmstrup P, Westergaard J. HIV infection and periodontal diseases. Periodontol 2000 1998;18:37–46.

Ishida CE, Ramos-e-Silva M. Cryosurgery in oral lesions. Int J Dermatol 1998;37:283–285.

Itin PH, Lautenschlager S. Viral lesions of the mouth in HIV-infected patients. Dermatology 1997;194:1–7.

Ives NJ, Gazzard BG, Easterbrook PJ. The changing pattern of AIDS-defining illnesses with introduction of highly active antiretroviral therapy (HAART) in a London clinic. J Infect 2001;42:134–139.

Jacobson JM, Greenspan JS, Spritzler J, et al. Thalidomide for the treatment of oral aphthous ulcers in patients with human immunodeficiency virus infection. National Institute of Allergy and Infectious Diseases AIDS Clinical Trials Group. N Engl J Med 1997;336:1487–1493.

Jones AC, Freedman PD, Phelan JA, Kerpel SM. Cytomegalovirus infection of the oral cavity. A report of six cases and review of the literature. Oral Surg Oral Med Oral Pathol 1993;75:76–85.

Khandwala A, Van Inwegen RG, Alfano MC. 5% Amlexanox oral paste, a new treatment for recurrent minor aphthous ulcers: I. Clinical demonstration of acceleration of healing and resolution of pain. Oral Surg Oral Med Oral Pathol Oral Radiol Endod 1997;83:222–230.

King MD, Reznik DA, O'Daniel SCM, et al. Human papillomavirus-associated oral warts among human immunodeficiency virus-seropositive patients in the era of highly active antiretroviral therapy: an emerging infection. Clin Infect Dis 2002;34:641–648.

Kreimer AR, Alberg AJ, Daniel R, et al. Oral human papillomavirus infection in adults is associated with sexual behavior and HIV serostatus. J Infect Dis 2004;189:686–698.

Linpiyawan R, Jittreprasert K, Sivayathorn A. Clinical trial: clotrimazole troche vs itraconazole oral solution in the treatment of oral candidiasis in AIDS patients. Int J Dermatol 2000;39:859–861.

Lozada-Nur F, Costa C. Podophyllum resin 25% for the treatment of oral hairy leukoplakia. A retrospective study. Oral Surg Oral Med Oral Pathol 1992; 73:555–558.

Lozada-Nur F, de Sanz S, Silverman S Jr, et al. Intraoral non-Hodgkins lymphoma in seven patients with acquired immunodeficiency syndrome. Oral Surg Oral Med Oral Pathol Oral Radiol Endod 1996;82:173–178.

Lozada-Nur F, Glick M, Schubert M, Silverberg I. Use of intralesional interferon-alpha for the treatment of recalcitrant oral warts in patients with AIDS: a report of 4 cases. Oral Surg Oral Med Oral Pathol Oral Radiol Endod 2001;92:617–622.

MacPhail LA, Greenspan D, Greenspan JS. Recurrent aphthous ulcers in association with HIV infection: diagnosis and treatment. Oral Surg Oral Med Oral Pathol 1992;73:283–288.

MacPhail LA, Greenspan JS. Oral ulcerations in HIV infections: investigation and pathogenesis. Oral Dis 1997;Suppl1:S190–193.

Mandel L, Hong J. HIV-associated parotid lymphoepithelial cysts. J Am Dent Assoc 1999;130:528–532.

Menon T, Umamheswari K, Kumarawamy N, et al. Efficacy of fluconazole and itraconazole in the treatment of oral candidiasis in HIV patients. Acta Trop 2001;80:151–154.

Moerman M, Danielides VG, Nousia CS, et al. Recurrent focal epithelial hyperplasia due to HPV 13 in an HIV-positive patient. Dermatology 2001;203:339–341.

Muzio LL, della Valle A, Mignogna MD, et al. The treatment of oral aphthous ulceration or erosive lichen planus with topical clobetasol propionate in 3 preparations: a clinical and pilot study on 54 patients. J Oral Pathol Med 2001;30:611–617.

Naesen SL, DeClercq E. Recent developments in herpesvirus therapy. Herpes 2001;8:12–16.

Narani N, Epstein JB. Classification of oral lesions in HIV infection. J Clin Periodontol 2001;28:137–145.

Navazesh M, Mulligan R, Komaroff E, et al. The prevalence of xerostomia and salivary gland hypofunction in a cohort of HIV-positive and at-risk women. J Dent Res 2000;79:1502–1507.

Newland JR. Oral and maxillofacial pathology case of the month. Condyloma acuminatum (venereal wart). Tex Dent J 2000;117:72,109.

Nicolatou O, Nikolatos G, Fisfis M, et al. Oral hairy leukoplakia in a patient with acute lymphocytic leukemia. Oral Dis 1999;5:76–79.

Novak MJ. Necrotizing ulcerative periodontitis. Ann Periodontol 1999;4:74–78.

Patel S, Mandel L. Parotid gland swelling in HIV diffuse infiltrative CD8 lymphocytosis syndrome. N Y State Dent J 2001; 67:22–23.

Patton LL, McKaig R, Strauss R, et al. Changing prevalence of oral manifestations of human immunodeficiency virus in the era of protease inhibitor therapy. Oral Surg Oral Med Oral Pathol Oral Radiol Endod 2000;89:299–304.

Piattelli A, Rubini C, Fioroni M, Iezzi T. Warty carcinoma of the oral mucosa in an HIV+ patient. Oral Oncol 2001;37:665–667.

Piluso S, Ficarra G, Lucatorto FM, et al. Causes of oral ulcers in HIV-infected patients: a study of 19 cases. Oral Surg Oral Med Oral Pathol Oral Radiol Endod 1996;82:166–172.

Powderly WG, Finkelstein DM, Feinberg J, et al. A randomized trial comparing fluconazole with clotrimazole troches for the prevention of fungal infections in patients with advanced immunodeficiency virus infection. N Engl J Med 1995;332:700–705.

Queiroz-Telles F, Silva N, Carvalho MM, et al. Evaluation of efficacy and safety of itraconazole oral solution for the treatment of oropharyngeal candidiasis in AIDS patients. Braz J Infect Dis 2001;5:60–66.

Redding SW, Farinacci GC, Smith JA, et al. A comparison between fluconazole tablets and clotrimazole troches for the treatment of thrush in HIV infection. Spec Care Dent 1992;12:24–27.

Redding SW, Kirkpatrick WR, Dib O, et al. The epidemiology of non-albicans Candida in oropharyngeal candidiasis in HIV patients. Spec Care Dent 2000;20:178–181.

Reichart PA. Oral ulcerations in HIV infection. Oral Dis 1997;Suppl1:S180–182.

Robinson PG. Treatment of HIV-associated periodontal diseases. Oral Dis 1997;3(Suppl1):S238–240.

Ryder MI. Periodontal management of HIV-infected patients. Periodontol 2000 2000;23:85–93.

Salmon-Ceron D. Cytomegalovirus infection: the point in 2001. HIV Med 2001;2:255–259.

Schmidt-Westhausen A, Grunewald T, Reichart PA, Pohle HD. Oral cryptococcosis in a patient with AIDS. A case report. Oral Dis 1995;1:61–62.

Schubert MM, Epstein JB, Lloid ME, Cooney E. Oral infections due to cytomegalovirus in immunocompromised patients. J Oral Pathol Med 1993;22:268–273.

Scully C, Laskaris G, Pindborg J, et al. Oral manifestations of HIV infection and their management. I. More common lesions. Oral Surg Oral Med Oral Pathol 1991;71:158–166.

Scully C, Porter S. Orofacial disease: update for the dental clinical team: 3. White lesions. Dent Update 1999;26:123–129.

Ship JA, Chavez EM, Doerr PA, et al. Recurrent aphthous stomatitis. Quintessence Int 2000;31:95–112.

Silverman S Jr, Gallo JW, McKnight ML, et al. Clinical characteristics and management responses in 85 HIV-infected patients with oral candidiasis. Oral Surg Oral Med Oral Pathol Oral Radiol Endod 1996;82:402–407.

Syrjanen S. Human papillomavirus infections and oral tumors. Med Microbiol Immunol 2003;192(3):123–128.

Syrjanens S, Leimola-Virtanen R, Schmidt-Westhausen A, Reichart PA. Oral ulcers in AIDS patients frequently associated with cytomegalovirus (CMV) and Epstein-Barr virus (EBV) infections. J Oral Pathol Med 1999;28:204–209.

Tappuni AR, Flemming GJ. The effect of antiretroviral therapy on the prevalence of oral manifestations in HIV-infected patients: a UK study. Oral Surg Oral Med Oral Pathol Oral Radiol Endod 2001;92:623–628.

Terai M, Takagi M, Matsukura T, Sata T. Oral wart associated with human papillomavirus type 2. J Oral Pathol Med 1999;28:137–140.

Vazquez JA. Therapeutic options for the management of oropharyngeal and esophageal candidiasis in HIV/AIDS patients. HIV Clin Trials 2000;1:47–59.

Younai FS, Marcus M, Freed JR, et al. Self-reported oral dryness and HIV disease in a national sample of patients receiving medical care. Oral Surg Oral Med Oral Pathol Oral Radiol Endod 2001;92:629–636.

Chapter 23

Skin Lesions

Chapter Objectives

1. List the three major types of skin cancer.

2. Describe the ABCD's of skin cancer.

3. List and discuss four causes of skin cancer.

4. List three ways to prevent skin cancer.

5. Describe several ways that clinicians can be instrumental in detecting skin cancer.

6. Describe several ways that clinicians can be instrumental in determining the origins of skin lesions and discuss why this is important.

7. List five diseases that have skin lesions as part of the disease state.

8. List five skin lesions that are benign but should be followed, measured, photographed, and documented.

9. List a skin lesion that is caused by *Candida*.

10. Discuss three skin diseases that are a part of a disease process and have oral lesions as well.

11. Describe three benign skin conditions that may be observed clinically but do not pose any major contagion factors.

12. List two diseases that may exhibit skin lesions and may be contagious.

13. Describe vitiligo and discuss the factors that may contribute to the disease state.

14. Discuss GVH disease and the skin characteristics that accompany the condition.

15. Compare and contrast comedone, nevi, and moles.

16. List the characteristics of scleroderma and describe the diseases often associated with scleroderma.

Chapter Outline

INTRODUCTION

This chapter provides the student and the practitioner with information related to the extraoral examination. The dental hygienist begins the pathology examination by observing, palpating, and thoroughly examining the external surfaces of the patient. Skin lesions are often evident on the exposed surfaces of the arms, legs, neck, face, and scalp regions. The clinician easily assesses this location, as these areas are the most visible during the dental appointment.

In some cases, long-standing lesions may either be premalignant or have changed into a cancerous state. Many patients have lesions removed and biopsies performed on a routine basis, since some patients tend to have more moles and develop skin lesions quickly. Patients who have had basal cell and squamous cell carcinoma have higher rates of melanoma and are advised to have new growth checked frequently. Additionally, a person who has more than 40 moles is at greater risk for any type of skin cancer. The patient in Figure 23.1 has multiple small facial scars from the removal of previous skin lesions on the forehead.

The hygienist may be the first person to inquire about a lesion and bring it to the attention of the patient. When diagnosed in an early stage, premalignant lesions can be quickly removed and will not cause the patient future

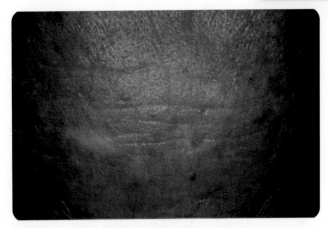

Figure 23.1. Previously removed skin lesions.

problems. Some skin discolorations may appear threatening, and they must be evaluated. A dermatologist is the best person to evaluate such lesions and often must biopsy the tissue to determine the exact nature of the lesion. In addition, some skin lesions may occur because of systemic conditions that are not connected to sun exposure but, rather, result from chronic disease states, radiation, viruses, or an undiagnosed disease that results in skin lesions. The hygienist is in a prime position to assist the patient in getting the treatment needed, in any case. Therefore, all lesions need to be evaluated and in most cases, when there is any question regarding the lesion, the patient needs to see a dermatologist. Detecting lesions early is of paramount importance to the patient so that early treatment can begin.

Statistics from the Skin Cancer Foundation (2006) predict that skin cancer will be diagnosed in more than a million people this year. By 2010, the melanoma rate is projected to rise to 1 in 50 Americans. Nationally, there are more new cases of skin cancer each year than the combined incidence of cancers of the breast, prostate, lung, and colon. Skin cancer is the number one cancer seen in men over the age of 50, and it has tripled in women under the age of 40. The risk factors for cancer in general are tobacco use, heavy alcohol use, physical inactivity, a poor diet, unprotected sun exposure including tanning beds, and exposure to carcinogens. The scale depicted in Table 23.1 is a modified burn index showing the susceptibility of an individual to sun damage based on the person's skin type.

Individuals in the type l and type ll categories are at a higher risk for developing skin cancer. When coupled with other risk factors, the individual's chances of developing a skin cancer increase. When counseling patients, it is important to determine where the individual falls on the burn index scale. The process of determining this factor also opens communication with the person.

Melanoma is the most common cancer in women aged 20–29 years and is second only to breast cancer in women aged 30–35 (Skin Cancer Foundation, 2006). One blistering sunburn during childhood greatly increases a person's chance of developing skin cancer. It is believed that the

Table 23.1   BURN INDEX

Skin Type	History of Past Sun Exposures
I	Person is pale, burns very easily, has never tanned, and may have blue or green eyes. The person is usually described as having a "porcelain complexion" with blonde or red hair
II	Person has a fair complexion and has tanned but gets a minimal tan; may have blue, gray, or green eyes
III	Person may still be fair complexioned, but burns; will go into a light tan
IV	Person has a lightly-tanned appearance, burns minimally to a moderate brown
V	Person has minimum brown skin, rarely burns
VI	Person has deep brown to black skin. This person never burns.

Modified from the Skin Cancer Foundation, 2007. http://www.skincancer.org/prevention/skin-types-and-at risk-groups.html

increased incidence and the increasingly young age of individuals diagnosed with melanoma has some correlation with tanning beds. Young adults are especially susceptible to the damaging rays of ultraviolet light, since their cells are dividing and changing more rapidly than those of adults. In a campaign directed toward teenage girls, the American Academy of Dermatology (October, 2006) issued a Public Service Announcement aimed at girls in the 12- to 14-year-old age group. This target population was selected because most have not starting using tanning beds at this stage of life. Tanning beds emit UVA (longer wavelengths that penetrate deeply into the tissues) and UVB (shorter wavelengths causing sunburns) radiation at levels that can be as much as 15 times stronger than the sun. On an average day, according to the American Academy of Dermatology (2006), more than 1 million people tan in tanning salons. Women and girls aged 16 to 49 years make up 70% of the total number using tanning beds. Ultraviolet light is a known risk factor for melanoma and basal cell and squamous cell carcinoma. Currently, only 25 states regulate youth access to tanning bed facilities. Problems have been compounded by the fact that the genitalia and the eyes are often not protected and are highly susceptible to the damaging radiation, since they are rarely exposed to intense ultraviolet rays. Melanomas are known to occur on the back of the legs and the thigh area and this area is often exposed during sunbathing by teens, especially.

The bulbs in tanning beds must be monitored and replaced frequently to keep the emitted UV levels at determined standards, and some facilities have been found to fall short of this requirement, thereby causing even more exposure to the customer. The advertisements for tanning salons often purport that tanning beds are "safe" and that they do not cause skin damage. This is false, and the ADA hopes to provide the correct information to those who use tanning salons and discourage this risky behavior. (See Clinical Protocol 10 for tips on reducing your risk for skin cancer.)

MALIGNANT SKIN LESIONS

There are three main types of skin cancer, named for the types of skin cells from which they develop. The most deadly form of skin cancer is melanoma; and fortunately, it is the least commonly found of the three types of skin cancer. The most commonly found skin cancer is basal cell. This type of cancer, consisting of malignant nests of basal cells, is usually very slow growing and typically does not spread. Basal cell carcinoma is commonly found on the hands, neck, and head. The second most commonly found skin cancer is squamous cell carcinoma, which is identified by malignant squamous epithelial cells. The three types of cancer are discussed in this section.

Basal Cell, Squamous Cell, and Melanoma

Basal cell and squamous cell carcinomas together account for most of the skin cancers diagnosed each year (see Chapter 4 for a more complete description), followed by melanoma, which accounts for 73% of skin cancer deaths. According to the American Cancer Association (2006), both basal cell carcinoma and squamous cell carcinoma have a better than 95% cure rate if detected and treated early. Figure 23.2 depicts an early basal cell carcinoma below the left eye. Basal cell carcinoma begins as a small, elevated lesion with rolled margins and often has a pearly, iridescent-type surface.

Basal cell carcinoma is often described as a nonhealing sore, a pink growth with rolled, elevated borders or a waxy type lesion. As seen in Figure 23.2, basal cell carcinoma occurs often in the upper two thirds of the face, including the eye area. The patient's glasses should always be removed to inspect the area protected by the eyeglass frame and the hairline. A dermatologist should evaluate any changes or growths, and the patient should be referred to someone board certified in dermatology in your area.

Figure 23.3 depicts a squamous cell carcinoma of the lower lip. The tissue of the lip has lost definition at the ver-

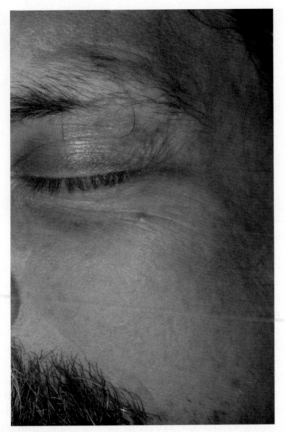

Figure 23.2. Basal cell carcinoma.

milion border and has obvious solar damage. Squamous cell carcinomas often have a roughened, scaly appearance and may appear ulcerated as they progress. The most vulnerable areas for these types of cancers would be the sun-exposed areas of the body. The face, head, neck, hands, legs, and arms are all exposed to sun, making these areas the most affected. The lower lip is often a prime area because of the angle to the sun. The upper lip is somewhat protected. Fair-skinned individuals with blonde or red hair and/or blue, green, or gray eyes are at increased risk. However, dark-skinned individuals do develop skin cancers as well and should be evaluated fully.

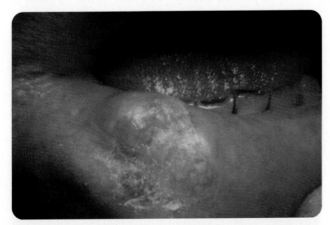

Figure 23.3. Squamous cell carcinoma. (Courtesy of Dr. John Jacoway.)

Women aged 20–29 (AAD, 2006) are especially affected by the most serious type of skin disease, the melanoma, because of its ability to spread quickly and to sometimes go unreported and unnoticed. Melanoma is the second most common cancer in women within this age group. The American Cancer Association (2006) reports that one American dies of melanoma almost ever hour—that is, every 67 minutes. The mortality rate for melanoma is highest in older Caucasian males. The melanoma may have a pigmented appearance such as brown or black mixed colors or it may be a flesh-colored lesion, pink, blue or white colored, with irregular surfaces. The flesh tones make the lesions more difficult to see, since they blend in with the surrounding surface. The oral melanoma is discussed in Chapter 15 under pigmented lesions. The flesh-tone melanoma is referred to as an amelanotic melanoma. Figure 23.4A shows a very early melanoma with mixed colors.

Melanomas are further described in the chapter on neoplasms, Chapter 5. More than 1 million new cases of skin cancer will be diagnosed in the United States this year, and one in five people will be diagnosed with skin cancer in their lifetime (American Cancer Society, 2006). In the United States, every 10 minutes someone is diagnosed with melanoma, and as mentioned above, someone else dies of it every hour. Although melanomas affect light-skinned individuals, dark-skinned individuals may develop these orally, on the soles of the feet, under nails, and on the palms of the hands. Because of the large amount of surrounding tissue that is removed to obtain clear margins, surgery is often extensive for even moderate-size melanomas. Figure 23.4B shows the scar that remained postsurgery for the removal of a melanoma on the upper leg of a 23-year-old female. This patient had at least four visits to tanning beds. The melanoma removed was 3 mm in diameter, but as seen in the figure, the amount of tissue that needed to be removed to get clear margins was extensive. The incision line reached 4 inches for the initial melanoma measuring 3 mm. Finding the melanoma in its earliest stages means a high cure rate, less-invasive surgery, and possibly avoidance of chemotherapy in some cases.

Skin changes are evaluated by what is termed the "ABCDs" of skin cancer (for more details, see "Neoplasia," Chapter 5). Essentially, any changes in the following criteria should be noted and referred to a dermatologist for further evaluation:

A. Asymmetry: A lack of uniformity in both sides of the suspected lesion
B. Border irregularity: Edges of the lesion may be blurred, notched, or ragged
C. Color variation: Lesion may show shades of tan, brown, black with red pigments or possibly white, blue, or black
D. Diameter: Noted when the lesion is more than 6 mm, or larger than a pencil eraser

If a patient has any of the above-mentioned ABCDs, the practitioner should suspect the possibility of cancer

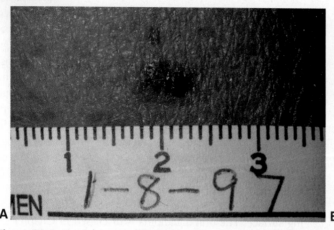

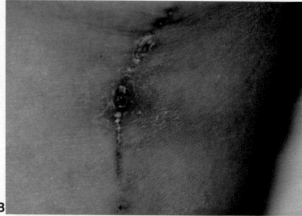

Figure 23.4. A. Melanoma. (Courtesy of Dr. Michael Brennan.) **B.** Melanoma removed from leg.

Digital photography is an excellent tool for capturing the status and documenting future changes. The images can be stored and used for comparison in future visits. This type of photography is easily transferred to another practice if the patient changes geographic locations. In addition, mole-mapping procedures are available that measure, record, and store data for future comparison.

Although the basal cell carcinoma, squamous cell carcinoma, and melanoma are the most commonly seen skin lesions, other types of skin lesions may require some investigative approaches to determine their classification. We present some other common types of skin lesions in this chapter because the possibility is real that hygienists will see them at some point in their clinical practice.

PREMALIGNANT SKIN LESIONS

Actinic Keratosis

Actinic keratosis is the most common type of precancerous skin lesion. Actinic keratoses, also called solar keratosis, are scaly or crusty patches appearing on the skin surface. The most common locations are the backs of the hands, the cheek, ear, forehead, and lower lip. It is necessary to remove the glasses of a patient so that the areas under the frames can be thoroughly evaluated for any lesions. The eyeglasses may be even more detrimental to the skin when they are metal, since they may intensify the reflection of the sun to the skin in that area. Living in a geographic location closer to the equator plays a role in the development of some skin lesions; however, even people in the colder climates may develop actinic keratosis as well as other types of skin lesions. For example, sunburned snow-ski instructors may be prone to developing skin lesions because of the amount of time that they spend in the sun. The snow also reflects the sun and intensifies
the ____ e even more.

____ y, the lesions associated with actinic keratosis
____ dry and rough textured but usually do not
____ as a typical characteristic. Figure 23.5 shows
____ th an early actinic keratosis skin lesion.

Clinicians must pay attention to these lesions because they may be the first step in the development of squamous cell carcinoma. The lesions occur because of long-term exposure to the sun. Often the lesions develop slowly and may wane, only to reappear later. Individuals who have multiple areas of actinic keratosis, have had substantial exposure to the sun, increasing their risk of developing all types of skin cancer. The usual treatment for actinic keratosis removal is cryosurgery, curettage and desiccation, laser surgery, photodynamic therapy, and topical medications. (See Clinical Protocol 10 for Sun Protection Guidelines.)

Actinic Cheilitis

Actinic cheilitis, or solar cheilosis, is another form of actinic keratosis that develops on the lips and may evolve into a type of squamous cell carcinoma that can spread rapidly to other parts of the body. Sun damage manifests clinically as fairly distinct stages of tissue destruction. The lips may appear scaly and crusted, with a loss of definition of the vermilion border of the lip (Fig. 23.6). The dental practitioner should recommend further evaluation, referral to a dermatologist, and the use of a lip balm with sunscreen. All patients should be advised to use lip balm or

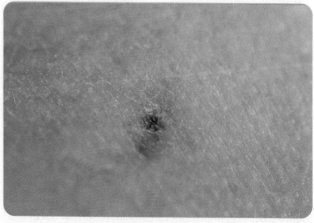

Figure 23.5. Actinic keratosis.

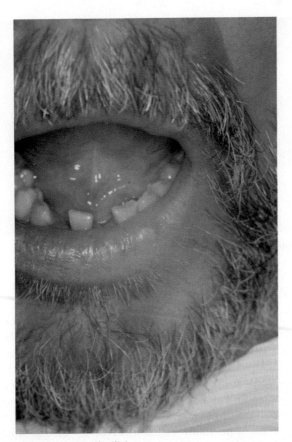

Figure 23.6. Actinic cheilitis.

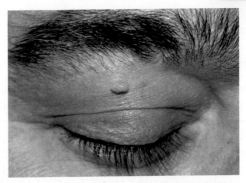

Figure 23.7. Acrochordon. (From Goodheart HP, MD. Goodheart's Photoguide of Common Skin Disorders, 2nd Edition. Philadelphia: Lippincott Williams & Wilkins, 2003.)

history of exposure to the sun and harsh elements. Comedones stem from solar damage and solar **elastosis**. **Favre-Racouchot disease** is a common disease characterized by solar elastosis and large open comedones and cysts in varying sizes. The disorder typically affects Caucasian men who spend a lot of time in the sun. The comedones may appear similar to those in acne without the inflammation that would usually occur with dermatologic problems. The orbital, temporal, and lateral canthi are prime locations for comedones. Tretinoin (vitamin A acid, retinoic acid) is used in the treatment because of the expulsion (decreases comedone formation) actions of the topical medication. Referral to a dermatologist is recommended.

lipstick with sunscreen. The newest lip balms that block the UVB sun rays are the most effective in protecting the lip area. The lower lip may appear wrinkled, uneven, and pigmented with multiple areas of discoloration, depending upon the level of destruction. As with other sun damage to the skin, the most vulnerable patients are those with fair-to-light skin. Smoking increases the risk of many cancers, but also increases the risk of actinic cheilitis because of the direct exposure of this area to chemicals and heat.

BENIGN SKIN LESIONS

Acrochordon

Acrochordons are skin tags that may be somewhat stalk-like or pedunculated. Skin tags are usually small, slender stalks of tissue that are typically flesh colored and blend in with the surrounding tissue (Fig. 23.7). These tags are benign and pose no problem for the patient, but should be noted in case of any future changes.

Comedones

Comedones are dilated hair follicles that are filled with keratin, bacteria, and sebum. In the case of open comedones, the lesions become trapped with a blackened mass of epithelial debris. Comedones are mentioned in this discussion to differentiate them from nevi. The patient usually has a

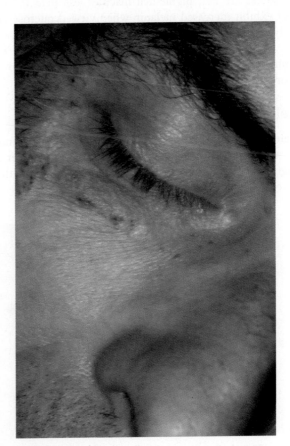

Figure 23.8. Comedones.

Figure 23.8 depicts blackened comedones in multiple areas around the lower area of the eye.

Eczema

Eczema is a general term for an inflammatory response of the skin to multiple agents and is often associated with hypersensitivity type 1 reactions. In Figure 23.9A, the patient has a contact eczema hypersensitivity response, as well as an inflammatory skin response (Fig. 23.9B). Occupational contact eczemas are commonly found in individuals who wash their hands frequently such as dental, medical, and laboratory workers. Additionally, individuals who have exposure to certain chemicals and multiple types of agents may exhibit eczema. In this particular case, the patient was reacting to the cherry flavoring agent in a lip balm. There are two forms of ectopic eczema, infantile and adult. The infantile type may exhibit more obvious ulcerative-type lesions and usually has some causative agent. An example would be rashes caused by diapers, skin medications, or candidiasis infections. Usual symptoms include dryness, pruritus, and inflammation. Topical steroids are prescribed in severe cases; however, most cases dissipate on their own.

Ephelides (Freckles)

Freckles are usually found in sun-exposed areas of skin. Ephelides are flat, pigmented macules less than 0.5 cm that exhibit increased melanin when viewed microscopically. Freckles tend to be found more commonly on people who have light complexions, and the ephelides become more intense with sun exposure. Most tend to be more prevalent in children and fade with adulthood.

Keloid

Keloids are hyperplastic scar tissue and are more common in African Americans. Keloids are covered in Chapter 3. Figure 23.10 depicts an African-American woman with a keloid on the forehead and on the nose.

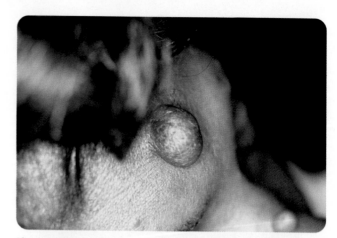
Figure 23.10. Keloid. (Courtesy of Dr. Carolyn Bentley.)

Solar Lentigo

Solar lentigo spots are benign macules caused by sun exposure. They are usually larger than freckles and fade more easily when sun exposure is diminished. Figure 23.11 depicts a lentigo spot on the arm of a patient. When they occur periorally, disorders such as Addison's disease (Chapter 7), Laugier-Hunziker (Chapter 15), and Peutz-Jeghers syndrome (Chapter 10) may be considered. These spots are sometimes called liver spots or age spots. Lentigos are benign and vary in number with the individual and the amount of cumulative sun exposure.

Milia

Milia (plural of milium) are small subepidermal keratinous cysts (also called epidermal inclusion cysts) that develop usually on the eyelid or facial surfaces. They may be removed for cosmetic reasons or may sometimes dissolve on their own, since they are close to the skin surface. Often the cysts will be expelled during normal face washing. Figure 23.12 shows small white milia found on the patient's forehead.

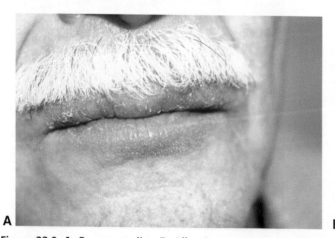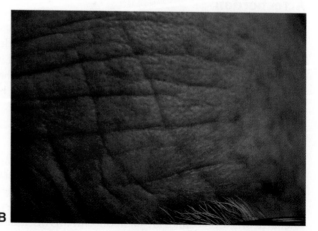
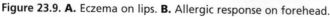
Figure 23.9. A. Eczema on lips. **B.** Allergic response on forehead.

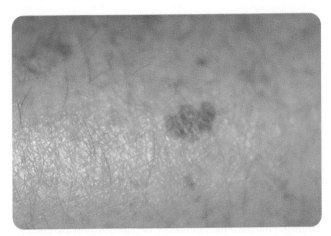

Figure 23.11. Solar lentigo.

Nevi

Acquired melanocytic nevi (plural; sing., *nevus*), commonly called *moles,* may be visible on the face, neck region, and virtually any part of the skin seen by the practitioner. Figure 23.13 is a classic nevus on the neck. A mole is a collection of nevus cells in the dermis or the epithelium, with a variation of types of nevi. The nevi are classified into junctional and compound types. Nevi usually have a smooth surface, sometimes pebbled, and may be flesh colored or pigmented, ranging in size from 0.1 to 0.6 mm. Moles usually begin in childhood and may increase in adulthood, with removal when there is an abnormal appearance or some questionable characteristic. More than 50 moles may be associated with an increased risk of skin cancer. Sometimes changes can be subtle, and extraoral photography and mole mapping (digitally documenting all moles) is very important.

Perlèche (Angular Cheilitis or Angular Stomatitis)

Perlèche occurs at the commissures of the mouth, and these skin lesions may appear red and crusted and sometimes as open wounds. The lesions are caused by *Candida,* loss of dimension due to aging, and may be involved in vitamin B deficiencies in older populations as well. The le-

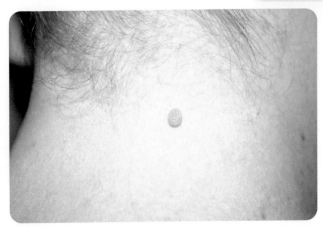

Figure 23.13. Nevus.

sions result from saliva infected with *Candida* resting in the folds of skin at the commissures. Figure 23.14 depicts *Candida* at the commissures with an erythematous area visible. Perlèche is commonly found in the elderly and especially edentulous patients.

Pityriasis Rosea

Pityriasis is an inflammatory dermatosis of unknown etiology. Some studies suggest that an infective agent may be responsible, but no conclusive evidence exists to support any viral or bacterial agent. The condition is self-limiting, pruritic, and reported most commonly in the spring and fall. Most affected are individuals between the ages of 10 and 29 (Chuh et al., 2006). The lesions are typically red to pink, with oval or round shapes and average from 2 to 10 cm. The center part of the lesion has been described as a deeper salmon color. Figure 23.15 shows an oval pityriasis lesion on the patient's back exhibiting a darker external halo.

Poison Oak

Poison oak causes a skin reaction after exposure, producing multiple vesicle-like lesions. Poison oak belongs to the

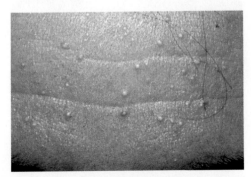

Figure 23.12. Milia. (From Goodheart HP, MD. Goodheart's Photoguide of Common Skin Disorders, 2nd Edition. Philadelphia: Lippincott Williams & Wilkins, 2003.)

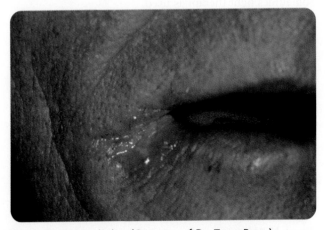

Figure 23.14. Perlèche. (Courtesy of Dr. Terry Rees.)

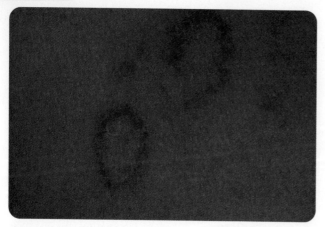

Figure 23.15. Pityriasis.

species of plant called the toxicodendron family, which includes poison oak, poison sumac, and poison ivy. Contact with poison oak, poison ivy, or poison sumac often produces an allergic reaction such as the one seen in Figure 23.16.

Psoriasis

Psoriasis affects approximately 2.6% of the United States population (Regezi, 2003) and usually occurs in younger adults. The dental hygienist can expect to see the skin disorder at some point clinically. Psoriasis has a classic appearance of red, plaquelike lesions covered with a white, thin scale that has a pearly, iridescent characteristic surrounding the lesions. The condition may have many different forms, but commonly exhibits a scaly, pearllike appearance. Removal of the scales may produce bleeding. Figure 23.17 depicts an area behind the ear that exhibits scaling. Psoriasis is often episodic, with periods of exacerbation (increased severity) and quiescence (inactive state). Pruritus (itching) is a common complaint. Several factors appear to be involved in the occurrence of psoriasis: a genetic predisposition, environmental factors, and certain stimuli such as trauma, infections, and sun exposure. Treatment varies and includes the use of corticosteroids, coal tar products, and other topical agents. Sometimes light therapy is used.

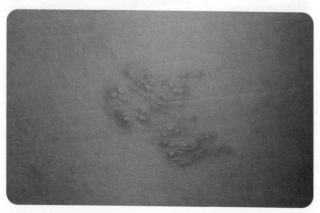

Figure 23.16. Poison oak.

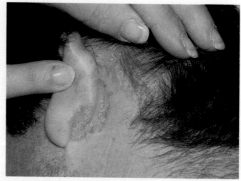

Figure 23.17. Psoriasis. (From Goodheart HP, MD. Goodheart's Photoguide of Common Skin Disorders, 2nd Edition. Philadelphia: Lippincott Williams & Wilkins, 2003.)

Rhinophyma

Rhinophyma is seen on the nose, and the sebaceous glands are enlarged and appear swollen, with increased fibrosis and vascularity. Seen more in males and often called "hammer nose," the enlarged glands are referred to as rhinophyma. **Telangiectasia**, or enlarged capillaries, may also be present, with obvious dilated capillaries visible. Figure 23.18 depicts the enlarged glands of the nose on a male patient.

Rosacea

Rosacea is typically seen on the nose and cheek areas and exhibits redness with chronic vascular and follicular dilation. Figure 23.19 depicts a cheek area that exhibits rosacea with a reddened skin area. The sebaceous glands may be hyperplastic, and the pustules may be erythematous. Rosacea is characteristic of some systemic diseases, such as lupus, which exhibits the chronic butterfly rash in the malar area.

Seborrheic Keratoses

Seborrheic keratoses will vary from light brown to black and may appear as multiple or singular lesions. The le-

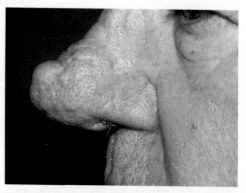

Figure 23.18. Rhinophyma. (From Goodheart HP, MD. Goodheart's Photoguide of Common Skin Disorders, 2nd Edition. Philadelphia: Lippincott Williams & Wilkins, 2003.)

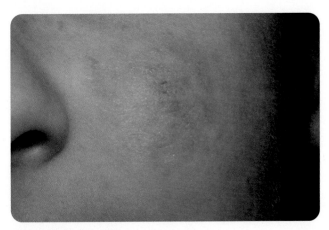

Figure 23.19. Rosacea.

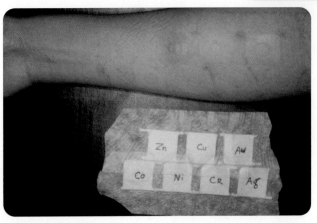

Figure 23.21. Urticaria. (Courtesy of Dr. Peter Jacobsen.)

sions often appear in middle age and increase as the person ages. Because of the corrugated appearance of the growths, they may be confused with warts. Seborrheic keratosis is characterized by the overproduction of sebum by the sebaceous glands, causing overproduction of the horny layer of the skin.

Figure 23.20 depicts the forehead of a patient who has a multiple area of raised, pigmented seborrheic keratosis. The lesions usually do not require treatment, but they may be removed with cryotherapy or curettage and electrodesiccation. Once removed, they do not usually return.

Urticaria

Urticaria are also known as hives or allergic reactions and are covered thoroughly in Chapter 4. The clinician may notice hives in a patient who is reacting to a substance, insect, medication, the sun (sometimes called sun poisoning), excitement, or possibly a systemic disease. A wheal is a plaque or papule produced because of edema within the skin. The wheals may be slightly reddened and may be coalescing or single. Figure 23-21 depicts skin reactions

to certain metals such as zinc, gold, nickel, chromium, and silver. The lesions are produced because of histamine production or allergy testing. The treatment is often antihistamines, corticosteroids, epinephrine, and identification of the offending substance.

Xanthelasma

In xanthelasma, the lower eyelids often exhibit a pale yellow-orange raised area that is usually in the corner of the eye (Fig. 23.22). The lesions are benign and are only removed for cosmetic reasons when there is a large noticeable discoloration. On examination, the lesion may appear as a cyst or other skin lesion. The lesions are predominately lipid material, are benign, and pose no problem to the patient. The papules have been associated with hyperlipidemia and with low-density lipoproteins.

DISEASES ASSOCIATED WITH SKIN LESIONS

Certain disorders may also have oral skin lesions as part of the infection or disease. The diseases listed below have cutaneous manifestations, and the skin component may often be seen before any other systemic reactions. The dental hygienist may notice a lesion and question the pa-

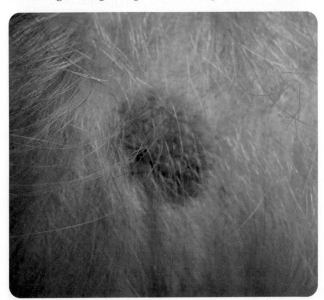

Figure 23.20. Seborrheic keratoses.

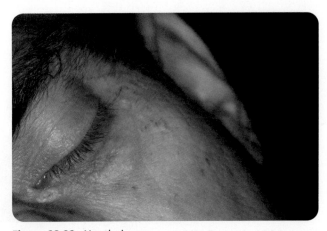

Figure 23.22. Xanthelasma.

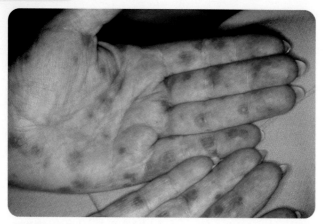

Figure 23.23. Erythema multiforme. (Courtesy of Dr. Peter Jacobsen.)

tient before he or she is even aware that a systemic infection is occurring.

Erythema multiforme

Erythema multiforme is caused by a drug sensitivity or possibly by exposure to any of the following: herpes simplex infection, mycoplasma, tuberculosis, or histoplasmosis. In severe cases, the patient may be treated with systemic corticosteroids. The severe form (discussed in Chapter 12) is termed Steven-Johnson syndrome. Most often, the lesions subside within a few weeks. Oral lesions are reported in up to 50% of cases (Regezi et al., 2003). Erythema-multiforme is covered in Chapter 12. Figure 23.23 shows the hand and arm area of a patient with the classic target or iris lesions.

Graft versus Host Disease

Graft versus host disease (GVHD) primarily occurs in association with bone marrow transplants, although it may occasionally follow solid organ transplantation. Essentially the grafted bone marrow recognizes the tissues of the host as foreign and attacks them. GVHD occurs in up to 45% of bone marrow patients, and the oral cavity may be involved 80% of the time (Imanguli et al., 2006). It can occur as an acute reaction within days of the engraftment or as a

chronic condition months to years later. GVHD may affect the liver and other organs, but skin and oral mucosa is often involved as well. Figure 23.24A depicts the arm area of an African American with GVHD exhibiting a loss of pigmentation in areas of the skin causing a spotted appearance. Figure 23-24B shows the facial area of the same patient, exhibiting a loss of pigmentation on the face and the lips, causing a diffuse, spotted appearance. Skin lesions may be similar to those found in lupus erythematosus, scleroderma, or lichen planus. Loss of pigmentation (vitiligo) is a relatively common skin manifestation of chronic GVHD. Oral manifestations include lesions similar to lichen planus, lupus erythematosus, or nonspecific mucosal ulcerations.

Impetigo

Impetigo is highly contagious and is caused by infection with *Staphylococcus aureus* and streptococci organisms. Nonbullous impetigo is the most common pediatric skin infection and usually starts in a traumatized area. The lesion usually begins as an erythematous papule that becomes pustular and ruptures with a yellow, crusted appearance. The lesions may also be in a bullous form that accounts for only about 30% of cases (Edlich et al., 2005). Figure 23.25 shows typical lesions related to impetigo around the nose and mouth of a child. Impetigo is predominately seen in children and groups that are in close proximity such as children in daycare centers. Topical and systemic antibiotics are necessary. Dental treatment should be postponed because of the highly contagious nature of the disorder and the fact that it will spread to other parts of the face and body of the patient.

Lichen Planus

Lichen planus is both an oral and cutaneous disorder that produces a variation of mucosal disturbances such as ulceration, plaques, erosion, and skin lesions. Both the red and white forms of oral lichen planus are discussed above in Chapters 13 and 14, respectively. In this chapter, we mention the skin lesions related to lichen planus that a practitioner may discover during a routine examination.

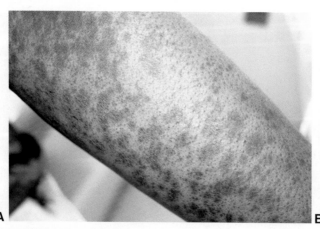
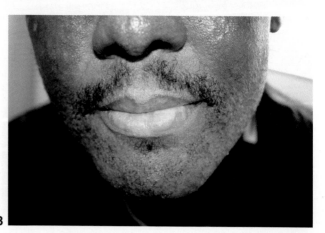

Figure 23.24. A and **B.** GVHD.

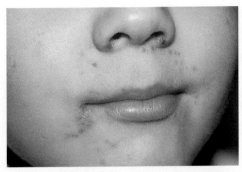

Figure 23.25. Impetigo. (From Goodheart HP, MD. Goodheart's Photoguide of Common Skin Disorders, 2nd Edition. Philadelphia: Lippincott Williams & Wilkins, 2003.)

Although lichen planus is most often noted intraorally, some patients may have external lesions as well. Approximately 5 to 45% of those with lichen planus have both oral and cutaneous lesions at some point in time (Plemons et al. 1999). Additionally, other mucosal diseases such as pemphigus and pemphigoid may exhibit skin lesions as well. These types of skin lesions have a different appearance from that of lichen planus in most cases but can appear similar in some instances. Some skin lesions may be so subtle that they are often not noticed or recorded as lichen planus. When lichen planus appears on the skin, the lesions appear as keratotic, purple, pruritic plaques that occur most frequently on flexor surfaces as seen in Figure 23.26A, depicting a female with lichen planus on the lips, and Figure 23.26B showing lichen planus lesions on the arms with pink to purple raised plaques.

Lupus

Lupus erythematosus is an autoimmune disease described as an inflammatory connective tissue disease. Lupus is covered in more detail in Chapter 12 on ulcers and erosive lesions. Skin lesions related to systemic and discoid lupus may be recognized as having the classic "butterfly rash" that is often found across the nose and malar processes. The skin involvement may be in the scalp region as in

Figure 23.27A showing a patient with systemic lupus erythematosus who has scalp lesions and wears a wig to cover the area. In Figure 23.27B, the patient exhibits cutaneous lesions below the right eye. Sometimes oral tissues may be affected as well. Systemic lupus erythematosus is very serious and may affect vital organs.

Sarcoidosis

Sarcoidosis is a granulomatous disease of unknown cause often affecting African Americans. Sarcoidosis is a systemic disease affecting multiple organs, skin, eyes, and especially targeting the lungs, exhibiting interstitial fibrosis. The disease causes the formation of granulomas composed of epithelioid and multinucleated giant cells. Cutaneous lesions occur in about 25% of cases (Fatahzadeh et al., 2006), with skin and eye lesions apparent. Figure 23-28 shows a male with facial skin involvement exhibiting pronounced, raised lesions on the nose and around the lip area. Enlargement of the salivary glands is often the first characteristic that is noticed in the development of sarcoidosis, and xerostomia is commonly reported by patients. (Sarcoidosis is covered in Chapter 17.)

Scleroderma

Scleroderma has an unknown etiology, but is classified as an immune dysfunction disease. Normally affecting women (4:1) and usually occurring in middle age, scleroderma may occur in children as well (Laxer and Zulian, 2006). The disease may occur in two forms: a generalized progressive systemic form and a diffuse cutaneous form. Both forms manifest with progressive thickening and tightening of the skin in all areas. The lungs, skin, gastrointestinal tract, musculoskeletal system, heart, and kidney are affected by fibrosis and extensive collagen production. Typically, the disease occurs in conjunction with rheumatoid arthritis, lupus erythematosus, dermatomyositis, and/or Sjögren syndrome. **Raynaud's phenomenon** is found in conjunction with the above-mentioned diseases and is characterized by numbness and pallor of the fingers, toes, and nose due to intermittent lack of

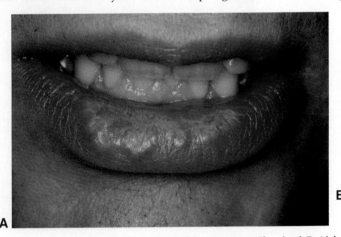

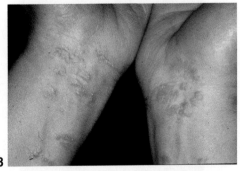

Figure 23.26. A. Lichen planus (Courtesy of Dr. Summer Shapiro.) **B.** Lichen planus (Courtesy of Dr. Terry Rees.)

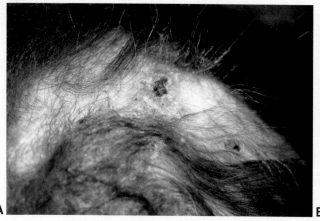
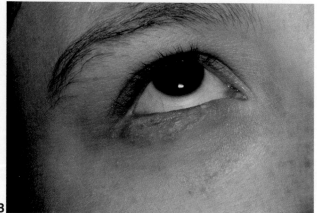

A   **B**

Figure 23.27. A and **B.** Lupus.

blood flow. Major organs are affected with fibrosis, and the skin is usually first noticed. The skin becomes less mobile, exhibits rigidity and becomes tightly elastic. The thickening or hardening of the skin is termed **sclerodactyly**. The fingers become shortened and stiff and exhibit fibrosis. The localized type of scleroderma is known as morphea. Figure 23.29 shows the hands of a patient with sclerodactyly, with fingers in a rigid posture.

The oral structures become rigid and cause the perioral tissues to become constricted, thereby limiting the opening of the mouth and esophagus (Ebert, 2006). This can cause the patient major difficulty with oral hygiene and eating. The disease can also cause resorption of the facial bones and fibrosis of the salivary glands, leading to xerostomia and contributing to an increase in caries. Telangiectasia increases the risk of spontaneous internal bleeding and fibrosis of the esophagus, causing difficulty in swallowing with eventual destruction of the esophageal wall.

Vitiligo

Vitiligo is an autoimmune disorder that is characterized by a lighter appearance of the tissue due to loss of pigment and destruction of melanocytes. The disorder involves 1% of the world population (Whitton et al., 2006), with varying degrees of melanocyte destruction. The cause of the disease is unknown, but exposure to chemical substances is suspected, with the largest class of chemicals being phenolic/catecholic derivatives. Other causes suggested are deficiency in an unidentified melanocyte growth factor, alterations in the mechanisms of the melanocyte, and breakdown in free radical defense in the dermis. Figure 23.30A shows vitiligo with loss of pigmentation on the hands of an African-American male patient. Figure 23.30B shows the back and shoulder area of a Caucasian female with vitiligo. The contrast of the loss of pigmentation is, of course, not as great in the Caucasian woman. The disease occurs in both males and females, usually beginning in the second decade of life.

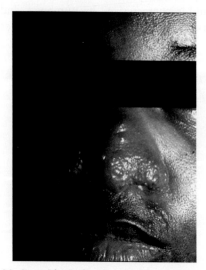

Figure 23.28. Sarcoidosis. (Courtesy of Dr. Terry Rees.)

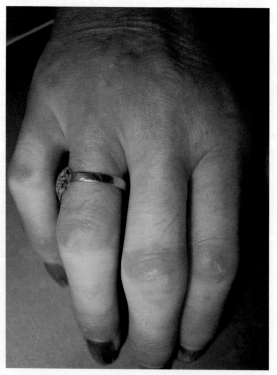

Figure 23.29. Sclerodactyly. (Image provided by Stedman's.)

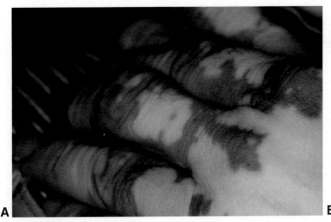 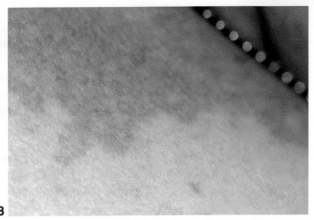

Figure 23.30. A and **B.** Vitiligo.

Warts

Warts are a common name for verrucae vulgaris and may be referred to as plantar warts, flat warts, or often just warts. These lesions are benign and caused by various strains of the human papillomaviruses (HPV). Warts appear as papillary lesions and are usually difficult to remove because of their ability to spread. When found on the fingers, the virus is sometimes transferred to other areas of the body such as the face, lips, nose, and genitalia. Over 70 types have been identified. Cervical cancer related to HPV is the most significant factor in women. Most external lesions regress spontaneously, but some may need other means such as surgical excision, cryosurgery, or application of certain acids.

SUMMARY

The dental office is in a unique position for both detecting and monitoring premalignant and malignant skin lesions. As discussed throughout the chapters, many diseases have oral manifestations before any other sign of disease is present. An added benefit of screenings in the dental practice is that we may be the only practitioners that the patient visits for years. Routine dental visits have increased in the past decades, and the dental hygienist and dentist may be the key healthcare providers who treat the patient most frequently. The increased dental visits may be due to social factors or pressures related to the public awareness and the wish to have a nice smile and a healthy mouth. We should be aware that we could be the only persons who may screen and evaluate the patient for skin cancer as well. If dental offices make this routine, many early cancers and disease states can be detected, and the patients may be referred to a dermatologist or other healthcare provider for treatment early before the disease progresses.

Signs of Skin Cancer:

- Asymmetry
- Border irregularity
- Color varied
- Diameter greater than 6 mm
- A noted change in any skin lesion
- A mole or lesion that does not heal
- Bleeding within or around a mole or any growth

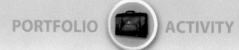

PORTFOLIO ACTIVITY

1. Develop your own set of skin lesion slides to use as examples when talking with patients and for future reference. Consider making a permanent record of existing skin lesions of your patients for future comparison on recall appointments.
2. Develop a set of educational materials related to the prevention of sun damage, which can be given to patients. Use self-examinations for monitoring changes in new and existing lesions. A list of dermatologists in your area should be included in the packet of materials along with a list of the web sites mentioned in this chapter.
3. Have your office order/purchase a variety of skin product samples that could be given to patients seen in your office. Having an assortment of various sam-

ples of quality skin lotions, self-tanning products, and creams on hand for the patient to try would provide a beneficial service. Patients are more likely to buy suggested products that are readily available, and they are more willing to try samples first. Some offices offer products such as lip balms with the office logo and number on the balm. You could then make suggestions to the patient or to the parents of children.
4. Your office may want to consider "Mole Mapping" to assist the patients. The company providing this service is called Digital Derm and can be viewed at *www.digitalderm.com* The patient's mole information, size, and slide may be stored digitally on a CD to be compared at each visit.

INTERNET RESOURCES

http://www.aad.org
http://www.nci.nih.gov
http://www.mpip.org
http://www.aad.orgcancer-information@uiowa.edu
http://www.cancer.org
http://www.skincancer.org
http://www.bad.org.uk/patients

http://www.cancer.gov/cancerinformation
http://www.melanoma.org
http://www.skincarephysicians.com/skincancernet/index.html
http://www.digitalderm.com
http://www.cdc.gov/ChooseYourCover/qanda.htm
http://www.epa.gov/sunwise/uvindex.html

Critical Thinking Activity

Study the image and note and describe the lips of this patient.

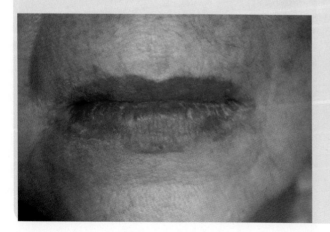

Sun damage is apparent for this patient because of:

- The loss of the definition of the vermillion border on the lower lip
- The tissue is crusted and not smooth surfaced as would normally be seen in healthy tissue.

The student would want to ask

- What is the sun exposure history
- Does she use a sunscreen and a lip balm with a sunscreen of at least SPF15
- How long has changed her lipstick recently-this may be a factor in an allergic-type response to a cosmetic or a dental product.
- Does she bite or lick her lip constantly. The student would want her response but also evaluate whether she

Critical Thinking Activity *(continued)*

is actually biting, chewing or licking the lips during the conversation.

- Vaseline on the lips would be relevant to any dental treatment since the lips are dry and crusted. Any manipulation will cause them to bleed.

This patient is probably very self-conscious about the appearance of her llips. The lips appear read, crusted and somewhat ulcerated. Sometimes patients can cause the lips to become irritated with a history of biting, chewing and licking the lips. In addition, the frequent use of lip balm, especially those with flavors such as cherry, can cause an irritation such as the slide for the case study. Some medications may also cause such a response. A careful evaluation of all factors must be considered and sometimes the process of elimination of certain products and behavioral modifica-

tion will be needed.

Do you think that she has sun damage? If so why? What are you noting that would be characteristic?

What would you want to ask her?

What can you tell by her appearance in the figure?

What would you do before you start any type of dental procedure?

Do you think she would be uncomfortable and suffer any pain from the lips?

Do you think she would have any emotional conflict with her appearance?

Are there any types of diseases that you would want to ask about when you take her medical history?

What do you think are the possibilities regarding an etiology?

APPLICATION

The extraoral screening for skin lesions and external signs of disease are important in early cancer and disease prevention, recognition, and treatment. Making your office known for such screening promotes the office and reflects the importance your office places on both intra- and extraoral cancer screening. (Perhaps with some type of button logo worn by the office that could also be used in newsletters.) Any type of promotion for the office would be a good way to have all the office members vested in a common goal. This could include assistants, office managers, and receptionists. The Oral Cancer Foundation at *http://www.oralcancer.org* offers such buttons as those seen in Figure 23.31. Your office could design your own or perhaps order a type that has been designed by the oral cancer foundation such as "I Save Lives." The logo that is chosen could even be displayed on letterhead, web sites, and perhaps the bags that are used for dental products given to the patient.

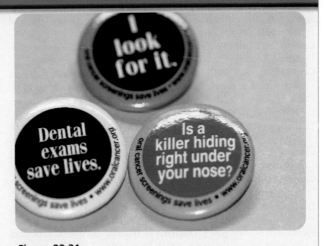

Figure 23.31.

Case Study

Please refer to slide 23.4B

Your receptionist has just returned to work this afternoon with a great tan. She has in her hand some brochures with free coupons from the tanning salon two blocks away. Her intent is to distribute these to patients and to leave them in the waiting area. Your practice is a family practice and many of your patients are 10-20 years of age.

What would you say to the receptionist regarding tanning beds?

- What would you tell the receptionist about tanning beds and about skin cancer that may help to justify why she cannot place such brochures in the office? Refer to information within the chapter.
- Use the slide 23.4B to demonstrate the extent of the damage caused by a melanoma. Remember that the patient used a tanning bed at least four times.

REFERENCES

American Cancer Society's. 2006 Facts and Figures. 2006.

Axell T, Rundquist L. Oral lichen planus—a demographic study. Community Dent Oral Epidemiol 1987;15;52–56.

Barabino G, Canepa M, Ragonesi M, Fiallo P. Persistent acantholytic dermatosis of the lip related to solar damage. Oral Surg Oral Med Oral Pathol Oral Radiol Endod 2003;95:90–93.

Batal H, Chou LL, Cottrell DA. Sarcoidosis: medical and dental implications. Oral Surg Oral Med Oral Pathol Oral Radiol Endod 1999;88:386–390.

Boissy RE, Manga P. On the etiology of contact/occupational vitiligo. Pigment Cell Res 2004;17;(3):208–214.

Bourrain JL. Occupational contact urticaria. Clin Rev Allergy Immunol 2006;30(1):39–46.

Cawson RA, Odell EW. Essentials of oral pathology and oral medicine. 6th ed. London: Churchill Livingstone–Harcourt Brace, 1998.

Cawson RA, Binnie WH, Eveson JW. Color atlas of oral disease—clinical and pathologic correlations. 2nd ed. London: Wolfe Publishing, 1994.

Ebert EC. Esophageal disease in scleroderma. J Clin Gastroenterol 2006;40(9):769–775.

Eisen D. Lynch DP. The mouth—diagnosis and treatment. St. Louis: Mosby, 1998.

Chuh A, Lee A, Zawar V, et al. Pityriasis rosea—an update. Indian J Dermatol Venereol Leprol 2005;71(5):311–315.

Cooper M. Diseases of the epidermis: pityriasis rosea, lichen planus, keratosis pilaris. Dermatol Nurs 2005;17:6, 457–458.

Edlich RF, Winters KL, Britt LD, Long WB. Bacterial diseases of the skin. J Long Term Eff Med Implants 2005;15(5):499–510.

Fatahzadeh M, Rinaggio J. Diagnosis of systemic sarcoidosis prompted by orofacial manifestations. JADA 2006;137:54–60.

Hood AF, Kwan TH, Mihm MC, Horn TD. Dermatopathology. 2nd ed. Boston: Little, Brown & Co., 1993.

Imanguli M, Pavletic SZ, Guadagnini JP, et al., Chronic graft versus host disease of oral mucosa: review of available therapies. Oral Surg Med Oral Pathol Oral Radiol Endod 2006;101:177–185.

Langlais R., Miller C. Color atlas of common oral diseases. Baltimore: Lippincott Williams & Wilkins, 2003.

Laxer RM, Zulian F. Localized scleroderma. Curr Opin Rheumatol 2006;18(6):606–613.

Miller RL. Gould AR, Bernstein ML. Cinnamon-induced stomatitis venenata. Oral Surg Oral Med Oral Pathol 1992;73:708–716.

Neville BW, Damm DD, Allen CM, Bouquot JE. Oral & maxillofacial pathology. Philadelphia: WB Saunders, 1995.

Ortonne JP, Bose SK. Vitiligo: where do we stand? Pigment Cell Res 1993;6(2):61–72.

Parsad D, Kanwar AJ, Kumar B. Psoralen—ultraviolet A vs narrow-band ultraviolet B phototherapy for the treatment of vitiligo. J Eur Acad Dermatol Venereol 2006;20(2):175–177.

Patterson WM, Fox MD, Schwartz RA. Favre-Racouchot disease. Int J Dermatol 2004;43(3):167–169.

Plemons JM, Gonzales TS, Burkhart NW. Vesiculobullous diseases of the oral cavity. Periodontology 2000. 1999;21.158–175.

Pickett F, Gurenlian J. The medical history: clinical implications and emergency prevention in dental settings. Baltimore: Lippincott Williams & Wilkins, 2005.

Porth CM. Essentials of pathophysiology. Baltimore: Lippincott Williams & Wilkins, 2004.

Regezi J, Sciubba J, Jordan R. Oral pathology—clinical pathologic correlations. 4th ed. St. Louis: WB Saunders, 2003.

Rivera A, Tyring SK. Therapy of cutaneous human papillomavirus infections. Dermatol Ther 2004;17(6):441–448.

Rubin, E. Essential pathology. 3rd ed. Baltimore: Lippincott Williams & Wilkins, 2001.

Scully C, Eisen D, Carrozzo M. Management of oral lichen planus. Am J Clin Dermatol 2000;1(5) 287–306.

Scully C. Handbook of oral disease—diagnosis and management. London: Martin Duntz Ltd. The Livery House Publishers, 1999.

Stedman's medical dictionary. 27th ed. Baltimore: Lippincott Williams & Wilkins, 2000.

Sugerman PB, Savage NW. Oral lichen planus: causes, diagnosis and management. Aust Dent J 2002;47:(4):290–297.

Ulmansky M, Michelle R, Azaz B. Oral psoriasis: report of six new cases. J Oral Pathol Med 1995;24:42–45.

Whitton M, Ashcroft D, Barrett CW, Gonzalez U. Interventions for vitiligo. Cochrane Database Syst Rev 2006;(1):CD003263.

Wilkins EM, Clinical practice of the dental hygienist. 9th ed. Baltimore: Lippincott Williams & Wilkins, 2005.

Clinical Protocols

CLINICAL PROTOCOL 1

Supplies for a Cytology Smear May Be Used for Suspected HSV or Candida

- Tongue blade
- Spatula
- Box of glass pathology slides
- Pencil
- Can of hair spray/or purchase special fixative agent
- Mailing containers

1. Pencil in the name of the person on the slide edge.
2. Lightly scrape the suspected area with either tongue blade of the spatula.
3. Lightly place the scraped substance on the slide.
4. Lightly spray with hair spray to fix the slide.
5. Have a slide box, cardboard box, or holder for mailing that will not get damaged.
6. Mail slide to an oral pathologist for evaluation. The nearest dental school will provide the name of a facility where your cytology smear can be processed.

Courtesy of Dr. Valerie Murrah,
University of North Carolina School of Dentistry.

CLINICAL PROTOCOL 2

How to Apply Topical Corticosteroids in the Mouth

GEL, OINTMENT, CREAM

Your doctor has prescribed a topical corticosteroid gel, ointment, or cream for periodic application to your mouth sores. Please follow his/her instructions as written on the prescription box regarding how many times you should apply the medication daily.

It is important to make sure that one of these applications occurs just before bedtime in the evening. The medication probably stays in place longer at that time because saliva flow diminishes when you are asleep.

Whenever you can, it will help if you gently blot the mouth sores dry just before you apply the medication. Do not rub them dry, just blot using gauze. This also will help keep the medication in place for a longer period of time.

When you apply the topical corticosteroid, try to avoid rubbing it in place using a back-and-forth motion, because that motion may rub the "skin" surface away. Instead "dab" the medication into place.

Remember that more is not better. All you need to do is apply a thin coating of the medication. If you do this, it will stay in place better, last longer, and will be safer to use.

RINSE

Use as often as directed for as long as directed. After use, expectorate but do not ingest other liquids for thirty minutes.

SPRAY

Direct spray toward mouth sores as directed. After use, do not ingest water or other liquids for thirty minutes.

From The International Oral Lichen Planus Support Group
www.tambcd.edu/lichen,
Dr. T. D. Rees,-contributor.

CLINICAL PROTOCOL 3

Maintenance Appointment Guidelines for the Mucosal Disorder Patient

- Patients should have professional cleanings every 2-3 months. Periodontal patients many need to be seen every 2 months, depending upon the patient's status and periodontal health.
- Careful scaling of all teeth should be performed with as little disruption of the tissue as possible. When significant periodontal pocketing is present, multiple appointments with gentle scaling and debridement are preferable to conventional deep scaling and root planing.
- All soft tissue areas should be evaluated. Findings should be described and recorded, with any suspicious areas being reevaluated. Careful evaluation for *Candida* is suggested; especially for patients who are using topical corticosteroids.
- The practitioner should note any areas that are in contact with sharp edges, crowns, or restorative materials.
- Tissue areas that do not respond to treatment may need further evaluation and possibly future biopsy.

- Ultrasonic scalers should not be used for extensive subgingival debridement to minimize irritation to the tissue.
- Polishing paste that is gritty or coarse should not be used because of irritation to the tissue both above and below the gingival margin.
- Mouth rinses containing alcohol should be avoided to prevent patient discomfort and tissue irritation.
- Air polishers are too disruptive to the tissues and should not be used.
- Any polishing of the teeth should be performed using a mild paste such as Biotene toothpaste and can be applied with a prophy cup. Simply brushing the teeth with the paste in the dental office will be of some benefit.
- We recommend toothpaste without additives, such as sodium laurel sulfate and flavor-free products, for home care with the use of a soft bristle brush. Paste without many additives can be tolerated by most patients. It is also highly effective in patients with xerostomia.
- Patients should be instructed to discontinue the use of chewing gum, candy, mints, toothpastes, or mouth rinses that contain flavoring agents such as wintergreen, peppermint, spearmint, and cinnamon.
- Periodic photographs both initially and for follow-up appointments are suggested. This allows better evaluation of treatment progress or lack of progress.

Adapted from: International Oral Lichen Support Group Web Site www.tambcd.edu/lichen Drs. Rees and Burkhart, 2007.

CLINICAL PROTOCOL 4

For Patients with Xerostomia

I. Salivary glands

1. Gustatory stimulation (sugar-free candies)
2. Mechanical stimulation
   a. Sugar-free chewing gum (fruit flavors)
   b. Food (apples, carrots, celery, etc)
3. Pharmacologic stimuli (Require prescription)
   a. Salagen (pilocarpine HCl), MGI Pharma, Inc.
   b. Evoxac (cevimeline HCl), Daiichi Pharmaceutical Co. Ltd.
4. Salivary substitutes may be helpful in patients with damage of salivary glands
   a. Mouth-Kote[a] (Parnell Pharmaceuticals)
   b. Optimoist[a] (Colgate-Palmolive Co.)
   c. Oral Balance (Laclede Professional Products)
   d. Salivart (Xenex Laboratories, Inc.)
   e. Numoisyn (Align Pharmaceutical)
   f. Oasis (GlaxoSmithKline)

[a] *Both contain citric acid and could potentially cause softening of the teeth.*
Note: Patients should also maintain adequate level of hydration.

II. Teeth

1. Maintain meticulous oral hygiene
2. Frequent dental visits
3. Daily use of prescription fluoride

III. Oral mucosa

1. Treatment of oral candidiasis with oral nystatin
2. Avoid excessive use of cinnamon and mint

Provided by Ibtisam Al-Hashimi, BDS, MS, PhD. Director, Salivary Dysfunction Clinic, Department of Periodontics, Baylor College of Dentistry, 3302 Gaston Avenue, Dallas, TX 75246.

CLINICAL PROTOCOL 5

Clinical Protocol Treatment for *Candida*

HISTORY OF THE PATIENT: INITIAL MEDICAL EVALUATION OF THE PATIENT

1. Evaluate the medical history of the patient for contributing factors to the presence of candidiasis (endocrine abnormalities, diabetes, HIV, pregnancy, etc.)
2. Initial dental evaluation of the patient for possible oral causative factors for candidiasis: (xerostomia, poor oral hygiene, radiation therapy, aging, inadequate denture retention, etc.)
3. Symptomatology (evaluate for the presence of burning or soreness of the oral mucosa, etc.)

CLINICAL APPEARANCE:

Forms of *Candida*: observe and note what form/forms of *Candida* may be exhibited in the patient (pseudomembranous, chronic atrophic, angular cheilitis, etc.)

Diagnostic Tools

Culturing of *Candida*

1. Test tubes filled with 10 mL of diluted saline are used to culture saliva.
2. The patient rinses with the entire solution in one test tube for 1 minute.
3. The patient expectorates all of the solution back into the test tube.
4. The salivary specimens are sent to the microbiology laboratory for analysis.
5. Culture results are separated into 3 species of *Candida*.
6. Patients are notified in about 4 days of their culture results.

Exfoliative Cytology

1. Take a tongue depressor and roll it over the area of the tongue considered to be a site of candidiasis.
2. Place the specimen gathered on the tongue depressor on a microscope slide and smear the specimen on the slide evenly.

3. Fix the specimen to the slide with a cell fixative solution.

4. Write the patient's name on the frosted end of the slide in pencil.

5. Send the specimen to the pathology laboratory for staining and evaluation.

TREATMENT OF INTRAORAL *CANDIDA*:

Various medications are used for the treatment of intraoral candidiasis. Three common medicaments include nystatin oral suspension, clotrimazole (Mycelex) and fluconazole (Diflucan). Nystatin ointment can be used at the corners of the mouth for the treatment of angular cheilitis.

Nystatin oral suspension (Mycostatin): topical agent for localized treatment for patients whose immune system is not compromised
Disp: 240 mL
Sig: 1 tsp. 4× daily for 2 minutes each time and expectorate. Use for 16 days

Mycelex tablets (clotrimazole)
Disp: 70 tabs
Sig: Dissolve 1 tab on the tongue 5× daily for 14 days

Diflucan is used for florid/disseminated candidiasis or for patients who have an immune system that is compromised.
Diflucan (fluconazole):
Disp: 16 tabs (100-mg tabs)
Sig: Take 200 mg on day 1; take 100 mg daily for 14 days

Nystatin ointment
Disp: 15-g tube
Sig: apply to the corners of the mouth 3–4× daily for the treatment of angular cheilitis

Treatment of Dentures:

1. Chlorhexidine is an antibacterial with some antifungal properties.

    Use of chlorhexidine gluconate 0.12%
    Place denture in chlorhexidine gluconate solution for 1–2 minutes twice daily.
    Remember to treat both the denture and the oral tissues. (The denture will act as a reservoir for *Candida* and reinfect the tissues if they are not treated concurrently.)

2. The following can also be performed in the treatment of dentures:

    Instruct patients to leave their dentures out at nighttime and to soak the denture in a 1% sodium hypochlorite solution for 15 minutes. Make sure that they completely rinse the denture under running water for at least 2 minutes before bedtime.

Prepared by: Dr. Celeste Abraham, Assistant Clinical Professor, Baylor College of Dentistry, TAMHSC, Dallas, Texas. Faculty in The Stomatology Center and The Department of Periodontics.

CLINICAL PROTOCOL 6

Clinical Protocol for Treatment for Sensitivity to Flavoring Agents

Mints, gums, and candies to be avoided are those that have the various mints (mint, spearmint, peppermint) or cinnamon listed on their labels as well as the following:

Some food products containing cinnamon

Canned or packet soups
Canned meat with sauces
Curries
Chinese food
Canned vegetables in sauce
Store made cakes or biscuits
Cola drinks
Carbonated beverages
Alcoholic drinks such as vermouth and gin
Pickles
Ketchup
Chocolates
Powdered aspirin

Toothpastes containing cinnamon:

Aim
Close-Up
Regular Crest
Crest Mint
Crest Tartar Control
Colgate Tartar Control
Gleem

Toothpastes that do not contain cinnamon:

Biotene
Aqua-Fresh
Pepsodent
Colgate with MFP
Ultrabrite
Tom's Natural

Common irritants in toothpaste

Cinnamon aldehyde
Cinnamic acid
Menthol
Alcohol
Boric acid
Surfactants
Flavoring agents
Benzoyl alcohol
Carbamide peroxide
Sodium lauryl sulfate

Avoid chewing gum products that have mints or cinnamon. Some examples are

Big Red
Trident Freshmint
Trident Peppermint

Altoids Mint
Altoids Cinnamon
Ice Breakers Hot Cinnamon
Ice Breakers Cool Mint

Benzoates (benzoic acid, sodium benzoate, propyl 4-hydroxybenzoate) are also preservatives found in foods, carbonated beverages, sauces, fruit products, and toothpastes. They can cause reactions in the oral mucosa similar to those of cinnamon-containing products. Most toothpastes contain benzoates; some toothpastes that have no benzoates are Crest and MacCleans Fresh Mint.

There are several steps to take when you have a patient whom you suspect has sensitivity to various flavoring agents found in toothpastes, mouth rinses, gums, and food products.

Elimination diets, keeping a food diary, as well as patch testing and intraoral biopsies are important in ruling out allergies to flavoring products. Patch testing is useful to distinguish irritant reactions from allergic reactions.

1. It is advisable to first remove/eliminate the causative agent, if that agent is known.
2. The use of intraoral topical steroids may be required.
3. Patients may be referred to a dermatologist for the evaluation of possible skin disorders and for patch testing. Patches with the suspected allergen are placed on small disks and evaluated at intervals of 48 and 72 hours. The results are evaluated as doubtful, weak, strong, or extreme reactions.
4. Patients may be advised to avoid foods that irritate the mouth, such as spicy foods that may contain preservatives such as cinnamon.
5. Patients may be advised to avoid soft drinks, candies, mints, and chewing gums in case allergy to flavoring agents is suspected.
6. Patients may be asked to keep a food diary and list all the foods that they ingest over a period of 1-2 weeks. They must also list the dentifrice they are using, any snacks that they may eat between meals, any alcoholic drinks they use, etc.
7. A biopsy to rule out other oral lesions may be required if there is no resolution after a few recall appointments.

Prepared by: Dr. Celeste Abraham, Assistant Clinical Professor, Baylor College of Dentistry, TAMHSC, Dallas, Texas. Faculty in The Stomatology Center and The Department of Periodontics.

Adapted from handouts of the Stomatology Center, Baylor College of Dentistry, Dallas, Texas and from the handbook Non-plaque-related Diseases of the Periodontium (Terry D. Rees 2005).

CLINICAL PROTOCOL 7

Patient Education: Recommendations for Recurrent Herpes Labialis

Proper diagnosis of recurrent herpes labialis (RHL) is important to help with treatment and prevention. A diary of the nature of the outbreak can help identify a triggering event. Location, appearance, symptoms such as duration, type and severity of pain, exposure to cold air, sun, stress (emotional or physical), types of dental treatment, fever and infections, and, in some cases, allergies are helpful elements to include.

- Itching, tingling, or burning may precede the eruption of vesicles. The reactivation of virus from the nerves occurs repeatedly in the same location. It is rare that a patient has RHL in more than one area.
- Typically, there is a cluster of vesicles as the virus comes to the surface. The surface of the vesicle ruptures easily within several hours, leading to a weeping of fluid that contains virus particles and can spread the infection to the patient's partner or other sites. The area then progresses to a crust or scab, with or without bleeding. Most patients heal within 7 to 10 days of the vesicle formation.
- Topical antiviral cream (1% penciclovir) or ointment (5% acyclovir) are helpful for some patients. Patients should apply the ointment to the area every 2 hours while awake. For some patients, this may prevent the vesicle formation. In others, it reduces the duration and may make the lesions less infectious (patients should continue application every 2 hours for up to 1 week). These prescription topical agents also keep the crust moist and flexible so it is less likely to crack and bleed, and therefore is less painful.
- Over-the-counter docosanol 10% (Abreva, GlaxoSmithKline) helps some patients. Patients should apply this agent to the area five times daily until healed.
- Patients should wash hands frequently and always after manipulation of these areas. A cotton tip applicator may be helpful to apply the cream or ointment. Some preparations come in a tube with a narrow applicator tip that allows more precise placement, but the tube should be discarded after the episode so as not to infect another area.
- The systemic antiviral valacyclovir has been approved to prevent RHL. Eight 500-mg tablets should be prescribed. Patients should be instructed to take 4 tablets when the first symptoms are noticed; they then should take 4 tablets 12 hours after the first dose is ingested. This is a very time-sensitive prescription and patients should have the tablets in their possession; this usually

is only prescribed for patients who have had a clear history of recurrence, with episodes that occur more than 6 times per year.

- Use of lip balm with SPF15 sunscreen or higher may help patients whose episodes are stimulated by sun exposure.
- Routine dental treatment should be deferred during the vesicle and crust stages, for the patient's comfort as well as for reducing the spread of infection. Proper infection control is essential to protect the clinician as well as other patients.

Prepared by: Dr. Wendy S. Hupp, DMD, Assistant Professor of Oral Medicine, Department of Diagnostic Sciences, Prosthodontics, Restorative Dentistry, University of Louisville School of Dentistry

CLINICAL PROTOCOL 8

Clinical Protocol for Patients with Intraoral Ulcers (Recurrent Intraoral Herpes, Recurrent Aphthous Ulcers, or Traumatic Ulcers)

Understanding the cause of intraoral ulcers helps to prevent recurrences and to select the best treatment. A diary of the nature of the ulcer helps to distinguish between aphthous and traumatic ulcers and recurrent herpes. Information that is helpful to determine the diagnosis includes location, appearance, symptoms such as duration, type and severity of pain, and "triggers" such as cold air, sun exposure, stress, dental treatment, fever and infections, and, in some cases, allergies. All patients who have intraoral ulcers may choose to defer dental treatment until they are more comfortable.

- Recurrent aphthous ulcers (RAU) usually start to appear in the teen years and most commonly are solitary round or oval lesions on movable tissue; they have a red halo and a yellow to white covering, are quite painful, and heal within 2 weeks without scarring
- RAU may be more frequent in patients during high stressful periods, such as during a woman's menstrual period or during an emotional situation.
- RAU are caused by the immune cells called T-lymphocytes that lead to a limited destruction; therefore, treatment should include some type of immune modulator, such as topical steroids (see Clinical Protocol #2). In some patients, the early use of steroids can actually prevent the RAU from becoming very severe, but over use of topical or systemic steroids may lead to candidal infection or medication side effects.

- Palliative treatment should be suggested for patients to help manage the symptoms. Warm saline and bicarbonate rinses are helpful: ½ teaspoon of table salt and ½ teaspoon of sodium bicarbonate (baking soda) in 8 ounces of warm water, swished and held in the mouth until the warmth dissipates, then expectorate the solution. This can be used after meals in place of tooth brushing during the most painful time. Another product called Orabase Soothe'n'seal (Colgate, no prescription needed) works for up to about 6 hours. It is similar to super glue and helps by covering up the nerves, even providing some protection from further injury. It is likely that this coating allows the ulcer to heal a little faster. Other topical anesthetics may be too caustic; while easing the pain, they may actually delay healing. Viscous lidocaine mixed with diphenhydramine elixir and an antacid liquid such as Maalox (Novartis Consumer Health) or Kaopectate (Pfizer Consumer Healthcare) can also be used. The pharmacist must mix these three liquids in equal parts, then the patient can swish a teaspoonful for 30 to 60 seconds and spit before meals. Caution the patient that this may lead to difficulty swallowing because the mouth is numb.
- Traumatic ulcers (TU) can occur at any time and anywhere in the mouth, but can be confused with RAU when they are present on movable tissue. They are usually linear or with irregular edges, with a yellow to white covering, and variably with a red halo
- Trauma occurs from broken fillings or rough edges of teeth, extreme temperatures (e.g., hot food or drinks, very cold foods), eating implements, misuse of medications (e.g., an aspirin tablet applied to the tissue or overuse of topical anesthetics), or other chemicals that may cause burns or allergic reactions. A food diary is helpful in diagnosing some patients, including use of any toothpaste, mouthwash, bleaching products, chewing gum or candies, and condiments such as cinnamon that are placed into the mouth.
- TU may heal faster with the use of topical steroids once the cause is removed.
- See palliative treatment above.
- Recurrent intraoral herpes occurs on non-movable tissue, most commonly on the hard palate in the premolar region (see section on Herpes Labialis). There is a clear demarcation at the midline as the virus follows a nerve, and the same area is affected repeatedly.
- Dental treatment is commonly the stimulus for recurrence, including injections and tissue manipulation during scaling and curettage.
- Vesicles are often missed because the covering is very delicate; the ulcerations that follow are shallow and multiple, but may coalesce to form a larger, irregularly shaped lesion that has a yellow to white covering and a red halo. These lesions often become painful, but the pa-

tient may confuse the pain with that of the dental treatment that initiated the recurrence.

- Recurrent intraoral herpes is best treated by prevention, perhaps with systemic antiviral medications just before the manipulation of the tissue. Topical antiviral preparations are not helpful. At the first sign of itching, tingling, or burning, valacyclovir 2000 mg should be taken, repeating the same dose 12 hours later. This 1-day treatment is also used to treat recurrent herpes labialis.
- Once the ulcers have occurred, the same palliative measures for RAU and TU can be used (see above). Topical steroids should not be used for herpetic lesions in the early stages.

Prepared by: Dr. Wendy S. Hupp, DMD, Assistant Professor of Oral Medicine, Department of Diagnostic Sciences, Prosthodontics, Restorative Dentistry, University of Louisville School of Dentistry

CLINICAL PROTOCOL 9

Prevention of Further Oral Tissue Damage in Patients with Eating Disorders

- Carefully monitor the amount of enamel loss by using models and intraoral photographs.
- Provide patients with custom trays and 1.1% neutral fluoride gel (Prevident[a]). Patients can use the trays for 5 minutes daily. A good time is while taking a shower.
- After vomiting, rinsing with 1 tsp of baking soda mixed with 8 oz of water will help neutralize the hydrochloric stomach acids that damage the enamel.
- Daily rinses with 0.05% fluoride (such as Act[b]) will help harden the enamel against acid dissolution.
- Rinse with just water after vomiting (if baking soda and water is not available).
- Do not brush the teeth for at least 1 hour after vomiting. Rinsing after vomiting is crucial to minimize enamel loss.
- Instruction of proper tooth brushing methods using a soft-bristle toothbrush is important to minimize enamel loss.
- Instruct patients to use a tongue cleaner and to brush the tongue thoroughly to remove acid residue that collects in the papillae after vomiting.
- Encourage patients to drink water throughout the day to decrease the acid content of the mouth.
- Minimize the use of abrasive materials in professional dental hygiene procedures related to scaling and polishing practices.
- Providing education for healthy snack foods is crucial. Foods such as cheese, fruits, vegetables, and other nonacidic, non-sugar-containing foods are important to good oral and general health.
- Encourage saliva flow with the use of sugarless gum and mints, especially those sweetened with xylitol.
- Suggest that patients drink through a straw when drinking any acidic beverage such as fruit juice or carbonated beverages.

[a] Colgate Oral Pharmaceuticals, Inc.

[b] Johnson & Johnson Distributed by Personal Products Company. Division of McNeil-PPC, Inc., Skilman, New Jersey.

Adapted from: Burkhart, N. Roberts M, Alexander M, Dodds A. Communicating effectively with patients suspected of having bulimia nervosa. J Am Dent Assoc 2005;136:1517.

CLINICAL PROTOCOL 10

UVA Protection-Advising Your Patients

- Sun avoidance is the best defense. Remember that sunscreens reduce the damaging effects, but do not eliminate them.
- Use a broad-spectrum protection sunscreen of at least an SPF #15 (Sun Protection Factor) and apply approximately 1 ounce, 20 to 30 minutes before going out into the sun.
- Reapply every 4 to 5 hours, and always reapply after going in water. When going in the water, use a waterproof sunscreen and reapply after 50 minutes if you have been in the water for that amount of time. Reapply if you perspire a lot.
- Ultraviolet B (UVB) light is primarily responsible for tanning and burning. Ultraviolet A (UVA) is light that penetrates deep into the tissue (these are especially emitted in tanning beds and greatly damage connective tissue).
- Active ingredients of a sunscreen should contain titanium dioxide, zinc oxide or avobenzone (Parasol 1789). Titanium dioxide and zinc oxide protect against both UVB and UVA, and Tinosorb and Mexoryl SX are options.
- Be aware that concrete, snow and water can reflect up to 85% of the sun's rays exposing you to more than double the normal amount.
- Seek shade between 10:00 AM and 4:00 PM, which is when the ultraviolet light is the most intense. Even cloud cover allows 80% of UV rays to pass through. The UV Index is on a 0 to 10+ scale, and special care should be taken when the index is 5+. Remember that the shorter your shadow, the more damaging the sun's rays.
- Wear a wide-brimmed hat that has been specially treated to block the sun's rays. Wear opaque clothing

specially treated to protect the skin (one that has a UPF [ultraviolet protection factor] of 30 or more), and buy large beach umbrellas that are specially protected to block the sun's rays completely at 100%.

- Never use tanning beds—the exposure emits mostly UVA rays, which penetrate deep into the tissues and cause considerable tissue damage and premature aging.
- Consider using sunless self-tanning lotions.
- Use a lip balm containing PABA (para-aminobenzoic acid) an active ingredient and at least an SPF of 15.
- Wear sunglasses with UV-blocking capacity.
- Know the ABCDs of skin cancer.
- Teach children good skin care—PASS IT ON!
- Perform skin self-exams monthly using a hand mirror and search for any skin spots that have changed color, size, or shape.
- Ask your hair salon or stylist to check the scalp and hairline for any discoloration or lesions while shampooing your hair.
- Be evaluated by your dermatologist at least once a year or every 6 months if you have a history of skin cancer, especially melanoma.
- Cloudy days do not protect you from sun damage, dark skin does not protect you, and a good tan does not protect you from further damage.
- REMEMBER THAT EARLY DETECTION IS THE KEY!
- SEE YOUR DERMATOLOGIST!
- NEVER BE SUNBURNED—THIS IS THE BEST DEFENSE.

Prepared by Nancy Burkhart, RDH, M.Ed., Ed.D. April, 2007.

CLINICAL PROTOCOL 11

Suggestions for Training the Patient To Do an Oral Cancer Self-Examination

1. When you perform your intraoral examination, give the patients a large mirror and show them what you are seeing. Point out the normal anatomy and any atypical findings that you may see so that they will know what is normal for them (e.g., benign migratory glossitis, Fordyce's granules, and tori or exostoses).
2. Instruct patients that they are looking for any of the following signs or symptoms of cancer. In most cases, these symptoms should be present for approximately 2 weeks; however, anything that a patient is concerned about should be brought to the attention of a medical or dental professional as soon as possible.

Reprinted with permission from the American Society of Clinical Oncology; signs and symptoms of oral cancer from www.plwc.org.

- Sore in the mouth or on the lip that does not heal (the most common symptom)
- Red or white patch on any oral tissues, tongue, tonsil, or lining of the mouth
- Irritation, lump, or thick patch in the mouth, neck, or throat
- Persistent sore throat, or a feeling that something is caught in the throat
- Hoarseness or change in the voice
- Numbness in the tongue or mouth
- Pain or bleeding in the mouth that does not resolve
- Difficulty chewing, swallowing, or moving the jaws or tongue
- Ear and/or jaw pain
- Chronic bad breath
- Changes in speech
- Loosening of teeth or toothache
- Dentures that no longer fit
- Unexplained weight loss
- Fatigue
- Fever of unknown origin, especially when prolonged; this is usually a sign of paraneoplastic syndromes and indicative of advanced disease.
- Loss of appetite, especially when prolonged (anorexia); similar to fever, this is usually a sign of advanced disease.

3. The following are suggestions for instructing the patient how to do the self-examination:
   - Find a mirror in a well lighted area; do not use a mirror that you need to hold unless you have no other option.
   - Have a flashlight with a strong beam available for use.
   - Start by directing the flash light beam toward the back of the throat by bouncing the light off of the mirror into the throat area.
   - Look at the roof of the mouth
   - Stretch the cheeks out from the teeth and look at the lips
   - Put the tongue on the roof of the mouth and look at the floor of the mouth
   - Stick the tongue out or hold it and look at the top, both sides, and the bottom
4. Any suspicious findings should be brought to the attention of a medical or dental professional. The self-examination should be preformed once a month.

Prepared by Leslie DeLong, RDH, MHA.

CLINICAL PROTOCOL 12

Adjunctive Oral Premalignant Screening Devices

The essential part of any form of early detection begins with the clinical exam of the patient, including a careful assessment of the health history, a lifestyle factor evaluation and, ultimately, the extraoral and intraoral dental exam. Dental students and dental hygiene students are taught that the clinician must search for an explanation for any persistent lesion that appears to be of abnormal color or size, or exhibits any unusual characteristics. A dilemma develops when a lesion is detected that does not appear to be threatening, but that also has no known etiology. Lesions such as this may be associated with an injury or a benign condition, or they may contain dysplastic cells and be the clinical manifestation of the early stages of premalignant or malignant growth. The newest cancer screening devices/techniques can help the clinician identify lesions that have a higher degree of suspicion, and therefore present with a more urgent need for a definitive diagnosis. These devices/techniques are considered to be adjuncts to, not substitutes for, a tissue biopsy. They should help the clinician and the patient with their decision to either: (1) proceed with a referral, (2) perform a biopsy, or (3) monitor the lesion. However, it should be noted, that while a report that is positive for dysplasia or malignancy indicates the immediate need for a biopsy, a negative report does not mean that the lesion is necessarily innocuous, and may leave the clinician and the patient with additional uncertainty as to the need for a biopsy.

EXFOLIATIVE CYTOLOGY

Exfoliative cytology has been performed for many years. It is the basis for the Pap test that women are familiar with and it has been used in the oral cavity to help determine if a biopsy is necessary. Historically, this procedure was performed with a moist tongue depressor that scraped surface cells off the lesion. In 1999, a technique using a patented spiral stiff nylon bristle brush was introduced, and termed "the brush biopsy."

BRUSH BIOPSY

Materials for performing the "Brush Biopsy" are obtained from the company that developed and markets the system, and that will eventually examine the specimen and report the findings to the dentist.

Materials in the kit include:
- Brush
- Clear glass slide with UPC code
- A fixative liquid
- Plastic slide container
- Form for patient and tissue information
- Mailer box for return of the specimen.

Procedure:
- The cells for the specimen are obtained by twirling a patented spiral-shaped, stiff nylon brush into the lesion.
  - Apply enough pressure to the lesion that you note a slight bend in the brush.
  - Continue to twirl the brush on the lesion until pinpoint spots of bleeding are observed. This is supposed to indicate that cells from the entire thickness of the epithelium have been gathered in the specimen.
- Transfer the collected cells immediately to the slide provided in the kit. The surface of the brush that was used to obtain the sample should be rotated on the slide. Continue to rotate the brush on the slide until an observable film is seen on the surface of the slide.
  - If no film is seen, repeat the technique on the lesion with the same brush.
- Apply the liquid fixative to the slide immediately after you have determined that you have an adequate sample. Do not worry about excess fixative that runs off the slide. Let dry for approximately 15 to 20 minutes.
- Place the slide in the container provided and follow the instructions to submit the sample for testing.

LIQUID-BASED CYTOLOGY

One reported problem inherent in the technique described above is most of the cells collected on the brush are often thrown away with the brush. A new technique that is being used by many hospitals and obstetrics-gynecological practices may also eventually be considered for use in the mouth. This technique uses a similar type of brush to collect a sample of cells, but instead of transferring the cells onto a glass slide, the brush is twirled in a container that holds a preservative liquid. By using this method, as many of the cells as possible are collected. The plastic brush handle is then cut and the plastic brush is placed in the container. The container with the specimen and preservative liquid is sent for testing. This technique is supposed to yield a better representative collection of the cells in the lesion. In addition, the cells are filtered out from other debris included in the sample, resulting in a qualitatively superior sample to examine and interpret. This procedure has been shown to decrease the false-positive and false-negative reports observed with the traditional exfoliative cytology technique.

TOLUIDINE BLUE VITAL STAINING

This technique was first introduced in the early 1970s with varying degrees of acceptance and has been used more or less ever since. It recently has been the object of several studies, and its use appears to be increasing once again. Toluidine blue is a basic metachromatic vital dye that stains the nuclear material of cells that are undergoing increased DNA synthesis, such as malignant cells (and atypical reactive cells). This is being used not only to help determine a degree of suspicion with regard to a specific lesion, but to also guide clinicians while they determine the best area from which to remove tissue during a biopsy of a lesion (i.e., marker system).

Materials:
- 1% toluidine blue dye
- Water
- 1% acetic acid solution.

Procedure:

- Rinse the mouth with water twice, for approximately 20 seconds each time, to remove debris.
- Rinse the mouth with 1% acetic acid solution, for approximately 20 seconds, to remove saliva.
- Gently dry the area.
- Apply the toluidine blue dye to the high-risk areas or to a specific lesion.
- Rinse with 1% acetic acid for 1 minute to clear excess stain.
- Rinse with water.

Interpretation:

Expertise is required to interpret the true staining from inconsequential diffuse film or mechanical retention of the stain (e.g., filiform papillae of the tongue). This procedure is more than 90% accurate in identifying lesions that are dysplastic or malignant*.

CHEMILUMINESCENCE (VIZILITE® PLUS, ZILA PHARMACEUTICAL, PHOENIX, AZ)

This system uses a chemical light to identify abnormal areas and a form of toluidine blue (i.e., Tolonium chloride) to mark these areas.

Materials:

- Small bottle of 1% raspberry-flavored acetic acid solution (vinegar)
- Chemical light source
- Toluidine blue dye (TBlue630®)

Chemiluminescent procedure:

- Rinse the mouth with the acetic acid solution for 1 minute and expectorate.
- Activate the light source by breaking the inner vial and shaking the capsule to mix the chemicals.
- Assemble the light stick following instructions.
- Dim the room lights and look for white appearing lesions or areas.

Interpretation:

- Normal epithelium absorbs the device's light and appears dark.
- Abnormal cells will reflect the light and appear white.
- Once the suspicious areas are identified, you can use the toluidine blue dye to further mark the lesion for subsequent removal, partial or total.

Precautions

- ViziLite® Plus should not be used for pregnant women or children. Other precautions are noted in the manufacturer's instructions.

DIRECT OPTICAL FLUORESCENCE VISUALIZATION TECHNOLOGY (VELscope™)

The VELscope™ handpiece emits a safe blue light into the mouth, which stimulates the fluorophores with the mucosa tissues, causing them to emit a fluorescent green glow. Special optical filters in the handpiece allow the clinician to view the different fluorescence responses of healthy versus abnormal oral tissue.

Materials:

- VELscopeTM handpiece/unit

Procedure:

- Turn off ambient lights and direct the unit light at the oral tissues, observing the fluorescence response.
- The healthy oral mucosal tissue will appear bright green, while suspicious regions are identified by a loss of fluorescence and will appear dark.

From: Silverman S, Migliorati C, Barbosa J. Adjunctive techniques in oral cancer detection. Dimensions of Dental Hygiene 2006; 4(9):28.

Prepared by: Dr. Michael Kahn, Chairman and Professor of Oral and Maxillofacial Pathology, Tufts University School of Dental Medicine

CLINICAL PROTOCOL 13

Recommendations for Alleviating the Oral Symptoms of Mucositis

- Remove any prosthetic appliances during episodes of mucositis.
- For lesions that do not resolve, evaluate the patient orally for a secondary bacterial or yeast infection.
- Keep the oral tissues moist in the presence of xerostomia (refer to Clinical Protocol 4).
  - Increase fluid intake.
    - Sip on water frequently.
    - Suck on ice chips.
  - Use sugar-free candy or gum (products containing xylitol are excellent for stimulating saliva and inhibiting the growth of oral bacteria).
- Use oral rinses to soothe tissues and maintain hydration. Avoid any rinse containing alcohol or other astringents.
  - ½ tsp. baking soda, 1 qt. water—neutralizes acids after vomiting, dissolves thick saliva, soothes tissues, and dislodges debris; use once every 2 hours, or as needed
  - ½ tsp salt, 8 oz. water—helps moisturize tissues, reduce irritation, and removes thick saliva and debris
- Use topical anesthetics and/or systemic pain medications for pain control.
  - Topical anesthetics should be used as soon as possible to manage mild to moderate pain and should continue to be used in conjunction with systemic pain relievers for moderate to severe pain.
    - Avoid accidental mucosal injury.
    - Do not eat or perform oral hygiene procedures while anesthetized.
    - Avoid using on the soft palate or rear of the mouth.
    - Examples
      - Lidocaine: viscous gel, jelly, ointment, solution
      - Benzocaine: gel, ointment, spray

- Compounded rinse: Lidocaine, Benadryl, Amphojel, Nystatin, and sometimes a topical steroid. The ingredients in these rinses vary according to the individual prescriber.
- Systemic analgesics
  - NSAIDs
    - Acetaminophen
    - Ibuprofen
    - Naproxen
  - Opioids
    - Codeine
    - Oxycodone
    - Morphine
- Therapy should be based on the level of pain that is present and will be different for every individual.

Prepared by Leslie DeLong, RDH, MHA.

Used with permission from Rankin KV, Jones DL, Redding SW, eds. Oral Health in Cancer Therapy, second edition. Texas Cancer Council, 2004:43–52.

CLINICAL PROTOCOL 14

Post-Operative Instructions for Oral Surgery Patients

You have just had a dental extraction, an oral surgery procedure. The following instructions, which may be modified by your doctor, will help you recover from this procedure as you heal over the next several days:

1. Bleeding: Applying firm pressure, continue to bite on the gauze pack for 1 hour. Do not chew on the packing; if you have to talk, do so with clenched teeth. At the end of 1 hour, remove the gauze and, if you are still bleeding or oozing, replace it with gauze that has been given to you, biting on it for 30 minutes. If bleeding still persists, wrap a tea bag in fresh gauze, moisten it, and bite on it for another 30 minutes. If this does not solve the problem, call the office or go to a hospital emergency room.

2. Rinsing/Spitting: Do not rinse or spit for the rest of the day. This is very important, as rinsing or spitting can dislodge the clot, causing renewed bleeding and other complications. Just swallow instead; you will be swallowing the same saliva you have swallowed for years. You may swallow a little bit of blood that is mixed with the saliva; do not worry about it, it will not hurt you.

3. Swelling: Use an ice pack to minimize swelling, 20 minutes on and 20 minutes off for the rest of the day. You can easily make an ice pack out of a bag of frozen peas; just bang on the bag to loosen the peas, then wrap it in a towel and apply it so that it molds to the side of your face. Do not use ice for more than 24

hours, and never apply heat to your face unless your doctor tells you to.

4. Medication: You may take over-the-counter medication that you usually take for pain, and your doctor may have prescribed a stronger medication, such as a narcotic. The sooner you take pain medicine after surgery, the more effective it will be. Try to take it at regular intervals, before your pain returns, so that you remain as pain-free as possible during the postoperative period. Always swallow the medication; do not let it dissolve in your mouth next to the surgical site. You may also have been prescribed an antibiotic; take it as directed, and try not to miss any doses. If you do miss a dose, do not double up; just take the missed dose as soon as you remember it, then resume the prescribed schedule (See "A word about antibiotics" at the end of these instructions).

5. Eating: After you remove the gauze, and there is no more bleeding, you may eat anything you desire on the other side of your mouth. For the first few days, you may be more comfortable eating soft foods such as cool soup, applesauce, mashed potatoes, baby food, milkshakes, yogurt, and ice cream. It is important to maintain a good nutritional intake, as this is essential for rapid and proper healing. Do not worry if you accidentally chew on the extraction side; you will not do any damage, as your body will quickly remind you of your recent surgery.

6. Drinking: Avoid drinking through a straw, especially if you have had an upper back tooth removed. Sometimes the roots of these teeth are very close to your sinuses, and drinking through a straw can cause complications. Your doctor will tell you if other precautions are necessary.

7. Smoking: Above all, if you smoke, DO NOT SMOKE for at least 1 week after surgery. If you had an open wound on your hand, you would not blow smoke into it, would you? Similarly, you now have an open wound in your mouth, and your body needs all the TLC you can give it to help you heal. Do not make its job harder by smoking!

8. Oral Hygiene: It is very important that you keep your mouth clean. Starting this evening, brush and floss your teeth as you normally do, but avoid the surgical site; and remember to rinse the toothpaste from your mouth very gently with a small amount of cool water. You should be able to resume brushing the surgical area within a day or two. If it hurts to brush gently, just cleanse the area with a moistened gauze pad.

9. Irrigation: Starting tomorrow, rinse your mouth with warm salt water. This is one of the best things you can do to help you heal and feel better as soon as possible, and you cannot do it too often! Rinse as follows: fill a drinking glass with very warm water and stir in half a teaspoon of table salt. Rinse with a small amount of this mixture, bathing the surgical site. Be gentle; it is not

necessary to rinse vigorously. When the water cools off, spit it out and take another portion. Do this until you have used up the entire glass. Repeat every hour while you are awake, and continue for 5 to 7 days.

10. Sutures: Your doctor may have placed sutures (stitches) over the surgical site to enable your body to heal faster. If the sutures are made of a resorbable material ("gut"), they will dissolve in approximately 7 to 21 days, depending on the type used, and you should not need a follow-up visit. If a non-resorbable suture was used (e.g., silk, nylon), you will have been given an appointment to return to the office in 5 to 7 days to have them removed. This will also give your doctor a chance to check on your progress, so it is imperative that you keep this appointment.

A word about antibiotics: If you have been given an antibiotic, it is very important that you take it as directed to treat your infection caused by "bad" bacteria. Antibiotics must be taken regularly, usually every 6 hours by the clock, and should be taken until they are all gone. Do not share them with anyone else, and do not save some for another time. Antibiotics may cause gastrointestinal (GI) distress, which can be avoided by eating a cup (4–8 ounces depending on the container) of yogurt, 20 to 30 minutes after each dose. It does not matter what brand or flavor of yogurt you choose; it can be with or without fruit; fat-free or not. What is important is that it has live cultures, and it will indicate "with active cultures," or "with live cultures" on the container. Do not use yogurt that is sterilized or does not have the "culture" statement on the package—it will not protect you from GI distress! The reason for this is that antibiotics, as they go through your GI tract, can destroy the "good" bacteria needed for proper digestion and, if these are not replaced, you may experience distress (pain, gas, diarrhea). The live cultures replace the good bacteria that are normally present. Some antibiotics are more likely to cause distress than others, but if you have been prescribed clindamycin or Cleocin® (Pfizer, New York, NY), it is very important to eat the yogurt, as described above, after every dose. Your doctor will advise you of any additional precautions concerning antibiotics or any medicine prescribed for you.

Good luck with your recovery! These instructions were written with your welfare and comfort in mind. If you follow them carefully, you will minimize postoperative problems. If you have questions or concerns, experience swelling or severe pain after the second day, or develop a fever over 101°, do not hesitate to call the office. If it is after hours, your doctor or a doctor on-call can be reached through the answering service.

Written July 2006, by: A. Michael Krakow, D.M.D., M.S., M.F.S.

Clinical Associate Professor of Oral Medicine and Attending, Department of Dental Medicine, University Hospital, University of Medicine and Dentistry of New Jersey

CLINICAL PROTOCOL 15

Office Protocol For Identifying Suspected Family Violence

REMEMBER—Office safety planning must be a part of the office protocol before any intervention in suspected family violence.

STEPS IN IDENTIFICATION OF SUSPECTED FAMILY VIOLENCE

1. **General physical assessment of the patient.** Although general physical examinations may not be appropriate in the dental setting, be aware of obvious physical traits that may indicate family violence (e.g. difficulty in walking or sitting, physical signs that may be consistent with the use of force, delay in seeking treatment, general neglect, financial neglect)
2. **Behavior assessment.** Judge the patient's behavior against the demeanor of patient's of similar maturity in similar situations.
3. **Health histories.** If you suspect child maltreatment, it can be useful to obtain more than one history, one from the child and one separately from the adult. If you suspect intimate partner violence or elder abuse and neglect, also try to separate the patient from any suspected perpetrator to conduct the history.
4. **Orofacial examination.** Look for signs of violence, such as multiple injuries or bruises, injuries in different stages of healing, or oral signs of sexually transmitted diseases.
5. Consultation. If indicated, consult with the child's physician about the patient's needs or your suspicions.

STEPS IN REPORTING SUSPECTED CHILD ABUSE OR NEGLECT

1. Documentation. Carefully document any findings of suspected abuse or neglect in the patient's record.
2. Witness. Have another individual witness the examination, note and co-sign the records concerning suspected child abuse or neglect.
3. Report. Call the appropriate child protective services (CPS) or law enforcement agency in your area, consistent with state law. Make the report as soon as possible without compromising the child's dental care.

The telephone number for reporting is _____.

4. Necessary information. Have the following information available when you make the report:
   - name and address of the child and parents or other persons having care and custody of the child;
   - child's age

- name(s) of any siblings
- nature of the child's condition, including any evidence of previous injuries or disabilities; and,
- any other information that you believe might be helpful in establishing the cause of such abuse or neglect and the identity of the person believed to have caused such abuse or neglect.

DEALING WITH SUSPECTED INTIMATE PARTNER VIOLENCE OR ELDER ABUSE AND NEGLECT

Reporting adult victims of family violence may or may not be appropriate. State laws vary considerably on mandated reporting of adult victims of family violence, and safety issues will affect your decision to intervene. Consult local authorities on reporting requirements for adults and the elderly who may be victims. Ensure that you protect both patient's confidentiality and the health and safety of both the patient and your office staff.

Lynn Douglas Mouden, DDS, MPH; PO Box 1437, Little Rock, AR 72203; 501-661-2595; fax 501-661-2055; e-mail: Lynn.Mouden@arkansas.gov

CLINICAL PROTOCOL 16

Diabetes Care Guidelines

OVERVIEW

The attainment of optimal oral health outcomes in patients with diabetes is determined by the level of the patient's adherence to their prescribed medical therapy (diabetes self-management) and the presence of medical complications resulting from diabetes. The role of the dental professional is to reinforce the basic principals of diabetes care, recognize medical and dental complications of this disease, and ultimately improve the patient's quality of life.

MEDICAL HISTORY EVALUATION:

1. Is the patient adherent to medical recommendations for care of their diabetes?
   - Patients should self-monitor blood sugar 2 to 4 times a day (80–120 mg/dL before meals; 100–140 mg/dL at bedtime). Note: Ideally, diabetes medications should keep blood sugars within these ranges.
   - Medications should be taken as prescribed by their physician.
   - Patients should undergo yearly updates of basic diabetes self-management education.
2. Questions that will help to determine the patient's level of control of their disease.
   - How are you feeling today?
   - What type of diabetes do you have and when were you diagnosed?
   - When was your last visit to your physician (diabetes) and how often do you go?
   - From which healthcare providers do you seek care on a regular basis?
   - What medications (prescription and over-the-counter) do you take?
   - Are you taking the medications as they were prescribed for you?
   - Do you know your glycosylated hemoglobin value (normal range: 4.5-6.5%; obtained 2-4 times per year)?
   - Do you smoke or use tobacco products? If so, how much?
   - How often do you check your blood sugar and what was the most recent value?
   - Have you had a hemoglobin A1c test done and what was the value?
   - Have you had any problems with low or high blood sugar levels recently?
   - Have you had any heart or vascular problems?
   - When did you last have a dilated eye exam? (yearly)
   - Do you have pain or cramps in your legs at any time?
   - Do you have any open sores, numbness, pain, tingling, or coldness in your feet? If so, how often and where?
   - Do you have any trouble swallowing?
   - If you take insulin injections, where do you administer them? (important to rotate sites)
3. Emphasize that proper diabetes management leads to better oral health, which will positively impact the patient's overall health.
4. After obtaining or updating the medical history, determine whether there are medical issues that warrant immediate care prior to elective dental procedures being performed.
5. Medical referral is appropriate if there are serious issues related to the patient's diabetes care, self-care regimen, or if the patient presents with problems not previously noted or diagnosed.

ORAL ASSESSMENT:

1. Salivary glands
   - Look for swellings in glands
   - Assess salivary flow and quality of saliva
2. Periodontal examination
   - Gingival assessment for bleeding and clinical signs of disease
   - Full mouth probing on initial examination and annually thereafter
3. Examine all tooth surfaces
   - Caries
   - Erosions
   - Abfractions
   - Other abnormalities
4. Examine soft tissues for pathology
5. Evaluate the patient's hands for problems that would interfere with dental self-care regimens

DENTAL TREATMENT MODIFICATIONS:

The decision to obtain a medical consultation, postpone treatment, or modify treatment should be based on the patients' level of disease control, as evidenced by their answers to the questions above. The goal in cases where consultation, postponement or modifications are indicated is to improve the patient's glycemic control and minimize the risk of an emergency during dental procedures. If patients have good control of their disease, no modifications are necessary during routine dental treatment. In all instances, balance treatment needs with patients' medical status and their motivation and ability to follow dental self-care recommendations <u>without</u> limitations.

The following are examples of modifications that may be indicated for scaling and root planning or other invasive dental procedures including oral and periodontal surgery:

- Schedule patients for morning appointments after they have taken their medications and have eaten.
- Prepare patients in advance for dietary changes that may be associated with dental procedures that have the potential to affect their ability to eat. Diabetes educators or dietitians can recommend various diets that will conform to post-treatment requirements and provide proper nutrition for the patient.
- Consider antibiotic prophylaxis if the patient's blood glucose level exceeds 200 mg/dL (use AHA recommendations or consult with the physician).
- Do not attempt to adjust insulin doses for routine dental treatment. Any adjustment to insulin doses should be done only after consultation with the patient's physician and/or core diabetes team member.

Diabetes Resources for Dental Professionals
National Institute of Diabetes, Digestive, and Kidney Disorders
www.niddk.gov
Centers for Disease Control and Prevention, Division of Diabetes
Translation www.cdc.gov/diabetes
National Diabetes Education Program www.ndep.nih.gov
Patient education materials
Healthcare professional materials (Working Together to Manage Diabetes: A Guide for Pharmacists, Podiatrists, Optometrists, and Dental Professionals, Primer and poster)
Awareness Campaigns
American Diabetes Association www.diabetes.org
Prepared by: Frank Varon, DDS, Omaha, Nebraska

CLINICAL PROTOCOL 17

Management of the Patient with Heart Disease

Cardiovascular disease continues to be the leading cause of death in the United States, although a greatly increased number of individuals are living relatively normal lives despite the presence of one or more manifestation of this condition. It is beyond the scope of this section to fully address the nature of various heart conditions and principles of dental management of patients with the conditions. The reader should review one of several oral medicine texts that discuss cardiovascular diseases and their management in detail. However, we will attempt to outline certain general principles that apply to dental management of individuals with various forms of this disease.

VALVULAR HEART DISEASE/HEART MURMUR

1. Heart damage from conditions such as rheumatic heart disease, congenital heart defects, systemic lupus erythematosus, mitral valve prolapse, and others may place individuals at increased risk of developing infectious endocarditis (IE), a life-threatening infection. However, there is minimal evidence associating bacteremias produced during dental treatment with episodes of infectious endocarditis to a greater extent than that associated with bacteremias induced by normal oral functions such as chewing, toothbrushing, and flossing. Consequently, the American Heart Association (AHA) has recently (2007) updated their recommendations regarding dental considerations in patients at risk for infectious endocarditis. Prophylactic antibiotic coverage is recommended for individuals with valvular heart disease only if they have a history of infectious endocarditis or if they have a prosthetic cardiac valve.

2. For patients at risk (those with a history of infectious endocarditis or who have a prosthetic cardiac valve), some authorities believe that IE sometimes may occur following dental treatment. Consequently, certain steps are appropriate in dental management of these individuals.

3. Prophylactic antibiotic coverage is recommended for at-risk patients for all dental treatment procedures that involve manipulation of gingival tissue or the periapical region of teeth or perforation of oral mucosa. According to these recommendations, only a few specific dental procedures do not require prophylaxis. These include routine anesthetic injections through noninfected tissue, taking dental radiographs, placement of removable prosthodontic or orthodontic appliances, adjustment of orthodontic appliances, placement of orthodontic brackets, shedding of deciduous teeth, and bleeding from trauma to the lips or oral mucosa. Use the current antibiotic guidelines established by the AHA in 2007, which are very similar to previous guidelines. The AHA emphasizes that IE is best prevented by insuring maximal periodontal and dental health through maintaining effective oral hygiene and frequent office recall intervals.

NOTE: AHA Guidelines available at website: DOI: 10.1161/CIRCULATIONAHA.106.183095. Hard copy will be published in *Circulation* 2007. Meanwhile a single reprint is available by calling 800-242-8721 (United States only), Reprint #71-0407.

4. Occasionally, prophylactic antibiotic may be inadvertently omitted during a dental procedure. In this event, prophylactic antibiotics may still be effective if administered within the first 2 hours following the procedure.

5. Medical consultation may be indicated to determine the nature of the patient's risk during dental treatment. If immediate dental treatment must be administered before medical consultation, use the AHA recommendations for prophylactic antibiotic coverage during dental emergency treatment.

CONGENITAL HEART DEFECTS

1. Heart defects that are present at birth can affect any part or function of the heart. Today, surgical correction of these defects is often quite successful, but patients may continue to be at risk for complications during dental treatment. Consequently, medical consultation is imperative to determine the true nature of the patient's health status.

2. Prophylactic antibiotic coverage may be required if the risk of infectious endocarditis persists. It is recommended if cyanotic congenital heart disease, including shunts and conduits, is present for 6 months following successful repair with a prosthetic patch or device. Patients with incompletely repaired defects require antibiotic pre-medication, as do patients with congenital heart defects who have experienced infectious endocarditis or who have received a prosthetic valve at any point in their lives.

3. Be aware of the patient's drug and medical history and be alert for any signs or symptoms that may indicate the continuing presence of a heart defect.

ISCHEMIC HEART DISEASES (CORONARY ARTERY DISEASE)

1. Partial blockage of heart arteries (atheroma) may impair blood supply to the heart, leading to pain on exertion (angina) or death (myocardial infarction). Patients with this condition are at risk of serious complications during dental treatment, and medical consultation is imperative prior to elective dental therapy. Practitioners must remain alert for signs or symptoms of developing ischemic heart disease during dental treatment.

2. Vasoconstrictors in local anesthetics (epinephrine or its equivalent) may be needed to obtain effective local anesthesia. However, most authorities recommend limiting total epinephrine to that contained in two to three carpules of local anesthetic with 1:100,000 epinephrine (0.02 mg per carpule) or its equivalent in individuals with ischemic heart disease. There does not appear to be any advantage in substituting levonordefrin for epinephrine, and intraosseous or intraligamental injections should be avoided. The use of vasoconstrictors on retraction cord is contraindicated.

3. An office stress reduction protocol is essential. Dental therapy should be administered in a calm and relaxing atmosphere, and conscious sedation techniques should be considered. Profound dental anesthesia is very important and procedures should be kept short.

4. In the event that a patient experiences an ischemic attack during dental treatment, the dental procedure should be terminated and the patient should be placed in a semi-supine position; 100% oxygen should be administered and vital signs monitored. If necessary, nitroglycerin 0.2-0.4 mg should be administered and repeated if needed. In severe office emergencies, the Emergency Medical System should be activated and, if necessary, external cardiac defibrillation administered by trained office personnel.

HYPERTROPHIC CARDIOMYOPATHY

1. Hypertrophic cardiomyopathy is a genetically derived heart enlargement that may go undetected for many years. The enlargement may impair normal heart function and, as a result, some affected individuals may experience unexpected sudden cardiac arrest, often during exercise or stressful situations. Dental patients who report a history of this condition should be referred to their physician for medical consultation to determine their health status and to insure that dental therapy can be safely performed.

2. Patients with hypertrophic cardiomyopathy are at some risk of developing infectious endocarditis, but according to the recent recommendations of the AHA, prophylactic antibiotic coverage is not required for dental treatment unless the individual has a history of infectious endocarditis or a prosthetic heart valve. In this event, appropriate antibiotic prophylaxis should be administered in keeping with the recommendations of the AHA.

3. A dental office stress-reduction protocol should be followed as described above.

4. If a patient becomes symptomatic during dental treatment (e.g., syncope, chest pains, arrhythmia, loss of consciousness), the procedure should be terminated and the Emergency Medical System activated. Nitroglycerin and other vasodilating drugs are contraindicated in these patients, but 100% oxygen and appropriate cardiopulmonary resuscitation should be performed if necessary.

CARDIAC ARRHYTHMIAS

1. Abnormal heart rhythms can be induced by any condition that influences normal electrical impulses to the heart muscle. Arrhythmias may range from a slow heart beat (bradycardia) to a rapid beat (tachycardia), loss of atrial rhythm (atrial fibrillation), or loss of ventricular rhythm (ventricular fibrillation). Individuals who experience atrial fibrillation are at increased risk for stroke, while ventricular fibrillation

can result in death. Medical consultation is required for any patient who reports a history of significant cardiac arrhythmias or who shows signs or symptoms of the condition.

2. Local anesthetics containing vasoconstrictors should be limited to two to three carpules of anesthetic containing 1:100,000 epinephrine or its equivalent. Local anesthetic should be administered slowly, and no vasoconstricting agent should be used on retraction cords.

3. Prophylactic antibiotic coverage is not required for dental treatment based solely on a history of cardiac arrhythmias. However, complications of the patient's heart condition may create an indication for its use.

4. An interoffice stress reduction protocol should be followed as described above.

5. Cardiac pacemakers are often used today to control cardiac arrhythmias, and an increasing number of individuals with life-threatening ventricular arrhythmias are being treated by placement of automatic implanted cardioverter defibrillators (AICD). The presence of these devices does not represent a contraindication to dental treatment, nor does it require prophylactic antibiotic coverage. However, older AICDs (more than 10 years old) sometimes may be disrupted by electromagnetic currents and caution should be taken with the use of electrosurgical devices and magnetorestrictive ultrasonic instruments.

6. AICD patients will receive an electrical shock if their device is activated. Consequently, the patient's experience with the device should be discussed in advance. Most devices are not activated for several seconds after the beginning of the arrhythmia, and patients should be asked to forewarn the dental staff if they perceive a possible pending electrical shock. The treatment procedure should be suspended and all dental items removed, when possible, before the shock. A mouth prop should be considered for use with these patients to minimize the risk of injury to them or the dental practitioner. Under most circumstances, the patient will return to normal rhythm after the shock. If this does not occur, the Emergency Medical System should be activated and cardiopulmonary resuscitation initiated if needed.

CONGESTIVE HEART FAILURE

1. Congestive heart failure occurs when a weakened heart muscle is no longer able to pump adequate quantities of oxygenated blood to the body. It may be caused by any of the conditions discussed above, and it results in fluid accumulation in the lungs along with kidney failure. Consequently, affected individuals may experience shortness of breath, peripheral edema, angina, cyanosis, and chronic fatigue. Despite the serious life-threatening nature of the condition, current cardiology treatment modalities may signifi-

cantly prolong life. Many individuals with congestive heart failure can be expected to seek dental care when needed.

2. Medical consultation is imperative to determine a patient's overall health status. Patients with severe congestive heart failure are not candidates for routine dental care, but many others are. Antibiotic prophylaxis may be indicated depending on the etiologic factors associated with heart failure. When antibiotics are indicated, the recommendations of the AHA can be followed.

3. Medications used in the treatment of heart failure sometimes may induce gingival overgrowth or a spontaneous dry cough that may interfere with routine dental treatment.

4. Stress-reduction protocols are indicated for dental treatment, as described above.

5. The dental practitioner must remain alert for signs or symptoms of cardiac crisis, and must be prepared to activate the Emergency Medical System and administer cardiopulmonary resuscitation if needed. Prophylactic antibiotic coverage is not required for dental treatment unless the patient has a history of infectious endocarditis, a prosthetic heart valve, or prophylaxis is requested by the physician.

THE SURGICALLY CORRECTED HEART

1. Surgical correction of congenital heart defects, valvular stenosis, or occluded coronary arteries has become a standard of care in cardiology, and heart transplantation is an acceptable treatment option. Medical consultation is important to determine the cardiac treatment outcomes for dental patients who report such surgical procedures. Prophylactic antibiotic therapy is not required for dental treatment in patients who have had successful heart surgery such as correction of minor congenital defects and coronary artery bypass grafts. However, patients with artificial heart valves or partially repaired congenital defects will require antibiotic prophylaxis using AHA guidelines.

2. It is important to be aware that severe periodontal disease may predispose patients to recurrence of their original heart condition such as coronary artery occlusion or stroke.

CORONARY ARTERY STENTS

1. Placement of coronary artery stents has become increasingly common in the management of individuals with coronary artery disease. Individuals receiving these stents may remain on anticoagulant medication for life. Consequently, medical consultation may be necessary to determine any necessary dental treatment precautions.

2. Antibiotic prophylaxis is not required based solely on the presence of coronary artery stents following a 4- to 6-week healing period. In most instances, no re-

duction in anticoagulant therapy is required for routine dental procedures, including periodontal surgery and extractions.

HEART TRANSPLANTATION

1. Heart transplants are currently being used to manage a variety of cardiovascular conditions. Improvements in protocols to insure good donor-patient tissue matches, improved surgical techniques, and the use of immunosuppressant drugs to prevent organ rejection have markedly increased the success rate. However, transplants are not without complications, and medical consultation is essential before performing dental therapy. Ongoing close medical-dental coordination is important to ensure that the dentist is aware of any developing condition that may adversely affect rendering safe and effective dental care.

2. Gingival enlargement may occur as a side effect of anti-rejection drugs such as cyclosporine, and immunosuppressant drugs may cause an individual to be more susceptible to opportunistic oral infections, osteoporosis, or avascular osteonecrosis.

3. In general, prophylactic antibiotic coverage is not required for dental treatment after a normal healing period of up to 6 months. However, the AHA recommends antibiotic prophylaxis for heart transplant recipients if they develop cardiac valvulopathy. Organ recipients who do not achieve maximal cardiac function or who require extensive immunosuppressive therapy may remain at risk of life-threatening infections. Consequently, consultation with the patient's physician is recommended. In most cases, the antibiotic guidelines recommended by the AHA probably would be appropriate unless more stringent antibiotic coverage is requested by the cardiologist.

4. Optimal periodontal and dental health is extremely important for transplant recipients. It should be noted that immunosuppressive medications may mask the usual signs and symptoms of oral infections, so very careful dental/periodontal examination is indicated. Meticulous oral hygiene measures and frequent maintenance recall visits help to insure prevention or early detection of developing dental or periodontal problems.

5. Due to loss of innervation to transplanted hearts, patients may experience "silent" painless myocardial infarction, so close monitoring of vital signs in imperative.

Prepared by: Dr. Terry Rees, Professor, Baylor College of Dentistry, Department of Periodontics, TAMHSC, Dallas, Texas.

Ablated (ablation): Removed completely.

Acanthosis: Thickening of the epithelium.

Acrochordon: Acrochordons are commonly referred to as skin tags. Skin tags are usually flesh colored, benign, and pose no risk to the person.

Actinic cheilitis: The term actinic denotes solar involvement, and cheilitis denotes inflammation of the lip. The term actinic cheilitis is solar damage, and these tissue changes in the lip region are considered a premalignant condition.

Actinic keratosis: A premalignant condition involving the sun-exposed areas of skin, resulting in a "wart-like" lesion forming a hyperkeratotic surface.

Albers-Schönberg disease (osteopetrosis): A rare bone disease affecting the skeleton, and resulting in an absence of bone resorption due to reduced osteoclastic activity.

Aneurysmal bone cyst: The aneurysmal bone cyst is considered a pseudocyst in that it appears as a cyst but, unlike the epithelial-lined true cyst, the aneurysmal bone cyst does not have the epithelial-lined lumen.

Ankylosis: The stiffening of a joint as the result of abnormal bone fusion; to become joined or consolidated.

Anogenital: Relating to the anus and genitals.

Antifungal: Agent used to destroy or inhibit the growth of fungi.

Atopic/atopy: Genetically linked hypersensitivity to environmental allergens

Atrophic: Tissue demonstrating thinning of the epithelium.

Autoinoculation: The self-induced transferring of a virus from one part of the body to another.

Autosomal: Pertaining to any of the ordinary two paired chromosomes (in contrast to the sex chromosomes) that make up the genetic material of an individual.

Basal cell carcinoma: Basal cell carcinoma of the skin is the most common skin cancer. The cancer evolves from the basal cell layer of the epidermis, resulting in invading nests and strands of neoplastic basal cells.

Bohn's nodules (gingival cyst of the newborn or dental lamina cysts of the newborn): Tiny nodules along the junction of the hard and soft palate and along dental ridges that are derived from epithelial remnants.

Botryoid odontogenic cyst: A variant of the periodontal lateral cyst that is seen as a multilocular, grape-like cluster of cysts with the exact characteristics of the periodontal lateral cyst.

Callous: Over-production of keratin on the skin as a result of friction.

Caseous necrosis: A term denoting a necrotic tissue resembling cheese that is made of a mixture of protein and fat. Caseous granulomas are typically found in tuberculosis.

CD4 Count: A measure of the number of helper T cells per cubic millimeter of blood; used to analyze the prognosis of patients infected with HIV.

Cementoblastoma (or true cementoma): A true neoplasm of cementoblast. The lesions may produce pain and the tooth remains vital. The cementoblastoma is attached to the tooth root and appears radiographically as an opaque calcified mass.

Cheilitis: Inflammation of the lips or of a lip, with redness and the production of fissures radiating from the angles of the mouth.

Coagulation necrosis: Necrosis of cells in which cellular outlines are maintained.

Coloboma: An absence or defect of some portion of the tissues of the eye.

Comedones: Inflamed, dilated hair follicles filled with keratin, bacteria, and sebum. Comedones may be open to the outer skin surface or they may be closed. Another common name for them would be whiteheads or blackheads.

Coronal: Pertaining to the crown portion of a tooth.

Cyst: A pathologic cavity lined by epithelium and surrounded by a fibrous cyst wall.

Depapillated: Atrophy with loss of filiform papillae of the dorsal tongue.

Dominant: A trait that is manifest in an individual even though the characteristic is present on only one of the paired sets of chromosomes. For example, an individual with one blue eyed gene and one brown eyed gene would have brown eyes since brown eyes are dominant over blue eyes.

Dysplasia (epithelial): Cytological changes the epithelium goes through prior to becoming malignant.

Ectoderm: The outermost of the three germ layers present in the developing embryo. From it, the skin, nails, hair, glands, nervous system, and teeth, among other structures, are developed.

Eczema: Generic term denoting the inflammatory conditions of the skin.

Electrodesiccation: A high-frequency electrocurrent is used to seal off blood vessel supply to the skin.

Elastosis: Degeneration of collagen fibers, making the tissue more expansive.

Endosteal: A term used to denote the layer of endosteum lining the inner surface of the bone.

Ephelides: Commonly known as freckles.

Epithelial rests: The remains of the epithelial root sheath that cover the roots during root development. These rests are small clusters of cells that are left during tooth formation and later remain in the periodontal ligament. One of the theories for cyst development states that inflammation in the bone can stimulate rests of odontogenic epithelium to proliferate and become cystic.

Erythema multiforme: Presents as an eruption of papules, macules with the classic target lesion appearance or Iris-type appearance. Erythema multiforme may have multiple appearances and is caused by a hypersensitivity reaction or the herpes simplex virus.

Erythroleukoplakia: Premalignant or malignant lesion consisting of erythroplakia and leukoplakia.

Exophytic: Growing outward. Used of a tumor or an oral lesion.

Favre-Racouchot disease: Is a common disease characterized by solar elastosis and large open comedones and cysts in varying sizes. The disorder typically affects Caucasian men who spend a lot of time in the sun.

Florid cementoosseous dysplasia: Form of dysplasia seen on a radiograph with varying degrees of radiolucent and radiopaque appearance depending on the degree of calcification. The lesion may have a ground glass appearance.

Focal cementoosseous dysplasia: Dysplasia usually seen on a radiograph with varying degrees of radiolucent and radiopaque appearance depending on the degree of calcification. The calcification progresses with the age of the lesion. Focal cementoosseous dysplasia is a reactive process and the tooth is vital.

Focal sclerosing osteomyelitis (condensing osteitis): A reaction to some type of trauma or an inflammatory reaction to some stimulus. Focal sclerosing osteomyelitis usually involves pulpal inflammation and necrosis of the pulp, resulting in sclerotic bone in an isolated area.

Follicular: Pertaining to the tissues surrounding the developing tooth bud.

Gardner's syndrome: An autosomal dominant disease characterized by gastrointestinal polyps that develop in the colon, stomach, and upper intestine. The syndrome includes the osteoma and sometimes odontomas, epidermoid cysts, supernumerary teeth, other benign tumors of the skin and soft tissues, and multiple polyps.

Gastroesophageal reflux: Backward flow of the acidic contents of the stomach through the muscle sphincter into the esophagus. If severe, stomach contents may regurgitate into the oral cavity.

Genokeratosis: Inherited disorders of the skin and oral mucosa.

Graft vs. host disease: Graft vs. host disease may occur after the initial organ or tissue has been transplanted into the host. The patient may suffer skin lesions, ulcerations that may vary in number, and multiple sites may be affected. The ulcerations may occur both orally and on the skin surfaces.

Hamartoma: A focal malformation that resembles a neoplasm, grossly and even microscopically, but results from faulty development in an organ; composed of an abnormal mixture of tissue elements, or an abnormal proportion of a single element growing at the same rate as normal components. (Stedman's 2000)

Heterozygous: Having two different genes form at any specific site on a paired set of chromosomes. For example, an individual with one blue eyed gene and one brown eyed gene would be heterozygous.

Hiatal hernia: Protrusion of a portion of the stomach through the hole in the diaphragm through which the esophagus normally passes. This condition predisposes an individual to gastroesophageal reflux.

Homozygous: Having the same gene forms at any specific site on a paired set of chromosomes. For example, an individual with two blue eyed genes would be homozygous for blue eyes. Likewise, an individual with two brown eyed genes would be homozygous for brown eyes.

Human papillomavirus, low-risk: Low-risk human papillomaviruses are associated with benign lesions and are not likely to cause the infected cells to undergo a malignant transformation.

Human papillomavirus, high-risk: High-risk human papillomaviruses are associated with an increased risk of primary malignancy or of malignant transformation of a benign lesion.

Hyperkeratosis: Over production of keratin.

Hyperplastic: An abnormal increase in the number of cells in an organ or a tissue with consequent enlargement.

Hyphae: Elongated form of *Candida albicans*.

Idiopathic: Of unknown cause.

Impetigo: Caused by the bacterial organism *Streptococci* or by *Staphylococcus aureus*. Impetigo is highly contagious, and is often observed in day care centers.

Intralesional: Introduced into or performed within a lesion.

Keratolytic: Relating to or causing keratolysis (breakdown of keratin).

Keloid: Excessive hyperplastic scars that are reactions to trauma. Keloids are sometimes painful lesions on the face, arms, and legs. The African American population is affected more frequently.

Keratinization: The process whereby epithelial cells lose water and become hard.

Keratinocyte: An epithelial cell that produces keratin, other proteins, and sterols. It is formed at the basal layer from undifferentiated cells and then undergoes progressive changes as it moves toward the surface layer of the skin, where it eventually exfoliates.

Kindred: A group of related persons; a family. In genetics, multiple generations of a family unit carrying a genetically transmitted characteristic that is used for study of the abnormality.

Koebner phenomenon: Ability of a disease to affect chronically irritated tissue.

Koilocyte: A vacuolated pyknotic epithelial cell that has either a clear cytoplasm or a perinuclear halo, and that tends to be associated with certain human papillomavirus infections.

Leukoplakia: Premalignant lesion presenting as a white plaque without distinguishing clinical features.

Lichen planus: Lichen resembles the mossy plant known to grow on rocks with a lacy spreading of the plant. Lichen planus is a disease of unknown cause that may affect both the skin and the oral tissues. Six types of lichen are identified orally, and up to 45% of patients may have both oral and cutaneous lesions. Lichen planus is classified as a cell-mediated immune response.

Lumen: The space in the interior of a tubular structure.

Lupus: Lupus erythematosus is an autoimmune type of disease and is also referred to as discoid lupus when the skin is affected. Systemic lupus erythematosus affects major organs, and the disease is termed systemic lupus when systems of the body are affected. Lupus found on the skin exhibits follicular plugging, telangiectasia, hyperkeratosis, and atrophic plaques.

Lymphadenopathy: A chronic, abnormal enlargement of the lymph nodes usually associated with disease.

Macule: An area that is usually distinguished by a color different from that of the surrounding tissue. It is flat and does not protrude above the surface of the normal tissue (e.g., freckles).

Melanoma: The third most occurring skin cancer. Melanoma is caused by malignant cells that are capable of producing melanin and may originate from a pigmented nevus. Melanomas have the ability to spread to other organs within the body in later stages.

Metastatic calcifications: Calcification that is occurring in non-osseous tissue that is not degenerated or necrotic. The cells of these organs secrete acid materials and, under certain conditions (e.g., in instances of hypercalcemia), the alteration in pH causes precipitation of calcium salts in these sites.

Milia: Benign cysts that are commonly found on the skin. The cysts may be expelled through normal skin care regimens, and are often noticed around the eye area.

Mitosoid figures: Cells in which the nuclear DNA has fragmented, resulting in a cell that looks like it is undergoing mitosis.

Morbidity: Rate of disease.

Mortality: Death rate.

Necrosis: Death of cells or tissues through injury or disease, especially in a localized area of the body.

Nevoid basal cell carcinoma syndrome: This syndrome is an inherited, autosomal dominant disorder with a male predilection. Characteristics include nevoid basal cell carcinoma, jaw cysts, congenital skeletal anomalies, ectopic calcifications, and palmar and plantar pits, nevi, or small basal cell carcinomas on cutaneous areas.

Nevus (nevi, pl.): A benign overgrowth of melanin-forming cells. The nevi may be classified as junctional, compound, or intramucosal in structure. The classification is determined by the proximity to the basal cell layer. Another name for the common nevus is the mole.

Non-vital tooth: A tooth in which the pulp is not long-living; the tooth will test negative when a pulp-testing device is used on the surface of the tooth.

Nuclear hyperchromatism: Cytological feature of malignancy or premalignancy.

Odontogenic cysts: Cysts with an epithelial lining that is formed from the remnants of the tooth-forming organ, the rests of Malassez (rests of the root sheath of Hertwig), glands of Serres (rests of the dental lamina), and reduced enamel epithelium (remnants of the enamel organ).

Odontoma: Developmental anomalies that are hamartomas. In the case of odontomas, the tissue is a mixture of enamel, dentin, cementum, and pulp.

Osteoma: A benign tumor consisting of mature compact or cancellous bone. Osteomas may be classified as either periosteal, which occurs on the surface of bone, or as endosteal, which occurs in the bone.

Osteopetrosis: Also referred to as Albers-Schönberg disease (See definition on page 559).

Papilloma: A benign exophytic papillary growth of stratified squamous epithelium.

Paradental cyst: Cyst derived from the reduced enamel epithelium thought to be a variant of the dentigerous cyst, which is usually found at the bifurcation areas of molars.

Parafunctional: Characterized by abnormal function.

Parakeratotic/parakeratosis: An abnormal formation of keratin cells in the stratum corneum that have retained their nuclei, may contain abnormal keratin, and contain too much water, causing swelling of the cell.

Pathognomonic: Specifically distinctive or characteristic of a disease that allows nearly instant recognition.

Penetrance/penetrant: The frequency with which a heritable trait is manifested by an individual that has the gene form associated with causing the disease.

Percussion: Striking a tooth with short, sharp blows as a diagnostic tool to attempt to elicit pain.

Periapical cementoosseous dysplasia (cementoma): A lesion that is usually seen on a radiograph with varying degrees of radiolucent and radiopaque appearance depending on the degree of calcification. The calcification progresses with the age of the lesion, and the tooth is vital.

Periapical granuloma (dental granuloma, apical periodontitis): The result of necrotic pulp tissue and by-products resulting from an inflammatory process that has damaged the tissue at the apex of the tooth. The etiology may be trauma, injury to the pulp through dental procedures, caries, periodontal disease that has affected the root area severely, and fractures to the tooth.

Periosteal: A term that relates to the periosteum or the thick fibrous membrane covering the entire surface of a bone.

Perlèche: Also termed angular cheilitis, the folds and angles of the mouth become inflamed from normal aging and skin sagging, causing the pooling of saliva in the corners of the mouth. The inflammation may be compounded by licking the area constantly and Candida may grow in the moist folds.

Phleboliths: A calcified deposit in a venus wall.

Pityriasis: Dermatologic response resulting in oval-shaped lesions with reddened outlined plaques that have central salmon-colored appearances. Pityriasis usually occurs on the trunk of the body, with the lesions following creases in the skin. The condition is self-limiting and usually dissipates on its own. The cause is unknown, but may be found after the use of some medications.

Plaque: An area with a flat surface and raised edges.

Poison oak: Causes a skin reaction after exposure, producing multiple vesicle-like lesions. Poison oak belongs to the species of plant called the Toxicodendron family, which includes poison oak, poison sumac, and poison ivy.

Polyposis: The presence of several polyps. Adenomatous coli or familial adenomatous are terms used in relation to the presence of malignant polyp development in Gardener's syndrome.

"Precystic" epithelial proliferation: The rests that remain during tooth development become stimulated and are said to proliferate. The rests begins to grow and start to circle in order to wall off from the existing tissue during in this earliest stage of cyst development.

Premalignant lesion: A specific clinical alteration in tissue that predisposes to the development of oral cancer.

Primordial cyst: A variant of the odontogenic keratocyst that technically develops in place of the existing tooth or before any calcification of the tooth. Odontogenic keratocysts can be associated with impacted third molars and develop with no association to third molars.

Premalignant lesion: A specific clinical alteration in tissue that predisposes to a high likelihood of malignant degeneration.

Prophylactic: Tending to ward off or prevent a disease process or condition from occurring.

Pruritic: Itchy.

Pseudocysts: Lesions that have an accumulation of fluid in a cyst-like structure, but they do not have an epithelial lining.

Pseudomembrane: Build-up of tissue or debris on the surface mucosa, which wipes off.

Psoriasis: A dermatologic condition with a strong hereditary component. The conditions may have many different forms, as well as severity, but commonly exhibit a scaly, silver-like appearance. Removal of the scales may produce bleeding. Psoriasis is usually found in younger individuals, but may persist throughout life with periods of exacerbation and remission.

Pyknotic: A degenerative state of the cell nucleus.

Radicular: Pertaining to the root of a tooth.

Radicular cyst: A cyst that is always associated with a nonvital tooth, with common causes being caries, trauma, or periodontal disease. The inflammatory process and necrosis of the pulp causes the epithelial proliferation that a cyst needs to develop.

Raynaud's phenomenon: Characterized by numbness and pallor of the fingers, toes, and nose due to intermittent lack of blood flow to the fingers.

Recessive: A trait that must be present on both members of the paired set of chromosomes in order for the individual to manifest that trait. For example, an individual must have two blue eyed genes in order to manifest blue eyes because blue eyes are a recessive trait.

Recalcitrant: Markedly resistant to a form of therapy.

Reservoir: Substance or living host within which an organism can multiply and develop and potentially be transmitted to a susceptible host.

Residual cysts: Cysts that develop after the stimulating inflammatory products have been removed from a previous cyst. Some byproducts may remain and stimulate the development of a new cyst.

Rests of Malassez: Refers to the epithelial remains of the Hertwig's root sheath in the periodontal ligament.

Rests of Serres: Refers to the odontogenic rests with remnants of the dental lamina that originate from the connection between the mucosa and the enamel organ.

Retromolar trigone: The soft tissue area posterior to the mandibular molars that extends toward the pharynx.

Reverse smoking: Method of smoking tobacco in which the lit end is placed in the mouth when the smoke is inhaled.

Rosacea: Chronic vascular and follicular dilation involving the nose and cheeks. The sebaceous glands may be hyperplastic and the pustules may be erythematous in nature. Rosacea is also noted as a characteristic in some systemic diseases, such as lupus, which exhibits the chronic butterfly rash in the malar area.

Sarcoidosis: Systemic disease affecting multiple organs, skin, and eyes, and especially targets the lungs, exhibiting interstitial fibrosis. The disease causes the formation of granulomas composed of epithelioid and multinucleated giant cells.

Sclerodactyly: Thickening or hardening of the skin and is associated with scleroderma. The fingertips become shortened and thickened.

Scleroderma: Immune dysfunction that is characterized by fibrosis of the skin, organs, and collagen. Several disease states are associated with scleroderma, such as Sjögren's syndrome, Raynaud's phenomenon, and rheumatoid arthritis.

Seborrheic keratosis: Characterized by the over-production of sebum by the sebaceous glands, causing an over-production of the horny layer of the skin.

Sequestrum: Refers to a fragment of bone that has broken away from the healthy tissue in the surrounding area.

Solar lentigo: Lentigos are benign macules that are larger than freckles and usually occur on sun-exposed skin. The melanin and the melanocytes are increased in the basal cell layer.

Speckled leukoplakia: Non-homogeneous form of leukoplakia characterized by small, whitish nodular elevations with an erythematous base.

Squamous cell carcinoma: Squamous cell carcinoma is the second most common skin cancer, with proliferation of malignant squamous cells. The lesions are typically rough in appearance with a scaling and crusty surface. The lip is commonly a prime area for squamous cell carcinoma.

Stellate reticulum: One of the layers of the developing enamel organ. It must be present in order for the formation of enamel to progress.

Tensile strength: The resistance of a material to a force tending to tear it apart; the ability of a material to deform and return to normal without breaking or tearing.

Tonsilloliths: A concretion in a tonsil crypt.

Troche: Medication in lozenge form.

Urticaria (hives): Characterized by pruritic wheals that occur when a person has been exposed to a source causing hypersensitivity within the body. The resulting wheals may cause extreme itching and will vary in size depending on the sensitivity of the individual.

Vacuolated: Clearing of the cytoplasm of a cell.

Venereal disease (sexually transmitted disease): Due to or propagated by sexual contact.

Verrucous leukoplakia: Non-homogeneous form of leukoplakia characterized by irregularity of the surface.

Vesiculobullous: Diseases characterized by fluid-filled blisters.

Viral load: The concentration of a virus, such as HIV, in the blood.

Vitiligo: Autoimmune response causing the loss of melanocytes in certain skin areas. The skin surface becomes devoid of pigmentation and appears white in color.

Warts (verrucous vulgaris): A wart is produced by the human papillomavirus, with varying types of the virus. The surfaces will vary depending on the location and the strain of the virus. The warts are usually removed by freezing, burning, or the use of various acids.

Wickhams striae: Interlacing white lines characteristic of lichen planus.

Xanthelasma: Characterized by yellow plaques and are especially noticeable when located on the eyelids and below the eye at the medial canthus. The papules have been associated with hyperlipidemia and low-density lipoproteins.

Xerostomia: Abnormal dryness of the mouth.

X-linked: A trait that is carried on the X (female) chromosome.

Index

Page numbers followed by f denote figures; those followed by t denote tables

A

Abdominal aortic aneurysm, 184–185, 185f
Abfraction, 253, 482
Ablated (ablation), 357
Abnormalities of the teeth, 480–481
    alterations in color of teeth,
        509–512, 509f, 511f
    alterations in number of teeth,
        487–492, 488f, 489f, 490f,
        491f, 492f
    alterations in shape of teeth,
        493–501, 494f, 495f, 496f,
        497f, 498f, 499f, 500f, 501f
    alterations in size of teeth,
        492–493, 493f
    alterations in the structure of teeth,
        501–509, 502f, 503f, 504f,
        505f, 506f, 507f, 508f, 509f
    crowns, 494–498, 494f, 495f, 496f,
        497f
    developmental, 487–512
    inflammatory conditions, 484–487,
        485f, 487f
    postdevelopmental, 481–487
    roots, 498–501, 498f, 499f, 500f,
        501f
    traumatic conditions, 481–484,
        482f, 483f
Abrasions, 13, 482–483, 482f
Abscess, inflammation and abscess
    formation, 43, 53, 54f
Abuse and neglect, oral injuries in, 22–25,
    24f, 25f
Acantholysis, 286
Acanthosis, 353
Acanthosis nigricans, 168, 168f
Accessory cusps, 494–495, 495f
Accessory roots, 498, 498f
Acidosis, 167
Acinic cell carcinoma, 413, 413f
Acquired bleeding disorders, 230
Acquired immune deficiency syndrome
    (AIDS), 67, 75, 86
    actinomycosis and, 301, 302
    hemophilia and, 232
    herpes simplex virus and, 274
    lymphomas and, 223, 224
    necrotizing ulcerative gingivitis
        and, 307
    oral manifestations in HIV/AIDS
        patients, 517–523, 517f, 518f,
        519f, 520f, 521f, 522f, 523f
    syphilis and, 303

Acrochordon, 531, 531f
Acromegaly, 83, 153–154, 154f
Actinic cheilitis, 530–531, 531f
Actinic keratosis, 95, 96, 355f, 530, 530f
Actinomycosis, 301–302, 301f
Active immunity, 67
Acute adrenal insufficiency, 73, 161
Acute atrophic candidiasis, 331
Acute inflammatory process
    acute inflammation, defined, 43
    amplification phase, 43, 46–47,
        48f
    initiation phase, 43, 44–46, 46f,
        46t, 47f
    phases of, 43–47
    termination phase, 43–44, 44t, 45f,
        47
Acute lymphoblastic leukemia, 225t
Acute lymphonodular pharyngitis, 284
Acute myeloblastic leukemia (AML), 225t
Acute osteomyelitis, 429, 462
Acute pseudomembranous candidiasis,
    349–350, 350f
Addison's disease, 159–160, 160f, 161f,
    532
Adenocarcinoma, 314, 419, 419f
Adenohypophysis, 148
Adenoid cystic carcinoma, 414–415, 414f
Adenomatoid odontogenic tumor, 472,
    473f
Adhesion, 44t, 45f, 46, 46f
Adjuvant therapy, 413
Adrenal crisis, 161
Adrenal gland disorders, 159–164, 160f,
    160t, 161f, 162f
Adrenocortical insufficiency, 159–160f,
    161f
Advanced glycation end products, 166
Age, 31
Agenesis, 111, 112
Agranulocytes, 47–49, 49f
Agranulocytosis, 219–220f
Albers-Schönberg disease, 449, 449f
Alcohol-related birth defects, 113
Alcohol-related neurodevelopmental dis-
    order, 113
Alcoholism
    and diffuse parotid enlargement,
        404
    fetal alcohol syndrome, 113–114,
        114f
Alleles, 118
Allergic contact dermatitis, 73, 73f
Allergic stomatitis, 71

Allergies, contact, 288
Alopecia, 93
Alternative pathway, 51
Alveolar osteitis, 58
Amalgam tattoos, 14, 14f, 364–366, 365f
Amelanotic melanoma, 376, 376f
Ameloblastic fibroma, 474–475, 474f
Ameloblastomas, 431–432, 431f
Amelogenesis imperfecta, 502–503, 503f
American Academy of Dermatology, 528
American Cancer Society
    basal cell carcinoma, data on, 94,
        528
    breast cancer, data on, 99–100
    cervical cancer, data on, 391
    colorectal cancer, data on, 103
    Hodgkin's lymphoma, data on,
        221, 222
    lung cancer, data on, 102
    melanoma, data on, 97, 98–99,
        529
    multiple myeloma, data on, 227
    non-Hodgkin's lymphomas, data
        on, 222
    oral cancer, data on, 6, 320
    prostate cancer, data on, 101–102
    squamous cell carcinoma, data on,
        95–96, 314
American Dental Association, 261
American Diabetes Association, 164, 167
American Heart Association
    congenital heart defects, data on,
        192
    diet recommendations, 37
    Marfan syndrome recommenda-
        tions, 131
    medications for prophylactic
        antibiotic regimens, 195, 196t
    venous thrombosis, data on, 186
American Joint Committee on Cancer, 89
American Lung Association, 246, 247
American Parkinson Disease Association,
    252
Amyloid, 228
Anaphylactic reactions, 69–70
Anaplasia, 89, 89f
Anemia, 90, 212f, 212t
    aplastic, 218, 219
    associated with chronic
        diseases/disorders, 218, 218t
    hemolytic, 216, 510–511
    iron deficiency, 211–213, 213f
    megaloblastic, 215–216, 216f
    pernicious, 215